Oxford Specialty Training:
Training in Anaesthesia

Oxford Specialty Training: Training in Anaesthesia

Edited by

Catherine Spoors

Specialist Registrar in Anaesthesia and
Intensive Care Medicine,
Bart's and the London School of Anaesthesia,
London

Kevin Kiff

Consultant in Anaesthesia and
Intensive Care Medicine,
Broomfield Hospital,
Chelmsford

Series Editor

Matthew D. Gardiner

Research Fellow in Plastic and
Reconstructive Surgery,
Kennedy Institute of Rheumatology Division,
Imperial College London,
London

OXFORD
UNIVERSITY PRESS

OXFORD

UNIVERSITY PRESS

Great Clarendon Street, Oxford OX2 6DP

Oxford University Press is a department of the University of Oxford.
It furthers the University's objective of excellence in research, scholarship,
and education by publishing worldwide in

Oxford New York

Auckland Cape Town Dar es Salaam Hong Kong Karachi
Kuala Lumpur Madrid Melbourne Mexico City Nairobi
New Delhi Shanghai Taipei Toronto

With offices in

Argentina Austria Brazil Chile Czech Republic France Greece
Guatemala Hungary Italy Japan Poland Portugal Singapore
South Korea Switzerland Thailand Turkey Ukraine Vietnam

Oxford is a registered trade mark of Oxford University Press
in the UK and in certain other countries

Published in the United States
by Oxford University Press Inc., New York

British Library Cataloguing in Publication Data

Data available

Library of Congress Cataloging in Publication Data

Data available

Typeset by Glyph International, Bangalore, India
Printed in Italy
on acid-free paper by
LEGO SpA – Lavis TN

ISBN 978-0-19-922726-6

1 3 5 7 9 10 8 6 4 2

Oxford University Press makes no representation, express or implied,
that the drug dosages in this book are correct. Readers must therefore
always check the product information and clinical procedures with the
most up-to-date published product information and data sheets provided
by the manufacturers and the most recent codes of conduct and safety
regulations. The authors and publishers do not accept responsibility or
legal liability for any errors in the text or for the misuse or misapplication
of material in this work. Except where otherwise stated, drug dosages
and recommendations are for the non-pregnant adult who is not
breastfeeding.

Foreword

This is the first edition of a book which will undoubtedly see further editions and become enormously popular with those sitting the Primary FRCA, their teachers and, quite possibly, their examiners.

The editors and authors, trainees and consultants, have worked as a team to produce an imaginative new textbook that follows the College's curriculum and assessment techniques. It is imaginatively and vividly illustrated with a huge number of practical examples that show trainees exactly what to do, and diagrams that will help enormously in examinations.

Although the e-Learning Anaesthesia project also covers the content of the curriculum, many still prefer the written word for learning and revising; this book fulfils that need admirably.

Dr Peter Nightingale
Consultant in Anaesthesia & Intensive Care
University Hospital of South Manchester

v

Series Preface

The recent upheaval in training and education has left junior doctors much to contend with, including a new career structure, online curricula, and workplace-based assessments. The need for resources that reflect these changes is great. Other books have become outmoded and although the Internet offers access to boundless medical material, little is tailored to the needs of specialty trainees. Fear not, change is coming; the *Oxford Specialty Training Series* has arrived. The Series encompasses core specialty books as well as basic science and revision texts that directly follow their respective Royal College curriculum.

Training in Anaesthesia exemplifies their compact, but comprehensive style. It has self-contained double-page spreads with a clear layout incorporating high quality illustrations. These features make information easy to access and digest. In addition, the editorial team and contributing authors are drawn from both trainees and senior clinicians to ensure the content is both relevant and of a high standard.

The *Oxford Specialty Training Series* will see you through the first few years of training whether on the ward, in the clinic, or revising for exams. I am confident that it will get you off to a great start in your chosen specialty.

Matthew D. Gardiner
Series Editor

Visit our website for details of forthcoming self-assessment titles www.oup.com/uk/medicine/osf

Preface

'The art of life is the art of avoiding pain; and he is the best pilot, who steers clearest of the rocks and shoals with which it is beset.' **Thomas Jefferson**

Our intention in editing this volume has been to adopt an integrated approach to the provision of information, presenting basic scientific principles and their clinical applications together. *Training in Anaesthesia* is aimed at anaesthesia trainees approaching the Primary FRCA Examination, but we hope that we do more than provide an examination primer. We have tried to see trainees and their patients in a clinical setting, and to give information and practical advice, which will be of use in day-to-day practice.

Each chapter, and the book as a whole, represents a collaboration between consultants and trainees, in order to provide a dual perspective on the material. We have tried to consider what the teachers want to teach, and what the learners need to learn.

In common with the other volumes of the Oxford Specialty Training series, *Training in Anaesthesia* presents its topics as a series of double-page spreads. The anaesthetic curriculum is a daunting one, and we hope that readers will find this format helpful in planning and tackling revision. We have tried to avoid needless repetition of material, but readers should bear in mind that anaesthesia is itself a blended specialism — principles explored in a chapter on one area of practice usually have applications in others.

Anaesthetics trainees need an extensive knowledge of drugs. We have presented information on drugs in an easily accessed tabular format, to facilitate comparison and contrast. Please note that drug doses have been checked exhaustively, but readers should always double-check with the British National Formulary and product literature.

We hope that our work in this book will evolve with the needs of trainees, and the comments of readers — negative and positive — will help us to develop our approach. All feedback is welcome; therefore, comments should be sent to ost@oup.com.

Special thanks must go to: our contributors - we thank you for your tireless work and expertise; Andy Sandland, Marionne Cronin, and Fiona Goodgame (among others) at Oxford University Press, whose encouragement and advice were our guiding lights; Mike Clegg for giving up so much free time to our IT support; the armies of anonymous reviewers whose names we do not know but whose words of wisdom have been invaluable; and to our colleagues and friends for their kindness and help.

Finally, to our families, Michelle, Rebecca, Sophie, Eleanor, Robbie, and Alice; Alan, Margaret and Mike. Your unwavering support, loyalty and love must sometimes have seemed to escape unnoticed. We failed to thank you often; we tested your last shreds of patience. Even now, the enormity of our gratitude robs us of any more articulate way to express it: thank you, thank you, thank you.

Kevin Kiff
Catherine Spoors

Contents

Detailed contents

Abbreviations

α-MSH	α-melanocyte stimulating hormone
2,3-DPG	2,3-diphosphoglycerate
5-HT	serotonin (5-hydroxytryptamine)
AAA	abdominal aortic aneurysm
ABG	areterial blood gas
ABG	arterial blood gas
ACA	anterior cerebral artery
ACE	angiotensin-converting enzyme
ACh	acetylcholine
ACS	acute coronary syndrome
ACTH	adrenocorticotrophic hormone
ADH	antidiuretic hormone
ADP	adenosine diphosphate
ADR	adverse drug reaction
AEP	auditory evoked potential
AF	atrial fibrillation
AG	anion gap
AHTR	acute haemolytic transfusion reaction
AIDS	acquired immune deficiency syndrome
ALF	acute liver failure
ALI	acute lung injury
AMI	acute myocardial infarction
AMS	acute mountain sickness
ANOVA	analysis of variance
ANP	atrial natriuretic peptide
AP	anteroposterior, action potential
APC	antigen presenting cell
APH	ante-partum haemorrhage
APL	adjustable pressure-limiting (valve)
APS	Acute Pain Service
APTT	activated partial thromboplastin time
AQP-2	aquaporin-2
ARDS	adult respiratory distress syndrome
ARF	acute renal failure
ASA	American Society of Anesthesiologists
ASD	atrial septal defect
ASIS	anterior superior iliac spine
AT	anaerobic threshold
AT-III	antithrombin III
ATN	acute tubular necrosis
ATP	adenosine triphosphate
AUC	area under the concentration–time curve
AV	atrioventricular, arteriovenous
AVNRT	AV node re-entry tachycardia
AVP	arginine vasopressin
AVRT	AV re-entry tachycardia
BBS	bicarbonate buffer system
BBV	blood-borne virus
BD	twice daily
BE	base excess
BIS	bispectral index

BMI	body mass index
BMR	basal metabolic rate
BNP	brain natriuretic peptide
BP	blood pressure
BSI	bloodstream infection
BVM	bag–valve–mask
CABG	coronary artery bypass graft
CAD	coronary artery disease
CAI	carbonic anhydrase inhibitor
CAL	chronic airflow limitation
cAMP	cyclic adenosine monophosphate
CAP	community-acquired pneumonia
CBD	common bile duct
CBF	cerebral blood flow
CC	closing capacity
CCF	congestive cardiac failure
CCK	cholecystokinin
CCT	cortical collecting tubule
CD	collecting duct
cGMP	cyclic 3',5'-guanosine monophosphate
CHCT	caffeine–halothane contracture test
CHD	common hepatic duct
CI	cardiac index
$CMRO_2$	cerebral metabolic rate
CMV	controlled mandatory ventilation, cytomegalovirus
CNT	connecting tubular
CO	cardiac output, carbon monoxide
COMT	catechol-O-methyl transferase
COPA	cuffed oral pharyngeal airway
COPD	chronic obstructive pulmonary disease
COX	cyclo-oxygenase
CPAP	continuous positive airways pressure
CPP	cerebral perfusion pressure
CPR	cardiopulmonary resuscitation
CPX	cardiopulmonary exercise (testing)
CRC-BSI	catheter-related bloodstream infection
CRF	corticotrophin-releasing factor
CRH	corticotrophin-releasing hormone
CSE	combined spinal–epidural
CSF	cerebrospinal fluid
CSHT	context-sensitive half-time
CSM	cerebral state monitor
CSW	cerebral salt wasting
CT	computed tomography
CTPA	computed tomographic pulmonary angiography
CTZ	chemoreceptor trigger zone
CV	circulating volume, closing volume
CVA	cerebrovascular accident
CVC	central venous catheter
CVLM	caudal ventrolateral medulla
CVP	central venous pressure

CVR	cerebral vascular resistance
CVS	cardiovascular system
CXR	chest X-ray
CYP	cytochrome P450
DA	ductus arteriosus
Da	dalton(s)
DAG	diacylglycerol
DBP	diastolic blood pressure
DBS	double-burst stimulation
DCT	distal convoluted tubule
DIC	disseminated intravascular coagulation
DKA	diabetic ketoacidosis
DLG	dorsal lateral geniculate
DMR	depolarizing muscle relaxant
DOA	depth of anaesthesia
DRG	dorsal respiratory group
DVT	deep vein thrombosis
ECF	extracellular fluid
ECG	electrocardiogram
ED	effective dose
EDHF	endothelium-derived hyperpolarization factor
EF	ejection fraction
eGFR	estimated glomerular filtration rate
ELISA	enzyme-linked immunosorbent assay
EMI	electromagnetic interference, erythema multiforme
EMLA	eutectic mixture of local anaesthetic
ENT	ear, nose, and throat
EPP	end-plate potential, equal pressure point
EPSP	excitatory postsynaptic potential
ER	endoplasmic reticulum
ERCP	endoscopic retrograde cholangiography
ERPC	evacuation of retained products of conception
ERV	expiratory reserve volume
$EtCO_2$	end-tidal carbon dioxide
ETT	endotracheal tube
FAST	focused assessment sonography for trauma
FDP	fibrin degradation product
FEV_1	forced expiratory volume in 1 second
FF	filtration fraction
FFA	free fatty acid
FFP	fresh frozen plasma
FGF	fresh gas flow
FPM	first-pass metabolism
FRC	functional residual capacity
FSH	follicle-stimulating hormone
FVC	forced vital capacity
G1P	glucose-1-phosphate
G6P	glucose-6-phosphate
G6PD	glucose-6-phosphate dehydrogenase
GA	general anaesthesia
GABA	gamma aminobutyric acid
GCS	Glasgow Coma Scale
GCSF	granulocyte colony-stimulating factor
GDM	gestational diabetes mellitus
GFR	glomerular filtration rate
GH	growth hormone
GHRH	growth-hormone-releasing hormone
GIT	gastrointestinal tract

GnRH	gonadotrophin-releasing hormone
GORD	gastro-oesophageal reflux disease
GPCR	G-protein coupled receptors
GRP	gastrin-releasing peptide
GTN	glyceryl trinitrate
GVHD	graft-versus-host disease
HAART	highly active anti-retroviral therapy
HACE	high-altitude cerebral oedema
HAFOE	high air flow oxygen enrichment
HAPE	high-altitude pulmonary oedema
Hb	haemoglobin
HbS	sickle haemoglobin
HCAI	healthcare-associated infections
hCG	human chorionic gonadotrophin
Hct	haematocrit
HDL	high-density lipid
HDU	high-dependency unit
HELLP	haemolysis, elevated liver enzymes, and low platelets
HES	hydroxyethyl starch
HH	Henderson–Hasselbalch
HITS	heparin-induced thrombocytopenia syndrome
HIV	human immunodeficiency virus
HLA	human lymphocyte antigen
HME	heat and moisture exchanger
HOCM	hypertrophic obstructive cardiomyopathy
HPS	hepatopulmonary syndrome
HPV	hypoxic pulmonary vasoconstriction
HR	heart rate
hr	hour(s)
HSV	herpes simplex virus
HUS	haemolytic uraemia syndrome
IABP	intra-aortic balloon pump,
IAP	intra-abdominal pressure
ICD	implantable cardioverter defibrillator
ICF	intracellular fluid
ICG	impedance cardiography
ICP	intracranial pressure
ICU	intensive care unit
IE	infective endocarditis
IF	intrinsic factor
IFV	interstitial fluid volume
Ig	immunoglobulin
IGT	impaired glucose tolerance
IHD	ischaemic heart disease
IJV	internal jugular vein
IL	interleukin
ILMA	intubating laryngeal mask airway
IM	intramuscular
INR	international normalized ratio
IO	intra-osseous
IOP	intra-ocular pressure
IPPV	intermittent positive-pressure ventilation
IPSP	inhibitory postsynaptic potential
IQR	interquartile range
IR	infrared
ISA	intrinsic sympathomimetic activity
ISF	interstitial fluid
ISO	International Standards Organization

ITP	inisitol triphosphate, idiopathic thrombocytopenic purpura
IV	intravenous
IVC	inferior vena cava
JG	juxtaglomerular
JGA	juxtaglomerular apparatus
JVD	jugular venous distension
JVP	jugular venous pressure
L	litre(s)
LA	local anaesthetic
LBBB	left bundle branch block
LC	locus coeruleus
LDL	low-density lipid
LED	light-emitting diode
LFT	liver function test
LH	luteinizing hormone
LMA	laryngeal mask airway
LMWH	low molecular weight heparin
LOR	loss-of-resistance
LOS	lower oesophageal sphincter
LSCS	lower segment Caesarian section
LTOT	long-term oxygen therapy
LV	left ventricular
LVED	left ventricular end-diastolic
LVEF	left ventricular ejection fraction
MAC	minimum alveolar concentration, membrane attack complex
MAO	monoamine oxidase
MAOI	monoamine oxidase inhibitor
MAP	mean arterial pressure
MBC	minimum bactericidal concentration
MBL	mannose-binding lectin
MCA	middle cerebral artery
mcg	microgram(s)
MDR	multidrug-resistant
MEPP	miniature end-plate potential
mEq	milli-equivalent
MET	metabolic equivalent
MH	malignant hyperthermia
MHC	major histocompatibility complex
MI	myocardial infarction
MIC	minimum inhibitory concentration
MLCK	myosin light-chain kinase
MLT	microlaryngoscopy tube
MMC	migrating motor complex
MMEF	maximum mid-expiratory flow
MOH	major obstetric haemorrhage
MRI	magnetic resonance imaging
MRSA	methicillin-resistant *Staphylococcus aureus*
MS	multiple sclerosis
MSFP	mean systemic filling pressure
MUGA	multiple-gated acquisition
MV	minute volume
MW	molecular weight
nAChR	nicotinic acetyl choline receptor
NAQBI	N-acetyl-p-aminobenzoquinoneimine
NCA	nurse-controlled analgesia
NDMB	non-depolarizing muscular blocker
NDMR	non-depolarizing muscle relaxant

NGT	nasogastric tube
NIBP	non-invasive blood pressure
NIST	non-interchangeable screw-thread unit
NIV	non-invasive ventilation
NK	natural killer
NMDA	N-methyl-D-aspartate
NMJ	neuromuscular junction
NNH	number needed to harm
NNT	number needed to treat
NO	nitric oxide
NOR	noradrenaline
NOS	nitric oxide synthetase
NPY	neuropeptide Y
NRM	nucleus raphe magnus
NS	nociceptive-specific
NSAID	non-steroidal anti-inflammatory drug
NTS	nucleus tractus solitarius
OBA	oral bioavailability
ODC	oxygen dissociation curve
OSA	obstructive sleep apnoea
OSAHS	obstructive sleep apnoea–hypopnoea syndrome
PA	postero-anterior
PABA	para-aminobenzoate
PAF	platelet-activating factor
PAFC	pulmonary artery flotation catheter
PAG	periaqueductal grey
PAH	para-amino hippurate
PAI	plasminogen activator inhibitor
PAMP	pathogen-associated molecular pattern
PAOP	pulmonary artery occlusion pressure
PAR	protease-activated receptor
PCA	patient-controlled anaesthesia, posterior cerebral artery
PCEA	patient-controlled epidural analgesia
PcoA	posterior communicating artery
PCR	polymerase chain reaction
PCT	proximal convoluted tubule
PCV	pressure-controlled ventilation
PDA	patent ductus arteriosus
PDGF	platelet-derived growth factor
PDPH	post-dural puncture headache
PE	pulmonary embolism
PEA	pulseless electrical activity
PEEP	positive end-expiratory pressure
PEFR	peak expiratory flow rate
PEP	post-exposure prophylaxis
PF	platelet factor
PFT	pulmonary function test
PG	prostaglandin
PIH	pregnancy-induced hypertension
PK	pharmacokinetic
PKA	protein kinase A
PKC	protein kinase C
PLC	phospholipase C
PMGV	piped medical gases and vacuum (systems)
PN	parenteral nutrition
PNMT	phenylethalanolamine-N-methyltransferase
PNS	peripheral nervous system
PO	by mouth
POCD	postoperative cognitive dysfunction

POD	postoperative delirium
POMC	pro-opiomelanocortin
PONV	postoperative nausea and vomiting
PPH	post-partum haemorrhage
PPI	proton pump inhibitor
ppm	parts per million
PPV	pulse pressure variation
PR	per rectum
PRN	as required
PSIS	posterior superior iliac spine
PSV	pressure support ventilation
PT	pubic tubercle, prothrombin time
PTC	post-tetanic count
PTH	parathyroid hormone
PTU	propylthiouracil
PVC	polyvinyl chloride
PVD	peripheral vascular disease
PVR	pulmonary vascular resistance
RA	regional anaesthesia
RAAS	renin–angiotensin–aldosterone system
RAr	rapidly adapting stretch receptor
RAS	reticular activating system
RBBB	right bundle branch block
RBC	red blood cell
RBF	regional blood flow
RCA	right coronary artery, root cause analysis
rhAPC	recombinant activated protein C
RhD	rhesus D
RMP	resting membrane potential
rms	root mean square
RPF	renal plasma flow
RQ	respiratory quotient
RR	respiratory rate
RS	respiratory system
RSI	rapid sequence induction
RTA	road traffic accident
RV	residual volume, right ventricular
RVLM	rostral ventrolateral medulla
SA	sino-atrial
SAN	sinoatrial node
SAR	slowly adapting stretch receptor
SBP	systolic blood pressure
SD	standard deviation
SIADH	syndrome of inappropriate antidiuretic hormone secretion
SID	strong ion difference
SIMV	synchronized intermittent mandatory ventilation
SIRS	systemic inflammatory response syndrome
SJS	Stevens–Johnson syndrome
SLE	systemic lupus erythematosus
SMR	standardized mortality ratio
SNRI	selective noradrenaline re-uptake inhibitor
SP	surfactant protein
SR	sarcoplasmic reticulum
SSI	surgical site infection
SSRI	selective serotonin re-uptake inhibitor
StAR	steroidogenic acute regulatory protein
STEMI	ST-segment elevation myocardial infarction
SV	stroke volume
SVC	superior vena cava
SVP	saturated vapour presure
SVR	stroke–volume ratio, systemic vascular resistance
SVT	supraventricular tachycardia
SVV	stroke volume variation
TAFI	thrombin-activatable fibrinolysis inhibitor
TAL	thick ascending limb
TBI	traumatic brain injury
TBW	total body water
TCA	tricyclic antidepressant, tricarboxylic acid cycle
TCI	target-controlled infusion
TCR	T-cell receptor
TDS	three times daily
TEN	toxic epidermal necrolysis
TENS	transcutaneous electrical nerve stimulation
TF	tissue factor
TFPI	tissue factor pathway inhibitor
TFT	thyroid function test
TIPPS	transjugular intra-hepatic portosystemic shunt
TIVA	total intravenous anaesthesia
TLC	total lung capacity
TNF	tumour necrosis factor
TOE	transoesophageal echocardiography
TOF	train-of-four
TOFC	train-of-four count
tPA	tissue-type plasminogen activator
TRH	thyrotrophin-releasing hormone
TSH	thyroid-stimulating hormone
TTP	thrombotic thrombocytopenic purpura
TURP	transurethral resection of prostate
TV	tidal volume
U&E	urea and electrolytes
UA	unstable angina
URTI	upper respiratory tract infection
UTI	urinary tract infection
VAE	venous air embolism
VAP	ventilator-associated pneumonia
VCV	volume-controlled ventilation
VF	ventricular fibrillation
VIE	vacuum-insulated evaporator
VIP	vasoactive intestinal polypeptide
VMA	vanillylmandelic acid
VRG	ventral respiratory group
VSD	ventricular septal defect
VSM	vascular smooth muscle
VT	ventricular tachycardia
vWD	von Willebrand disease
vWF	von Willebrand factor
WBC	white blood cell
WDR	wide dynamic range
WHO	World Health Organization
WOB	work of breathing
WPW	Wolff–Parkinson–White

Abbreviations which do not appear above are defined where they appear in the text.

Contributors

Mark C Blunt
Consultant in Anaesthesia and Critical Care
Queen Elizabeth Hospital, King's Lynn
Recovery

Davinia Bennet
Consultant Anaesthetist, Liver Transplant Anaesthesia
Queen Elizabeth Hospital,
Liver & GI tract physiology, pharmacology & medicine

Peter Bromley
Consultant Anaesthetist
Birmingham Children's Hospital,
Honorary Consultant Anaesthetist
University Hospitals Birmingham,
Honorary Senior Lecturer, Medical Sciences
University of Birmingham, Birmingham
Liver & GI tract physiology, pharmacology & medicine

Shane N Campbell
Clinical Fellow, Anaesthetics & ICU
Newham University Hospital Trust, London
Cardiovascular physiology, pharmacology & medicine

Jo Challands
Consultant Paediatric Anaesthetist
Barts and the London NHS Trust, London
Paediatric anaesthesia & analgesia

Linda Chigaru
Pain physiology, pharmacology & medicine

Arnwald Choi
Consultant Anaesthetist
John Radcliffe Hospital, Oxford
Maintenance of anaesthesia

Jake Collins
Consultant anaesthetist & intensive care medicine
Broomfield Hospital, Chelmsford
Trauma

Garth LJ Dixon
Consultant Medical Microbiologist
Great Ormond Street Hospital, London
Microbiology & infection control

John Durcan
Consultant in Anaesthetics & Intensive Care
Mid Essex NHS Hospitals Trust, Chelmsford
Body compartments & fluid balance

Tom Durcan
Consultant Anaesthetist
Broomfield Hospital, Chelmsford
Pain physiology, pharmacology & medicine

Barry Mark Featherstone
Anaesthetics Specialist Registrar
Guy's and St Thomas' Hospital, London
Pain physiology, pharmacology & medicine

Mala C Greamspet
ST4 trainee
Bristol Royal Infirmary, Bristol
The anaesthetic room: checks & equipment

Nick Huddy
Consultant Anaesthetist
Broomfield Hospital, Chelmsford
Induction of anaesthesia
Maintenance of anaesthesia

Sonia J. Hudson
Consultant in Anaesthesia / Intensive Care Medicine
Broomfield Hospital, Chelmsford
Endocrine physiology, pharmacology & medicine

Huw Steven Jenkins
Consultant Physician, Respiratory Medicine
Broomfield Hospital, Chelmsford
Respiratory physiology, pharmacology & medicine

Ellen Makings
Consultant in Anaesthesia & Intensive Care
Broomfield Hospital, Chelmsford
HDU & ICU care

Krishore Maney
SpR Anaesthetics
Barts and The London NHS Trust, London
Neurological physiology, pharmacology & medicine

Jonathan Mason
Specialist Registrar Anaesthetics
Oxford Radcliffe NHS Trust, Oxford
Emergencies

VK Melachuri
Consultant Anaesthetist
Tameside Hospital NHS Foundation Trust, Lancashire
Pre-operative assessment

Mike O'Connor
Consultant Anaesthetist
The Princess Margaret Hospital, Windsor
The anaesthetic room: checks & equipment

Breda O'Neill
Paediatric Anaesthetic Research Fellow
Barts and The London NHS Trust,
Great Ormond St Hospital for Children, London
Paediatric anaesthesia & analgesia

Mark Peters
Consultant in Paediatric and Neonatal Intensive Care
Great Ormond Street Hospital, London
Haematology & immunology

Jay Rahharkrishnan
Essential concepts in physiology & pharmacology
Maths for the anaesthetist

Elspeth Reid
Consultant anaesthetist
Broomfield Hospital, Chelmsford
Obstetric anaesthesia & analgesia

Matthew Rowland
SpR Anaesthetics
John Radcliffe Hospital, Oxford
Muscle physiology & pharmacology

Alasdair Short
Consultant Physician
Intensive Care Medicine, Broomfield Hospital, Chelmsford
Renal physiology, pharmacology & medicine

Clare V. Taylor
SpR Anaesthetics
Barts and the London Hospitals, London
Applied anatomy, regional anaesthesia & practical procedures

Christopher Toner
Consultant in Anaesthetics and Intensive Care
William Harvey Hospital, Ashford
Emergencies

Anil Visram
Consultant Anaesthetist
Barts and The London NHS Trust, London
Neurological physiology, pharmacology & medicine

Stuart Withington
Director of Critical Care
Newham University Hospital NHS Trust, London
Cardiovascular physiology, pharmacology & medicine

Pamela Winton
Specialist Registrar Anaesthetics and Intensive Care
Wessex School of Anaesthesia
Obstetric anaesthesia & analgesia

James D. A. Wood
Specialist Registrar in Anaesthetics and ICM
Guy's and St Thomas' NHS Trust, London
Muscle physiology & pharmacology

Chris Wright
Consultant Anaesthetist
Broomfield Hospital, Chelmsford
Pre-operative assessment
Epidural & spinal anaesthesia

Sarah I Yarham
SpR Anaesthesia
Queen Elizabeth Hospital, Norfolk
Recovery

Additional Material

Quention Sayer
Regional Medical Affairs Manager
UK, Ireland, Africa
The BOC Group, plc

Hannah Stockley
Specialist Registrar in Radiology
Manchester Radiology Training Scheme

Tom Newton
Specialist Registrar in Radiology
Manchester Radiology Training Scheme

Chapter 1

Preoperative assessment

1

1.1 Preoperative assessment

The preoperative assessment is the first opportunity for the anaesthetist to meet the patient before surgery. A preoperative assessment has several goals. These include:

- Developing a rapport with the patient
- Taking an anaesthetic history and performing an examination
- Detecting and assessing concomitant disease
- Identifying and reducing risk
- Appropriate premedication prescription
- Discussing and planning anaesthetic technique
- Explanation of and consent for anaesthetic procedures.

Anaesthetic history

It is vital to take account of previous anaesthesia, not only of the patient but also of immediate family members. Patients may be aware of previous anaesthetic difficulties such as difficult intubation, postoperative nausea and vomiting, anaphylaxis, or unexpected ICU admission. Previous anaesthetic records should be scrutinized.

Past problems may cause anxiety in a patient presenting for another anaesthetic. Try to allay any worries regarding anaesthesia, pain control, and PONV.

Family history

Family history of anaesthetic problems is important. There are a handful of hereditary conditions which can cause life-threatening anaesthetic complications. In the anaesthetic-naive patient (or family), these will only declare themselves after induction. These conditions include:

- Malignant hyperthermia (Section 22.20)
- Suxamethonium apnoea (Section 8.4)
- Acute porphyrias.

Patients with genetic disorders, with or without physical anomalies, present unique challenges to the anaesthetist. It is important to research risk factors and potential complications before administration of an anaesthetic. Patients themselves may have a wealth of information relating to the condition.

Medical history

Aside from the problem requiring surgery, most patients will not arrive with a 'presenting complaint' affecting anaesthesia. However, many will harbour medical problems which will influence anaesthetic and surgical risk. A thorough previous medical history, medication history, and social history, should unearth old problems; a good systemic inquiry will evaluate current symptoms. Most abnormalities relevant to anaesthesia are easily detected by careful history and physical examination. Do not forget to enquire about gastro-oesophageal reflux, smoking, alcohol, recreational drugs, and heart problems which may require antibiotic prophylaxis, although the role for endocarditis prophylaxis for most procedures is currently in question. The cardiovascular and respiratory systems are of particular importance, and their assessment is discussed in more detail in the next few pages.

Drug history and allergies

Most of the patient's own drugs should be continued until the morning of surgery. However, certain medications need to be stopped a few days prior to surgery (e.g. anticoagulants). Medication strategy during the patient's admission needs to be planned (e.g. insulin therapy during an expected period of reduced oral intake). Table 1.1 lists some common interactions between drugs and anaesthetic agents.

Some common drugs exhibit significant interactions with anaesthetic agents. It is important to be aware of these in order to anticipate problems. Most hospitals have local guidelines regarding which medications should be omitted prior to surgery. However, it is imperative to be guided by the clinical status of the patient and the type of surgery. For example, it is reasonable to continue ACE inhibitors for a normo- or hypertensive patient undergoing minor surgery, but not for a patient due to undergo major abdominal surgery with an epidural.

Table 1.1 Drug interactions with anaesthetic agents

	Class of drug	Drug interaction
Cardiac	β-blockers	Negative ionotropic effects can precipitate severe hypotension and severe bradycardia
	ACE inhibitors	Vasodilatory action may precipitate severe hypotension
	α-agonists (clonidine)	Causes hypotension when used in conjunction with many IV and inhalational anaesthetic agents
	Calcium-channel blockers	Vasodilatory properties can result in severe hypotension in the presence of anaesthetic agents
	Diuretics	Can cause electrolyte disturbances and potentiate arrhythmias with inhalational agents
CNS	Monoamine oxidase inhibitors	Can potentate hypertensive episodes when used in conjunction with pressor agents.
	Tricyclic antidepressants	Can cause arrhythmias with various anaesthetic agents
	Benzodiazepines	Can potentiate the sedative effects of anaesthetic agents
Other	NSAIDs	Variable antiplatelet function
	Aminoglycosides	Can potentiate muscle relaxants
	Oestrogen therapies	Increase risk of thrombosis

Allergy history

Any drug can theoretically cause allergy. The most frequently implicated agents from anaesthetic practice are:

- Thiopentone
- Suxamethonium
- Non-depolarizing muscle relaxants
- Ester local anaesthetics
- Opioids
- Antibiotics
- Plasma expanders
- Latex (gloves, urinary catheters etc.)
- Iodine (skin preparation for invasive procedures).

Detailed preoperative assessment and history are essential for the subsequent safe administration of anaesthetics. Involvement of the allergy clinic may be useful in identifying the causative agent. Referral to specialist centres may also be needed for more detailed analysis of the degree of sensitivity.

Other anaesthetic considerations

The state of the patient's dentition (including loose teeth, caps, crowns, and dentures) needs to be assessed, and the starvation time must be ascertained.

Investigations

During the history-taking and examination, decisions about investigations should take place. Routine laboratory testing of patients who are apparently healthy on clinical examination and history is invariably a waste of resources. Investigations are necessary only if the results of such tests would influence the management of the patient.

In order to reduce the volume of tests being performed, guidelines have been produced by various groups such as the Royal College of Anaesthetists, the Association of Anaesthetists, the Royal College of Radiologists, NICE, etc. Reproduction of all these guidelines would take a book in itself; however, the advice is broadly summarized in Table 1.2.

⊕ Table 1.2 Preoperative investigations: a guide

Urinalysis

Can actually be performed on every patient. It is an inexpensive test, and will occasionally pick up undiagnosed diabetes or urinary tract infection.

Full blood count (FBC)

This should be contemplated in the following groups:

- Males >50 years of age
- All menstruating females
- Haematological history
- Major surgery
- Afro-Caribbeans.

Urea and electrolytes (U&E)

Indications for measuring urea and electrolytes are:

- >50 years of age
- Diuretic therapy
- Renal disease
- Adrenal disease
- Systemic corticosteroid therapy
- Digoxin therapy
- Fluid shifts: dehydration, vomiting, bowel prep, metabolic disease
- Diabetes
- Major surgery.

Estimated glomerular filtration rate (eGFR) is derived from the serum creatinine. It can be a useful test as it may reveal more minor degrees of renal impairment, which may warrant the avoidance of drugs and/or anaesthetic techniques which may adversely affect renal function.

Liver function tests (LFTs)

LFTs are usually required only in those with:

- Hepatic disease or history of jaundice
- Abnormal nutritional state or metabolic disease
- Excessive alcohol intake
- Therapy with hepatotoxic drugs
- History of IV drug abuse.

Blood glucose

- History of diabetes
- Abnormal urinalysis
- Current systemic corticosteroid therapy
- Adrenal disease

Clotting studies

Coagulation studies (e.g. APTT, INR) are required if:

- Personal or family history of bleeding disorders
- Taking anticoagulants
- Known liver disease.

Haemoglobinopathy

Patients with suspected haemoglobinopathy must first have their haemoglobin concentration measured, followed by haemoglobin electrophoresis.

Sickledex, often undertaken prior to emergency surgery, merely identifies the presence of HbS. It does not determine the type of sickle cell abnormality e.g. trait, disease or combination haemoglobinopathy (Section 15.2).

Therapeutic drug monitoring

Some medications are subject to therapeutic drug monitoring. Measurement of levels is not usually required unless signs of sub-therapeutic dosage or side effects are present.

- Theophylline
- Digoxin
- Lithium
- Carbamazepine.

Thyroid function tests (TFTs)

Only in patients who exhibit signs of hyper- or hypothyroidism, or if thyroid therapy has changed recently.

Arterial blood gas (ABG)

These are required in patients who have:

- Severe respiratory disease
- Dyspnoea at rest
- Thoracotomy planned.

ABG analysis can also be invaluable in sick patients or those undergoing major surgery, e.g. to avoid hypoxia and oxygen toxicity, detect acid–base abnormalities, guide fluid replacement, and identify electrolyte disturbances

Chest X-ray

This investigation actually influences management fairly infrequently in anaesthetic practice. It should be considered in the following situations:

- Cardiovascular/respiratory disease (if no previous X-ray in last 12 months)
- New respiratory symptoms
- Possible metastases
- Recent immigrant from area where tuberculosis is endemic
- Age >60 years.

Pulmonary function tests (PFTs)

These should be considered in all patients with:

- Dyspnoea at rest or on mild to moderate exertion
- Wheeze at time of assessment
- Planned thoracotomy.

Electrocardiogram (ECG)

Should be considered in the following groups:

- History of cardiac disease
- Suspected cardiac disease
- Hypertension
- Arrthymias or palpitations
- Patients >50 years of age.

Echocardiogram

Should be considered if there is:

- A previously undiagnosed murmur
- Symptoms and signs of cardiac disease including shortness of breath, angina, arrhythmias, or heart failure
- Known cardiac disease without a recent (<12 months) echocardiogram, particularly if symptoms have progressed.

Other investigations

Cervical spine X-rays can be useful in known difficult intubations, patients with rheumatoid arthritis, or Down's syndrome patients. Classically, thoracic inlet views have been used pre-thyroid surgery.

The airway assessment forms an integral part of any anaesthetic evaluation. It starts with a thorough history, including a review of the case notes. The airway should then be examined: soft tissues, bony structures, teeth, neck and jaw movements, and airway patency.

Check anaesthetic notes for previous difficulties and ask patients whether they are aware of any anaesthetic problems.

Radiotherapy to the mouth, airway, or neck has long-lasting effects and it is important to identify. Swelling or scarring of tissues can lead to anatomical distortion, limited mouth opening, or poor neck movement.

Three questions should be considered during the airway assessment and subsequent planning of anaesthesia.

- Is the patient likely to be difficult to ventilate with a bag-and-mask system?
- Is the patient likely to be difficult to intubate?
- Is the airway at risk of soiling?

As a rule of thumb, if the answer to two out of the three questions is 'yes', consideration should be given to special airway techniques such as awake fibreoptic intubation.

Predicting difficult ventilation

Factors indicating that bag–valve–mask ventilation may be difficult fall into three categories:

Difficulty forming a seal between mask and face: edentulous (tend to lack facial structural support), beards, facial deformities.

Reduced thoracic compliance: obesity, pregnancy, abdominal distension, severe musculoskeletal disease, restrictive lung disease.

Difficulty maintaining a patent airway with simple adjuncts: excess tissue in the pharynx or larynx (e.g. fat, tumour, thyroid goitre, large tongue); sleep apnoea (airway known to collapse during sleep); tempo-ro-mandibular joint disease (standard jaw-thrust manoeuvres may be ineffective); cervical spine immobilization (cannot perform head-tilt/chin-lift manoeuvres).

Predicting difficult intubation

There are several tests and scoring systems that can help predict a difficult intubation. The most commonly used is the Mallampati score (see Figure 1.1). None is particularly accurate on its own, but in combination they may help to identify difficult airway anatomy. The following clinical features raise the possibility of a difficult intubation:

- Body habitus: obesity, large breasts, short muscular neck
- Dentition: prominent upper incisors
- Facial morphology: receding jaw, high-arched palate, facial deformity (including congenital syndromes such as Pierre Robin or Klippel–Feil)
- Limited neck movement, especially neck extension
- Limited mouth opening (less than three finger breadths)
- Oropharyngeal infection or tumour
- Stridor (present at assessment or reported on history)
- Previous thyroid or cervical spine surgery.

Wilson risk score

Wilson's score incorporates various aspects of airway assessment to attempt to predict intubation difficulty. Five variables are considered:

- Weight
- Head and neck movement
- Temporomandibular joint movement (lower teeth can be protruded in front of upper teeth)
- Receding mandible
- Prominent overbite.

Each is given a score between 0 and 2, with a maximum of 10. Using a cut-off of 2 or more gives a specificity of 90% (the false negative rate is low) but sensitivity of only 40% (a high false-positive rate). Increasing the cut-off value to 3 or 4 increases sensitivity but at the expense of specificity: the test then fails to predict 50% of difficult intubations. Also, assessment of many of the components is highly subjective.

Other measures of difficult intubation

Thyromental distance

This is a measure of the distance between the upper edge of the thyroid cartilage and the chin, with the head fully extended. A short thyromental distance is associated with a high anterior larynx: <6cm may predict a difficult intubation, whereas >7cm is usually associated with an easy intubation.

Horizontal length of mandible

Horizontal mandibular length >9cm is suggestive of good laryngoscopic view, because of the large potential space for forward displacement of the tongue.

Mandibulohyoid distance

This is the vertical distance between the anterior edge of the hyoid and the mandible vertically above (measured by lateral X-ray). A distance >6cm predicts difficult intubation, as it suggests that more of the tongue is present in the hypopharynx. This must be displaced at laryngoscopy.

Cervical spine movements

The effect of mobility of the atlanto-occipital and atlanto-axial joints on ease of intubation is probably underestimated. It may be best assessed by asking the patient to extend their head with the neck in full flexion (as if taking the first sip from a very full glass). Extension of the head on an immobile atlanto-axial joint results in an exaggerated cervical spine lordosis. This pushes the larynx forward and impairs the laryngoscopic view.

Prayer sign

Inability to place both the palms flat together with the wrists at 90° suggests difficult intubation. This is probably a reflection of generalized musculoskeletal immobility, possibly limiting atlanto-axial and cervical extension. It may be more common in diabetics.

Risk of aspiration

On induction of anaesthesia with most agents, the lower oesophageal sphincter relaxes. In certain patients this may lead to passive regurgitation of food into the oropharynx. The oro- or nasopharynx may also be contaminated with debris or blood. Anaesthetized patients have obtunded airway reflexes, so regurgitated material be aspirated into the airway. The following factors increase risk of aspiration:

Upper airway
- Epistaxis or oropharyngeal bleeding
- Loose teeth
- Pharyngeal pouch

Oesophagus
- Achalasia
- Strictures

Full stomach
- Recent oral intake (Section 1.9) or upper airway bleeding
- Delayed gastric emptying (even if starved): pain, trauma, anxiety—especially in children.
- Drugs (e.g. opioids)
- Distal bowel obstruction or pathology, gastrointestinal haemorrhage.
- Labour

Lower oesophageal sphincter incompetence
- Hiatus hernia
- Pregnancy
- History of gastro-oesophageal reflux
- Drugs (atropine, opioid analgesics)

Raised intra-abdominal pressure
- Abdominal distension
- Pregnancy
- Lithotomy/head-down positioning
- Obesity

✚ **Mallampati score**

This test is performed with the patient in the sitting position, head neutral. The patient is instructed to open their mouth as wide as possible and stick their tongue right out. The classification is assigned based on the pharyngeal structures visible (see below). A class 1 view is associated with a grade 1 intubation >99% of the time. A class 4 view is associated with grade 3 or 4 intubations 100% of the time. However, the interpretation of other grades is difficult, and the test fails to predict over 50% of difficult intubations.

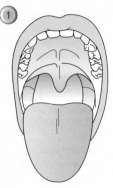 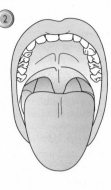 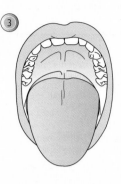 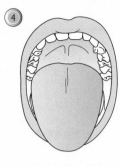

Class 1

Visualization of soft palate, fauces, uvula, anterior and posterior pillars

Class 2

Visualization of soft palate, fauces, and uvula

Class 3

Visualization of soft palate and base of uvula

Class 4

Soft palate not visible at all

Fig. 1.1

Most respiratory problems relevant to anaesthesia are readily appreciable on history and examination. If problems are identified, investigations are necessary to evaluate their severity and likely impact on the anaesthetic outcome.

History

The respiratory history should explicitly enquire about the following.

Dyspnoea

Note the onset, severity, and pattern. Is it associated with exertion? What is the effort tolerance? Is it worse when lying flat?

Cough

What is its duration? Has it changed in character? What time of day is it worse (asthmatics cough more at night)? Is it worse after food or drink (aspiration or reflux)?

Sputum

What is its character (colour, amount, frequency, changes)? Is there evidence of haemoptysis?

Wheeze

Are there known precipitants? What is the frequency of attacks? Is the asthma stable, or worsening? Has the patient ever been hospitalized or admitted to ICU? Are there current symptoms of respiratory infection?

Chest pain

If associated with respiratory disease, this type of pain is often localized to the chest wall, and may be pleuritic in nature. This might indicate underlying infection or the presence of pleural inflammation.

Other questions should determine the presence of fevers, night sweats, or symptoms of obstructive sleep apnoea (snoring, daytime somnolence, morning headaches) or aspiration (morning cough or sore throat, postural heartburn or reflux). Enquiry should also ascertain previous respiratory surgery or illnesses including pneumonia, pulmonary embolism, and tuberculosis.

Medications

The frequency of use of inhalers gives a clue to the pattern of disease: they are used more with worsening or unstable disease. In particular, enquire about steroid use. Around 20% of adult asthmatics and 5% of children with asthma are sensitive to NSAIDs. It is essential to establish whether this is the case, although the problem is under-reported on patient interview.

Examination

General inspection

Undress the patient to the waist. Note the respiratory rate, pattern of breathing, and use of accessory muscles in order to judge the effort of breathing. Central cyanosis may be detected by looking at the tongue. Listen for audible stridor, wheeze, hoarseness of voice and cough. Note the presence of any supplemental oxygen.

Hands and face

Clubbing is associated with a variety of pulmonary problems (lung cancer, chronic suppurative lung disease, pulmonary fibrosis). Tar staining of the fingers demonstrates current smoking. Wasting of the small muscles of the hand may indicate brachial plexus compression by an apical lung tumour. Hypoxia and hypercapnia cause tachycardia.

Horner's syndrome (partial ptosis, pupil constriction, and absence of sweating) is due to the loss of sympathetic supply to that side of the face. It may be caused by a tumour compressing the sympathetic chain in the neck. Inspect the tongue, pharynx, and nose.

Neck

Gently palpate to assess the position of the trachea (Figure 1.2). Assess for tracheal tug.

Chest

Inspection, palpation, percussion, and auscultation should be performed at both the front and back of the patient. The key is always to compare each side with the other, to identify asymmetry.

Inspection

Observe for thoracic shape and scars. Assess the symmetry of expansion (note: pathology is always on the side with decreased movement). Note the pattern of respiration.

Palpation

Palpate for equal chest movement and assess the apex beat; this may be difficult to feel in the hyperexpanded chest, and displacement may indicate mediastinal shift. Gentle AP and lateral compression of the thorax may identify occult rib fractures.

Tactile vocal fremitus is felt with the bony ulnar border of the hand (Figure 1.3).

Percussion

Percussion technique is shown in Figure 1.4. The feel and sound of percussion are as follows:

Stony dull	Fluid (e.g. pleural effusion)
Dull	Solid structure (e.g. liver, consolidated lung)
Resonant	Normal lung
Hyper-resonant	Gas-filled structure (e.g. pneumothorax)

A dull note over the liver starts at the sixth rib in the mid-clavicular line; if lower, this suggests hyperinflation.

Auscultation

Assess the quality and strength of the breath sounds and note the presence of extra sounds. Always compare one side with the other.

Normal breath sounds are louder and longer in inspiration, with no gap between inspiration and expiration.

Bronchial breathing has a different quality and is due to turbulent flow in larger airways (listen over your own trachea to hear the characteristic noise). There is a gap between inspiration and expiration.

Wheeze has a musical sighing quality and is due to narrowing of the small airways. It is usually louder on expiration. True inspiratory wheeze implies severe airways narrowing.

Crackles and crepitations are heard when unstable collapsed alveoli snap open during inspiration. Early inspiratory crackles suggest small airways disease, whereas late inspiratory crackles are a feature of alveolar pathology. Crackles may be:

- Fine (like peeling Velcro)—characteristic of pulmonary fibrosis
- Fine/medium—left ventricular failure
- Coarse—when secretions pool in the lungs.

A *pleural rub* is said to sound like footsteps crunching on snow. It is non-specific but indicates that the pleura are thickened or roughened by disease (e.g. inflammation, malignancy, pulmonary infarction).

Vocal resonance is assessed by listening over the lungs while the patient repeats 'ninety-nine'. These words become more audible and loud over solid areas (much as a knock on a table sounds very loud when your ear is pressed to the tabletop). It conveys the same clinical information as tactile vocal resonance, and signs need to be interpreted while bearing in mind the likely side of the abnormality, as demonstrated by the rest of the examination.

Focused systemic examination

Look for signs of cor pulmonale (right heart failure with peripheral oedema due to pulmonary hypertensive lung disease). Listen to the heart sounds for the pulmonary component of the S2; if louder than the aortic sound, pulmonary hypertension is likely. Palpate the abdomen for liver ptosis from hyperinflated lungs, or hepatomegaly from metastatic disease. Examine the calves for signs of DVT.

Look at the **observations chart** for oxygen saturations, temperature, and peak flow. Ask to see a sputum sample.

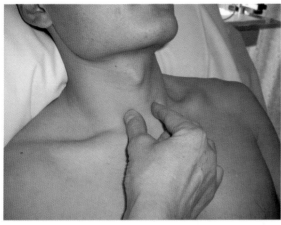

Fig. 1.2 Palpation of the trachea to determine its position relative to the midline. Tracheal deviation may be due to 'pull' (e.g. towards fibrosis) or 'push' (e.g. away from a pneumothorax or effusion). The remainder of the examination should reveal which side is abnormal.

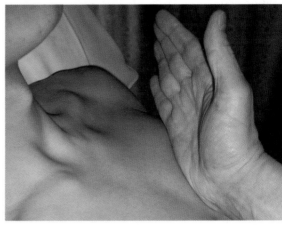

Fig. 1.3 Assessment of tactile vocal fremitus. The sensation of vibration is pathologically increased over areas of consolidation where sound waves travel more efficiently. It is decreased or absent over areas of pneumothorax or pleural effusion.

➕ **Box 1.4 Percussion of the chest wall**

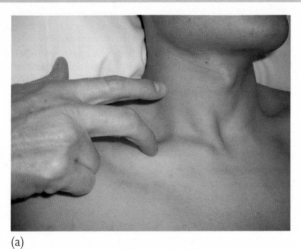

(a)

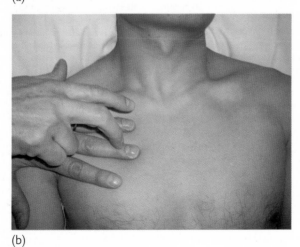

(b)

Fig. 1.4 Percussion of the chest wall. The tip of the plexor finger strikes the DIP joint of the pleximeter finger held flat in a rib space. The front, back, and both axillae should be assessed. Do not forget to percuss the supraclavicular fossa (lung apex) and the clavicle, which is percussed directly without the pleximeter finger. Compare both sides of the chest at each stage.

Tests of lung function can be performed at the bedside or consulting room, in the physiology laboratory, in the ICU, or in the field in research settings. They are useful in:

- Preoperative assessment
- Diagnosis of respiratory and other conditions
- Monitoring progression of disease and response to treatment
- Assessment of industrial injury and epidemiological research.

Peak expiratory flow rate

The peak expiratory flow rate (PEFR), also known as peak flow, is the maximal flow rate that can be developed by forced expiratory effort following full inspiration. It is measured by simple hand-held devices used at the bedside or at home. PEFR variability aids in the diagnosis of asthma. It is particularly useful in the assessment of severity of exacerbations and response to treatment in asthma.

Maximal mid-expiratory flow (MMEF)

Maximal flow rate between 25% and 75% of a forced exhalation from TLC. It is indicative of small airways performance.

Maximal mouth inspiratory pressure

This is measured from residual volume (RV). A forceful inspiration is sustained with maximal effort followed by a release upon fatigue. The best 1 sec average is used as an indication of inspiratory muscle strength.

Spirometry

Spirometry means 'the measuring of breath'. After maximal inspiration, a single forced complete expiration is recorded. FEV_1 is the volume recorded after 1 sec and is usually around 80% of FVC. This is a very simple and useful test that is used widely in clinical practice. It is robust and repeatable but effort-dependent. Spirometry defines the two key types of ventilatory defect:

- Obstructive   Reduced FEV_1/FVC ratio.
- Restrictive   Both FEV_1 and FVC reduced; FEV_1/FVC ratio normal or increased.

Reversibility of airways obstruction (suggestive of asthma rather than COPD) can be assessed by repeating spirometry after a dose of an inhaled bronchodilator such as salbutamol. Reversibility is defined by an increase in FEV_1 >200 ml or 15%.

Measurement of lung volumes

A diagram of lung volumes with normal values is shown (Figure 1.5). Most of these values can be measured by spirometric techniques. However, (RV) cannot be measured by spirometry. Instead it is deduced by subtracting ERV from FRC, measured by one of two techniques.

- **Whole-body plethysmography**
  In this technique the patient sits in an airtight box, and the increased box pressure of inspiration is measured (Figure 1.6). This provides a more accurate measure of total gas volume in the lung (see above), but is less commonly available than helium dilution. Whole-body plesythmography is also used for measurement of airway resistance.

- **Closed-circuit gas dilution**
  Dilution of helium in a closed-circuit spirometer (Figure 1.7) allows measurement of alveolar volume. This method is straightforward but can be inaccurate due to gas trapping in small airways disease, or with bullae in COPD. Helium will not diffuse into these spaces.

Clinically, abnormal lung volumes can affect both ventilatory capacity and gas exchange. Increased volumes are usually seen in emphysema and small airways disease, whereas reduced lung volumes are present in many causes of restrictive defects, such as interstitial disease, and after pneumonectomy.

RV/TLC ratio

The ratio of RV to TLC is used as a marker of hyperinflation of the chest, as seen with COPD.

 ## Case studies

The following examples demonstrate how lung function testing aids diagnosis and measures response to treatment. Table 1.3 summarises the lung function abnormalities seen with various diseases.

COPD/emphysema, moderate severity

A 58-year-old male smoker presented to his GP after an episode of winter bronchitis, complaining of persistent dyspnoea and wheeze. Examination revealed quiet breath sounds with expiratory rhonchi. Chest X-ray showed hyperexpanded lung fields with bullous changes. At the respiratory clinic he was noted to have airways obstruction: FEV_1 0.8L, FVC 2.2L—ratio 0.36.

There was no significant response to inhaled bronchodilator. Flow-volume loop showed very low mid-expiratory flow rates.

Lung volume assessment confirmed hyperexpansion with elevated RV and RV/TLC ratio. Transfer factor (K_{CO}) was reduced at 45% of predicted. Arterial blood gases at room air showed PaO_2 8.7kPa.

Asthma

A 58-year-old male smoker presented to his GP after an episode of winter bronchitis, complaining of persistent dyspnoea and wheeze. Examination revealed expiratory rhonchi. Chest X-ray showed hyperexpanded lung fields. At the respiratory clinic he was noted to have airways obstruction: FEV_1 0.8L, FVC 2.2L—ratio 0.36.

There was a moderate response to bronchodilator—17% increase in FEV_1. Lung volume assessment confirmed moderate hyperexpansion with elevated RV and RV/TLC ratio. Transfer factor (K_{CO}) normal. After 6 weeks treatment with inhaled steroids his symptoms had improved considerably: FEV_1 2.2L, FVC 3.4L—ratio 0.65.

Pulmonary fibrosis

A 58-year-old male smoker presented to his GP after an episode of winter bronchitis, complaining of persistent dyspnoea and dry cough. Examination revealed bilateral fine inspiratory crepitations. Chest X-ray was normal. At the respiratory clinic he was noted to have a restrictive defect: FEV_1 1.7L, FVC 1.9L—ratio 0.89

There was no response to bronchodilator. Lung volume assessment showed reduced RV and TLC, indicating reduced lung volumes. Transfer factor (K_{CO}) was reduced at 28% of predicted. CT scan of chest showed interstitial changes in both lungs

Restrictive defect and type 2 failure due to obesity

A 58 year-old male smoker presented to his GP after an episode of winter bronchitis, complaining of persistent dyspnoea and wheeze. Examination revealed quiet breath sounds and possible rhonchi. Chest X-ray was normal. At the respiratory clinic he was noted to have a restrictive defect: FEV_1 1.7L, FVC 1.9L—ratio 0.89.

There was no response to bronchodilator. Lung volume assessment showed reduced RV and TLC, indicating reduced lung volumes. Transfer factor (K_{CO}) was normal. BMI was 42. Arterial blood gases at room air showed PaO_2 8.7kPa, $PaCO_2$ 6.7 kPa.

Restrictive defect and type 2 respiratory failure due to respiratory muscle weakness—motor neuron disease

A 58-year-old male smoker presented to his GP after an episode of winter bronchitis, complaining of persistent dyspnoea. Examination revealed quiet breath sounds. Fasciculations were noted. Chest X-ray was normal. At the respiratory clinic he was noted to have a restrictive defect: FEV_1 1.7L, FVC 1.9L—ratio 0.89.

There was no response to bronchodilator. Lung volume assessment showed reduced RV and TLC, indicating reduced lung volumes. Transfer factor (K_{CO}) was normal. BMI was 28. Arterial blood gases at room air showed PaO_2 8.7 kPa, $PaCO_2$ 6.7 kPa. Maximal mouth inspiratory pressure was reduced, indicative of impaired effort.

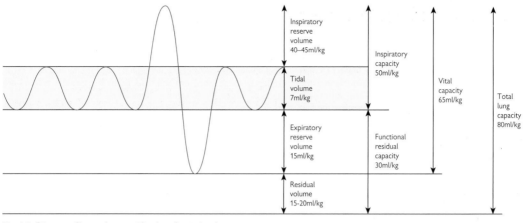

Fig. 1.5 Diagram of lung volumes with values for each volume

	FEV$_1$	FVC	FEV$_1$/FVC	Bronchodilator response	MMEF	RV	K$_{CO}$
Asthma	Normal or ↓	Normal or ↓	Normal or ↓	Yes	Normal or ↓	Normal	Normal
Small airways disease	Reduced	Normal or ↓	↓	Yes	↓	↑	Normal
Emphysema	Reduced	Normal or ↓	↓	No	↓	↑	↓
Pulmonary fibrosis	Normal or ↓	↓	↑	No	Normal or ↓	↓	↓
Obesity	Normal or ↓	Normal or ↓	Normal or ↑	No	Normal	↓	Normal
Kyphoscoliosis	Normal or ↓	↓	↑	No	Normal	↓	Normal
Respiratory muscle disease	Normal or ↓	↓	↑	No	Normal	↓	Normal
Pneumonectomy	↓	↓	Normal	No	Normal	↓	Normal

⊕ **Table 1.3 Common medical conditions and lung function testing**

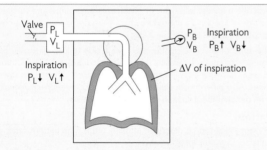

Fig. 1.6 Measurement of FRC by body plethysmography. From FRC, inspiration is taken against a closed valve. Because inspiration is obstructed in this manner, the total volume of gas in the lungs (and the box) remains the same, and so their pressure and volume will change inversely, according to Boyle's law.

The pressure and volume of the box are measured before and after inspiration, with the change in volume denoted as ΔV. The pressure of the lung (airway pressure at the lips) before and after inspiration is also measured. The volume of the lung at FRC can then be calculated. Gas contained within a pneumothorax will be measured as part of the FRC.

	At rest		Inspiration
Boyle's Law	P_1V_1	=	P_2V_2
Box	$P_{B1}V_{B1}$	=	$P_{B2}(V_{B1}-\Delta V)$
Lung	$P_{L3}FRC$	=	$P_{L4}(FRC+\Delta V)$

Solving simultaneous equations, $\mathbf{FRC} = \dfrac{P_{L4}(P_{B2}V_{B1}-P_{B1}V_{B1})}{P_{B2}(P_{L3}-P_{L4})}$.

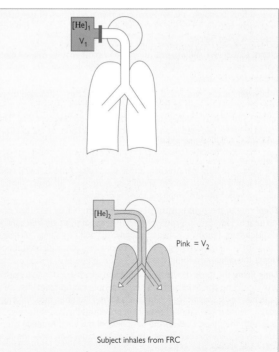

Subject inhales from FRC

Fig. 1.7 Measurement of FRC by dilution. This method will not detect gas hidden behind obstructed airways since it will only measure the volume of communicating gases. The concentrations of helium ([He]$_1$ and [He]$_2$) are measured:

$$V_1 \times [He]_1 = (V_1 + FRC) \times [He]_2$$

When interpreting a chest X-ray, it is important to take a systematic approach. First, check the patient name and number. Make sure that you are looking at the correct film by verifying the date and time of the study. Then review the film in a structured fashion. Look at previous films also, especially in difficult cases. Finally, always correlate the film to how ill or well the patient is.

Film quality

View: PA erect is the standard view, but requires the patient to stand upright. If this is not possible, an AP view (semi-erect or supine) is performed. This tends to magnify the cardiac outline. The scapulae are projected over the lung fields in an AP view.

Penetration: underpenetrated films appear white, and the thoracic vertebrae cannot be seen through the heart (the body of T4 should be clearly visible). Overpenetrated films appear dark, with poor visualization of the lung fields.

Rotation: check that the thoracic spine aligns between the clavicles. Both clavicles should form the same angle with the line of the spinous processes. Rotated films may distort the cardiac shadow and make one lung field appear darker than the other.

Inspiration: chest X-rays should be taken in full inspiration. If inspiration is adequate, it should be possible to see ten posterior or six anterior ribs. Poorly inspired films give a hazy view of the lung bases which may be mistaken for basal atelectasis or even pleural effusion.

Artefacts: sharply defined shadows projected across different tissues (e.g. lung field and cardiac shadow, diaphragm, and chest wall) are likely to be artefactual. Endotracheal tubes, central venous catheters, nasogastric tubes, or other indwelling devices should be assessed for position.

Key areas for inspection

All areas should be systematically inspected twice: once from a distance (1–2m), and once close up. Do not settle for the first abnormality you find: complete the systematic examination in full. A suggested approach, starting from the heart and working outwards to the soft tissues, is given below.

Heart: size, shape, and margins of heart and great vessels. The cardiothoracic ratio should be 50% or less. Check the contours for unusual prominence or shape.

Mediastinum: the mediastinal contour should be clear (although there may be some haziness at the cardiophrenic angles, right hilum, and apices). Other hazy patches suggest pathology in the adjacent lung. The mediastinum is widened in aortic aneurysm, dissection, or transection, thymoma, or lymphadenopathy.

Hila: size, shape, density. The left hilum is up to 2.5cm higher than the right. The right paratracheal stripe (comprising the tracheal wall, parietal and visceral pleura) should be <5mm on an erect film. It appears widened with lymphadenopathy or other masses.

Diaphragms: the right is usually higher than left, but by less than one rib space. Elevation suggests phrenic nerve paralysis or mechanical displacement ('push', e.g. hepatomegaly, or 'pull', e.g. lung collapse). Look for tenting, flattening, and loss of outline (consolidation). Look under the diaphragm for free air.

Lung fields: the lungs should have should be symmetrical in vascularity, and should be visible behind the heart. Identify the horizonal fissure if possible. Look specifically for focal shadows. (Number, size, location, shape, density? Cavitation? Present on previous films?) Compare each side with the other. Look at the periphery of the lung. A pneumothorax can be distinguished from a bulla as the latter will have the lung edge outside the area of lucency.

Review the vascular pattern. Normally there is little vascularity in the outer 2cm of the lung fields, but this pattern can be distinguished from a pneumothorax by absence of a lung edge. There is poor vascularity in areas of emphysema, bullae, and massive pulmonary embolus (a rare sign). Upper lobe diversion (prominent upper zone vessels) can be seen in left ventricular failure, and may be accompanied by hilar shadowing (bat's wing appearance), Kerley B lines, pleural effusions, and cardiomegaly. Large (early on) and then 'pruned' pulmonary arteries are signs of chronic pulmonary hypertension.

Lobar collapse may cause significant respiratory compromise, but can be difficult to identify on a chest x-ray. Figures 1.8, 1.9, 1.10, 1.11, and 1.12 demonstrate the patterns typical of each type.

Pleura: look for thickening, effusions, pneumothorax (radiolucency with a defined lung edge), effusion (may represent exudate, transudate, blood, or pus), haemopneumothorax (identified by a flat air–fluid level rather than a meniscus), and masses. Pleural masses tend to have partly sharp, partly ill-defined margins.

Bone: examine all the bones closely, tracing the outline of each. This approach should identify lytic lesions or fractures. The presence of a rib fracture should prompt a careful review of the lung edges to rule out a pneumothorax. The overall lucency of the bone may give clues about generalized osteopenia. Check for kyphosis and scoliosis, and consider how these may affect the lungs.

Soft tissue: examination of the soft tissues may reveal obesity, masses, previous surgery (e.g. mastectomy or amputation), or surgical emphysema (Figure 1.13).

Review areas: tThe following seven areas should always be double-checked at the end of the inspection: the apices, costophrenic angles, cardiophrenic angles, lung edges, lung hila, under and behind the hemidiaphragms, and behind the heart.

How to describe abnormalities

Abnormalities on chest X-rays fall into four groups: abnormal lucency, abnormal opacity, abnormal size, or displacement. Having categorized the abnormality, it then remains to describe its distribution, pattern, and relation to other structures.

Distribution

Describe the side: left, right, or bilateral. Always check and re-check the side of a lesion if a procedure (e.g. a chest drain) or surgery is contemplated on the basis of the X-ray.

The zone of the abnormality may give a clue to the diagnosis. For example, sarcoidosis is usually seen in a mid to upper zone distribution, whereas fibrosing alveolitis more commonly affects the mid to lower zones. Also differentiate central distribution (e.g. pulmonary oedema) from peripheral distribution (e.g. fibrosing alveolitis).

Pattern

Abnormalities can be described in many terms. The pattern can give valuable diagnostic information.

Alveolar shadowing (consolidation) is characterized by fluffy shadowing with vague borders and air bronchograms. It often follows a lobar or segmental distribution. It represents filling of the alveolar spaces with fluid. This may be pus (pneumonia), blood (pulmonary contusion or infarction), or transudate (severe pulmonary oedema).

Interstitial infiltrate may be linear (reticular), nodular, miliary, or reticulonodular. These patterns indicate interstitial pathology, e.g. pulmonary fibrosis.

Coin lesions are discrete shadows within the lung fields. They may be solid or show cavitation or calcification. They may represent tumour, abscess, granuloma, or focal consolidation.

Relation to other structures

The silhouette sign occurs when an area of shadowing abuts another organ. Their two silhouettes appear to merge and the normal border is obscured. For example, right lower lobe consolidation obliterates the diaphragm but preserves the heart border, whereas middle lobe consolidation will obscure the heart border without loss of the diaphragmatic shadow.

A lateral chest X-ray can often help to localize lesions visible on a PA or AP view.

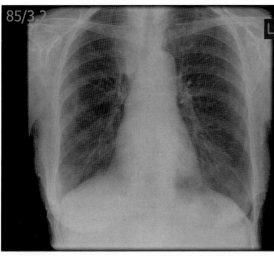

Fig. 1.8 A right upper lobe collapse. Note the upward shift of the right hilum and the opacity at the right apex. This is frequently seen in intubated children if the ETT migrates into the right main bronchus and occludes the right upper lobe bronchus.

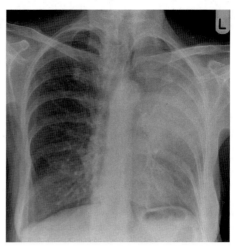

Fig. 1.11 Left upper lobe collapse. There is a general haze over the left lung field, denser in the upper zone: the "veil" sign. Note the upwards movement of the horizontal fissure. The aorta is sharply outlined on the left.

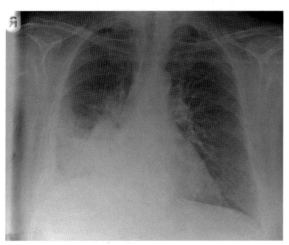

Fig. 1.9 Right middle lobe collapse. Note the downward movement of the horizontal fissure. The opacity obscures the right heart border, indicating that the shadow abuts the heart. However, the diaphragm shadow is preserved.

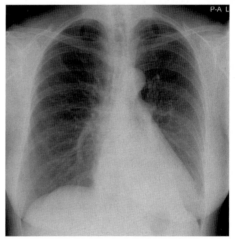

Fig. 1.12 Left lower lobe collapse. The collapsed lobe appears as a sail-shaped shadow behind the heart, and the lung hilum is dragged downwards.

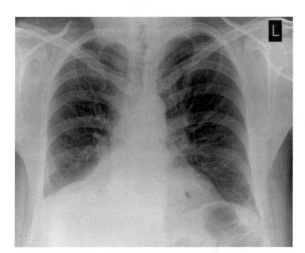

Fig. 1.10 Right lower lobe collapse. Since the lower lobe abuts the diaphragm, the diaphragmatic border is lost whereas the right heart border is preserved. Contrast this with the middle lobe collapse above.

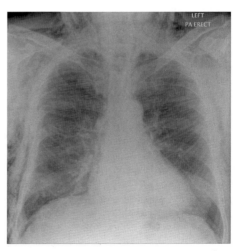

Fig. 1.13 Severe surgical emphysema and pneumomediastinum. There is air within the soft tissues of the chest wall, which appear to be lifted away from the ribs. The fascicles of the pectoral muscles are outlined by air. The pneumomediastinum is visible most clearly at the right heart border.

Most abnormalities relevant to anaesthesia can be found on careful history and examination. The following is a summary of clinical assessment.

History

Previous cardiac problems

CVS disease impacts on anaesthetic outcome, and so a history of hypertension, MI, angina, rhythm disturbances, murmurs, or rheumatic fever is important to discover. Recent cardiac surgery or percutaneous interventions (angioplasty, stenting) and associated antiplatelet therapy may also influence anaesthetic technique.

Chest pain

The onset, character, and radiation provoking and relieving factors should be noted. Ischaemic chest pain is characteristically dull, central, and heavy in nature, with radiation to the arms or neck.

Dyspnoea

Whether the patient becomes short of breath (at rest or on exercise) is important. Recent changes to exercise tolerance should be noted, since deterioration is associated with worsening myocardial performance or treatment failure. Paroxysmal nocturnal dyspnoea, cough, wheeze, and pink frothy sputum suggest pulmonary oedema.

Palpitations

Enquire about rate, rhythm, and duration. Ascertain whether the dysrhythmia causes associated symptoms (e.g. pre-syncope, blackouts, dyspnoea, chest pain).

General enquiries should include weight loss, fatigue, sleep, and appetite.

Medications

Antihypertensives, anti-anginals, anticoagulants, or anti-arrhythmics all potentially interact with anaesthetic agents. Compliance with these medications should be considered. With most patients presenting on the day of surgery, the most recent dose of such medicines is important. This is especially true with aspirin and clopidogrel, each of which might impact on anaesthetic technique.

Social history

Smoking, alcohol, and level of functional ability should be assessed objectively and recorded, e.g. can the patient climb stairs unaided?

Examination

General visual inspection

The chest should be exposed and the patient sat back at 45°. Features of CVS disease should be noted, including dyspnoea at rest, cyanosis, pallor, cachexia, and the malar flush of mitral valve disease.

Hands

The hands should be examined for clubbing a feature of cyanotic heart disease, endocarditis, and atrial myxoma. Osler's nodes, Janeway lesions, and splinter haemorrhages may also be seen with infective endocarditis.

Pulse

Examine the pulse for rate, rhythm, volume, and character. A collapsing pulse, seen with aortic regurgitation, is indicated by energetic pulsation against flat fingers held across the radial pulse with the patient's arm raised above the level of the heart. A slow-rising pulse is a sign of aortic stenosis. Radio-femoral delay is a feature of aortic coarctation. Pulsus alternans, where volume varies between pulsations, is a feature of left ventricular failure.

Blood pressure

The blood pressure should be measured. In general, isolated diastolic pressures of <110mmHg or isolated systolic measurements of <200mmHg can be tolerated for most types of surgery. However, they mandate further investigation and treatment.

Neck

Observe for pulsations and scars. Vigorous carotid pulsation is a feature of aortic regurgitation and aortic coarctation. Palpate carotid pulses for character.

JVP

The height reflects CVP. It is measured from the sternal angle with the patient semi recumbent at 45°, although more accurately it should be referenced against the right atrium, which is about 5cm below this. *(Hint: if the external neck veins are empty, the JVP cannot be raised.)* The pulsations may give a clue about right heart function.

Precordium

Inspect for scars, pulsations, and pacemaker boxes. The apex beat may be visible in slim healthy people: other visible pulsations are probably abnormal.

Palpate the apex, and assess its character and position. The normal apex beat is in the fifth intercostal space, mid-clavicular line. A displaced apex usually indicates cardiomegaly, but importantly may also indicate mediastinal shift (e.g. in pneumothorax). A tapping character indicates a calcified stenotic mitral valve and a double impulse is a sign of hypertrophic obstructive cardiomyopathy (HOCM).

Feel for a parasternal heave left of the sternum. If present, it indicates right ventricular enlargement. Palpate over the apex, left para-sternal area, and aortic and pulmonary areas for thrills (vibrations caused by turbulent flow). Thrills are nearly always pathological.

Auscultation

Low-pitched diastolic murmurs and third heart sounds are sought with the bell, and higher-pitched systolic murmurs and fourth heart sounds with the diaphragm. Murmurs should be timed by the apex beat or carotid pulse. Figures 1.14, 1.15, and 1.16 demonstrate ausculation of the aortic area, apex, and pulmonary area.

The first heart sound

This indicates closure of mitral and tricuspid valves, and the start of ventricular systole. It is:

- Loud in tricuspid or mitral stenosis or reduced diastolic filling time (e.g. tachycardia)
- Soft in prolonged diastolic filling, tricuspid or mitral regurgitation, or delayed LV systole (e.g. left bundle branch block).

The second heart sound

This signals the closure of the aortic and pulmonary valves. During inspiration, the negative intrathoracic pressure increases venous return. The right heart takes longer to eject this extra volume, leading to delayed pulmonary closure and 'splitting' of the second heart sound. The splitting of S2 is also altered by posture.

- Aortic component is loud with a hyperdynamic circulation and in hypertension; it is soft in aortic regurgitation.
- Pulmonary component is loud in pulmonary hypertension.
- Wide fixed splitting occurs in ASD. Pressures equalize in the atria with flow across the ASD. RV preload is increased in both inspiration and expiration and so the splitting is maintained.
- With LBBB, the LV contracts later and so the pulmonary sound precedes the aortic. This is known as paradoxical splitting.

Additional heart sounds

These usually indicate ventricular diastolic dysfunction (poor ventricular compliance). The third sound results from tensing of the chordae tendinae during during early ventricular filling. Vibration of the ventricular wall during atrial contraction causes the fourth heart sound.

Pericarditis is associated with a friction rub, said to sound like footsteps on snow.

Murmurs

Murmurs are usually caused by turbulent blood flow. The characteristics of common murmurs are shown opposite. However, the diagnosis of a new murmur in an adult warrants further investigation including echocardiography, since clinical evaluation is subjective and unreliable.

Focused systemic examination

Right heart failure: palpate the liver for hepatomegaly and determine whether it is pulsatile (seen in tricuspid regurgitation). Examine for ankle oedema and and palpate for sacral oedema.

Left heart failure: auscultate the lung bases for pulmonary oedema.

⊕ Cardiac risk stratification

In addition to general scoring systems such as the ASA grade, several scoring systems exist specifically to predict cardiac events in the peri-operative period. The most widely used is the Goldman cardiac risk index.

Goldman cardiac index

The Goldman cardiac index was developed in 1977 to identify patients at risk of perioperative cardiovascular complications. It scores nine different variables with a total possible score of 53.

Clinical feature	Points
Third heart sound or elevated JVP	11
MI in past 6 months	10
ECG: rhythm other than sinus	7
ECG: ventricular ectopic beats	7
Age >70 years	5
Emergency operation	4
Thoracic, abdominal, or aortic surgery	3
Aortic stenosis	3
Poor medical condition	3

From the total score, patients are stratified for risk of major cardiovascular complication (MI, cardiogenic pulmonary oedema, ventricular tachycardia) or death:

- 0–5: 0.7% severe cardiovascular complication, 0.2% mortality
- 6–25: 17% severe cardiovascular complication, 4% mortality
- >25: 22% severe cardiovascular complication 56% mortality

Various modifications of the score exist, including the **Detsky score**. This assigns three levels of risk to each parameter (5, 10, or 20 points), including three further risk factors: MI at any time, unstable angina within 6 months, or poor LV function. The maximum score is 120, with risk stratified into three levels:

- 0–15, low risk
- 20–30, medium risk
- >30, high risk.

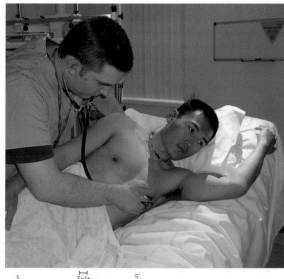

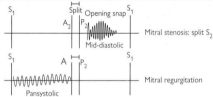

Fig. 1.15 Auscultation of the mitral area. The patient lies on his/her left side, in expiration. Mitral stensosis is heard over the apex and the murmur of regurgitation usually radiates to the axilla.

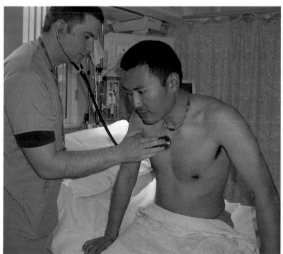

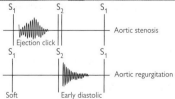

Fig. 1.14 Auscultation of the aortic area. Aortic stenosis is heard in the aortic area with radiation into the neck. The murmur of aortic regurgitation is heard best along the left sternal edge. Both should be listened for with the patient leaning forward in expiration.

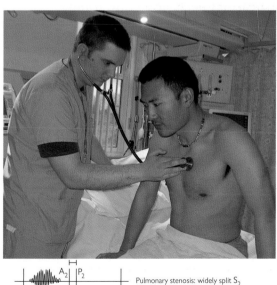

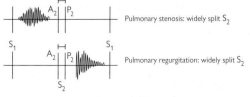

Fig. 1.16 Auscultation of the pulmonary area: the patient sits forward and maintains inspiration (increased pulmonary blood flow).

Pulmonary stenosis is usually a congenital condition diagnosed during childhood. In adults, pulmonary regurgitation is often due to pulmonary hypertension.

1.7 Assessment of cardiac function

The cardiac function of most patients can be adequately assessed by history, examination, and ECG analysis (Section 10.16). However, some patients require further evaluation to exclude or diagnose cardiac pathology, in order to instigate treatment, assess response, and stratify risk. Some of the more advanced cardiac function assessments are described below.

Exercise testing

The evaluation of chest pain can be very difficult. It is possible to have a normal resting ECG with considerable narrowing of the coronary arteries. Exercise testing was developed in the 1950s with the Bruce protocol published in 1963. It is now a well-established technique and can be used in the following circumstances:

- Assessing a clinical diagnosis of angina
- Risk stratification after myocardial infarction
- Risk stratification in patients with HOCM
- Evaluation of revascularization procedures or treatment
- Evaluation of exercise tolerance and cardiac function
- Assessment of cardiopulmonary function in patients with dilated cardiomyopathy or heart failure
- Assessment of treatment for arrhythmia
- Assessment of those in high-risk occupations (e.g. airline pilots).

Dobutamine stress echocardiography can be used when the patient is unable to use a treadmill or exercise bike (e.g. because of claudication or musculoskeletal problems).

Exercise testing has a sensitivity of 78% and a specificity of 70% in detecting coronary artery disease: a negative test does not completely rule out disease.

A positive test at a low workload is a poor prognostic sign and indicates the need for urgent further investigation (e.g. coronary angiography) and treatment.

Myocardial perfusion scintigraphy

Myocardial perfusion scintigraphy ('thallium scanning') should follow an equivocal or inadequate exercise test. This is especially useful where respiratory or musculoskeletal disease prevents a full exercise test. In the elderly, thallium scanning produces slightly more reliable results than exercise testing.

The technique uses a potassium analogue, thallium-201, to demonstrate areas of poorly perfused myocardium. The investigation consists of a standard exercise test with continuous ECG and blood pressure monitoring. At peak exercise the thallium-201 is injected intravenously.

Areas of myocardium that are well perfused take up high levels of thallium, while ischaemic areas appear as scintigraphic defects in the immediate post-exercise exposures. Repeat imaging with the gamma camera at 2–4 hr post-exercise permits reassessment of the scintigraphic defects. If the defect has resolved, the area was relatively ischaemic but still viable, but if the defect persists, the area has infarcted.

Echocardiography

Echocardiography is a non-invasive method for imaging the heart. It is based on ultrasound. There are various echocardiographic techniques:

- M (motion) mode, in which the ultrasound beam is aimed manually at selected cardiac structures to give a graphic recording of their positions and movements.
- A more recent development uses electromechanical or electronic techniques to scan the ultrasound beam rapidly across the heart to produce two-dimensional (2D mode or B mode) tomographic images of selected cardiac Sections. This gives more information than the M mode about the shape of the heart and also shows the spatial relationships of its structures during the cardiac cycle.

- Colour flow Doppler studies of blood flow in the heart can be used to construct a colour map of local blood flow in chambers and around valves. In this way, a non-invasive semi-quantitative estimate of regurgitant and stenotic valves can be made.

A comprehensive echocardiographic examination, utilizing both M-mode and 2D recordings, provides a great deal of information about cardiac anatomy and function. This has major diagnostic value.

Cardiopulmonary exercise (CPX) testing

The major determinant of perioperative mortality is the ability of the heart to increase its output in response to surgical stress. Poor ventricular function and myocardial ischaemia pose the highest risk in combination. Studies with CPX testing show that, without cardiac failure, ischaemia alone has little effect on perioperative mortality.

ECG treadmill studies focus on detection of ischaemia. CPX detects this too, but also measures gas exchange, from which a series of inferences can be made, including ventricular function, respiratory function, and cellular function.

CPX is cheap and non-invasive and evaluates both the cardiovascular and respiratory systems, making it ideal for investigation of the patient with exertional dyspnoea. It is also used to assess fitness of athletes and evaluate patients for cardiac transplantation. The aim of CPX testing is to determine the patient's anaerobic threshold (AT) (Figure 1.17)

The test takes 1 hr to perform and requires minimal preparation, and so may be performed on an outpatient basis. It is extremely safe, with very few patients suffering myocardial ischaemia. ECG and respiratory function tests are integral to CPX assessment.

AT may be evaluated even in poorly motivated patients, and it occurs well before maximum aerobic capacity (VO_{2max}). AT is easily obtained in elderly patients as the measurement does not require great physical stress. Increasing age produces a reduction in AT that is more dependent on disease and fitness than on age alone.

Following major surgery, basal oxygen consumption is 40% greater than usual. Cardiac output will have to be proportionally greater. Patients unable to achieve an AT of 8.5–11.5ml/min/kg (290–390ml/m^2) on CPX may be unable to increase cardiac output enough post surgery to compensate for the higher oxygen requirement. Cardiovascular mortality is higher in patients with an AT <11ml/min/kg (see Table 1.4).

MUGA scan

Multiple gated acquisition scanning (MUGA) is a nuclear medicine test to evaluate the function of the heart. It provides a movie-like image of the beating heart, allowing determination of the health of the heart's major pumping chambers. In myocardial infarction or other myocardial diseases, this scan can help pinpoint the position and degree of myocardial damage. MUGA scans are also used to assess heart function prior to and during certain chemotherapies (e.g. adriamycin) that have known cardiac effects.

Stannous (tin) ions are injected into the patient's bloodstream to make the red cells 'sticky'. An IV injection of radioactive [^{99m}Tc]pertechnetate labels the red blood cells *in vivo* and the radiation is detected by a gamma camera. The patient's heart beat is used to 'gate' the acquisition of a series of images of the heart (usually 16), one at each stage of the cardiac cycle. The resulting images show the blood pool in the chambers of the heart. The images can be digitally analysed to calculate the ejection fraction.

- The scan provides a reliable estimation of left ventricular ejection fraction (LVEF). LVEF is simply the proportion of blood that is expelled from the left ventricle with each heart beat. A normal LVEF is 0.5 (i.e. 50%) or greater.
- However, it has not been shown to be a valid screening test for prediction of postoperative cardiac events. Furthermore, it correlates poorly with peak exercise capacity and oxygen uptake.

The Bruce protocol

This is very widely used and has been extensively validated. There are seven stages of 3min each so that a complete test takes 21 min.

The level of exercise is estimated in METs. In stage 1 the patient walks at 1.7mph (2.7km/h) up a 10% incline. Energy consumption is estimated to be 4.8 METs during this stage. The speed and incline increase with each stage. The information from an exercise tolerance test can be used to advise the patient on what activities and exercise levels are reasonable.

Ideally, for an adequate test the patient should achieve 85% of maximum heart rate. Maximum heart rate is approximately 220 – age in years for men, and 210 – age in years for women.

Abnormalities during testing

An abnormal ST segment response is when there is a horizontal (planar) or down-sloping depression of >1 mm. T-wave elevation of >1 mm in leads without Q waves is also abnormal. It suggests severe coronary artery disease and poor prognosis.

Extrasystoles induced by exercise are of no significance for coronary artery disease.

Stopping the test

Patients rarely exercise for the full 21min of the Bruce protocol but completion of 9–12min of exercise or reaching 85% of the predicted $HR_{maximum}$ is usually satisfactory.

The test is terminated when diagnostic criteria have been met or when the patient's condition prevents continuation. After the exercise has ended the recording continues for up to 15min. ST segment changes or arrhythmias may occur during the recovery period even if they were not present during exercise.

The following findings suggest high probability of coronary artery disease:

- Horizontal ST segment depression of <2 mm
- Down-sloping ST segment depression
- Early positive findings within 6min
- Persistence of ST depression for more than 6min after stopping
- ST segment depression in five or more leads
- Hypotension with exercise.

The following are contraindications to performing the test:

- Acute myocardial infarction in the previous 4–6 days
- Unstable angina with rest pain in the previous 48 hr
- Uncontrolled heart failure
- Acute myocarditis or pericarditis
- Acute systemic infection
- Deep vein thrombosis is likely to shift and cause a pulmonary embolism
- Uncontrolled hypertension with a systolic blood pressure >220mmHg or diastolic >120mmHg
- Severe aortic stenosis can cause sudden death on exercise
- Severe hypertrophic obstructive cardiomyopathy.

CPX testing

Baseline values are measured at rest before exercise. The patient then pedals a bicycle ergometer at 55–65 rpm until the end of the test.

With a zero watt bicycle, the flywheel is assisted electrically to reduce the load further. This is termed 'unloaded cycling'. The first 3min of exercise are performed without external load on the ergometer; after 3min, the load is increased towards the maximum predicted work rate for that patient (a 'ramp protocol').

The test is designed to last about 6min after the unloaded cycling stage.

The test is stopped if the patient reaches maximum work rate or if there is symptom limitation to the test (develops some form of distress or significant ECG change).

Oxygen and carbon dioxide concentrations and tidal volume are measured on a breath-by-breath basis. The tidal volume is multiplied by the respiratory rate to give minute volume, and thus VO_2 (total oxygen uptake) and VCO_2 (total carbon dioxide excretion) can be calculated.

The software is configured for continuous display of oxygen uptake, carbon dioxide output, work rate in watts, and other cardiorespiratory parameters.

Table 1.4 Grades of heart failure as determined by CPX		
Cardiac failure assessment	VO_2 max (ml/min/kg)	AT (ml/min/kg)
None	>20	>14
Mild	16–19.9	11–13.9
Moderate	10–15.9	8–10.9
Severe	<10	<8

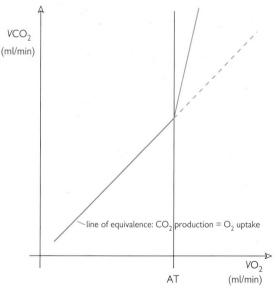

Fig. 1.17 Anaerobic threshold (AT) as determined by CPX. Aerobic metabolism supplies the majority of ATP up to the anaerobic threshold. Although anaerobic production of ATP commences at this point, it supplements aerobic metabolism, which does not stop. CPX detects the change from aerobic to partial anaerobic metabolism. At AT, the production of CO_2 relative to the consumption of O_2 increases. The onset of anaerobic respiration increases lactate production, which is buffered by bicarbonate: for each 1mmol/l increase in lactate, bicarbonate will fall by a similar amount. CO_2 is produced in excess, as demonstrated by the AT.

The term 'anaesthetic risk' is often used to describe the overall risk of mortality and morbidity from surgery. In fact, the incidence of death within 30 days attributable *solely* to anaesthesia is around 1:185,000. Studies have shown that the main anaesthetic factors increasing risk to patients are:

- Poor preoperative assessment
- Inadequate staff / poor supervision of junior staff
- Inadequate postoperative care.

The overall risk for any procedure may be much higher, but it is important to realize that this comprises patient, surgical, and anaesthetic factors.

The assessment of risk during the preoperative assessment has several purposes:

- Planning anaesthetic technique to avoid specific problems (e.g. difficult intubation, anaphylaxis, malignant hyperpyrexia)
- Identifying the need for optimization of medical status
- Giving information to patients about morbidity and mortality, to allow informed consent for anaesthesia and surgery
- Determining the most suitable environment for perioperative care.

Scoring systems

Numerous tools and scoring systems exist for assessing operative risk.

ASA physical status classification

The American Society of Anesthesiologists (ASA) originally introduced this description of the preoperative state of a patient. Despite its simplicity, it remains a useful tool that can be applied to all patients. There are five categories (addition of the postscript E indicates an emergency operation):

I	Healthy patient
II	Mild systemic disease, with no functional limitation
III	Moderate systemic disease, with definite functional limitation
IV	Severe systemic disease that is a constant threat to life
V	A moribund patient who is not expected to live for 24hr, with or without the operation

A further category (ASA VI) was added in 1983, denoting a brain-dead patient whose organs are being harvested for transplant.

There are some risk factors that the ASA classification does not take into account. These include age, expected airway difficulty, anaesthetist experience, pregnancy, obesity, and smoking. Nevertheless it remains the most widely adopted risk assessment score, partly because it is so simple and quick to apply. It is also used in many clinical trials and studies to standardize patients.

Mortality rates after anaesthesia and surgery for each ASA category are as follows:

I	0.1%
II	0.2%
III	1.8%
IV	7.8%
V	9.4%

New York Heart Association classification

This divides patients into four groups, according to their functional status.

Class 1	No functional limitation
Class 2	Slight functional limitation. Fatigue, palpitations, dyspnoea or angina on ordinary physical activity, but asymptomatic at rest
Class 3	Marked functional limitation. Symptoms on less than ordinary activity, but asymptomatic at rest
Class 4	Inability to perform any physical activity, with or without symptoms at rest

Cardiovascular risk increases with decreasing effort tolerance.

Metabolic equivalents (METs)

The MET is a unit of oxygen consumption. One MET equates to an oxygen uptake of 3.5ml/min/kg. Multiples of this are used to estimate a patient's effort tolerance and $VO_{2\ max}$ (Section 1.7).

1 MET	Eating, washing
3 MET	100m walk on flat, light housework
4 MET	Climb one flight of stairs, walk uphill
6 MET	Run for a bus
10 MET	Strenuous sport, e.g. tennis, football
20 MET	Elite athletic performance

The significance of $VO_{2\ max}$ is simple: postoperatively, oxygen uptake increases. The degree of increase varies depending on factors such as the type of operation, presence of sepsis, extent of tissue injury, vomiting, and shivering. Pain alone can cause oxygen consumption to reach 7ml/min/kg (2 METs); this is equivalent to a short walk. The ability of the patient to meet this increased metabolic demand is the basis of the CPX test (Section 1.7) and is the most reliable predictor of outcome from surgery. Patients unable to meet a 4-MET demand are at increased perioperative and long-term risk of cardiovascular complications.

Other systems

Other scoring systems have been developed for specific subsets of patients and types of surgery. They include the Goldman cardiac risk index (Section 1.6), the liver failure score, the European System for Cardiac Operative Risk Evaluation (EuroSCORE), used in cardiac surgery, and the Vascular Physiological and Operative Severity Score for the enUmeration of Mortality and morbidity (V-POSSUM), used in vascular surgery.

Scoring systems are used in the critical care environment for prognostication and clinical research. Such systems include Acute Physiology And Chronic Health Evaluation II (APACHE II) and Sepsis-related Organ Failure Assessment (SOFA). See Section 23.1 for further details.

Other factors that influence outcome following anaesthesia include:

- ASA >3 (accounts for 84% of perioperative deaths)
- Presence of cardiac failure
- High cardiac risk index
- Pulmonary disease
- Pulmonary pathology seen on chest X-ray
- ECG abnormalities.

Prediction of outcome is an important part of anaesthetic practice. Systems capable of identifying individuals at risk are at present still in their infancy. It is worth emphasizing that anaesthesic outcome cannot be considered in isolation but must include surgical, patient, and social factors.

⊙ Case study

A 59-year-old man presents for anterior resection for rectal carcinoma. He had a myocardial infarction 2 months ago, treated with thrombolysis and percutaneous stenting.

Current medications include aspirin, clopidogrel, metoprolol, enalapril, furosemide, and simvastatin.

He gives a history of shortness of breath on climbing one flight of stairs. He suffers from mild ankle swelling and sleeps with two or three pillows. He denies ongoing angina.

He is an ex-smoker of 30 pack-years and a social drinker. He is retired and lives with his wife.

On examination, he is comfortable at rest. Pulse is 55 bpm (regular); blood pressure is 130/82mmHg. He has no basal crepitations and heart sounds are normal.

How would you investigate this patient further?

ECG: Q waves anteriorly

U&E: sodium 135mmol/l, potassium 4.8mmol/l, creatinine 135μmol/l, urea 7.7mmol/l

Chest X-ray: hyperinflated lung fields; cardiothoracic ratio 50%.

Lung function tests: FEV_1 0.8L, FVC 2.2L (ratio 0.36)

There was no significant response to inhaled bronchodilator. Flow–volume loops showed very low mid-expiratory flow rates.

Lung volume assessment confirmed hyperexpansion with elevated RV and RV/TLC ratio. Transfer factor (K_{CO}) was reduced to 45% of predicted.

ABG: mild hypoxia (pH 7.39, PO_2 9.0, CO_2 4.5)

CPX testing: anaerobic threshold 10ml/min/k

The history and investigations indicate an increased perioperative risk of mortality. However, surgery in this case cannot be significantly delayed. The decision was made to admit the patient electively to the ICU perioperatively for invasive monitoring, including cardiac output assessment.

His recent coronary stenting required ongoing antiplatelet therapy, and so epidural analgesia carried an increased risk. Instead, systemic analgesia was used. He was managed in theatre with the aim of maintaining HR, MAP, and CO within 20% of their baseline preoperative values. This approach is associated with a reduction in cardiovascular causes of perioperative death.

⊕ Consent for anaesthesia

Most UK centres do not require written consent forms for anaesthetic procedures which are undertaken as part of broader surgical treatment. Nevertheless, respect for patients' autonomy is a central pillar of medical practice. Voluntary and informed consent must be obtained (and documented) from all competent patients prior to anaesthesia, even if this does not take the form of a written agreement. It is the responsibility of the anaesthetist treating the patient to gain such consent. Some procedures (such as nerve blocks in chronic pain patients) are considered primary interventions, and these do require written consent.

All patients should be assumed to be competent unless proven otherwise. Pain, illness, drugs, or emergency situations do not necessarily render a patient incompetent to give or withhold consent. Refusal of treatment by a competent adult is legally binding, even if it appears irrational or ill-considered. In some situations, however, the patient may not have capacity to consent (e.g. because of unconsciousness), and in these circumstances emergency life- or health-saving treatment may be provided in the best interests of the patient. Provision for less urgent interventions in adult patients without capacity is described in Section 21.4.

Wherever possible, patients should be provided with written information well in advance of their anaesthetic. It is often difficult to balance the provision of sufficient information with the need to reassure the patient. On the other hand, it is unacceptable to withhold information from patients because it may deter them from accepting a procedure. The rule of thumb is that the patient should be warned of any common (approximately 1%) and any serious hazards, taking into account their circumstances. The question to ask is: 'What would *this particular* patient view as relevant when deciding which (if any) treatment to accept?' For example, an edentulous patient does not need to be warned about damage to teeth, whereas such damage may be a particularly significant concern for a professional model. It is also important to estimate the extra risk posed by the patient's pre-existing medical state and to discuss this. While describing any risks inherent in anaesthesia, it may help to tell the patient about any steps which will be taken to minimize these risks.

Competent patients have the right to qualify their consent in advance, e.g. to refuse blood products in the event of haemorrhage. Such qualifications are binding, and the anaesthetist may only refuse to treat the patient if no additional harm is likely to come to them because of the refusal. If the treatment is urgently necessary, the anaesthetist should proceed while still being bound by the patient's wishes. If the treatment is less urgent, reasonable attempts to find another anaesthetist willing to treat the patient should be made.

Consent must be given voluntarily, without coercion. It is essential to give patients time to consider their options, ask questions, and come to a conclusion without pressure. For this reason, it is unacceptable for the preoperative consultation to occur in the anaesthetic room immediately before the procedure (although this may sometimes be unavoidable in cases of extreme urgency).

Further reading

Consent for Anaesthesia (revised edn). Association of Anaesthetists of Great Britain and Ireland, London, 2006.

Premedication

Premedicaton refers to the administration of drugs preoperatively, to aid the process of anaesthesia. Despite the many indications, premedication is not used as much as in previous years. Reasons for this include:

- Lack of evidence of efficacy for anxiolysis
- Admission on the day of surgery
- More day stay procedures
- Difficult timing of drug administration
- Excessive postoperative sedation associated with premedication
- Pain from IM injection
- A dry mouth at induction is no longer considered desirable
- Improvements in anaesthetic drugs and techniques.

Indications for premedication

Anxiolysis

There is understandably a high incidence of anxiety in surgical patients, and an inverse relationship exists between anxiety and smoothness of induction of anaesthesia.

Some of the anxiety should have been allayed during the preoperative visit, or in the assessment clinic. This has been shown to be the most effective mode of patient anxiolysis. However, in some patients, pharmacological means (e.g. benzodiazepines) may be beneficial, albeit with some placebo effect.

Anti-sialagogue action

Some anaesthetists still prescribe anticholinergic drugs preoperatively to reduce secretions. However, modern anaesthetic drugs stimulate salivation to only a minor degree.

There are still some specific cases where drying is necessary, such as fibreoptic intubation and when using ketamine.

Analgesia

Prescribing paracetamol and NSAIDs prior to paediatric surgery helps to achieve adequate analgesia postoperatively.

Pre-emptive analgesia is used in day stay surgery, but there is little evidence that it is effective for paracetamol, NSAIDs, local anaesthetic, or opioids. Total doses are the same whether the drugs are given pre- or postoperatively.

Anti-emesis

Nausea and vomiting are still very common postoperatively. Occasionally, anti-emetics are given preoperatively for very short procedures, but have been found to be more effective when given intraoperatively.

Other methods of anti-emesis, such as acupressure and acupuncture, can be used preoperatively (Section 17.10).

Amnesia

In some circumstances it may be appropriate to induce amnesia preoperatively, e.g. for children or for surgery when multiple visits to theatre are required. Anterograde amnesia is commonly experienced after administration of benzodiazepines.

Reduction in volume and pH of gastric contents

This is used for patients who are at risk of vomiting or regurgitating gastric contents.

Metoclopramide may increase gastric emptying. The pH of gastric contents can be increased by the use of antacids such as omeprazole, ranitidine, and sodium citrate.

Particulate antacids and alginates (e.g. Gaviscon) should not be used, because they can cause lung injury when aspirated.

Attenuation of vagal reflexes

The administration of anticholinergics can inhibit the vagal bradycardia seen with:

- Surgical manoeuvres such as traction on eye muscles in ophthalmic surgery, cervical dilatation in gynaecology, and peritoneal stretch in laparoscopic surgery
- Repeated suxamethonium administration.

Reduction of sympathetic responses

Induction of anaesthesia and tracheal intubation can evoke a significant sympathetic response. This may be of little consequence in an otherwise fit individual; however, in a patient with cardiovascular disease it is less desirable.

Premedication with β-blockers in combination with anxiolytics and local anaesthesia to the airway at time of induction is commonly used. The administration of β-blockers to patients with CVS disease undergoing non-cardiac surgery is controversial (Section 10.11).

Preoperative starvation

In general, a period of starvation is required before surgery in all but life-threatening situations. It must be stressed that the period of preoperative starvation does not preclude administration of tablets with a small amount of water. The Association of Anaesthetists of Great Britain and Ireland (AAGBI) recommends:

- 6 hr for solid food, infant formula, or other milk
- 4 hr for breast milk
- 2 hr for clear non-particulate and non-carbonated fluids.

The chewing of gum is controversial. A practical approach is to consider it as an oral fluid and restrict it for 2 hr preoperatively. The greater danger is that the gum acts as foreign body, potentially blocking the airway.

It is important that patients who are vulnerable to dehydration should be monitored during this period and should be not left for long periods without hydration. They may require intravenous fluid therapy. These groups include:

- The elderly
- Patients who have undergone bowel preparation
- Sick patients
- Children
- Breastfeeding mothers
- Patients with chronic renal failure and obligatory urine losses.

Further reading

Preoperative Assessment: The Role of the Anaesthetist. Association of Anaesthetists of Great Britain and Ireland, London, 2001.

Chapter 2

The anaesthetic room: checks and equipment

19

2.1 The anaesthetic machine

It is important to establish a familiar and thorough routine for checking an anaesthetic machine. The schematic opposite (Figure 2.1) shows the overall layout of the machine. This page describes the checking procedure (as laid down by the Association of Anaesthetists of Great Britain and Ireland). The following pages discuss the component parts in turn.

Checking the machine

The following checks should be made prior to each operating session. In addition, checks 2, 6 and 9 (monitoring, breathing system, and ancillary equipment) should be made prior to each new patient during a session.[1]

1. **Check that the anaesthetic machine is connected to the electricity supply (if appropriate) and switched on.**

   Note: Some anaesthetic workstations may enter an integral self-test programme when switched on; those functions tested by such a programme need not be retested.

   - Take note of any information or labelling on the anaesthetic machine referring to the current status of the machine. Particular attention should be paid to recent servicing. Servicing labels should be placed into the service logbook for the machine. If not attached/tethered to the machine, any service logbook must carry an identifier of the machine serial number.

2. **Check that all monitoring devices, in particular the oxygen analyser, pulse oximeter and capnograph, are functioning and have appropriate alarm limits.**

   - Check the integrity of the gas-sampling line: security of attachment, lack of kinks, obstruction or breaks in the line. Test system by monitoring the rise and fall of an added measurable gas or vapour to the system. Check for presence of and integrity of any gas sampling return line.
   - Check that an appropriate frequency of recording non-invasive blood pressure is selected and that an appropriate patient size has been selected (adult or paediatric).
   - Some monitors need to be in stand-by mode to avoid unnecessary alarms before being connected to the patient.

3. **Check with a 'tug test' that each pipeline is correctly inserted into the appropriate gas supply terminal.**

   - Check that the anaesthetic machine is connected to a pipeline supply of oxygen of adequate pressure (400kPa for the UK), and that an adequate reserve cylinder supply of oxygen is available (at least half full, or greater if back-up cylinder supplies not immediately available).
   - Check that adequate supplies of other gases (nitrous oxide, air) are available and connected as appropriate.
   - Check that all pipeline pressure gauges in use on the anaesthetic machine indicate 400–500kPa.

   Note: Carbon dioxide cylinders should not be present on the anaesthetic machine unless requested by the anaesthetist. A blanking plug should be fitted to any empty cylinder yoke.

4. **Check the operation of flowmeters (where fitted).**

   - Check that each flow valve operates smoothly and that the bobbin moves freely throughout its range.
   - Check that the anti-hypoxia device is working correctly.
   - Check the operation of the emergency oxygen bypass control.

5. **Check the vaporizer(s).**

   - Check that each vaporizer is adequately, but not over, filled.
   - Check that each vaporizer is correctly seated on the back bar, locked in position, and does not appear to be tilting to one side.
   - Check the vaporizer for leaks (with vaporizer on and off) by temporarily occluding the common gas outlet.
   - Turn the vaporizer(s) off when checks are completed.
   - Repeat the leak test immediately after changing any vaporizer.

6. **Check the breathing system to be employed.**

   Note: A new single-use bacterial/viral filter and angle-piece/catheter mount must be used for each patient. Packaging should not be removed until point of use.

   - Inspect the system for correct configuration. All connections should be secured by 'push and twist'.
   - Perform a pressure leak test on the breathing system by occluding the patient-end and compressing the reservoir bag. Bain-type coaxial systems should have the inner tube compressed for the leak test.
   - Check the correct operation of all valves, including unidirectional valves within a circle, and all exhaust valves.
   - Check for patency and flow of gas through the whole breathing system including the filter and angle-piece/catheter mount.

7. **Check that the ventilator is configured appropriately for its intended use.**

   - Check that the ventilator tubing is correctly configured and securely attached.
   - Set the controls for use and ensure that an adequate pressure is generated during the inspiratory phase.
   - Check the pressure relief valve functions.
   - Check that the disconnect alarms function correctly.
   - Ensure that an alternative means to ventilate the patient's lungs is available (see check 10).

8. **Check that the anaesthetic gas scavenging system is switched on and is functioning correctly.**

   - Check that the tubing is attached to the appropriate exhaust port of the breathing system, ventilator, or workstation.

9. **Check that all ancillary equipment which may be needed is present and working.**

   - This includes laryngoscopes, intubation aids, intubation forceps, bougies, etc. and appropriately sized facemasks, airways, tracheal tubes and connectors, which must be checked for patency.
   - Check that the suction apparatus is functioning and that all connectors are secure.
   - Check that the patient trolley, bed, or operating table can be rapidly tilted head down.

10. **Check that an alternative means of ventilating the patient is immediately available (e.g. self-inflating bag and oxygen cylinder).**

    - Check that the self-inflating bag and cylinder of oxygen are functioning correctly and the cylinder contains an adequate supply of oxygen.

11. **Recording.**

    - Sign and date the logbook kept with the anaesthetic machine to confirm the machine has been checked.
    - Record on each patient's anaesthetic chart that the anaesthetic machine, breathing system and monitoring has been checked.

[1] Association of Anaesthetists of Great Britain and Ireland 2004. Reproduced with permission.

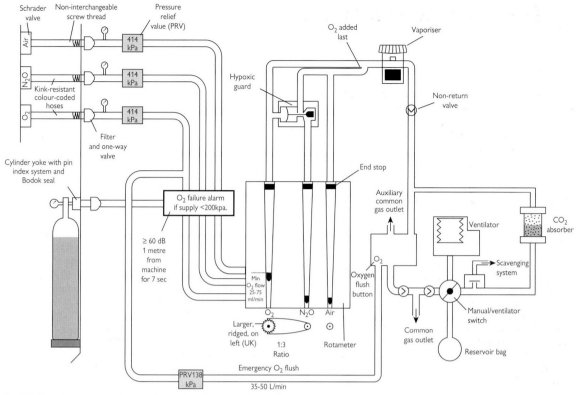

Fig. 2.1 Overview of an anaesthetic machine with circle system. For simplicity only one cylinder is attached. The anaesthetic machine includes numerous features, which are described in the following sections. The chief functions of the anaesthetic machine are: to plumb into medical gas supplies; measure and regulate gas pressures; set gas flows; add vapours; and deliver the mixture to the patient. The machine must also be designed to minimize risk to the patient, operating room staff, and the machine itself. Monitoring equipment is usually integrated into modern machines.

➜ Anaesthetic machine checks

A major contributory cause of anaesthetic mishaps has been the use of anaesthetic machines and/or breathing systems that had not been adequately checked beforehand by an anaesthetist. Checking the correct functioning of anaesthetic equipment before use is a mandatory procedure.

It is the responsibility of Department of Anaesthesia (if present) to ensure that all personnel are trained in the use and checking of relevant equipment. Trained staff must routinely check the machine according to the checklist and manufacturer guidelines, and maintain a record.

The checking procedure is applicable to all anaesthetic machines and should take only a few minutes to perform. It is not intended to replace any pre-anaesthetic checking procedures issued by manufacturers, but be used in conjunction with them. Some modern anaesthetic machines have an integral self-testing cycle when the machine is switched on. Checks should not be so superficial that their value is doubtful, nor so detailed that the procedure is impracticable.

All machines must be fully serviced at regular intervals and a service record maintained. The 'first user' check after servicing is important, in order to check for errors which are liable to occur after reassembly of machine parts.

The laminated checklist should be attached to each anaesthetic machine and used to assist in the routine checking of anaesthetic equipment.

Anaesthetic gases in common use include oxygen, compressed air, nitrous oxide, and entonox. Helium is occasionally valuable (its low density reduces turbulent flow and hence the work of breathing in airway obstruction). Carbon dioxide is rarely used. Xenon may be a useful anaesthetic gas in future, although at present expense prohibits widespread use.

The behaviour of gases is governed by the three **gas laws** (see opposite). These describe the relationships between pressure, volume, and temperature of gases. The gas laws combine to form the **ideal gas law.**

Oxygen

Manufacture and storage

Hospitals: industrial manufacture by fractional distillation of liquid air and storage in a VIE or cylinders (see below).

Home: cylinders (as above); alternatively, oxygen concentrators can be used. These use zeolite to absorb nitrogen from air, producing about 90% oxygen.

Vacuum insulated evaporator

The vacuum-insulated evaporator (VIE) (Figure 2.2) is used for the bulk storage and supply of oxygen in larger institutions. It contains liquid oxygen in equilibrium with oxygen vapour.

Structure (Figure 2.3)

- **Container:** the outer and inner metal shells are separated by a vacuum, which acts as an insulator
- **Blow-off safety valve (V):** opens at 1500–1700kPa (15–17 bar)
- **Control valve (C):** opens during excess demand
- **Superheaters:** made of copper tubing
- **Pressure regulator (R)**
- **Weighing device** to indicate the contents (more recently, a differential transducer measures pressure at the base of the cylinder)
- **Non-interchangeable filling system** to enable liquid oxygen to be filled from the supply truck

Function

Liquid oxygen is stored below its critical temperature (−150 to −180°C) at a pressure of 5-10 bar (the saturated vapour pressure (SVP) of oxygen at this temperature; see Section 2.8.

The low temperature of the vessel is maintained by the loss of latent heat of vaporization (Section 4.11) as oxygen is used, as well as the insulating vacuum.

As liquid oxygen evaporates, the vapour passes through a superheater and pressure regulator, to enter the hospital pipeline at around 400kPa.

During periods of low oxygen use, or hot weather, the pressure in the VIE may rise (since the SVP of oxygen increases with temperature). The safety valve opens and oxygen gas escapes to the environment. Loss of latent heat of vaporization re-cools the interior.

During high oxygen demand, or cold weather, the pressure in the VIE may fall (since the SVP of oxygen decreases with temperature) The control valve opens, and liquid oxygen passes through a vaporizer to the superheaters and the main pipeline.

Hazards

A VIE is sited away from buildings. There are non-combustible surfaces where leakage of liquid oxygen might occur. Liquid oxygen can cause cryogenic burns.

Oxygen cylinder manifold

A cylinder manifold is used for bulk storage. In smaller institutions it may be the main oxygen supply; in larger organizations it is used as back-up in case of problems with the VIE.

The cylinders have black bodies with white shoulders, and contain gaseous oxygen at 137 bar (13,700kPa or 2000psi).

Structure

- The system consists of two **supply banks:** primary and secondary, of large J size oxygen cylinders connected by a pair of regulators.
- All cylinders have a **non-return valve,** a **blow-off valve** and a **pressure regulator.**

Function

When the primary ('duty' or 'running') bank is on, all the cylinders in the bank are switched on. The bank in use is set at a higher pressure so that the second bank is not used simultaneously.

The oxygen passes through a pressure regulator to a pipeline pressure of 4 bar (400kPa).

When the primary bank is nearly exhausted, the pressure falls below that of the secondary bank, which takes over. An alarm light alerts the operator about the changeover.

Hazards

A cylinder manifold should be accessible to authorized personnel only. It should not be exposed to electric power lines or flammable substances.

Oxygen cylinders on the anaesthetic machine

These are a back-up supply. Like the manifold, the cylinder has a black body with white shoulders and contains gaseous oxygen at 137 bar (13,700kPa or 2000psi).

Compressed air

The composition of compressed air (dry) is: 78.1% nitrogen, 21.0% oxygen, 0.9% argon, 0.3% carbon dioxide, and trace neon, helium, methane, krypton, hydrogen, nitrous oxide, and xenon.

Storage

Compressed air may be supplied by a central compressor, a cylinder manifold, or individual cylinders. Cylinders have grey bodies with black-and-white quartered shoulders and a pressure of 137 bar.

Uses

- Anaesthetic use, at a supply pressure of 4 bar (400kPa).
- To operate surgical tools, at a supply pressure of 7 bar (700kPa).

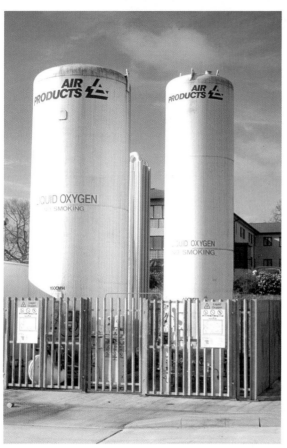

Fig. 2.2 A vacuum-insulated evaporator (VIE). Note the non-combustible hard standing – and 'no smoking' signs!

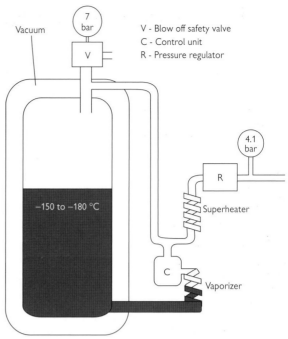

Vacuum

7 bar

V - Blow off safety valve
C - Control unit
R - Pressure regulator

4.1 bar

R

Superheater

−150 to −180 °C

C

Vaporizer

Fig. 2.3 Schematic diagram of the inside of a VIE.

The gas laws

Boyle's law

At a constant temperature, the volume of a given mass of gas is inversely proportional to the absolute pressure

$P \propto 1/V$ or $PV = $ constant

This law can be used to calculate the volume of gas obtainable from a gas-filled cylinder (oxygen, air, entonox) when opened to the atmosphere:

A full, size E (4.7L) cylinder contains oxygen at 137 bar. When its entire contents are released to the atmosphere (1 bar), the volume of oxygen will be $137/1 \times 4.7 = 644$L. This could deliver oxygen at a rate of 10L/min for just over an hour (64.4min).

Note that this calculation does not apply to vapour-containing cylinders (nitrous oxide, carbon dioxide; Section 2.5)

Charles' law

At a constant pressure, the volume of a given mass of gas is directly proportional to the absolute temperature

$V \propto T$ or $V/T = $ constant

Note the use of the absolute temperature scale. A balloon warmed from 10°C to 20°C does not double in size, as the *absolute* temperature change is from 283K to 293K.

Third law (Gay Lussac's law)

At constant volume, the pressure of a given mass of gas is directly proportional to the absolute temperature

$P \propto T$ or $P/T = $ constant

Ideal gas law

This combines the three gas laws

$PV = nRT$

n is the number of moles of gas (**Avogadro's hypothesis:** equal volumes of gases, at the same temperature and pressure, contain the same number of molecules).

R is the ideal gas constant: 8.31m3 Pa/K/mol or 0.082L atm/K/mol.

The ideal gas law (*not* Boyle's law, as is commonly quoted) allows us to determine how full a cylinder is. The cylinder volume is constant; therefore at any given temperature, the pressure in the cylinder is directly proportional to the number of gas molecules present. Again, this does not apply to vapour-containing cylinders (Section 2.5)

Dalton's law of partial pressure

In a mixture of gases, the pressure exerted by each gas is the same as it would exert if it alone occupied the container

If a gas mixture contains 40% oxygen at atmospheric pressure (101.3kPa), the partial pressure of oxygen (PO_2) is 40.5kPa.

Nitrous oxide

Manufacture

Nitrous oxide (N_2O) is manufactured commercially by heating ammonium nitrate to 250°C. This results in a number of impurities, including nitrogen, nitric acid, nitric oxide, nitrogen dioxide, and ammonia. As cooling occurs, the ammonia and nitric acid combine to re-form ammonium nitrate. The remaining impurities are removed by passage through a series of scrubbers, compressors, driers, and expanders.

Storage

Nitrous oxide in cylinders stored at room temperature (15°C) is a liquid in equilibrium with its vapour at 45 bar (4500kPa, the SVP of nitrous oxide at this temperature). The nitrous oxide main supply is from manifolds (similar to the oxygen manifolds described in Section 2.2). There may also be cylinders on the anaesthetic machine.

Entonox

Entonox is a compressed gas mixture, containing 50% oxygen and 50% nitrous oxide *by volume*.

Manufacture and storage

The critical temperature and pressure of one gas may be affected by mixture with another. When gaseous oxygen is bubbled through liquid nitrous oxide, there is vaporization of liquid to form a gaseous O_2–N_2O mixture (the **Poynting effect**). It is stored as a gas at 137 bar in cylinders with a blue body and blue-and-white quartered shoulders.

Entonox inhalation apparatus (Figure 2.4)

Structure

- **Entonox cylinder**—blue with blue-and-white quartered shoulders.
- A **two-stage valve** clamped directly onto the pin index cylinder. This contains a first-stage pressure regulating valve, and a second-stage demand valve (Figure 2.5).
- A **mask or mouthpiece** through which the patient inhales.

Function

The patient's inspiratory effort deflects a sensitive diaphragm in the demand valve, allowing gas to flow. Minimal inspiratory effort is needed to achieve a high flow rate, making this an efficient demand valve. Gas flow ceases at the end of the inspiratory effort.

Entonox takes 30 seconds to act, and continues acting for approximately 60 seconds after inhalation has ceased.

Uses

- Obstetric analgesia
- Analgesia for trauma and minor procedures

Hazards

Liquefaction and separation of contents occur when the temperature of the cylinder falls below −5°C (the pseudocritical temperature). This may result in:

- A liquid mixture containing mostly nitrous oxide with about 20% oxygen dissolved in it
- A gas mixture of high oxygen concentration above the liquid.

Separation can be reversed by storing cylinders horizontally (to increase the surface area between liquid and vapour) for about 24 hr at a temperature of 5°C or above.

Entonox must be avoided in conditions where nitrous oxide is contraindicated, such as pneumothorax. Prolonged exposure can lead to bone marrow suppression by nitrous oxide.

Carbon dioxide

The presence of carbon dioxide cylinders on anaesthetic machines is rare, and not recommended. Carbon dioxide was commonly used in the days before capnography to stimulate respiration after the use of intermittent positive-pressure ventilation. It may still occasionally be encountered (for example in exams, where its prompt removal from the anaesthetic machine is advised).

Manufacture

As a by-product of fermentation, or hydrogen manufacture.

Storage

Cylinders: stored at room temperature (15°C) as a liquid in equilibrium with its vapour at 50 bar (the SVP of carbon dioxide at this temperature).

Helium

Helium is more viscous but less dense than nitrogen. Its reduced density leads to an increased flow rate under conditions of turbulence, and it is used to reduce the work of breathing in upper airways obstruction. It is not as useful in small airways obstruction, since its higher viscosity tends to reduce flow (Poiseuille equation; Section 2.7). However, it can be useful in the diagnosis of small airways disease because the flow–volume loops of helium–oxygen and nitrogen–oxygen are more similar in small airways disease than in normal lungs. The reduced density of the mixture also results in higher-frequency vocal sounds, giving rise to characteristic voice changes when helium is inhaled.

Helium is not absorbed to any significant degree across the pulmonary capillary membrane. It is used in dilution methods of measuring lung volumes (Section 1.4).

Manufacture

Helium is manufactured by fractional distillation of natural gas. It is present in air at a concentration of 5.2 ppm, but its concentration in natural gas can be up to 7%.

Storage

Pure helium is stored as a gas at 137 bar in brown cylinders with brown shoulders.

Heliox, a mixture of 79% helium and 21% oxygen, is supplied at a pressure of 137 bar in white cylinders with brown-and-white quartered shoulders.

Xenon

Xenon is a noble gas: a colourless, odourless, and chemically inert gas whose atoms possess complete outer electron shells. It is an anaesthetic agent, with MAC of 71%.

Xenon has a favourable pharmacokinetic profile when used as an inhalational anaesthetic: its low blood/gas solubility (partition coefficient 0.14) gives a rapid uptake and offset of effect. Unlike nitrous oxide, xenon is not a greenhouse gas. However, its relatively high MAC limits the amount of oxygen which can be co-administered during anaesthesia. It is also very costly.

Manufacture

Xenon is purified from liquid air by fractional distillation. It can also be extracted by adsorption onto activated charcoal. As it is present only in trace amounts in the atmosphere (0.086 ppm), production yields are low. Recycling by adsorption is possible.

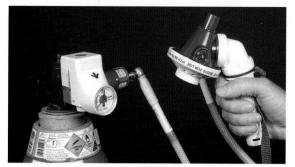

Fig. 2.4 Entonox apparatus.

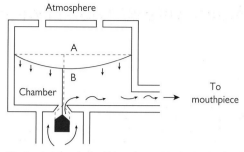

Atmosphere

A

B

Chamber

To
mouthpiece

Fig. 2.5 A demand valve. When the pressure in the chamber falls below atmospheric, the diaphragm moves from position A to position B, allowing gas to flow.

Table 2.1 Properties of anaesthetic gases

	Oxygen	Air	Nitrous oxide	Entonox	Helium	Carbon dioxide	Xenon
Formula	O_2	78% N_2; 21% O_2	N_2O	O_2:N_2O 50/50 by vol	He	CO_2	Xe
MW (Da)	32	29 (average)	44	38 (average)	4	44	131
Manufacture	Fractional distillation of liquid air	Compression, filtering and drying	Thermal decomposition of ammonium nitrate	Bubbling oxygen through nitrous oxide	Fractional distillation of natural gas	By-product of hydrogen manufacture, fermentation, and combustion	Fractional distillation of liquid air; adsorption on activated charcoal
Boiling point at 1atm	−183.1°C	−194.4°C	−88.6°C	−	−269°C	−78.5°C (sublimes)	−106.6°C
Critical temperature*	−118.4°C	−140°C	36.5°C	−5°C (pseudocritical)	−268°C	31°C	16.6°C
Critical pressure†	50.8 bar	39 bar	72.5 bar	−	2.24 bar	77 bar	57.6 bar
State at 1atm/15°C	Gas	Gas	Vapour (gaseous >36.5°C)	Gas	Gas	Sublimate (gas >31°C)	Gas
Density at 1atm/15°C	1.3 g/L	1.2g/L	1.9g/L	1.6g/L	0.17g/L	1.9g/L	5.9g/L

*The critical temperature of a gas is the temperature above which it cannot be liquefied no matter how much pressure is applied.

†The critical pressure of a gas is its SVP at its critical temperature. See Section 2.8 for further discussion of SVP.

In the UK, most hospitals have piped medical gases and vacuum (PMGV) systems for oxygen, nitrous oxide, compressed air, and medical vacuum. Some hospitals also have piped entonox.

Piped medical gas supply

The pipeline network carries medical gases from central bulk storage sites to hose outlets at a pressure of 4 bar (400kPa).

Structure

- **Central supply:** VIE or cylinder manifolds (Section 2.2).
- **Pipes:** high-grade copper alloy to prevent degradation of gases, degreased to prevent explosion. Labelled at regular intervals.
- **Valves:** lever-operated, non-lubricated. In accessible glass units, to control supply to individual theatres or departments.
- **Terminal outlet connections:** specifically labelled, shaped and colour-coded. Non-interchangeable **Schrader sockets** ensure connection with only the correct probe of the corresponding hose. The specificity of Schrader probes is conferred by a unique collar which only fits the corresponding socket (Figures 2.6, 2.7 & 2.8).
- **Flexible hoses:** colour coded and labelled. Made of two-core braided plastic with antistatic and bacteriostatic properties. Non-kinking construction.
- The hoses are connected to the anaesthetic machine by a **non-interchangeable screw-thread unit (NIST).** This unit consists of a probe unique to each gas, and a nut to screw the assembly onto the machine. A stainless steel ferrule is crimped over the tail of the NIST to seal the connection and prevent its removal.

Hazards and safety tests

Pipelines for different gases are manufactured in different sections of the factory.

Low-pressure alarms detect gas failure.

Tug tests—see Section 2.1 A tug test checks that the pipeline is securely connected to the correct outlet.

Vacuum system and suction

Vacuum systems are used to provide suction. It is recommended that a separate vacuum system be used for anaesthetic gas scavenging, incorporating reservoirs open to air (Figure 2.9A).

Structure

- **Central processor:** generates a sub-atmospheric pressure of 67kPa, and can accommodate airflows of 40L/min.
- **Terminal outlet:** a labelled self-sealing yellow valve which accepts a Schrader probe with indexing collar to prevent misconnection.
- **Flexible hoses:** colour-coded (yellow) with a specific Schrader probe connection.
- **Vacuum control regulator unit:** between the reservoir and the vacuum source.
  - Allows adjustment of the vacuum applied to the suction tubing.
  - Acts as a variable orifice (either directly, or by a spring acting on a diaphragm) to adjust the force of vacuum, which is indicated on a gauge.
  - Contains a filter and float valve to provide protection from particulate matter.
- **Reservoir** of sufficient size to contain the suctioned material, but not so large that it increases the time taken for the vacuum to build up.
  - Usually constructed of clear material, and graduated to permit assessment of aspirate volume.
  - Disposable liners are used, to reduce staff exposure to potentially infective material.

- **Suction apparatus:** tubing constructed of semi-rigid plastic to minimize kinking, with a smooth internal surface to limit resistance to flow. Of sufficient length to ensure laminar flow.
- **Nozzle** with a smooth tip to prevent tissue damage. Multiple holes allow continuation of suction should one hole become blocked.

Anaesthetic gas scavenging

Scavenging of anaesthetic gases prevents them from building up within the operating theatre and its environs. Scavenging flows are typically 80L/min, adequate to remove all expired gases.

Classification

Open vs. non-open systems: open systems involve no connection to the expiratory valve, whereas other systems enclose the expiratory valve within the exhaust port of the system (Figure 2.9B).

Passive vs. active systems: passive systems are powered by the patient's expiratory effort. Active systems employ a vacuum system to remove gases. It is important that active systems are open to air (usually at the reservoir), so that in case of obstruction or malfunction, the airway is not subjected to excessive positive or negative pressure, but will instead equilibrate with atmospheric pressure (this 'air-break' is a concept similar to earthing in electrical systems; Figure 2.9B).

Structure

- **Exhaust port:** the point at which the excess gases enter the system. Its input is via the expiratory valve or limb of the breathing system.
- **Transfer hoses:** wide (30mm) hoses and connectors.
- **Receiving system:** this includes the open-ended reservoir described above, as well as a flow indicator.
- **Disposal system:** a suction pump or fan which exhausts to the exterior (away from windows or air inlets).

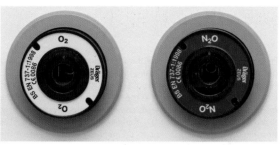

Fig. 2.6 Schrader outlets. Each is designed to fit the Schrader probe with the corresponding indexing collar.

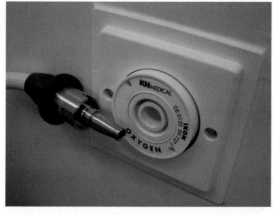

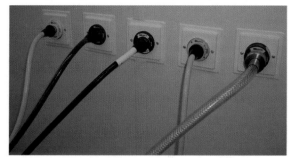

Fig. 2.8 Schrader outlets with hoses connected. From left to right: oxygen, nitrous oxide, air, vacuum, scavenging. Scavenging outlets do not have Schrader valves.

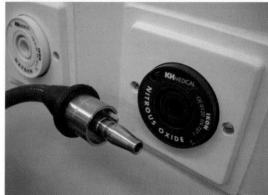

Fig. 2.7 Oxygen (top) and nitrous oxide (bottom) Schrader probes.

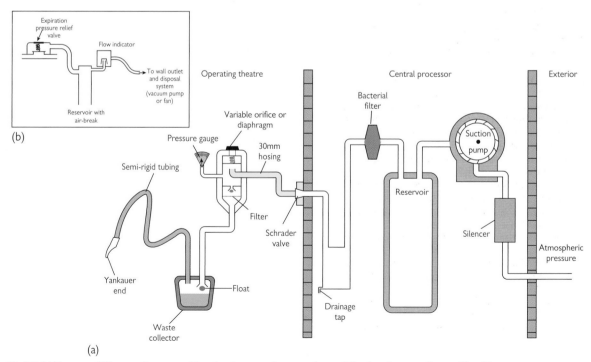

Fig. 2.9 (a) Vacuum and (b) scavenging systems. Note that the scavenging system has an air break at the reservoir to avoid applying extreme pressures to the patient's airway.

2.5 Cylinders

Cylinders contain compressed gas or liquid–vapour mixtures under pressure.

Structure
- Anaesthetic machine cylinders are made of molybdenum steel.
- Light-weight cylinders used for transport are often made of aluminium alloy with a fibreglass covering in epoxy resin matrix.
- Cylinders are constructed as a seamless tube and consist of a body, shoulder, and neck.

Characteristics
Cylinders are manufactured in different sizes from A, the smallest, to J, the largest. The cylinders on the anaesthetic machine are usually size E, and size J cylinders make up manifolds.

The cylinder body is colour coded, depending on the gas inside (Table 2.2), and engraved with:
- Test pressure
- Date of last test performed
- Chemical symbol of contents
- Tare weight (weight of the empty cylinder).

The cylinder is labelled with the name and symbol of the gas it contains, and its volume, pressure, and minimum purity. The label gives additional information relating to storage, use, and safety.

The cylinder valve fits into the neck via a screw thread. The junction between the cylinder and valve melts in intense heat (fusible), allowing escape of gas and minimizing the risk of explosions. Cylinders for domiciliary use have a multi-flow valve, with fixed preset flows.

Between the neck and cylinder valve is a plastic disc, the colour and shape of which denote the year in which the cylinder was last examined.

Cylinder valves are made of brass, and screw into the cylinder neck. There are four types of valve:
- Pin index valve block
- Bullnose valve
- Hand-wheel valve
- Star valve.

A **pin index** is used on cylinders attached to an anaesthetic machine to prevent the fitting of an incorrect gas to the yoke. Pins (metal prongs) project from the yoke to insert into corresponding holes in the cylinder valve block. A **Bodok seal,** an aluminium-rimmed neoprene washer, prevents any gas leak between the outlet on the valve block and the yoke.

Testing of cylinders
Destructive testing of one cylinder per 100:
- Tensile strength: during manufacture, one in every 100 cylinders is cut into strips and tested for its yield point.
- Flattening, bend and impact tests are also carried out in one cylinder in every 100.

Regular testing of all cylinders:
- Hydraulic (i.e. liquid) pressure test: this is done every 5 years by exposure to a pressure of about 150% of the operating pressure. Liquid is used because a pressure test using a gas would carry the risk of sudden expansion of the gas (Boyle's law) if the cylinder failed. This might result in an explosion.
- Internal endoscopic inspection.
- Test date details are recorded on the plastic disc between the cylinder valve and the neck, and engraved onto the cylinder body.

Filling
Medical gases are stored either as gas (O_2 and air), or as a mixture of liquid and vapour (N_2O and CO_2). The pressure within the cylinder can be assessed using a Bourdon gauge (Section 2.6).

For a cylinder containing gas alone, the absolute quantity of gas remaining (in moles) can be calculated using the ideal gas law (Section 2.2). Applying the law predicts that the quantity of gas left is linearly related to the cylinder pressure, as long as the temperature and volume of the cylinder do not change. This leads some people to believe, wrongly, that they are applying Boyle's law. Remember that Boyle's law applies to a fixed quantity of gas, not to an emptying cylinder where the amount of gas remaining is changing.

However, Boyle's law can be used to determine the equivalent volume, at atmospheric pressure, of a given (fixed) amount of gas in the cylinder. This requires the volume and pressure of the cylinder to be known, and the temperature of the system to remain constant. Do not forget to use the absolute pressure (Section 2.6), not the gauge pressure, in the calculation (e.g. if the gauge reads 57 bar, the absolute pressure is 57 bar + atmospheric pressure = 57 + 1 = 58 bar).

For cylinders containing liquid and gas, the pressure shows the **saturated vapour pressure** of the contents, not the degree of filling. The SVP does not change with the volume of liquid remaining; this can only be determined by weighing the cylinder and subtracting the empty (tare) weight. Once the liquid is exhausted, the contents will behave as a gas, and the pressure will fall as the cylinder empties (Figure 2.11(a)).

During continuous N_2O use, the liquid within the cylinder cools because of loss of latent heat of vaporization. Condensation or ice may form on the outside of the cylinder, and the pressure drops (because of the fall in SVP with the drop in temperature of the liquid; Figure 2.11(b)). Once the gas flow is turned off, the cylinder temperature returns to ambient and the gauge pressure rises again.

Liquid is less compressible than gas, so to prevent explosions cylinders are only partially filled with liquid. The **filling ratio** is important when manufacturers fill liquid-containing cylinders. It is given by

$$\frac{\text{the mass of liquid contained in the cylinder}}{\text{the mass of water that it would hold if filled to the top}}$$

The filling ratios for both N_2O and CO_2 are 0.75 in temperate climates and 0.67 in the tropics.

Table 2.2 The characteristics of different cylinders

	Body colour	Shoulder colour	Contains	Pressure when full (bar)*	Pin index
Oxygen	Black	White	Gas	137	2,5
Nitrous oxide	Blue	Blue	Liquid and vapour	45	3,5
Entonox	Blue	White/blue quarters	Gas	137	7
Air	Grey	White/black quarters	Gas	137	1,5
Carbon dioxide	Grey	Grey	Liquid and vapour	50	2,6/1,6
Oxygen/helium	Black	White/brown quarters	Gas	137	4,6/2,4

*Note that all gas-containing cylinders are filled to 137 bar; the pressure in vapour-containing cylinders is the SVP of the liquid at room temperature (15°C).

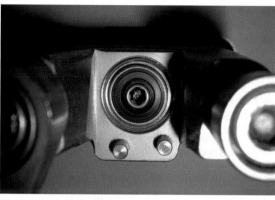

(a)

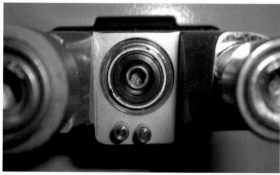

(b)

Fig. 2.10 Pin index valve blocks on the anaesthetic machine. (a) shows the attachment for an air cylinder, with the pins in the 1 and 5 positions (numbered from right to left on the machine cylinder yoke). (b) shows the yoke for a nitrous oxide cylinder, with the pins in the 3 and 5 positions.

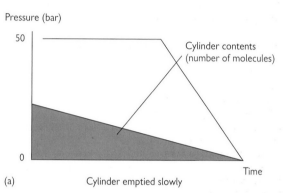

(a) Cylinder emptied slowly

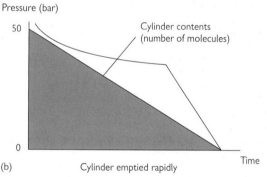

(b) Cylinder emptied rapidly

Fig. 2.11 Graphs of the emptying of a vapour-containing cylinder (e.g. nitrous oxide). (a) When the cylinder is emptied slowly, the temperature is able to equilibrate with the ambient temperature: the pressure of the vapour stays constant until the liquid phase is exhausted. (b) When the cylinder is emptied more rapidly, loss of the latent heat of vaporization causes the cylinder to cool. This affects the saturated vapour pressure of the contents, and the pressure falls even though the liquid phase has not been used up.

Table 2.3 Cylinder sizes

Size	C	D	E	F	G	J
Approx. internal volume (L)	1.25	2.5	5	10	25	50
Oxygen capacity when full (L)	170	340	680	1360	3400	6800

2.6 Pressure, pressure measurement, and regulation

Pressure

Pressure is the force distributed over a surface. It is expressed as **force per unit area**:

$$P = \frac{F}{a}$$

The SI unit of pressure is the Pascal (Pa), but this is so small that many pressures are expressed as kilopascals (kPa).

Atmospheric pressure at the Earth's surface is due to the gravitational force exerted on air molecules. The pressure depends on air density, which varies with altitude and weather conditions, but is taken as 101.325kPa as standard.

1 atmosphere pressure equals:

- 101.325kPa (SI system).
- 760mmHg (until relatively recently, blood pressure was measured with a mercury sphygmomanometer).
- 1035cmH$_2$O (the low pressures of respiratory function were measured with water manometers. Still relevant when thinking about the physics of chest drains).
- 1 bar (useful for high pressures, e.g. oxygen cylinders; and weather forecasting, where millibars are used).
- 15 pounds per square inch (psi), largely relegated to the filling of car tyres. Gas-containing cylinders are often filled to 137 bar, as a hangover from the days when imperial units were used: 137 bar is about 2000 psi.

For perspective, it is useful to think about familiar pressures in another set of units. How many of us could quote our blood pressure in SI units? (120/75 mmHg ≈ 16/10kPa).

'Gauge' and 'absolute' pressures

A full oxygen cylinder has a **gauge pressure** of 137 bar (read from a pressure gauge). When the cylinder is empty, the gauge records 0kPa (0 bar), but the cylinder still contains oxygen at atmospheric pressure (101kPa or 1 bar). Therefore the **absolute pressure** in the empty cylinder is 1 bar, and in the full cylinder it is 138 bar (atmospheric pressure plus an extra 137 bar).

Absolute pressure is the pressure relative to a vacuum. It is the gauge pressure plus atmospheric pressure.

For practical purposes, we use gauge pressure readings in gas cylinder pressures and physiological pressures such as blood pressure.

Pressure measurement

Low pressures—**fluid-filled manometers** (Figure 2.12). Pressure (*P*) is expressed as height (*h*) of liquid.

- Water: 1035cmH$_2$O = 1 atm, so used for very low pressures such as respiratory pressures.
- Mercury: 760mmHg = 1 atm, so used for rather higher pressures, such as blood pressure or atmospheric pressure.

Higher pressures—**aneroids** (non-fluid containing).

- Diaphragm pressure gauges, typically used to measure atmospheric pressures (barometers).
- Bourdon gauges (Figure 2.13), used to measure high pressures. Can also be used as thermometers (usually for very high temperatures—Charles' law (Section 2.2).

Pressure regulators

Pressure regulators are also called pressure-reducing valves. They are located between the cylinder and the anaesthetic machine.

Uses

- Reduce variable cylinder pressure to a constant delivery pressure of 400kPa (or other preset pressure).
- Ensure constant flow despite variations of temperature and pressure (e.g. reduction of cylinder contents with use).
- Protect components of the anaesthetic machine downstream of their position from pressure surges.

Structure (Figures 2.14 & 2.15)

- **Two chambers:** one high pressure (P) and the other low pressure (p).
- **Valve (v)** of area a.
- **Diaphragm (area A):** attached to an adjustable spring in the low-pressure chamber. The diaphragm is made of rubber/neoprene (for low-pressure regulators) or metal (for high-pressure regulators).

Function

- Gas enters the high-pressure chamber P through an inlet and acts on the valve (area a).
- The high pressure of the gas tends to close the valve. This is balanced by the elastic recoil of the diaphragm and the tension in the spring (adjustable). Since the force F within the spring and diaphragm is constant, the pressure of the gas in the low-pressure chamber p, which is now acting on a larger area A (of the diaphragm) is reduced.
- The gas then passes to the outlet at a constant pressure of 400kPa.
- As the pressure P falls when the cylinder empties, the valve v opens further to maintain a constant flow at the outlet, i.e. p rises (Figure 2.15).

Safety mechanisms and faults

- A one-way valve prevents backflow and loss of gas if a cylinder is not connected.
- The diaphragm can rupture or leak, leading to a hissing noise and escape of gas.
- Dirt can cause damage to the valve and its seating.

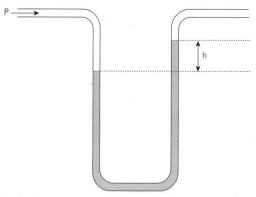

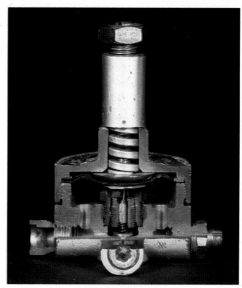

Fig. 2.12 A liquid manometer. As pressure P increases, the difference in height h between the two columns of liquid rises proportionally. Note that the fluid column is open to the atmosphere.

Fig. 2.14 Photograph of a pressure regulator

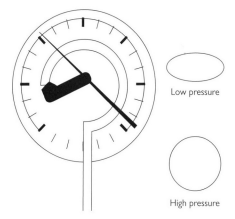

Low pressure

High pressure

Cross section through tube

Fig. 2.13 A Bourdon gauge. As the pressure builds, the cross-sectional shape changes from flattened to round, and the gauge unfurls slightly.

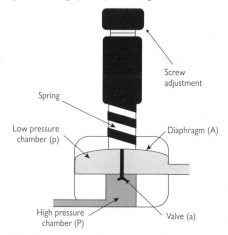

Screw adjustment

Spring

Low pressure chamber (p)

Diaphragm (A)

High pressure chamber (P)

Valve (a)

Fig. 2.15 Cross-section of a pressure regulator.

→ The Système International d'Unités

The *Système International d'Unités*, known by the abbreviation SI, is the modern metric system of measurement. It has seven base units (mnemonic: Kevin Sleeps As Mr. Kipling Makes Cakes):

Mass (kilogram, kg): the mass of the international prototype of the kilogram held at Sèvres, Paris.

Time (second, s): based on the frequency of radiation from the transition between two levels of the ground state of caesium-133.

Electric current (ampere, A): based on the current which produces a force of 2×10^{-7} Newton per metre of length, between two parallel conductors, 1 metre apart in a vacuum.

Length (metre, m:) the distance travelled by light in a vacuum in 1/300th of a second.

Temperature (kelvin, K): the interval of this scale is the same as that of the Celsius scale, for ease of comparison. Absolute zero is defined as 1/273.16th of the thermodynamic temperature of the triple point of water. Since the Kelvin scale relates to a zero point, it is a ratio scale; whereas the Celsius scale, which measures an interval between the ice point and boiling point of water, is an interval scale.

Amount of substance (mole, mol): the amount of substance which contains as many particles as there are atoms in 0.012 kilograms of carbon-12.

Luminous intensity (candelas, c:): based on the luminous intensity of a black body at a specified temperature.

These are often called **fundamental** units. However, the metre and candela are not truly fundamental as they are derived from other units.

Derived units

Derived units are defined in terms of the seven base units. Some common examples are given below

Area	square metre	m^2	Frequency	hertz (Hz)	s^{-1}
Volume	cubic metre	m^3	Force	newton (N)	Mass × acceleration
Density	kilogram per cubic metre	kgm^{-3} or kg/m^3	Pressure	pascal (Pa)	Force divided by area
Acceleration	metre per second squared	ms^{-2} or m/s^2	Work (energy)	joule (J)	Force × distance
Velocity	metre per second	ms^{-1} or m/s	Power	watt (W)	Rate of work

Flow

Flow is defined as the volume of a fluid (gas or liquid) passing a point in unit time. It is measured in litres per minute, millilitres per second, etc.

Types of flow

Laminar flow

The particles in the fluid follow parallel lines of flow. These lines of flow can be visualized as 'sheets' and are known as streamlines. The flow is greatest is the centre (twice the mean flow) and becomes slower towards the side of the tube (approaching zero at the walls).

Laminar flow, Q, is described by the **Hagen–Poiseuille equation:**

$$Q = \frac{(P_2 - P_1)\ \pi r^4}{8\eta l}$$

$P_2 - P_1$ = pressure change

r = radius

η (eta) = viscosity

l = length

r = radius of cylinder.

Turbulent flow

The particles move in swirls and eddies. The transition from laminar to turbulent flow is given by the **Reynolds number.** This is a dimensionless number, expressing the ratio of inertial to viscous forces within the system.

$$\text{Reynolds number} = \frac{v \rho d}{\eta}$$

v = mean velocity

ρ (rho) = density

d = diameter

η = viscosity

Below a Reynolds number of 2000 flow tends to be laminar; above 4000 the critical velocity is exceeded and flow becomes turbulent. Between the two, flow is mixed.

Turbulent flow is likely to be encountered when there is an sudden increase in flow, or when there are constrictions or bends.

Rotameters

Rotameters are **variable-orifice constant-pressure flowmeters** (Figure 2.16). They are most commonly encountered in anaesthetic machines and on wall outlets for oxygen.

Structure

- **Flow control knobs:** colour- and touch-coded (Figure 2.7).
- **Needle valves.**
- **Glass or plastic tube** with varying inner diameter—wider at the top and narrower at the bottom (variable orifice). The tubes are encased in a transparent cover, and are calibrated according to the gas passing through them.
- A lightweight **bobbin,** often with a dot to demonstrate rotation.

Function

The flow control opens the needle valve.

There is a constant pressure gradient across the bobbin. As the flow varies, the bobbin sits in the tube at the position where the Hagen–Poiseuille equation is satisfied. As the gas flow increases, the bobbin moves up and the annular space (area around the bobbin) increases.

- At lower flow rates, the annulus is long and narrow (length > diameter) and behaves like a tube. The main property governing gas flow is the gas viscosity.
- At very high flow rates, the annulus is short and wide (diameter > length) and behaves like an orifice. The main property governing gas flow is the gas density.

The bobbin has notches or flutes cut into it so that when gas flows, the bobbin spins. The dot confirms that the bobbin is spinning freely and is not stuck.

Safety features

Arrangement of flowmeters: if oxygen were the first flowmeter in the arrangement and a subsequent tube were broken, the oxygen could leak out, allowing a hypoxic mixture to be delivered. This is prevented by adding oxygen to the back bar last (by the arrangement of the flowmeters or internal piping) (Figure 2.1)

The flow control knobs are colour- and touch-coded (the oxygen knob is white, is always on the left in the UK, has larger ridges, and protrudes further than the others (Figure 2.17).

Most models ensure that a minimum oxygen flow (usually 250ml/min) is present when the machine is switched on.

There is an interlink mechanism to prevent delivery of nitrous oxide without oxygen. When the nitrous knob is turned, the oxygen knob is engaged as well so that hypoxic mixtures cannot be delivered. It is recommended that no machine is able to deliver a mixture with <25% oxygen.

A wire stop at the top on the rotameter prevents the bobbin from disappearing from sight.

The glass tubes are sprayed with antistatic material to prevent static build-up and sticking of the components.

Accuracy

Calibration is from the lowest accurate point, not zero. Accuracy is ±2%

Potential sources of inaccuracy

- Pressure rises at the common gas outlet are transmitted back to the gas above the bobbin, resulting in a falsely low reading.
- Rotameters are calibrated for the specific gas viscosity and density. If other gases are used, the readings are incorrect.
- If the tube is not vertical, the reading is affected.
- Dirt and static electricity can disrupt the mechanism.
- A defect in the top sealing washer will allow delivery of varying flow rates.
- Atmospheric pressure affects density; very low atmospheric pressure causes over-reading at high flows.
- Temperature affects density and viscosity. Increased temperature causes decreased density and increased viscosity.

Other gas flowmeters

The rotameter is a **variable-orifice constant-pressure flowmeter**. Other flowmeters of this type include the Wright peak flowmeter, where the expiratory flow causes a vane to rotate, opening a slit-like orifice in the device to a variable degree The more portable cylindrical peak flow meter works on the same principle (Figure 2.18).

There are many other types of flowmeter. Some examples include the following.

Constant-orifice differential pressure flowmeters, such as the Fleisch pneumotachograph (Figure 2.19), are used for machine and respiratory gas flow measurement. The pressure drop across a constant orifice is measured, and the Hagen–Poiseuille equation is applied to calculate flow. The orifice should be a tube structure to ensure laminar flow. Using a gauze screen across the orifice has the effect of converting it into numerous tiny tubes to achieve this. The pressure transducer can electronically calculate the area under the flow–time curve to measure volumes during the respiratory cycle.

Inferential flowmeters, such as the (unidirectional) Wright's respirometer, measure flow to infer volume. This has a vane which is rotated by a periodic gas flow (such as respiration). The movement of the vane is detected by a set of gears which move a gauge to display the tidal volume. The vane does not move when the flow is reversed, and so the machine can only measure inspiratory or expiratory volumes.

Positive displacement flowmeters: these mechanical flowmeters repeatedly entrap gas in a container before releasing the contents downstream. This allows them to measure total volumetric flow over the entire diameter through which the gas is flowing. 'Slippage' refers to gas which escapes through the mechanism without being measured.

Fluidic flowmeters rely on dynamic instability of the gas. Fixed vanes can induce a swirl, causing rotation of a movable vane. This can be detected optically and is used on some machines to measure exhaled volumes and flows. Vortex-shedding flowmeters place an obstruction in the gas flow, and the frequency of shedding of the resultant vortices is proportional to flow.

Ultrasonic flowmeters measure gas flow using the 'transit-time' principle. The time taken for a pulse of ultrasound to pass through a gas varies with flow.

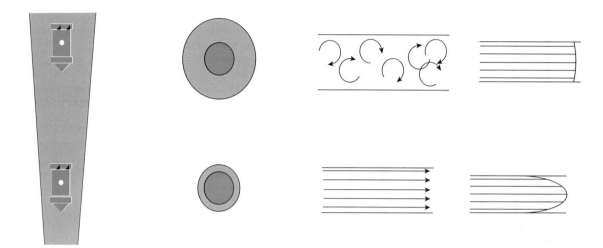

Viewed from in front   Viewed from above   Particle direction   Flow velocity profile

Fig. 2.16 Turbulent (top) and laminar (bottom) flow in rotameters. Note the differences in the way the particles move, and the flow velocity profiles between the two types.

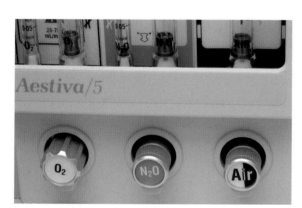

Fig. 2.17 Rotameter controls. Note that the oxygen knob is on the left, and is larger and more ridged than the others. This picture also demonstrates the machine's obligatory basal oxygen flow (the small oxygen bobbin cannot return to zero).

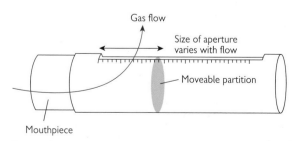

Fig. 2.18 Principle of action of the compact peak flowmeter.

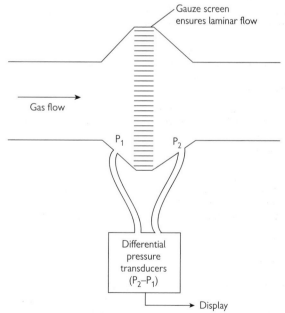

Fig. 2.19 Principle of action of the Fleisch pneumotachograph.

2.8 Vaporizers

Vaporizers produce a controlled and predictable concentration of anaesthetic vapour in the fresh gas flow (FGF). Output is expressed as the percentage of saturated vapour in the gas flow. All vaporizers have a tendency to cool with use as liquid vaporizes, and this tends to reduce the output by decreasing the saturated vapour pressure of the anaesthetic agent.

Classification

Vaporizing system
- Drawover
- Plenum
- Measured flow

Location
- Outside the breathing system—vaporizer outside circuit (VOC).
- Within breathing system—vaporizer inside circuit (VIC). Only drawover vaporizers can be used within a breathing system; they are uncommon in the UK.

Drawover vaporizers

Structure
- Low-resistance devices of simple construction.
- Powered by the patient's own inspiration.
- Performance is variable; they cannot be accurately calibrated.

Function
Mostly found in locations where there is no compressed gas supply (developing nations, portable military equipment).

They can also be used inside a circle system. Figure 2.21 is a photograph of a Goldman vaporizer, one variety of drawover system.

Plenum vaporizers

Most vaporizers in the UK are plenum vaporizers.

Structure (Figure 2.23)
- **Chambers:** a bypass chamber and a vaporizing chamber which has wicks or baffles to increase the surface area of vaporization and ensure saturation of the gas flow with the vapour.
- A **control** to split the gas flow between the two chambers.

Function
High-resistance devices; they require a pressurized gas source to push gas through the vaporizer. Therefore they can only be used outside the breathing circuit.

The FGF is split into two streams. One flows through the vaporizing chamber, while the other bypasses it. The ratio of the bypass to vaporizing stream is the **splitting ratio.** This can be adjusted, and determines the final concentration of gas. If the FGF is 10L/min and 1L passes through the chamber, the splitting ratio is 9:1 (i.e. (10 − 1)/1 = 9).

The vapour concentration in the chamber is given by:

$$\textbf{(SVP/atmospheric pressure)} \times \textbf{100\%}$$

The concentration for sevoflurane at 20°C would be (22.7/101.3) × 100 = 22.4%.

The concentration in the final gas flow is given by the concentration in the chamber/(splitting ratio + 1). For example, to give a final concentration of 2.2%, the gas from the chamber must be diluted tenfold, i.e. a tenth of the gas flow should go through the chamber, giving a splitting ratio of 9:1.

Factors affecting the vapour concentration
Temperature: as the liquid vaporizes, it cools (due to uptake of latent heat of vaporization). SVP drops, resulting in a reduced delivered vapour concentration. This can be prevented as follows.
- **Temperature stabilization:** the vaporizer is made of a dense metal with high specific heat capacity and thermal conductivity. This jacket acts as a heat reservoir (sink).

- **Temperature compensation** devices, including bimetallic strips in Tec models (temperature-compensated) or pressure transducers in Aladin vaporizers (see below).

Pumping effect: there can be an increased vaporizer output if gas already loaded with vapour is pushed back into the vaporizer. This can happen if a downstream ventilator produces back pressure. The effect is minimized as follows.
- Increasing the resistance to flow through the vaporizer and bypass.
- Lengthening the retrograde path of the gas flow.
- Placing a non-return valve downstream of the vaporizer.

Safety features
- Tec vaporizers are mounted on the back bar using the Selectatec system (Figure 2.22). This prevents accidental usage of more than one vaporizer at a time by an interlock system.
- Vaporizers are filled using non-interchangeable connectors.

Measured-flow vaporizers

(Even less memorably known as **dual-circuit gas–vapour blenders**). These are mostly used for desflurane (Figure 2.24).

The boiling point of desflurane is 22.5°C—close to room temperature. Near the boiling point, SVP varies greatly with small changes in temperature; thus a plenum vaporizer would produce an unpredictable output.

In the measured-flow vaporizer, the vaporizing chamber is heated to 39°C, producing complete vaporization of desflurane and a pressure of 2 bar.

The FGF does not enter the vaporization chamber. The vapour is added to the FGF via a metered output.

A few anaesthetic machines use measured-flow vaporizers for other agents. Aladin cassettes can only fit one vaporizer into the machine at a time (Figure 2.24).

→ Gases and vapours

A gas is the gaseous form of a substance above its critical temperature; it can never coexist with its liquid form.

A vapour is the gaseous form of a substance below its critical temperature, it can coexist with its liquid form.

The terms are often used loosely.

Saturated vapour pressure

Saturated vapour pressure is one of the colligative properties of a solution. If a liquid is kept within a closed container,

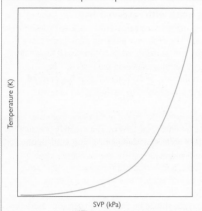

Fig. 2.20 A typical graph of SVP vs. temperature

particles escape to the space above the liquid until equilibrium is established between the particles leaving the liquid and those returning. These particles exert a pressure—the saturated vapour pressure (SVP).

The SVP of a given liquid depends only on its temperature. Ambient pressure, composition of the atmosphere, surface area exposed, size of container, etc. have *no effect* on SVP.

SVP has many important implications for anaesthesia: vaporizers, cylinder pressures (Section 2.5), the alveolar gas equation (Section 13.11), and altitude medicine (Section 13.17).

Evaporation

The average energy of the particles within the liquid is directly dependent on the temperature (the higher the temperature, the higher the average energy). The particles on the surface of the liquid can achieve enough energy to escape the surface – evaporation.

Boiling

The temperature at which the saturated vapour pressure of the liquid equals that of the atmospheric pressure is the boiling point of the liquid. Molecules from throughout the liquid (not just the surface) enter the vapour phase.

Sublimation

Solids can also lose particles from their surface to form vapour directly, a process called 'sublimation' (as opposed to evaporation). Sublimation is the direct change from solid to vapour (or vice versa) without going through the liquid stage (e.g. solid carbon dioxide).

35

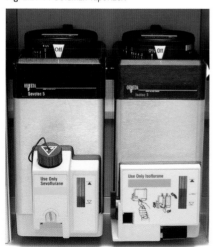

Fig. 2.21 A Goldman vaporizer.

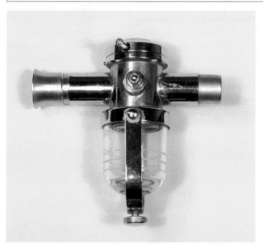

Fig. 2.22 Tec 5 series vaporizers: sevoflurane (left) and isoflurane (right).

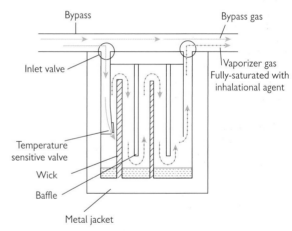

Fig. 2.23 Schematic showing the structure of a plenum vaporizer.

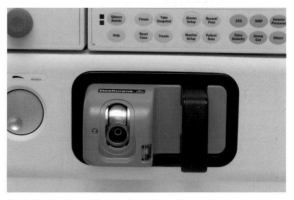

Fig. 2.24 A measured-flow (desflurane) vaporizer.

2.9 Oxygen delivery systems

Oxygen delivery systems can be classified as fixed- and variable-performance devices. A variable-performance device delivers a varying concentration of oxygen, depending on the phase of the respiratory cycle. A fixed-performance device delivers a constant concentration of oxygen throughout the respiratory cycle.

Variable-performance devices

Variable-performance devices tend to deliver oxygen at fixed flow rates. To exclude atmospheric gas completely, such devices would require the FGF to exceed the patient's inspiratory flow throughout the whole respiratory cycle. In quiet breathing, peak inspiratory flow may be 30L/min; for a deep breath it may be hundreds of litres per minute. Flows of this magnitude would be wasteful, and the patient would feel rather windswept.

Therefore the FiO$_2$ delivered by variable-performance devices changes throughout the inspiratory cycle (Figure 2.25) and depends on the ratio of delivered to inspiratory flow, and a number of other factors (see below).

Simple facemasks

Simple masks are plastic moulded devices designed to fit to the patient's face (Figure 2.26). They are generally held in place by elastic bands or straps. They deliver a variable concentration of oxygen to the patient. They contain side vents which can entrain air during inspiration, and also vent exhaled gases. The FiO$_2$ delivered depends on:

- Oxygen flow rate (usually 5–12L/min).
- The patient's inspiratory flow rate (demand) compared with the oxygen flow rate (supply). When demand exceeds the supply there is air dilution through the side vents.
- Respiratory rate and duration of the expiratory pause. During this pause, the mask fills with oxygen, which is available for the next breath. With increased respiratory rates, the pause is lost and the patient rebreathes expired gas.

Simple masks are usually easily available, and are used when a moderate oxygen concentration is required for the short term—medium concentration (MC) masks.

Nasal cannulae

Nasal cannulae are soft disposable plastic prongs placed in the nostrils. They are more comfortable and less claustrophobic than facemasks. However, they can cause dryness and trauma to the nasal mucosa. Flows greater than 4L/min are uncomfortable and require humidification. Usually the flow is limited to <4L/min. The FiO$_2$ delivered is proportional to the oxygen flow, and also depends on the degree of air dilution.

Nasal cannulae can be used to reasonable effect even if the patient is mouth breathing. The air flow through the oropharynx entrains oxygen from the nasopharynx. The obvious exception to this rule is when the nasal passages are blocked.

Fixed-performance devices

The Earth's atmosphere acts as a fixed-performance device with an FiO$_2$ of 0.21. A hyperbaric oxygen chamber also displays fixed performance. Other systems, designed to be more convenient for everyday use, include the following.

High air flow oxygen enrichment device

High air flow oxygen enrichment (HAFOE) devices or Venturi masks use the Bernoulli principle (Figure 2.27) to create a constant ratio of entrained air to delivered oxygen.

- Oxygen flows through a restricted orifice (Venturi device) at high velocity. Even though the delivered flow may seem modest (e.g. 10L/min from wall supply), the constriction ensures that the oxygen is accelerated to very high speed, ensuring total flows in excess of the patient's peak inspiratory flow.

- The oxygen entrains air by the Bernoulli principle (low lateral pressure) and jet entrainment (shear forces). The smaller the orifice, the greater is the oxygen velocity and the more air is entrained.
- The high flow rate and large mask volume prevent rebreathing.
- The devices are colour-coded, and the recommended oxygen flow rate is marked. Delivered FiO$_2$ varies from 24% to 60%.

Non-rebreathing mask with reservoir bag

The non-rebreathing mask is a clear plastic mask with inspiratory and expiratory valves. The reservoir allows a peak inspiratory flow (35L/min) greater than can be delivered by conventional flowmeters.

- One-way valves: an inspiratory valve on the reservoir bag and expiratory valves in the side vents. The reservoir bag must be filled prior to use; this is achieved by occluding the one-way inspiratory valve.
- Inspiration: the inspiratory valve opens and oxygen from the reservoir bag and inlet enters the airway. The negative pressure causes the expiratory valve to occlude, preventing air dilution.
- Expiration: the positive pressure opens the expiratory valve to vent the expired gases, and occludes the inspiratory valve so that expired gases cannot enter the reservoir bag (hence 'non-rebreathing').
- The flow rate of oxygen should be enough to keep the reservoir bag from collapsing on patient effort.
- The FiO$_2$ delivered can be up to 0.85.

Anaesthetic breathing systems

Anaesthetic breathing systems deliver oxygen and other gases and vapours from the anaesthetic machine to the patient. Various types are available, with different efficiencies and design features. See Sections 2.10 and 2.11 for further details.

Other fixed-performance devices

Other fixed-performance devices include head boxes and incubators. These are more commonly encountered in paediatric practice.

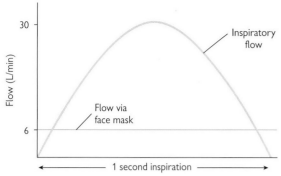

Fig. 2.25 Comparison of inspiratory flow with delivered oxygen flow during a single inspiration, with a variable-performance oxygen device *in situ*. At the very beginning and end of inspiration, when inspiratory flow is lower, all the inspired gas is oxygen delivered from the mask. However, throughout most of the inspiratory cycle, entrained air exceeds delivered oxygen, and at peak inspiration four times as much air is entrained from the atmosphere as oxygen is delivered from the mask.

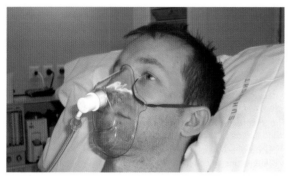

Fig. 2.26 A simple variable-performance facemask. The performance can be improved by adding inspiratory and expiratory valves and a reservoir bag, and using high oxygen flows. Note the misting of the mask, which occurs on expiration.

Bernoulli principle

The Bernouilli principle hinges on the fact that the total energy (potential + kinetic) of a system remains constant. Gas or fluid flow through a constriction increases velocity (kinetic energy). Therefore pressure (potential energy) falls.

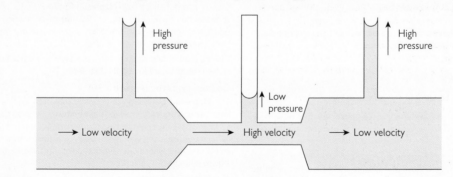

Fig. 2.27

Venturi effect

A venturi (a constrictor) is the practical application of the Bernouilli principle. It uses a constriction to accelerate gas, reducing the pressure immediately next to the gas stream. Air (or another fluid substance) is drawn into the area of low pressure. Venturi devices have a number of other applications, including nebulizers and jet ventilation.

Jet entrainment

This is the phenomenon where a fast-moving stream of gas drags adjacent stationary gas with it by shear forces.

The debate over whether HAFOE masks work on the Bernouilli principle, the jet entrainment principle, or a mixture of both has not been resolved.

Breathing systems deliver a fresh gas flow (FGF) of oxygen/air and inhalational agents from the anaesthetic machine to the patient. They also cater for removal of exhaled CO_2.

Classification

There are two main ways of classifying breathing systems.

Based on prevention of **rebreathing** (inhaling one's own previously exhaled carbon dioxide):

- **Non-rebreathing systems** with valves—self-inflating resuscitation bags
- Systems with the **potential for rebreathing,** minimized by the design of the system—Mapleson systems
- Systems with **carbon dioxide absorption:** circle systems (and historically, to-and-fro systems).

Based on the **boundaries** of the system:

- **Open**—no boundary and no dead space, e.g. at the beginning of a gas induction, with the breathing circuit not in contact with the patient.
- **Semi-open**—partial boundary between the airway and atmosphere, e.g. ether dripped onto a gentleman's silk handkerchief.
- **Semi-closed**—fully bounded, prevents entry of atmospheric air but vents excess fresh gas, e.g. Mapleson systems; circle system at high flows.
- **Closed**—no venting of excess gas, e.g. circle system at very low flows.

This is a functional classification. A circle system used for gas induction might initially be an open system; with a secure airway and high gas flows it would be a semi-closed system; while at low flows it may become a closed system.

Non-rebreathing valve systems

Self-inflating resuscitation bags (e.g. Ambu-bag). Used to ventilate in the absence of a gas supply to inflate the bag, in emergencies and during transport.

Structure

- **Self expanding compressible bag** with an inlet valve and port for oxygen.
- **Unidirectional valves:** there are a number of types—spring disc valves, fish mouth valves and flap valves.
- **Oxygen reservoir.**

Function (Figure 2.28)

Non-rebreathing valves allow fresh gas to enter the patient during inspiration, with occlusion of the expiratory pathway.

During expiration, the exhaled gases leave via the now open expiratory path, whilst the inspiratory limb is occluded by the valve mechanism.

Fresh gas flow (FGF) rate must be at least equal to the patient's minute volume. With an oxygen flow of 15L/min, the FiO_2 of inspired gas approaches 40% (variable-performance device).

With an oxygen reservoir on the inspiratory limb, the FiO_2 can approach 100% (fixed performance) if (a) the size of the reservoir is greater than the volume of the bag, and (b) oxygen flow is greater than the patient's minute volume.

Systems with rebreathing potential

The Mapleson classification (Figure 2.29) ranks breathing systems in order of their efficiency (FGF requirement) during spontaneous ventilation (A being the most efficient). The original classification described A–E; F was added later, as a modification of the E system. When learning the configurations, it can help to think about the reservoir position: afferent, junctional, or efferent.

Afferent reservoir systems

As already discussed, a simple tube system would have to deliver flows greater than the patient's peak inspiratory flow in order to exclude atmospheric gas. Taking the FGF through a reservoir (**Mapleson A** or **Magill system**) means that the system has to match volumes, not flows (this is a general property of reservoirs). In the Mapleson A, a reservoir bag at the machine end connects via a hose to the facemask. The expiratory valve is at the patient end.

In IPPV, the valve opens during (positive pressure) inspiration. Fresh gas is lost; the system is relatively inefficient.

However, in spontaneous breathing, the valve opens during expiration and gas from the lungs escapes. If the FGF equals the minute volume, the gas lost on each cycle will be the tidal volume. If the FGF is reduced, the first gas exhaled (the dead-space gas, *which has not taken part in respiratory exchange and does not contain carbon dioxide*) will enter the reservoir. Only CO_2-containing alveolar gas will be lost through the valve. In theory, the FGF can be reduced to match the alveolar minute volume: $(V_T - V_D) \times f$ (Section 2.11).

Junctional reservoir systems

Junctional reservoir systems have both the FGF and the adjustable pressure-limiting (APL) valve at the patient end. (The **Mapleson B** system is a more cumbersome version of the Mapleson C, described below, and is not in routine clinical use).

The **Mapleson C** breathing system is sometimes (incorrectly) called a Waters circuit, to which it bears a superficial resemblance (see Section 2.11).

It is interesting to compare the Mapleson C with self-inflating bags, which are used in similar circumstances. The Mapleson C requires a high-pressure gas source to function at all, and needs very high flow rates to prevent re-breathing. This may be particularly important in situations where controlling $PaCO_2$ is important, such as head injury.

Efferent reservoir systems (T-pieces)

The reservoir in the **Mapleson E** or **Ayer's T-piece** consists of a simple open tube. Positive pressure ventilation can be provided by intermittently occluding the reservoir. There is no APL valve and the FGF is taken in at the patient end.

Adding an open-ended bag (**Mapleson F**) allows easier observation of spontaneous ventilation and application of controlled ventilation. Again, this system is valveless, offering low expiratory resistance; it is commonly used for children (<30kg).

Closing the bag and adding a valve increases resistance but makes the system easier to use for adults (**Mapleson D**).

Coaxial systems (Figure 2.30)

The **Mapleson D** system can be made coaxial by leading the afferent limb through the efferent limb (**Bain system**). Because the flow in the inner limb is from a compressed source, resistance is not a limiting factor and the breathing system can be long, making it suitable for use in an MRI scanner where one wishes to keep the anaesthetic machine at a distance from the patient.

The **Mapleson A** sytem can be made coaxial by extending the tubing leading to the valve (the efferent limb), and then leading this back though the centre of the afferent limb (**Lack system**). Because the flow in the inner limb is powered by the patient's passive expiration, resistance is important and these breathing systems are short and fat. They are not in common clinical use.

Hybrid systems

These coaxial (or collateral with the limbs in parallel), systems use a switch to change between Mapleson A and D modes. The Mapleson A mode is relatively efficient for spontaneous breathing while the D mode is relatively efficient for IPPV. The most common example is the Humphrey ADE system, which can also be connected to a ventilator and CO_2 absorption system.

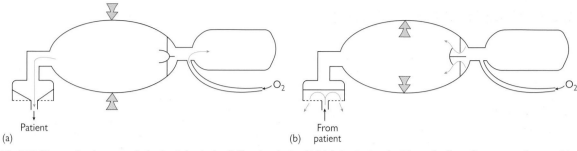

Fig. 2.28 Diagram showing a resuscitation bag in inspiration (left) and expiration (right). In inspiration, the fishmouth valve at the patient end opens while the bag filling valve closes. The reverse occurs in expiration, and the exhaled gases are vented via the expiration ports. (The expiration ports are covered by flap valves (not shown) to prevent entrainment of air during inspiration).

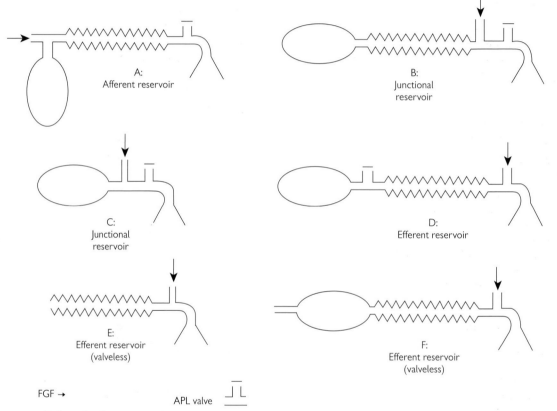

A:
Afferent reservoir

B:
Junctional
reservoir

C:
Junctional
reservoir

D:
Efferent reservoir

E:
Efferent reservoir
(valveless)

F:
Efferent reservoir
(valveless)

FGF →

APL valve

Fig. 2.29 Mapleson classification.

✚ How to check a Bain circuit

If a leak develops between the inner tubing and the outer lumen of the Bain circuit, a huge increase in apparatus dead space is likely to cause rebreathing and dilution of anaesthetic fresh gas, some of which will escape via the APL valve.

Firstly, perform a visual inspection for cracks or disconnections in the tubing.

Exclude a leak between the inner and outer tubes: occlude the inner tube with a little finger or 2ml syringe. This should lead to back-pressure within the anaesthetic circuit, detectable by pressure gauges and a dip of the bobbin in the rotameter. *The reservoir bag should not fill.* Alternatively, depress the oxygen flush with the end of the circuit open. This causes a Venturi effect at the patient end if the tube is intact: The reservoir bag will be seen to collapse as this occurs.

Check the outer tube. Occlusion of the tube should lead to inflation of the reservoir bag, with no evidence of air leak.

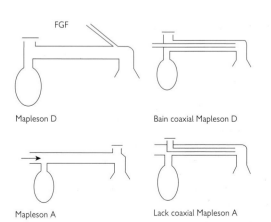

FGF

Mapleson D

Bain coaxial Mapleson D

Mapleson A

Lack coaxial Mapleson A

Fig. 2.30 Converting a breathing system into a coaxial version makes it less bulky and easier to use. A Mapleson D converts into a Bain circuit, while a Mapleson A becomes a Lack circuit.

2.11 Breathing systems II

Systems with CO_2 absorption

Breathing systems with CO_2 absorption can be very efficient, allowing recirculation of exhaled warm humidified gases, with the removal of CO_2 by soda lime. The circle absorber system is commonly used.

Circle systems

In a circle system, the patient is connected via a Y-piece to the inspiratory and expiratory corrugated hoses. Unidirectional valves ensure one-way flow around the breathing system. A circle system comprises several essential components: there are over 30 possible arrangements. Figure 2.31 shows one possible configuration.

Components

- Inspiratory and expiratory hoses
- Two unidirectional valves
- Reservoir bag
- Gas inlet
- APL valve
- CO_2 absorber
- Switch to throw absorber in or out of circle

Vaporizers with high internal resistance (e.g. plenum type) are commonly mounted outside the circle (VOC) on the back bar to introduce inhalational agent to the FGF. Vaporizers in the circle (VIC) must have low resistance to gas flow (drawover design, e.g. Goldman vaporizer).

Using the circle system

High flows are used initially to flush and prime the breathing system, de-nitrogenate the lungs and allow for initial high anaesthetic uptake. The FGF in the system can then be reduced to low flow rates. This is very economical, and minimizes atmospheric pollution from scavenging.

The flow rate is increased if changes to the gas composition in the circle are required (e.g. at the end of surgery when 100% oxygen is delivered).

To-and-fro systems

These are no longer used, but are included here for completeness. The Waters canister bears a superficial resemblance to a Mapleson C system with a soda lime canister, but it is actually an absorption system. Several problems have led to its demise.

- The exothermic soda lime reaction occurs close to the patient's head, with a risk of burns.
- The soda lime can form channels, allowing gas to pass through without contact with the soda lime.
- Soda lime dust can be inhaled.
- The soda lime closest to patient becomes exhausted first, and so the apparatus dead space increases.

Soda lime

Soda lime is incorporated into circle breathing systems for removal of expired CO_2. Flow through the canister is directed by one-way valves (visible to the user). Soda lime contains the following.

- 80% calcium hydroxide
- 4% sodium hydroxide: hygroscopic (binds water) and improves reactivity. This is regenerated every reaction cycle, so only a small amount is required.
- A small proportion of potassium hydroxide
- 14–20% water
- Silica (to maintain a granular structure)
- pH-sensitive indicator dye.

The reaction between CO_2 and soda lime has two stages:

$$CO_2 + 2NaOH \rightarrow Na_2CO_3 + H_2O$$

$$Na_2CO_3 + Ca(OH)_2 \rightarrow 2NaOH + CaCO_3.$$

The reaction is exothermic (produces heat), and also yields water. This has the benefit of warming and humidifying the gas, limiting respiratory heat loss from the patient (Section 4.12). The process also changes pH, allowing use of indicator dyes to show exhausted granules (Figure 2.32).

Granule size is important: it must be small enough to allow adequate surface area contact, but large enough to maintain uniform airflow (i.e. avoid either obstructing the breathing system or creating channels which bypass the soda lime). Most systems use granules of 4–8 mesh (i.e. they can pass through a mesh containing 4–8 openings per liner inch; i.e. 16–64 per square inch.).

Baralyme

An alternative to soda lime, baralyme contains 80% calcium hydroxide and 20% barium octahydrate. The reaction with reaction is less exothermic, and the mixture is more stable in dry climates. Some inhalational agents may produce carbon monoxide when passed over warm dry baralyme.

About 10% of heat loss of a patient is from the respiratory tract—a small proportion compared with heat loss due to evaporation from wounds and contact with the cold environment. However, respiratory heat loss may be relevant in smaller children.

The specific heat capacity, (energy required to raise the temperature of 1kg of a substance by 1°C) of gases is about 1000 times less than that of liquids; it is far more important to humidify gases than warm them. Two-thirds of lost respiratory heat is used to humidify dry gases.

It is also important to humidify the fresh gas as this may maintain normal ciliary function in the trachea and help to prevent drying of secretions in the airway (which can cause destruction of the airway epithelium and atelectasis).

Efficiency of breathing systems

Each breathing circuit has its own characteristics which may make it more useful for spontaneous ventilation, controlled ventilation, paediatric use, remote use (e.g. in the MRI scanner), or other clinical scenarios. Table 2.4 shows the efficiency of the various circuits during spontaneous and controlled ventilation. In most cases, an increase in efficiency for controlled ventilation comes at the cost of a decrease in efficiency for spontaneous breathing. The notable exception is the circle system, which can be extremely efficient for all ventilatory modes at low flows.

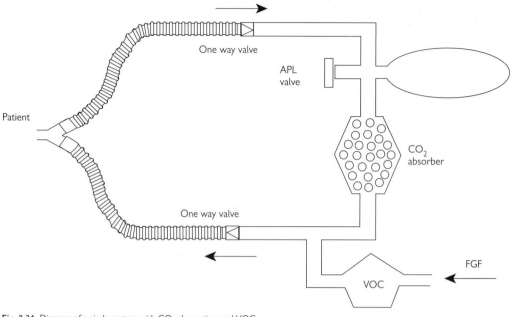

Fig. 2.31 Diagram of a circle system with CO_2 absorption and VOC.

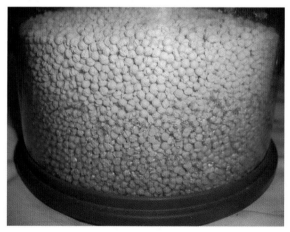

Fig. 2.32 Soda lime canister. Note the colour change.

Table 2.4 **Fresh gas flow in breathing systems**						
	A	**B**	**C**	**D**	**E and F**	**Circle**
Spontaneous breathing	In theory, alveolar minute volume; in practice, minute volume	2–3× minute volume	2–3× minute volume	2–3× minute volume	2–3× minute volume	*In theory*, only the patient's oxygen consumption (once primed with fresh gas and volatile)
Intermittent positive-pressure ventilation	2–3× minute volume	2–3× minute volume	2–3× minute volume	70–100ml/kg/min	200–300 ml/kg/min	
Note that the difference in FGFs for IPPV between the D and the E systems is because the E system is used in paediatric practice. Children have a relatively higher minute volume than adults because of their higher metabolic rate.						

2.12 Ventilators

There are many types of mechanical ventilator. They differ in the modes of ventilation allowed, the capacity to set target parameters, and interaction with the patient's own respiratory efforts.

Classification

There are various ways of classifying ventilators. The following is a useful structure.

Modern ventilators utilize two basic patterns of inspiratory gas flow. With **pressure generation**, a constant pressure is provided for the duration of inspiration. This pattern is used to deliver 'pressure control' ventilation.

Flow generation is used to deliver constant flow until a pre-set tidal volume is reached. This is 'volume control' ventilation.

Control of flow

Pressure control

These deliver a constant pressure during the inspiratory phase, which expands the lungs. The volume delivered will depend on the compliance of the patient's respiratory system. The system has the advantage that the pressure applied will never exceed the preset value, avoiding barotrauma. However, changes in resistance and compliance can cause dramatic changes to the tidal volume delivered. This risks:

- hypoventilation (if compliance suddenly falls, e.g. during the pneumoperitoneum in laparoscopic surgery), or
- large tidal volumes and volutrauma if the compliance increases for any reason.

Pressure-controlled ventilators can compensate to a certain extent for leaks in the system. Traditionally, pressure generators were used in theatre (more concern about leaks, less about lung disease).

Volume control

These can compensate for changes in patient compliance (e.g. lung disease) but not for leaks in the system.

Traditionally, flow generators were used in the ICU (more concern about providing adequate minute volumes in the face of lung disease, less concern about leaks).

This distinction is widely quoted and important to understand, but in practice it is more important to think of the practicalities of ventilating patients: where the ventilator is to be used, how it cycles from inspiration to expiration, and the mode of ventilation.

Cycling

- **Volume cycling:** phase of ventilation changes when a preset inspiratory volume is reached.
- **Pressure cycling:** the change occurs when a preset pressure is reached during inspiration.
- **Time cycling:** the change occurs when a set inspiratory time is reached.
- **Flow cycling:** the change occurs when a particular flow is reached during inspiration or expiration. Inspiratory flow during the expiratory phase of ventilation can be used as an indicator that the patient is taking spontaneous breaths (allowing the ventilator to synchronize with the patient). A drop-off in flow during the inspiratory phase signifies that the patient is nearing the end of inspiration, giving the cue for the ventilator to cycle into expiration.

Place of use

- **Anaesthetic ventilators:** theatres and anaesthetic rooms. Robust and relatively simple.
- **Intensive care ventilators:** designed to cope with changing resistance and compliance, and to help manage weaning.
- **Transport ventilators:** light and portable.

Function (method of delivering ventilation)

- **Minute volume divider** (MV=FGF/TV), e.g. Manley MP3
- **Time-cycled pressure generator**
- **Intermittent blower** (powered by driving gas independent of FGF), e.g. Penlon Nuffield 200
- **Time-cycled flow generator**
- **Bag squeezer** (fresh gas enters bellows and a driving gas into the surrounding gas-tight chamber squeezes the bellows), e.g. Ohmeda Aestiva 7900

Modes of ventilation commonly found in anaesthetic ventilators

Controlled mandatory ventilation (CMV) or intermittent positive-pressure ventilation (IPPV), where the ventilator simply delivers breaths according to the parameters set:

- **Pressure-controlled ventilation (PCV)**—time cycled, pressure preset
- **Volume controlled ventilation (VCV)**—time cycled, volume preset.

Synchronized modes, where the ventilator detects spontaneous breaths and coordinates its delivery with these:

- **Pressure support ventilation (PSV)**—spontaneous breaths are detected and assisted by ventilator gas flow to achieve a preset pressure. Flow cycled.
- **Synchronized intermittent mandatory ventilation (SIMV)**— a background of controlled (mandatory) breaths delivers a target minute volume (These mandatory breaths may be pressure or volume controlled). It also allows (and may assist) spontaneous breaths.

On modern anaesthetic machines each of these (or similar modes) can often be selected on a software menu controlled via microprocessors.

Over recent years, ventilators have become much more sophisticated. Anaesthetic ventilators routinely provide the modes above, while ICU ventilators provide a wider range of options (Section 23.3).

Examples of parameters that can be set on modern ventilators include:

- Fractional inspired oxygen concentration
- Tidal/minute volume, peak airway pressure
- Respiratory rate
- I:E ratio (inspiratory time to expiratory time)
- PEEP (positive end expiratory pressure)
- Alarms for apnoea and upper/lower limits (tidal/minute volume, peak airway pressure).

Pressure generator

Flow generator

P_{aw}

Flow

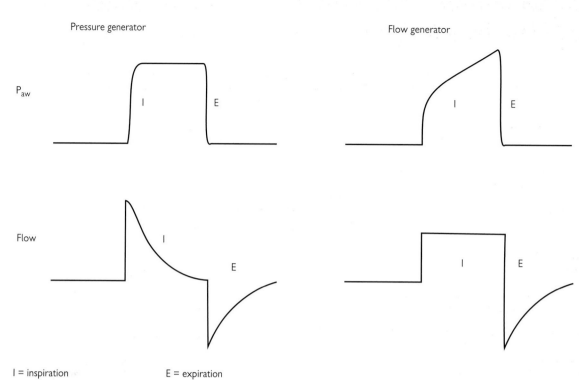

I = inspiration   E = expiration

Fig. 2.33 Ventilator types.

There are many different types of airway device and each has a specific role. They may be used as adjuncts to manual airway control, to maintain the airway during surgery, to protect against aspiration, to facilitate IPPV, to manipulate the lungs (e.g. double-lumen tube), or to regain airway control in an emergency situation. For techniques of airway control, see Sections 3.1 and 3.2.

Facemasks

Anaesthetic facemasks (Figure 2.34) can be made of transparent plastic or silicone rubber. Most have an air-filled cuff around the rim to distribute pressure evenly over the patient's face and achieve an air-tight seal. The mask has a standard 22mm connector to allow the attachment of a catheter mount and breathing circuit. Endoscopy masks (Figure 2.34b) have an offset connection and a self-sealing hole, which allows passage of a fibreoptic laryngoscope. The use of nasal masks is described in Section 3.3.

Sizing

The upper part of a correctly sized mask should lie over the bridge of the nose when the lower cuff is in the cleft between the chin and lower lip.

Basic airway adjuncts

If simple manoeuvres fail to clear the airway, it is likely that an artificial airway of some form will be required.

Oropharyngeal (Guedel) airway

Oral airways (Figure 2.35) are rigid and usually plastic. They have a flange, a thickened bite area, a curve (to fit the soft palate), a channel, and a blunt pharyngeal end. They come in a variety of sizes. Some are split to allow extraction of a fibreoptic laryngoscope (e.g. the Berman airway).

Sizing

The airway should be placed against the cheek of the patient and should measure from the patient's incisors to the angle of the mandible.

Function

The airway is inserted upside down and rotated through 180° as it passes back (adults). It is inserted directly and without rotation in children since this reduces the risk of airway trauma and bleeding.

Hazards

- Vomiting (if pharyngeal reflexes are intact)
- Damage to teeth or oropharynx
- Incorrect sizing can worsen airway obstruction

Nasopharyngeal airway

Nasal airways (Figure 2.36) are soft hollow malleable plastic bevelled tubes. They have a flanged end, and usually a safety pin to prevent the airway slipping in too far. (Alternatively an endotracheal tube of the correct size can be cut to the required length, with a safety pin). They are better tolerated than oral airways if pharyngeal reflexes are not completely obtunded. They are especially useful in patients who cannot open their mouths.

Sizing

Traditionally the airway is compared with the patient's little finger, but there is a lack of correlation between this and the diameter of the internal nose. A Portex size 6 for adult females and size 7 for adult males is usually appropriate. When placed against the cheek of the patient it should measure from the tip of the nose to the tragus of the ear.

Function

The airway is inserted perpendicularly to the face along the floor of the larger nostril (preferably sprayed with local anaesthetic and vasoconstrictor). The concave curve should be towards the ear on the same side as the nostril: during insertion it will rotate to fit the floor of the nose.

Hazards

- May create a false passage: avoid in basal skull fractures, nasal deformities or polyps.
- Bleeding (coagulopathy, nasal polyps or deformities, over-forceful insertion).

- Can provoke vomiting.
- Insertion may provoke laryngospasm.

Supraglottic airways

Laryngeal mask

The laryngeal mask airway (LMA) was developed by Brain in the early 1980s. The basic structure includes a shaft, an elliptical inflatable cuff, and a pilot balloon with self-sealing valve. Two bars may be present to prevent obstruction by the epiglottis. There are now a large number of different variations (Figures 2.37, 2.38 and 2.39).

The LMA has been proven to be a safe, easy to use, hands-free airway device. Muscle relaxants and laryngoscopy are not required, and there is little haemodynamic disturbance on insertion. There is minimal risk of major tissue or dental damage, and the emergence is smooth and controlled.

Sizing

See table opposite for sizing of the LMA.

Function

When in position, the opening in the LMA sits over the laryngeal inlet. The cuff forms a seal with the pharyngeal tissues. The LMA is ideally suited to spontaneously ventilating patients; many patients are also suitable for IPPV via an LMA, as long as a good seal is achieved.

Hazards

- Malposition and airway leak (often resolved by re-introducing, inflating, deflating, or using a different size)
- Airway pathology (placement may be difficult)
- Does not protect against aspiration (in fact may funnel regurgitated material into the trachea). LMAs should not be used in patients at risk of regurgitation.

Other complications include minor bleeding, sore throat, tongue paraesthesia, nerve palsies (recurrent laryngeal nerve, hypoglossal, lingual), arytenoid dislocation, uvular bruising, epiglottitis.

Other types of LMA

Proseal

This is the design of choice for positive-pressure ventilation via the LMA. The double-cuff design allows much higher seal pressures (up to $30cmH_2O$). It also incorporates a gastric channel, down which a gastric tube may be passed. Higher up the tube, a bite guard is included.

Reusable/disposable LMA

Disposable LMAs were introduced around 2000. Because of the theoretical risk of transmission of prions by reusable LMAs, the Royal College of Anaesthetists recommends disposables for use in adenoidectomy, tonsillectomy, or other cases where the device may come into direct contact with lymphoid tissue.

Flexible LMA

Flexible LMAs (also known as reinforced or armoured LMAs) have the same cuff as a standard LMA, but the shaft is smaller, reinforced with wire, and flexible. They are useful in procedures where the surgeon and anaesthetist are competing for access to the upper airway or face. The wire coil reduces the chance of kinking, and the flexible tube allows the shaft to be positioned away from the surgical field, without displacing the cuff within the airway.

Intubating LMA

The intubating LMA is a rigid, anatomically curved LMA with a shaft wide enough to accept a size 8.0 cuffed ETT. The shaft is shorter than standard LMAs to facilitate passage of the ETT beyond the vocal cords. A version with a fibreoptic system for visualizing structures immediately beyond the aperture of the mask is now available.

Cuffed oral pharyngeal airway

These are cuffed oral airways. When in place, a connector protrudes from the mouth and a circuit can be attached. They generally do not maintain the airway as well as an LMA and are rarely used.

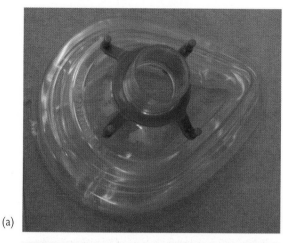

(a)

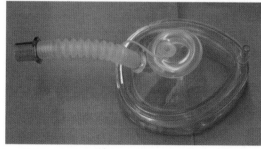

(b)

Fig. 2.34 (a) A standard anaesthetic facemask. (b) An endoscopy mask has a sealable port and an offset connector to accommodate a fibreoptic laryngoscope.

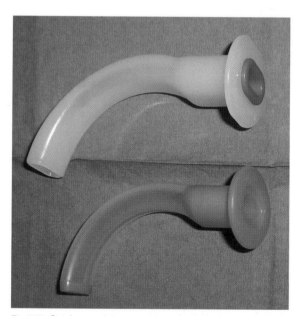

Fig. 2.35 Oropharyngeal airways.

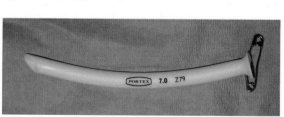

Fig. 2.36 A nasopharyngeal airway. Note the safety pin.

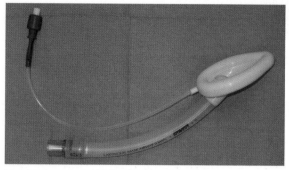

Fig. 2.37 A standard LMA. This device can be used in a wide range of elective surgical procedures and in resuscitation.

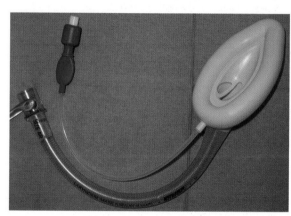

Fig. 2.38 A flexible ('armoured') LMA.

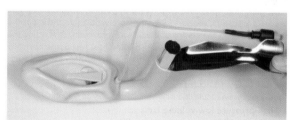

Fig. 2.39 An intubating LMA. As well as acting as an LMA, a wide short rigid angled shaft allows the passage of an 8.0mm cuffed ETT. A handle enables one-handed insertion, removal, and adjustment of the LMA. A vertical bar (in place of the two aperture bars) elevates the epiglottis as the ETT is passed. Originally developed for resuscitation, this is now largely used in failed intubation.

Endotracheal tubes

Endotracheal tubes (ETTs) come in a variety of pre-formed shapes and sizes (Figures 2.40, 2.41, 2.42, 2.43, 2.44 and 2.45).

Most are single use, disposable, and sterile packed. They are made of implant-tested thermosensitive polyvinyl chloride (PVC) or silicone, and are latex free.

Standard oral ETTs should have a curve of 12°–16°, and usually a left-facing bevel at an angle of 30°–45°. The tube can be cut to the required length. Cuffed tubes have a pilot tube to inflate the balloon, which emerges proximally.

At the proximal end, ETTs have a standard 15mm International Standards Organization (ISO) connector. At the distal end there is often a Murphy eye—a small opening on the right lateral tube tip, designed to allow ventilation if the bevel of the ETT lodges against the airway wall. However, the Murphy eye has been shown to reduce the reliability of chest auscultation in detecting endobronchial intubation. If present, it should be at least 80% of the cross-sectional area of the tube and located opposite the bevel.

ETTs have a radio-opaque line along their length to allow visualization on X-ray. They also have various markings on them:

- Manufacturer's logo
- **ID**—internal diameter in millimetres
- **ED**—external diameter in millimetres
- Length marking in centimetres from the distal end
- **IT**—implant tested (the material has been tested for allergic reaction by implantation into animals)
- **Z-79**—representing the room number at the ISO of the committee governing standards for ETTs.

Cuffed or uncuffed?

Most adults are intubated with cuffed endotracheal tubes. The cuff prevents aspiration, allows positive-pressure ventilation, and keeps the tip of the ETT in the centre of the airway, preventing it abutting the tracheal wall. Capillary pressure in the tracheal mucosa is normally about 25–30mmHg, and tube cuff pressure higher than this can cause ischaemia. Cuffs can be inflated with water, anaesthetic gas mixture (to prevent N_2O shifts changing the cuff pressure), or air. The pressure should just prevent a leak during ventilation, and be <30mmHg.

- **High-pressure low-volume cuffs** can develop very high pressures, particularly if used with N_2O, which diffuses into the balloon.
- **High-volume low-pressure cuffs** were developed to try to reduce this risk by minimizing the pressure at any one point. However, the larger cuff is less effective at preventing aspiration, is bulkier (more difficult to pass and can cause trauma), and can potentially affect a larger mucosal area if capillary pressure is exceeded.

Sizing

Usually, size 8.0mm and 9.0mm internal diameters are used for men and women, respectively. There is evidence that smaller ETTs reduce the incidence of sore throat.

Hazards

- Manufacturing defects.
- Cuff herniation can occlude the bevelled opening.
- Obstruction by secretions or foreign bodies.
- Tearing of the cuff on the patient's teeth.
- Laryngeal trauma, especially after difficult intubation.
- Nasal intubation may provoke bleeding.

Stylets and gum elastic bougies

It may be difficult to visualize the larynx and/or to manoeuvre the tip of the ETT into the laryngeal opening. Stylets can impose a particular shape onto the ETT to aid intubation. Bougies are passed through the laryngeal inlet, allowing the ETT to be railroaded over. See Figure 2.46.

Stylets

The stylet is a single-use device available in variable sizes. It has a flexible aluminium wire shaft, sheathed in PVC. This should be passed down the lumen of the ETT (but not protruding from the tip) prior to intubation. The proximal end should be folded over the ETT to prevent advancement of the stylet. The ETT can then be moulded into a J-shaped curve, allowing better manoeuvrability of the tip into the larynx. Once the tip is through the cords, the stylet should be removed and the ETT advanced into the trachea.

The lightwand is a stylet with a light at its tip. When passed through the vocal cords, a well-circumscribed light is seen transilluminating the trachea (with oesophageal placement, the light is much more diffuse). A darkened room may be necessary in order to use a lightwand effectively.

Gum elastic bougies

These are soft flexible plastic guides of variable length. With the help of the laryngoscope as normal, the bougie is introduced through the laryngeal inlet. A series of 'clicks' may be felt as the tip runs over the inside of the tracheal rings. When introduced to about 10cm below the cords, the ETT should be threaded over the bougie and gently advanced. The ETT can stick at the laryngeal opening; rotating the ETT anticlockwise, while gently advancing, will usually overcome this.

Airway exchange catheters

These appear similar to gum elastic bougies, but they are hollow. The lumen can be used for short-term ventilation via a special adapter, or in some cases (e.g. Aintree intubation catheter, Arndt airway exchange catheter) can accept a fibreoptic laryngoscope.

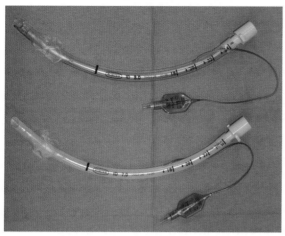

Fig. 2.40 Standard ETT with (top) or without (bottom) the Murphy eye.

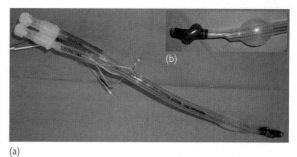

(a)

Fig. 2.43 Double-lumen tubes are used for single-lung ventilation. They may be right- or left-sided (the version shown here is right-sided). They have a tracheal and a bronchial lumen which can be used separately, with separate cuffs, for isolating each lung. This allows easier access for intrathoracic surgery.

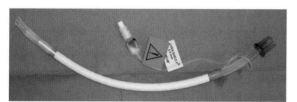

Fig. 2.41 Laser-resistant ETTs are made of stainless steel or silicone with aluminium and Teflon wrap. Some have two cuffs in case one is damaged (these should be inflated with saline).

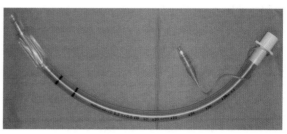

Fig. 2.44 Armoured tubes have a wire spiral running through the length of the tube. Used in head and neck surgery.

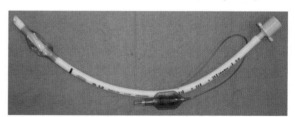

Fig. 2.45 Microlaryngoscopy tubes (MLTs) have a small diameter but a large cuff, to allow visualization of larynx.

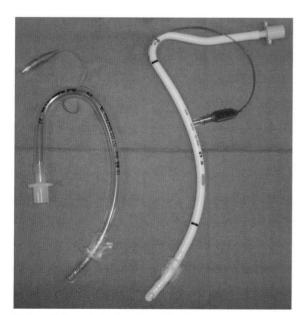

Fig. 2.42 Preformed tubes: RAE (Ring, Adair, Elwyn) tubes may be 'south-facing' (pointing towards the chin) (left) or 'north-facing' (towards the forehead) (right). They may be shaped for nasal use, as is the north-facing version shown (right). An over-large size may lead to inadvertent endobronchial intubation.

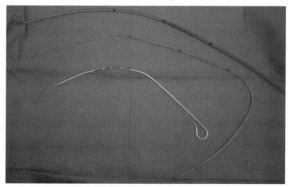

Fig. 2.46 Gum elastic bougies (top and middle), and a stylet (bottom). The top of the stylet is folded over to prevent its advancing beyond the tip of the endotracheal tube.

47

Direct laryngoscope

Structure

The standard assembly of a laryngoscope is a handle containing a battery, a light source, and a blade. The blade can detach from the handle and may be reusable or disposable.

- **Handle:** usually steel, containing the batteries for the device. 'All-in-one' plastic laryngoscopes are available for single use. Short ('stubby') handles can be used where insertion of the blade is difficult because of impingement (e.g. large breasts, surgical corset, pectus carinatum, or the hand of the assistant providing cricoid pressure).
- **Light source:** this may be from a bulb in the blade; alternatively many modern laryngoscopes contain a bulb in the handle whose light is transmitted via a fibreoptic connection to the front of the blade.
- **Blade:** the blade of the laryngoscope determines its fit in the oropharynx. Numerous different designs are available (see below).

Function

The blade is introduced into the right side of the patient's mouth, sweeping the tongue away to the left as it is advanced. Usually the tip of the blade rests in the vallecula and lifts the base of the tongue. This in turn lifts the epiglottis to reveal the larynx. In neonates and infants, the blade is used to pick up the epiglottis, which is large and floppy, in order to view the cords. (A left-sided version is available for patients with right-sided facial or oropharyngeal pathology which would make use of the standard right-sided blade difficult).

Uses

- Tracheal intubation.
- Inspection of the airway (e.g. after shared airway cases).
- Can help with placement of LMAs in some patients.

Hazards

There is a risk of trauma to the lips, teeth, tongue, oropharynx, and larynx. The light source may fail and so a spare handle should always be available. Laryngoscope blades have been known to snap during use, exposing sharp edges.

Trauma to the airway may result in the introduction of infective agents. There is a theoretical risk of prion transmission in adenoidectomy, tonsillectomy, or where the device may come into contact with lymphoid tissue; disposable blades should be used.

The oropharynx and larynx are very sensitive. Use of a laryngoscope is extremely stimulating and the patient may cough, gag, or vomit if not adequately anaesthetized. Tachycardia and hypertension are common during laryngoscopy.

Blades

Macintosh blade (Figure 2.47)

This is the most commonly used blade in adults. It is curved to follow the contour of the oropharynx. There are two versions: the American, which has a straighter tip, and the English, with a more uniform curve over its whole length. An L-shaped profile allows better visualization of the larynx. The blade has a blunt, slightly bulbous tip to reduce trauma and elevate the larynx. The American version is available in sizes 0–4 (neonate to large adult), and the English version in sizes 1–5 (infant to extra-large adult).

McCoy blade/Flexiblade

These blades are designed to give better elevation of the base of the tongue. They can be attached to standard handles, and are essentially hinged Macintosh blades with a lever to activate the hinge mechanism. They are useful in difficult intubation situations (particularly in grade 3 views where the epiglottis is visible but the cords are not). See Figure 2.48.

Polio blade

The polio blade was originally developed for use on patients ventilated by 'iron lungs' (negative-pressure ventilators). The blade resembles a Macintosh blade but is set at an angle of 120° to the handle of the laryngoscope. This avoids handle impingement on the patient's chest or other obstacle. Note: laryngoscopy technique is modified when using the polio blade, and takes practice. An alternative approach is to use a stubby handle (Figure 2.48)

Miller blade

The Miller blade is designed for paediatric practice. It has the L-shaped profile of the Macintosh, but is straight rather than curved. It is designed to pick up the epiglottis and lift it.

Fibreoptic intubating bronchoscope

A fibreoptic intubating bronchoscope (Figure 2.49) is a device which allows indirect visualization of the larynx. An ETT can then be railroaded over the instrument and its position confirmed. This procedure can be perfomed under general anaesthetic, or in certain patients, awake (Section 3.5).

Structure

- A **light source** with a cable to transmit light to the instrument.
- The **control unit,** consisting of an eyepiece (this may be linked to an external screen via a cable), control knob, and focusing ring.
- A **suction channel**—this can also be used for insufflating oxygen, or instilling saline (for airway lavage) or local anaesthetics.
- A **flexible cord,** consisting of around glass fibre bundles. Each fibre is 5–20µm in diameter, and a bundle consists of 10,000–15,000 fibres. Cords vary in size; typically they are around 4mm but ultra-thin cords for paediatric practice are available (e.g. 2.2mm diameter, accommodating a size 2.5 ETT).

Function

There are various airway adjuncts modified for use with the fibreoptic laryngoscope, including facemasks, oropharyngeal airways, and airway exchange catheters. Each fibre is coated with a layer of glass, which has a different refractive index from the fibre itself. This coating optically insulates the fibre, ensuring total internal reflection of light as it travels down the cord. The fibres are extremely thin and are lubricated—this allows the cord to be flexible. The control knob can flex the tip of the cord (through an angle of up to 240°). The fibres have exactly the same spatial arrangement throughout the cord, so the image seen at the eyepiece is the same as that at the tip of the cord.

Uses

- Tracheal intubation (oral or nasal) – in difficult airway cases
- Inspection of the airway (laryngoscopy, bronchoscopy)
- Confirmation of tube placement (endotracheal, double-lumen, endobronchial. or tracheostomy tubes)
- Tracheobronchial lavage and toilet
- Endotracheal visualization during tracheostomy

Hazards

There is a risk of cross-infection if the instrument is not properly cleaned. After use, the suction channel should be immediately and thoroughly flushed before the 'scope is sent off for cleaning. Fibreoptic bronchoscopes are fragile and break easily.

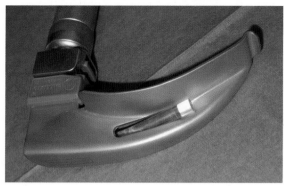

Fig. 2.47 A standard laryngoscope handle with Macintosh blade (UK version).

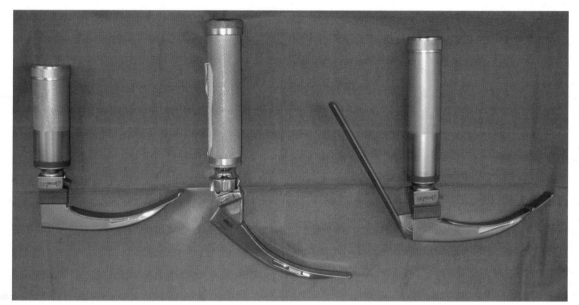

Fig. 2.48 Laryngoscopes designed to assist with difficult intubation. From left to right: stubby handle (with Macintosh blade), polio blade, McCoy blade.

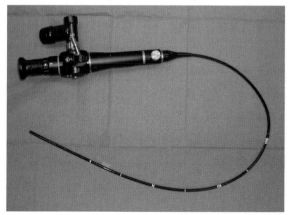

Fig. 2.49 A fibreoptic bronchoscope.

Chapter 3

The anaesthetic room: induction of anaesthesia

51

3.1 Preparation for induction of anaesthesia

Adequate and appropriate preparation is essential to ensure patient safety and the efficient running of a list.

In routine practice, anaesthesia is induced either in an anaesthetic room with dedicated equipment, or in the operating theatre itself. Important factors to consider are:

- Transfer of patient from bed to operating table
- Temporary disconnection of monitoring and anaesthetic circuit
- Proximity of senior help and back-up.

Factors favouring induction in theatre
Patient
- Morbidly obese patient (to minimize transfers)
- Infection control, e.g. MRSA (to minimize potential contamination)
- Pregnancy (operating table easier to tilt than bed).

Surgery
- Emergency or unstable patient (e.g. ruptured aortic aneurysm, emergency Caesarean section), to minimize induction to surgery time and allow uninterrupted monitoring
- Day surgery (for quicker patient turnover).

Preparing anaesthetic drugs

Multiple drugs are used during induction, maintenance and emergence. All drugs should be checked for:
- The correct drug name
- The dose or dilution
- A valid expiry date
- Labelling.

Gases and volatile agents, particularly oxygen, should also be checked for availability, delivery, and reserve supply.

Drugs should be drawn up using strict no-touch aseptic techniques. Figure 3.1 outlines the different drug classes with examples, and current standard background colour for syringe labelling.

Equipment

For each patient, all the equipment required for the planned anaesthetic (including emergency equipment) should be available, checked, and ready for use. A range of sizes should also be available.

There may be a need for additional specific equipment. This should be obtained and checked prior to induction. Examples are:
- Fibreoptic laryngoscope.
- Drug infusion devices.
- Ultrasound imaging device.

Patient arrival and communication

Preoperative assessment should have informed the patient about the plan for induction of anaesthesia. It is important to continue a professional approach at all times.
- Introduce anaesthetic team members and their role.
- Minimize unnecessary noise, talking, and personnel.
- Explain procedures such as application of monitoring, awake regional anaesthesia.
- Warn about potential discomfort, e.g. IV access.

The patient may arrive on a bed or trolley; this should be checked for head-down tilt prior to induction.

Preoperative checks
A preoperative checklist should be completed in accordance with local guidelines. The following information should be recorded.
- Name
- Date of birth
- Hospital ID number
- Patient ID/allergy bracelet check
- Signed consent form
- Planned operation
- Side and site of operation (marked if applicable)
- Marking of surgical site (if applicable)
- Allergies
- Dentition
- Starvation for solids/fluids
- Removal of jewellery
- Metal prostheses.

Monitoring

Minimum standards of monitoring are laid down by the Association of Anaesthetists of Great Britain and Ireland (2000). They comprise:
- Continuous presence of anaesthetist
- Pulse oximeter
- Non-invasive blood pressure (NIBP)
- ECG
- Capnograph
- Vapour analyser
- Availability of nerve stimulator
- Availability of temperature measurement.

Monitoring should be in place, and a set of observations taken, prior to the induction of anaesthesia.

Vascular access

Insertion of secure IV access is essential for all patients undergoing anaesthesia. The timing, location, number, and type depends on the clinical scenario. The box opposite outlines some options during major haemorrhage.

Roles of IV access
- Drugs: anaesthetic drugs (induction and maintenance); emergency drugs; other IV drugs.
- Fluids: fluid resuscitation; intraoperative fluids; postoperative fluids.
- Monitoring (arterial and central venous access)
- Blood sampling (arterial and central venous access)

Difficult IV access
This may be predictable: examine previous anaesthetic charts and notes for difficulties with vascular access, and sites used for cannula insertion. Ask the patient where previous phlebotomy or cannulation has been successful.

During preoperative assessment, look for potential sites and mark them. Ensure that these sites are covered appropriately with topical local anaesthetic if appropriate. Encourage the patient to keep warm while waiting to come to theatre.

If peripheral IV cannulation is unobtainable, consider access via the external jugular vein or a central venous cannula. Record successful sites of access for future reference.

Call for help if prolonged and numerous attempts are unsuccessful for difficult IV access. An inhalational induction may be necessary; consider a second anaesthetist to help with the insertion of an IV cannula after induction.

Intra-arterial blood pressure monitoring (Section 4.6)
This may be indicated prior to induction in some patients (e.g. those with a labile haemodynamic status or cardiovascular disease, which may be adversely affected during induction).

Induction agents

> **Propofol**
> ....mg/ml.

Examples:
Propofol
Thiopental (Thiopentone)
Ketamine
Etomidate

Hypnotics

> **Midazolam**
> ....mg/ml.

Examples:
Midazolam
Diazepam
Lorazepam

Anti-emetics

> **Ondansetron**
> ....mg/ml.

Examples:
Ondansetron
Cyclizine
Metoclopramide

Narcotics

> **Fentanyl**
> ....micrograms/ml.

Examples:
Fentanyl
Morphine
Diamorphine
Alfentanil
Remifentanil
Codeine Phosphate

Narcotic antagonist

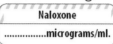
> **Naloxone**
> ....micrograms/ml.

Example:
Naloxone

Anticholinergic agents

> **Atropine**
> ....micrograms/ml.

Examples:
Atropine
Glycopyrronium

Muscle relaxants

> **Vecuronium**
> ....mg/ml.

Examples: (Non-depolarising)
Vecuronium
Atracurium
Cis-atracurium
Rocuronium
Pancuronium

Muscle relaxants

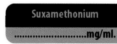
> **Suxamethonium**
> ....mg/ml.

Example: (Depolarising)
Suxamethonium

Relaxant antagonist

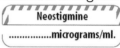
> **Neostigmine**
> ....micrograms/ml.

Example:
Neostigmine

Vasopressors

> **Adrenaline**
> ....micrograms/ml.

Example:
Adrenaline

Vasopressors

> **Ephedrine**
> ....mg/ml.

Examples:
Ephedrine
Metaraminol
Phenylephrine
Noradrenaline
Dopamine

Hypotensive agent

> **Labetalol**
> ....mg/ml.

Examples:
Labetalol
Glyceryl trinitrate
Phentolamine
Nitroprusside

Local anaesthetics

> **Lidocaine**
> ....%.

Examples:
Lidocaine
Bupivacaine
Ropivacaine

Miscellaneous

> **Heparin**
> ....units/ml.

Examples:
Heparin
Dexamethasone
Insulin
Antibiotics

Miscellaneous

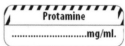
> **Protamine**
> ....mg/ml.

(Antagonists)
Examples:
Protamine

Fig. 3.1 Drug labelling.

---

❶ Vascular access for major haemorrhage

Consider:

Two large-bore (14G) peripheral cannulae in proximal veins, e.g. antecubital fossa. In the unstable patient, these should be inserted under local anaesthetic before induction.

Central venous cannula for monitoring (or fluid and drug infusion if no peripheral access obtainable).

High-flow large-bore central venous cannula.

Intra-arterial blood pressure monitoring.

Pressure infusion device, e.g. inflatable pressure bag.

Fluid warmer, e.g. Hotline®.

Rapid infuser device, e.g. Level 1®.

Drugs used during induction

Multiple drugs will be used during induction, maintenance, and emergence from anaesthesia. It is essential to understand the different classes of anaesthetic drugs, their pharmacodynamic and pharmacokinetic properties, and the potential for drug interactions. Many drugs have several roles during the anaesthetic. For example, hypnotic agents and opioids can act as co-induction agents (reducing the dose of induction agent required), as well as playing their traditional anxiolytic and analgesic roles.

IV and inhalational induction

General anaesthesia can be induced by either an IV or an inhalational technique. The choice will depend on patient factors, as well as the anaesthetist's experience and preference. It is important to become familiar with each technique. The diagram opposite shows the sequence of events in each type; steps in grey are common to both.

IV induction

IV induction is the most commonly used technique for general anaesthesia. Unless there is an immediate indication for large-bore IV access (e.g. ongoing resuscitation), the smallest possible cannula should be used. Further IV access can be obtained, if required, once the patient is anaesthetized. This avoids unnecessary discomfort.

Indications
- Rapid sequence induction
- 'Default' choice for most anaesthetists

Advantages
- Common and familiar technique
- Rapid induction time
- Excitatory phase is minimal
- IV access may be used to give other drugs

Disadvantages
- IV access must be obtained anyway
- Induction agent may be painful on injection
- Risk of extravasation injury
- Risk of inadvertent intra-arterial injection
- Potential for rapid loss of airway control.

Inhalational induction

Although inhalational induction is more common in paediatric anaesthesia, it is a useful technique that can be used for many patients

Indications
Paediatrics and those with needle phobia
- Avoids IV cannulation in awake patient

Partial airway obstruction or potential difficult airway
- Maintains spontaneous ventilation until airway control is ensured
- It is preferable to obtain IV access prior to induction

Advantages
- IV cannulation is deferred until anaesthesia is established
- Spontaneous ventilation is maintained

Disadvantages
- Unfamiliar to inexperienced anaesthetist
- Slow induction time
- Increased excitement phase
- Facemask may be unpleasant or frightening
- May be directly irritant to airway
- Risk of apnoea or obstructed airway with no IV access
- Difficult to scavenge; pollution with volatile agent is likely.

Stages of anaesthesia

Stages of inhalational anaesthesia using ether were described by Guedel in 1937. There are four, with stage 3 (surgical anaesthesia) being divided into four 'phases'. The stages are largely of historical interest and are rarely seen with the rapid action of modern anaesthetic agents.

Stage 1
During stage 1, voluntary control of eyeball movements is lost. The eyelash reflex is preserved and muscular tone is normal, becoming increased just at the end.

Stage 2
This is the excitatory phase, when the patient becomes tense and appears restless. Coughing, gagging, and breath-holding are common, and there is a risk of vomiting. The pupils are dilated, although the eyelash reflex is lost.

Stage 3
Stage 3 represents surgical anaesthesia. Breathing is regular until phase 4, but overall becomes shallower.
- *Phase 1* Breathing is deep and rapid, the pupils are of intermediate size, and the muscles become more relaxed. There may still be swallowing, coughing, and retching. Involuntary ocular movements occur but are lost at the beginning of phase 2.
- *Phase 2* Breathing becomes shallower. The pupils gradually dilate. The response to a surgical stimulus is attenuated and then disappears.
- *Phase 3* Tidal volumes reduce as the intercostal muscles lose power. $PaCO_2$ rises as the patient hypoventilates. There is no response to a surgical stimulus. Phase 3 is the correct level for maintenance of anaesthesia.
- *Phase 4* Diaphragmatic paralysis occurs and the patient becomes apnoeic. Laryngeal reflexes are lost during this phase.

Stage 4
Stage 4 is the deepest stage of anaesthesia and represents toxicity: the patient remains apnoeic, and cardiorespiratory depression will lead to death unless counter-measures are taken.

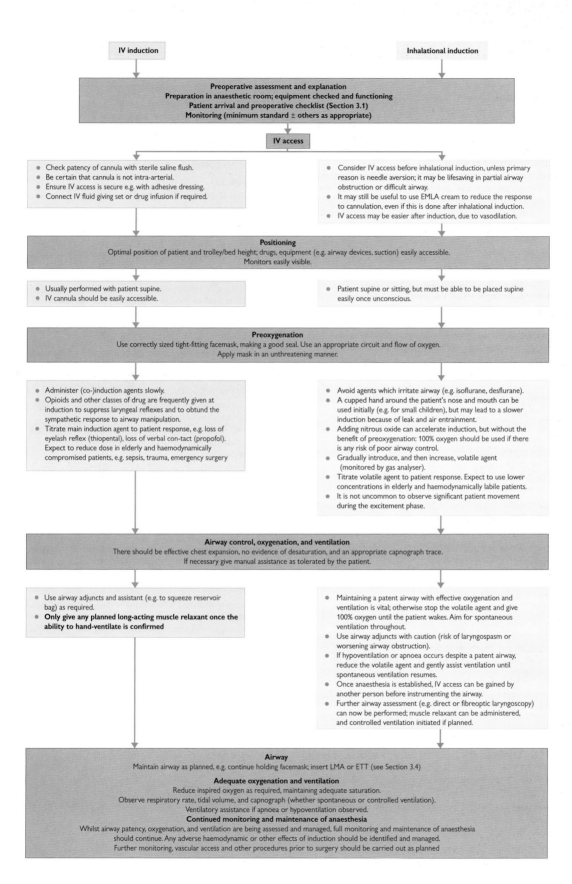

IV induction

Inhalational induction

Preoperative assessment and explanation
Preparation in anaesthetic room; equipment checked and functioning
Patient arrival and preoperative checklist (Section 3.1)
Monitoring (minimum standard ± others as appropriate)

IV access

- Check patency of cannula with sterile saline flush.
- Be certain that cannula is not intra-arterial.
- Ensure IV access is secure e.g. with adhesive dressing.
- Connect IV fluid giving set or drug infusion if required.

- Consider IV access before inhalational induction, unless primary reason is needle aversion; it may be lifesaving in partial airway obstruction or difficult airway.
- It may still be useful to use EMLA cream to reduce the response to cannulation, even if this is done after inhalational induction.
- IV access may be easier after induction, due to vasodilation.

Positioning
Optimal position of patient and trolley/bed height; drugs, equipment (e.g. airway devices, suction) easily accessible.
Monitors easily visible.

- Usually performed with patient supine.
- IV cannula should be easily accessible.

- Patient supine or sitting, but must be able to be placed supine easily once unconscious.

Preoxygenation
Use correctly sized tight-fitting facemask, making a good seal. Use an appropriate circuit and flow of oxygen.
Apply mask in an unthreatening manner.

- Administer (co-)induction agents slowly.
- Opioids and other classes of drug are frequently given at induction to suppress laryngeal reflexes and to obtund the sympathetic response to airway manipulation.
- Titrate main induction agent to patient response, e.g. loss of eyelash reflex (thiopental), loss of verbal con-tact (propofol). Expect to reduce dose in elderly and haemodynamically compromised patients, e.g. sepsis, trauma, emergency surgery

- Avoid agents which irritate airway (e.g. isoflurane, desflurane).
- A cupped hand around the patient's nose and mouth can be used initially (e.g. for small children), but may lead to a slower induction because of leak and air entrainment.
- Adding nitrous oxide can accelerate induction, but without the benefit of preoxygenation: 100% oxygen should be used if there is any risk of poor airway control.
- Gradually introduce, and then increase, volatile agent (monitored by gas analyser).
- Titrate volatile agent to patient response. Expect to use lower concentrations in elderly and haemodynamically labile patients.
- It is not uncommon to observe significant patient movement during the excitement phase.

Airway control, oxygenation, and ventilation
There should be effective chest expansion, no evidence of desaturation, and an appropriate capnograph trace.
If necessary give manual assistance as tolerated by the patient.

- Use airway adjuncts and assistant (e.g. to squeeze reservoir bag) as required.
- **Only give any planned long-acting muscle relaxant once the ability to hand-ventilate is confirmed**

- Maintaining a patent airway with effective oxygenation and ventilation is vital; otherwise stop the volatile agent and give 100% oxygen until the patient wakes. Aim for spontaneous ventilation throughout.
- Use airway adjuncts with caution (risk of laryngospasm or worsening airway obstruction).
- If hypoventilation or apnoea occurs despite a patent airway, reduce the volatile agent and gently assist ventilation until spontaneous ventilation resumes.
- Once anaesthesia is established, IV access can be gained by another person before instrumenting the airway.
- Further airway assessment (e.g. direct or fibreoptic laryngoscopy) can now be performed; muscle relaxant can be administered, and controlled ventilation initiated if planned.

Airway
Maintain airway as planned, e.g. continue holding facemask; insert LMA or ETT (see Section 3.4)

Adequate oxygenation and ventilation
Reduce inspired oxygen as required, maintaining adequate saturation.
Observe respiratory rate, tidal volume, and capnograph (whether spontaneous or controlled ventilation).
Ventilatory assistance if apnoea or hypoventilation observed.

Continued monitoring and maintenance of anaesthesia
Whilst airway patency, oxygenation, and ventilation are being assessed and managed, full monitoring and maintenance of anaesthesia should continue. Any adverse haemodynamic or other effects of induction should be identified and managed.
Further monitoring, vascular access and other procedures prior to surgery should be carried out as planned

During a period of unconsciousness, a patient requires a patent and secure airway. There are various ways of achieving this: holding a facemask (with or without simple airway adjuncts), or using a laryngeal mask airway or endotracheal tube. The devices available are described in Chapter 2.

Unobstructed breathing (Figure 3.2a)

In normal unobstructed breathing in the supine position, during inspiration the diaphragm contracts and descends. This compresses the abdominal contents, and the anterior abdominal wall rises. The descent of the diaphragm develops a negative pressure in the chest and air is drawn in. The anterior chest wall rises with the abdominal wall.

Expiration is a passive process, where the diaphragm relaxes. The abdominal and chest walls fall.

Obstructed breathing (Figure 3.2b)

As a patient becomes unconscious, the unsupported airway will collapse and obstruct. Recognition of the obstructed airway should become second nature to the anaesthetist.

In a patient with an obstructed upper airway, descent of the diaphragm still compresses the abdominal contents, causing the abdominal wall to rise. Negative pressure develops in the chest, but no air can enter. Instead, the anterior chest wall is drawn inwards and appears to fall as the abdominal wall rises.

In expiration, as the diaphragm relaxes, the dome ascends and the abdominal wall falls. The negative pressure in the chest diminishes and returns to its rest position.

This 'seesawing' of the abdominal and chest walls is characteristic of obstructed respiration.

Opening the airway

To open the airway, two manoeuvres are used: the head tilt/chin lift, and the jaw thrust (Figures 3.3a and b).

Head tilt–chin lift

This manoeuvre flexes the cervical spine, and extends the atlanto-occipital joint. The position achieved is known as 'sniffing the morning air'.

Standing at the head of the patient, hold the occiput in one hand and gently tilt the head backwards. The chin can be lifted by stabilizing it with the fingers of the other hand.

This manoeuvre is not appropriate for patients with suspected unstable cervical spine injury (Section 23.2) or those with neck problems or rheumatoid arthritis. *(Caveat: even in these cases, establishing a patent airway is always the highest priority).* In these patients, or where the chin lift and tilt has failed to clear the airway, a jaw thrust should be used (Figure 3.4).

Jaw thrust

This clears the airway by bringing the tongue, which is attached to the mandible, forward. It can be performed by the anaesthetist standing at the head of the patient, or by an assistant standing to the side.

The index fingers are placed under the angle of the mandible. The thumbs, placed on the body of the mandible, open the mouth. The index fingers pull the mandible forwards. Gentle counter-pressure on the maxilla with the heel of the hand prevents movement of the cervical spine, if necessary.

If the head tilt–chin lift or jaw thrust do not clear the airway, basic adjuncts such as oropharyngeal and nasopharyngeal airways (Section 2.13) can be used in addition.

Use of a facemask

Maintaining the airway with a mask is one of the most important skills to acquire in anaesthesia. Impeccable technique is needed to achieve optimal oxygenation and ventilation, to prevent unnecessary spillage of anaesthetic gases, and to avoid inflating the stomach with gas during bag–valve–mask ventilation.

Technique (Figure 3.5)

The lower border of the mask sits in the groove between the lower lip and chin. The mask is held between the thumb and index fingers. The little finger hooks behind the angle of the mandible, with the ring and middle fingers fanned along it. These fingers pull upwards on the jaw, maintaining the open airway. The upper part of the mask rests on the bridge of the nose, forming an airtight seal.

Tips

- Sometimes it is easier to have the middle finger on the mask to stabilize it rather than on the jaw. This depends on the size of your hands and of the patient.
- Although the thumb and index finger push the mask onto the face, the overall force is upwards, supporting the jaw.
- The lips should remain parted (particularly important if the nose is blocked, e.g. by nasal polyps).
- Pressure must not be applied to the soft tissues as this can cause airway obstruction (especially in children).
- If the patient is very large (or the anaesthetist's hands are small), it may be necessary to use both hands.
- In patients with beards, achieving a seal can be difficult. Suggested remedies include cutting a hole in a defibrillator gel pad or occlusive dressing, and placing it over the mouth.
- If your ring finger is placed carefully, you can feel the pulse of the mandibular artery.

Bag–valve–mask ventilation

Using the mask as described above, squeeze the reservoir bag on the breathing circuit gently, so that the chest wall rises. The airway must be maintained for expiration. Watch for the chest wall to fall again. With practice, the mask can be held with one hand. If there are difficulties, the mask can be held with both hands and the assistant can squeeze the bag.

Nasal mask

In the past much dental anaesthesia was performed in the dental chair in hospital outpatients and dental surgeries. This is now relatively uncommon, although some anaesthetists do use the technique, usually for the removal of anterior deciduous teeth in children. After induction, the anaesthetic gas mixture is administered through a nasal mask, e.g. a Goldman mask ± a nasopharyngeal airway. Obviously this allows a totally unprotected oropharyngeal airway, and the dental practitioner should pack the mouth to prevent any teeth, root fragments, or blood from entering the airway. This packing itself may obstruct the airway, so extreme care must be taken.

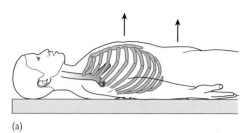
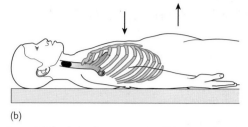

(a) (b)

Fig. 3.2 Normal and obstructed respiration. In normal respiration (a), the chest and abdominal walls move together. If the upper airway is obstructed (b), there is 'see-sawing' of the chest and abdominal walls.

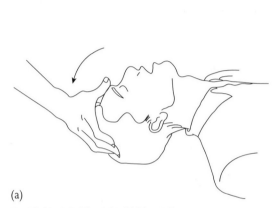
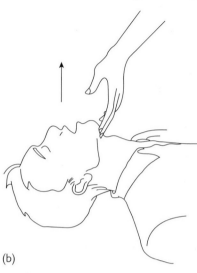

(a) (b)

Fig. 3.3 Head tilt (a) and chin lift (b) techniques.

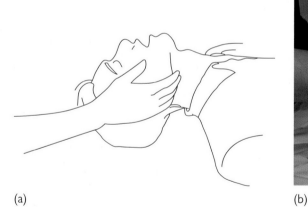
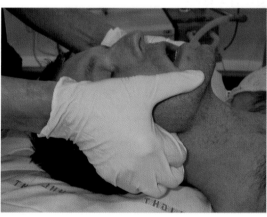

(a) (b)

Fig. 3.4 Jaw thrust diagram (a) and photo (b)

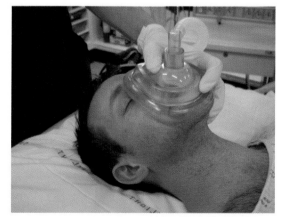

Fig. 3.5 Facemask technique.

Insertion of an LMA

The back of the cuff is lubricated. The head is tilted to extend the head and flex the neck. The mouth is opened and the LMA introduced, aperture downwards (Figure 3.6).

After manoeuvring around the teeth, gentle pressure is used to slide the LMA along first the hard and then the soft palates, and then downwards (trying to keep it on the posterior pharyngeal wall). It helps to lift the jaw forward as it passes down to prevent the epiglottis folding over. It should come to rest against the inferior constrictor of the pharynx. The black line faces the upper lip.

The cuff is inflated (initially with about half the maximum cuff volume) to obtain an adequate seal.

In spontaneously breathing patients, respiration should be quiet and unobstructed. In apnoeic patients, manual ventilation should be easy with no leaks or obstruction. A normal capnograph trace should be seen after successful insertion.

Intubation

Indications for intubation include:
- Anaesthetic and/or surgical preference
- Airway protection (e.g. if risk of aspiration)
- Need for positive-pressure ventilation with high airway pressures (e.g. laparoscopy, asthma)
- Failure of oxygenation by other means
- Compromised airway (obtunded consciousness, obstruction, trauma)
- Resuscitation (cardiac arrest, coma (GCS ,8), etc)

Oral intubation

Technique

The mouth is opened and the laryngoscope, held in the left hand, is introduced into the right-hand side, sweeping the tongue to the left. The blade is carefully advanced in a curling motion, following the surface of the tongue back until the epiglottis is visualized. The tip of the laryngoscope should lie in the valecula (between the epiglottis and the base of the tongue). The laryngoscope is then lifted, being careful not to lever on the upper teeth. Lifting the epiglottis should reveal the glottic opening and vocal cords. The anaesthetic assistant may manipulate the glottis externally to improve the view. The ETT should be passed using the right hand. The tip is advanced between the vocal cords until the black marker is just through. The laryngoscope is carefully removed.

Grades of intubation

In 1984, Cormack and Lehane classified the best view obtained at laryngoscopy with a standard Macintosh laryngoscope blade (Figure 3.7).
- *Grade I:* visualization of entire laryngeal aperture.
- *Grade II:* visualization of posterior laryngeal aperture.
- *Grade III:* visualization of epiglottis only.
- *Grade IV:* not even the epiglottis is visible.

This system standardizes nomenclature for difficult intubation and allows accurate communication via medical records.

Nasal intubation

Indications for nasal intubation include:
- Need for unhindered surgical access to the mouth or face
- Oral route not possible (e.g. trismus, plans to wire the jaw shut)
- Fibreoptic intubation (most commonly used route)
- Longer-term intubation, especially in children (better tolerated and easier to nurse).

Nasal tubes are longer and narrower than oral tubes.

Assessment

It is common for one nostril to be larger than the other because of a deviated septum. Patients are often acutely aware of which side is clearer. A visual inspection should be made, and the patient can be asked to occlude first one nostril and then the other while taking deep breaths through the nose.

The nostril is often sprayed with a vasoconstrictor prior to intubation, to shrink the mucosal vessels and decrease bleeding. As for nasal airways (Section 2.13) nasal intubation should not be performed on patients with evidence of basal skull fracture. Similarly, nasal ETTs should be used with extreme caution in patients with intranasal pathology or clotting abnormalities.

Technique

The tip of the nasal ETT should be passed into the post-nasal space via the chosen nostril. The laryngoscope is introduced as for oral intubation and the vocal cords visualized. The nasal ETT can then be passed simply by advancing (the anaesthetic assistant may be asked to manipulate the glottis externally to improve the line of intubation) or Magill's forceps can be used to introduce the tip of the ETT into the larynx. Sometimes a nasal ETT gets stuck at this point, but anticlockwise rotation whilst gently advancing will usually overcome this.

Awake intubation

This technique is used in cases of expected airway difficulty. See Section 3.5 for a brief outline.

Confirmation of ETT placement

After any intubation, the following must be confirmed (see Table 3.1):
- Bilateral chest movement on lung inflation
- Bilateral breath sounds on auscultation
- Absence of sounds over stomach
- Sustained oxygenation
- Capnograph trace sustained for six breaths.

It is important to remember that even after successful intubation, the ETT may become displaced (either down a main bronchus or out of the trachea) or obstructed (because of external pressure, e.g. kinking, or blockage by secretions). The ETT should be verified after every patient transfer. It is one of the first things to check if problems of any kind arise during anaesthesia.

Nasogastric tubes

Nasogastric (NG) tubes are sometimes required. They can be difficult to pass after an ETT has been placed. If possible (as long as there is no risk of aspiration and the patient is stable), they should be positioned before intubation under direct vision using Magill's forceps. Various strategies have been proposed if an ETT has already been passed:
- Visualize the oesophagus with a laryngoscope and use Magill's forceps to feed the tube.
- Pass the NG tube down a longitudinally cut nasal ETT positioned in oesophagus.
- Place the index and middle fingers in the mouth on either side of the tongue, and lift the tongue and larynx.
- Deflate ETT cuff (only if not an aspiration risk).

To confirm placement, tube aspirate can be tested with pH paper (normal gastric pH is 1–4) or an X-ray performed. Injecting air while auscultating at the epigastrium is not recommended, as it is less accurate.

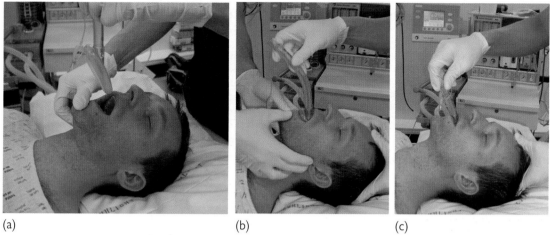

(a)   (b)   (c)

Fig. 3.6 LMA placement:
(a) Open the patient's mouth. Hold the LMA with the lumen facing the patient's feet.
(b) Insert the LMA into the patient's mouth. Asking your assistant to perform a jaw thrust often helps the device to slide over the tongue.
(c) Steady, gentle downward pressure manoeuvres the LMA into place. The cuff should be inflated and the LMA 'rises' into position

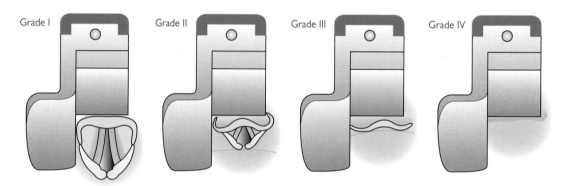

Fig. 3.7 Cormack and Lehane grades of intubation.

Table 3.1 Tests of ETT position						
	Chest movement		**Breath sounds**		**Capnograph trace**	**Sounds over stomach**
	Left	Right	Left	Right		
Oesophageal	No	No	No	No	No	Yes
Left main bronchus	Yes	No	Yes	No	Yes	No
Right main bronchus	No	Yes	No	Yes	Yes	No
Trachea	**Yes**	**Yes**	**Yes**	**Yes**	**Yes**	**No**

3.5 Induction in special circumstances

Some patients present special challenges for induction. These include acutely unstable patients and those with potential airway difficulties. It is essential to think out the induction technique carefully in advance. The plan must include appropriate alternative strategies for use if complications occur. In cases of airway difficulty, whether expected or not, the priority is oxygenation of the patient, regardless of how this is achieved.

The anticipated difficult airway

Both IV and inhalational techniques can be used to induce anaesthesia in the difficult airway. The key questions are:

Is airway control with mask ventilation expected to be difficult?
Are laryngoscopy and intubation anticipated to be difficult?
Is the patient at risk of aspiration?

All expected difficult airways should be discussed with a senior anaesthetist, and help should be immediately available. This point cannot be overemphasized.

Examine previous anaesthetic charts and notes for any previous difficulties with airway management, relevant investigations, and how the induction and airway management were eventually dealt with. Consider difficult airway algorithms such as those produced by the Difficult Airway Society (Section 22.2).

A 'difficult airway trolley' is available in many departments, and contains useful equipment such as:

- McCoy laryngoscope
- Short-handled laryngoscope
- Polio or variable-angle laryngoscope blade
- Ventilation-exchange bougie
- Intubating LMA
- Cricothyroidotomy cannulation set and high-pressure ventilation system.

It is vital to familiarize yourself with your local difficult airway equipment and guidelines. Practice the use of this equipment during normal inductions as often as you are able.

Awake intubation

Awake intubation has the advantage that spontaneous ventilation is maintained until the airway is secure. Meticulous preparation is necessary and includes the administration of an anti-sialogogue (e.g. glycopyrrolate) well in advance. The airway is anaesthetized topically (again, several methods can be used). The patient is usually sedated, but care must be taken not to induce anaesthesia inadvertently.

The most usual method of awake intubation uses the fibreoptic laryngoscope. However, other approaches, such as blind nasal intubation or even direct laryngoscopy, are practised. All awake intubation techniques require experienced anaesthetic and assisting personnel, and full patient cooperation.

The fibreoptic laryngoscope can be used on anaesthetized patients. It is useful in cases of likely difficult intubation, where mask ventilation is expected to be easy and the patient is not at special risk of aspiration.

Rapid sequence induction

Rapid sequence induction (RSI) is an IV induction technique for patients at risk of regurgitation and aspiration, but who are not predicted to be difficult to intubate. Factors which increase the risk of regurgitation and aspiration during induction of anaesthesia include the following.

Incompetent lower oesophageal sphincter
- Hiatus hernia, gastro-oesophageal reflux disease
- Pregnancy (from 16 weeks' gestation to 48 hr post-delivery)

Reduced gastric emptying
- Recent trauma, opiates, alcohol
- Abdominal pathology
- Bowel obstruction, peritonitis
- Reduced conscious level
- Metabolic disease/disturbance, e.g. diabetes, renal failure

The ideal RSI
An ideal RSI should include:

- Rapid induction of anaesthesia with immediate muscle relaxation, laryngoscopy, and passage of ETT (to minimize time during which the airway is unprotected).
- No need for manual ventilation of the lungs prior to intubation (avoids inflation of the stomach).
- No hypoxaemia during period of apnoea.
- Measures to minimize the risk of regurgitation during muscle relaxation, prior to securing the airway.
- The option to wake the patient rapidly and safely if unable to intubate.

Performance of RSI

Assessment, preparation, explanation, and trained assistance are required, as with any induction of anaesthesia. One extra person is needed (e.g. a ward nurse), who can go for help should problems arise.

Equipment and drugs should be checked and accessible. In case of regurgitation during induction, suction should be on and tucked under the pillow, and the bed or trolley must be checked for head-down tilt.

The patient must be thoroughly preoxygenated prior to induction (for 3–5min, or end-tidal oxygen concentration of ˜0.85). This pulmonary denitrogenation can significantly increase time from apnoea to desaturation. The actual time to desaturation depends on factors such as: FRC, ventilation prior to apnoea, oxygen consumption, and airway patency during apnoea (oxygen can passively diffuse to the alveoli during apnoea as long as the airway remains patent).

A fast-acting IV induction agent (classically thiopental) is given, followed by rapid-acting muscle relaxant (classically suxamethonium). Cricoid pressure (10N force) is applied by the assistant, and increased to 30N as soon as the patient is unconscious.

As soon as muscle relaxation occurs, direct laryngoscopy and intubation are performed. The ETT cuff is inflated and ETT placement is confirmed by gentle ventilation, observing for chest movement, capnography, and bilateral breath sounds (and absence of sounds over the epigastrium).

Cricoid pressure is removed only after confirmed placement of the ETT. If the ETT has to be adjusted later (e.g. migrates into a main bronchus), cricoid pressure should be reapplied.

Potential hazards during induction

The period between an awake and an anaesthetized patient (or vice versa) can be associated with many complications. It is important to be aware of these problems, to try to prevent their occurrence. Should they happen, they should be identified early, and actively managed.

- Difficult or failed intubation (Section 25.3)
- Laryngospasm (Section 25.4)
- Haemodynamic instability (Sections 25.14–25.17)
- Adverse drug reactions (Section 25.20)

Cricoid pressure

The surface anatomy of the cricoid ring is shown in Figure 3.8.

Palpate the thyroid cartilage (Adam's apple). Just below its lower border is an indentation. Continue to run your finger down in the midline; the next firm structure is the cricoid cartilage. It is situated at the C6 level. The triangular-shaped membrane between the two cartilages is the cricothyroid membrane, another important structure (it is the point of insertion of an emergency surgical airway) (Section 6.4).

The cricoid cartilage is the only complete cartilaginous ring in the upper airway (the thyroid cartilage and tracheal rings are deficient posteriorly). Pressure applied to the cricoid is transmitted effectively to the oesophagus, which lies immediately posterior to it.

Cricoid pressure was formally described in 1961 by B.A. Sellick, and is still occasionally termed 'Sellick's manoeuvre'. The assistant identifies the cricoid, and uses his/her thumb and index fingers (± the middle finger) to apply direct posterior pressure to the cartilage (Figure 3.9). Applying the correct 30N force takes practice; only trained personnel should perform the manoeuvre. Sometimes a two-handed technique is employed, where the non-dominant hand supports the neck.

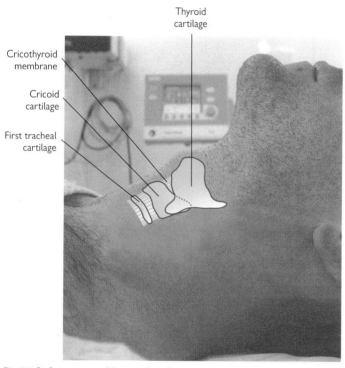

Fig. 3.8 Surface anatomy of the cricoid cartilage.

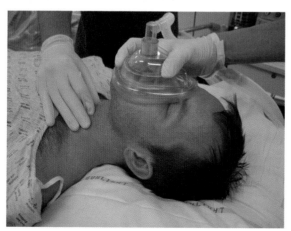

Fig. 3.9 Application of cricoid pressure during a rapid sequence induction.

Chapter 4

The operating theatre environment

Meticulous care of the unconscious patient is essential to avoid injury (particularly to nerves and soft tissues) during transfer and positioning.

Patient transfer

After induction, the patient may need to be transferred onto the operating table and eventually back to the trolley/bed. Transferring a patient incorrectly can lead to injury to both patient and staff. Local guidelines and manual handling procedures may be in place. The important principles are listed below.

- Team leader to organize individual staff roles and timing of manoeuvres.
- Appropriate equipment, e.g. Patslide®, hoist.
- Appropriate technique during transfer.
- Secure and avoid displacement of:
  - Airway device e.g. ETT, LMA
  - Vascular access and infusion lines
  - Monitoring devices
  - Urinary catheter, chest/surgical drains.
- Restore and check function and position of any ventilation circuit, monitoring or infusion, which may be temporarily disconnected for the transfer.
- Spinal precautions and log-rolling should be used as appropriate.
- Pre-existing joint instability requires care (e.g. rheumatoid arthritis and atlanto-axial instability).
- Special care should be taken with extremities (fingers can become trapped between the bed and operating table!).
- Special considerations are required for the obese patient:
  - Check weight restriction of table
  - Induce anaesthesia on operating table in correct position for surgery if possible
  - Ensure enough staff available if manoeuvring required.
- Ensure patient is safe and secure in final position.

Some trolleys are designed for the multiple roles of anaesthesia, surgery and recovery, and avoid the need for multiple transfers. These are often used in day surgery units, aiding rapid and efficient turnover of patients.

Environmental control in the operating theatre

Management of temperature, humidity, and air composition is important in maintaining a safe environment in the operating theatre complex.

Temperature

The operating room usually maintained at 22–24°C. This is important for staff comfort, but primarily it is to minimize heat loss from patients to avoid hypothermia. This is especially important for paediatrics and burns patients, and in prolonged surgery. Various other methods are employed.

- **Passive:** theatre temperature, insulation (sheets, insulating padding).
- **Active:** warmed IV fluids, forced air warming blanket, heated mattresses, overhead radiant heaters, increasing the ambient temperature.

Humidity

The operating room is usually maintained at 50–60% relative humidity (see Section 4.12). Above this level, it is uncomfortable for workers, but if the air is too dry there is a risk of sparking from electrical equipment.

Atmosphere:

Air changes

At least 20 air changes per hour are recommended in order to remove excess anaesthetic gases. Increased effectiveness of ventilation may be required for infection control (e.g. for joint replacement surgery). This can be achieved with laminar flow systems.

Scavenging

Scavenging minimizes potential health risks to staff and the possibility of reduced performance from inhalation of accumulated waste/expired anaesthetic gases. See Section 2.4 for details.

Nerve and soft tissue protection

It is important to assess and document pre-existing nerve or soft tissue injury. It is also vital to assess factors that increase risk of injury during surgery (see below). A plan for minimizing this risk should be made, and appropriate equipment made available.

An accurate and complete record of measures taken to minimize risk of injury to the patient during transfers and positioning is essential; it may be assumed that no steps were taken to prevent injury if there is no written evidence from medical notes.

Peripheral nerve injury

This may be transient or permanent. The onset of symptoms may be delayed. Nerve injury can be associated with general or regional anaesthesia. The ulnar nerve is most commonly involved, followed by the brachial plexus and spinal cord. Often the exact cause is not identified. Mechanisms include stretch, compression, ischaemia, and metabolic disturbance. Risk factors include:

- Old age
- Diabetes mellitus
- Pre-existing neuropathy
- Tourniquet with long tourniquet time (see opposite)
- Surgical retractors
- Malpositioning of patient
- Musculoskeletal abnormalities
- Reduced proprioception and nociception during regional anaesthesia.

Prevention:

- Ask patient to adopt the operative position while awake during preoperative assessment to identify any problems.
- Careful/modified positioning (liaise with surgeon).
- Padding of vulnerable areas.

Ocular injury

Again, this may be transient or permanent.

Mechanisms include:

- Corneal abrasions by direct trauma (most common; decreased tear production under general anaesthesia contributes)
- Ischaemic optic neuropathy.

Increased risk:

- Elderly
- Pre-existing hypertension
- Diabetes
- Prolonged hypotension
- Prone position
- Direct pressure on globe
- Long duration of surgery

Prevention:

- Ensure eyelids are fully closed (e.g. tape).
- Lubrication and padding as appropriate (e.g. during prone position, or if the surgical field is close to the eyes).

Soft tissue injury and pressure sores

Prolonged pressure over an area of soft tissue can lead to ischaemia, with skin and tissue necrosis.

Increased risk

- Elderly
- Long duration of surgery
- Poor condition of skin (e.g. malnutrition)

Prevention

- Optimal positioning
- Appropriate padding of pressure areas
- Regular assessment
- Early postoperative mobilization

✚ Use of tourniquets

By mechanical compression, tourniquets reduce arterial circulation to, and venous drainage from, a limb. They are used to improve the surgical field, to limit blood loss, and in IV regional anaesthesia. The equipment includes padding and tape, a special pneumatic tourniquet, a supply of compressed gas, and a pressure regulator and display.

Application of a tourniquet

Apply an appropriately sized cuff above the surgical site, using soft padding underneath (Figure 4.1). Aim for even pressure, and ensure that the skin is not pinched. Use adhesive tape as a barrier to surgical skin preparation solutions (which can cause chemical burns if they soak through the padding).

Exsanguination of limb may be passive (by elevation) or active (Esmarch bandage or Rhys-Davies exsanguinator).

Once the limb is exsanguinated just prior to surgery, inflate the cuff. Typical inflation pressures are:

- Lower limb: ≥100mmHg above systolic BP (usually around 300mmHg)
- Upper limb: ≥50mmHg above systolic BP (usually around 250mmHg).

Limit inflation time to ≤2hr. If surgery is prolonged, consider deflation for 10min every 2hr to allow reperfusion. Longer ischaemic times increase the risk of nerve and soft tissue damage. Record inflation and deflation times on the anaesthetic chart.

Absolute contraindications:

- Presence of AV fistula
- Compromised limb circulation
- Previous vascular surgery to limb.

Relative contraindications:

- Sickle cell disease or trait (optimize acid–base status, oxygenation, hydration, temperature prior to use)
- History of DVT.

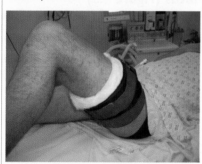

Fig. 4.1 Generous padding should be used when applying a tourniquet to avoid nerve and soft tissue injury.

Systemic effects and complications

Cardiovascular

- ↑ preload and SVR: transient ↑ CVP and BP.
- ↑ HR and BP after 30-60min (tourniquet pain); may not respond to analgesics or increasing depth of anaesthesia.
- ↓ SVR and venous return on deflation, during reperfusion.
- Application may dislodge intravascular material leading to venous or arterial emboli.

Haematological

- Systemic hypercoaguability
- May precipitate sickling in susceptible individuals

Metabolism

- >30min, anaerobic metabolism may lead to metabolic acidosis, hypoxia, hypercarbia, and tachycardia.

Respiratory

- Transient ↑ $EtCO_2$ and O_2 consumption on deflation.

CNS

- Pain (awake patients may not tolerate prolonged usage).

✚ Lasers

A laser (light amplification by the stimulation of emitted radiation) produces a high-energy non-divergent beam of light.

Within a lasing medium, stable atoms are excited by a pumping source. When an excited atom returns to ground state, spontaneous emission of a photon occurs. If the pumping source energy is reapplied to an already excited atom, stimulated emission of two photons can occur.

The emitted photons are parallel, in phase and monochromatic (single wavelength).

The process is amplified via mirrors (positive feedback).

Examples of medical laser use

CO_2	Bloodless cutting, vaporizer
Argon	Small vessel coagulation, e.g. retina
NdYAG	Deep tissue cutting and coagulation

Laser safety

Local guidelines for safe laser use and procedures for managing emergencies (e.g. burns, fire) should be in place. The correct type of laser and adequate training of staff are essential.

The operator should take responsibility for safety during use e.g. verbal or automatic audible warning when activated.

Eye protection (laser-type specific) for patient and staff should be provided and worn. Information and protection warnings should be prominently displayed outside the theatre; doors should be locked and windows covered.

Minimize risk of injury to patient and staff:

Avoid burns to skin
  to retina, cornea, lens of eye
  to airway
  to surgical drapes

Airway surgery

Use O_2/air, relatively low FiO_2
Non-reflective instruments, non-flammable ETT

Airway fire

Switch off laser, flood site with saline

Disconnect breathing circuit temporarily, remove ETT if possible, and ventilate with BVM

Inspect airway and reintubate

Risk of ALI: sedate, ventilate, humidified O_2, reassess airway.

4.2 Patient positioning

Final positioning of the anaesthetized patient allows good surgical access, whilst minimizing the risk of injury. Always verify the airway and check ETT position after any postural change. Physiological effects depend on the position, and may be beneficial or adverse.

Supine (Figure 4.2)

Used for many procedures. The arms may be by the sides (wrapped or with padded supports), on arm boards (shoulder abduction <90°, forearms pronated), or resting on the abdomen or chest.

Cardiovascular
- Initial ↑ cardiac output (redistribution of venous blood; ↑ venous return); rarely, may compromise a patient with very poor cardiac reserve.
- IVC compression (e.g. in pregnancy, obesity) can lead to ↓ BP (consider left lateral tilt).

Respiratory
- ↓ FRC and pulmonary compliance (cephalad movement of abdominal contents splints the diaphragm).
- ↑ V/Q mismatch.
- ↑ Risk of regurgitation/aspiration.

Pressure/problem areas
- Occiput
- Elbows (care with ulnar nerve protection)
- Knees (avoid hyperextension)
- Sacrum, heels, greater trochanter of femur

Head-down tilt (Trendelenburg)

Used, e.g., for pelvic surgery. The severity of problems increases with the degree of tilt. Use a non-slip mattress if available. As for supine position, plus:

Cardiovascular
- Initial increase of venous return.
- Higher ventilation pressures may subsequently reduce venous return.

Respiratory
- Risk of displacement of ETT during positioning.
- Oedema of head and neck, *including the larynx*.
- Further ↓ FRC and pulmonary compliance.
- Risk of atelectasis.
- Passive oesophageal reflux; risk of aspiration on re-positioning.

CNS
- Increase in ICP and IOP.

Head-up tilt (reverse Trendelenburg)

Used for head and neck, upper GIT, and shoulder surgery. As for supine, plus:

Cardiovascular
- Postural hypotension.
- Risk of venous air embolism (VAE).
- Increased head and neck venous drainage.

Respiratory
- Potentially beneficial: reduced airway pressures during IPPV, increased lung compliance and FRC.
- Decreased risk of passive regurgitation/ aspiration

CNS
- Reduced ICP and IOP

Lithotomy (Lloyd-Davies)

Used for lower GIT, urological, and gynaecological surgery.

Cardiovascular
- Leg elevation increases venous return and SVR.
- Hypotension may occur on lowering legs.

Respiratory
- Relative caudal displacement of ETT during positioning—risk of endobronchial intubation.
- Further ↓ FRC and pulmonary compliance.
- Risk of atelectasis.
- Passive oesophageal reflux, risk of aspiration.

Pressure/problem areas
- Arms by side can risk digit entrapment.
- Sciatic/obturator nerve stretch and femoral nerve compression if hips are flexed >90°.
- Common peroneal and saphenous nerve compression against supports.
- Calf compression leading to risk of venous thrombo-embolism and/or compartment syndrome (↑ risk with long-duration surgery).

Lateral decubitus (Figure 4.3)

Used for hip, thoracic, and renal surgery. 'Right lateral' means that the patient's right side is lowest.

Respiratory
- IPPV: dependent lung relatively under-ventilated and over-perfused (and vice versa for uppermost lung).

CNS
- Risk of corneal abrasions/pressure on lower eye.

Pressure/problem areas
- Ensure adequate lateral support for head and neck.
- Support shoulders and pelvis to prevent rolling.
- Avoid pressure on abdomen.
- Dependent arm: nerve compression, ischaemia.
- High risk of corneal abrasions and pressure on dependent eye.
- Padding between legs to protect common peroneal and saphenous nerves.
- **Ensure correct side for surgery is accessed.**

Prone (Figure 4.4)

Used in calcaneal, varicose vein, and spinal surgery. Ensure a well-secured airway (e.g. reinforced ETT) and vascular access before positioning. Figure 4.5. shows the type of eye protection and tube strapping which may be used.

Respiratory
- FRC is reduced.
- There may be improved V/Q matching.

CNS
- Increased IOP; eyes should be padded, with no direct pressure.

Pressure/problem areas
- Neck (avoid hyperextension and flexion).
- Eyes and nose (cushioned support, e.g. gel horseshoe).
- Breasts (position medially) and genitalia.
- Dorsal feet, knees, elbows.
- Brachial plexus (maintaining some anterior flexion, simultaneously abduct and externally rotate both arms to <90°); avoid pressure on axilla.
- Forearm supports to protect ulnar nerve.
- Support for chest and pelvis to avoid pressure on abdomen. High intra-abdominal pressures lead to IVC compression and ↓ cardiac output, and ↓ pulmonary compliance.

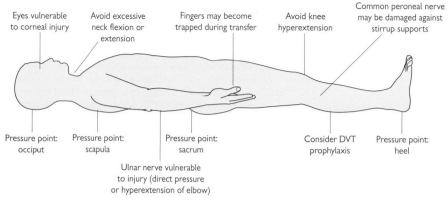

Fig. 4.2 The supine position. Although this is the most straightforward position for surgery, there are still a number of risks to the unconscious patient, which must be avoided.

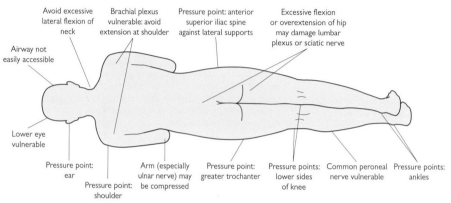

Fig. 4.3 Lateral position. It is very important to stabilize the patient in the lateral position to prevent falls and injury. Various methods can be employed, including padded poles and supports and vacuum mattresses.

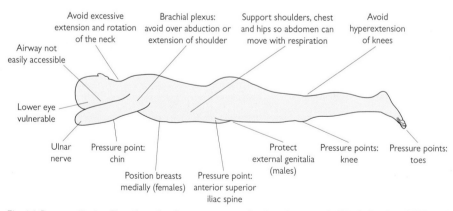

Fig. 4.4 Prone positioning. Once the patient is prone, access to the airway is extremely difficult. Reinforced ETTs and generous application of tape and tube ties is recommended. Eye protection is also extremely important.

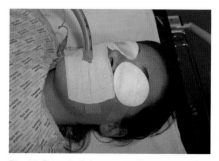

Fig. 4.5 Eye taping/tube strapping for prone positioning.

Once the airway has been established at the beginning of anaesthesia, it must be monitored closely. The anaesthetist must remain constantly vigilant for signs of an impending problem and be ready to react promptly and appropriately.

Whenever the patient is moved, the position of the head changed, or the airway manipulated or instrumented, a check should be performed. This should confirm that the patient still has a patent clear airway which is connected via a patent breathing system to the anaesthetic machine.

The shared airway

The challenge of the shared airway involves a huge amount of cooperation between surgeon and anaesthetist. If at any point during the surgery the airway becomes obstructed or compromised, the surgeon must stop operating until the airway is cleared. At the end of surgery, the airway should always be inspected for blood, foreign material, and packs, *even if the surgeon has already done this*.

Where the airway is likely to be contaminated (e.g. by blood, saliva, fluids, or foreign bodies), it is vital that the trachea and lungs are protected. This can be achieved in a number of ways.

Endotracheal tube

Endotracheal intubation remains the gold standard method of protecting the airway from foreign substances. This usually involves the administration of a muscle relaxant to the patient prior to intubation, but can also be achieved with local anaesthesia, with local anaesthesia and sedation, or by generous doses of anaesthetic agent and short-acting opioids.

Microlaryngoscopy tube

A microlaryngosopy tube (MLT; Figure 4.6) is used when the surgeon requires access to the vocal cords. It is narrow, presenting a large resistance to breathing. MLTs are sometimes useful in the management of difficult airways, when standard sized ETTs are too large to pass through the glottis.

Pharyngeal pack

Many anaesthetists insert a pharyngeal pack ('throat pack') around the base of the tube if copious amounts of blood, saliva, or other fluids are likely to collect. This helps to prevent them bypassing the ETT or being swallowed. There is no evidence that pharyngeal packs reduce the incidence of PONV; moreover, the incidence of sore throat is probably increased and there is always the risk of leaving the pack in. The pack may then obstruct the airway after extubation.

Tips for the safe use of throat packs

- *It is the responsibility of whoever inserted the pack to remove it.*
- Insertion and removal of packs should be recorded on the anaesthetic sheet.
- A sticker can be put on the patient, indicating they have a pack inserted in the airway.
- If possible, the tail of the pack should hang out of the mouth and/or be secured to the airway.
- The ends of the throat pack can be knotted to verify that it has been removed intact.
- *Always perform a laryngoscopy at end of shared cases.*

Laryngeal mask airways

LMAs have been used for shared airway work since the early 1990s, when an armoured version was released. They are useful for procedures such as tonsillectomy, removal of teeth, nasal surgery, and surface surgery of the mouth cavity. They are not appropriate for cases such as laryngoscopy or microlaryngoscopy, where they hinder surgical access. Special care should be taken when using LMAs for this work as they are easier to dislodge than ETTs and can obstruct (e.g. when the mouth gag is positioned in tonsillectomy). Flexible laryngoscopy can be performed thorough a LMA, using a catheter mount which has a silicone diaphragm with an aperture for the scope. This approach has the advantage that vocal cord movement can be viewed (see Table 4.1).

Nasal mask

In the past nasal masks were frequently used with an anteriorly placed oral pack for the removal of teeth. After gaseous or IV induction a nasal mask is held over the nose with or without a nasal airway. The mouth gag is inserted and a pack is carefully placed to prevent any foreign material from falling into the airway, whilst at the same time not obstructing it. The patient is kept asleep via this airway until the procedure is completed. This used to be done in the dental surgery but is now confined to hospitals and larger centres.

Jet ventilation

When performing a bronchoscopy the surgeon requires uninterrupted access to the airway and there is no room for an ETT. In this case oxygenation can be maintained by insufflation of oxygen and air, using a Sanders Injector (Figure 4.7). This consists of a handle with a trigger attached to a high-pressure (4 bar) oxygen outlet. Modern versions have a pressure gauge and tap to adjust the delivery pressure. The end usually comprises a Luer lock which attaches to a port on the bronchoscope such that as the oxygen is flushed down the scope, air is entrained. Dangers include barotrauma, pneumothorax, and eye contamination of the endoscopist. There should be a clear opening to the atmosphere to allow the escape of gas. When oxygenation is maintained in this way, the patient cannot be kept anaesthetized by inhalational anaesthetics, and either an intermittent injection of a hypnotic or an infusion technique such as total intravenous anaesthesia (TIVA) (Section 7.14) must be used.

Tracheostomy

In cases where the patient's airway is likely to obstruct, or extreme difficulty with a shared airway is envisaged, an elective tracheostomy may be performed. This can be done either under general or local anaesthetic, depending on the circumstances. When a tracheostomy has been performed and access to the head and neck is required by the surgeon, a Montandon ETT (Figure 4.8) can be used.

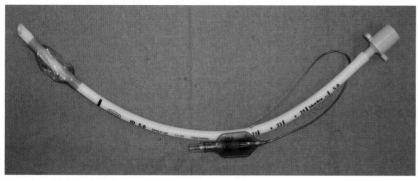

Fig. 4.6 A microlaryngoscopy tube.

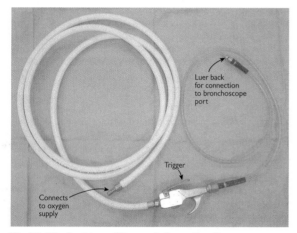

Fig. 4.7 A Sanders injector. This uses the Bernouilli and/or jet entrainment principles to deliver oxygen to the alveoli. Expiration is passive via the upper airway. The chest should rise as the trigger is pulled, and must be allowed to fall before the next breath is delivered to avoid barotrauma and pneumothorax.

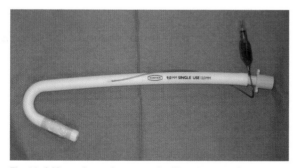

Fig. 4.8 A Montandon tracheostomy tube. This tube is used for ventilation through a tracheostome. Its length keeps the bulk of the breathing circut away from the head and neck, improving surgical access.

Table 4.1	**LMA vs. ETT for shared airway work**	
	LMA	**Tracheal Tube**
Advantages	Fewer haemodynamic changes during airway manipulation Avoidance of muscle relaxants and reversing agents: lower risk of anaphylaxis/MH/suxamethonium apnoea Less traumatic: decreased incidence of sore throat, damage to teeth, etc. Less airway irritation (coughing, bronchospasm) Better extubating conditions	Secure airway Good access Airway protected until awake
Disadvantages	Less secure airway Can encroach on surgical view Can distort anatomy Failure rate (approx. 2%)	Failed intubation Haemodynamic responses

4.4 Maintenance of anaesthesia

It is important to maintain anaesthesia at a level that minimizes adverse effects while preventing awareness.

A number of factors normally maintain 'wakefulness:' these include cortical and brainstem activity, and sensory input including nociception and muscle spindle feedback. Reducing these inputs by the use of a number of different types of agent produces balanced anaesthesia (Figure 4.10).

Drugs

Sedatives

Sedatives such as benzodiazepines can be given as premedication or at induction to allay anxiety, smooth induction, and decrease the requirement for hypnotics during maintenance of anaesthesia. α-adrenergic neuron blockers such as clonidine are sometimes used pre- and intra-operatively as sedatives, but also act synergistically with analgesics.

Hypnotics

Hypnotics are drugs that induce general anaesthesia, and include propofol, thiopental, etomidate, and inhalational agents.

Muscle relaxants

In the past suxamethonium was used as an infusion throughout surgery, but is associated with a number of side effects and is now rarely used for this purpose. The longer-acting non-depolarizing muscle relaxants are used nowadays (Section 8.5). They have an onset time of 1–3min and last 5–60min. They can be monitored by the use of neuromuscular blockade monitoring (Section 8.6).

Anti-emetics

It is important to have made a preoperative assessment of the likelihood of the patient suffering postoperative nausea and vomiting (PONV) (Section 17.10). If the risk of PONV is high, prophylactic measures should be taken. These include:

- Maintenance of normal physiological parameters
- IV fluid 20ml/kg
- Avoidance of nitrous oxide
- Avoidance of opioids (e.g. by using paracetamol, NSAIDs, and nerve blocks)
- TIVA (Section 7.14)
- Anti-emetics (single, double, or triple therapy).

Analgesia

Nitrous oxide

Nitrous oxide has analgesic properties as well as being hypnotic. It cannot be used as the sole anaesthetic agent because of lack of potency. Its use may reduce the risk of awareness, but it may be associated with PONV and has various other effects (Section 7.16).

Simple analgesia and non-steroidal anti-inflammatory drugs

Paracetamol and several NSAIDs are available as IV preparations, making them ideal for administration during anaesthesia.

Opioids

A wide variety of opioids can be used during anaesthesia, ranging from the ultra-short-acting remifentanil, through the short-acting alfentanil and fentanyl, to the longer-acting diamorphine and morphine. They are not hypnotic agents in their own right, but their use will tend to decrease the amount of hypnotic required by reducing nociception and pain.

Local and regional anaesthesia

Nociceptive pathways can be interrupted or modulated at any point from the peripheral nociceptor to the brain. Local anaesthetics and other drugs can be applied to these nerve pathways at various points (Figure 4.9) If the nerve block is effective, the patient can undergo surgery awake, under sedation, or under a very 'light' anaesthetic.

When the patient is being 'lightly' anaesthetized with a regional block, care should be taken that the surgical field does not stray outside the anaesthetized area. Other procedures (e.g. airway manipulation, nasopharyngeal temperature probe placement) may cause stimulation or precipitate awareness, and so the anaesthetic should be deepened appropriately to cover these.

Ventilation during anaesthesia

Following induction of anaesthesia and satisfactory control of a patent airway, ventilation must be continued. Either spontaneous or controlled ventilation may be used: whichever method is chosen, effective oxygenation and ventilation should be confirmed prior to the start of surgery. The advantages and disadvantages of each method are shown in Table 4.2. Factors to assess include oxygen saturation, capnography, and tidal volume (TV). Spirometry can help to assess the compliance of the lungs (Section 13.5). In spontaneous ventilation, the respiratory rate (RR) and pattern of breathing can also be observed.

The fresh gas flow should be appropriate to the breathing system and size of patient, to prevent rebreathing (Section 2.11).

Spontaneous ventilation

Factors that favour spontaneous ventilation

Patient factors

- Good preoperative respiratory function; no significant obstructive or restrictive lung disease

Surgical factors

- Superficial minor surgical procedure
- Short or medium duration of surgery
- Assessment of vocal cord mobility (ENT)
- Foreign body airway obstruction (positive-pressure ventilation may force the foreign object further into the airway)
- Inability to control $PaCO_2$—hypercapnia may adversely affect ICP and IOP
- Increased depth of anaesthesia may be required in intubated patients

Controlled ventilation

Respiration can be controlled during anaesthesia via intermittent positive-pressure ventilation (IPPV). This can be carried out via a facemask, LMA, or ETT.

During IPPV it is still important to assess for effective oxygenation and ventilation. The clinical effect should correlate with delivered ventilation (whether manual or mechanical). For example, if high airway pressure is required for an adequate TV in a patient with normal lungs, the problem should be investigated and corrected (common causes include obstruction within the breathing system and movement of the ETT into a main bronchus).

Although neuromuscular blockade is commonly used to provide profound muscle relaxation, deep anaesthesia with or without the use of opioids can be used to allow controlled ventilation.

Factors that favour controlled ventilation

Patient factors

- Poor respiratory function or reserve
- Obesity
- Hypoventilation due to deep anaesthesia or opioids

Surgical factors

- Profound muscle relaxation required (e.g. intra-abdominal surgery)
- Close control of $PaCO_2$ required (e.g. control of ICP or IOP)
- Long duration of surgery
- Pneumoperitoneum
- Prolonged head-down tilt or lithotomy position
- Cardiothoracic surgery

Methods of controlled ventilation

- Hand ventilation via a breathing system can allow the anaesthetist to assess lung compliance (the 'feel' of the reservoir bag).
- Mechanical ventilators can ventilate accurately to a given set of parameters. Various modes of ventilation are available with modern machines (Section 2.12).

Table 4.2 **Spontaneous vs. controlled ventilation**		
	Spontaneous	Controlled
Advantages	Respiratory rate can be observed Avoids use of muscle relaxant (risk of incomplete reversal, awareness, anaphylaxis etc).	Fine control of respiratory parameters, e.g. TV, RR, minute volume, I:E ratio, PEEP Reduced work of breathing for the patient
Disadvantages	Anaesthesia and the supine position can reduce the FRC; this can lead to lower airway collapse and increased work of breathing May be difficult to apply effective PEEP High resistance in airway or anaesthetic circuit can lead to increased work of breathing (especially in small children, or with a small-diameter ETT and a breathing system filter)	May be more difficult to assess for inadvertent awareness under anaesthesia as the patient is paralysed and the respiratory rate imposed Risk of inadvertent residual paralysis if muscle relaxant used IPPV via facemask or LMA can lead to gastric insufflation and risk of regurgitation.

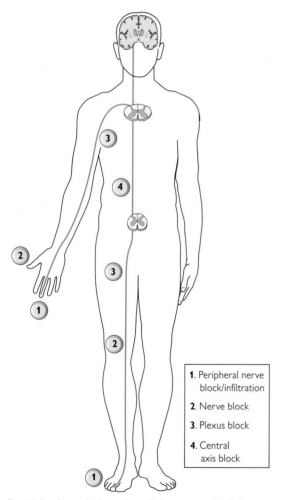

1. Peripheral nerve block/infiltration
2. Nerve block
3. Plexus block
4. Central axis block

Fig. 4.9 Local anaesthetics can be applied at various points in the nervous system to halt pain transmission from the periphery to the centre.

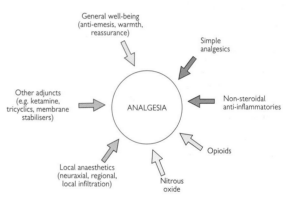

Fig. 4.10 Many different approaches can be used to provide overall analgesia in the perioperative period. This multimodal approach is more effective than the use of a single agent.

4.5 Bioelectrical potential recording and the ECG

The use of patient monitoring to complement clinical observation improves safety in anaesthesia. However, clinical observation remains paramount, and when machines fail there is little alternative. The old adage holds true: 'the best monitor is the one between your ears… as long as it is switched on.'

Recording bioelectrical potentials

Bioelectrical potentials arise from small membrane currents within excitable tissues (muscle and nerve). The potentials created by excitable membranes are of the order of about 100mV. However, attenuation in tissues results in much smaller potentials at the body surface: the ECG potential is around 1–2 mV when measured at the chest wall. Other bioelectrical potentials detectable at the body surface include the electroencephalogram (EEG) and the electromyogram (EMG).

The process of recording bioelectrical potentials involves:

- Detection
- Transduction
- Amplification
- Processing
- Display.

Detection

Detection and transduction of bioelectrical potentials is achieved by the use of electrodes applied to the skin. Electrodes can be in the form of needles or gel pads consisting of a metal disc coupled to the skin by a conducting gel. The electrode is designed to reduce skin impedance (*Note:* deliberately applying points of electrical contact with reduced skin impedance unavoidably puts the patient at risk of electric shock if equipment is faulty or basic principles of electrical safety (Section 4.14) are not applied). The most common type of pad has a silver–silver chloride electrode with a chloride gel, surrounded by an adhesive patch. The gel becomes polarized if a potential is applied to it, and this creates a small current which is transmitted via a metal wire to the processing unit.

Transduction

Transduction of bioelectrical potentials is also performed by the skin electrode. Other types of transducer are used in different monitoring systems; examples include piezoelectric crystals in invasive blood pressure measurement, and thermistors in temperature probes.

Amplification

The signal that arrives at the processor consists of the small bioelectrical potential together with a large amount of interference (e.g. mains electricity, movement artefact). The amplification apparatus for any given signal is designed specifically to extract and amplify the correct signal, while reducing interference. The ability of an amplifier to do this is referred to as the **signal-to-noise ratio**.

The gain of a system is a logarithmic measure of its output/input ratio (i.e. the size of the signal produced compared with the size of the signal detected). It describes the sensitivity of the system, and should be matched to the size of the signal to be detected (the voltage range). If the gain is too high, small voltages that are not part of the signal will be amplified alongside it, creating noise; if the gain is inadequate, the amplifier will not detect the signal itself.

The **bandwidth** of an amplifier is the range of wave frequencies to which it will respond. This needs to be wide enough to accommodate the frequencies contained within the signal, but excessive bandwidth increases interference as extraneous frequencies are also amplified.

The frequency and voltage ranges of amplifiers suitable for processing the ECG, EMG, and EEG are shown in Table 4.3.

Processing

One of the main functions of signal processing is to remove interference from the signal.

Since body surface electrodes are designed to work together to compare potentials at various points on the body surface, one step in the processing of the signal is to discard any waveform that is identical in all leads (e.g. mains current). This is called **common mode rejection**. A further way of removing interference is **averaging,** where repetitive waveforms are compared over a few cycles. Random noise is reduced as it tends to average out to zero.

Display

Display of bioelectrical potentials involves a second transduction process: the electrical signal from the amplifier and processing unit must be converted into another energy form. Examples include kinetic energy (the movement of a beam of electrons in a cathode ray tube, or of a pen on a scroll of paper) and sound (the beeping of the pulse oximeter). Further processing can allow the display of numerical parameters which may be coupled to warning lights or alarms.

Stimulation of bioelectrical potentials

As well as being recorded, bioelectrical potentials can be stimulated by the application of potential differences across tissues. Examples include defibrillation, cardiac pacing, electroconvulsive therapy, and nerve stimulation for nerve blocks or neuromuscular junction monitoring.

ECG

The standard three-electrode ECG position usually observes lead II for heart rate and arrhythmias. A five-electrode ECG or three-electrode CM5 configuration (Figure 4.11) can also detect left ventricular ischaemia. The ECG monitor should always be connected to the patient before induction of anaesthesia or institution of a regional block. This gives a baseline trace, allowing detection of changes in its appearance during anaesthesia.

The ECG detects bioelectrical potentials arising from the heart. It does not provide information about the mechanical function of the heart, and cannot be used to assess cardiac output or blood pressure.

The bandwidth required for ECG analysis is 0.05–100Hz. Paper recording, with a standard size (1cm = 1mV) and paper speed (25mm/s) is commonplace on the wards. In theatre the signal is usually digitized and displayed on a cathode ray tube monitor.

Algorithms in the monitor software can be used to calculate various properties of the ECG waveform. The programmes can identify R waves, allowing the R–R interval and thus the heart rate (1/R–R interval) to be calculated. More advanced algorithms can be used to identify ST changes and arrhythmias on the digitized ECG waveform.

Table 4.3 Frequency and voltage ranges of bioelectrical potentials

	Frequency range (Hz)	Voltage range
ECG	0.5–100	0.1–1mV
EMG	1–1000	10µV–50mV
EEG	1–60	1–100µV

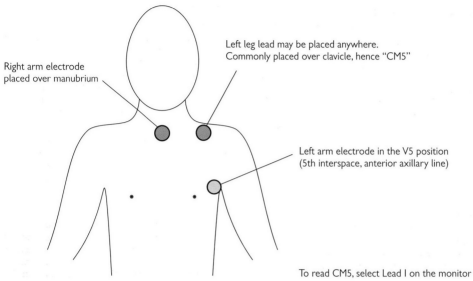

Right arm electrode placed over manubrium

Left leg lead may be placed anywhere. Commonly placed over clavicle, hence "CM5"

Left arm electrode in the V5 position (5th interspace, anterior axillary line)

To read CM5, select Lead I on the monitor

Fig. 4.11 In the CM5 configuration, the right arm (red) lead is placed at the suprasternal notch, the left arm (yellow) lead is placed at the V5 position, and the left leg (green) lead is at the left shoulder. Displaying lead I on the monitor gives a trace which best detects left ventricular ischaemia.

Monitoring of blood pressure (BP) is now routine during all procedures and critical care periods. Blood pressure is usually measured either non-invasively, using a pressure cuff, or invasively by means of an intravascular catheter.

Non-invasive blood pressure monitoring

Auscultatory techniques
The blood pressure cuff was developed by Riva-Rocci in 1896. It is inflated until distal arterial pulsation disappears. When released, BP is measured by auscultation of Korotkoff sounds. Initial tapping sounds (Korotkoff I) represent systolic BP. Sounds may quieten or disappear and become louder again. When the sounds disappear (Korotkoff V), this corresponds to diastolic BP.

Oscillometric techniques
The majority of modern non-invasive blood pressure monitors use oscillometry (measurement of the oscillations caused by the arterial pressure pulse). These oscillations are the result of the direct mechanical coupling of the occlusive cuff to the artery.

Automated oscillometry uses a microprocessor to inflate and deflate the cuff, and a transducer to detect arterial pulsations. Systolic BP = onset of rapidly increasing oscillations. Mean arterial pressure (MAP) = maximum oscillation at the lowest cuff pressure. Diastolic BP = onset of rapidly decreasing oscillations (or calculated via MAP = diastolic BP + one-third pulse pressure).

Unlike auscultatory techniques, which measure systolic and diastolic but estimate MAP, oscillometric devices measure the mean but estimate systolic and diastolic.

Different devices employ different algorithms of measurement. Although there is reasonable agreement between machines from different manufacturers, their results may not be identical. Newer devices measure oscillometrically but have a back-up auscultatory method of measurement, which is used when the former technique fails. These are used mainly in the assessment of hypertension in the community.

An appropriately sized cuff should be used to minimize error. It should cover >2/3 of the upper arm and the bladder width should be 40% of the arm mid-circumference. Too small a cuff will over-read, too large will under-read.

These devices are sensitive to patient movement and do not allow measurement validation. Readings may be inaccurate at low systolic BP (<60mmHg) or in the presence of arrhythmias. There may be a tourniquet effect if IV access or a pulse oximeter is placed on the same arm.

Invasive intravascular pressure monitoring

Intravascular pressures commonly measured include the following.

Arterial pressure
In patients monitored with an arterial catheter, the arterial pressure wave provides information on heart rate and pulse volume, an indication of contractility, and a useful estimate of heart filling. In addition, intermittent sampling or intravascular electrodes permit arterial blood gas analysis.

Central venous pressure
Central venous pressure (CVP) can be measured with a simple manometer containing normal saline, although it is usually done with a transducer system similar to the arterial apparatus. The intravascular catheter can be inserted into a neck or arm vein and advanced into the SVC, or via a femoral vein to the IVC (the latter is much less accurate, as it reflects changes in intra-abdominal as well as intravascular pressure). The CVP waveform consists of three waves and two descents (Figure 4.12).

- The **a wave** reflects **a**trial systole.
- The **c wave** reflects **c**losure of the AV (tricuspid) valve.
- The **v wave** reflects **v**entricular systole.
- The **x descent** reflects atrial rela**x**ation.
- The **y descent** reflects atrial empt**y**ing.

The mean CVP is a reflection of right atrial filling pressure: an index of right-heart preload. It is raised in right heart failure and fluid overload, and is reduced in hypovolaemia.

If there is a suspected discrepancy between left- and right-heart function, a pulmonary artery catheter can be used to measure pulmonary capillary wedge pressure (an index of left atrial filling pressure and left-heart preload; Section 10.7).

Central venous catheterization is indicated prior to operations likely to involve large fluid shifts (including haemorrhage), inotropic support, postoperative haemofiltration, or parenteral nutrition, or where there are concerns about cardiac failure.

Physical principles
Intravascular pressures are usually measured using a fluid-filled catheter connected to a semiconductor pressure transducer (which converts the pressure wave into an electic signal). The model describing the physical behaviour of such a system is a simple mass–spring system. When the mass is displaced and then released, a characteristic movement called simple harmonic motion is obtained.

Resonance
Resonance is the tendency of a system to oscillate at maximum amplitude at a particular frequency. This frequency is known as the system's resonant (or natural) frequency. In order to reproduce any waveform accurately, without resonant waves being set up, the resonant frequency of the measurement system must be higher than that of the system which it is trying to measure. For the human cardiovascular system, the natural frequency of the measurement system should be at least 45Hz.

Damping
Damping is any effect, either deliberately introduced or inherent, that tends to reduce the amplitude of oscillations in an oscillatory system. When measuring intravascular pressures, the transducer is hydraulically connected to the vessel by a fluid-containing system which is subject to frictional resistance, creating a damping effect.

Critical damping is the minimum damping that results in non-periodic motion of a system under free vibration. An ideal system should be about 70% critically damped (Figure 4.13). Over-damping can be produced by the insertion of additional three-way taps or the introduction of small air bubbles anywhere in the catheter–transducer system.

Zeroing
The hydraulic pressures measured by invasive systems are expressed in mmHg (arterial) or cmH_2O (CVP). This measurement must be referenced to a fixed zero point within the system. The transducer is set at the level of the right atrium (the mid-axillary line in a supine subject). The atmospheric pressure at this point is recorded and the apparatus is calibrated with this as its zero point. For subsequent measurements to be accurate, the transducer must be level with the zero point. This is particularly important when the pressure measured is small (e.g. the CVP).

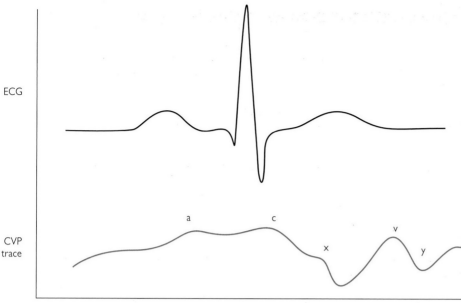

Fig. 4.12 The CVP trace, with reference to the ECG. The a wave occurs due to atrial systole; the c wave is a reverberation from the closure of the tricuspid valve. The x descent is a drop in pressure as the atrium relaxes and expands. However, during this relaxation, forward flow through the system (driven by left ventricular systole) gives rise to the v wave. As ventricular diastole begins, the ventricle relaxes and this opens the tricuspid valve. The atrium empties passively at first, giving the y descent, before contracting to start the cycle again with another a wave.

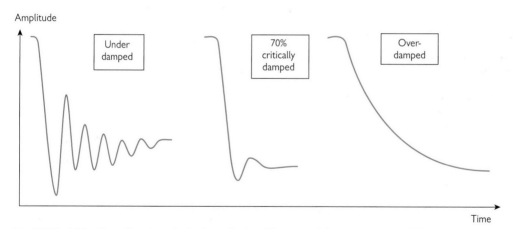

Fig. 4.13 The left-hand trace illustrates an 'under-damped' system. It has responded to a square wave applied at, or near, the resonant frequency by becoming grossly over-amplified. In contrast, a 'critically damped' system is shown on the right. Here, the system has accurately recorded the initial and final changes in pressure without oscillation, but the response is too slow to record rapid changes in pressure. The middle trace, a system which is 70% critically damped, represents the best compromise. Here the overshoot during oscillation is about 7%, but the response amplitude is accurate at frequencies up to 70% of the natural frequency.

Monitoring inspired and expired respiratory gases and vapours is essential to ensure adequate oxygenation and ventilation, and the appropriate delivery of anaesthetic vapours. Monitoring should include analysis of:

- oxygen (Section 4.8)
- CO_2
- nitrous oxide
- volatile agent.

Molecules with at least two dissimilar atoms are known as diatomic. Diatomic molecules (e.g. CO_2, N_2O, volatile anaesthetics) absorb infrared light. By Beer's law (Section 4.8), this property can be used to measure their concentration in samples.

Each gas absorbs infrared best at a particular wavelengths. Absorbance curves can be constructed for all the anaesthetic gases and vapours, similar to absorbance curves of oxy- and deoxyhaemoglobin (Section 4.8). By considering which gases are likely to be in a sample and choosing different infrared wavelengths (obtainable by passing 'raw' infrared light through filters), it is possible to minimize interference between measurement of individual gases.

Capnography

Capnography is the measurement of the end-tidal partial pressure of CO_2 ($P_{ET}CO_2$). It gives a continuous visual display.

CO_2 is measured by infrared absorption spectrometry (Figure 4.14). Two beams of infrared light at a specific wavelength are passed across two chambers (the sample and reference chambers). Carbon dioxide absorbs infrared; the amount absorbed is proportional to its concentration. The infrared beams pass through each chamber and hit photoelectric cells, which measure the light intensity. This allows real-time continuous accurate waveforms to be produced. In patients without significant pulmonary disease, the end-tidal CO_2 should give a close estimate of pulmonary arteriolar CO_2 partial pressure (P_aCO_2), after the gradient of about 0.5 kPa is taken into account. However, since some expired gas comes from unperfused alveoli, there is always a slight discrepancy, even in normal lungs. This is exaggerated where there is significant V/Q mismatch.

Capnography is a useful monitor in many situations.

Routine monitoring of CO_2

- Operating theatre
- ICU
- Transport
- Sedation
- Recovery

Detection of airway, respiratory, and circulatory problems

- Correct ETT placement (it does not exclude endobronchial intubation)
- Disconnection
- Airway obstruction
- Pulmonary embolism
- Rebreathing
- Falls in cardiac output
- Malignant hyperpyrexia
- Cardiopulmonary resuscitation (adequacy of chest compressions, correct ETT placement).

There are two main types of capnograph: mainstream and sidestream.

Sidestream capnograph

This uses a narrow (1.2mm) sampling tube to deliver gases to the sample chamber at a constant rate (e.g. 150ml/min). It is usually attached to the heat and moisture exchanger (Section 4.12), and should be as close to the patient's trachea as possible for accurate readings. The tubing must be impermeable to CO_2, and some tubes are designed to remove water vapour (or else a water trap is present before the sampling chamber).

The sampling chamber often contains filters that can change the infrared wavelength applied to the sample, allowing measurement of other gases such as anaesthetic vapours.

An exhaust port vents the sampled gas to the theatre scavenging system, the atmosphere, or back to the breathing system.

The system should have a delay of less than 3.8sec to be acceptable for clinical use.

Mainstream capnograph

In a mainstream capnograph, the sample chamber itself is incorporated into the breathing system so that it lies in the patient's gas stream. It is heated (41°C) to prevent condensation. There is no delay in the measurement, but the device can only measure CO_2 and increases dead space.

Capnograms (Figure 4.15)

Normal ETCO₂ trace

- Phase 1: dead-space phase. As the patient breathes out, the first part represents anatomical dead-space gas, which contains no CO_2.
- Phase 2: mixture of anatomical and alveolar dead-space phase. Gas from the alveoli, which has been involved in gas exchange, is mixed with dead-space gas and the CO_2 concentration rises until pure alveolar gas is detected.
- Phase 3: alveolar plateau phase. This is practically all alveolar gas. It usually has a positive up-slope since CO_2 is being continuously excreted into the alveoli. In addition, alveoli with low V/Q ratios tend to empty late.
- Phase 4: inspiratory phase. The CO_2 falls to zero as fresh gas is inhaled.

The α-*angle* is the angle between phase 2 and phase 3, and is supposed to represent the V/Q status of the lungs.

The β-*angle* is the angle between phase 3 and phase 4, and can be used to assess the extent of rebreathing.

Inhalational agent monitoring

Monitoring of inhalational agents and nitrous oxide is also by infrared absorption spectrometry. The infrared filters are mounted on a rotating disc. By rapid sequencing through different wavelengths, simultaneous measurement of all the gases of interest in the sample is possible. (The intermittent signal is also easier to amplify). Again, a reference chamber is used in order to prevent variation in the performance of the system being interpreted as a change in gas.

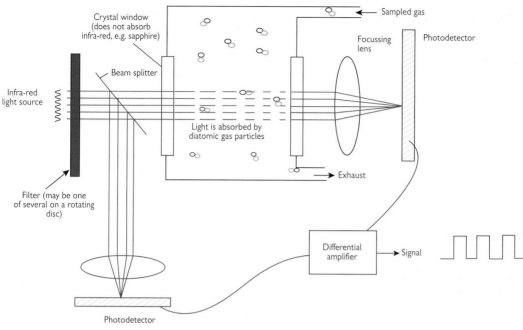

Fig. 4.14 Infrared absorption spectrometry.

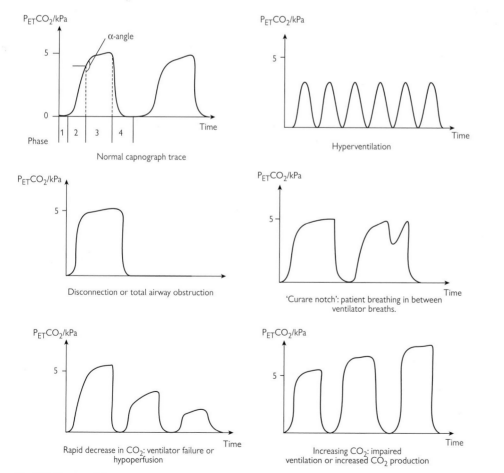

Fig. 4.15 Capnograph traces.

4.8 Oxygen monitoring

An oxygen molecule possesses two identical atoms and therefore is unsuitable for infrared absorption spectrometry. However, oxygen has unpaired outer-shell electrons and is highly reactive, giving rise to some interesting properties which can be exploited for measuring its concentration or partial pressure.

Paramagnetic oxygen analyser

The paramagnetic oxygen analyser takes advantage of the fact that oxygen is a paramagnetic gas; since it contains two electrons in unpaired orbits, it is attracted into a magnetic field. Most other gases of relevance in anaesthesia are weakly diamagnetic (repelled by a magnetic field).

Older paramagnetic devices use two dumb-bells containing nitrogen (weakly diamagnetic), suspended on a wire in a magnetic field. Oxygen entering the chamber displaces the dumb-bells (which rotate around the wire) as it is attracted into the magnetic field. The position of the reflected light beam is detected by photodiodes, calibrated to give the percentage of oxygen.

Alternatively, an opposing current can be applied to restore the dumb-bell to its resting position (null deflection). In the null deflection system, the current required is directly proportional to the partial pressure of oxygen. This method is extremely accurate (e.g. 0.1%).

Modern paramagnetic devices use a differential pressure transducer diaphragm, with a reference gas on one side and the sample gas on the other. A pulsed magnetic field is applied downstream of the transducer. Oxygen atoms from the sample gas are drawn in, reducing pressure on the side of the diaphragm facing the stream which is richer in oxygen. The resulting pressure pulses are transduced into an alternating current whose amplitude measures the oxygen content of the sample gas (Figure 4.16).

Polarographic (Clark) electrode

The Clark electrode is used in blood gas machines, but can also be used to analyse gas mixtures. It consists of two half-cells separated by a salt bridge (Figure 4.17). The components are:
- Silver/silver chloride anode (**A**g at the **A**node)
- Platinum cathode (platinum is a strong catalyst for the dissociation and reassociation of water)
- Aqueous electrolyte solution (e.g. KCl)
- Power source providing a constant potential difference (0.6V)
- Ammeter.

The sample is separated from the platinum cathode by an oxygen-permeable membrane because protein deposits on the cathode can prevent its functioning. Electrons are formed at the silver electrode:

$$Ag \rightarrow Ag^+ + e^-$$

Oxygen diffuses to the platinum cathode, where electrons (which originate from the silver electrode, leaving silver ions) combine with oxygen and water to give hydroxyl ions:

$$O_2 + 4e^- + 2H_2O \rightarrow 4(OH)^-$$

Within the electrolyte solution, KCl gives chloride to the silver ions (creating AgCl) and picks up the hydroxyl ions (making KOH). This completes the circuit, allowing current to flow. The rate-limiting step is the availability of oxygen at the platinum electrode, and so the size of the current is proportional to the partial pressure of oxygen in the sample.

Transcutaneous and intravascular oxygen electrodes
The polarographic electrode can be miniaturized for use within arterial catheters or adapted for transcutaneous measurement. Intravascular measurement is more accurate than transdermal measurement but does not replace the need for blood gases as only the oxygen partial pressure is measured and not the pH, PCO_2, etc.

Transdermal oxygen measurement involves local heating of the skin to 43°C in order to induce vasodilatation and allow reading. There is a risk of burns, and the electrode position should be changed every few hours. The device is less accurate than those which read directly from blood. Response time is up to a minute.

Fuel cell

Again, this consists of two half-cells and a salt bridge (Figure 4.18). However, the reaction with oxygen occurs spontaneously and so the fuel cell does not require a power source: in fact, it is a power source in itself (hence the name). The components are:
- Lead anode
- Gold mesh cathode (separated from the sample by an oxygen-permeable membrane)
- Aqueous potassium hydroxide (KOH) solution
- Ammeter
- Thermistor (for temperature compensation).

The reaction at the gold cathode is identical to that in the polarographic electrode:

$$O_2 + 4e^- + 2H_2O \rightarrow 4(OH)^-$$

The reaction at the lead anode is

$$Pb + 2(OH)^- \rightarrow PbO_2 + H_2O + 2e^-$$

Like the polarographic electrode, the current registered on the ammeter is a measure of the partial pressure of oxygen present.

The fuel cell is small, light, and portable. However, it can be damaged by nitrous oxide as this releases nitrogen at the lead anode which can pressurize the cell. Like a battery, the fuel cell will expire: the more oxygen to which it is exposed, the faster this will occur.

Pulse oximetry

Although pulse oximetry does not measure oxygen partial pressure or concentration directly, it is used to assess the percentage of arterial haemoglobin combined with oxygen. Assessment of arterial oxygenation state and heart rate can be made via a continuous visual display. An audible tone, which alters in pitch and rate, can alert the anaesthetist to changes in both. The physical principle behind the device is the Beer–Lambert law, comprised of two parts. Figure 4.19 demonstrates the effects of concentration and path length on absorption.
- *Beer's law:* the absorption A of light transmitted through a substance is proportional to the concentration C of the substance.
- *Lambert's law:* the absorption of transmitted light is proportional to the thickness of the substance (or path length L).

Combining these two laws gives the Beer–Lambert law:

$$A = \varepsilon LC,$$

where ε is a constant called the extinction coefficient.

The pulse oximeter exploits the differences between the absorption spectra for oxy- and deoxyhaemoglobin (Figure 4.20). Oxyhaemoglobin absorbs more infrared light (940nm) and deoxyhaemoglobin absorbs more red light (660nm). When light at these two wavelengths is shone through haemoglobin-containing solutions, it is possible to solve simultaneous equations to calculate the relative proportions of oxy- and deoxygenated forms, giving a percentage oxygen saturation.

The light is emitted by two separate LEDs, one transmitting the red light (660nm) and the other the infrared component (940nm). Sensors measure the absorption of transmitted light across the tissue. The sensor itself detects the light, but not its wavelength, and so the machine has to 'know' which of the LEDs is flashing. The sequence also contains a pause to analyse ambient light, and the 'red–infrared–pause' pattern is repeated.

The signal obtained when ambient light has been filtered consists of a DC and an AC component. The DC part arises from skin, muscle, bone, and venous blood flow. The AC component of the signal comes from arterial blood flow causing tiny pulsatile changes in the thickness of the tissue. A microprocessor analyses the data by filtering out the ambient light and DC components, and amplifying the AC component before averaging it over a few seconds. As well as calculating the oxygen saturation, this AC signal also gives a characteristic blood flow waveform (plethysmography).

Limitations include falsely low readings with peripheral vasoconstriction or hypoperfusion, methaemoglobinaemia, dyes (e.g. methylene blue, indocyanine green), and some nail varnishes. Falsely high readings may occur with carboxyhaemoglobinaemia. Values under 70% are inaccurate, as the data are extrapolated rather than experimentally determined.

▶ Beware of time lag between clinical desaturation and low oximeter reading. Response times may be >60sec with a finger probe and >10sec with an ear probe.

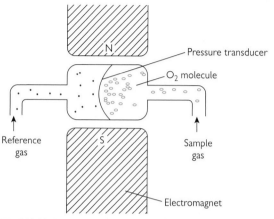

Fig. 4.16 Modern paramagnetic oxygen analyser.

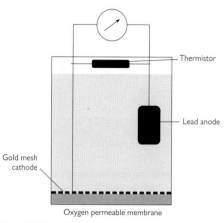

Fig. 4.18 Fuel cell.

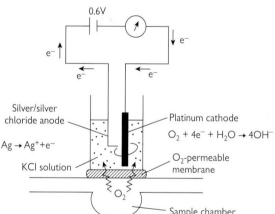

Fig. 4.17 Clark electrode.

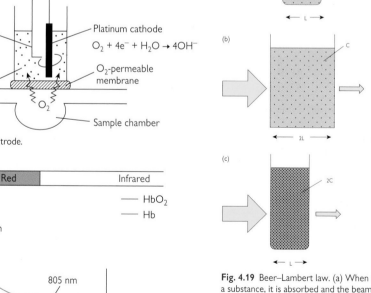

Fig. 4.19 Beer–Lambert law. (a) When light of intensity I_0 passes through a substance, it is absorbed and the beam exiting the substance has a reduced intensity, I_1. (b) If the path length L doubles, twice the light absorption occurs with a proportional reduction in I_1. (c) If the concentration C of the substance doubles, twice the absorption occurs, and again I_1 is reduced proportionally.

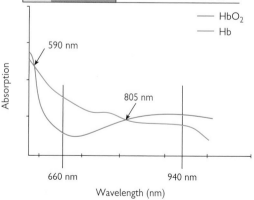

Fig. 4.20 Absorption graphs and isosbestic points. An isobestic point is the wavelength at which two substances absorb light to the same extent (590nm and 805nm for oxyhaemoglobin and deoxyhaemoglobin, respectively). Light at these wavelengths is unable to distinguish between oxy- and deoxyhaemoglobin, but can be used to quantify the total haemoglobin in a solution. This is the basis for some near-patient haemoglobin estimation devices.

4.9 Awareness and depth of anaesthesia monitoring

Definition

Awareness represents the inadvertent return to consciousness during a supposed general anaesthetic, with or without recall. The important factors, in terms of the severity of adverse after-effects, appear to be:

- Whether there is recall
- Whether the patient is in pain
- Whether patient is paralysed.

Classification of awareness

- Conscious awareness with spontaneous recall (explicit)
- Conscious awareness with amnesia
- Dreaming or unconscious awareness with amnesia
- No awareness

Incidence

Dreaming around the time of operation is common (60%). In the 1960s the incidence of awareness was around 1–2%. This fell to about 0.2% during the 1990s and now stands at about 0.13%.

Cause

The cause of awareness is the failure to deliver adequate anaesthesia. This can be a deliberate risk–benefit decision (as in the sick, the elderly, or major haemorrhage), accidental, or due to equipment malfunction (ventilators, vaporizers, infusion devices). Patients are more likely to have recall if the experience is painful or personal remarks have been made.

Risk factors

- Types of surgery: cardiac (1/100), obstetric (1/250 for LSCS under GA), major trauma (1/20), bronchoscopy
- Major haemorrhage
- Sick or unstable (avoid adverse effects of anaesthetic agents by reducing dose; risk–benefit decision)
- Muscle relaxants (twice as likely to suffer awareness)
- Substance abuse (higher anaesthetic and analgesic requirements)
- Past history of awareness
- Omission of N_2O from inhalational anaesthesia

Prevention

Above all vigilance is the key. There MUST be thorough anaesthetic machine and equipment checking and monitoring. It is poor practice to make personal or inappropriate comments even when the patient is supposedly anaesthetized. If the patient is maintained at MAC ≥1.0 (adjusted for age), spontaneous recall is *virtually* eliminated.

Treatment of suspected awareness

Quickly deepen the anaesthetic either with an IV hypnotic or by increasing the inhalational agent. Some authorities advocate the use of benzodiazepines for their amnesic properties, but there is no evidence of a retrograde action. Then you must try to discover why the potential awareness has occurred. Check all anaesthetic delivery equipment, vaporizers, and ventilator. Good records are essential (ideally a computerized record system). If you suspect that a patient may have been aware, you should inform a senior anaesthetist. Visit the patient postoperatively, with a witness, when they are awake enough to be interviewed. Take the patient seriously if they have been affected, and obtain a detailed account of the event to distinguish between dreaming and awareness. It is essential to express sympathy and apologize. Visit the patient daily during their hospital stay, always with a witness. Inform the GP. The patient may require referral for counselling.

Depth of anaesthesia (DOA) monitors

In the past a number of physiological parameters have been used as a measure of patients being too 'lightly' anaesthetized. These include movement, increase in heart rate or blood pressure, hyperventilation, sweating, lacrimation, and increase in pupil size. These have now been shown to be unreliable measures of depth of anaesthesia, as they are neither sensitive nor specific. They may be masked or exaggerated by drugs and diseases, e.g. β-blockers, neuromuscular blockers, vagolytics, hyperthyroidism, autonomic neuropathy (e.g. diabetes).

If the correct level of anaesthesia for the particular procedure can be achieved, this will reduce amount of anaesthetic required, decrease cardiovascular responses to anaesthesia and surgery, and reduce the costs of anaesthesia.

Isolated forearm technique (IFT)

First described by M.E. Tunstall, some would regard this as the 'gold standard', while others feel that it is of historical interest only. The patient's forearm is 'isolated' by a tourniquet inflated above arterial pressure before muscle relaxant is given. After the patient is anaesthetized he/she is asked to do some simple tasks (e.g. 'bend your thumb'). A number of patients have given appropriate responses to the commands, indicating apparent awareness. However, many of these have no recollection at later interview, making interpretation difficult.

Bispectral index (BIS)

BIS is the system that shows the most promise at present and has been most widely evaluated. BIS monitors record the raw EEG, which alters with anaesthesia, and after processing produces a dimensionless number from 0–100, which is an index of probability that the patient is aware (Figure 4.21). BIS is a good measure of the hypnotic effect of drugs and estimates the level of sedation over the preceding 15–60sec. It does not predict movement in response to surgical stimulus, but does correlate with the probability of recall/awareness. The B-Aware Trial and Swedish Awareness Follow-up Trial 2 (SAFE-2) showed an 80% reduction in awareness when adjusting the BIS score between 40 and 60 in normal and 'at-risk' groups. The majority of the cases of awareness in these trials actually had BIS scores above the recommended 60 during their intubation.

Auditory evoked potential (AEP)

This works on similar principle to BIS but looks at the electrophysiological response of the CNS to a repeated auditory stimulus. It measures changes in the latency and amplitude of the processed waveform, which vary with depth of anaesthesia (Figure 4.22).

Entropy

This depth of anaesthesia monitor quantifies the irregularity of a signal. As anaesthesia deepens, EEG entropy decreases. The M Entropy monitor calculates two measures of spectral entropy. State entropy (SE) is derived from the EEG 'power' in the range 0–30Hz (the range of frequencies associated with cortical activity) and response entropy (RE) is derived from the activity in the range 0–44Hz. The entropy difference (ED) between these two readings, e.g. activity in the 30–44Hz range, represents the frequencies seen with facial muscle activity.

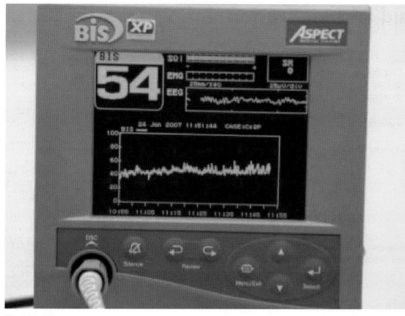

Fig. 4.21 BIS monitor.

Amplitude/μV

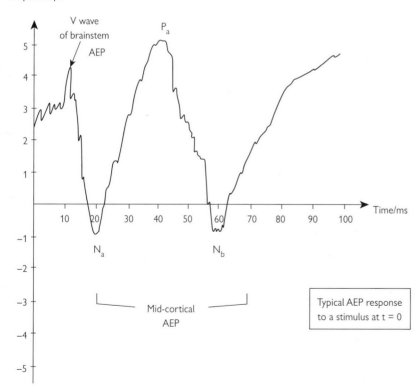

Fig. 4.22 Auditory evoked potentials.

4.10 Aspects of fluid administration during anaesthesia

All patients presenting for surgery must have an assessment (see Chapter 11) of fluid volume status prior to going to theatre, as they may require volume replacement prior to their anaesthetic. It is important to consider the major compartments separately.

- Intravascular volume
- ECF volume, judged by Na^+ content and the presence of peripheral oedema
- ICF volume, inferred from measurement of tonicity and $[Na^+]$

Volume deficits or excess may be expected in:

- Emergency cases
- After prolonged starvation
- Those who have had bowel preparation
- Those with inappropriate fluid prescription and administration.

During an operation a patient will have a number of fluid requirements. These include basal fluid and electrolyte requirements, replacement of body fluid losses, replacement of drug-induced redistribution (anaesthetic vasodilators or central neuraxial blocks), and replacement of blood losses. Replacement of 'third-space' losses is contentious and discussed in further detail in Section 11.8.

As a rule, electrolyte and fluid loss should be replaced with appropriate isotonic crystalloid. If intravascular losses are replaced by crystalloid, three times the amount of loss must be given, as it will rapidly leave the vascular compartment and redistribute throughout the ECF.

Blood loss should be replaced with synthetic colloid/blood as appropriate.

Basal requirements

The basal fluid and electrolyte requirements of a patient are normally given in the form of an isotonic crystalloid such as Hartmann's. The replacement volume will vary with the individual's weight, age, and sex, and will depend on assessment of the ECF and tonicity.

Children

The '4–2–1' method can be used to estimate basal fluid requirements. The formula is:

- 4ml/kg/hr for the first 10kg of body weight
- 2ml/kg/hr for the second 10 kg
- 1ml/kg/hr thereafter.

For example, a child weighing 26kg will need $(4 \times 10) + (2 \times 10) + (6 \times 1) = 66$ml/hr. This formula, which corrects for the relatively greater fluid requirements of smaller children, can also be applied to adults: a normal male (weight 70kg) will require $(4 \times 10) + (2 \times 10) + (50 \times 1) = 110$ml/hr = 2.64L in 24h.

It is important to emphasise that all calculated regimes are merely guides that require interpretation in light of clinical findings.

Blood loss estimation

Blood loss can be extremely difficult to estimate, especially when it is spilt onto drapes or the floor or lost in washout. Nowadays, transfusion is reserved for patients whose haemoglobin levels have fallen below or are likely to fall below 7–8g/dl, or who have significant cardiovascular disease (i.e. they require a higher haemoglobin to prevent ischaemia). Accurate estimation of haemoglobin is now relatively easy; as well as laboratory measures, arterial blood gas machines and near-patient devices (see below) can be used.

Perioperative cell salvage

With the decreasing availability of blood, fears of infection acquired from blood transfusion, and risk of allergic reaction to allogenic blood, there is increasing interest in autotransfusion. Where a reasonable amount of blood is likely to be lost, it is possible to collect the patient's blood and re-infuse it either directly or after centrifugal washing. This is possible during many types of surgery and also postoperatively (e.g. after knee surgery, blood is collected from the drain and can be re-infused without washing; there is a time limit of about 6hr). It cannot be used when the blood may have mixed with bacteria.

The advantages of autotransfusion after cell salvage are:

- No cross-match required
- No risk of new infection from blood
- No risk of immune reaction to blood
- Cost savings
- May be acceptable to some Jehovah's Witnesses.

Infusion devices

At times it is necessary to infuse fluids rapidly. Various methods are available to achieve this.

- Hand syringing: this is useful in paediatrics, where volumes are small and it is important to measure accurately.
- Pressure bag: this contains a pump system similar to a manual sphygmomanometer. The fluid bag can be placed within it and the bag inflated by hand to pressures up to 300mmHg.
- Rapid infusor: these machines (e.g. Level 1® warmer, Figure 4.23) have two compartments into which the fluid bags are placed. These compartments contain automated pressure bags. The Level 1® also warms the fluid as it is given and can infuse at rates of 75–30,000ml/hr.

Near-patient testing

HemoCue®

The HemoCue® (Figure 4.24) is a portable system for haemoglobin concentration analysis which consists of a dual-wavelength (570 and 880nm) photometer-based system. This works on broadly the same principle as the pulse oximeter (Section 4.8), with the dual photometer allowing correction for leucocytosis, lipaemia, and other sources of turbidity. It has an accuracy of ±1.5% over the range 0–25.6g/dl.

Blood is drawn into the cuvette and mixed with sodium deoxycholate. This breaks down the erythrocyte membrane, releasing haemoglobin. Sodium nitrite then converts the haem iron from ferrous (2^+) to ferric (3^+) form, giving methaemoglobin. This combines with azide to form azidemethaemoglobin, which is measured.

It is simple, lightweight, and quick, and requires only 20μL of blood. As long as the lens is kept clean and calibrated regularly, it is extremely accurate.

i-STAT®

i-STAT® (Figure 4.25) is a hand-held system which can provides various blood analyses using as little as two drops of blood which are added to the cartridge. The advanced biosensor allows different tests by simply changing the cartridge, which the i-STAT® module recognizes by its 'tag'. The results are printable or downloadable. It is simple, easy to use, and entirely portable.

Hemochron®

The Hemochron® is a device used to measure activated clotting time. It is used when rapid assessment of heparinization is required (e.g. cardiothoracic surgery). Whole blood is placed in the test tube which is warmed and gently rotated. Within this test tube is a ferrous metallic bar; as the clot forms, this stops moving freely and the change in its motion is detected by a magnetic sensor.

Thromboelastogram

The thromboelastogram (TEG) plots the viscoelastic properties of a clot against time. From this plot it is possible to assess the interaction between platelets, fibrinogen and clotting factors.

Different coagulation abnormalities give characteristic traces. This method is a near-patient real-time measure of clotting, clot characteristics, and clot lysis. See Section 15.8 for further details.

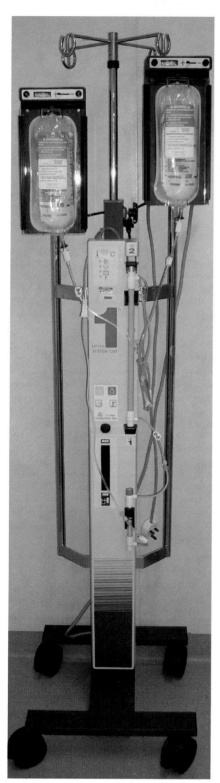

Fig. 4.23 A Level 1® infusor. This is used when rapid infusion of large volumes of fluid is necessary (e.g. in major haemorrhage).

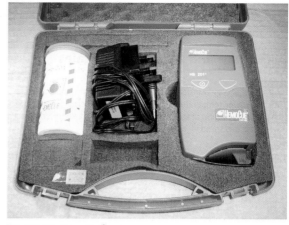

Fig. 4.24 The HemoCue® system

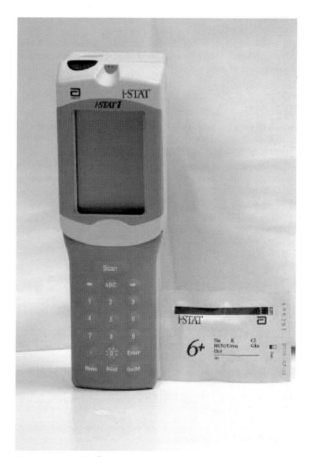

Fig. 4.25 The i-STAT® system

4.11 Temperature

Definitions and temperature scales

Heat

Heat is the energy transferred from a body at high temperature to a body at a lower temperature. It is a measure of internal kinetic energy (the vibratory motion of atoms within a substance). Like other forms of energy, it is measured in joules (J).

Temperature

Temperature is a measure of heat within a system. Various linear scales are used to define it. Any linear scale requires at least two fixed points between which a fundamental interval can be assigned. The most commonly used temperature scale in everyday use is the **Celsius scale,** and the **absolute (Kelvin) scale** is important in physics. Weather reports often still include the old-fashioned Fahrenheit scale.

The Celsius scale

The Celsius scale takes the ice and boiling points of water as its fixed points. It is measured in degrees Celsius (°C).

The **ice point of water** is the temperature at which ice and air-saturated water are in equilibrium at standard atmospheric pressure (101.3kPa). This is designated 0°C.

The **steam point of water** is the temperature where the saturated vapour pressure of pure water equals standard atmospheric pressure. This is designated 100°C.

The fundamental interval of the Celsius scale has been assigned the value of **1/100th the temperature change between the ice and steam points of pure water**.

The absolute scale

The absolute scale takes as its fixed points 'absolute zero' and the triple point of water. It is measured in kelvins (K).

Absolute zero has never been measured, but is defined theoretically as the point at which particles within a substance have the minimum possible internal energy: 'zero-point' energy.

The **triple point of water** is the single temperature and pressure combination where pure water, pure water vapour, and pure ice can exist in equilibrium. It occurs at 0.01°C and 611Pa (0.006 atm).

The scale preserves the same fundamental interval as the Celsius scale (for ease of comparison). Therefore absolute zero is defined as 1/273.16th the thermodynamic temperature of the triple point of water. It follows that:

- Absolute zero = −273.15K
- 0°C = 273.15K
- Triple point of water = 0.01°C = 273.16K

Laws of thermodynamics

Thermodynamic processes are governed by four laws

Zeroth law: If two thermodynamic systems are each in equilibrium with a third, then they are in equilibrium with each other.

First law: Energy is conserved; it can be changed from one form to another but cannot be created or destroyed.

Second law: Entropy. The disorder of a system tends to increase with time (think of your desk!).

Third law: As a system approaches absolute zero temperature, all processes cease and the entropy of the system approaches a minimum.

States of matter: solid, liquid, and gas

The usual sequence of transition with increasing temperature is solid → liquid → gas. However, some materials (e.g. carbon dioxide) can change directly from solid to gas if the pressure is low enough; this process is called sublimation. Some important temperatures for a substance include:

- Freezing point—the temperature at which a liquid turns into a solid
- Boiling point—the temperature at which a liquid turns into a gas
- Critical temperature—the temperature above which a substance cannot be liquefied, no matter how much pressure is applied to it
  - O_2: −119°C
  - N_2O: 36.5°C
  - CO_2: 31°C.

For a substance to change its state, energy is needed. This energy is consumed by the change of state without raising the temperature of the substance, and is called latent heat.

- **Latent heat of fusion** is the energy required to transform a solid into a liquid. Ice at 0°C is changed into liquid water, also at 0°C.
- **Latent heat of vaporization** is the energy required to transform a liquid into a gas or vapour.

Adiabatic processes

In an adiabatic process, no energy is gained or lost by the system. This occurs if the process happens so quickly that there is no time to transfer heat, or if the system is very well insulated from its surroundings. Therefore changes in one type of energy affect temperature.

- **Adiabatic heating** If a gas is compressed rapidly, it heats up. This may occur in anaesthetic machine pipes if a cylinder is opened quickly, and has been the cause of explosions.
- **Adiabatic cooling** If gas expands rapidly, energy is required to overcome van der Waals forces of attraction between molecules and therefore the temperature falls. This principle is used in the cryoprobe, a device which emits a stream of compressed gas to cause freezing of superficial skin lesions.

Measuring temperature

Many different devices can be used to measure temperature. They can be classified as non-electrical or electrical.

Non-electrical

- *Touch:* this can be used as an extremely crude but rapid assessment of temperature, and requires no equipment.
- *LCD thermometer:* this consists of a line of cells containing liquid crystal, a substance whose order falls between that of solid and liquid. At the temperature specific to the liquid crystal medium, thermal motion destroys the delicate liquid crystal structure, changing the colour. This gives a relatively coarse assessment of temperature.
- *Liquid-filled thermometers (mercury, alcohol):* these are used for accurate assessment of the temperature of adults or children in hospital or the home. However, mercury thermometers are made of glass; and mercury is a toxic substance. These thermometers have largely been phased out in hospitals. Alcohol thermometers are used for recording low temperatures (e.g. severe hypothermia).

- **Gas-filled thermometers:** the hydrogen thermometer consists of a syringe filled with hydrogen gas, which expands to calibrated lines as the temperature increases. It is extremely accurate and is used in the laboratory setting. Bourdon gauges (Section 2.6) can be used to measure (very high) temperatures, although their response is slow and they are not particularly accurate.
- **Bimetallic strip:** this consists of two dissimilar metals bonded together, which expand to different degrees with increasing temperature. The unequal expansion causes the structure to bend. Bimetallic strips are used in vaporizers for temperature compensation (as the temperature of the liquid in the sump falls, the bimetallic strip mechanism allows a higher gas flow over the vapour). They can also be used as thermostats, but have a slow response time.
- **Infrared thermometer:** all surfaces emit infrared radiation—the hotter they are, the more they emit. These devices are used on wards to measure tympanic membrane temperature (which should reflect core temperature). There are two possible problems: first, the probe must be aimed accurately at the tympanic membrane, and secondly the ear must be clear of wax.

Electrical

- **Resistance thermometer:** this consists of a platinum wire in which resistance increases with temperature. Resistance thermometers require a Wheatstone bridge to operate (Section 4.13) but offer great stability and accuracy.
- **Thermistor:** this consists of a semiconductor metal oxide bead. The resistance of the bead falls exponentially as the temperature rises. The thermometer can be very small, and gives an accurate rapid response.
- **Thermocouple:** electrons in different metals have different energy levels. When dissimilar metals are brought into contact, the electrons move from the higher to the lower energy level, producing a small current. This is known as the Seebeck effect. The current changes with temperature, and can be measured. One junction is held at a reference temperature, and the other at the temperature to be measured. This is a very accurate and cheap thermometer, with a rapid response time. However, it requires a power supply.

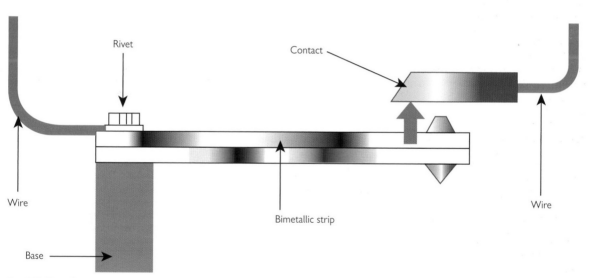

Fig. 4.26 Bimetallic strip

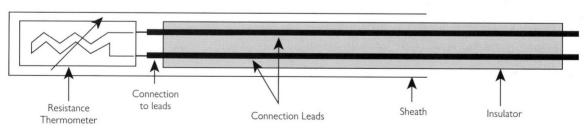

Fig. 4.27 Resistance thermometer

4.12 Humidity

Definitions

Absolute humidity
The mass of water vapour in a given volume of gas. Expressed as mg/L or g/mm^3.

Relative humidity
The amount of water vapour expressed as a percentage of the amount the gas would hold if fully saturated.

Dew point
As air cools, it can hold less water vapour. The temperature at which a mass of air is 100% saturated (so that water condenses) is called the dew point.

Measurement of humidity

A device that measures humidity is known as a hygrometer. Various principles can be utilized to measure humidity:

Hair hygrometer
Natural fibres relax when the air is wet, and this changes the length of a hair. A horsehair attached to a sprung pointer lengthens and contracts and causes the position of the pointer to change, indicating the level of humidity (Figure 4.28).

Wet and dry bulb thermometer
This apparatus exploits the principle that evaporation causes cooling. Evaporation of liquid requires heat energy. As higher-energy molecules leave the surface of a liquid, lower-energy molecules are left behind and the liquid cools. In the wet and dry bulb thermometer, the wet bulb is attached to a wick immersed in water. The lower the humidity, the more water evaporates, cooling the wet bulb. The dry bulb measures atmospheric temperature for reference. The temperature difference between the wet and dry bulbs is looked up in a table to find the humidity of the air at the specified atmospheric temperature (Figure 4.30).

Dewpoint hygrometer
Dewpoint hygrometers use an optoelectronic mechanism to detect condensation on a chilled mirror surface as the air is cooled to its dew point.

A more traditional version of the same principle is **Regnault's hygrometer** (Figure 4.29), where air is bubbled through ether in a silvered tube to produce cooling (again, loss of latent heat of evaporation). As the temperature falls to the dew point, condensation occurs on the silver tube and the temperature is read from a thermometer immersed in the ether. At this point the cooled air is saturated. Tables are consulted to find the amount of water vapour in the air so that its relative humidity prior to cooling can be calculated.

Humidity in the respiratory tract

It is important to humidify fresh gas delivered to the patient, as this helps to maintain normal ciliary function in the trachea, and prevents drying of secretions in the airway (which can cause destruction of the airway epithelium and atelectasis).

About 10% of a patient's heat loss occurs from the respiratory tract. Around two-thirds of this heat is used in the humidification of dry gases. Although the influence of respiration is relatively small when compared with the heat loss from wounds and contact with a cold environment, respiratory heat loss may be relevant in smaller children.

The specific heat capacity (energy required to raise the temperature of 1kg of a substance by 1°C) of gases is tiny—about 1000 times less than the specific heat capacity of a liquid. As water evaporates into the respiratory tract, the latent heat of vaporization results in significant patient cooling. To reduce heat loss from the respiratory tract, it is far more important to humidify gases than to warm them.

Heat and Moisture Exchangers (HME)
HMEs are usually single use, hygroscopic material (e.g. paper, cellulose, ceramic) in a plastic casing (Figure 4.31). They work on either the hygroscopic or condensation principle. The condenser humidifier consists of a matrix of substance, usually corrugated paper, positioned between the patient and the anaesthetic tubing. During expiration the water vapour condenses on the matrix (which is warmed by the latent heat of condensation) and during inspiration the dry fresh gas is humidified as it passes through the wet matrix. These devices are cheap, easy to use, about 50–70% efficient. They often double as bacterial filters (either depth filter, or 0.2 μm screen). They take a few minutes to saturate before working properly.

Hot water baths
Water is heated up to 60°C in a small bath, over which passes the fresh gas. A thermostat controls the heating element. These devices are able to humidify gas up to about 80%, even at high flows. However, there are a few problems associated with their use:

- They may require heated wires along the tubing to prevent recondensation and pooling, making the equipment heavy and bulky.
- Drowning is a risk: active humidification at high temperature may cause oversaturation of the lungs with water.
- It is possible to scald the patient and cause airway burns.
- The bath may become colonized by bacteria: care must be taken to keep them clean.
- These are more expensive and need regular servicing and cleaning.

Nebulizers
Many nebulizers employ a Venturi system, which utilizes the Bernoulli principle (Section 2.9). Gas is passed through a Venturi constriction (a small orifice, which accelerates the gas); and the liquid to be nebulised is entrained. Some designs incorporate an anvil, which sits in the path of the entrained droplets. When the liquid hits the anvil it is dispersed into much smaller droplets. These nebulizers require a driving gas. Gas-driven nebulisers are shown in Figures 4.32 and 4.33

Ultrasonic nebulizers use a plate vibrating at around 3 MHz. Water dropped onto this plate is broken into droplets around 1–2 μm in diameter (droplets of <1 μm will travel to the alveoli themselves). These are extremely efficient nebulizers but they pose a risk of oversaturation of the airways, especially in children.

Some designs incorporate a micro-mesh through which the fluid streams, enabling the production of smaller droplets. These devices are very susceptible to contamination by dust and other particles.

Spinning-disc nebulizers use a motorized rotating plate, which throws out droplets by centrifugal force. They require an electrical power supply.

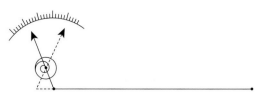

Fig. 4.28 Principle of action of horse hair hygrometer.

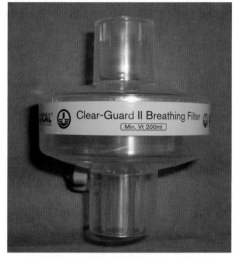

Fig. 4.31 Heat and moisture exchanger.

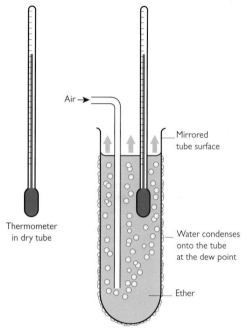

Air →

Mirrored tube surface

Water condenses onto the tube at the dew point

Thermometer in dry tube

Ether

Fig. 4.29 Regnault's hygrometer.

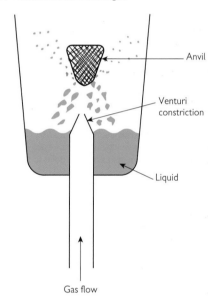

Anvil

Venturi constriction

Liquid

Gas flow

Fig. 4.32 Principle of action of the gas-driven nebulizer.

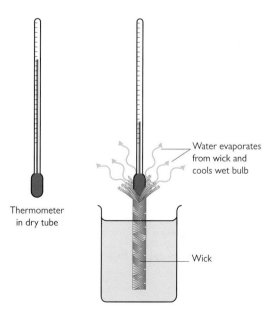

Water evaporates from wick and cools wet bulb

Thermometer in dry tube

Wick

Fig. 4.30 Wet and dry bulb thermometer.

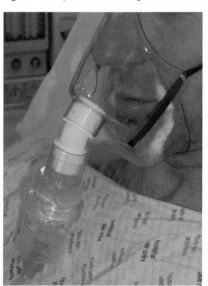

Fig. 4.33 A gas-driven nebulizer.

Electrical energy is transferred by the movement of electrons in a conducting medium.

Definitions and equations

Current

The transfer of electrical energy is known as current, I. The SI unit of current is the ampere (A), and is defined by the magnetic force developed by a current: one ampere is the current which, when flowing in two infinitely long parallel conductors of negligible cross-sectional area, one metre apart, in a vacuum, produces a force between them of 2×10^{-7} newtons per metre of their length.

Charge

An electrical charge Q is obtained when a material builds up an excess (negative charge) or deficit (positive charge) of electrons. The unit of charge is the coulomb (C), which is defined as the quantity of electric charge carried past a point when a current of one ampere flows for one second:

$$Q = It$$

where t is time in seconds. This is equivalent to 6.24×10^{18} electrons.

Potential difference

Potential difference (PD) V is the driving force behind the flow of electricity. When electricity flows, electrical potential is converted into other forms of energy W such as heat, light, and kinetic energy. The PD beween two points in a circuit is the amount of energy converted when unit charge passes from one point to the other. (By convention, earth has a potential of zero). The unit of PD is the volt (V), defined as the PD between two points in which one joule of energy is converted when one Coulomb of charge passes from one point to the other:

$$W = QV$$

Resistance

The resistance R of a conductor is defined as the ratio of the PD V across it to the current I flowing through it. The unit is the ohm (Ω) which is defined as the resistance of a conductor when a PD of one volt causes a current flow of one ampere. This relationship is called Ohm's law:

$$R = \frac{V}{I}$$

Many devices make use of changes in resistance for measurement (see strain gauges and semiconductors below). The sensitivity of these circuits can be improved by using a Wheatstone bridge, a 'balanced null-deflection' circuit (Figure 4.34). In its simplest form, it consists of an arrangement of three known resistances (R_3 is a variable resistor which can be adjusted) and a semiconductor or strain gauge (R_4). It also requires a galvanometer and a power source. R_3 is adjusted until the galvanometer reads zero (hence null deflection). At this point $R_1/R_2 = R_3/R_4$. The resistance R_4 can be calculated and correlated with whatever property is being measured.

Capacitance

Capacitance C is a charge given to an isolated conductor, and can be considered as being stored on that conductor. The unit of capacitance is the farad (F), which is defined the capacitance of an isolated conductor when one Coulomb of charge causes a change of one volt in PD:

$$C = \frac{Q}{V}$$

A defibrillator contains a large capacitor. This builds up an electrical charge, before discharging across the patient's heart.

Direct and alternating current

In direct current (DC), the flow of electrons is in one direction only. In alternating current (AC), the flow of electrons forms a sine wave. The overall magnitude of the current is in fact zero, but the energy converted can be calculated by using the root mean square (rms) of the current (Figure 4.35). UK mains current is alternating, with a peak voltage of 340V. This has an rms value of 240V, and therefore is equivalent to a direct current with a PD of 240V. Hence UK mains current is described as 240V.

Capacitors offer resistance to DC, since current flow ceases once the capacitor is charged. However, in a circuit carrying AC, the capacitor is rapidly charging and discharging in opposite directions, and offers little impedance to current flow.

Electrical properties of materials

Conductors can transfer electrons easily: they are usually metals whose outer electrons are loosely bound and free to move. Water conducts electricity by hydrolysis: when an electrical current is applied, it splits into OH^- and H^+ ions, and these move towards the cathode (positive electrode) and anode (negative electrode), respectively. Pure water is actually a fairly poor conductor, but its conductance can be increased dramatically by the presence of ions such as Na^+ and Cl^-. It follows that body fluids and salt-containing solutions such as Hartmann's are excellent conductors.

Certain factors alter the conductivity of metal wires. One is the tension within the wire, which tends to stretch it and reduce its diameter. This property gives rise to the strain gauge, which can be used to quantify forces acting along the axis of the wire.

Insulators are materials with tightly bound electrons; they do not transfer electrical energy easily. Insulating layers of plastic are used to coat electrical wires to isolate them electrically from the environment.

Semiconductors are materials with intermediate electron binding. They conduct electricity only when extra energy is added, e.g. heat (thermistors) or light (photodetectors).

Electricity, magnetic fields, and motion

A current-carrying conductor behaves as a magnet, and when placed in a perpendicular magnetic field, it experiences a force. The direction of current, field, and motion (thrust) can be determined by Fleming's left-hand (motor) rule (Figure 4.36). This is the principle behind the deflection of a moving-coil ammeter (galvanometer), which measures current.

Similarly, a magnetic field can induce a current in a conductor moving perpendicularly through it. This current will generate a magnetic field opposing the flux change causing it. In the case of induced current, the directions of field, motion, and current can be determined by Fleming's right-hand rule (Figure 4.36). This phenomenon provides the basis for the electromagnetic flowmeter, where blood (a conductor) passes through a magnetic field and the current across the vessel is measured.

Earthing

The earth, by convention, is considered to be a point of zero electrical potential. Current travels to it, along the gradient of potential difference. Electricity is supplied via live and neutral wires, with a connection between the neutral and earth at the supply end, and between the apparatus and earth at the user end. In the event of a fault in the circuit, the energy passes to earth, and this current should be large enough to melt the fuse in the plug. If there is an inadvertent contact between the electrical supply (e.g. via faulty insulation) and earth at the user end, there is a risk of electric shock. See Box 4.1.

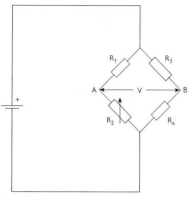

Fig. 4.34 Wheatstone bridge.

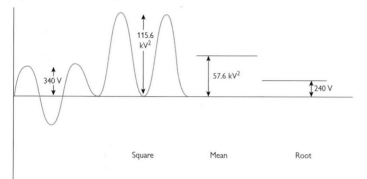

Fig. 4.35 DC vs. AC current and rms analysis.

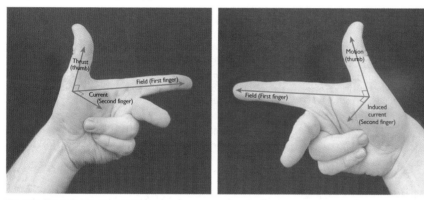

Fig. 4.36 Fleming's left- and right-hand rules.

Box 4.1 Earthing of equipment

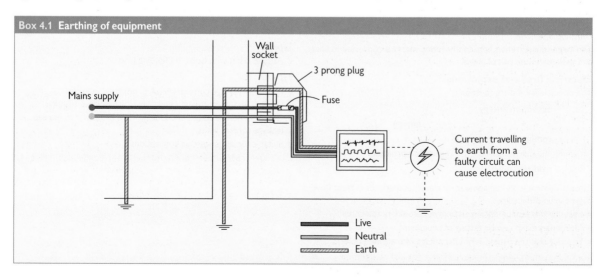

4.14 Electrical safety

Ensuring safety for both patients and staff involves the understanding and recognition of potential hazards inherent in electrical equipment. Anaesthetized patients are exposed to a number of electrical risks: their skin impedence is reduced by gel electrodes and sterilizing solutions, they are linked by metal wires to electrical equipment, they are connected to fluids hung on metal drip stands, and they are placed on beds with metal parts, to name a few.

Hazards of electricity

UK mains electricity consists of AC at 240V, with a frequency of 50Hz. The main hazards of electricity are electrocution (particularly cardiac arrhythmias), burns, and fire/explosion. The current is the important factor, and is determined by the resistance (or impedance for AC current) and potential difference across an object or person ($I = V/R$). Dry skin impedance is typically around 10kΩ, but can be reduced markedly by moisture (this is why a gel is used to improve electrical contact of ECG electrodes). Therefore mains voltage gives rise to a current of about 25mA if touched with a dry hand.

Electrocution and burns
The effects of electrocution increase with the current:
- 1 mA: tingling sensation.
- 5 mA: pain.
- 15 mA: local muscle spasm.
- 50 mA: generalized muscle spasm (including respiratory muscles).
- 80 mA: ventricular fibrillation (currents of a few amps are needed for the tonic myocardial contraction brought about by defibrillation).

Other factors affecting the risk of injury include the following.

Current pathway
Pathways across the heart (e.g. hand-to-hand) increase the risk of VF.

Current density
Current density J is calculated by dividing the current by the area of contact ($J = I/A$). High current densities increase the risk of local electrocution and burns; this principle is utilized in the design of diathermy equipment. **Microshock** describes the phenomenon of very low currents (of the order of 100μA) causing fibrillation if applied directly to a small area of myocardium (e.g. via a central line tip touching the endocardium). The timing of these currents is important: an 'R on T' type shock is particularly dangerous.

Current type and frequency
The risk of arrhythmias and muscle spasm increases with alternating current and is also affected by frequency: mains frequency (50Hz) is particularly dangerous, whereas the high frequencies used in diathermy (e.g. 100kHz) are much less so.

Duration of current
The longer the current is applied, the more energy is converted to heat and the greater the risk of burns.

Electrical fires and explosions
The principle behind combustion is:

$$\begin{array}{c}
\textit{activation energy} \\
+ \\
\textit{combustible agent} \\
+ \\
\textit{oxidizing agent}
\end{array}
\quad = \quad
\begin{array}{c}
\textit{energy} \\
+ \\
\textit{reaction products}
\end{array}$$

The activation energy can come from electrical sparks or current flow. Risks can be reduced by:
- Ensuring that equipment meets appropriate safety standards
- Maintenance and regular testing of equipment
- Ensuring that the patient is not in contact with earthed objects

- Minimizing generation of static electricity, e.g. antistatic equipment and footwear, maintain relative humidity >50%.

Note: only powder (blue label) or CO_2 (black label) fire extinguishers are suitable for electrical fires.

Isolated patient circuits

Isolated ('floating') circuits are designed to separate patients from mains electricity (Figure 4.39) Although the equipment can be powered by the mains, any component attached to the patient draws power from a transformer. A transformer uses two coils of wire wrapped around iron cores. These are in proximity, but not touching. An electric current passing through the first coil will create a magnetic field, which induces a current in the second coil without the need for direct electrical contact. This arrangement gives some protection from faults (e.g. power surges) in the mains part of the equipment, and limits leakage currents in the equipment. However, even an isolated circuit can cause electrocution if the patient is inadvertently earthed by another route.

Transformers can also be used to alter the potential difference supplied to a piece of equipment, stepping up or down depending on the design.

Classification of equipment

Electrical equipment is subject to strict quality standards and is classified according to the protection it affords against electric shock. Most monitoring equipment is type B or BF (or better).

Class I (insulated + earthed)
- Accessible conducting parts (e.g. metal handles) are insulated from the live wire and earthed.
- If live current passes to these parts, there is a low-resistance fuse to earth, which melts and breaks the circuit.

Class II (double insulated)
- Accessible conducting parts have double or reinforced insulation from the live supply.
- An earth wire is not required.

Class III (internally powered or SELV)
- Voltage <24V via a battery or safety extra low voltage (SELV) transformer.
- Although risks are reduced, the risk of microshock remains.

Type B
- Maximum leakage current of 100μA under normal conditions (500μA with single fault).
- Standards are for the earthed equipment as a whole.
- Not safe for direct cardiac connections.

Type BF
- As type B but with isolated ('floating') circuit.

Type CF
- Maximum leakage current <10μA in normal conditions (<50μA under single-fault conditions), plus isolated circuit.
- Components are tested individually; none is allowed to exceed leakage current limits.
- Suitable for direct cardiac connections.

✚ Surgical diathermy

Diathermy uses electrical current to produce localized heat. This can either cause coagulation of vessels, or cut through tissue. The current density is extremely high at the tip of the instrument, as the contact area is small. The current density at the grounding plate (Figure 4.40) is much lower, since the area of the plate is large. Therefore heating and burning effects occur only at the instrument tip.

Safety features and hazards

- High-frequency (0.5–1MHz) current reduces risk of arrhythmias.
- Diathermy circuit is usually isolated/floating.
- Needs good contact between the patient and grounding plate. Patchy contact increases current density and may cause burns.
- Electromagnetic waves produced can affect ECG monitoring and cardiac pacemaker function (especially monopolar).

Monopolar diathermy

- High current density at instrument tip
- Low current density at patient plate (large surface area, reduced heat production and risk of burns)
- High power for cutting

Bipolar diathermy

- Current flow from one side of forceps to the other
- Patient's body not part of circuit
- Low power for better coagulation effect

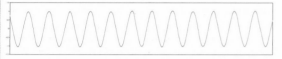

Fig. 4.37 Cutting diathermy: continuous sine wave.

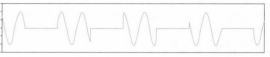

Fig. 4.38 Coagulation diathermy: non-continuous sine wave.

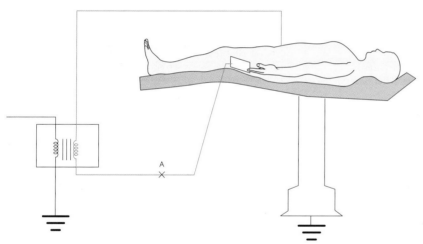

Fig. 4.39 Isolated patient circuit. If the circuit is broken (e.g. at point A), current flow ceases. However, inadvertent earthing of the patient (for example, via metallic parts on the operating table) can provide a route for current flow. This puts the patient (and theatre staff!) at risk of electric shock.

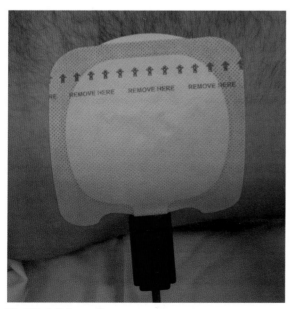

Fig. 4.40 A diathermy plate.

Pacemakers were originally used to prevent death from asystole or severe bradycardia. The most common indication is acquired atrio-ventricular block (e.g. third-degree heart block with bradycardia or long periods of asystole, symptomatic second-degree heart block, sinus node dysfunction with symptomatic bradycardia).

More recently, device capabilities and indications for pacing have expanded dramatically to include heart failure, cardiomyopathy, and tachyarrhythmias.

Permanent pacemakers deliver impulses of up to 4 mV, lasting for <1ms, via a pacing lead to cardiac muscle. They contain lithium iodine batteries (>10 year battery life) and have a titanium casing to reduce electromagnetic interference.

Radiofrequency programmable devices allow data analysis and adjustments at the bedside. Rate adaptability can detect changes in heart rate by movement sensor (piezoelectric crystal) or minute volume sensor (transthoracic impedance).

MRI scanning is contraindicated after insertion. A chest X-ray with a pacemaker is shown in Figure 4.41.

Pacemaker codes

Pacemakers have a three-, four-, or five-letter code depending on their functions (letters 1–3 describe anti-bradyarrhythmia functions only) (Table 4.4).

Advanced pacemaker functions

Cardiac resynchronization therapy (biventricular pacing)

Multiple leads/pacing sites can reduce inter/intraventricular asynchrony in moderate to severe heart failure

ICDs

Utilize algorithms to sense and manage ventricular tachycardias and fibrillation. Responses include observation, anti-tachycardia pacing, low-energy synchronized shock, and high-energy unsynchronized shock.

ICD codes:

Chamber shocked	O/A/V/D (see Table 4.4)
Anti-tachycardia pacing	O/A/V/D (see Table 4.4)
Anti-tachycardia detection	E (ECG)/H (haemodynamic)
Pacing chamber	O/A/V/D (see Table 4.4)

Preoperative assessment

Preoperative work-up involves liaison with cardiologists, cardiac technicians, and the surgeon, as well as evaluation of the patient. The patient should have an information card which identifies the make of pacemaker, indication for insertion, time and place of insertion, mode, rate, cardiologist, and nature of the leads. Additional work-up should cover:

- Last pacemaker check (should have been within last year): function satisfactory? Battery life? Pacing thresholds appropriate? Degree of pacemaker dependency?
- Full cardiovascular history, current symptoms, examination. Any cardiac symptoms should be evaluated by a cardiologist prior to anaesthesia.
- Ensure electrolyte abnormalities are corrected.
- ECG (NB: some ECG machines remove pacing spikes, and may not give an accurate picture of pacemaker dependency). Figure 4.42 shows a paced ECG.
- Whether any programme adjustment is necessary preoperatively?
- How the pacemaker will respond to a magnet (see below).
- Likely use of electocautery or diathermy? Exact site of surgery?
- Contingency plan if pacemaker or ICD fails or malfunctions.

Intraoperative management

The greatest intraoperative concern is electromagnetic interference (EMI). This has unpredictable effects, which may include inappropriate inhibition/triggering, reprogramming, and damage to circuitry.

Electromagnetic waves between 0 and 10^{11}Hz may cause interference (diathermy uses waves of the order of 10^{6}Hz and radiofrequency ablation is at around 10^{5}Hz, not forgetting AC current at 50Hz).

All anti-tachyarrhythmia functions (pacing and shock) should be disabled by the cardiac technician preoperatively in case they are inadvertently triggered. These functions should be reinstated before the patient goes back to the ward.

An external defibrillator should be available throughout surgery and in recovery. If used, this carries a high risk of damage/reprogramming. Place the pads far from the device (>10cm).

Diathermy: bipolar diathermy is preferred. Monopolar diathermy should be avoided. If it must be used, it should be in short bursts for the minimum possible time, and the grounding plate should be far from the device. As well as interference, diathermy may cause heating of the pacemaker wires. If this results in myocardial burn, contact between the pacemaker and the heart is impaired.

A pacemaker magnet should be available (although its routine use is not recommended). Often, this switches the pacemaker to an asynchronous ventricular pacing mode and is used in emergencies (e.g. if excessive interference causes loss of pacemaker function and cardiovascular compromise). However, some modern programmable pacemakers respond in other ways to the magnet: the magnet may open the reprogramming channel, and outside sources of interference may then change the pacemaker functions unpredictably. It is essential to know how the pacemaker will respond to magnetization prior to surgery.

External wires (e.g. central lines, oesophageal temperature probes) may pass near the pacemaker, increasing the risk of current flow in the pacemaker wires and myocardial microshock (Section 4.14).

Postoperative management

All pacemaker functions should be restored to normal, and the pacemaker checked. Any adverse events should be carefully documented. A coronary care bed may be appropriate if problems have arisen.

Defibrillators

Defibrillators are used to apply a short direct current across the myocardium to terminate arrhythmias. The intention of defibrillation is to stop the heart's electrical activity momentarily in the hope that normal sinus rhyhm will resume.

A diagram of a defibrillator circuit is shown in Figure 4.43. The central component of a defibrillator is a capacitor. This is used to store the required charge before discharging across the patient's heart. Other components include a transformer (to step up the mains voltage), a rectifier (to convert mains AC current into DC current, allowing charge to accumulate on the capacitor), a switch for defibrillation itself, and an inductor which alters the waveform pattern of current delivery.

There also needs to be a connection to the patient. With external defibrillators, this is via a set of two paddles. Skin impedance must be overcome, so gel pads can be put onto the chest or hands-free paddles incorporating adhesive and gel can be used.

A defibrillator system typically delivers a current of 50A into a resistance of 50Ω. Since $V = IR$, the voltage required is 2.5kV.

The defibrillator is set to deliver a particular energy (in joules(J)). The energy used depends on the clinical scenario. The need for defibrillation must be balanced against potential damage resulting from a high-energy current passing through the heart; this can result in burns and myocardial scarring.

- Emergency defibrillation (VF, pulseless VT): 200–360J.
- Elective or semi-elective cardioversion (AF, VT with pulse): 50–150J depending on response.
- Internal defibrillation during cardiothoracic surgery: 10–25J.
- Implantable internal defibrillator: 25J.

Table 4.4 Pacemaker codes

First letter	Second letter	Third letter	Fourth letter	Fifth letter
Paced chamber	Sensed chamber	Response to detected impulse	Programmable functions	Active anti-tachyarrhythmia function
O = nil	O = nil	O = no sensing function	O = none	O = none
A = atria	A = atria	I = inhibited	R = rate modulation (adaptive rate pacing)	D = dual (pace + shock)
V = ventricles	V = ventricles	T = triggered	M = multi-programmable	S = shock
D = dual chamber	D = dual chamber	D = dual	P = simple programmimg	P = pace
			C = communicating	

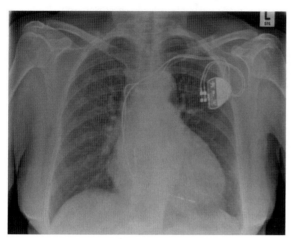

Fig. 4.41 Chest X-ray showing a pacemaker.

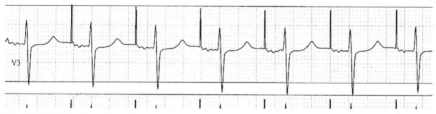

Fig. 4.42 ECG showing pacing spikes.

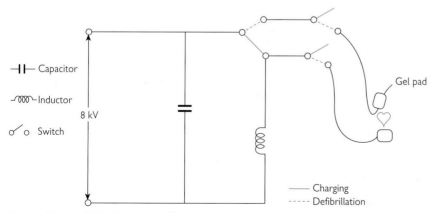

Fig. 4.43 Diagram of defibrillator circuit. The capacitor stores the charge. During defibrillation, the inductor modifies the shape of the current pulse. Skin impedance is reduced by conducting gel pads.

The importance of good preoperative assessment along with the processes of induction and maintenance of anaesthesia using appropriate drugs, equipment, and clinical monitoring have been discussed. It is also important to make a contemporaneous, detailed, and legible record of this information in addition to any unusual, unplanned, or untoward events. A sample anaesthetic chart is shown in Figure 4.44.

Why?

Keeping an anaesthetic record can serve several functions.

Current clinical care

Anaesthetists and other medical staff can review all aspects of anaesthetic assessment and management.

This can aid handing over care to an anaesthetic colleague or to recovery staff for post-anaesthetic care.

Trends in physiological change and responses to management can be visualized from the charted observations.

The chart may incorporate prompts/checklists to act as reminders to improve practice.

Future source of clinical information

Adverse events that occurred intraoperatively can be reviewed with regard to monitoring for further postoperative events and subsequent management.

A history of potential or actual difficulties in any part of previous anaesthetic care and how they were managed is extremely useful to help avoid or plan for similar situations, e.g. unexpected difficult intubation, anaphylaxis.

Warning or hazard flags can highlight these patients early in the care pathway.

Education and training

The processes of recording and reviewing all aspects of patient care can help in training and maintaining a logbook of experience.

Audit and research

Retrieving data from anaesthetic records can be used for assessing the quality of patient care and analysis for research purposes to help improve clinical practice.

Medico-legal aspects

As with all medical documents and notes, records should be accurate, legible and complete.

Recording should be contemporaneous because memory of events can deteriorate over time.

During medico-legal review, the quality of record-keeping may be judged as a reflection of the quality of clinical care given.

What?

The Royal College of Anaesthetists has recommended a data set for the content of the anaesthetic record chart. There is no national standardized chart and there are variations in presentation, size, and content. However, all charts should be able to serve the functions described above, appropriate to the anaesthesia, surgery, and peri-operative care carried out within a particular department.

The suggested anaesthetic record set includes the following.

Preoperative information

Patient identity (name, date of birth, gender, hospital ID number).

Assessment and risk factors including:

- Medication, known allergies
- Previous anaesthetic history
- Potential problems e.g. airway, IV access
- Dentition (warning of potential damage/loss of loose teeth or prostheses)
- Results of investigations
- Cardiorespiratory functional assessment
- ASA status
- Urgency (elective scheduled, urgent, emergency).

Perioperative information

Checks (e.g. NBM, consent)

Place and time (e.g. induction, start of surgery, tourniquet)

Personnel (names and grades, duty consultant informed?)

Operation planned/performed

Apparatus (equipment used, checks performed)

Vital signs recording/charting

Drugs and fluids

- Dose, concentration, volume, route, time, ?warmed
- Cannulation site, size

Airway and breathing system

- Airway type, size, shape, route, technique
- Breathing system
- Ventilation mode, parameters
- Difficulties encountered and their management

Regional anaesthesia

- Consent (specify risks and benefits)
- Block performed
- Entry site, needle used, catheter
- Location aids, e.g. ultrasound-guided

Patient positioning and attachments

- Special positions, limb positioning
- Protection of pressure areas
- Temperature control
- Thromboprophylaxis

Postoperative instructions

- Airway instructions, oxygen, drugs, fluids, analgesia
- Monitoring

Untoward events

- Abnormalities, critical incidents
- Context, cause, effect, management

Hazard flags

When and how?

Records should be kept and filed appropriately in the medical notes for all aspects of anaesthetic management, e.g. sedation, regional anaesthesia, general anaesthesia, monitored patient transfers requiring anaesthetic cover.

Anaesthetic records can be manually written charts, a computerized system which can automatically collate data from monitors, or a combination of both. Computerized records can still require a significant amount of time for data entry via a keyboard.

Although record-keeping during a critical incident is particularly useful for retrospective analysis, the priority should be direct patient care.

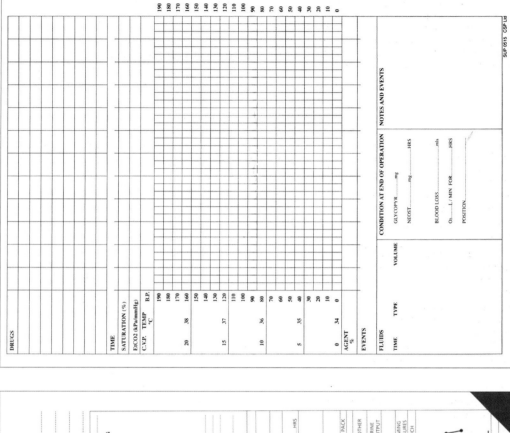

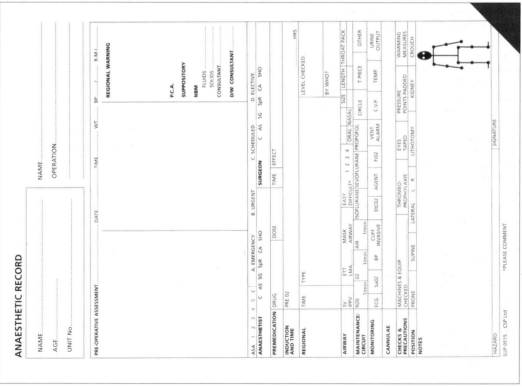

Fig. 4.44 An anaesthetic chart.

Laparoscopic surgery involves pressurized gas insufflation of the peritoneal cavity, usually using CO_2. The extent of surgery can range from a simple inspection of the abdominal contents (diagnostic or staging laparoscopy) to prolonged and extensive operations (e.g. major bowel resection, nephrectomy, oesophagectomy, liver resection).

Various positions for surgery are used including Trendelenburg (for easier visualization of the pelvic organs), reverse Trendelenburg (for surgery on the upper abdominal organs), and lithotomy.

Advantages of laparoscopic surgery

- Lower morbidity/mortality compared with open procedure.
- Reduced tissue trauma/damage and stress response.
- Reduced postoperative analgesic requirement.
- Improved postoperative respiratory function.
- Earlier mobilization and discharge.
- Less scarring, improved cosmetic result.
- Improved patient satisfaction.

Disadvantages of laparoscopic surgery

- Risk of damage/trauma due to trochar.
- Duration of surgery may be prolonged.
- Requires specialist equipment.
- Potential for conversion to open procedure.
- Has its own special complications (see below).

Anaesthetic considerations

An ETT is usually recommended, although some anaesthetists will use an LMA. It is important to consider risk of reflux and lung compliance. If an LMA is used, an excellent seal must be achieved.

Minimize gastric insufflation with bag–valve–mask ventilation. Consider NGT insertion to decompress the stomach, particularly with upper abdominal procedures (e.g. laparoscopic cholecystectomy).

Good muscle relaxation is usually required.

Monitor and manage cardiovascular and respiratory system changes (see below).

Establishing the pneumoperitoneum

Usually, the surgeon identifies the peritoneal cavity by dissection at the umbilicus or by use of a small needle. An initial 4–6L/min gas flow raises the intra-abdominal pressure (IAP) to 10-20mmHg, followed by a flow of 200–400ml/min to maintain the IAP. A trochar is used to open up several port sites, allowing insertion of the camera and instruments.

Usual maximum IAP: 14mmHg for abdominal surgery

25mmHg for pelvic surgery.

Particular attention must be paid while the pneumoperitoneum is being established, as several complications may occur at this time.

Respiratory:

- Risk of ETT displacement (particularly bronchial intubation), with upward shift of thoracic organs.
- Increased IAP reduces thoracic compliance and increases airway pressures. Tidal volume and ventilation decrease if ventilation is not adjusted appropriately.
- ↓FRC, basal atelectasis, and ↑V/Q mismatch may lead to hypoxia.
- Gas may be insufflated into a vessel, causing a pulmonary gas embolus (may be massive).
- Pneumothorax may occur.
- Risk of regurgitation of stomach contents.
- CO_2 is absorbed, leading to ↑P_aCO_2.

Cardiovascular

- Peritoneal stretch can stimulate an intense vagally mediated, bradycardia.
- Initial ↑cardiac output due to ↑venous return.
- Later, ↓cardiac output due to ↓venous return and myocardial contractility (particularly if patient hypovloaemic).
- ↑IAP causes ↑SVR, catecholamine release and afterload.
- MAP may increase or decrease, depending on the balance of the above factors.
- Poor cardiac reserve can lead to tachycardia, ↓coronary blood flow, and cardiac ischaemia.
- Major abdominal vessels may be injured by the trochar, leading to severe haemorrhage.

If acute complications are encountered, ask the surgeon to release the pneumoperitoneum. Subsequent management depends on the problem.

Chapter 5

Recovery

5.1 The recovery room

The recovery room provides an environment for managing emergence from anaesthesia. Patients are monitored one-to-one, immediate problems are managed, and finally they are prepared for transfer back to the ward. Standards for the provision of immediate postoperative recovery have been recommended by the AAGBI (Table 5.1).

Transferring patients to recovery

The anaesthetist is responsible for safe transfer to the recovery room. Recovery staff should be contacted prior to transfer. Monitoring is discretionary; factors such as the proximity of recovery and the patient's clinical state should be considered. Supplemental oxygen should be given to all patients during the journey to the recovery room.

Equipment and personnel

The recovery room should be in a central position in the theatre complex. There should be at least two recovery beds for every theatre in order to ensure availability of recovery room space. A typical recovery bed space is shown in Figure 5.1.

There are clearly defined regulations that stipulate how a recovery room should be constructed and to what standard. It should have a non-recirculating ventilation system (16 air changes per hour) to cope with exhaled anaesthetic gases. It should have pipeline outlets for suction, oxygen, and air.

A variety of oxygen delivery facemasks should be available at each space, together with a Mapleson C circuit. This circuit is useful when assessing appropriateness for, and performing, extubation. In addition to pulse oximetry and NIBP monitoring, an ECG monitor, nerve stimulator, capnograph, and thermometer should be immediately available. Each bed space should contain a sharps bin, aprons, and gel for hand-cleaning between patients.

The recovery room should have full resuscitation equipment, immediate availability of emergency drugs and fluids, and spare (full) cylinders of oxygen for use in the event of pipeline failure. There should be means of ventilating the lungs with a self-inflating bag (with reservoir), and the facilities should cater for the use of an anaesthetic machine.

Recovery staff should be appropriately trained (e.g. in resuscitation, airway skills, recognition of surgical complications, and IV drug and fluid administration). Two staff members must be present when a patient who does not fulfil criteria for ward discharge is in recovery. In addition, an anaesthetist supernumerary to theatre requirements should be immediately available.

Handover

The anaesthetist should give a formal handover to an appropriately trained member of recovery staff. This should include:

- The patient's name
- A brief description of preoperative status
- Known allergies
- Details of the operation (including any complications)
- Details of the anaesthetic (including any complications)
- A clear plan of management (including specific airway instructions, and administration of analgesics, other medication, and fluids in the immediate postoperative period and on the ward).

It is also important to state who to contact if there are any concerns.

Monitoring

Appropriate standards of monitoring should be maintained until the patient is fully recovered from anaesthesia. Ideally, there should be compatibility between operating theatre, recovery room, and ward equipment.

Clinical observation should be supplemented by a *minimum* of pulse oximetry and non-invasive blood pressure measurement.

Information to be recorded at regular intervals during the recovery period includes:

- Respiratory rate
- Oxygen saturations and oxygen administration
- Heart rate and rhythm
- Blood pressure
- Conscious level
- IV fluid and drug administration
- Other parameters depending on the situation, e.g. urine output, surgical drainage, temperature, end-tidal CO_2, CVP, GCS.

Airway management in recovery

Some facilities cater for the removal of LMAs. However, tracheal extubation is the responsibility of the anaesthetist. Whether this occurs in theatre or recovery, it must happen before the anaesthetist leaves the patient. Situations where extubation may be problematic are listed opposite.

Timing of extubation

The safest time to extubate a patient is when he/she is fully awake, obeying commands, and literally trying to take out the endotracheal tube. Before extubation, 100% oxygen should be given for several minutes. The following must always be considered:

Adequacy of ventilation: defined as a normal respiratory rate for the patient, with tidal volumes of 5–10ml/kg.

Presence of protective reflexes: signs of protective reflexes include gagging and coughing on the endotracheal tube. However, the patient remains at risk of aspiration if the conscious level and peripheral/respiratory muscle function have not returned to normal.

Reversal of neuromuscular blockade: even with return of adequate ventilation, substantial paralysis may still be present. A better clinical assessment is the ability to hold a sustained muscle contraction (such as lifting the head off the bed for 5sec or a handgrip). Signs of inadequate reversal include tachycardia, lacrimation, and uncoordinated 'jerky' muscle movements. Awake patients feel extremely anxious, and complain of a feeling of not being able to breathe.

A potential residual block should be confirmed with a nerve stimulator (either TOF or DBS; Section 8.6), and one additional dose of reversal administered. If the problem persists, the patient should be re-anaesthetized and ventilated to allow time for the relaxant to wear off. If suxamethonium apnoea is a possibility, arrangements will have to be made for several hours' ventilation (e.g. in ICU).

Table 5.1 Key recommendations for immediate post operative recovery (AAGBI Guidelines, September 2002)
Handover from anaesthetist to appropriately trained nurse/staff
Agreed discharge from recovery to the ward in place
Effective emergency call system
At least two staff members should be present when any patient is in recovery
All staff should have appropriate training
Patients should be nursed one-to-one until the airway is fully controlled and there is cardiovascular stability
Removal of the ETT is the responsibility of the anaesthetist
A recovery room/ area should exist in all areas where anaesthetics are given
Special areas should be present for children
Dignity and privacy for patients should be maintained at all times
If patients are kept in recovery because of ICU overspill, the responsibility for their care lies with ICU
Audit and critical incident systems must be in place

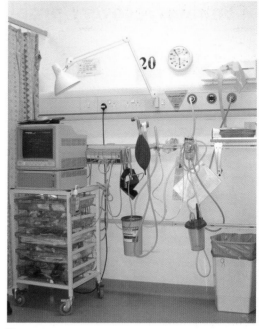

Fig. 5.1 Recovery bed space.

⊕ Special considerations during extubation

Initial rapid sequence induction: aspiration of stomach contents via an NG tube should be considered. Patients should always be extubated fully awake.

Initial difficult intubation: patients should be extubated awake, with difficult airway drugs and equipment immediately available.

Obese patients: the work of breathing is increased, and FRC is reduced. Closing capacity exceeds the FRC, leading to airway closure. Increased oxygen demand and reduced reserve leads to early desaturation. Thoracic compliance can be decreased by over 30% by the heavy chest wall and splinted diaphragm. Obstructive sleep apnoea (OSA) is much more common; this may cause derangements in normal CO_2 drive. Sitting the patient up prior to extubation can reduce diaphragmatic splinting and the work of breathing. Patients with OSA may require postoperative CPAP. They should be encouraged to bring their usual CPAP machine to hospital.

Irritable airways: pre-existing respiratory disease, including upper respiratory tract infection, carries a higher incidence of coughing, laryngospasm, and bronchospasm on awakening. This is exacerbated by manipulation of the airway. Smokers also have increased airway reactivity; mucus production is increased, with a reduction in mucociliary clearance. This can lead to plugging and collapse of airways. The incidence of airway irritation can be reduced with the use of less irritant volatile agents, such as sevoflurane.

Neurological and muscular disease may lead to altered respiratory drive. Protective airway reflexes may be depressed. Many neuromuscular diseases (e.g. motor neuron disease, muscular dystrophy, dystrophia myotonica, myasthenia gravis) affect the action of muscle relaxants.

Prolonged surgery can give rise to basal atelectasis and impaired gas exchange, especially if the patient has spent time head-down. These patients may benefit from recruitment manoeuvres prior to extubation.

'Deep' extubation: there are circumstances when extubation of the trachea when the patient is still deeply anaesthetized may be appropriate, to avoid coughing (e.g. in neurosurgery). This is usually done in theatre, with equipment for re-intubation immediately available. Anaesthetic is deepened, muscle relaxation is reversed, and the anaesthetic is carefully lightened to establish spontaneous ventilation. The anaesthetic is deepened a second time to obtund the laryngeal reflexes. The pharynx is carefully suctioned and the ETT removed. Manual airway support or a supraglottic airway is then required until return of consciousness.

5.2 Common recovery problems

Nausea and vomiting

Postoperative nausea and vomiting (PONV) is a common perioperative complication (30–50% of cases). The presence of risk factors (Section 17.10) should have prompted the use of anti-emetics intraoperatively. PONV incidence is also reduced by good pain control and hydration.

Significant or uncontrolled PONV can lead to:
- Failure of oral medication
- Electrolyte imbalances and dehydration
- Increased oxygen demand with retching
- Tension on suture lines
- Pulmonary aspiration if airway reflexes are depressed
- Wound haematomas
- Amplification of pain
- Prolonged hospital stay, or admission from day surgery
- Embarrassment and distress, reluctance to undergo further procedures.

Management

Prescribe postoperative anti-emetics for all patients on a PRN basis.

There is evidence that combination prophylaxis, using drugs with different mechanisms of action, can markedly reduce the incidence of PONV compared with single agents. There is a lack of data for the treatment of established PONV, but anti-emetic monotherapy has a significant failure rate; it seems logical to use drugs that work on different receptors. It is important to treat nausea and vomiting promptly in recovery. The single most effective drug is ondansetron. Medical and surgical causes (e.g. hypotension, pain) must be sought and corrected.

Pain

Postoperative pain and nausea often occur simultaneously. Pain is a well-known cause of nausea, and of course opiate analgesia has side effects of nausea and vomiting. Therefore it is important that a multimodal approach to both analgesia and anti-emesis be taken to target as many areas as possible. As mentioned previously, patients who receive opiate analgesia intraoperatively should be given an anti-emetic, even if no other risk are factors present. Simple analgesia such as paracetamol and NSAIDs (unless contraindicated) should be given as part of the anaesthetic technique and regularly postoperatively to avoid excessive use of opiates.

The WHO analgesic ladder (Section 7.30) takes a stepwise approach to pain, where the next rung is used if the current one is not effective. Postoperative pain must be considered differently, as it starts at peak intensity and improves over time. Analgesia may be started at a higher level and gradually stepped down. Adjuvant therapy (e.g. NSAIDS, tricylic antidepressants) can be used at all three levels.

Difficulty can be anticipated in chronic pain patients, and those with opioid dependency. It is useful to liaise with the chronic and acute pain teams to help manage these patients both in recovery and on the ward. As a rule, the need for analgesia because of the surgery undertaken should be addressed in addition to the normal requirement/intake. It is particularly useful with these patients to consider the use of local anaesthetics and regional techniques where possible.

Sore throat

Sore throat is particularly associated with:
- Artificial airways (up to 90% of cases of endotracheal intubation; 5% of cases with an LMA)
- Throat surgery (e.g. tonsillectomy, thyroid surgery)
- Traumatic laryngoscopy
- Multiple intubation attempts
- Use of stylets, bougies, throat packs, and NGTs
- Anticholinergic premedication
- Use of suxamethonium
- Unhumidified gases

It is more common in females. Lubrication of airway devices does not reduce the incidence of sore throat.

Management

Analgesia, humidified oxygen. Most airway-associated sore throats resolve within 24 hr.

Postoperative confusion

This is often a multifactorial phenomenon. Things to take into consideration include the age and premorbid state of the patient, the length and type of operation and intraoperative events. More organic factors to consider include hypoxia, hypotension/hypovolaemia, hypo/hypercarbia, hypothermia, an early presentation of sepsis, or a cerebral event.

Management

It is important to examine the patient systematically and manage by correcting any problems (hypoxia, hypotension etc) simultaneously. In many cases, reassurance and directly asking the problem can help the patient: for example, a patient waking up pain-free with good analgesia may be distressed by a urinary catheter.

Shivering

It is important not to underestimate the impact that shivering can have on certain patients. Severe shivering may increase the basal metabolic rate and oxygen requirements five- to tenfold (i.e. from 300ml/min to 1.5–3L/min). In patients with ischaemic heart disease, where the oxygen supply and demand relationship is critical, this could cause angina or a myocardial infarction. It is important to note the patient's past medical history, and whether there is any history of diabetes or epilepsy; hypoglycaemia or fits can give a similar presentation and must be excluded.

Management

Give high-flow oxygen; measure the vital signs, core temperature, and blood glucose. The patient needs to be reassured and gently warmed (if required) with blankets and a forced air warmer. A 12-lead ECG should be taken if there is any concern about cardiac ischaemia. Pethidine 20-25mg IV may be beneficial in refractory cases.

Specific discharge issues

Oxygen

Oxygen for the immediate postoperative period should be prescribed if the patient has undergone prolonged or major surgery, or has ischaemic heart disease (note that the peak incidence of postoperative myocardial infarction is at 72 hr post surgery). Oxygen should also be prescribed if there has been, or is likely to be, a problem with desaturation in the perioperative period or significant blood loss, or the patient has ongoing opioid analgesia (including epidural and patient-controlled analgesia).

Care should be taken with the small minority of patients in whom increased oxygen delivery precipitates hypercarbia (Section 13.3). These patients are best looked after in a high-dependency unit or ICU after all except minor surgery.

Fluids

A fluid regimen for the next 24 hr must also be prescribed. This should account for maintenance fluids and anticipated insensible losses, and take into account the type of surgery and the anticipated length of time to eating and drinking. In general, Hartmann's solution is the most 'physiological' fluid to use. However, it may not meet the patient's potassium requirements, particularly if losses from the bowel (e.g. via NGT) are likely to be ongoing. It is useful to prescribe the use of a colloid to be given rapidly on the ward if the parameters of urine output or systolic blood pressure fall below acceptable limits.

Regional anaesthesia in the postoperative period

Central neuraxial block

Each hospital will have its own protocol for looking after these patients on the ward. Patients with an epidural *in situ* should be identified to the acute pain service. It is important to monitor the adequacy of analgesia by regularly assessing the height of the block and the patient's ability to cough and deep breathe. Blood pressure measurements should be taken regularly (initially every 15min), with a system in place to give colloid boluses when required to counteract the effects of the vasodil-atation. The degree of motor block should also be noted, and high-lighted if this becomes a persistent problem. It is useful to hand over the likely duration to recovery of function. Bladder care is also very important, as urinary retention is common.

Limb blocks

It is important to hand over the anticipated duration of the block and have background analgesia such as paracetamol/NSAIDs initiated in anticipation of the block wearing off. Stronger breakthrough analgesia should also be prescribed on a PRN or patient-controlled basis.

Day stay

The criteria for the discharge of day-stay patients will again be hospital dependent. Anaesthetists working in day units should use techniques that permit the patient to undergo the surgical procedure with minimum stress, and the maximum chance of an early discharge. Analgesia is paramount and must be long lasting; but nausea and vomiting must be minimized.

There are both medical and social aspects of the discharge to consider. Medically, discharge criteria are the same as for ward patients, plus the patient must be able to eat, drink, and void urine. Social criteria for discharge include:

- Having a responsible adult able and willing to care for the patient for at least the first 24 hr
- Easy access to a telephone
- A home situation compatible with postoperative care (i.e. satisfactory heating, lighting, kitchen, bathroom, and toilet facilities)
- Easy transport back to hospital in case of problems.

Clear written and verbal postoperative instructions should be given together with a supply of analgesic medication with a list of possible side effects and instructions. Guidance should be given for follow-up care (e.g. the removal of sutures) and contact numbers given for any concerns. Where regional techniques have been used, it is acceptable to discharge a patient home with a numb limb if he/she is advised about expected duration of the block, and how to prevent accidental damage to the limb.

Further reading

Immediate Post Anaesthetic Recovery. Association of Anaesthetists of Great Britain and Ireland, London, 2002.

Recommendations for Standards of Monitoring During Anaesthesia and Recovery. Association of Anaesthetists of Great Britain and Ireland, London, 2007.

➕ Discharge from the recovery room

Discharge from the recovery room is the responsibility of the anaesthetist. The nurse involved in the patient's immediate postoperative care may discharge patients, provided that guidelines have been successfully followed. If any discharge criterion is not fulfilled, the patient should be assessed by the anaesthetist. If there is no improvement after simple management interventions, an admission to a higher-dependency area should be considered.

Before discharge to the ward, the patient should be:

- Awake and orientated (in keeping with premorbid state).
- Maintaining a patent airway independently.
- Breathing adequately, with satisfactory oxygenation. Oxygen should be prescribed as per local policy.
- Cardiovascularly stable with parameters (including urine output, if measured) close to the patient's preoperative state. There should be no ongoing bleeding, and good peripheral perfusion.
- Pain-free, with appropriate analgesia prescribed for the ward.
- Not nauseated, again with appropriate anti-emetics prescribed for the ward.
- Normothermic (within acceptable limits).

The trained member of staff responsible for the patient during their stay in recovery should hand over directly to the member of staff responsible for caring for the patient on the ward. It is good practice to follow up all patients on the ward before leaving the hospital. Patients who have had unexpected anaesthetic problems may need to have further follow-up arranged.

Recovery units will follow a range of protocols with these goals in mind. These may differ according to the surgical specialty (e.g. GCS monitoring is emphasized in neurosurgical patients).

Some patients are not expected to meet the above discharge criteria (e.g. those with significant respiratory compromise, requiring intraoperative inotropes, or unable to be extubated immediately postoperatively). Arrangements should have been made as early as possible for these patients to be managed in an appropriate high-dependency unit or ICU.

Chapter 6

Applied anatomy

6.1 Introduction to regional anaesthesia

Regional anaesthesia (RA) refers to a group of techniques:
- Topical anaesthesia
- Infiltration of local anaesthetics
- Peripheral nerve blocks
- Central neuraxial blockade
- IV regional anaesthesia
- Sympathetic nerve blocks.

These techniques can be used either as adjuncts to general anaesthesia (GA) or as the sole anaesthesic technique.

In addition to the obvious benefits of good intra- and postoperative analgesia, when used alone RA preserves the airway, produces less respiratory and cardiovascular depression, and allows the patient to communicate and cooperate. RA also attenuates the stress response to surgery and reduces postoperative complications such as chest infection and DVT. There is inconclusive evidence that it produces improved wound healing.

Combined GA and RA

This technique provides good intra- and postoperative analgesia. It also provides comfort for the patient during long procedures. Occasionally, the operation lasts longer than the block and sometimes RA provides inadequate blockade; additional GA reduces the impact of these problems.

Ideally, RA is performed before induction. This reduces the risk of nerve damage since the patient is able to report pain or paraesthesia. In practice some blocks are performed with the patient asleep because of patient or anaesthetist choice. In this case the risks must be clearly discussed with the patient and documented in the notes.

Problems
- A muscle relaxant should not be used as part of the GA technique before using a nerve stimulator to locate the nerve!
- Hypotension may be a problem with a joint technique as a good block will stop the usual stimulation from surgical incision.

Complications of RA

Although RA is generally safe, there are several risks to consider.
- Nerve damage from:
  - Direct trauma from the needle
  - Intraneural injection.
- Positioning of the patient.
- Trauma to blood vessels and haemorrhage.
- Infection at the site of injection.
- Local anaesthetic toxicity.
- Excessive spread of local anaesthetic, e.g. total spinal, blockade of adjacent nerves including the phrenic nerve.
- Failure of block.
- Hypotension.

Contraindications to regional blockade

There are very few absolute contraindications to RA and many of the relative contraindications depend on the type of block to be performed. There are also contraindications specific to particular types of block that will be discussed later.

Absolute contraindications
- Patient refusal
- Infection at the site
- Local anaesthetic allergy

Relative contraindications
- Clotting disorder/anticoagulation
- Systemic sepsis
- Distorted anatomy
- Trauma within area of blockade: development of compartment syndrome could pass undetected
- Neurological disease.

Consent for regional blockade

The patient should give consent in advance of the procedure. Ideally they should be given leaflets and information regarding the procedure and this should explain the process, risks, and benefits. The anaesthetic room is not considered an acceptable place or time for providing patients with large volumes of new information.

Consent should also involve a thorough explanation of:
- What will happen, what they will feel and when
- What will happen in the case of full or partial failure of the block
- What will happen afterwards, i.e. when and how feeling will come back
- What precautions they need to take postoperatively, e.g. foot protection, arm support, or walking support
- Whether they will be awake/asleep for both performance of the block and the operation itself
- What the alternative options are.

This should all be documented in the patient record. At present there is no requirement for a separate formal consent for regional anaesthesia when it is done to facilitate another procedure.

Recent AAGBI Guidelines state that the nature of information given to the patient should be determined by the question: 'What would this patient regard as relevant when coming to a decision about which of the available options to accept?' For complications, this would usually involve discussion about frequently occurring risks, i.e. those with an incidence of greater than 1 in 100. Additionally, less frequent but serious risks that may affect the patient's decision should also be anticipated. The patient should be encouraged to ask any other pertinent questions.

Performing the block

List planning and regional blockade
Some blocks take up to 45min to take effect, so planning the block is important for efficient list management. Preventing delays requires good communication and organization between theatre and recovery staff, surgeons, and anaesthetists.

It is useful to have a spare room within the theatre suite that can be used for the performance of regional techniques and assessment of their efficacy. In the absence of such a luxury, patients are often 'blocked' and then kept in recovery whilst the anaesthesia develops. Therefore block failure can be assessed prior to induction.

Monitoring, safety, and approach
The same standards of monitoring and documentation apply to both GA and RA. The patient should have a working IV cannula, supplemental oxygen, and full resuscitation and airway equipment immediately available. The presence of a trained assistant is mandatory.

On a practical level this usually means the anaesthetic room, theatre, or other critical care facility should be used; these rooms also provide adequate space and light to facilitate successful block placement.

Following blockade, the patient should be closely observed.

Methods of sedation

Many patients prefer not to be awake for either the block or the procedure and sedation is a good compromise. There are many recipes, the most popular being midazolam or propofol infusion.

If sedation is used, oxygen should be given via a facemask or 'nasal specs'. The patient should be fully monitored and closely observed since airway obstruction, cardiovascular depression, and respiratory depression are possible.

Positioning of patients

The same careful attention to detail and padding of pressure points as for GA should be applied to patients undergoing RA. The only difference is that awake patients will soon tell you that they are uncomfortable. Repositioning the patient intraoperatively is often difficult, so spending time getting it right at the start is worth the effort.

Communication and reassurance

Having a regional technique performed whilst awake can be frightening and uncomfortable, particularly in the absence of proper explanation. Good communication is key, and this starts with the process of consent. It is important that the patient has full trust and understanding in you and the block that you are performing. This is especially true if it is to be their only form of anaesthesia.

Ensure that the patient is in as comfortable a position as possible for both the block and the operative procedure. Talk through what will be happening around them in the theatre environment and who all the people are.

Explain exactly what you are about to do at each stage and what sensations they should expect. Ensure that someone is present throughout for the patient to talk to if they so wish and encourage them to report any uncomfortable feelings.

Be careful to document the extent of the block, whether or not the patient was comfortable throughout the procedure and whether any additional analgesia or anaesthesia was required.

⊕ Procedure

Prepare the patient: obtain consent, position, and clean the skin.

Attach the positive electrode to skin about 20cm from the site of injection and the negative electrode to the needle. Remember 'negative to needle, positive to patient'.

After piercing the skin, turn the machine to 1–2 mA and advance slowly towards the nerve until twitches are seen. When the appropriate twitch is seen, gradually reduce the current until the twitch disappears and note this value. If it is:
- \>1mA—the needle is unlikely to be near the nerve.
- 0.5–1mA—it is usually close enough for nerve block.
- <0.4mA—there is a possibility of intraneural placement so withdraw slightly and try again.

Inject the local anaesthetic using a two-person immobile-needle technique. The twitch will disappear immediately on injection of the solution because of displacement of the nerve.

Choice and injection of the local anaesthetic

Once the block needle is in the correct position, the local anaesthetic should be injected only after careful aspiration: repeat aspiration should be performed after every 5ml bolus to reduce the chance of intravascular injection.

There should be no pain or resistance on injection of the local anaesthetic solution. If this occurs, stop injecting and withdraw the needle since it may be intraneural. Performing the block with the patient awake allows the patient to report pain on injection.

Care should be taken not to exceed the toxic dose. Adrenaline is sometimes added to local anaesthetic solutions to produce vasoconstriction and reduce systemic absorption, improving the block duration. However, adrenaline-containing solutions should not be used on extremities and their end-arteries, e.g. finger or penis.

CVS toxicity is an important consideration for all regional techniques but especially in intravenous regional anaesthesia (Section 6.6).

→ Use of a nerve stimulator for peripheral nerve blockade

The use of nerve stimulators and more recently ultrasound technology has improved the accuracy and safety of these techniques and hence their popularity.

There are many identification techniques, e.g. loss of resistance, landmarks, paraesthesia, measured advancement, and ultrasound. However, the most popular aid is the peripheral nerve stimulator. It is similar to that used to assess peripheral neuromuscular blockade, although specific devices should be used for regional anaesthesia.

The nerve stimulator provides a small current to stimulate nerves and hence produce muscular contraction. A sound knowledge of the anatomy of the nerve to be blocked and the muscle groups it supplies are still imperative.

→ Components of nerve block needles

Bevel types
- Short blunt bevel: more resistance but better operator feedback; do not cut nerve fibres. These are the most popular type for nerve blocks.
- Long sharp bevel: less resistance and easier to pass but will cut nerve fibres.

Needles can be insulated or non-insulated (see Figure 6.1).
- Insulated: Teflon coated with only tip exposed. Current is localized at the tip, allowing localization with a smaller current.
- Non-insulated: current passes along the whole shaft; nerves can be stimulated by the shaft with inaccurate placement of LA.

50, 100, and 150mm lengths are available.

22G is considered the optimal gauge (others are available).

Side port with a transparent hub and tubing for injection.

Electrical connection to nerve stimulator.

→ Features of a nerve stimulator

- Constant current output. The impedance of the needle tissues and wires varies 20-fold and the device should automatically compensate for this.
- Current meter.
- Current intensity control and display.
- Short pulse width. This will cause less pain for the awake patient.
- Stimulating frequency. Both 1Hz and 2Hz are frequently used.
- Disconnect indicator. This is essential and helps prevent nerve injury.

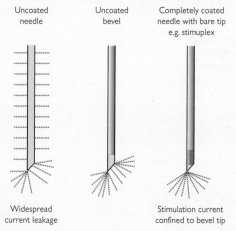

| Uncoated needle | Uncoated bevel | Completely coated needle with bare tip e.g. stimuplex |

Widespread current leakage · Stimulation current confined to bevel tip

Fig. 6.1 Current density.

105

The mouth

The oral cavity is bounded by the hard palate, the anterior two-thirds of the tongue and the alveolar arch and teeth anteriorly. The vestibule is the gap between the outer surface of the teeth, the mucosa over the gums, and the inner surfaces of the lips and cheeks.

A coronal section of the mouth and tongue is shown in Figure 6.2.

Salivary glands

All the glands produce saliva, which is essential for the breakdown of food. There are three major pairs of salivary glands in the mouth.

- The **parotid glands**—the largest pair—lies just behind the angle of the jaw, below and in front of the ears.
- The **submandibular glands,** which lie between the mandible, skin and mylohyoid muscle.
- The **sublingual glands,** which lie deep in the floor of the mouth.

In addition to these, smaller salivary glands are distributed throughout the mouth.

The stratified squamous mucosal membrane of the hard palate is directly connected to the underlying periosteum. The membrane thickens laterally due to the presence of small palatine salivary glands.

The pharynx

The nasopharynx, oropharynx and laryngopharynx make up the pharynx. There are four layers:

- The **mucosal layer** is mainly stratified squamous (although the nasopharynx is lined by ciliated columnar epithelium).
- The **submucosa (fibrous layer)** is thick superiorly, forming the pharyngobasilar fascia. This fills the space between the superior constrictor and the base of the skull. Elsewhere the fibrous layer is thinner, although it thickens again in the oropharynx to form the sheath surrounding the tonsils.
- The **muscular layer.** The superior, middle and inferior constrictor muscles, together with palatopharyngeus, stylopharyngeus and salpingopharyngeus, form this layer that controls deglutition and aids the production of speech. The structure of the constrictors is shown in Figure 6.7; they have been described as resembling a stack of beakers, each inside the next
- The **fascial layer** is the outermost, thinnest, and most delicate.

The oropharynx

The palatoglossal arches, soft palate, and dorsum of the tongue signal the beginning of the oropharynx, and this extends to the tip of the epiglottis.

There are five muscles of the soft palate:

- **Tensor palati.** The tendon of tensor palati forms the tough aponeurosis of the soft palate, attached to the posterior edge of the hard palate.
- **Levator palati**
- **Palatoglossus**
- **Palatopharyngeus**
- **Muscularis uvulae.**

The palatal structures close off the nasopharynx from the oral cavity during swallowing and speaking. This is aided by contraction of superior constrictor, which forms a physical barrier of contracted muscle along the back and side walls of the oropharynx.

Tonsils

The tonsils lie between the anterior pillar (palatoglossus), the posterior pillar (palatopharyngeus) and the tongue below.

They consist of lymphoid tissue covered by stratified squamous epithelium with up to 20 tonsillar pits visible in each. The deeper border is marked by the fibrous layer which separates the tonsil from the superior constrictor muscle.

The lymphoid tissue often extends into the base of the tongue, behind the faucal pillars and into the soft palate. Together with the adenoids, these extensions make up Waldeyer's ring.

The majority of blood is supplied by the tonsillar branch of the facial artery and venous drainage passes via the paratonsillar vein into the pharyngeal plexus beyond the pharyngeal wall. Lymphatic drainage is to the upper deep cervical nodes.

The nerve supply is complex, with branches from IX, the palatine branch of V and the mandibular branch of VII. For this reason, anaesthesia is best accomplished topically or with infiltration, rather than multiple nerve blocks.

The nose and nasopharynx

The nose consists of bone, cartilage and fibro-fatty tissue, The central cartilage of the septum provides the central support. A coronal section is shown in Figure 6.3, with the structure of the walls in Figure 6.4.

There are four, loosely symmetrical groups of sinuses: maxillary, frontal, ethmoid and sphenoid. They all drain into the nasal cavity. Most begin to develop at 7 or 8 years, and mature after puberty.

The maxillary sinus is pyramid-shaped, and its base forms the lateral wall of the nasal cavity. Bulges in the inferior aspect are formed by the 1st and 2nd molars, and this explains the association between dental and maxillary sepsis. The superior aspect forms the floor of the orbit. Drainage is dependent upon the efficiency of the cilliary lining, since the ostium is unfortunately located high along its medial wall.

Lateral wall

Within the nose, three turbinates (conchae) each overlie a meatal opening of a paranasal sinus. Additionally, the nasolacrimal duct drains through the lateral wall. The nerves of the lateral wall are shown in Figure 6.5

Septum

The septum is formed by the vomer, the septal cartilage and the perpendicular plate of the ethmoid. The nerves of the septum are shown in Figure 6.6. Anterior septal deviation is common and results from often trivial injury in childhood. It does not manifest until after puberty.

Clinical relevance

The nasal airway or nasal endotracheal tube are passed along the floor of the nasal cavity below the inferior concha, to avoid obstruction of the tube by the other conchae. It should be kept as lateral as possible as there is a rich arterial supply to the anterior part of the septum, which is rich in capillaries (Kieselbach area). Nasal intubation with any device is contraindicated when there is any suspicion of fracture of the cribriform plate.

Infections of the nasal cavity may be caused by long-standing cannulation, and may spread to the:

- Anterior cranial fossa through the cribriform plate.
- Nasopharynx and retropharyngeal soft tissues.
- Middle ear through the phayryngo-tympanic tube.
- Paranasal sinuses through the various apertures.
- Maxillary sinus. Most commonly infected because the ostia are small and located high on their superior medial wall, an area that does not drain well.
- Ethmoidal cells. An infection here can cause visual problems following penetration the fragile medial wall of the orbit.

Moffat's solution

Moffat's solution is used for topical anaesthesia and vasoconstriction of the nasal cavity. It is prepared by mixing:

- 3ml 8.4% sodium bicarbonate
- 2ml 10% cocaine
- 1ml 1:1000 adrenaline (1mg).

There are different ways of ensuring the solution anaesthetises the anterior ethmoidal nerves and the short and long sphenopalatine nerves. A good method is to extend the head and neck with pillows under the shoulders, thus allowing the sphenopalatine fossa to collect the solution. It is also imperative to allow enough time for it to work: 5min in this position produces excellent vasoconstriction and anaesthesia for operations within the nasal cavity.

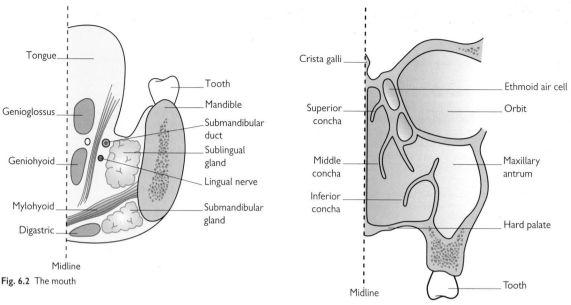

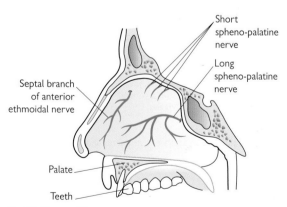

Fig. 6.2 The mouth

Fig. 6.3 Coronal view of the nose.

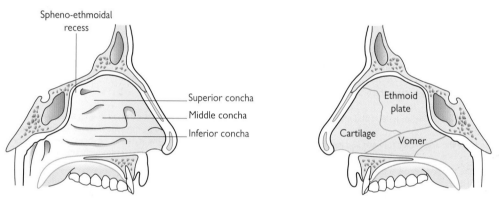

Fig. 6.4 The lateral wall and ostia. This bony labyrinth is made up of the ethmoid above, the palatine bone behind, and the maxilla anteriorly.

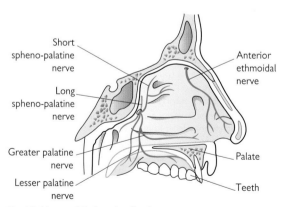

Fig. 6.5 Nerves of the lateral wall and ostia.

Fig. 6.6 Nerves of the septum.

6.3 The larynx

The larynx protects the lungs from soiling and is an organ of speech.

Cartilages
The larynx is a fibrocartilaginous structure made up of six different cartilages.

- **Epiglottis**. A broad leaf-like structure attached at its lower end to the back of the thyroid cartilage. Superiorly projects upwards and backwards behind both the hyoid and the tongue. Its mucosa is reflected anteriorly in the mid-line as the glosso-epiglottic fold and laterally as the pharyngo-epiglottic fold. The valleculae lie as valleys outside the lateral folds.
- **Thyroid**. Shield-like, consisting of two laminae that meet in the mid-line with the thyroid notch superiorly. The inferior horns articulate with the cricoid below.
- **Cricoid**. The only complete ring. It articulates with both the thyroid and arytenoid cartilages. The 'signet' part of the ring lies posteriorly.
- **Arytenoid** (two). Three-sided pyramid. Both sit on the cricoid and together control the tension of the vocal cords.
- **Corniculate** (two). Together with the cuneiform they sit in the aryepiglottic fold.
- **Cuneiform** (two).

Muscles
Intrinsic
These alter the tension of the cords during speech (Figure 6.7). They also open the cords during inspiration and close them during swallowing.

- **Posterior cricoarytenoid:** this externally rotates the arytenoids and is the ONLY abductor of the cords.
- **Lateral cricoarytenoid:** this internally rotates the arytenoid and abducts the cords, closing the glottis.
- **Interarytenoid:** this is the only unpaired muscle. It abducts the cords and closes the glottis.
- **Thyroarytenoid:** these draw the arytenoids forward and relax (shorten) the vocal cords.
- **Vocalis:** these arise from the thyroarytenoid muscle and may alter the tension of the vocal cord.
- **Cricothyroid:** contraction lifts the cricoid anteriorly, towards the thyroid cartilage above. This tilts the arytenoids backwards, thus lengthening the vocal cords (Figure 6.9).

Abductors of the cords	Posterior cricoarytenoid
Adductors of the cords	Lateral cricoarytenoid Interarytenoid
Sphincter action	Aryepiglottic muscles (extension of the Interarytenoid muscle) Thyroepiglottic muscles (extension of the Thyroarytenoid muscles)
Cord tension regulators	Cricothyroids Thyroarytenoids Vocales

Extrinsic
These attach the larynx to adjacent structures and help to elevate or depress it (Figure 6.8a).

- **Sternothyroid**
- **Thyrohyoid**
- **Inferior constrictor**

Ligaments
Extrinsic ligaments connect the larynx to adjacent structures and the intrinsic ligaments connect the laryngeal cartilages.

Extrinsic
- Thyrohyoid membrane: this connects the upper borders of the thyroid laminae and superior horns to the hyoid bone. The thickened midline part is the median thyrohyoid ligament, and the posterior free borders form the lateral thyrohyoid ligaments.
- Three paired folds connect the epiglottis to surrounding structures: the aryepiglottic folds to the arytenoids, the median glossoepiglottic folds to the tongue, and the lateral glossoepiglottic folds to the pharynx. In addition, the hyoepiglottic and thyroepiglottic ligaments attach it to the hyoid bone and thyroid cartilage, respectively.
- The cricotracheal ligament connects the cricoid cartilage to the first tracheal ring.

Intrinsic
- Quadrangular membrane: this extends between the epiglottis and the arytenoid cartilage. The upper border is the aryepiglottic fold (the two folds border the laryngeal inlet, shown in Figure 6.10), and the lower border is the vestibular fold or false cord.
- Cricothyroid ligament: this joins the cricoid and thyroid cartilages. The lateral portion arises from the arch of the cricoid cartilage, and attaches anteriorly to the junction of the thyroid laminae, and posteriorly to the vocal process of the arytenoid. Its thickened upper border forms the cricovocal ligament (vocal fold or cord).

Blood supply
The superior laryngeal artery accompanies the internal branch of the superior laryngeal nerve to supply the inner structures of the larynx. The inferior laryngeal artery follows the route of the recurrent laryngeal nerve.

The laryngeal nerves
Superior laryngeal nerve
This arises from the inferior vagal ganglion and crosses the greater cornu of the hyoid before dividing into the internal laryngeal nerve (sensory and autonomic) and the external laryngeal nerve (motor). The internal nerve pierces the thyrohyoid membrane to supply the mucosa down to the cords.

Paralysis of the superior laryngeal nerve causes anaesthesia of the superior laryngeal mucosa; the protective mechanism designed to keep foreign bodies out of the larynx is inactive and aspiration is a risk. Injury to the external branch of the superior laryngeal nerve can occur during thyroid surgery as it accompanies the superior thyroid artery, which is usually ligated during surgery.

This injury causes paralysis of the cricothyroid muscle and so prevents tone modulation; the patient is unable to vary the length and tension of the vocal fold. This can be disastrous for opera singers.

The inferior laryngeal nerves
These are the continuation of the recurrent laryngeal nerve; this is the primary motor nerve of the larynx, and damage will cause paralysis of the vocal folds. Injury to the recurrent laryngeal nerve may be caused by aneurysm of the arch of aorta or operations on the neck.

Injury of one recurrent laryngeal nerve causes hoarseness as the paralysed vocal fold cannot adduct to meet the normal vocal fold. Within weeks the contralateral fold crosses the midline to compensate.

Bilateral recurrent nerve damage causes a lost voice; the vocal folds are in a position that is slightly narrower than the usual neutral respiratory position. They cannot be adducted for phonation or abducted to increase respiration and therefore produce inspiratory stridor during exercise.

Local anaesthesia for airway procedures

Topical
Instrumentation of the nasopharynx and larynx requires appropriate anaesthesia. It is very convenient to provide aerosolized 4% lidocaine (±1% phenylephrine) given via a standard oxygen-driven nebulizer. The safe dose of lidocaine for airway anaesthesia is 7mg/kg.

Alternatively, local anaesthetic and vasoconstrictor can be sprayed to anaesthetize the proximal nasal airway. As the endoscope is advanced, further boluses of LA are sprayed under direct vision via the injector channel, producing anaesthesia exactly where it is needed.

Injection of 2ml 4% lidocaine through the cricothyroid membrane during inspiration is sometimes used to provide anaesthesia of the recurrent laryngeal nerve, trachea, and glottis, since the topical solution is coughed proximally. The major drawback with this technique is that it is often associated with significant bleeding within the trachea, which obscures the view through the bronchoscope.

Blocks for specific nerves are rarely used.

- Glossopharyngeal: submucosal infiltration behind tonsillar pillars.
- Superior laryngeal nerve: walk off the greater cornua of the hyoid and penetrate the thyrohyoid membrane. Perform bilaterally.

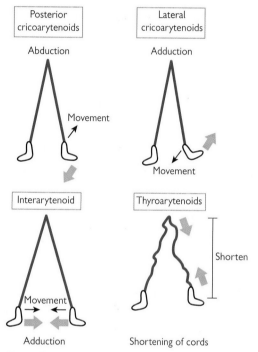

Fig. 6.7 Cord movements: intrinsic muscles (recurrent laryngeal nerve).

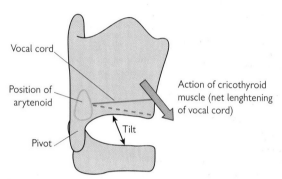

Fig. 6.9 Extrinsic muscles of the larynx (superior laryngeal nerve).

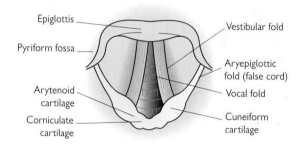

Fig. 6.10 The view at laryngoscopy.

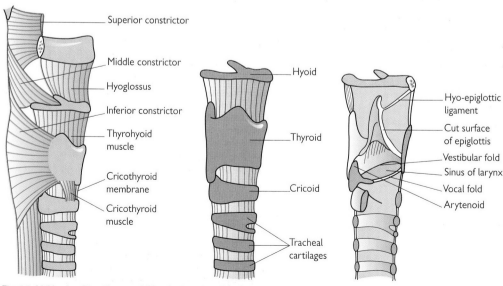

Fig. 6.8 (a) Muscles, (b)cartilages, and (c) sagittal section of the larynx.

6.4 The surgical airway

The surgical airway may be an elective procedure or performed as an emergency.

The percutaneous route of insertion has become the method of choice for elective tracheostomy tube insertion in the ICU.

Emergency cricothyroidotomy with a definitive airway allows ventilation and airway protection to the same standards as oral intubation. It is performed in the 'can't intubate can't ventilate' situation when neither oral nor nasal intubation is possible.

Needle cricocothyroidotomy is used when no other method of oxygenation is possible. It is a temporizing measure only.

Elective: percutaneous tracheostomy

This technique is performed most commonly for intensive care patients requiring prolonged ventilation as it assists with weaning from mechanical ventilation, improves patient comfort, and allows better oral care and bronchial toilet. However, it is also used to give prophylactic relief of airway obstruction or to protect against aspiration.

The technique should not be confused with emergency cricothyroidotomy: this is performed when a definitive airway is urgently required but conventional oral or nasal intubation is impossible.

Equipment needed

- LA with adrenaline
- Skin prep, syringes/needles, surgical blade
- Tracheostomy insertion kit
- Appropriate size of tracheostomy tube (± one size)
- Immediately available airway equipment
- Capnograph as part of full patient monitoring
- Bronchoscope (optional)

Preparation

- Ensure consent and give sedation/GA as appropriate.
- At least three, trained personnel are needed: one for tracheostomy insertion, one assistant, and one anaesthetist.
- The patient should be positioned supine, with neck hyperextension (using a pillow or towel under shoulders).
- Ventilate with 100% O_2 for at least 5min.
- Withdraw the ETT to just above the cords (under direct vision).

Technique (Figure 6.11)

Using full aseptic technique, palpate trachea and locate space between cricoid and first or first/second tracheal cartilages; infiltrate LA.

Hold trachea between two fingers, ensure midline positioning and absence of overlying veins, and make a horizontal skin incision between the two rings about 2cm long. Perform blunt dissection down to tracheal rings.

Take a syringe half-filled with saline and a cannula. Aiming slightly caudad, insert the cannula between the rings whilst constantly aspirating. Stop when air is aspirated; this signifies that the needle tip is in the trachea. Feed the cannula over the needle into the trachea. Withdraw the needle and again check cannula position by aspirating air into a syringe.

Pass the wire into the trachea. Remove the cannula. Dilate the tracheotomy using either a single or serial dilation kit over the wire. Insert the tracheostomy tube, inflate cuff, and check adequate ventilation.

Secure the tube with tapes. Order a check CXR.

Tips

Choose level based on the patient's anatomy and clinical preference. A high approach, between first and second rings, avoids the thyroid isthmus but has a higher incidence of tracheal stenosis. A low approach, between second and third tracheal rings, reduces risk of tracheal stenosis; this is the preferred level.

If the anatomy is difficult or distorted in any way, a surgical tracheostomy is safer.

A bronchoscope is often used to check positioning at each step, although this has not been shown to improve outcome or reduce the rate of complications.

Emergency procedures

Surgical cricothyroidotomy

The skin is cleaned rapidly and the landmarks identified. All equipment to be used should be checked prior to use. Full patient monitoring should also be used, including capnography.

An incision is made through the skin over the cricothyroid membrane and a second one through this membrane. The handle of the scalpel is inserted through the hole in the cricothyroid membrane and rotated 90°. This will open it sufficiently to allow the introduction of a cuffed ETT or tracheostomy tube. Once inserted, the cuff of the tube is inflated, the position checked, and ventilation begun.

Needle cricothyroidotomy

This technique is used for emergency oxygen administration in the 'can't intubate, can't ventilate' situation. The cricothyroid membrane is chosen for its relative avascularity and ease of identification.

This is not considered a definitive airway procedure; it only buys time and must be followed by another method of securing the airway.

There are specifically designed cricothyroidotomy kits; however, these are not always easily available and equipment found in all anaesthetic rooms can be used as a DIY kit (Figure 6.12).

Technique

Extend the neck and identify cricothyroid membrane between cricoid and thyroid cartilages. Hold secure between two fingers.

The 14G or 16G cannula (or other crycothrotomy device) is advanced through the cricothyroid membrane in the caudad direction. A saline-filled syringe attached to the cannula is aspirated continuously. When air is aspirated, the needle is in the trachea; the cannula may be advanced over the needle. When fully advanced, ensure that air can still be aspirated from cannula. Secure this in position. Oxygen may be administered through this by using the following.

- A size 3.5 ETT tracheal tube connector will fit the Luer lock end of the cannula, allowing connection of a standard 15mm ventilator circuit.
- Similarly, a 2ml syringe will fit the Luer lock end and this will snugly receive an 8mm ETT connector and therefore connection of a standard 15mm ventilator circuit fitting (see Figure 6.12).
- A 10 ml syringe barrel intubated with a cuffed ETT.

Oxygenation options

- Jet injector (high pressure). This is rarely available in the emergency setting.
- Anaesthetic breathing system and reservoir bag (low pressure).
- Simple green oxygen tubing can be attached to a 2ml syringe fitted to the end of the cannula. 15L/min O_2 is passed through this tubing; intermittent occlusion of a hole cut in its side allows gas inflation of the chest. This technique does not provide adequate ventilation and CO_2 levels will rise significantly within 30min. Expired gas is not exhaled via the cricothyroid cannula and exits through the partially obstructed airway. Watch for kinking of the tube (high pressures/ no ventilation) and migration of the cannula (subcutaneous emphysema/difficulty ventilating).

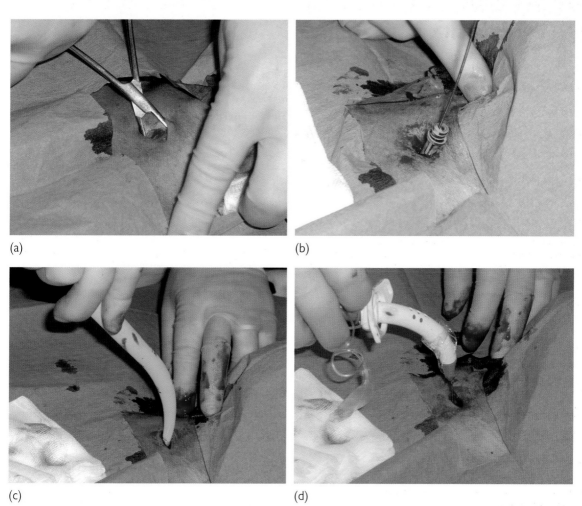

(a)

(b)

(c)

(d)

Fig. 6.11 Percutaneous tracheostomy. (a) Following horizontal incision in a skin crease below the level of the cricoid cartilage, blunt dissection is performed down to the pre-tracheal fascia. (b) With the distal guide wire within the trachea, the first stiff dilator enlarges the hole made between the cricoid and first tracheal cartilage rings. (c) This dilator enlarges the hole to allow introduction of the tracheostomy tube. (d) The tracheostomy tube is carried into the trachea over an introducer, itself guided by its wire.

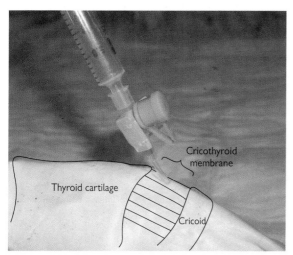

Fig. 6.12 Emergency needle cricothyroidotomy: the cannula should be placed caudally through the cricothyroid membrane.

6.5 Peripheral cannulation

Obtaining access to the peripheral circulation allows sampling of blood and infusion of fluids and IV medications. It is one of the most basic tasks for the anaesthetist, yet it can also be one of the most challenging and important. Obtaining adequately sized and placed IV access is imperative for the smooth running of all cases in theatre and for the treatment and monitoring of ITU patients.

Contraindications

Massive limb oedema, burns, or peripheral trauma alter venous return. IV cannulae will be difficult to site in such limbs and suffer significantly reduced rates of fluid flow. Similarly, for the patient with severe abdominal trauma, it is prudent to first attempt cannulation in the upper limb.

Other situations to avoid include:

- Cannulation of an area of cellulite: there is a risk of inoculating the circulation with bacteria.
- An AV fistula is precious. Its high luminal pressure affects the rates of IV fluid administration and it is likely to be damaged by administration of medications.
- A mastectomy with axillary clearance is often associated with inadequate rates of flow if the ipsilateral arm is used.

Complications

Peripheral cannulae are potential sites for local thrombophlebitis and, more seriously, systemic infection. To prevent this, cannulae should be inspected daily for signs of redness of overlying skin, pain, or fluctuance. Any suspect cannulae should be changed immediately, and all cannulae should be removed as soon as they are no longer necessary. It is also common for the IV sites to leak interstitially.

Migration of the cannula out of vein and extravasation of fluids or drugs can cause subcutaneous oedema and local irritation or necrosis.

Suitability of sites

The suitability of a site for vascular access depends on the situation for which it is required. It is usually based on the adequacy of the patient's veins, site of the surgery, speed with which fluid needs to be given, and whether or not central venous access is required.

In trauma patients, it is common to first use the median cubital vein because it will accommodate a large-bore IV and is easy to hit.

Peripheral sites:

- Back of the hand: easy visibility, less kinking. Most popular site.
- Antecubital fossa (Figure 6.14): large visible veins, but easily kinked and occluded. Uncomfortable for the patient.
- Feet/ankles: more difficult. Painful; venous stasis more common.

Equipment

All necessary equipment should be prepared, assembled, and available at the bedside prior to starting the IV. Basic equipment:

- Gloves and protective equipment
- Appropirate size catheter 14–25G IV catheter
- Non-latex tourniquet
- Alcohol swab to clean the skin
- Tape
- IV bag with giving set flushed and ready or saline lock
- Sharps container.

To prepare the IV line, protective caps are removed from the fluid bag and the spiked end of the IV tubing. The regulating clamp for the IV line should be closed. The spiked end of the giving set is inserted into its port on the IV bag whilst holding the IV bag upside down.

The bag should be hung from the IV pole and the drip chamber filled halfway. The regulating clamp should be opened to 'flush' the line and remove air bubbles prior to connection of the giving set to the patient.

Universal precautions

Gloves must be worn during cannulation. If the risk of blood splatter is high, the operator should consider face and eye protection and use of a gown.

Sharps should be disposed of in accordance with hospital policy. This will mean immediate disposal of the sharp into an adjacent sharps container.

Tips for insertion of IV cannulae

- Optimize venous filling after tourniquet application by using gravity, gentle slapping or squeezing of the hand, asking the patient to open and close fist, or immersing hand in warm water. Ideally, choose a prominent straight vein with no bifurcations over the length of the cannula and not over a joint.
- IVs are generally started at the most peripheral site that is available and appropriate for the situation. If you puncture a proximal vein first, and then start an IV distal to that site, the fluid will leak proximally.
- Advancement of the cannula into the vein should be smooth and not painful. If it is not, it may not be correctly placed. Other signs of incorrect placement include difficulty in flushing, tissuing at the end of the cannula, and painful injection.
- Do not try to reinsert the needle after it has been withdrawn from the cannula as this can lead to shearing of the plastic sheath.
- Recapping needles, putting catheters back into their sheath, or dropping sharps to the floor (an unfortunately common practice in trauma) should be strictly avoided. Recapping of needles is one of the most common causes of preventable needle-stick injuries in healthcare workers.

Removing the IV

Shut off the IV by closing the roller camp. Remove the tape and dressing from the tubing and cannula. Place a dressing over the IV site and remove the cannula from the arm. Secure the new dressing with tape.

Technique for intravenous injection

- Use a no-touch technique and universal precautions.
- Flush cannula to ensure patency.
- Check for patient allergies.
- Check drug type, dose, concentration, and expiry; inject as per timing and dilution recommended by manufacturer.
- Flush cannula again after use and before injecting another drug.
- Record the dose and time of drug on either drug or anaesthetic chart.

Characteristics of intravenous cannulae

There are many different types and makes of peripheral IV cannulae. They all look slightly different but have the same basic characteristics. The most important aspect to note is the large increase in flow rates seen as the gauge of the cannula decreases (i.e. the diameter increases). Peripheral cannulae are colour-coded according to their gauge (Figure 6.13).

Basic features

- Needle with attached transparent hub
- Plastic cannula with hub for Luer lock attachment
- Additional injection port (not on all cannulae)

Flow characteristics and colour coding

Measured using British Standard: distilled water at 22°C, under pressure of 10kPa connected via 110cm of tubing of internal diameter 4mm.

Gauge	Flow rate	Colour
24G	13–24ml/min	yellow
22G	23–42ml/min	blue
20G	40–80ml/min	pink
18G	75–120ml/min	green
16G	130–220ml/min	grey
14G	250–360ml/min	orange.

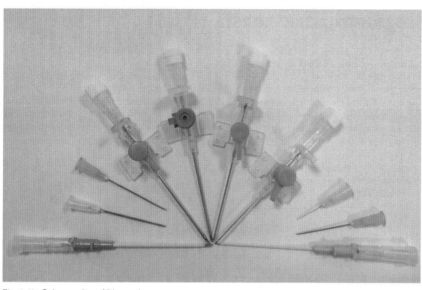

Fig. 6.13 Colour coding of IV cannulae.

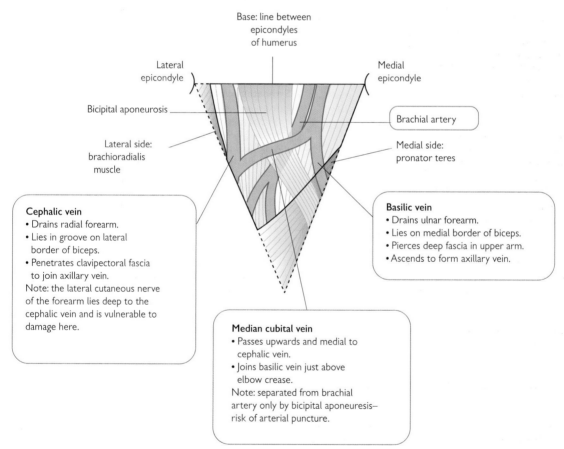

Base: line between
epicondyles
of humerus

Lateral
epicondyle

Medial
epicondyle

Bicipital aponeurosis

Brachial artery

Lateral side:
brachioradialis
muscle

Medial side:
pronator teres

Cephalic vein
• Drains radial forearm.
• Lies in groove on lateral
  border of biceps.
• Penetrates clavipectoral fascia
  to join axillary vein.
Note: the lateral cutaneous nerve
of the forearm lies deep to the
cephalic vein and is vulnerable to
damage here.

Basilic vein
• Drains ulnar forearm.
• Lies on medial border of biceps.
• Pierces deep fascia in upper arm.
• Ascends to form axillary vein.

Median cubital vein
• Passes upwards and medial to
  cephalic vein.
• Joins basilic vein just above
  elbow crease.
Note: separated from brachial
artery only by bicipital aponeuresis—
risk of arterial puncture.

Fig. 6.14 Structures in the (right) antecubital fossa. The antecubital fossa is an intermuscular depression which lies at the crease of the elbow joint. It is an important area as veins, arteries, and nerves pass through it superficially on their way to the forearm and are easily cannulated. However, there are significant risks of arterial puncture (brachial artery) and nerve damage (lateral cutaneous nerve of the forearm) in this area.

6.6 Intravenous regional anaesthesia (IVRA)

IVRA was first described by August Bier for forearm anaesthesia (Bier's block), which remains the most widely used IVRA application. However, it can also be used on the lower limb and for sympathetic nerve blocks in chronic pain.

The technique involves IV injection of local anaesthetic into an extremity which has been isolated by a tourniquet. Anaesthesia is thought to result from diffusion of local anaesthetic from the venous system into local nerve endings.

Unlike most regional anaesthesia techniques, IVRA requires little knowledge of anatomy and is therefore simple yet reliable. However, it is potentially dangerous, especially in inexperienced hands, as escape of the local anaesthetic into the systemic circulation can lead to toxicity.

Choice of local anaesthetic
This decision is based mainly on the relative cardiotoxicity of the various agents. Dilute solutions are used.

Prilocaine is thought to be the safest and is usually the agent of choice: 0.5%, maximum of 6mg/kg or up to 300mg.

Lidocaine is also used: 0.5% without adrenaline, maximum 3mg/kg or 250mg.

Bupivicaine, laevobupivicaine, and ropivicaine should not be used because of their unfavourable cardiovascular effects.

The local anaesthetic should be injected slowly to avoid the risk of forcing the solution past the tourniquet.

Volume: 40–60ml (depending on size of patient/arm).

Biers block of the forearm

Uses
- Manipulation of minor fractures
- Minor forearm/hand surgery
- NB: only use if the operation expected to last <30min

Preparation
- Thorough preparation and checking of equipment is especially important in this technique because of the potential for local anaesthetic toxicity.
- Check both cuffs of the tourniquet for leaks.
- As with any regional technique, ensure that full monitoring and resuscitation equipment are immediately available and working.
- Obtain consent and check that the patient is starved.

Technique
- Insert two IV cannulae, one into the arm to be blocked (for local anaesthetic injection) and one into another site which will be outside the tourniquet (safety cannula).
- Exsanguinate the limb (elevate or use Esmark bandage or similar).
- Apply the tourniquet proximally to the arm requiring blockade, ensuring adequate padding under the tourniquet to protect from pinching or bruising.
- Inflate the cuff to around twice the patients systolic BP (i.e. usually to around 100mmHg above systolic).
- Check for absence of the radial pulse.
- Inject local anaesthetic slowly into the cannula on that limb.
- Motor and sensory block should occur within 5–10min.
- The tourniquet can be deflated only after a minimum of 20min after injection of lidocaine or 15 min after prilocaine.

Tips
The duration of this block is usually limited to around 40min by the discomfort caused to the patient by the tourniquet. This can be extended by using a double tourniquet (Figure 6.15), first anaesthetizing the area under the lower cuff. First, deflate the lower cuff, ensuring the upper cuff is inflated. Then after 5–10min inflate the lower cuff and deflate the upper cuff.

This block is often inadequate for bony surgery.

Complications
- Systemic local anaesthetic toxicity.
- Pressure damage from the tourniquet.
- Failure.

Contraindications
- Prepubertal children (intra-osseous vessels may allow the local anaesthetic to enter the systemic circulation).
- Sickle cell anaemia.

Cautions
- Obese patients or those with fat arms.
- Hypertension (systolic BP>200mmHg).
- Peripheral vascular disease.

Other IVRA techniques

Lower leg block
A similar technique can be used for minor surgery or fracture manipulation of the lower leg. Larger volumes of local anaesthetic will be required.

Sympathetic nerve block (guanethidine)
Indications
- Chronic pain, e.g. for treatment of complex regional pain syndromes
- Peripheral vascular disease
- Acute vascular disorders: post-traumatic vasospasm; acute arterial or venous occlusion; cold injury; inadvertent intra-arterial injection of drugs, e.g. thiopentone or contaminated drugs of abuse
- Chronic vasospastic conditions: Raynaud's syndrome; acrocyanosis; livedo reticularis; sequelae of spinal cord injury or disease (e.g. polio)
- Chronic obliterative arterial diseases: thromboangiitis obliterans (Buerger's disease); atherosclerosis
- Perioperative purposes: microvascular surgery; arteriovenous fistula formation for dialysis

Guanethidine is an adrenergic neuron blocking drug which prevents the release of noradrenaline from postganglionic adrenergic neurons. Guanethidine is rapidly taken up from the venous system by the peripheral nerves during the 20min that a tourniquet is applied to the affected limb. It has an immediate action locally on the peripheral sympathetic nerves. During the next 24hr, the guanethidine is transported by the peripheral nerves to the dorsal root ganglion in the spinal cord, where it contributes further to the sympathetic block centrally.

Technique
- As for Bier's block of the forearm.
- 10–25mg of guanethidine in 20ml of saline (for the arm); local anaesthetic (lidocaine or prilocaine) also often added.
- Tourniquet can be deflated after 20min.

Caution
Hypotension can occur up to several hours later.

Technique

The block should be performed in an area with suitable resuscitation equipment and where trained assistants are available. The patient should be fasted for 4hr beforehand. Two IV lines are inserted, one into the affected limb, and one (spare) in the back of a hand. The first line is used to inject the guanethidine–local anaesthetic mixture, and the second line acts as emergency venous access, should the need arise. Vital signs monitoring is used throughout to measure heart rate, blood pressure, and oxygen saturation. IV sedation is used for patient comfort, and can be supplemented with entonox. The upper part of the affected limb is wrapped in gauze to protect it, and a tourniquet is applied. Excessive blood is gently squeezed out of the affected limb using an exsanguinator. The tourniquet is inflated to about 100mmHg higher than the patient's systolic BP and held at that pressure by a gas-powered machine.

The guanethidine mixture is injected slowly into the exsanguinated arm via the IV line, and the tourniquet is kept in place for 20min.

Commonly used mixtures

- Arm: guanethidine 20mg + 25ml 0.5% lidocaine or 0.5% prilocaine
- Leg: guanethidine 30 mg + 30ml 0.5% lidocaine or 0.5% prilocaine.

While the touniquet is inflated, the affected limb will slowly become numb from the combination of the LA and the lack of blood flow. After 20min, the tourniquet is slowly deflated, allowing blood to return to the affected limb. During this time, all the guanethidine and LA should have been absorbed by the peripheral nerves.

Complications

Major

If the tourniquet deflates before 20min and before all the LA and guanethidine has been absorbed, significant amounts of both drugs can escape into the systemic circulation. Depending on the dose, this can cause hypotension (guanethidine) or cardiac arrest (lidocaine).

If the injection pressure rises too high when the mixture is initially injected, some of the drug can escape into the systemic circulation through blood vessels that travel through bone, therefore avoiding the tourniquet. Thus it is important not to inject too quickly or with too high a volume.

Unstable asthmatics can develop severe wheezing on tourniquet deflation because of the effects of traces of guanethidine leaking into the circulation and causing bronchoconstriction of the airways. This is usually managed with bronchodilators and steroids.

Minor

Allergic reactions to guanethidine can occur, causing an itchy rash in the affected limb. Most settle spontaneously but some require treatment with steroids and antihistamines.

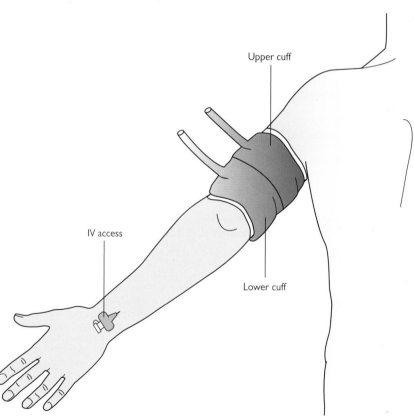

Fig. 6.15 IVRA and the double cuff

The great veins of the neck, in particular the internal jugular vein (IJV), are popular sites for central venous access as they allow monitoring of central venous pressure and risks of infection and occlusion are less than the femoral route. However, these techniques have several major complications, especially in inexperienced hands. Therefore the current recommendation is to use ultrasound guidance for elective placement of central venous cannulae at these sites.

A diagram of the thoracic inlet is shown in Figure 6.16. It is clear that a number of important structures should be avoided during procedures in this territory. Figure 6.17 shows the large veins of the neck.

Approaches

Internal jugular vein

The right internal jugular is usually the first choice for placement as the SVC and right atrium are most directly aligned with it. High approaches reduce the risk of pneumothorax but increase the risk of arterial puncture. The reverse is true of a low approach.

It is a reliable technique which is relatively easy to perform. However, both the insertion and subsequent positioning of the line are uncomfortable for the patient. The site is associated with a lower incidence of complications than the subclavian approach. If arterial puncture has occurred, this should prevent the operator from trying the other side.

Anatomy

The sigmoid venous sinus passes through the mastoid portion of the temporal bone, emerging from the base of the skull via the jugular foramen. It passes vertically down through the neck within the carotid sheath. The vein initially lies posterior to the internal carotid artery rotating around it as it descends, becoming lateral and then anterolateral to the artery. It joins the subclavian vein behind the sternal end of the clavicle to enter the chest as the innominate vein.

Subclavian vein

This approach is more comfortable for the patient and easier to keep clean, but it is more difficult to perform and has a greater risk of pneumothorax and haemothorax. If the artery is punctured direct pressure cannot be applied to stop the bleeding.

The SCV drains blood from the arm and is the continuation of the axillary vein. It begins at the lower border of the first rib. Initially the vein arches upwards across the first rib and then inclines medially downwards and slightly forwards across the scalenus anterior muscle to enter the thorax. It joins the IJV behind the sternoclavicular joint.

General technique of insertion

- Explain the procedure to the (conscious) patient.
- All equipment should be present and checked prior to use. Remember to flush all CVP lumens to ensure their patency and absence of damage.
- Aseptic technique should be used, including the use of adequate sized drapes.
- Place the patient in a head-down position since this will distend large veins and reduce the risk of air embolism.
- Infiltrate with local anaesthetic if the patient is awake.
- Using a combination of landmarks and ultrasound guidance, insert the needle into the appropriate area and advance, aspirating constantly. Often blood is aspirated on the way out rather than as the needle is advanced.
- When venous non-pulsatile blood is aspirated, the guidewire is inserted through the needle using the Seldinger technique. Remember to watch the ECG for arrhythmias. If these occur, pull back the wire a few cm. (Clearly, more serious arrhythmias such as VF require abandonment of the procedure and resuscitation).
- Make a small nick in the skin with a blade, remove the needle, and dilate the vein using the dilator.
- Holding the guidewire at all times remove the dilator and insert the CVP line over the wire to the estimated correct length.

- Ensure that blood can be aspirated from all lumens and flush with saline.
- Suture the line in place and cover with a dressing.
- Give written instructions as to how to use the line and whom to contact in the event of a problem.
- Request a CXR (should usually be done before use).

What to look for on the CXR

- Absence of pneumothorax/haemothorax.
- Correct positioning: the tip should lie at the junction of the SVC and the right atrium (tip too high—risk of thrombosis; tip too low—risk of arrhythmias and myocardial erosion).

Complications

Early

- Pneumothorax/haemothorax
- Air embolism
- Cardiac dysrhythmia
- Carotid artery puncture or cannulation
- Thoracic duct injury
- Nerve injury
- Local haemorrhage/haematoma
- Catheter embolus

Late

- Infection
- Venous thrombosis
- Perforation of the atrial wall with ensuing tamponade
- Hydrothorax

Care of the central venous catheter

- Use an aseptic technique for catheter insertion.
- Use a dry sterile dressing to cover the entry site.
- Secure the line well to prevent movement, since this increases the risks of infection and clot formation.
- Change the catheter if there are signs of infection at the site or features of generalized sepsis.
- The catheter should be removed as soon as it is no longer needed since duration of insertion is proportional to the risks of sepsis and thrombosis.
- There is no evidence that the routine changing of CVP lines reduces risk. Indeed, repeated cannulation attempts worsen patient outcomes.

Ultrasound guidance

The use of ultrasound guidance has been promoted as a method for reducing the risk of complications during central venous line insertion. An ultrasound probe is used to localize the position and depth of the vein (Figure 6.18). The introducer needle is visualized as it passes through the skin and into the vessel.

Use of this technique for internal jugular catheterization reduces the number of mechanical complications and catheter placement failures. However, it has had mixed results for the subclavian approach. The clavicle makes ultrasound-guided catheterization of the subclavian more difficult and less reliable than landmark-based techniques.

The ultrasound-guided technique is relatively new and its introduction requires training. NICE have stated that all CVP lines should be inserted with ultrasound guidance. In hospitals where staff are trained and there is adequate provision of equipment, the use of ultrasound guidance should be routinely considered for insertion of all internal jugular venous lines.

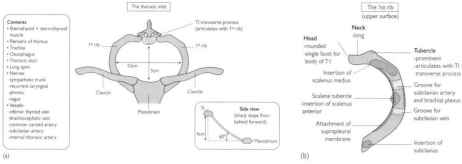

Contents
- Sternohyoid + sternothyroid muscle
- Remains of thymus
- Trachea
- Oesophagus
- Thoracic duct
- Lung apex
- Nerves
  - sympathetic trunk
  - recurrent laryngeal
  - phrenic
  - vagus
- Vessels
  - inferior thyroid vein
  - brachiocephalic vein
  - common carotid artery
  - subclavian artery
  - internal thoracic artery

(a)

The thoracic inlet

T1 transverse process (articulates with 1st rib)
1st rib
1st rib
10cm
5cm
Clavicle
Clavicle
Manubrium

Side view
(sharp slope from behind forward)
T1
4cm
60°
Manubrium

(b)

The 1st rib
(upper surface)

Neck
-long

Head
-rounded
-single facet for body of T1

Tubercle
-prominent
-articulates with T1 transverse process

Insertion of scalenus medius

Groove for subclavian artery and brachial plexus

Scalene tubercle
-insertion of scalenus anterior

Groove for subclavian vein

Attachment of suprapleural membrane

Insertion of subclavius

Fig. 6.16 The thoracic inlet and first rib. These are of anaesthetic interest because of their relations to the brachial plexus, the major vessels, and the apices of the lungs. The thoracic inlet in particular is a narrow space through which many important structures pass; enlargement or damage of any of these can have disastrous consequences.

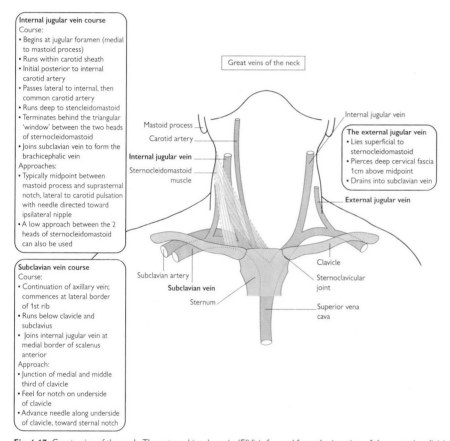

Internal jugular vein course
Course:
- Begins at jugular foramen (medial to mastoid process)
- Runs within carotid sheath
- Initial posterior to internal carotid artery
- Passes lateral to internal, then common carotid artery
- Runs deep to stencleidomastoid
- Terminates behind the triangular 'window' between the two heads of sternocleidomastoid
- Joins subclavian vein to form the brachicephalic vein

Approaches:
- Typically midpoint between mastoid process and suprasternal notch, lateral to carotid pulsation with needle directed toward ipsilateral nipple
- A low approach between the 2 heads of sternocleidomastoid can also be used

Subclavian vein course
Course:
- Continuation of axillary vein; commences at lateral border of 1st rib
- Runs below clavicle and subclavius
- Joins internal jugular vein at medial border of scalenus anterior

Approach:
- Junction of medial and middle third of clavicle
- Feel for notch on underside of clavicle
- Advance needle along underside of clavicle, toward sternal notch

Great veins of the neck

Mastoid process
Carotid artery
Internal jugular vein
Sternocleidomastoid muscle
Subclavian artery
Subclavian vein
Sternum

Internal jugular vein

The external jugular vein
- Lies superficial to sternocleidomastoid
- Pierces deep cervical fascia 1cm above midpoint
- Drains into subclavian vein

External jugular vein

Clavicle
Sternoclavicular joint
Superior vena cava

Fig. 6.17 Great veins of the neck. The external jugular vein (EJV) is formed from the junction of the posterior division of the posterior facial vein and the posterior auricular vein. It passes down the neck from the angle of the mandible and crosses sternocleidomastoid obliquely, passing through the clavipectoral fascia to join the subclavian vein. The EJV is useful for emergency IV fluid administration and in cardiac arrests, when the carotid pulsation cannot be felt. Its tortuous anatomy, especially below the clavicle, usually precludes is use for central venous access.

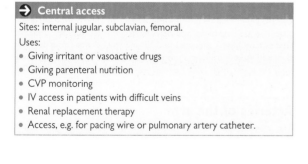

→ Central access

Sites: internal jugular, subclavian, femoral.

Uses:
- Giving irritant or vasoactive drugs
- Giving parenteral nutrition
- CVP monitoring
- IV access in patients with difficult veins
- Renal replacement therapy
- Access, e.g. for pacing wire or pulmonary artery catheter.

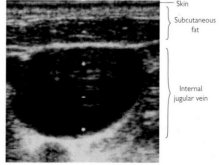

Skin
Subcutaneous fat
Internal jugular vein

Fig. 6.18 Ultrasound image of the internal jugular vein.

6.8 Upper limb anatomy and blocks

The brachial plexus and nerves of the arm

The brachial plexus is of importance because of the many approaches through which it can be blocked and the avoidance of damage to the branches during patient positioning.

It is formed from the anterior primary rami of C5 to T1 and consists of roots, trunks, division, cords, and finally nerves which go on to supply the arm (Figure 6.19). A diagram of the dermatomes of the arm is shown in Figure 6.56.

The five roots emerge from the intervertebral foramina and then pass through the anterior triangle of the neck between the scalenus anterior and medius muscles and across the base of the posterior triangle as three trunks (upper, middle and lower).

When the trunks have crossed the first rib, behind the clavicle, each divides into anterior and posterior divisions.

The six divisions then pass to the axilla where they join to form the lateral, medial, and posterior cords (named for their relation to the axillary artery).

The lateral cord is formed from the anterior divisions of the upper and middle trunks. It gives off a branch to the median nerve and then becomes the musculocutaneous nerve.

The medial cord is the continuation of the anterior division of the lower trunk. Its terminal branch is the ulnar nerve.

The posterior cord is formed from the posterior divisions of all three trunks. Its terminal branches are the radial and axillary nerves.

(NB: remember to think of the arm in the anatomical position when reading and picturing the course of these nerves).

The radial nerve (C5–8, T1)
Course

The radial nerve is formed from the posterior cord, posterior to the axillary artery, and passes between the long and medial heads of the triceps into the posterior compartment of the arm. It spirals around the lower third of the humerus and into the anterior compartment of the arm where it lies between the brachialis and the brachioradialis. It ends at the lateral epicondyle of the humerus by dividing into the superficial nerve and the posterior interosseous nerve.

Supplies

- Sensory: dorsal surface of the hand, base of the thumb
- Motor: triceps, brachialis and brachioradialis, extensors of the wrist and hand
- Articular: the elbow

The median nerve (C5–T1)
Course

The lateral and medial heads are formed from the lateral and medial cord, respectively, and unite in front of the axillary artery. The nerve runs initially lateral to the brachial artery crossing to the medial side at the midpoint of the upper arm. It then descends to the antecubital fossa and passes into the forearm. At the wrist it lies between the palmaris longus and flexor carpi radialis. It then enters the hand under the flexor retinaculum.

Supplies

- Sensory: thenar eminence of the palm and the palmar surface of the radial 3½ digits and their tips
- Motor: superficial fexors of the forearm, muscles of the thenar eminence and the lateral two lumbricles (LOAF—**L**ateral two lumbricles, **O**pponens pollicis, **A**bductor policis brevis, **F**lexor digitorum brevis)
- Articular: wrist and elbow

The ulnar nerve (C7–T1)
Course

The ulnar nerve is formed from the medial cord, and lies initially in the extensor compartment of the upper arm medial to the axillary and the brachial artery. It descends on the anterior aspect of the triceps then passes behind the medial epicondyle in the ulnar groove. It passes between the heads of flexor carpi ulnaris and then lies medially on the capsule of the elbow joint. It passes through the forearm on the flexor digitorum profundis to the wrist where it lies medial to the ulnar artery. It enters the hand above the flexor retinaculum lateral to the pisiform.

Supplies

- Motor: flexor carpi ulnaris, flexor digitorum profundus, hypothenar muscles and all the small muscles of the hand except 'LOAF' (see median nerve)
- Sensory: doral and palmar aspects of the medial side of the hand and medial 1½ fingers
- Articular: elbow and wrist

The musculocutaneous nerve (C5-7)
Course

Continuation of the lateral cord lying lateral to the axillary artery. It pierces the coracobrachialis and then descends between the biceps and brachialis. It pierces the deep fascia of the anticubital fossa and then continues as the lateral cutaneous nerve of the forearm.

Supplies

- Sensory: radial aspect of forearm
- Motor: coracobrachialis, biceps, brachialis
- Articular: elbow joint

Ultrasound assistance in regional anaesthesia

Valuable features of this technique include:

- Real-time guidance of the needle towards the target nerve
- Observation of local anaesthetic spread.

Nerve localization by ultrasound can be combined with nerve stimulation. Both tools are valuable and complementary, are not mutually exclusive, and in combination provide both anatomical and functional information.

The quality of ultrasound image is dependent on many factors:

- The quality of the ultrasound machine and transducers
- Appropriate transducer selection for each nerve location
- Knowledge of anatomy pertinent to the block
- Good coordination in order to track needle movements.

Optimal patient positioning and sterile technique are important. The block needle is aligned within the long axis of the ultrasound transducer. The needle should stay within the path of the ultrasound beam, and the needle shaft and tip should remain clearly visualized. This approach is especially useful when it is important to track the needle tip at all times.

Ultrasound-guided techniques are thought to improve the accuracy, success, and safety of regional anaesthesia. However, very few outcome studies have been conducted to date, and so evidence to support this is limited. Additionally, no study has examined the impact of ultrasound on nerve injury. More data are required to define the success and safety profile of ultrasound-guided peripheral nerve blocks.

Arteries of the arm

The main arteries of the arm are shown schematically in Figure 6.20.

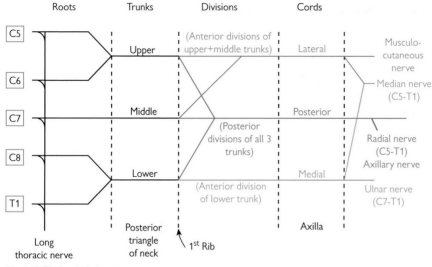

Fig. 6.19 The brachial plexus.

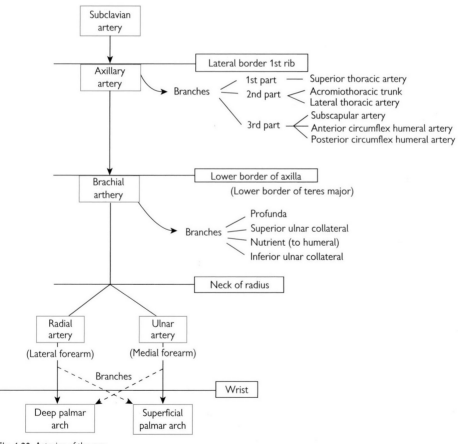

Fig. 6.20 Arteries of the arm.

6.9 Brachial plexus blockade

There are many different approaches to the brachial plexus, each having different indications and complications.

Blocks of the roots/trunks of the plexus in the neck, e.g. interscalene or supraclavicular, are good for upper arm and shoulder operations, especially in those patients for whom arm movement is difficult. However, they have many complications and they often miss the ulnar nerve, making them unsuitable for forearm or hand surgery.

The cords of the plexus can be blocked using an axillary nerve block, which is a good long-lasting block for hand surgey with few complications but often misses the musculocutaneous and intercostobrachial nerves. The anatomy of the axilla is shown in Figure 6.24.

In addition, there are also several techniques for blocking the nerves as they pass down the arm, e.g. mid-humeral, elbow, or wrist blocks. These are more rarely used as they require several injections to block all the nerves required. However, they can be useful for supplementation of other blocks or postoperative analgesia for minor surgery.

General principles

- As with all blocks, procedures should be carried out under aseptic conditions.
- Skilled help should be available and full monitoring in place.
- All resuscitation and anaesthetic equipment should be present, checked, and in good working order.

Interscalene block (Figure 6.21)

Indications
Shoulder or upper arm surgery, although with the low approach, elbow surgery may be appropriate.

NB: The upper approach often misses the ulnar nerve.

Position
Supine with the patient's head turned away from the side of procedure. Expose the arm in order to demonstrate which muscles contract following nerve stimulation.

Process
Locate the interscalene groove. This is found between the scalenus anterior and scalenus medius, lateral to the sternomastoid muscle. Ask the patient to lift their head from pillow whilst facing away; this demonstrates the posterior border of the SCM. Put your finger tips adjacent to this edge and roll your fingers posteriorly. The interscalene groove is a short distance behind the posterior border of the SCM. NB: The external jugular vein often overlies this groove.

Subcutaneous infiltration is usually unnecessary. If you do use it, remember that the plexus is very shallow at this point and LA beyond the skin may affect detection of an appropriate end-point.

Insert the needle perpendicularly into this groove, level with the cricoid (C6), heading slightly caudad, medial, and posterior.

Do not insert the needle more than 25mm since the rate of complications increases significantly at this depth. Take care to anchor your hands in position whilst the LA is being injected: this will ensure that the volume is not misplaced.

The block may be performed below this level, nearer the clavicle. The plexus is even more superficial here and the anatomy is reliable.

Depth
15–25mm.

End-points
- Deltoid, upper arm or forearm twitch. If in doubt, palpate to ensure it is those muscles contracting.
- If the diaphragm is stimulated, then the needle is too anterior.
- If trapezius is stimulated the needle is too posterior.

LA volume
30 ml

Complications
Phrenic nerve block (**never** do bilateral blocks; caution in patients with respiratory disease); extradural/intrathecal injection; puncture/injection of vessels of the neck; Horner's syndrome; vagal or recurrent laryngeal nerve block; pneumothorax; local infection; LA toxicity.

Supraclavicular block (Figure 6.22)

Indications
Elbow, forearm, and hand surgery.

Process
This block is almost identical to a low interscalene block in terms of process, dose of LA, and associated risk profile. Depth: 15–40mm.

End-points
Wrist and finger flexion/extension.

LA volume
30–40 ml.

Axillary block (Figures 6.23 and 6.24)

Indications
Elbow, forearm, and hand surgery.

NB This often misses the musculocutaneous and intercostobrachial nerves which lie outside the axillary sheath. It may need supplementation for tourniquet pain or for the missed area of skin on the radial forearm.

Position
Supine with the arm at 90° at the shoulder and elbow. Excessive abduction stretches the brachial plexus, making it easier to injure.

Process
At the insertion of pectoralis major (anterior axillary fold) feel for axillary artery pulsation.

Transarterial Insert the needle towards pulsation until arterial flashback is seen. Transfix the artery. Half the local anaesthetic should be injected behind and half in front of the artery in 5ml boluses, with careful aspiration after each injection

Multiple injections Locate each nerve above and below the artery using nerve stimulation, landmarks, or ultrasound guidance.

Mnemonic: 'M and M are tops'.
- Musculocutaneous and medial nerves are above the artery.
- Radial is behind.
- Ulnar is below.

Intercostobrachial nerve block

The intercostobrachial can be blocked by subcutaneous injection across the base of the axilla. This is not consistently blocked with the axillary brachial plexus block because it leaves the brachial plexus sheath proximally. This nerve covers a large area, and if unblocked may lead to pain in the forearm and biceps. Specific blockade is necessary for complete anesthesia. A separate injection above the artery and towards the coracobrachial muscle should provoke twitches of the biceps with nerve stimulation. 5ml of LA is injected.

Depth
1–2cm.

End-points
- Median: index/middlefinger flexion
- Ulnar: thumb adduction or little finger flexion
- Radial: thumb extension
- Musculocutaneous: elbow flexion

LA volume
40–50ml.

Complications
- Vascular injection
- Nerve damage

Tips

With failure of motor response, carefully and methodically reposition the palpating hand 1cm posterior or anterior to the original position.

Failure to stimulate a motor response should prompt needle withdrawal and a reassessment of the landmarks.

Remember:

* The most common reason for failure to obtain brachial plexus stimulation is a needle insertion which is too anterior.
* Ensure that the nerve stimulator is functional and properly connected.

Increasing the current intensity by >1.0 mA causes patient discomfort and does not help to localize the brachial plexus

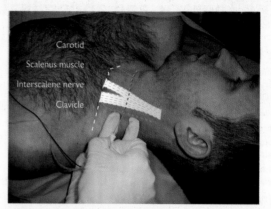

Fig. 6.21 Interscalene block.

Tips

Palpate the interscalene groove just above the clavicle; feel for the subclavian artery pulsation here. (NB: Only found in 50% of patients)

The brachial plexus crosses the clavicle at or near its mid-point. Because of the direction of the brachial plexus from medial to lateral as it descends, the higher in the supraclavicular area the more medial (closer to the SCM) the plexus is located.

Insert the needle into posterior part of the groove behind the artery.

With the needle lying against the neck and parallel to the midline, aim directly caudad toward ispilateral toe (do not angle medially).

The trunks descend in a steep downward direction, so increasing the distance laterally means that the needle might miss the plexus above the clavicle or miss the short trunks completely.

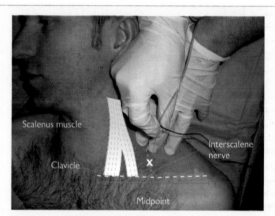

Fig. 6.22 Supraclavicular block.

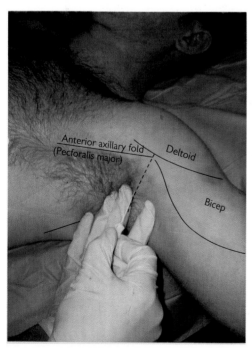

Fig. 6.23 Axillary block.

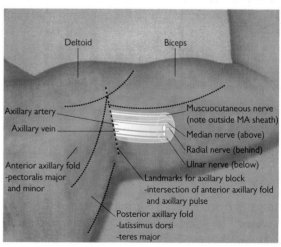

Fig. 6.24 Anatomy of the axilla.

The intercostal nerves

The intercostal nerves are formed as a continuation of the anterior primary rami of the spinal nerves of the thoracic segments T1–11 (T12 is called the subcostal nerve).

Supplies

- Sensory: skin over thorax, abdomen and medial upper arm.
- Motor: muscles of anterior abdominal wall (Figure 6.27) and intercostal spaces.

NB: Each nerve is also joined to a sympathetic ganglion by white and grey rami communicans.

The typical intercostal nerves (T3–6)

These nerves exit through the intervertebral foramen to lie initially between the posterior intercostal membrane and the pleura and then between the internal and innermost intercostal muscles.

They run as part of the neurovascular bundle in the intercostal groove under each rib (Figure 6.26). The nerve lies inferior to the artery and vein. They divide at the mid-axillary line to form a lateral and an anterior cutaneous branch (Figure 6.25).

The atypical intercostal nerves

1st This gives a large contribution to the brachial plexus, has no lateral cutaneous branch, and only a small anterior cutaneous branch.

2nd The lateral cutaneous branch is known as the intercostobrachial nerve and supplies the skin of the upper arm after crossing the axilla.

7th-11th These enter the abdominal wall between the diaphragm and transversus abdominis and penetrate the abdominal muscles to terminate in the overlying skin.

12th (subcostal) This passes behind the arcuate ligament, kidney, and colon to lie between transverses abdominis and internal oblique.

Dermatomes and levels for common operations

The block levels required for most operations can be worked out from the levels covered by the incision and the supply of tissues disrupted by surgery. Remember that although the parietal peritoneum is innervated in a dermatomal pattern, sensation from the viscera is conducted via afferent visceral fibres.

Laparotomy incisions can range from T6 to T12. Epidurals should be sited at T10–11 for lower abdominal procedures and T8–9 for upper abdominal procedures.

However, some operations need more extensive blocks than would initially be expected. Some common examples are:

- TURP: S4–T10 (urethra, prostate, and bladder neck S2–4; bladder T10–12)
- Testicular surgery: T10-S3 (sensory); L1–S3 (autonomic); T10–L4 (sympathetic); S1–S3 (parasympathetic)
- LSCS: S5–T4
- Labour: first stage T10–L1; second stage L1–S4.

Innervation of the inguinal region

The skin of the lower abdomen is supplied by L1 and L2 via the lumbar plexus together with a contribution from T12 (the subcostal nerve).

The iliohypogastric nerve (L1)

Course

It emerges from the lateral border of the psoas, pierces the internal oblique above and in front of ASIS, and runs deep to the external oblique, superior to the inguinal canal.

Supply

Sensation to suprapubic skin.

The ilio-ingunal nerve (L1)

Course

It arises from the lateral border of the psoas and lies below the internal oblique which it pierces before passing into the inguinal canal with the spermatic cord. It exits at the external inguinal ring.

Supplies

Sensory to skin of the upper thigh, root of penis/mons pubis, and scrotum/labia.

The genitofemoral nerve (L1,2)

Course

Emerges in front of psoas opposite L3–4, runs retroperitoneally down the psoas, and enters the thigh at the lateral end of the inguinal ligament. It divides above the inguinal ligament into genital and femoral branches.

The genital branch enters the inguinal canal via the deep inguinal ring.

The femoral branch passes below the inguinal ligament to enter the femoral sheath.

Supplies

Genital: cremaster and scrotal skin/ skin of mons and labia.

Femoral: skin over upper femoral triangle.

The inguinal canal

Represents the passage through the abdominal wall of the testis and the spermatic cord (or round ligament of the uterus). Lies above the inguinal ligament.

Components of the canal

Internal ring: the point at which the cord passes through the transversalis fascia.

External ring: the defect in the external oblique aponeurosis, site of exit of the cord from the canal.

Contents

- Spermatic cord (or round ligament)
- Ilio-inguinal nerve

Landmarks for suprapubic urinary and peritoneal lavage catheters

These are both inserted midline in the lower abdomen below the umbilicus.

For suprapubic urinary catheter insertion, first localize the bladder using ultrasound and then insert the catheter approximately 2cm above the symphisis pubis.

For diagnostic peritoneal lavage, first decompress the bladder and stomach with a urinary catheter and a gastric tube, respectively. The catheter should be inserted in the midline just below the umbilicus.

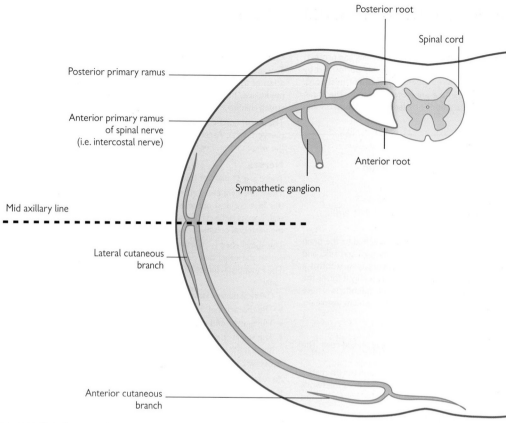

Fig. 6.25 Typical intercostal nerve.

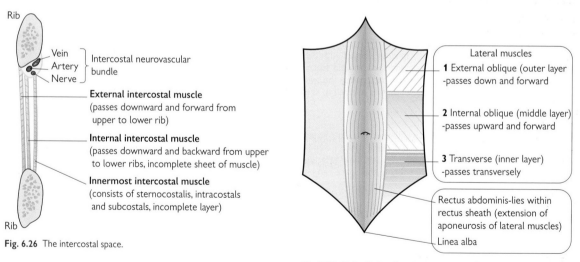

Fig. 6.26 The intercostal space.

Fig. 6.27 Abdominal wall anatomy.

6.11 The vertebral column

The vertebral column has a complex structure, containing and protecting the spinal cord. Neuraxial blockade is commonly performed by anaesthetists, and other procedures (such as facet joint injections, or lumbar drains) are also within the anaesthetist's remit. These can only be carried out safely with a sound knowledge of vertebral column anatomy.

Anatomy

Bones and ligaments of the vertebral column
See Figures 6.28 and 6.29

Meninges, subarachnoid and extradural spaces
The meninges envelop the central nervous system (Figure 6.30).

Pia mater
This is very delicate and is the innermost layer, attached to the brain and the spinal cord. It follows the contours of the gyri and sulci and cord, and it contains a network of capillaries. Posteriorly it forms a sheet (from the median sulcus) to meet the dura. Laterally it forms the ligamentum denticulatum and anteriorly the linea splendens. These also connect to the dura. Inferiorly it continues as the filum terminale, which pierces the dural sac to reach the coccyx.

Arachnoid mater
The arachnoid provides cushioning support for the brain and cord. The cord and brain arachnoid are continuous.

The subarachnoid space lies between the arachnoid and the pia mater, and contains the CSF. Within this space lies a delicate spongy network of connective tissue filaments that extend from the arachnoid and blend into the pia mater.

Dura mater
This is a thick and durable membrane. In the spinal canal, it is the extension of the inner layer of the cerebral dura: the outer cerebral layer terminates at the foramen magnum. It connects to the vertebral bodies of C2 and C3 and further along the canal to the posterior longitudinal ligaments via slender fibrous filaments. These filaments are often blamed for poor spread of epidural LA solutions.

The inner underside of the dura is usually in close contact with the thinner arachnoid, which overlies the brain and subarachnoid space. The arachnoid and the dura are easily separated, but because the two are so closely apposed, the interface between them is referred to as a potential space.

The extradural (epidural) space
Vertebral column dura mater (an extension of the cerebral inner layer) is fused with the foramen magnum. The extradural space extends down to the sacral hiatus and contains lymphatics, fat, small arteries, and a plexus of thin-walled veins. Nerve roots in this space can be anaesthetized with epidural techniques.

Cerebrospinal fluid and circulation
There is continuous circulation and absorption of CSF within the ventricles and the subarachnoid space.

The CSF is produced at 0.35ml/min (500ml/24hr) with a total volume of 150ml (it is replaced four times a day). CSF results from the filtration of plasma through fenestrated capillaries and active transport of water and dissolved substances through the epithelial cells of the blood–CSF barrier (choroid plexus) found in all ventricles. It escapes from the fourth ventricle via the median foramen of Magendie and the lateral foramina of Lushka.

Reabsorption of CSF takes place at the arachnoid villi and granulations of (primarily) the superior sagittal sinus. Reabsorption is determined by the difference between the CSF and the venous pressures.

Cord
The spinal cord begins superiorly at the foramen magnum as a continuation of the medulla oblongata. It terminates inferiorly at the conus medullaris. In the adult this corresponds to the L1 level and in the young child to the upper border of L3.

The spinal cord contains grey matter (nerve cells) and white matter (nerve fibres). Ascending and descending tracts are contained within the white matter. For further discussion see Sections 7.19, 7.20 and 7.24.

Nerves
There are 31 pairs of spinal nerves.

There are eight cervical nerves, although only seven cervical vertebrae: the first cervical nerve exits between the occiput and C1, and the eighth exits between C7 and T1. Subsequently each spinal nerve exits the vertebral column below its corresponding vertebra.

The spinal cord is shorter than the column, so spinal nerves descend within the canal before exiting through their intervertebral foramen. The most distal lumbar and sacral nerves travel the furthest within the canal.

- Cervical nerves leave the cord within the cervical region.
- The thoracic nerves leave the cord between T1 and T10.
- The lumbar and sacral nerves leave the cord between T11 and T12.
- The spinal cord ends around the level of the disc between T12 and L1.
- Below L1 the nerves are known as the cauda equina.

As each spinal nerve passes through the intervertebral foramen, it takes on a dural sleeve.

Blood supply
The posterior spinal arteries are derived from the posterior inferior cerebellar arteries and the anterior spinal artery from the vertebral artery (Figure 6.31).

The one anterior and two posterior spinal arteries anastomose and are assisted by segmental arteries that enter the canal through the intervertebral foramina. Segmental arteries are formed from:

- Radicular branches of the vertebral artery in the cervical region
- Radicular branches from the aorta in the thorax
- The radicularis magna (artery of Adamkiewicz) in the lumbar region.

The radicular branches are derived from the posterior intercostals that form directly from the aorta.

The anterior spinal artery lies on the anterior median fissure and supplies the anterior two thirds of the spinal cord.

Venous drainage is via anterior and posterior venous plexuses which drain along the nerve roots into segmental veins.

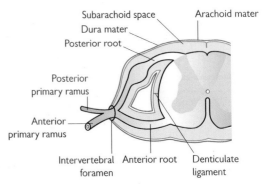

Fig. 6.30 Meningeal layers within the spinal canal

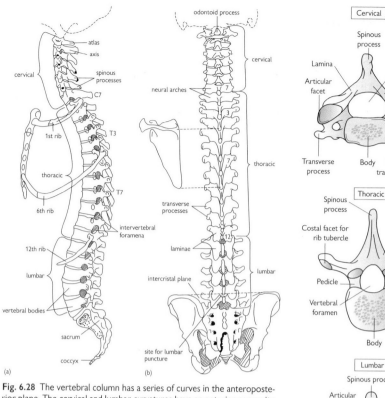

Fig. 6.28 The vertebral column has a series of curves in the anteroposterior plane. The cervical and lumbar curvatures have an anterior convexity (lordosis), and the thoracic and sacral curvatures have a posterior convexity (kyphosis). These curvatures influence the spread of local anaesthetic solutions according to their baricity.

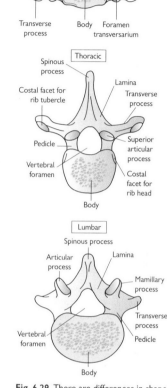

Fig. 6.29 There are differences in shape between vertebrae of the cervical, thoracic and lumbar regions. Furthermore, C1 and C2 are distinctly shaped, reflecting their specific functions.

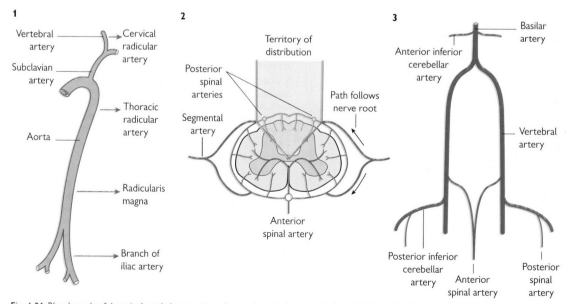

Fig. 6.31 Blood supply of the spinal cord: the anterior and posterior spinal arteries lie beneath the arachnoid mater. 21 pairs of segmental radicular arteries supply the nerve roots, and half of these contribute to the spinal arteries. The largest of these branches is the radicularis magna

6.12 Neuraxial blockade

Injection of small amounts of local anaesthesic into the cerebrospinal fluid (CSF) produces spinal anaesthesia. The injection is usually made below the level at which the spinal cord ends (L2). It is relatively easy to perform and provides excellent conditions for surgery below the umbilicus.

Epidural anaesthesia involves introducing local anaesthetic into the extradural space where it acts on the nerve roots. It is versatile and can be used for surgery, obstetrics and pain management.

Both can be used as the sole technique, the analgesic adjuvant to general anaesthesia, and for postoperative pain control in procedures from the chest to the lower limb. Use of local anaesthetic (LA) increases the potential for systemic side effects.

Advantages

- Patient satisfaction. The majority of patients are very happy with the technique and appreciate the rapid recovery and relative lack of side effects.
- Cost. In comparison, drugs and equipment for GA are expensive.
- The airway remains patent and the reflexes remain intact. There is less risk of loss of airway and aspiration.
- It affects the respiratory system much less and so is useful for the patient with respiratory dysfunction.
- There is less bleeding than with general anaesthesia. This is due to the lower BP and reduced vessel transmural pressure gradient.
- Splanchnic blood flow is increased, and this is thought to promote GI anastomotic healing.
- There is unopposed parasympathetic action. The vagus supplies the gut as far as the transverse colon and produces gut constriction with increased peristaltic activity.
- For diabetic patients there is a lower risk of unidentified hypoglycaemia and rapid return to normal food intake and drug regimens.
- There is outstanding muscle relaxation for lower abdominal and lower limb surgery.
- Postoperative DVT and PE are less common because of vasodilatation and improved local blood flow.
- It produces excellent perioperative pain relief that may be continued postoperatively.

Disadvantages

- It is not suitable for all types of surgery, e.g. head and neck.
- It may be technically difficult and sometimes impossible.
- Some patients are not psychologically suited to being awake during an operation.
- It often produces hypotension, which may adversely affect those with cardiovascular disease.
- There is a (small) risk of neuraxial infection.

Contraindications to neuraxial blockade

Most of these also apply to other forms of regional anaesthesia.

Patients may be apprehensive and initially state a preference for general anaesthesia, and refusal is an absolute contraindication. However, after a thorough explanation and discussion about the block, many agree to undergo blockade.

Patients with an abnormal clotting mechanism are at risk of developing a local haematoma that could compress the spinal cord. Those with abnormal tests of clotting function, a low platelet count, or patients with liver disease or receiving anticoagulant therapy are at risk.

Patients must be adequately volume resuscitated prior to performing neuraxial blockade. Sympathetic blockade invalidates the responses to hypovolaemia, producing catastrophic hypotension. Similarly, patients with fixed cardiac output states (aortic stenosis, hypertrophic obstructive cardiomyopathy, mitral stenosis, and complete heart block) cannot alter their cardiac output in response to vasodilatation, and sympathetic block might precipitate cardiovascular collapse.

Sepsis near the site of injection may allow infection into the epidural or subarachnoid space. The risk of a spinal or epidural abscess is also increased when the block is performed in a septicaemic patient.

Anatomical abnormalities might render the procedure impossible. Ankylosing spondylitis results in a calcified spinal column which prevents needle penetration of the appropriate space.

Active neurological disease is a relative contraindication. Careful assessment of the condition prior to the procedure is essential and clear documentation of the neurological deficit should be noted. In this way, alleged deterioration of neurological function following the block can be assessed objectively.

Raised intracranial pressure is an absolute contraindication as dural puncture could precipitate coning. Loss of CSF from the sub-arachnoid space lowers vertebral column CSF pressure and increases the gradient across the foramen magnum, precipitating movement of the brainstem.

Approach to neuraxial blockade

Preoperatively

Just like a general anaesthetic it is essential to visit the patient preoperatively, obtain a history, perform an examination, and consider what tests need to be done. Consent should be obtained following a full discussion about the pros and cons of the technique.

- Special consideration should be given to the cardiovascular status: a fixed cardiac output means that hypotension is likely.
- Examination of the back is important to determine conditions that would preclude a successful procedure.
- Clinical suspicion of coagulopathy mandates laboratory investigation.

In theatre

All anaesthetic equipment should be present and in good working order. Full resuscitation equipment should be checked and immediately available, and the presence of a trained assistant is essential. Standard monitoring (as a minimum) should be applied to the patient.

A large-bore IV cannula should be inserted and warmed fluids given through a blood giving set. The patient should be made as comfortable as possible.

Positioning the patient

Neuraxial blockade is most easily performed when there is maximum anterior flexion of the lumbar vertebrae.

This is best achieved with the patient sitting on the operating table resting their feet on a stool. With two pillows on their lap they can rest their forearms on their thighs and maintain a stable and comfortable position (Figure 6.32).

Alternatively, the procedure can be performed with the patient lying on their side with their hips and knees flexed (Figure 6.33). Using an assistant to help maintain either patient position is useful.

The anatomical landmarks for these procedures are important and contribute to the performance of a safe and successful block. Tuffier's line is an anatomical landmark which joins the two posterior superior iliac spines. This line passes through the body of the fourth lumbar vertebra. This forms the most common landmark to identify L3–4 and therefore any other interspace. The spinous processes demonstrate the midline.

The midline approach

This is the most commonly used technique (Figure 6.34). It is very important to identify the midline, otherwise problems will occur:

- Hitting a bony surface. This will be the lamina, the facet joint, or the spinous process. If it is the lamina, redirect to the midline. If it is the spinous process, point the needle either caudad (towards the tail) or cephalad (towards the head).
- Failure of identification of the ligamentum flavum. The needle tip is likely to be too lateral, missing the ligamentum flavum and the subarachnoid space. So remember: stay in the midline!

The paramedian technique (Figures 6.35, 6.36, and 6.37)

This is usually employed when the midline approach is unsuccessful. Clues that predict a difficult spinal are:

- Patients who are unable to flex the vertebral column.
- The elderly, where the interspinous muscle and ligaments have become calcified. It may be difficult to advance the thin spinal needle through these abnormal tissue layers.

How to perform paramedian needle insertion

The spinous process below the intended space is identified and the needle introduced 2cm paramedian to this. The needle should be directed slightly medial and cephalad. It will enter the ligamentum flavum, identified by its typically 'gripping' nature. If bone is encountered, the needle should be directed slightly more cephalad and walked off the laminae until the ligamentum flavum is found. The epidural or subarachnoid spaces can then be identified as for the midline approach.

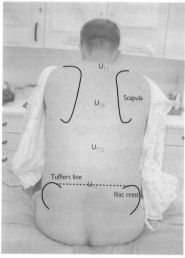

Fig. 6.32 Posterior view of the surface anatomy of the vertebral column

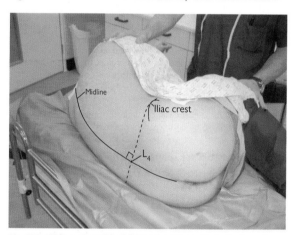

Fig. 6.33 Oblique view of the left lateral position with the lumbar spine convex posteriorly.

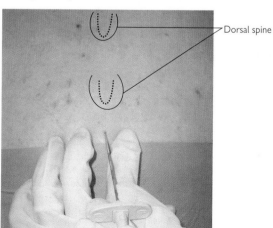

Fig. 6.34 Midline approach for neuraxial blockade

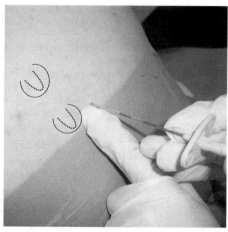

Fig. 6.35 Paramedian approach, starting at the skin surface lateral to the dorsal spine. As for the midline approach, this may be used for both epidural and SAB techniques.

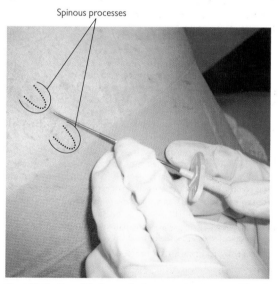

Fig. 6.36 Position of Tuohy needle demonstrating direction of insertion towards the midline and cephalad

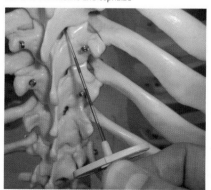

Fig. 6.37 Photograph of a Tuohy needle entering the epidural space having been walked off the lamina below

6.13 Sub-arachnoid blockade (SAB)

Appreciation of the patient's bony anatomy is important and appropriate spatial orientation will aid insertion.

Indications for SAB

Surgery above the umbilicus is accompanied by unpleasant visceral sensations that limit the acceptability of sole subarachnoid anaesthesia. However, it is good for the following:

- Urology: remember to ensure a block of at least T10 for operations that involve fluid distension of the bladder.
- Gynaecological surgery: open surgery that involves the peritoneum mandates blockade to at least T6.
- Obstetrics.
- Surgical procedures on the perineum and lower limb. This is useful for those with diabetes or significant respiratory disease.

Performing sub-arachnoid blockade

Position the patient, identify the desired interspinous space, and mark it with pen. Allow the patient to relax whilst you prepare.

Sterility is important: scrub, gown, and glove up carefully. The equipment should be checked on a sterile surface and the labels of injection substances should be reviewed with a trained assistant. Ensure sterile technique.

All intrathecal drugs should be aspirated with a filter needle. Draw up local anaesthesia for skin infiltration and neuraxial blockade. The use of different size syringes is a good way to differentiate between drugs.

Re-position the patient and clean their back with antiseptic solution. Repeat and allow the solution to dry. Remember to communicate with the patient at every stage.

Infiltrate the skin with local anaesthetic, using a 25G needle. Insert the introducer as far as the ligamentum flavum and take care not to puncture the dura. Insert the spinal needle through the introducer and advance slowly. Ensure the stylet is in place in order to prevent blockage with tissue or clot. It is imperative that the needle is kept in the midline and angled slightly cephalad. Otherwise, bony surfaces will distort the course of the needle.

There will be increased resistance as the needle enters the ligamentum flavum. There is a loss of resistance on reaching the epidural space, followed by another as the dura is pierced. CSF should flow when the stylet is removed. When CSF appears, take care not to alter the position of the needle as you attach the syringe (containing the solution for intrathecal injection). The needle is best stabilized by placing your non-dominant hand firmly against the patient's back and holding the hub of the spinal needle between the thumb and index finger.

Aspirate gently to ensure that the needle is still within the sub-arachnoid space and inject slowly. There should be no loss of solution during injection. Hyperbaric solutions are viscous, so there is often a little resistance to injection. This is especially apparent with the very fine gauge needles used for sub-arachnoid blockade.

When injection is complete, withdraw the needle syringe and introducer as one and apply dressing. Place the patient into the appropriate position and monitor closely.

Assessing the block

Some patients find describing sensation difficult. However, their clinical signs are very useful. If the patient cannot lift their legs the block is at least mid-lumbar.

Do not test for pain with sharp needles. Pain sensation travels in the same pathways as temperature appreciation, which may be assessed using ice or a swab soaked in alcohol.

- First, test in an unblocked area so that the patient appreciates normal sensation.
- Work up the body until the same sensation is produced, and document level of block. Repeat for both sides of the body.

A differential blockade will be produced. Sympathetic fibres are blocked for two segments above the sensory level and signs of motor blockade will be seen a few segments below it.

Factors affecting spread

A number of factors determine the extent of spread of local anaesthetic within the CSF:

- Baricity of LA solution, influenced by gravity.
- Position of the patient and spinal curvature.
- Concentration and volume of solution injected. Density of the block depends on the concentration of local anaesthetic used. Low-concentration solutions will tend to produce sensory blocks and higher concentrations will produce more motor blockade
- Larger volumes will produce a block over large areas and small volumes less so.
- Level of injection.
- Speed of injection. Slow injection will give predictable spread, whereas fast injections will produce eddy currents within the CSF with unpredictable spread.
- Direction of bevel. Anaesthetic will flow away from the bevel.
- Volume of the epidural space. The epidural space is congested with dilated epidural veins during pregnancy and similarly crowded with fat deposits in the obese. These conditions produce compression on the sub-arachnoid space and reduction in volume of the CSF. A given quantity of local anaesthetic solution will in theory spread further.
- When a patient is lying on their side the spinal cord is rarely truly horizontal. Male shoulders tend be to wider than their hips; therefore the spinal cord lies slightly head up. Female shoulders tend to be narrower than their hips; therefore the spinal cord lies slightly head down. These two factors will obviously affect spread; manipulation of the patient's bed will correct these variations.

Intrathecal local anaesthetic can continue to spread for up 15–20min after the injection, so modifying patient position will affect the level of blockade.

Local anaesthetics for spinal anaesthesia

Vials must be checked to make sure that they are preservative-free.

Hyperbaric solutions produce the most controlled blocks. These solutions are made by adding 7.5% dextrose to the local anaesthetic. Local anaesthetics are either heavier than (hyperbaric), lighter than (hypobaric), or have the same specific gravity as (isobaric) the CSF. Hyperbaric solutions tend to spread down (due to gravity) from the level of injection. Gravity has no influence on isobaric solutions. It is easier to predict the spread of hyperbaric solutions.

Bupivacaine (Marcain)

Hyperbaric 0.5% bupivicaine is the most commonly used agent, although plain is also used. Bupivicaine lasts longer than other LAs used (about 2–3hr).

Lidocaine (lignocaine) (Xylocaine)

Various concentrations are used, but the best results are with 5% heavy lidocaine. The duration of block is 45–90min. 2% lidocaine has a shorter duration of action.

Ropivacaine (Naropin)

A recently introduced long-acting agent. It is not currently licensed for intrathecal injection.

Pethidine

Has been used to provide spinal anaesthesia because of its local anaesthetic properties.

Special spinal anaesthesia techniques

Continuous spinal anaesthesia (CSA) is a method of producing and maintaining spinal anaesthesia. An initial injection of local anaesthetic into the subarachnoid space is followed by the placement of a catheter. SAB can be maintained with the addition of small doses of local anaesthetic via the catheter. The gauge of catheter may vary between 18G and 32G; however, most success is seen with a 20G catheter.

Advantages of this technique include duration of block and fewer cardiovascular problems (since the dose is titrated to the required level). Disadvantages include post-dural puncture headache (PDPH), risk of infection, and cauda equina syndrome.

Combined spinal epidural (CSE) anaesthesia is a regional technique that has the advantages of both spinal and epidural. It has a rapid onset and dense predictable block that lasts for a long time, providing continuous postoperative pain relief.

The needle-through-needle technique involves the identification of the epidural space as previously described. Once achieved, a long fine bore spinal needle (typically 25–27G) is passed through the Tuohy needle. The dura is punctured and an appropriate dose of local anaesthetic injected into the subarachnoid space. This needle is then withdrawn and the epidural catheter placed via the Tuohy needle in the conventional manner.

The technique carries the contraindications and complications of both individual procedures.

⊕ Different block heights

Mid-thoracic block

Produces a block to T4–T6. The patient should lie down immediately after lumbar puncture. 2.5–3ml of solution are needed.

Lumbar block

Produces a block to T10–T12. 2.0–2.5ml of solution are used.

Saddle block

Produces analgesia to S1. The patient is required to sit for 5min. 1ml of hyperbaric solution is all that is required.

Unilateral block

Small volumes of hyperbaric solution produce a block of variable height on the dependent side. True unilateral block is rare.

→ Types of spinal needle

Standard spinal needles are usually 25G and 90mm long. The length is suitable for most adult patients, although longer needles may be required for obese patients or for the combined spinal epidural technique.

Quincke tip needles tend to cut the longitudinal fibres of the dura. The conical or elliptical tip is associated with a lower incidence of PDPH.

Pencil-point needles separate the fibres. They provide a better feel and allow ease of identification of the anatomical layers encountered during insertion.

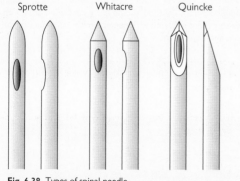

Sprotte   Whitacre   Quincke

Fig. 6.38 Types of spinal needle.

→ Equipment for neuraxial blockade

All equipment should be assembled in sterile conditions and checked prior to procedure (Figure 6.39). Sterile packs allow the skin to be cleaned, draped, and infiltrated with local anaesthesia. The type of dressing and method of taping the catheter in place are a matter of personal preference.

Modern epidural kits are pre-packed and usually contain:

- Modern plastic syringes with very low resistance for detection of the epidural space
- Catheters made of flexible plastic with a number of side holes at distal end
- Filter and Luer-lock catheter connection.

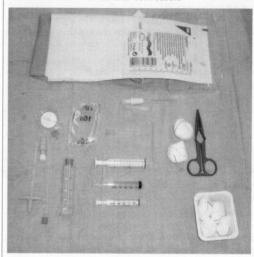

Fig. 6.39 Equipment for neuraxial blockade.

→ What anatomical layers do you encounter during SAB?

The layers are shown in Figure 6.40.

- Skin.
- Subcutaneous fat of variable thickness. May cause difficulty in identifying the interspinous space.
- Supraspinous ligament: C7 to sacrum. Joins tip of spinous processes together.
- Interspinous ligaments. Broad flat ligament running between the spinous processes.
- Ligamentum flavum. Thick (up to 1cm in midline) and mostly composed of elastic tissue. Runs vertically from lamina to lamina. Distinctive feeling when needle in ligament (gripped, gritty). Loss of resistance as needle leaves to enter epidural space.
- Epidural space. Contains fat, blood vessels, lymphatics, and nerve roots.
- The dura. Loss of resistance is felt as a 'click' as the needle pierces dura.
- Subarachnoid space. Contains spinal cord and nerve roots bathed within CSF.

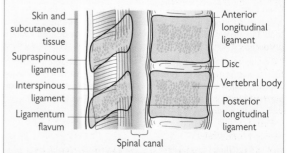

Skin and subcutaneous tissue — Anterior longitudinal ligament

Supraspinous ligament — Disc

Interspinous ligament — Vertebral body

Ligamentum flavum — Posterior longitudinal ligament

Spinal canal

Fig. 6.40 Anatomy encountered during sub-arachnoid blockade.

6.14 Epidural anaesthesia

Indications for epidural blockade

Epidural blockade is used either as the sole technique or as an adjunct to general anaesthesia for operations below the neck. It is also used as a method of pain relief postoperatively and in labour.

Procedure

The preliminary procedures are the same as for spinal anaesthesia and, again, the block is performed as a sterile technique.

There are various techniques for identifying the epidural space, which lies between the ligamentum flavum and dura. The space is very small and has to be identified immediately upon entry of the needle. Today, the majority of practitioners use the loss-of-resistance (LOR) method (to either saline or air).

As with spinal blockade, epidural blockade can be performed with the patient sitting or lying on their side. Again, there should be strict asepsis for the procedure.

The skin and deeper structures should be anaesthetized with LA as the Tuohy needle is large and can cause discomfort. The needle should be inserted and advanced through the supra- and interspinous ligaments in the midline with the bevel pointing cephalad. The ligamentum flavum will be identified by a gritty sensation of resistance. At this point remove stylet and connect the loss of resistance (LOR) syringe containing 5–10ml of sterile saline or air.

The needle should be stabilized by your non-dominant hand. Apply constant pressure on the plunger of the LOR syringe with your dominant thumb or thenar eminence. Advance the needle until the saline is injected easily; at this point the tip of the needle will be within the epidural space. Note the depth of the space from the markings on the Tuohy needle.

Removed the syringe and insert the catheter to the appropriate length. The catheter should pass freely and without obstruction; forcing it can result in dural puncture by the catheter itself. Knowing the depth of the space and the length of the Tuohy needle allows you to calculate the position of the catheter at the skin which results in 4cm of it remaining in the epidural space.

Remember to exclude intravascular and subarachnoid catheter placement. Neither blood nor CSF should flow back or be aspirated from the catheter in its final position. If this happens, repeat the procedure at another disc space.

Dress the device and secure carefully.

Test dose

This is typically 3ml 0.5% bupivicaine with adrenaline 1:200,000. This test is used to exclude catheter misplacement. Large volumes of local anaesthetic given intrathecally or IV may be catastrophic.

- Intrathecal catheter insertion would result in spinal anaesthesia. This might not be appreciated if the patient is concurrently undergoing general anaesthesia.
- If the catheter tip lies within an epidural vein, injection of the adrenaline bolus would cause an increase in heart rate. This will be appreciated even with an asleep patient. However, this is a non-specific sign.

Main dose

This is given after a negative test dose. Intermittent boluses of 5ml of local anaesthetic solution are administered until the desired effect is produced.

Maintanence of analgesia may be achieved with continuous infusion of local anaesthestic agents. Breakthrough pain is most quickly relieved with intermittent boluses, titrated to effect. Patient-controlled boluses and continuous infusion provide good quality analgesia.

Factors affecting spread

- Age. The narrower epidural space of increasing age increases vertical spread in the elderly.
- Site of injection. Volumes administered in the thorax produce a larger spread than in the lumbar region. This is due to the smaller calibre of the thoracic spinal canal.
- Body weight. Epidural fat reduces the room available for exogenous fluids causing larger spread of given LA volumes. Pregnancy causes dilatation of the epidural veins, with a similar effect.
- Height. Taller patients require larger volumes for the same effect.
- Baricity is not an important factor.

In general, 1–2ml of LA are required per segment to be blocked. Loss through the foramina limits vertical spread.

Spread and duration of block

Local anaesthetic agents

Epidural anaesthesia produces a band of segmental anaesthesia spreading both cephalad and caudally from the point of injection. It has a slower onset (15min) and is not as dense as spinal anaesthesia. The maximum effect is not seen for up to 45min.

LA concentration determines the block density. The extent of the block is determined by the the volume of LA solution.

Higher concentrations of LA increase the speed of onset and duration of blockade. The addition of adrenaline to the LA solution potentiates this since it reduces systemic absorption of the LA and maintains a higher concentration gradient for diffusion into nerve cells. Choice of drug, concentration, volume, and additives such as opioids depends on the indication.

Opioids

Epidural administration of opioids is common. They work in synergy with local anaesthetics, acting directly on opioid receptors on the spinal cord and CNS. Commonly used opioids include morphine, fentanyl, and diamorphine.

A low concentration of opioid and LA has been shown to be very successful in managing postoperative and labour pain. This combination can be administered by either slow infusion or intermittent boluses.

Opioids in the epidural space cause systemic effects such as respiratory depression and pruritis. The concentration of opioid should be reduced in patients with respiratory disease; these patients and those susceptible to the effects of opioids might be better off with only local anaesthetic epidural solutions.

Morphine can cause delayed respiratory depression. Its low lipid solubility means that although some binds to receptors in the spinal cord, some will remain in solution in the CSF. Circulation within the CSF transports this to the brainstem causing respiratory depression. This can happen up to 24hr after administration.

Because all opioids can cause respiratory depression, all patients with an opioid epidural infusion should be nursed in an area with a high nurse-to-patient ratio and with nurses familiar with epidurals and their actions and side effects.

➜ Epidural needle

The Tuohy needle (Figure 6.41), introduced in 1945, is the most commonly used epidural needle. It is made as 16G or 18G and is a standard 80mm long with markings at 1cm intervals along its length. Longer needles are available for procedures in the obese.

It has a blunt Huber tip which has a 15°–30° curve. This blunt tip helps push the dura away, 'tenting' it after the ligamentum flavum has been pierced.

Wings are attached at junction of the needle and hub to enable close control of the needle as it is advanced.

The associated epidural catheters are usually 18G or 20G.

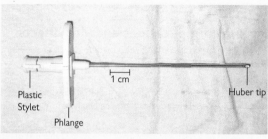

Fig. 6.41 Epidural needle.

➜ The sacrum

The sacrum (Figure 6.42) is wedge-shaped and concave anterior. It consists of five fused vertebrae, the arches of which form the roof of the sacral canal. The last laminar arch is missing, resulting in the sacral hiatus, with the deficient laminae known as the cornua. The hiatus is covered by the sacro-coccygeal ligamant The posterior sacral foramina are continuous with the extradural space of the canal.

The coccyx is formed by four rudimentary vertebrae. Its tip lies 5cm below the sacral hiatus.

Dose

The average volume of the sacral canal is 30–35ml. The dose for caudal anaesthesia is 20–30ml of 0.25–0.5% bupivicaine in young adults. This can be reduced in the elderly.

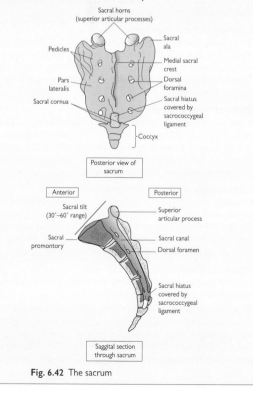

Fig. 6.42 The sacrum

✚ Caudal anaesthesia

Caudal anaesthesia is produced by the injection of LA (with or without adjuncts) into the extradural space through the sacral hiatus. It is easily performed but has a high failure rate because of the variations in the anatomy of the sacrum. It produces anaesthesia of the sacral and coccygeal nerve roots. Injection of large volumes of LA produces higher blocks but, again because of variations in anatomy, block height is unpredictable.

It is useful as an adjunct to general anaesthesia and for the provision of postoperative analgesia. It is very useful method of providing regional anaesthesia in children. The anatomical end-points are easier to identify in children and so it is very easy to perform and has a much higher success rate. By altering the volume, the block can be extended over a much wider anatomical area including up to the umbilicus. The greater spread in children is put down to the lower density of their epidural fat.

Complications

These are the same as for epidural anaesthesia but they are much less common. However, there are some rare reported complications such as insertion of needle into the rectum or the presenting part of the fetus during delivery.

Technique

Performed with the patient in the lateral position with the knees drawn up to the chest. The sacral hiatus is identified by drawing an equilateral triangle from the posterior superior iliac spines. The sacral cornua can be felt either side of the hiatus. See Figure 6.43.

Using an aseptic technique a 19-21G needle is directed in a slightly cranial direction through the hiatus. A click or loss of resistance is felt when the canal is entered and then the needle can be directed more cranially around 2cm. Further insertion may lead to dural puncture; the dura usually ends at S2.

After careful aspiration to make sure neither blood nor CSF can be aspirated, the local anaesthetic is injected. There should be no resistance. Resistance or pain on injection suggests that the needle tip is under the periosteum of the anterior wall of the canal.

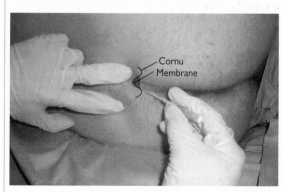

Fig. 6.43 Caudal block

6.15 Complications of SAB and epidural

SAB

Problems with the block

If the patient still has full motor function after 10min, the block has failed and the injection could not have been intrathecal.

Occasionally, a one-sided block is produced. With hyperbaric solutions, turn the patient onto the non-blocked side and tilt slightly head down. With an isobaric or hypobaric solution turn the patient onto the blocked side. These manoeuvres will increase the spread of solution to the unaffected side and improve symmetry.

Sometimes the resulting block is too low. With hyperbaric solutions, tilt the patient head down; the local anaesthetic will ascend the lumbar curvature. This effect is amplified by flattening the lordosis with a pillow under the knees. If isobaric solutions have been used, block height can be improved by turning the patient prone.

Do not put the patient head up if the block is too high.

Hypotension

This is the most common complication. It is the result of sympathetic blockade with vasodilatation and venous pooling below the level of the block. Less venous return reduces cardiac output and blood pressure. Compensatory tachycardia is common with blocks below T2. Nausea and vomiting are usually associated with hypotension.

The degree of hypotension depends on the extent of the sympathetic blockade, the intravascular volume, and the general cardiovascular reserve of the patient. Preloading with 250–500ml of fluid is beneficial. It allows venous return and cardiac output to be maintained.

Further hypotension can be treated with judicious use of vasoconstrictors and further fluid boluses. α_1-agonists cause peripheral vasoconstriction and maintain blood pressure. 0.5–1.0mg aliquots of metaraminol are commonly used.

Bradycardia

If sympathetic blockade reaches T2, cardio-accelerator fibres cannot oppose the action of the vagus nerve. The extent of the bradycardia is usually moderate and only 10–15% below baseline. However, severe braycardia and asystole have been reported.

Early recognition and prompt treatment are essential: consider a muscarinic antagonist, e.g. atropine.

Neurological conditions

Although not common, these are usually due to direct injury of a spinal nerve or the cord itself. They can be the result of physical damage from the needle or intraneural injection of local anaesthetic. Occasionally they are due to injection of inappropriate drugs or chemicals.

Damage of an epidural vein can lead to haematoma formation with subsequent spinal cord compression. This may not become evident until the block has worn off, which makes early detection and treatment (urgent decompression) more difficult.

Anterior spinal artery syndrome is not a form of direct nerve injury, but is most commonly seen in elderly patients following prolonged periods of hypotension. The syndrome is due to infarction of the spinal cord as a result of anterior spinal artery insufficiency. The clinical signs are predictable with knowledge of the anatomy of the spinal cord. It results in lower motor neuron signs at the level of injury. Below this level there will be spastic paraplegia with reduced temperature and pain sensation. However, since the posterior spinal artery remains unaffected, light touch, propioception, and vibration sensation will be preserved.

Backache

This is seen in up to 40% of patients following SAB but is also encountered in those who undergo general anaesthesia. It results from stretching of the ligaments of the anaesthetized vertebral column and responds to rest and simple analgesics.

Hearing loss

CSF leak reduces intracranial pressure and produces traction of the cranial nerves. It is self-limiting.

Infection

CNS infection associated with SAB is rare. Bacteraemic patients are at greater risk, although evaluation should be on an individual basis.

Urinary retention

Sacral autonomic fibres are the last to recover from blockade, leading to painful retention. Catheterization might be required.

Epidural complications and side effects

These are similar to those of SAB although they may occur significantly later, once continuous infusions are running.

Hypotension

This is especially common in pregnancy and requires prompt treatment with fluid and vasopressors. It may be heralded by nausea.

High block

This is caused by a relatively excessively large dose (Table 6.1) of local anaesthetic. It may present with hypotension, nausea, high sensory loss, high motor blockade, and weak hands. Difficulties in talking and breathing, and drowsiness, are also signs that should signify concern. Management is similar to that for total spinal (Section 19.8).

Total spinal

This occurs with inadvertent epidural needle placement or catheter migration into the subarachnoid space. Symptoms, signs, and treatments are similar to those for high block.

Local anaesthetic toxicity

This may be associated with large doses of LA. It is also caused by injection of LA into an epidural vein (it is vital to aspirate the catheter before use). Symptoms of toxicity include light-headedness, tinnitus, circumoral tingling, anxiety, confusion, tremor, convulsions, coma, and cardiorespiratory arrest. If recognized early, administration of the LA can be stopped. The treatment of established symptoms and signs is supportive. Cardiac arrest should be treated with intravenous lipid emulsion in addition to advanced life support.

Accidental dural puncture

This is easily recognized by immediate loss of CSF through epidural needle. It is seen in 1–2% of epidurals and the rate of complication is inversely related to the experience of the operator. It causes PDPH. Conservative management usually suffices, but occasionally blood patching is required.

Epidural haematoma

A rare but potentially catastrophic complication potentiated by bleeding diatheses. Bleeding from epidural veins can lead to the rapid development of a haematoma with compression of the spinal cord and nerves. The signs are often recognized postoperatively and late treatment is associated with poor outcome.

Local infection

A rare but again potentially catastrophic complication. Epidural abscess is a cause of spinal cord compression. A high index of suspicion is required since diagnosing cord compression in a patient with neuraxial blockade is difficult; signs of systemic illness or infection may be the only clue. Urgent surgical decompression is required.

Failure of block

Incorrect placement of the catheter the most common problem and related to the experience of anaesthetist.

Missed segments (dermatomes that remain unblocked) are not fully understood, but are most likely due to anatomical variations of epidural space. Unilateral blocks may develop because of the presence of a septum within the epidural space. Positioning the patient onto the missed side can sometimes improve spread, resulting in bilateral anaesthesia.

→ Post-dural puncture headache

- Due to CSF leak through dural puncture site with stretching of meninges.
- It is more severe when head up; pain is relieved by lying down
- Incidence 0.5–1%.
- Females > males.
- Young > old.
- Seen more frequently in pregnancy.
- Pencil-point needles reduce incidence significantly.
- Treatment: supportive or with a blood patch.
- Conservative; bed rest, oral or IV fluids. Sumatriptan, a migraine treatment that affects brain serotonin levels, may be useful. Abdominal binders increase venous pressure and reduce reabsorption of CSF. Hydration with caffeine solutions stimulates production of CSF.

✚ Blood patch

Should usually be performed only after at least 24hr of conservative treatment. One patch is 90% effective.

This is a two-person procedure and both should be gowned and gloved and employ strict aseptic technique. 15–20ml of autologous blood is injected into the epidural space at the same site above or below that of the dural puncture.

Once the epidural space has been identified, blood is taken from a peripheral vein. This should be passed in a sterile manner to the person performing the epidural. The blood is then injected into the epidural space. Pain may limit the amount injected. The needle should be flushed with a small amount of sterile saline as it is withdrawn. This ensures that the clot is separate from the skin and reduces its chances of contamination and subsequent epidural infection.

The blood is thought to seal the dura and prevent further leak, allowing recovery from headache. Relief has been reported immediately, but usually comes within 24hr. Repeat patching can be performed.

Complications of blood patching include pyrexia, root pain, backache, neck ache, tinnitus, and vertigo. However, these are rare.

✚ Post-operative care following neuraxial blockade

Following their operation the patient is admitted to the recovery unit. Before discharge from recovery the block level must be assessed. If it is persistently high, the patient must remain in recovery until block has reduced to an appropriate level and they have been seen by an anaesthetist.

Persistent hypotension requires anaesthetic assessment. Again, treatment is again aimed at improving venous return and cardiac output. Lifting the legs reduces venous pooling. IV fluids and vasoconstrictors might also be required.

Patients should be told to remain in bed until full power and sensation have returned to both legs. They should be assessed prior to mobilization. They should be monitored the same way as all post anaesthetic patients: respiration, pulse, blood pressure, sedation score, and pain score. Assessment of nausea and whether or not the patient is able to pass urine should be made.

IV access should be maintained until full recovery from the block.

Safe transfer of the patient from recovery to the ward

There should be individual hospital guidelines for the safe transfer and management of patients with epidurals to the postoperative ward.

- Nursing staff managing the epidural must have appropriate training and clinical skills to provide safe care.
- All epidural catheters must be inserted under aseptic conditions.
- The epidural programme is initiated by the anaesthetist and any future alteration should be done by appropriate staff such as an anaesthetist or acute pain team.
- IV access must be maintained for the duration of the epidural.
- Monitoring of RR, HR, BP, sedation score, pain assessment, nausea and vomiting, and motor function is essential.
- Monitoring should be recorded at 15min intervals for the first 2hr, 30min intervals for the next 2hr then every 1–2 hr thereafter.
- Integrity of the insertion point should be checked twice daily.
- Type of solution and running total should be recorded.
- Pressure points must be checked and degree of motor block assessed: a pressure-relieving mattress may be required.
- The acute pain team should assess the patient daily and wean them from the epidural appropriately.

Table 6.1 Considerations for epidural blockade for different types of surgery					
	Labour	LSCS	Hip/knee surgery	Abdominal surgery	Thoracic surgery
Level of needle insertion	L2–L4	L2–L4	L2–L4	T8–T10	T5–T7
Height of block required	T8–T9	T6–T7	T10	T7	Relevant area
Block type	Sensory	Motor, sensory	Motor, sensory	Sensory	Sensory
LA type concentration	Bupivicaine 0.1–0.25%	Bupivicaine 0.5%	Bupivicaine 0.5%	Bupivicaine 0.25–0.5%	Bupivicaine 0.25–0.5%
Opioid	Fentanyl	Fentanyl	Diamorphine	Diamorphine	Diamorphine
Infusion	0.1%, with 2mcg/ml fentanyl	Not necessary	Not necessary	0.1%, 0.1mg/ml diamorphine	0.1%, 0.1mg/ml diamorphine
Rate	0–15ml/hr			0–10ml/hr	0–6ml/hr

Arteries of the leg

The importance of the arterial supply of the limbs to anaesthetists lies primarily in their location for cannulation but also in the avoidance of their puncture during other procedures. It is also important to avoid their occlusion due to poor positioning of the anaesthetized patient. A schematic of the arteries of the leg is shown in Figure 6.44.

Large veins of the leg

These are divided into deep and superficial depending on their relationship to the deep fascia of the leg.

Deep veins

Accompany corresponding major arteries.

Superficial veins

Long saphenous vein Originates at the dorsum of foot. It passes in front of medial malleolus (NB: this is a reliable landmark and can be very useful for difficult or emergency IV access). It ascends over medial condyle of the tibia and femur and terminates at the saphenous opening (of the deep fascia), just below the inguinal ligament, and joins the femoral vein.

Short saphenous vein Originates at the ankle behind the lateral malleolus. Terminates in the popliteal vein.

Femoral vein and central venous access

This is very safe and especially useful in children requiring resuscitation where peripheral access has failed and intra-osseous access is difficult. It has minimal risk of serious complications. The femoral vein should not be used with pelvic or intra-abdominal injury. Remember that the femoral route is not a good choice for CVP monitoring since the intra-abdominal pressure significantly influences the result.

Technique

At the groin crease feel for the pulsation of the femoral artery 1–2 cm below the inguinal ligament. Insert the needle about 1cm medial to this point at an angle of 20°–30° to the skin. Aim rostrally.

In adults, blood will be aspirated 2–4cm from the skin. In small children the vein is more superficial, so reduce the elevation on the needle to 10°–15°.

The use of anatomical landmarks allows safe and successful placement of the catheter without the need for ultrasound guidance.

Advantages

Reliable landmarks.

No risks of neck or thoracic injury.

Disadvantages

Greater risk of infection.

More prone to kinking or dislodgement.

Nerves of the leg and foot

The lumbar and sacral plexuses supply the lower limb. Their nerves can be blocked in several different ways, some of which are described below. A thorough knowledge of the course of these nerves is important and will allow a variety of blocks to be used.

The lumbar plexus

The lumbar plexus (Figure 6.45) is mainly responsible for supplying the groin and anterior thigh region; the femoral nerve is its major branch.

It is made up of the anterior primary rami of L1–L4, although 50% have an additional contribution from T12. It lies in front of the lumbar vertebrae within psoas major.

The femoral nerve (L2,3,4)

Course

This is the major branch of the lumbar plexus. It enters the thigh beneath the inguinal ligament in the femoral triangle (Figure 6.46) where it is invested in the fascia iliaca (separating it from the femoral sheath; Figure 6.47). It divides into anterior and posterior divisions between the inguinal ligament and the base of the femoral triangle. Its major branch is the saphenous nerve which supplies the skin of the medial knee, lower leg, ankle and foot.

Supplies

- Sensory: anterior knee/thigh
- Motor: muscles of anterior thigh ie the knee flexors
- Articular: hip and knee

Obturator nerve (L2,3,4)

Course

Emerges at medial border of psoas at the pelvic brim, crosses down and forward to the obturator canal along the side-wall of the pelvis, where it divides into anterior and posterior branches.

Supplies

- Sensory: medial thigh
- Motor: anterior adductor compartment of thigh
- Articular: hip

Latenal cutaneous nerve of the thigh (L2,3)

Course

- Emerges at lateral border of psoas, enters the thigh at the lateral end of the inguinal ligament

Supplies

- Sensory: area of skin on anterolateral thigh

Femoral nerve block

Uses

Knee and anterior thigh surgery.

Position

Supine.

Landmarks/technique

Locate the groin crease (1cm below inguinal ligament). Insert needle 1cm lateral to the femoral pulse and 45° cephalad to a depth of 30–50mm (Figure 6.48).

Goal

Patellar twitch. Twitching of the sartorius muscle is the most common response to nerve stimulation. This results in a contraction across the thigh without movement of the patella. This is not reliable because the branches to sartorius may be outside the sheath. If the sartorius twitch occurs, redirect laterally and advance deeper.

Volume

10–30ml.

Fascia iliaca block

Position

Supine.

Landmarks/technique

Mark a point 1cm below the junction of outer and middle third of a line joining the anterior superior iliac spine and the pubic tubercle. Using a blunted needle pierce the skin at this point and then feel for two pops (fascia lata and fascia iliaca). Nerve stimulation is not needed.

Volume

20–30ml of local anaesthetic.

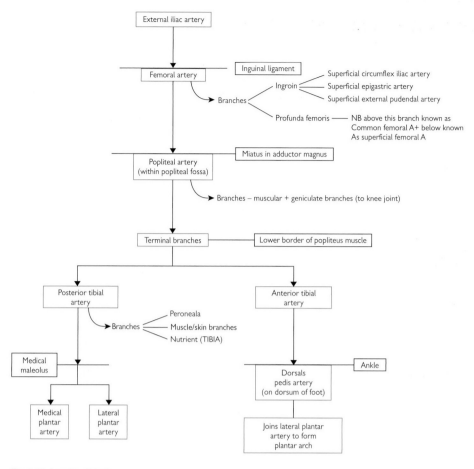

External iliac artery

Femoral artery — Inguinal ligament

Branches
- Ingroin
  - Superficial circumflex iliac artery
  - Superficial epigastric artery
  - Superficial external pudendal artery
- Profunda femoris — NB above this branch known as Common femoral A+ below known As superficial femoral A

Popliteal artery (within popliteal fossa) — Miatus in adductor magnus

Branches – muscular + geniculate branches (to knee joint)

Terminal branches — Lower border of popliteus muscle

Posterior tibial artery

Branches
- Peroneala
- Muscle/skin branches
- Nutrient (TIBIA)

Anterior tibial artery

Medical maleolus

Dorsals pedis artery (on dorsum of foot) — Ankle

Medical plantar artery

Lateral plantar artery

Joins lateral plantar artery to form plantar arch

Fig. 6.44 Arteries of the leg.

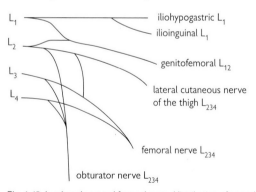

iliohypogastric L$_1$
ilioinguinal L$_1$
L$_1$
L$_2$
genitofemoral L$_{12}$
lateral cutaneous nerve of the thigh L$_{234}$
L$_3$
L$_4$
femoral nerve L$_{234}$
obturator nerve L$_{234}$

Fig. 6.45 Lumbar plexus and femoral nerve (distribution of anaesthesia)

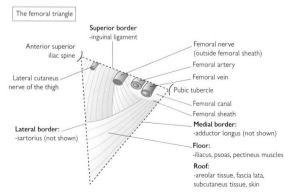

The femoral triangle

Superior border -inguinal ligament

Anterior superior iliac spine

Femoral nerve (outside femoral sheath)
Femoral artery
Femoral vein
Pubic tubercle
Femoral canal
Femoral sheath

Lateral cutaneous nerve of the thigh

Medial border: -adductor longus (not shown)

Lateral border: -sartorius (not shown)

Floor: -iliacus, psoas, pectineus muscles

Roof: -areolar tissue, fascia lata, subcutaneus tissue, skin

Fig. 6.46 The inguinal ligament and related anatomy.

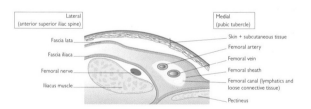

Lateral (anterior superior iliac spine)

Medial (pubic tubercle)

Fascia lata
Fascia iliaca
Femoral nerve
Iliacus muscle

Skin + subcutaneous tissue
Femoral artery
Femoral vein
Femoral sheath
Femoral canal (lymphatics and loose connective tissue)
Pectineus

Fig. 6.47 Relations of the femoral nerve at the groin.

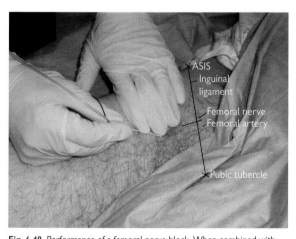

ASIS
Inguinal ligament
Femoral nerve
Femoral artery
Pubic tubercle

Fig. 6.48 Performance of a femoral nerve block. When combined with distal pressure it is known as a three-in-one block (femoral, lateral cutaneous nerve of the thigh and obturator). This provides analgesia for hip surgery.

The sacral plexus

- The sacral plexus (Figure 6.49) lies on the posterior wall of the pelvic cavity on the anterior surface of piriformis and deep to the pelvic fascia.
- Its major branches are the sciatic and the pudendal nerves.

The sacral plexus is mainly responsible for supplying the posterior thigh and lower leg, with the sciatic nerve being the major branch.

The sciatic nerve (L4–S3)

Course

This nerve is the major branch of the sacral plexus and the largest peripheral nerve in the body. It exits the pelvis posteriorly through the greater sciatic foramen and descends between the ischial tuberosity and the greater trochanter. Just proximal to or within the popliteal fossa it divides into the common peroneal and posterior tibial nerves.

Supplies

- Sensory: skin below the knee (except a sensory area of medial knee, lower leg, ankle and foot supplied by saphenous nerve)
- Motor: all muscles below the knee
- Articular: knee and all joints below the knee

Sciatic nerve block

Uses

- Ankle and foot surgery
- Knee and lower limb surgery (in combination with femoral block)

Anterior approach (Beck; Figure 6.50)

Position

Supine.

Landmarks/technique

Draw three lines:
- Anterior superior iliac spine (ASIS) to pubic tubercle (PT)
- Parallel line from the greater trochanter (GT)
- Perpendicular from the junction of the medial and middle third of the first line.

Insert needle at the intersection of lines 2 and 3. Direct posteriorly to hit the femur. When the bone has been reached, walk off medially approximately a further 2–3cm to a total depth of 80–100mm.

Goal

Ideally, inversion and dorsiflexion of foot.

Volume

10–20ml of local anaesthetic.

Classic posterior approach (Labat; Figure 6.51)

Position

Sims position (recovery position) operative side uppermost.

Landmarks/technique

Draw three lines:
- Posterior superior iliac spine (PSIS) to greater trochanter
- Sacral hiatus to greater trochanter
- Perpendicular line from mid-point of the first line

Insert needle perpendicularly at the intersection of lines 2 and 3.

Depth

50–100mm.

Goal and volume as above.

Posterior approach (alternative technique; Figure 6.52)

Position

Supine, leg flexed to 90° at hip and knee.

Landmarks/technique

Draw line from ischial tuberosity to greater trochanter. Insert needle at mid-point of this line, perpendicularly to skin.

Depth

60–100mm.

Goal and volume as above.

Nerves at the ankle

The nerves supplying the foot are all branches of the sciatic nerve, except the saphenous nerve (femoral).

There are two deep nerves that supply all the deep structures of the foot:
- Posterior tibial: supplies sole of foot
- Deep peroneal: sensory to first web space.

There are three superficial nerves (three S's):
- Superficial peroneal—sensation to dorsum of foot
- Sural—sensation to fifth toe and lateral border of foot
- Saphenous—sensation to medial border of foot/ankle.

Ankle block (Figure 6.53)

Uses

Surgery of the foot and toes. NB: an ankle block will not block the ankle joint.

Position

Supine with foot raised on a pillow.

Landmarks/technique

This technique requires a minimum of three puncture sites along a line connecting the maleoli and requires the operator to move around the foot for ease of injection.

- Deep peroneal (facing the sole of the foot). Between tendons of extensor hallucis longus and extensor digitorum longus (ask patient to dorsiflex foot) and lateral to dorsalis pedis pulse. Insert needle until it hits bone. Withdraw 1–2mm; inject 2–5ml; repeat with needle angled 30° lateral and medial to dorsalis pedis.
- Posterior tibial (facing medial aspect of ankle). Behind and distal to medial malleolus just posterior to posterior tibial pulse. Insert needle to bone; then inject as for deep peroneal.
- Superficial nerves are blocked with a subcutaneous injection in a circular line 3–4 finger-breadths above the malleoli (ensure a subcutaneous wheal). The nerves blocked are:
  • Superficial peroneal
  • Sural
  • Saphenous.

Volume

20–30 ml total.

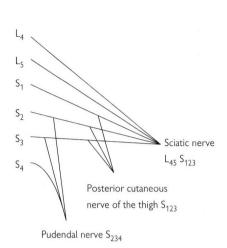

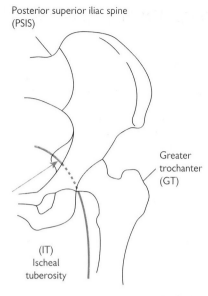

Posterior superior iliac spine (PSIS)

Greater trochanter (GT)

(IT) Ischeal tuberosity

Sciatic nerve L$_{45}$ S$_{123}$

L$_4$
L$_5$
S$_1$
S$_2$
S$_3$
S$_4$

Posterior cutaneous nerve of the thigh S$_{123}$

Pudendal nerve S$_{234}$

Fig. 6.49 Sacral plexus and course of the sciatic nerve.

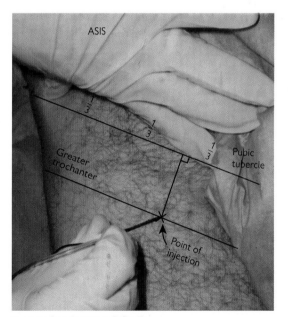

Fig. 6.50 Anterior approach (Beck).

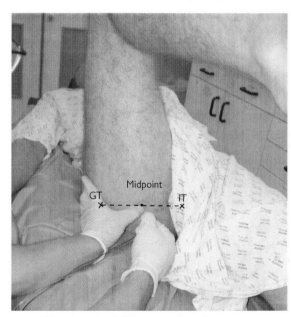

Fig. 6.52 Posterior approach (alternative technique).

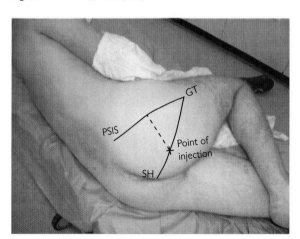

Fig. 6.51 Classic posterior approach (Labat).

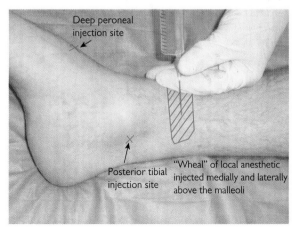

Fig. 6.53 The ankle block.

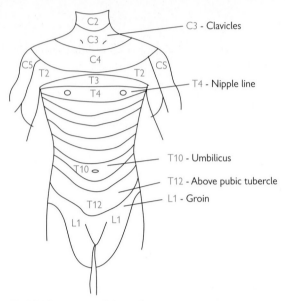

Fig. 6.54 Dermatomes of the trunk.

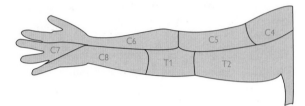

Fig. 6.56 Dermatomes of the arm.

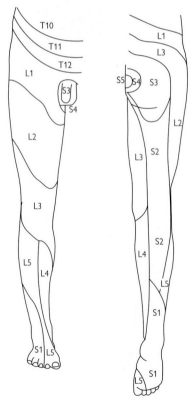

Fig. 6.55 Dermatomes of the leg.

Myotomes	
C5	Deltoid (lateral arm raise)
C6	Biceps, extensor carpi radialis longus and brevis (wrist extension)
C7	Triceps (elbow extension)
C8	Flexor digitorum profundum (middle finger flexion)
T1	Abductor digiti minimi (finger abduction)
L2	Iliopsoas (hip flexion)
L3/4	Quadriceps (knee extension)
L4/5/S1	Hamstrings (knee flexion)
L5	Tibialis anterior, extensor hallucis longus (ankle/big toe dorsiflexion)
S1	Gastrocnemius, soleus (plantar flexion)

Chapter 7

Central nervous system and pain

7.1 The brain

The brain develops from the hindbrain, midbrain, and forebrain.

The **hindbrain** gives rise to the medulla, pons, and cerebellum. It contains the vital respiratory and cardiac centres, and the nuclei for cranial nerves V–XIII. The cerebellum is concerned with balance and posture, with close affiliation to the vestibular apparatus, and also with the coordination of complex patterns of skilled movement.

The **midbrain** contains the nuclei for cranial nerves II and IV, and the centres for eye reflexes and auditory reflexes.

The **forebrain** develops into the thalamic structures and the cerebral hemispheres. The hemispheres are divided into cortical lobes, named after the cranial bones to which they are related: frontal, temporal, parietal, and occipital. The lobes are functional areas, not clearly demarcated structures.

There is structural and functional asymmetry between the hemispheres. The left hemisphere is involved in intellectual reasoning and language, while the right is concerned with spatial construction and emotion. Damage to Wernicke's area of the left temporal lobe causes significant speech defects in most people, whereas a similar lesion in the right temporal lobe will not cause a problem. In most right-handed people, the left hemisphere is dominant.

The hemispheres are connected by the corpus callosum, allowing integration of their functions. If the corpus callosum is completely Sectioned, a person will have two separate conscious portions of the brain, with the hemisphere best suited to a task directing behaviour.

Cerebral cortex

Different parts of the cortex perform different functions. The lobes of the cerebral cortex are shown in Figure 7.1.

The functional units can be divided into:

- **Primary** sensory and motor areas.
- **Higher order** sensory and motor areas, which process information from the various modalities.
- **Association areas** where information about different modalities is integrated to produce a more complete picture.

The lobes of the brain are anatomically separated by sulci or grooves. The two most important are:

- The **central sulcus** separating the frontal from the parietal lobe
- The **lateral sulcus**, which separates the frontal and parietal from the temporal lobes.

Frontal lobes

The **primary motor cortex** is in the frontal lobe, anterior to the central sulcus. It performs final cortical motor processing, and projects to contralateral motor neurons (see Section 7.21).

Anterior to the primary motor areas are the **supplemental** and **premotor areas**. These are higher-order processing areas. **Broca's area,** in the left frontal lobe, controls motor patterns of speech. Patients with lesions here can understand, but cannot speak or express ideas in writing (expressive dysphasia). Other higher-order processing areas control eye movements and skilled tasks.

The prefrontal association areas function in close association with the motor cortex to plan complex sequences of movements. They are also essential for abstract thought. An enormous amount of information about their role has been gained from patients with prefrontal lobotomy (for the treatment of psychotic depression). These patients cannot solve complex problems, are unable to learn to do parallel tasks, lose aggression and ambition, and are often disinhbited.

The prefrontal cortex was thought to be the site for the higher intellect (since it is much larger in humans than in apes). However, destruction of other areas of the brain is just as important in diminishing intellectual function.

Temporal lobes

The temporal lobe lies below the lateral sulcus. It is responsible for complex processing of sensory inputs. Temporal lobe epilepsy is characterized by complex auditory, visual, olfactory and visceral hallucinations. The temporal lobe also has association areas vital to learning, and lesions here may cause memory and personality changes.

Wernicke's area, located in the posterior part of the superior dominant temporal lobe, is one of the most important parts of the brain. The somatic, visual, and auditory association areas all coalesce in this region. Damage to Wernicke's area results in a person not being able to understand spoken or written ideas despite being able to hear and recognize different words (receptive dysphasia). Wernicke's area works closely with Broca's area, and disruption of the fibres between them leads to inability to repeat phrases, and frequent errors and substitutions in language (conductive dysphasia).

Parietal lobe

The parietal lobe lies behind the central sulcus and contains the **primary sensory** and **higher-order sensory areas**. It includes the parieto-occipito-temporal association area. This region analyses the spatial coordinates of the body, provides the initial processing of visual language (reading), and contains an area important for naming objects.

Damage to the parietal lobe can produce attention deficits, inability to make voluntary eye movements, constructional apraxia, disorders of spatial awareness, and problems with language.

Occipital lobe

The occipital lobe is concerned with vision and contains the visual cortex. Again, there is left–right asymmetry; the visual aspects of reading and writing are processed in the left occipital lobe; patients with lesions here have a visual field defect but also exhibit alexia (acquired dyslexia).

The limbic system

The limbic system (Figure 7.2) is located on the medial aspect of each temporal lobe and encircles the upper brainstem. Its functions include the coordination of behaviour and emotion. It has extensive interconnections with lower and higher centres, and is intimately involved with the hypothalamus.

Two of its important functions are:

- Learning and memory
- Processing of emotion.

Structures involved in memory include:

- The hippocampus
- The parahippocampal gyrus
- The fornix
- The mamillary bodies.

Lesions of the medial temporal lobe (e.g. caused by HSV encephalitis) produce profound defects in factual memory. Degeneration of the mammillary bodies (e.g. Wernicke–Korsakoff syndrome) results in memory disorders with anterograde amnesia.

Lesions in the amygdala disrupt motivational function, especially related to rewards of food and drink. When the amygdala is stimulated artificially, patients report strong feelings of fear.

Hypothalamus

The hypothalamus is important in many regulatory processes.

- **Cardiovascular regulation:** mediated by reticular regions of the pons and medulla.
- Control of **body temperature:** regulated by the anterior preoptic portion of the hypothalamus.
- **Water intake and excretion:** regulated by the hypothalamus in two ways. The thirst centre is located in the lateral hypothalamus; and fibres from the supraoptic nuclei project to the posterior pituitary where they secrete vasopressin. Vasopressin reduces water loss from the kidney (Section 12.4).
- A role in **hunger** and **appetite**.
- Control of **hormone secretion** from the pituitary gland.

→ Consciousness

Activity in the cerebrum is maintained by continuous transmission of nerve signals from the lower brain. These signals activate the cerebrum in two ways:

- Direct stimulation of areas of the brain.
- Activation of neurohumoral systems which release facilitatory or inhibitory neurocrine agents into selected areas of the brain.

The arousal or activity of the brain is mediated by the excitation of thalamocortical neurons and stems. These excitatory inputs arise from several areas.

- The **reticular activating system (RAS)** or bulboreticular facilitatory area in the brainstem transmits impulses to the thalamus, and from there to the cortex. Two major pathways are involved: a fast cholinergic pathway which activates the cerebrum for a few milliseconds, and slower pathways mediated by noradrenaline and serotonin, originating in many brainstem centres.
- **Somatosensory input** (particularly pain) increases the activity of the RAS. Lesions above the point where the trigeminal nerve enters the pons can produce a somnolent state, demonstrating the impact of somatosensory information on arousal.
- The **cortex** and adjacent **thalamic areas** also provide positive feedback, activating reverberating circuits to maintain alertness.

In the rat, four neurohumoral pathways also maintain alertness in the brain (Figure 7.3).

- The **noradrenergic circuit,** initiated in the locus coeruleus.
  This may have a role in REM sleep activity.
- The **dopaminergic system,** activated by neurons from the substantia nigra.
- The **serotonergic pathways** emerging from the midline raphe nuclei.
- The **gigantocellular neurons** in the reticular excitatory areas
  of the pons and mesencephalon secrete acetylcholine. Activation of these neurons leads to an acutely alert nervous system.

The site of anaesthetic action in the rat has been elucidated. All general anaesthetic agents attenuate sensory transmission to the cortex, although none has any significant action at the spinal level. They can broadly be differentiated into three groups, according to where they exert their major effect.

- The majority of anaesthetics, including the volatile agents and the barbiturates, principally affect the thalamic centres, with minor effects on the cortical neurons.
- The second group, which includes propofol and etomidate, does not reduce transmission in the thalamus but acts only at the cortical level.
- The third group, which includes benzodiazepines, affects thalamic and cortical areas but in a slightly different pattern from the first group.

Drugs can also effect neurohumeral pathways. α_2-adrenergic agonist drugs (e.g. clonidine) and central anticholinergic drugs (e.g. hyoscine) have anaesthetic effects which may be due to disruption of the neurohumoral component of alertness. The locus coeruleus (LC) is the major site for the hypnotic actions of clonidine and dexmedetomidine, both of which markedly reduce local noradrenaline concentrations.

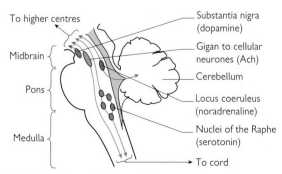

Fig. 7.1 Lobes of the brain. The temporal lobe is sited laterally and is not shown on this medial view.

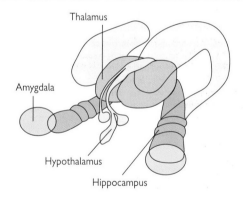

Fig. 7.2 The limbic system.

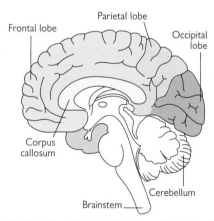

Fig. 7.3 Neurohumoral pathways of alertness.

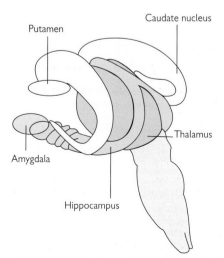

The brainstem consists of three parts: the **medulla,** the **pons,** and the **midbrain** (in caudal to rostral order). Although small, it is an extremely important Section of the CNS; not only do its tracts relay signals from the brain to the periphery and vice versa, but it contains control centres for the functions and processes vital to life. The brainstem, lying on the ventral surface of the brain, is shown in Figure 7.4. Lesions in the brainstem can have devastating clinical consequences. Tests of the brainstem are the basis for deciding whether a patient is brain-dead (Section 22.7).

The brainstem also contains the nuclei of cranial nerves III–XII (nerve I terminates in the olfactory bulb, and nerve II terminates in the thalamus and midbrain).

Brainstem nuclei

The sensory nuclei of the cranial nerves are distinct from the motor nuclei, in a similar fashion to that found in the horns of the spinal cord grey matter. The sensory nuclei are positioned laterally, whilst the motor nuclei are found medially (Figure 7.4).

There are three types of cranial nerve motor nuclei:

- **Somatic motor** nuclei project to striated muscles.
- **Branchial motor** nuclei supply muscles derived from embryonic branchial arches (muscles of the jaws and other craniofacial structures).
- **Visceral motor** nuclei project to smooth muscle and glands.

Most motor nuclei project to their targets via a single cranial nerve. In contrast, sensory nuclei usually receive inputs from several different nerves. The fibres intermingle in the periphery.

Major monoaminergic systems

There are three principle neurotransmitter systems in the brainstem.

Serotonergic neurons are the most numerous cells in the brainstem. They are located within the reticular activating system (see Section 7.1) and have widespread ascending and descending projections. Stimulation of the descending neurons results in increased excitability of spinal cord motor neurons and decreased pain perception (gate theory; see Sections 7.26 and 7.27). Ascending neurons project to all parts of the forebrain, and are generally excitatory.

Noradrenergic neurons are clustered in two areas:

- The **locus coeruleus**, a bluish area in the upper pons. These neurons are thought to be important in orientation and attention to sudden or unpleasant sensory stimuli. They have widespread projections to the ventral horn of the spinal cord, the sensory nuclei of the brainstem, the thalamus, the hippocampus, and the cerebellum. In addition, the locus ceruleus provides the main noradrenergic input to the cortex.
- In the **ventral lateral tegmentum**, noradrenergic neurons are more loosely arranged. They provide the chief noradrenergic input to the brainstem itself and the spinal cord. Importantly, they project onto sympathetic preganglionic cells in the intermediolateral grey matter of the cord, helping to integrate the autonomic response. Direct stimulation of the lateral tegmentum leads to profound parasympathetic responses (bradycardia, hypotension).

Dopaminergic neurons are highly organized, and categorized according to their projections within the brain:

- The **mesostriatal system** projects from the brainstem and globus pallidus, to the striatum (caudate nucleus and putamen). This pathway is involved in the extrapyramidal control of movement, and is affected in Parkinson's disease (Section 7.12).
- The **mesocortical** and **mesolimbic systems** project from the ventral tegmentum to the cortex and the limbic system, respectively. They are thought to play important roles in cognition. Many antipsychotics affect these neurons.

Brainstem lesions

There is rostral–caudal organization of the cranial nerve nuclei.

The *midbrain* contains nuclei for eye movements such as the occulomotor nuclei and the preganglionic parasympathetic innervation of the iris (Edinger–Westphal nuclei). Lesions here (e.g. aneurysms in the basilar artery or posterior part of the circle of Willis) will give rise to disturbances of eye movements.

The *pons* contains the sensory and motor nuclei that deal primarily with somatic sensation from the face, the muscles of facial expression and jaw movement, and abduction of the eye.

The **basal pontine syndrome** follows damage to the pontine arteries. Signs include ipsilateral inward deviation of the eye, paralysis of the face, and contralateral hemiparesis and loss of touch and position sense. (Note: destruction of cranial nerve nuclei or fibres produces lower motor neuron deficits, whereas interruption of the corticospinal tracts causes an upper motor neuron lesion.)

In the *medulla,* medial structures can be damaged by lesions of the anterior spinal artery or branches of the vertebral artery. Such injury produces medial medullary syndrome: hemiplegia, and contralateral loss of touch and position.

The lateral medulla is supplied by the posterior inferior cerebellar artery (Figure 7.26). The **lateral medullary syndrome** affects the spinal trigeminal nucleus and tract, causing:

- Ipsilateral loss of pain and temperature in the face
- Damage to the spinothalamic tract with contralateral loss of pain and temperature in the body
- Damage to the nucleus ambiguus leading to ipsilateral loss of gag reflex, dysphagia, dysphonia, and dysarthria
- Injury to the inferior cerebellar peduncle, producing ipsilateral ataxia
- Nystagmus, nausea, and vertigo due to destruction of the vestibular nucleus
- Possibly Horner's syndrome and vomiting due to lesions of the dorsal motor nucleus of vagus.

Effects of brainstem lesions on consciousness

Lesions within the brainstem cause altered consciousness, the severity of which is broadly related to tissue destruction in the ascending reticular activating system and associated nuclei such as the locus coeruleus and the midline raphe nuclei.

Lesions in the midbrain and the rostral pons usually cause coma.

More caudal lesions in the pons will normally not cause disturbances of consciousness but will have respiratory effects.

Medullary and high spinal cord lesions will not affect conscious level.

Effect of brainstem lesions on respiration

Midbrain Lesions occasionally lead to hyperventilation.

Pontine Lesions lead to a group of abnormalities called periodic breathing. These include *apneustic breathing*, where breathing is held in inspiration for several seconds, *ratchet breathing* which is characterized by a series of inspiratory 'steps' leading to apneustic breathing; and *cluster patterns*, where short periods of tachypnoea are followed by apnoea.

Medullary lesions can lead to irregular breathing patterns, such as Cheyne–Stokes respiration, Biot's ataxic breathing (breathing of variable rate and amplitude), or total apnoea.

Diagnosis of the anatomical site of injury from respiratory pattern alone is difficult in view of abnormalities of gas exchange and other associated complications (e.g. aspiration).

All three patterns of breathing can also be produced by higher lesions. Apneustic breathing has been described with hypoglycaemic coma and meningitis. The ataxic breathing of medullary damage can also occur with demyelinating diseases or viral meningitis.

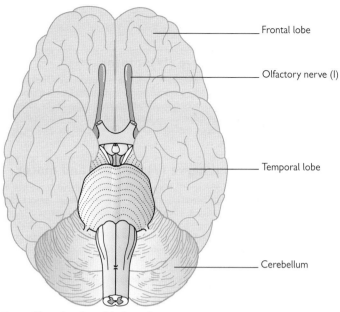

Fig. 7.4 Ventral surface of the brain demonstrating the relationship between the brainstem, cerebellum, and cerebrum.

- Frontal lobe
- Olfactory nerve (I)
- Temporal lobe
- Cerebellum

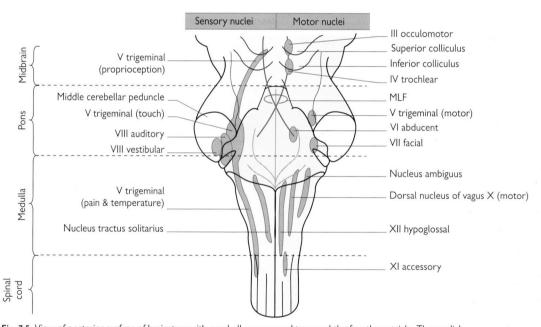

Sensory nuclei	Motor nuclei

Midbrain
Pons
Medulla
Spinal cord

- V trigeminal (proprioception)
- Middle cerebellar peduncle
- V trigeminal (touch)
- VIII auditory
- VIII vestibular
- V trigeminal (pain & temperature)
- Nucleus tractus solitarius

- III occulomotor
- Superior colliculus
- Inferior colliculus
- IV trochlear
- MLF
- V trigeminal (motor)
- VI abducent
- VII facial
- Nucleus ambiguus
- Dorsal nucleus of vagus X (motor)
- XII hypoglossal
- XI accessory

Fig. 7.5 View of posterior surface of brainstem with cerebellum removed to reveal the fourth ventricle. The medial longitudinal fasciculus (MLF) is the pathway that coordinates movements of the eyes.

The cranial nerves (Figure 7.6) have three main functions: they mediate the special senses (hearing, vision, olfaction, taste), they are motor and somatosensory to the head and neck; and (together with the sacral nerve roots) they provide parasympathetic control of visceral functions. Cranial nerves are either simple (sensory or motor) or complex (a combination of motor, sensory, and parasympathetic fibres).

Purely sensory nerves: I, II, and VIII. Nerves I (olfactory), II (optic), and VIII (vestibulocochlear) mediate olfaction, vision, and hearing/balance, respectively.

Purely motor nerves: III, IV, and VI; XI; and XII. Nerves III (oculomotor), IV (trochlear), and VI (abducent) move the eyeball. Nerve XI (accessory) innervates the sternocleidomastoid and trapezius. Nerve XII (hypoglossal) innervates the tongue muscles.

Mixed nerves: V, VII, IX, and X. Nerves V (trigeminal), VII (facial), IX (glossopharyngeal), and X (vagus) supply structures derived from embryonic branchial arches at the cranial end of the gut.

- The motor fibres of these nerves are responsible for movement of the mandible, face, pharynx and larynx.
- The sensory components convey somatic and visceral sensation from the face, nose, mouth, pharynx, and larynx (and in the case of X, visceral sensation from the thorax and abdomen).
- Cutaneous and oral sensation fibres are mostly contained in V, and pass to the trigeminal sensory nuclei in the brainstem.
- Visceral sensation reaches the brainstem via VII, IX, and X, passing to the nucleus of the solitary tract in the medulla.

Preganglionic parasympathetic fibres leave the brainstem in nerves III, VII, IX and X. Some fibres leave these nerves, and later travel with V to reach their destination.

Olfactory nerve (I): sensory

The fibres of the olfactory nerve arise from cell bodies in the olfactory epithelium. They pass into the skull through foramina in the cribriform plate. These fibres can be disrupted if the cribriform plate is fractured; anosmia may be a clue. Suspected plate fracture is a contraindication to insertion of a nasogastric tube or nasal airway.

Optic nerve (II): sensory

The cell bodies of optic nerve fibres reside in the retina. The nerve enters the skull via the optic canal; the medial halves decussate at the optic chiasm. As well as the special sense of vision, the nerve carries the afferent limb of the pupillary light reflex.

Oculomotor nerve (III): motor and parasympathetic

Motor and presynaptic parasympathetic fibres for the oculomotor nerve arise in the midbrain; the parasympathetic fibres synapse in the ciliary ganglion before passing with the rest of the nerve through the superior orbital fissure.

The nerve is motor to the superior, medial, and inferior recti, inferior oblique, and levator palpabrae superioris. If damaged, the eye points 'down and out', with ptosis.

The oculomotor nerve carries parasympathetic innervation (via the **Edinger–Westphal nucleus**) to the ciliary muscles of the eye for accommodation, and the sphincter of the iris for papillary constriction. Pupil size and reaction are important components of neurological observation. The presynaptic parasympathetic fibres are superficial in the nerve; loss of pupil response is an early sign of nerve compression, e.g. in impending uncal herniation. Oculomotor nerve damage can also occur due to pressure from aneurysms of the superior cerebellar and posterior cerebral arteries.

Trochlear nerve (IV): motor

The cell bodies of the trochlear nerve lie in the midbrain. The nerve is the only one to emerge from the posterior surface of the brainstem; it passes through the superior orbital fissure. It supplies the superior oblique muscle only. The classic presentation of a trochlear nerve palsy is double vision upon descending stairs. Patients will tend to dip their heads forwards.

Trigeminal nerve (V): sensory and motor

The trigeminal (Figure 7.7) is the principal sensory nerve of the face. It emerges from the lateral aspect of the pons, with a large sensory root and a small motor root. The motor root supplies the muscles of mastication.

The **trigeminal ganglion** houses the cell bodies of the sensory neurons. There are three sensory divisions (Figure 7.8).

Ophthalmic (Va)
Exits skull through superior orbital fissure.
Supplies cornea, upper conjunctiva, anterosuperior nasal cavity, paranasal sinuses, and anterior supratentorial dura mater.

Maxillary nerve (Vb)
Exits skull through the foramen rotundum.
Supplies sensation from skin of face over maxilla, upper lip, maxillary teeth, mucosa of nose and palate.

Mandibular nerve (Vc)
Exits via the foramen ovale.
Sensory to the skin over mandible (including lower lip), mandibular teeth, TMJ, and anterior two thirds of tongue (NB: taste in the anterior two thirds is carried by the chorda tympani from the VIIth nerve; Section 7.4)

Pathways to the brain

The three modalities of sensory information travelling in nerve V follow distinct pathways to the somatosensory cortex.

Pain and temperature fibres of the afferent tract of the trigeminal nerve synapse in the spinal trigeminal nucleus in the medulla. This extends into the cervical spinal cord and is continuous with the dorsal horn of the spinal grey matter. From the trigeminal nucleus, fibres decussate and ascend in the trigeminal lemniscus to the thalamus, and then the somatosensory cortex. (The pathway is very similar to the spinothalamic tract; Section 7.26).

Fibres carrying fine totuch and pressure impulses synapse in the pons, in the chief sensory nucleus of V. From here, second-order fibres decussate and ascend in the trigeminal lemniscus to the contralateral thalamus, although some fibres do not cross and ascend ipsilaterally.

Proprioception from the jaws and deep pressure sensation from the teeth and gums project to the mesencephalic nucleus in the upper pons. This nucleus is unique as it contains sensory cell bodies, which lie in the peripheral ganglia in other sensory fibres.

Some fibres synapse directly in the motor nucleus of V with the efferent fibres of Vc (supplying the muscles of mastication). These are the basis of the jaw reflex, which is tested by tapping the chin with a percussion hammer.

Abducent nerve (VI): motor

The abducent nerve fibres arise from cell bodies in the pons. The nerve has a very long course along the ventral surface of the pons, bends sharply over the petrous temporal bone, and traverses the cavernous sinus before passing into the superior orbital fissure. It is vulnerable to increased intracranial pressure; its dysfunction has little localizing value, especially if there is bilateral involvment.

The abducent nerve is motor to lateral rectus. Injury causes medial deviation of the eye, with diplopia in all directions of gaze except horizontal gaze to the opposite side.

Trigeminal neuralgia

The cell bodies of pain, temperature, and touch fibres from the trigeminal nerve lie in the trigeminal ganglion, within a pocket of dura (Meckel's cave) in the middle cranial fossa (Figure 7.8). Vascular compression of the ganglion may be responsible for trigeminal neuralgia, which is characterized by recurrent pain located to one side of the face and localized to one or more branches of the nerve. The pain is often triggered by light touch (allodynia). It can be treated by ablating or decompressing the ganglion. The herpes zoster virus can also affect the ganglion, giving rise to chronic post-herpetic neuralgia. Whilst trigeminal neuralgia more commonly affects the maxillary and mandibular divisions, herpes more often affects the ophthalmic division.

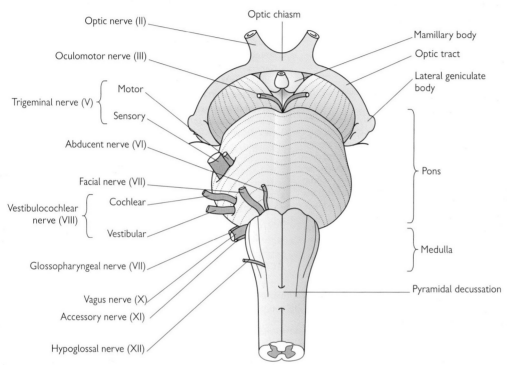

Fig. 7.6 Detail of the ventral surface of the brainstem showing the cranial nerves (which are omitted from the right-hand side of the diagram for clarity). The olfactory nerve filaments synapse at the olfactory bulb above the cribriform plate; from there the olfactory tracts pass directly back to the cortex and limbic system. The trochlear nerve leaves from the dorsal surface.

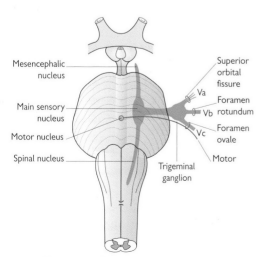

Fig. 7.7 Ventral view of brainstem showing position of trigeminal nuclei and relation to ganglion.

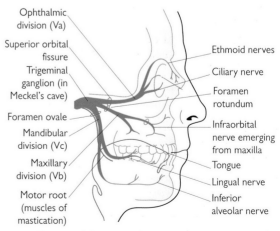

Fig. 7.8 Divisions of the trigeminal nerve.

Facial nerve (VII): motor, sensory, and parasympathetic

The facial nerve emerges from the junction of the pons and medulla as two roots: the motor and the intermediate (sensory and parasympathetic). The roots run separately through the internal acoustic meatus and the facial canal in the petrous temporal bone. They unite in the facial canal at the geniculate ganglion, and the nerve then travels through the middle ear and exits the skull via the stylomastoid foramen. Outside the skull, it runs within the parotid gland. It carries three types of fibre:

- *Motor fibres* (from the motor root) supply muscles of facial expression and scalp, stapedius, stylohyoid, and posterior belly of digastric.
- *Special sensory fibres*, via the chorda tympani, carry taste from the anterior two-thirds of the tongue and the palate.
- *Parasympathetic fibres* innervate the submandibular, sublingual, and lacrimal glands, and the glands of nose and palate.

The facial nerve is the most frequently paralysed cranial nerve. Lesions at its origin in the pons or near the geniculate ganglion can occur during reSection of tumours at the cerebellopontine angle. Injuries around the parotid region are common with trauma (e.g. forceps damage during obstetric delivery). Inflammation of the facial nerve can also occur in the stylomastoid foramen. These injuries produce a lower motor neuron pattern of injury, with total ipsilateral paralysis of all the muscles of facial expression (Figure 7.09). Upper motor neuron lesions of the face classically spare the forehead, as there is motor input from both hemispheres (Figure 7.10). In addition, the facial nerve can be affected by an idiopathic (Bell's) palsy.

Vestibulocochlear nerve (VIII): sensory

The vestibulocochlear nerve arises in the vestibular and cochlear nuclei in the pons. It emerges at the cerebellopontine angle, and crosses the subarachnoid space to enter the internal auditory meatus. It separates into its two separate elements (vestibular and cochlear), each of which pierces the temporal bone to enter the inner ear.

The **vestibular nerve** mediates sensation vital to balance, while the **cochlear nerve** carries the special sense of hearing. Although these nerves are essentially independent, they are frequently affected together because of their close anatomical relationship. Vestibulocochlear nerve injury (e.g. compression by acoustic neuroma) causes deafness, tinnitus, and vertigo.

Projections from the vestibular portion of the nerve to the lateral reticular formation of the medulla are important in nausea and vomiting (see Section 17.9).

Glossopharyngeal nerve (IX): motor, sensory, and parasympathetic

The glossopharyngeal nerve emerges from the lateral aspect of the medulla and leaves the cranium via the jugular foramen.

The nerve is motor to the stylopharyngeus muscle, sensory to the external ear (via the tympanic nerve), and also relays chemo- and baroreceptor afferents from the carotid sinus and taste from the posterior third of the tongue:

- The **carotid sinus nerve** relays afferents from the baroreceptors and chemoreceptors sensitive to oxygen and carbon dioxide. The central bodies of these nerves lie in the inferior petrosal ganglion near the jugular foramen, and synapse in the solitary nucleus. This information is integrated into reflex responses involving the reticular formation and hypothalamus, and affects respiration, blood pressure, and cardiac output.

- The **pharyngeal, tonsillar, and lingual nerves** transmit special sensory taste fibres to the posterior third of tongue.

Loss of nerve IX leads to absence of the gag reflex and loss of taste on the posterior one third of the tongue. The glossopharyngeal nerve is rarely injured in isolation, but may be involved by tumours adjacent to the jugular foramen (together with nerves X and XI) in jugular foramen syndrome (see opposite).

Vagus nerve (X): parasympathetic, sensory, and motor

This emerges as a series of 8–10 rootlets from the lateral aspect of the medulla. It leaves the skull via the jugular foramen. It contains many different types of fibre:

- *General sensory* from the auricle, external auditory meatus, and dura mater of the posterior cranial fossa.
- *Special sensory:* taste from the epiglottis and palate.
- *Visceral sensory:* sensation from base of tongue, pharynx, larynx, trachea, bronchi, heart, oesophagus, stomach, and intestine (to left colic flexure).
- *Motor* to the constrictor muscles of the pharynx (except stylopharyngeus), intrinsic muscle of the larynx, muscles of palate (except tensor veli palatini), and striated muscle in the superior two thirds of the oesophagus.
- *Visceral motor:* parasympathetic innervations to smooth muscle of trachea, bronchi, digestive tract, and cardiac muscle of heart.

Isolated lesions are uncommon. Injury to pharyngeal branches can cause dysphagia.

Accessory nerve (XI): motor

The accessory nerve has two roots: the cranial, from the nucleus ambiguus in the medulla, and the spinal, from spinal nuclei C1–C5. The nerve leaves the posterior cranial fossa between the vagus and the internal jugular vein, through the jugular foramen. It is motor to the sternocleidomastoid and trapezius muscles. Along with nerves IX, X, and XII, it may be involved in the jugular foramen syndrome.

Hypoglossal nerve (XII): motor

The cell bodies of the hypoglossal nerve are contained in the hypoglossal nucleus in the medulla. Numerous rootlets leave the anterolateral surface of the medulla, finally fusing into one nerve in the hypoglossal canal. Outside the skull the nerve runs lateral to the internal and external carotid arteries and the lingual artery. It passes over the greater cornu of the hyoid. The nerve runs forwards to supply the muscles of the floor of the mouth (hypoglossal means 'beneath the tongue'): the intrinsic muscles of the tongue—genioglossus, hyoglossus, and styloglossus. It also supplies the thyrohyoid and geniohyoid muscles.

Hypoglossal nerve palsies result in deviation of the tongue toward the side of the lesion (the shortening of genioglossus acts to 'push', not 'pull', the tongue forwards).

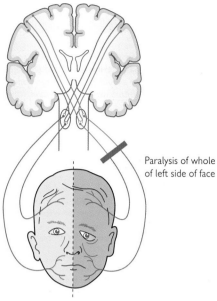

Paralysis of whole
of left side of face

Fig. 7.9 Lower motor neuron lesion of the facial nerve. This produces paralysis of the whole of the left side of the face.

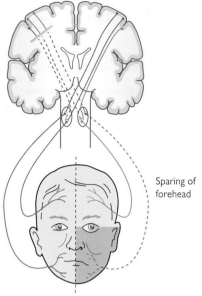

Sparing of
forehead

Fig. 7.10 Upper motor neuron lesion of the facial nerve. The bilateral innervation of the upper face means that only the lower face is affected.

→ Jugular foramen syndrome (Vernet's syndrome)

The jugular foramen and its relations are shown in Figure 7.11.

Neoplastic: paraganglioma, schwannoma, meningioma, and metastatic disease (haematological, nasopharyngeal carcinoma).

Non-neoplastic: Internal jugular vein thrombosis, aneurysm, osteomyelitis, cholesterol granuloma.

The clinical presentation of jugular foramen lesions depends on the size, extent, and pathology of the tumour.

Patients show signs of IX, X, and XI cranial nerve dysfunction and present with a wide range of bulbar and other cranial nerve signs. These include dysphagia, dysarthria, dysphonia, nasal regurgitation, ipsilateral trapezius and sternomastoid muscle weakness and atrophy, depressed gag reflex, palatal droop on the affected side with ipsilateral vocal cord paralysis and loss of taste on the posterior third of the tongue, and paresis of the soft palate, uvula, pharynx and larynx.

Some patients may present with neuralgia in the distribution of nerves IX and X. The causative lesions tend to grow slowly, and so the syndrome develops gradually and is well tolerated in most patients.

As a result, although imaging studies reveal extensive involvement of these neural structures, patients may have only subtle manifestation of their dysfunction.

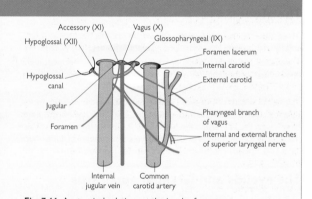

Fig. 7.11 Anatomical relations at the jugular foramen

7.5 The eye I

The circulation of the eye is via two systems; the dominant supply is from the uveal vessels, and the lesser is from the retinal vessels. Blood flow to the choroid is much larger than required for metabolism, and is thought to be important for temperature regulation of the retina.

The orbit

The pyramid-shaped orbit contains the visual apparatus, along with the nerves, muscles, and vessels vital to its function.

The orbit is formed by the **frontal bone**, the **zygoma**, the **maxilla**, and the **ethmoid bone**. It is commonly involved in anterior cranial fossa fractures. The boundaries of the orbit are as follows:

The medial walls of the orbits are parallel to one another. They are thin and easily damaged. Perforation of the medial wall (e.g. by a regional block needle!) can result in orbital infection. The medial wall contains the anterior and posterior lacrimal crests, between which lies the lacrimal sac.

The lateral walls do not reach as far forward as the medial walls, and so the eye is vulnerable from the side.

The roof of the orbit separates the eye from the frontal lobe; the frontal air sinuses can extend laterally above the eye.

The floor of the orbit separates the eye from the maxillary air sinus. The sphenoid air sinus lies behind the apex of the orbital cavity.

At the apex of the orbit are three entrances: the superior and inferior orbital fissures, and the optic canal. Their contents are described in Section 7.7. The anatomy is shown in Figure 7.13.

The orbital periosteum becomes continuous with the optic nerve sheath and dura mater at the back of the orbit.

The globe

The globe (Figure 7.12) contains the sensory retina, the focussing lens, and the mechanism for controlling incident light, the iris.

The wall of the globe is made up of three layers. The innermost is the retina; next comes the vascular layer (choroid, ciliary body and iris), and the outermost is the tough fibrous sclera.

The fascial sheath of the eye, Tenon's capsule, acts like a fluid pocket to allow low-friction eye movements. It is in two layers: the inner blends with the sclera, and the outer layer is pierced by the extraocular muscles. A sub-Tenon block uses a curved, blunt cannula to introduce local anaesthetic underneath Tenon's capsule (Section 7.6).

The eyelids and lacrimal apparatus

The eyelids are strengthened by fibrous tarsal plates. Three sets of muscles act on the eyelid.

- The **levator palpebrae superioris** is attached to the superior tarsal plate. It is innervated by cranial nerve III.
- **Muller's muscle** originates under the levator, and inserts into the upper tarsal border. It is smooth muscle, innervated by sympathetic fibres.
- The superficial tissues of the eyelid contain circular fibres of the **orbicularis oculi**, which is supplied by nerve VII. Local eye block anaesthetic placed behind the globe may not block nerve VII, and orbicularis oculi contraction can increase intra-ocular pressure, hindering surgery. The muscle is important in dilating the lacrimal sacs and providing a pumping action for tear drainage.

Because of the multiple nerves supplying the eyelid, many different conditions (involving nerve, muscle, and neuromuscular junction) can cause ptosis (drooping of the eyelid). Of particular interest is **Horner's syndrome**. This consists of partial ptosis, miosis, and anhydrosis, and is caused by interruption of the sympathetic pathways to the eye. A classic symptom of apical lung tumours infiltrating the sympathetic chain in the neck, Horner's syndrome is also a common complication of interscalene block.

The **lacrimal gland** is situated just inside the upper lateral margin of the orbit. The ducts pierce the conjunctiva, and tears wash across the eye and drain, via the superior and inferior lacrimal puncta, to the **lacrimal sac**. This drains into the **nasolacrimal duct** and ultimately the inferior meatus of the nose. Care should be taken not to damage the lacrimal sac during the medial compartment approach to retrobulbar and peribulbar blocks.

The extra-ocular muscles

Six muscles affect movement of the eye: the four rectus muscles, and the superior and inferior obliques. Their attachments and innervation at the apex of the orbit are shown in Figure 7.15. The superior oblique is supplied by nerve IV, the lateral rectus by nerve VI, and all others by nerve III. The nerves enter the muscles within the rectal muscle cone except for the trochlear (nerve IV), which innervates the superior oblique on its orbital surface. This is probably why the superior oblique is the most commonly missed muscle during a peribulbar or retrobulbar block.

Movements (Figure 7.14)

The rectus muscles all insert into the globe anterior to the coronal equator of the eye. The actions of the lateral and medial rectus muscles are simple: the lateral rectus abducts the eye, and the medial rectus adducts it. The superior and inferior recti elevate and depress the eye, respectively, but because of their insertions just medial to the axis of the globe, they both adduct the eye slightly.

The oblique muscles both insert posterior to the coronal equator. The superior oblique runs along the angle between the medial wall and roof of the orbit. Inside the orbital margin, its tendon passes through a fibrous pulley; it then passes backwards and laterally below the superior rectus to its insertion in the upper postero-medial quadrant of the eyeball. The muscle serves to depress and abduct the eye.

The inferior oblique is the only muscle that arises from the front of the orbital cavity. The muscle runs backwards and laterally below the inferior rectus and reaches an insertion near the superior oblique. It elevates and abducts.

Control of eye movements

Eye movements act to focus the fovea onto the target. The rapid movements that enable visualization of moving objects and the extraction of visual information during reading are called **saccadic eye movements**. Other eye movements include:

- **Smooth pursuit movements,** which are voluntary tracking movements.
- **Vergence movements** align the fovea of each eye when the head is rotated from its subject.
- **Vestibulo-ocular movements** stabilize the eyes relative to head movement.

The control of eye movements involves the frontal eye fields in the premotor cortex. They project to the superior colliculus; fibres from here project to the vertical and horizontal gaze centres in the brainstem. Connections via the fibres of the medial longitudinal fasciculus coordinate eye movements.

Visual pathways

Information supplied from the retina is relayed to many parts of the brain. Signals leave the retina through the optic nerve to the optic chiasm at the base of the brain. The fibres from the nasal half of the retina cross in the chiasm, so that the nasal fibres from one eye join the temporal fibres from the other. They form the optic tract. The optic tract fibres project to a number of structures.

- The primary visual pathway is from the retina to the **dorsal lateral geniculate (DLG)** nucleus in the thalamus. Fibres from here are transmitted via the internal capsule (optic radiation) and terminate in the primary visual cortex, along and within the calcarine fissure of the occipital lobe.
- The **pretectum** coordinates the pupillary light reflex. The fibres from the pretectum project to the Edinger–Westphal nucleus, which in turn sends preganglionic parasympathetic fibres to the ciliary ganglion.

- The **suprachiasmatic nucleus** of the hypothalamus is important for circadian rhythm coordination.
- The **superior colliculus** coordinates head and eye movements.

Visual field defect and localization of the site of injury

- Damage before the chiasm results of loss of vision in one eye.
- A chiasm lesion: bitemporal hemianopia, e.g. pituitary tumour
- Lesions in the pathway after the chiasm are rarely complete, since this pathway is divergent with fibres transmitted to several parts of the brain.

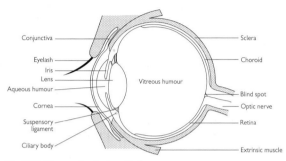

Fig. 7.12 The eye (sagittal section).

→ The pupillary light reflex

The light reflex (Figure 7.16) is useful in the diagnosis of comatose patients. Afferent input for the pupillary reflex is from the light-sensitive optic nerve. Afferent fibres travel to the pre-tectal nucleus. Here there is a relay to the Edinger-Westphal nucleus bilaterally, inducing an ipsilateral (direct) and contralateral (consensual) response. The efferent parasympathetic fibres travel via the oculomotor nerve to the ciliary ganglion, where they synapse and supply the iris.

The light reflex is **preserved** in metabolic or toxic coma. Even if the pupils are small, sufficient light will produce some reaction (except barbiturate and tricyclic antidepressant overdoses).

If pupils are **bilaterally unreactive**, the site of the lesion can be distinguished by the size of the pupil:

- Tectal lesions produce large fixed pupils which do not react to light but can still accommodate (the Argyll-Robertson pupil).
- Midbrain lesions produce mid-position pupils.
- Pontine lesions produce pinpoint pupils.

Bilateral unreactive pupils in a comatose patient are due to midbrain disease, bilateral nerve III palsy or intoxication.

A **unilateral unreactive pupil** may be due to an isolated nerve III lesion, but is normally due to external compression of nerve III by transtentorial herniation (Section 7.8).

Normally light shone in one eye will elicit constriction of the pupil in both eyes (the **consensual response**); the presence of a direct response but no consensual response suggests a problem with the efferent output from the Edinger–Westphal nucleus.

149

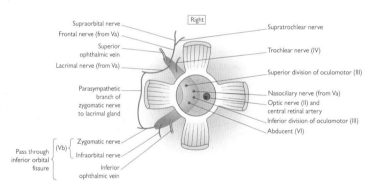

Fig. 7.13 Anatomy of the superior and inferior orbital fissures.

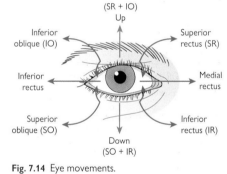

Fig. 7.14 Eye movements.

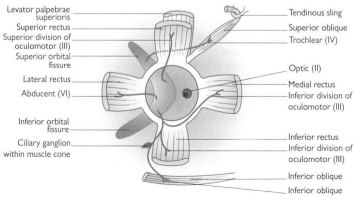

Fig. 7.15 Nerves and muscles at the apex of the orbit.

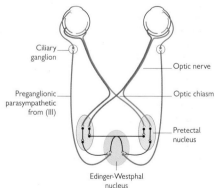

Fig. 7.16 The pupillary light reflex.

Intra-ocular pressure

During surgery, a rise in intra-ocular pressure (IOP) can exacerbate bleeding, and increase the chance of vitreous loss and lens prolapse. It is particularly important to avoid excessive IOP in penetrating globe injuries (see opposite).

The majority of the eyeball's volume comprises the intra-ocular fluid (aqueous and vitreous humours) and blood within the choroidal vessels. In front of the lens is the aqueous humour, which is freely flowing. Behind the lens is the more gelatinous vitreous humour.

Aqueous humour is continually being formed and absorbed. The balance of these processes controls the intra-ocular volume—and thus the intra-ocular pressure.

Aqueous humour is formed at a rate of 2ml/min by the ciliary processes, which project from the **ciliary body**. Formation is partly by ultrafiltration but mostly by active secretion. The fluid flows through the pupil into the anterior chamber. In the angle between the cornea and iris is a meshwork of trabeculae. Via these, aqueous humour flows into the **canal of Schlemm** (a very thin-walled vein) which empties into the extra-ocular veins.

Normal IOP is 10–25mmHg. Factors affecting IOP include altered choroidal venous volume, altered arterial blood pressure, altered intra-ocular fluid volumes, and extrinsic compression (see also Table 7.1).

Altered choroidal venous volume

Coughing, vomiting, positive pressure ventilation, head- or face-down positioning, and obstructed venous drainage all increase venous pressure within the eye. Hypercapnia raises IOP by two mechanisms: it dilates choroidal blood vessels, and also increases the release of carbonic anhydrase (important in aqueous humour formation). Hypoxia (PO_2 <8kPa) dilates vessels.

Altered arterial blood pressure

Below 90mmHg systolic, IOP is proportional to blood pressure. Autoregulation is similar to that in the brain (Section 7.9). Ketamine increases IOP due to its sympathomimetic actions.

Altered intra-ocular fluid volumes

Increasing absorption and decreasing production of aqueous humour can compensate for raised IOP. Vitreous humour volume is normally constant, but can be decreased by osmotic diuretics.

Absorption of aqueous humour is decreased if there is blockage of the trabecular meshwork (e.g. by debris from inflammatory cells or blood, or narrowing of the angle beween the cornea and iris). The consequent rise in intra-ocular pressure is acute glaucoma; it can compromise the blood supply to the optic nerve, resulting in blindness.

Extrinsic compression

Increased tone in the extra-ocular muscles can increase IOP. This can occur with the use of suxamethonium, but is transient (maximum at 2–4min, and returning to normal after 7min). Anaesthetic interventions, such as pressure on the eye from a mask, or large volumes of local anaesthesia within (retrobulbar) or outside (peribulbar) the muscle cone may increase IOP.

Autonomic control of the eye

Both sympathetic and parasympathetic fibres innervate the eye.

The parasympathetic preganglionic fibres stem from the **Edinger–Westphal nucleus** in the brainstem. They pass in nerve III to the **ciliary ganglion**, which lies behind the eye. The post-ganglionic fibres from the ciliary ganglion send fibres via the **ciliary nerves.** These nerves innervate the ciliary muscle which controls accommodation and the constricting sphincter of the iris.

The sympathetic fibres originate in the **intermedio-lateral horn cells** of the T1 segment of the spinal cord. They pass to the **superior cervical ganglion,** where they synapse with **post-ganglionic nerves**. These climb with the carotid artery and its branches to innervate the dilating radial fibres of the iris.

Ocular reflexes during surgery

Several alarming reflexes may occur during ophthalmic surgery.

- **Oculocardiac:** bradycardia or even sinus arrest on traction on the extra-ocular muscles. The afferent limb is via nerve V; unsurprisingly, the efferent is via nerve X. Common in squint surgery, especially in children. Vagolytics obtund the reflex.
- **Oculorespiratory:** the afferent limb of this reflex is via nerve V. This connects with the pneumotaxic centre in the pons, and the medullary respiratory centre. Shallow breathing, bradypnoea, or even respiratory arrest may occur. Common with squint surgery, and not responsive to anticholinergics.
- **Oculoemetic:** due to connections of the medial longitudinal bundle with vestibular nucleus. There is a high incidence of nausea and vomiting after squint surgery.

Regional anaesthesia of the eye

Peribulbar and sub-Tenon blocks are the most popular regional anaesthetics in eye surgery and has largely replaced retrobulbar blocks. Retrobulbar blockade is associated with a much higher incidence of complication and the need for an additional facial nerve block.

Perioperative care

Full monitoring should be used for all regional blockade.

Pressure area care and pillows are used to make the patient comfortable and reassurance administered by a dedicated observer. Patients should be encouraged to communicate silently: speaking alters the position of the face and eye, making surgery difficult.

Sedation is rarely required but additional oxygen may be used to reverse incidental hypoxia.

Complications of regional anaesthetic

Due to either the block or the agent used.

Intravascular injection and anaphylaxis
Retrobulbar haemorrhage

This is very rare with peribulbar injections. Noted as a sudden rise in IOP. The operation should be postponed. Subconjunctival haemorrhage is less of a problem and will be absorbed; surgery need not be postponed.

Subconjunctival oedema

This is seldom a problem since it dissipates with gentle pressure applied to the closed eye.

Perforation of the globe

Myopic eyes are longer but also thinner and so are more at risk of perforation. Noted as immediate pain with sudden loss of vision or vitreous haemorrhage.

Central spread of local anaesthetic

This is due to either retrograde arterial spread or direct injection into the dural cuff. May present within 5min with features of LA toxicity or contralateral blindness caused by reflux of the drug to the optic chiasma.

Oculocardiac reflex

Bradycardia that follows traction on the eye. May be a problem during perfomance of the block but not during surgery.

Optic nerve atrophy

This may be caused by direct damage to the optic nerve with vascular occlusion or haemorrhage of the central retinal artery.

Penetrating eye injury

When the globe of the eye has been penetrated, an increase in IOP may cause expulsion of intra-ocular contents and permanent damage.

Depending on the urgency of the operation (liaise with the surgical team), it is preferable to have the patient properly starved. As an emergency procedure, the patient may have a full stomach and require a rapid sequence induction. Senior anaesthetic input is required when planning anaesthesia.

Rapid sequence induction in penetrating eye injury

During pre-oxygenation, take care not to exert pressure on the eye with the facemask.

Suxamethonium is *theoretically* contraindicated as it causes a rise in IOP. However, it is important to weigh the risk to the eye against the risk of aspiration of gastric contents. If difficulties are anticipated, suxamethonium should be used to provide the best intubating conditions, despite the risk to the eye (in practice, this risk is minimized by the prior administration of an induction agent which reduces IOP, e.g. thiopental).

If there is no indication for a rapid sequence intubation (and assuming no anticipated airway problems), a generous dose of a non-depolarizing relaxant (e.g. vecuronium 0.15mg/kg) is appropriate. It is important to wait for this to take effect before intubation, since coughing or straining during laryngoscopy will increase IOP. An LMA can be used as an alternative in a properly starved patient, and this may help to avoid coughing and smooth recovery. However, once surgery has commenced, access to the airway may be awkward. When securing the airway, be careful to avoid pressure on neck veins with over-tight tube ties.

IPPV or spontaneous ventilation techniques can be used. IPPV allows better control of P_aCO_2 and allows the patient to be paralysed, minimizing coughing and straining. However, IPPV in itself can raise IOP, especially if high levels of positive end-expiratory pressure (PEEP) are used. In spontaneous ventilation, adequate depth of anaesthesia to prevent coughing is required, and this usually leads to hypoventilation and increased P_aCO_2.

Other strategies to consider include head-up tilt, hypotensive anaesthesia if appropriate, and avoidance of hypoxia and surges in blood pressure. Opioid analgesics may smooth extubation and prevent coughing; however, they may induce vomiting and so generous anti-emetic prophylaxis should be given.

Peribulbar blockade (Figure 7.17) and sub-Tenon block of the eye

Peribulbar block

Following IV cannulation, the conjunctival sac is anaesthetized with 3 drops of amethocaine 1%, repeated 3 times at 1min intervals.

The injection solution contains 5ml bupivacaine 0.75% plain plus 5ml lidocaine 2% with 1:200,000 adrenaline. Hyaluronidase 75 units improves diffusion of the LA within the orbit.

The patient is positioned supine, looking directly ahead and with the eyes in a neutral position.

The inferotemporal injection passes through an already anaesthetized conjunctiva. The needle is advanced without resistance, parallel to the orbital floor under the globe. When the needle tip is past the equator of the globe it should be angled slightly medial (20°) and cephalad (10° upwards), avoiding the wall of the orbit. With the needle 2.5cm below the skin and following negative aspiration, 5ml of solution is injected slowly. There should not be any resistance to injection, which would indicate possible extra-ocular muscle injection. During the injection the lower lid may fill with the anaesthetic mixture and there may be some conjunctival oedema.

This is repeated medially, and after passing through the medial canthal ligament, a further 5ml is injected. The eye is then closed with tape and placed under an oculopressor for 10min in order to ↓ IOP.

The signs of a successful block include ptosis, minimal eye movement in any direction, and inability to close the eye fully once opened.

LA outside the muscle cone might not completely abolish vision but only light perception might persist.

Sub-Tenon block

The sub-Tenon block carries a lower risk of globe perforation since a blunt cannula is used.

First, topical anaesthesia is applied to the eye. 5-6mm inferomedial to the limbus, the conjunctiva is raised with Moorfield's forceps. A small incision in the conjunctiva is made with scissors. The white, avascular Tenon's capsule is dissected off the vascular sclera. The sub-Tenon cannula is passed backwards around the globe, and local anaesthetic (approx 4ml) is injected. Hyaluronidase is often added, to aid the spread of solution. Gentle pressure is applied to the eye externally.

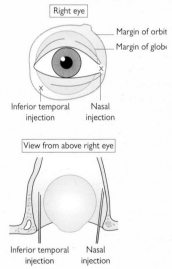

Fig. 7.17 Peribulbar blockade of the eye.

Table 7.1 Factors affecting intra-ocular pressure	
Increase	**Decrease**
Increased venous pressure	Decreased venous pressure
Coughing, straining	Hypovolaemia
Jugular compression	Head-up tilt
Head-down/face-down positions	Hypocarbia
Hypercarbia	Hypotension
Hypoxia	Intravenous induction agents (except
Hypertension	ketamine)
Increased aqueous humour	Inhalational agents (fall in IOP is
production or decreased resorption	proportional to
(e.g. acute glaucoma)	the inspired concentration
Extrinsic compression	Non-depolarizing muscle relaxants.
Suxamethonium	↓ aqueous volume: acetazolamide.
Ketamine	↓ vitreous volume: mannitol

7.7 The skull

The skull is made up of 22 bones (not including those of the inner ear). There are two types of bony structure in the cranium:

The **neurocranium** (Figures 7.18 and 7.19) comprises the flat bones of the vault of the skull. These are the **frontal, temporal, parietal,** and **occipital** bones. They form a bony armour to protect the brain. The flat bones are joined at fibrous sutures. The frontal and parietal bones are united by the coronal suture, the parietal bones meet at the midline sagittal suture, and the parietal and occipital bones meet at the lambdoid suture. The **bregma** is the site of the fused anterior fontanelle, and the **pterion** is an H-shaped pattern of sutures between the frontal, parietal, sphenoid, and temporal bones.

The **viscerocranium** comprises the bones around the base of the skull. The sensory organs for sight, smell, taste, hearing, and balance are contained within and supported by these bones. They also provide attachments for the muscles of facial expression. They house numerous passageways allowing nerves, vessels, and other structures to pass into and out of the skull.

Cranial fossae and holes in the skull

The cranial cavity is divided into three regions: the anterior, middle, and posterior fossae. The various openings into the skull are in bold; look at Figure 7.20 to identify them.

Anterior cranial fossa

The anterior cranial fossa is mainly surrounded by the frontal bone, which makes up its floor, anterior wall, and roof. It is bounded posteriorly by the sphenoid, and laterally by the pterion. In the midine, the ethmoid bone contributes to the floor. Between the frontal and ethmoid bones, the **foramen caecum** carries small veins from the nose to the superior sagittal sinus. The **cribriform plates** provide openings for the olfactory nerves, and the crista galli of the ethmoid projects upwards to give attachment to the falx cerebri (Section 7.8). The anterior cranial fossa contains the frontal lobes of the brain and the central olfactory apparatus.

Middle cranial fossa

The middle cranial fossa is butterfly-shaped, with the central portion made up of body of the sphenoid bone. This portion contains the pituitary fossa (or sella turcica) and the optic chiasm. The 'wings' of the butterfly are bounded by the sphenoid bone anteriorly, the squamous temporal bone laterally, and the petrous temporal bone infero-posteriorly. These Sections contain the temporal lobes. The middle cranial fossa has numerous openings:

Middle portion

The **optic canal** transmits the optic nerve from the back of the eye to the optic chiasm. The ophthalmic artery runs within the nerve.

Lateral portions

The **superior orbital fissure** transmits the oculomotor, trochlear, and abducent nerves (III, IV, and VI), the ophthalmic division of the trigeminal (Va, as separate lacrimal, frontal, and nasociliary branches), the ophthalmic veins, and branches of the middle meningeal and lacrimal arteries and their sympathetic fibres.

The **foramen rotundum** is tucked just below the inferomedial end of the superior orbital fissure, and transmits the maxillary division of the trigeminal nerve (Vb).

The **foramen ovale** runs through the greater wing of the sphenoid, carrying the mandibular division of the trigeminal nerve (Vc), the lesser petrosal nerve, and the accessory meningeal artery.

The foramen ovale and the **foramen spinosum** together resemble an exclamation mark, with the foramen spinosum forming the dot. The foramen spinosum carries the meningeal branch of Vc and the middle meningeal vessels.

Just lateral to the body of the sphenoid is the spiky **foramen lacerum**. The internal carotid artery enters behind and exits above (to run in the medial wall of the cavernous sinus); the greater petrosal nerve enters above/behind and runs forwards to enter the pterygoid canal. *The internal carotid does not directly traverse the foramen lacerum into the skull; it begins in the opening of the* **carotid canal** *(visible on the skull's external surface), and then turns 90° upwards to go through the lacerum. Note the trigeminal impression just behind and lateral.*

Posterior cranial fossa

The posterior cranial fossa is walled anteriorly by the petrous temporal bone and posteriorly by the occipital bone.

The **internal acoustic meatus** opens at the medial edge of the crest of the petrous temporal bone. It contains the facial and vestibulocochlear nerves (VII and VIII), and the labyrinthine artery.

The **jugular foramen** tucks in at the posterior border of the petrous temporal bone and exits in the slot between the petrous temporal and occipital bones. The sigmoid and inferior petrosal sinuses meet at the internal opening, running through to emerge as the internal jugular vein. The jugular foramen also contains the glossopharyngeal, vagus, and accessory nerves (IX, X, and XI).

The **hypoglossal canal** runs anterolaterally from just above the foramen magnum to emerge just medial to the jugular foramen. The hypoglossal nerve runs through it.

The **foramen magnum** cannot be missed. It contains the medulla and its covering meninges, the vertebral arteries, the anterior and posterior spinal arteries (and associated sympathetic nerves), and the spinal accessory nerve. The tectorial membrane (continuous with the posterior longitudinal ligament) and the atlanto-occipital membranes (anterior and posterior) are attached to the outer margins of the foramen magnum.

Exterior base of skull

More openings in the skull can be seen when looking at the external surface of its base.

The **incisive fossa** lies in the midline in the anterior hard palate and the **incisive canals** run into it from the floor of the nose above, each with its nasopalatine nerve and greater palatine vessels.

The **posterior nasal apertures** run from the posterior surface of the hard palate, forwards to the nose. The tiny **palatovaginal canals** open just behind, carrying the pharyngeal nerves and pharyngeal branch of the maxillary artery.

Passing through the **inferior orbital fissure** are: branches of Vb (infra-orbital and zygomatic); and veins draining to the pterygoid venous plexus.

The **stylomastoid foramen** lies just behind the styloid process. It carries the facial nerve away from the middle ear to emerge here.

The small **mastoid foramen** opens behind the mastoid process. It carries veins which connect the sigmoid sinus and occipital veins, and the meningeal branch of the occipital artery.

Skull fractures

The skull is liable to fracture at certain sites. The middle cranial fossa is the weakest compartment, with thin bones and multiple foramina. Commonly fractured areas include the pterion (as it is a confluence of several sutures), the sphenoid sinus, the cribriform plate, and the orbital roof in the anterior cranial fossa. Skull fractures are usually of limited clinical significance, although they do indicate the nature and force of injury. However, important skull fractures are as follows.

- Depressed skull fractures (Figure 7.21): may lead to secondary brain damage.
- Compound skull fractures: infection may occur if the fracture is associated with a skin breach.
- Pterion fractures: these are important because the middle meningeal artery lies deep to the pterion. Injury to this artery can produce extradural haemorrhage.

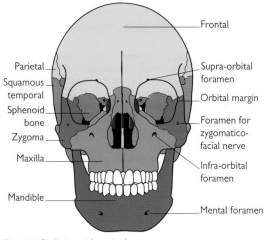

Fig. 7.18 Skull viewed from the front.

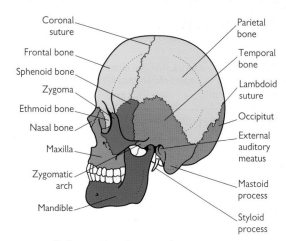

Fig. 7.19 Skull viewed from the side

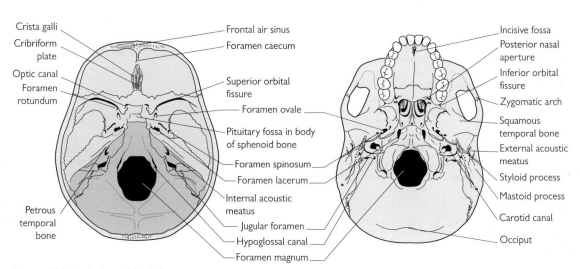

Fig. 7.20 Holes in the base of the skull.

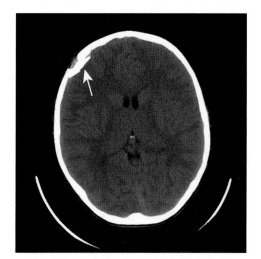

Fig. 7.21 CT scan of a depressed skull fracture (arrow).

Surrounding and supporting the brain are three tissue layers: the dura mater, the archnoid mater, and the pia mater. These are collectively known as the meninges.

The dura mater

The outermost layer is the **dura mater**, which is a two-layered membrane. The outer layer adheres closely to the skull; only the rupture of an artery disrupts this relationship. The inner layer of the dura is a strong fibrous layer, continuous with the dura of the spinal cord at the foramen magnum. The inner layer reflects away from the outer layer to form dural infoldings that divide the cranial cavity into compartments. The main dural infoldings are as follows.

The cerebral falx (falx cerebri) This sickle-shaped dural fold separates the right and left hemispheres. It is anchored anteriorly to the frontal crest (frontal bone) and crista galli (ethmoid bone), and posteriorly to internal occipital protuberance.

The cerebellar tentorium This is a cresent-shaped membrane which separates the occipital lobes of the cerebral hemispheres from the cerebellum (Figure 7.22). The falx cerebri attaches to the tentorium cerebeli in the midline, holding it up and giving it a tent-like appearance. The anteromedial border is free, leaving a gap called the tentorial notch. This notch separates the posterior and middle cranial fossae.

Two other smaller infoldings are the **cerebellar falx**, which separates the two lobes of the cerebellum, and the **sellar diaphragm**, a circular sheet suspended between the clinoid processes forming a partial roof over the pituitary fossa.

Space-occupying lesions may cause midline shift and herniation of the uncus of the temporal lobe through the tentorial notch. This flattens the midbrain and compresses the ipsilateral third nerve, giving rise to pupillary and occulomotor signs. There is compression of the posterior cerebral artery, leading to occipital lobe infarction.

The venous sinuses

In some regions the two layers of dura separate and are lined by endothelium to produce the **venous sinuses**. The venous sinuses are shown in Figure 7.22.

The sagittal sinuses

The **superior sagittal sinus** lies in the superior border of the falx cerebri (Figure 7.24). Blood drains into it from the dorsolateral veins of the cerebral hemispheres. At the occipital protuberance it turns to the right, becoming the **right transverse sinus**. The transverse sinus passes forward in the lateral attachment of the tentorium cerebelli to the edge of the petrous temporal bone. Here it curls down as the **right sigmoid sinus**, passing through the jugular foramen and becoming the **right internal jugular vein**.

The **inferior sagittal sinus** is in the midline of the inferior free margin of the falx cerebri (Figure 7.24). Together with blood from the **great cerebral vein** it forms the **straight sinus** at the tentorium falx. The straight sinus turns left, becoming the **left transverse sinus**.

The pattern on the right and left can sometimes be reversed. In most cases, the right-sided venous channels are larger than the left. Measuring oxygen saturation in the right internal jugular bulb gives a better indication of cerebral oxygen extraction than a measurement from the left.

The cavernous sinus

This is formed in the embryo. It is a confluence of several venous channels around the internal carotid artery as it enters the middle cranial fossa. The right and left cavernous sinuses lie on either side of the pituitary fossa, and communicate with the transverse sinuses and internal jugular veins through the **petrosal sinus**. Cranial nerves II, IV and Va pass through the cavernous sinus to the superior orbital fissure, and VI passes through the sinus on the internal carotid artery, also to pass through the superior orbital fissure (see Figure 7.23). The cavernous sinus is connected through various skull foramina to facial and other external veins. These connections can cause superficial infection to spread to the sinus, which can lead to cavernous sinus thrombosis.

The basilar and occipital sinuses

These communicate through the foramen magnum with the internal vertebral venous plexus. These veins do not have valves, and compression of the thorax or abdomen (as in coughing and straining) may force venous blood into the dural venous sinuses via this plexus. This increases blood volume and pressure within the skull. Similarly, infection and malignant disease may spread into the cerebral venous sinuses via these pathways.

Dural headache

Although brain tissue is insensible to pain, the dura is very sensitive. It is innervated by all three divisions of nerve V plus contributions from nerves X and XII. The nerve supply is particularly rich along the sagittal sinus and the cerebellar tentorium, and around the base of the skull. Tugging in any of these areas causes intense headache. Loss of CSF (e.g. from a dural puncture) causes a headache of this type as the brain sags and pulls on its dural supports. Other causes of dural headache include trauma or stretching to the dural blood vessels (the largest being the middle meningeal artery) and direct irritation (e.g. in meningitis).

Posterior fossa craniotomy is generally more painful than a supratentorial craniotomy, as there is disruption to the dura around the skull base.

The arachnoid and pia mater

The **arachnoid** is held against the inner layer of the dura by the pressure of CSF, which fills the space between the arachnoid and the pia. The dural walls of sinuses possess small defects, which allow the arachnoid to billow through. These are called **archnoid granulations** and are the sites of CSF reabsorption.

The **pia** is a thin highly vascular membrane; it adheres to the brain and follows its contours.

Trauma and bleeding into meningeal spaces

An **extradural haemorrhage** occurs when an artery ruptures (usually the middle meningeal, after a blow to the pterion). Blood collects between the external layer of dura and the calvarium. Typically, the history is of loss of consciousness, often followed by a lucid interval. There is a typical lentiform appearance on CT. The prognosis is good with timely intervention.

In a **subdural haematoma,** blood tracks into the space between the inner dural layer and the arachnoid. This is usually due to venous bleeding (often from a shearing injury of the superior cerebral vein as it enters the superior sagittal sinus, due to acceleration–deceleration forces associated with trauma).

A **subarachnoid haemorrhage,** where blood enters the CSF under the arachnoid mater, usually follows arterial bleeding (e.g. rupture of aneurysm in the circle of Willis).

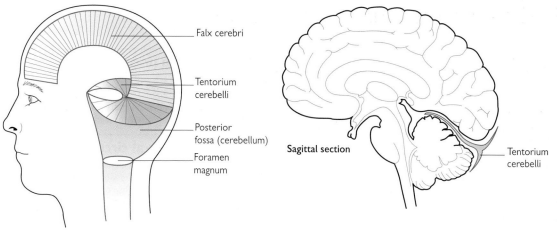

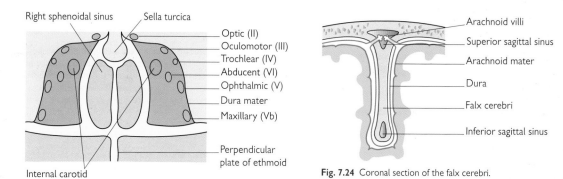

Fig. 7.22 The tentorium cerebelli separates the cerebellum from the occipital lobes above. In cases of raised intracranial pressure or space-occupying lesions within the skull, brain tissue may herniate around the free edge of the tentorium cerebelli, or down through the foramen magnum.

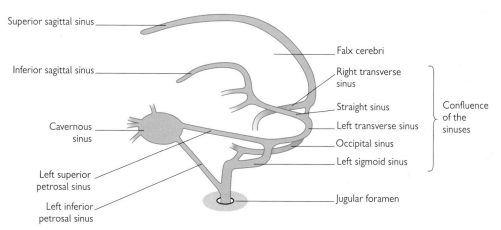

Fig. 7.23 Coronal section of the cavernous sinus.

Fig. 7.24 Coronal section of the falx cerebri.

Fig. 7.25 The venous sinuses.

7.9 Cerebral perfusion

The cerebral circulation

The brain is supplied by an anterior and a posterior circulation (Figure 7.26).

Anterior circulation

Formed from the paired **internal carotid arteries**. The left carotid comes directly off the arch of the aorta, while the right arises from the brachiocephalic artery.

At the top of the neck, the internal carotid enters the carotid canal in the temporal bone. After a series of bends, it enters the cranial cavity. In the middle cranial fossa it runs in the cavernous sinus, just medial to the abducent nerve (VI). It divides into the **anterior** and **middle cerebral arteries** (ACA and MCA, respectively). Before this terminal bifurcation, it gives rise to the **ophthalmic, hypophyseal**, and **posterior communicating arteries**. The posterior communicating artery (PcoA) connects the anterior and posterior circulations.

Posterior circulation

This is formed from the paired **vertebral arteries** (often unequal in size). These arise from the **subclavian arteries**, and ascend in the foramina of the transverse processes of the upper six cervical vertebrae. They join to form the single **basilar artery** at the lower border of the pons. The medulla is supplied directly by branches from the basilar artery. At the upper border of the pons, the basilar bifurcates into the two **posterior cerebral arteries** (PCAs). The two circulations anastomose to form the **circle of Willis**.

Arterial territories

Disruption to the blood supply of the brain is often due to rupture and haemorrhage, thrombus, or embolus. A knowledge of the arterial territories helps to identify the likely site of the disturbance:

The *MCA* supplies most of the dorsolateral surface of the frontal, parietal, and temporal cortex. MCA disruption leads to contralateral hemiplegia, contralateral hemiansethesia, homonymous hemianopia, and global aphasia.

The *ACA* supplies the optic chiasma, the frontal lobes, and the medial aspects of the parietal lobe. As the motor and sensory aspects of the lower limb are on the medial aspects of pre- and post-central gyri, disruption of the ACA results in contralateral lower limb dysfunction.

The *PCA* supplies the geniculate bodies and most of the visual cortex. Lesions here will lead to contralateral homonymous hemianopia.

Some areas of the brain are particularly vulnerable to vascular problems:

Emboli from the heart or internal carotid arteries most commonly enter the middle cerebral artery, with the effects described above.

The medial portion of the medulla is supplied by a single anterior spinal artery, formed by the joining of two branches from the vertebral artery. Compromise produces the medial medullary syndrome. (Section 7.2).

The posterior inferior cerebellar artery has a long tortuous course that is vulnerable to disruption. It provides the supply to the dorsolateral medulla and its disruption leads to the lateral medullary syndrome (Section 7.2).

Pontine vessels arising from the basilar arteries are end arteries, and so are vulnerable to disruption.

The basal ganglia, thalamus, and internal capsule rely on striate arteries for their blood supply. These branch from the proximal regions of the ACA, MCA (predominantly), and PCA. The striate arteries are end arteries, often at right angles to their feeding vessels and with much smaller internal diameters. Therefore they are susceptible to occlusion or rupture in patients with degenerative vascular changes. Haemorrhagic lesions of the striate arteries result in contralateral hemiplegia due to destruction of the descending motor fibres in the posterior limb of the internal capsule (Section 7.21). Contralateral hemianaesthesia may result if ascending thalamocortical fibres are destroyed (Section 7.22).

Cerebral perfusion pressure (CPP)

CPP is the pressure gradient across the cerebral circulation:

CPP = MAP – CVP or ICP (*whichever is the greater*).

When the ICP is greater than the CVP, the cerebral circulation can be considered to behave as a Starling resistor (Sections 13.10 and 13.13).

Control of the cerebral circulation

Normal CBF is 50ml/min/100g (i.e. 750ml/min), approximately 15% of the cardiac output. Flow rates vary little, allowing maintenance of normal brain function under variable systemic conditions. Cerebral blood flow (CBF) varies in an analogous manner to Ohm's law ($V = I \times R$; Section 4.13) and is determined by CPP and cerebral vascular resistance (CVR):

$$CBF = \frac{CPP}{CVR}$$

Baroreceptor mechanisms are designed to maintain a constant systemic driving pressure, allowing tissues to control their own rates of blood flow. Under normal circumstances, CPP is constant and CBF depends on the CVR. The following factors influence the CVR.

Metabolic autoregulation

This is an extremely important control mechanism for the cerebral circulation. When an area of brain is active, locally released vasodilator metabolites cause an increase in vessel calibre and therefore CBF. Anaesthetic agents reduce neuronal activity and CBF, whereas epilepsy (mass neuronal discharge) has the opposite effect. A graph of cerebral blood flow vs. metabolic activity (oxygen consumption) is shown in Figure 7.28.

Pressure autoregulation

This enables CBF to remain constant at MAP values of 50-150mmHg. Increased intravascular pressure tends to stretch vessels; they respond by contraction of smooth muscle. This reduces vessel diameter, increases CVR, and reduces CBF. The autoregulation curve is shown in Figure 7.29.

This mechanism takes a few minutes to occur, and is important in compensating for sudden changes in MAP. Chronic hypertension and chronic sympathetic stimulation will shift the curve to the right; these patients tolerate hypotension very poorly.

Response to carbon dioxide

The cerebral circulation is exquisitely sensitive to carbon dioxide; there is a roughly linear relationship between CBF and P_aCO_2 over a wide range (P_aCO_2 7–12 kPa) (Figure 7.30).

Hyperventilation (reduction in P_aCO_2) increases CVR and reduces the blood volume, and therefore the pressure, inside the skull. However, the vasoconstriction response lasts less than 6hr; bicarbonate crosses the BBB, returning interstitial pH to normal. Subsequent elevation (normalization) of PCO_2 then causes vasodilatation and worsening of ICP. This may explain why routine hyperventilation for head-injured patients results in worse outcomes.

Response to oxygen

Reduction in cerebral oxygen delivery results in vasodilatation. The graph is shown in Figure 7.31. The shape of the oxygen dissociation curve (Section 13.12) influences the shape of this graph: when saturations fall below 90%, oxygen content falls away sharply.

Nervous system control

The sympathetic system alters CVR by only a very small amount. However, it has a major influence on CBF by virtue of its effect on the performance of the systemic circulation, and therefore CPP.

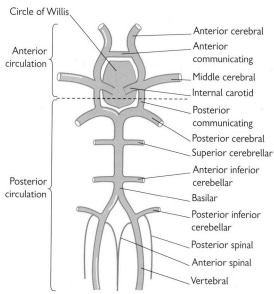

Fig. 7.26 The anterior and posterior circulations.

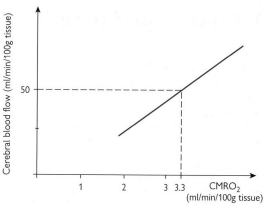

Fig. 7.28 Cerebral blood flow vs. cerebral metabolic rate.

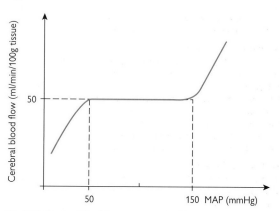

Fig. 7.29 Cerebral blood flow vs. mean arterial pressure.

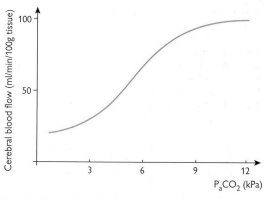

Fig. 7.30 Cerebral blood flow vs. P_aCO_2.

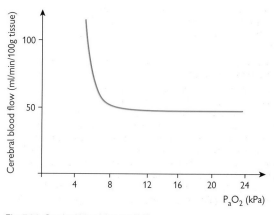

Fig. 7.31 Cerebral blood flow vs. P_aO_2.

→ The blood–brain barrier

Charged and polar macromolecules cannot pass into the ECF of the brain because of the presence of the blood-brain barrier (BBB). It provides a stable chemical environment for the neurons of the CNS.

What is the blood–brain barrier?

The BBB is formed by tight junctions (Figure 7.27) between the endothelial cells of the cerebral capillaries. Water-soluble molecules find this barrier impenetrable. In addition, endothelial cells contain monoamine oxidase and dopa decarboxylase; these metabolize amines before they can cross into the interstitium.

Circumventricular organs include the posterior pituitary, the chemoreceptor trigger zone, the pineal gland, the subfornical organ, and the organum vasulosum. These lie outside the BBB. They all have neuroendocrine functions and require access to the general circulation. They are the only parts to stain with trypan blue when injected IV.

CSF access

Oxygen, carbon dioxide, and all lipid-soluble substances pass through relatively easily. The transfer rate for water is significantly lower than that for other capillary beds. Glucose and amino acids cross via specific transporters. Electrolytes cross only very slowly, although sodium is actively secreted into the CSF during its formation.

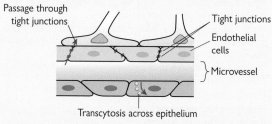

Fig. 7.27 Tight junctions consist of proteins, e.g. claudins, occludins and junctional adhesion molecules. They are anchored in the membranes of two adjacent cells and their interaction holds these cells together, preventing other molecules from passing between them. Tight junction proteins are connected to scaffold proteins; this allows the feedback (signal transduction and transcription) required for their regulation.

7.10 Cerebrospinal fluid, intracranial pressure, and head injury

Cerebrospinal fluid

The total volume of the CSF is about 130ml. The ventricular system (a series of irregularly shaped cavities within the brain) contains 30ml, and the subarachnoid space holds the rest (25ml intracranially, and 75ml around the spinal cord). The rate of formation is approximately 0.35ml/min (500ml/day), and the total CSF volume is replaced every 8-12hr. Its composition is shown opposite. The blood–CSF barrier is formed by tight junctions between choroid plexus epithelial cells.

CSF is produced by a process of active secretion by epithelial cells in the choroid plexus. Although the plexus is found in all four cerebral ventricles, most CSF is made in the **lateral ventricles**. It flows from there through the **interventricular foramen** (of Monro), into the **third ventricle**. It passes via the narrow **cerebral aqueduct** (of Sylvius) into the **fourth ventricle**. It leaves the ventricular system in the medulla, through the midline **median aperture** (foramen of Magendie) and paired **lateral apertures** (foramina of Luschka). CSF mainly drains back into the venous channels via **arachnoid villi**, although other pathways of absorption have been described. The main pathway of flow of CSF is shown in Figure 7.33.

Functions of the CSF

- Brain and spinal cord are rendered buoyant by the CSF in which they are suspended (the effective weight of the brain is reduced from 1.4kg to less than 50g).
- Provides nutrients for both neurons and glial cells.
- Vehicle for removal of waste products of cellular metabolism.
- Maintains the constancy of the ionic composition of the local microenvironment of the cells of the nervous system.
- May function as a transport system for biologically active substances (releasing factors, hormones, neurotransmitters).

Intracranial pressure (ICP)

Normal ICP is about 10–15mmHg (150–200mmH$_2$O). Values up to 8mmHg are considered normal in the first few months of life.

The pressure–volume relationship between ICP and cranial constituents (blood, CSF, and brain tissue) is explained by the **Monro–Kellie doctrine** (see opposite). The main intracranial volume buffer is CSF, and to a lesser extent blood. Compensatory mechanisms can maintain normal ICP for volume changes less than about 120 ml.

Symptoms and signs of raised ICP include headache, nausea, vomiting, ocular palsies, altered conscious level, and papilloedema. Late on, ICP can lead to Cushing's triad:

- Hypertension (increased systolic blood pressure with a widened pulse pressure)
- Bradycardia
- Abnormal respiration.

Head injury

Management is by an ABCDE approach, in line with ATLS recommendations. A patent airway, adequate ventilation and oxygenation, and maintenance of cardiovascular performance will minimize secondary insult to the brain.

Rapid assessment of 'Disability' involves determination of the GCS and inspection of the pupils for size and reaction. The latter is important in alerting the assessor to the possibility of significant intracranial pathology necessitating swift imaging and urgent neurosurgical referral.

CT scans are usually performed after completion of the primary survey if head injury is suspected. However, several points should be emphasized:

Patients should not be transferred if physiologically unstable. Their observations should be returning to normal and they should be showing signs of response to treatment before leaving the resuscitation room.

For ongoing haemorrhage resulting in continued shock, resuscitative surgery may be required before CNS imaging. Imaging should be performed immediately postoperatively.

All intubated head-injured patients should undergo CT imaging of both the cervical spine and the head. Adequate peg views are impossible following intubation, and this renders plain radiography redundant.

Imaging should take place with maintenance of full cervical protection. Transferring a patient in this manner can be difficult and is worth practising in advance.

Although modern CT scanning is fast, care must be taken to maintain clinical observation of the patient. Remember to assess the pupillary response regularly.

Referral to a specialist neurosurgical unit should be made early, with minimal delay before and during transportation. Use should be made of the time available prior to transfer.

Transfer strategies

- Maintenance of cerebral perfusion pressure above 70mmHg, with or without ICP monitoring. CBF is ultimately dependent on CPP.
- Maintenance of normal gas exchange. Mechanical ventilation may be required. Hyperventilation controls P_aCO_2 and cerebral blood volume. It can be used to control acutely elevated ICP, although the effect is temporary. In most circumstances, a P_aCO_2 at the lower end of the normal range is recommended.
- Maintenance of normal temperature. CBF is directly related to the cerebral metabolic rate (CMRO$_2$). Hyperthermia increases CMRO$_2$ and will increase ICP. However, the use of therapeutic hypothermia in head injury is controversial and it is not routinely performed.
- Maintenance of normoglycaemia and electrolyte balance.
- Avoidance of coughing and straining which might raise ICP.
- 15° head-up tilt and avoidance of compression of the neck veins (e.g. by endotracheal tube ties or CVP line dressings). This will aid venous drainage and prevent elevation of ICP.
- Mannitol or barbiturates may be used to reduce ICP in specific circumstances. Steroids are useful only if raised ICP is caused by tumour.

Indications for referral to a neurosurgical unit

A patient with a head injury should be discussed with a neurosurgeon when:

- CT scan in a general hospital shows a recent intracranial lesion.
- When a patient fulfils the criteria for CT scanning but cannot be scanned within an appropriate period.
- When a patient has clinical features that suggest that neurosurgical assessment, monitoring, or management is appropriate, irrespective of CT scan findings.
- Persistent coma (GCS 8/15 or less) after initial resuscitation.
- Confusion persisting for more than 4 hr.
- Deterioration in conscious level after admission.
- Progressive focal neurological signs.
- A seizure without full recovery.
- Depressed skull facture.
- Definite or suspected penetrating injury.
- CSF leak, or other sign of basal fracture.

Further reading

Early management of patients with a head injury: Scottish Intercollegiate Guidelines Network 2000. http://www.sign.ac.uk

→ Causes of raised ICP

Mass effect: tumor, haematomas, abscesses.

Generalized brain swelling: ischaemic states, acute liver failure, hypertensive encephalopathy.

Increase in venous pressure: venous sinus thrombosis, obstruction of superior mediastinal or jugular veins.

Hydrocephalus: obstruction to CSF flow and/or absorption (e.g. subarachnoid haemorrhage, tumour, bacterial meningitis,); increased CSF production (e.g. choroid plexus tumour, meningitis).

→ Composition of CSF

The composition of CSF differs from that of plasma.

Appearance	Clear colourless
pH	7.32
Specific gravity	1.004–1.007g/cm^3
Osmolality	290mosm/kgH$_2$O
Protein	0.3g/L
Glucose	4.8mmol/L
PCO_2	6.6kPa

→ *Monro–Kellie doctrine*

Brain	85% of intracranial volume
Blood	10% of intracranial volume
CSF	5% of intracranial volume

The skull is a rigid box; fluids are incompressible. Therefore any increase in intracranial volume will result in an increase in ICP. The initial compensation is by movement of CSF out of the skull to surround the spinal cord. This is followed by a small reduction of blood volume. When the compensatory mechanisms are exhausted, the pressure will rise abruptly (Figure 7.32).

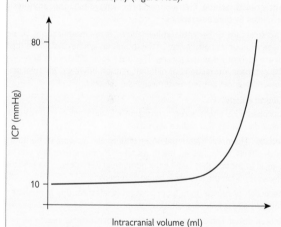

Fig. 7.32 Cerebral elastance curve. Once compensatory mechanisms for accommodating extra intracranial volume (e.g. arterial bleed, tumour) are exhausted, intracranial pressure rises rapidly.

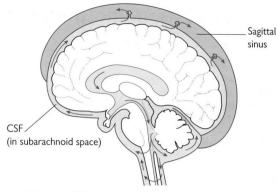

Sagittal sinus

CSF (in subarachnoid space)

Fig. 7.33 Flow of CSF.

✚ Glasgow Coma Scale

The GCS is derived from three parameters:

Best eye response
1 No eye opening
2 Eye opening to pain
3 Eye opening to verbal stimulus
4 Eye opening spontaneously

Best verbal response
1 No verbal response
2 Incomprehensible sounds
3 Inappropriate words
4 Confused speech
5 Oriented

Best motor response
1 No motor response
2 Extension to pain
3 Abnormal flexion to pain
4 Withdrawal from pain
5 Localizing to pain
6 Obeys commands

GCS is scored between 3 and 15. It is important to break the score into its components, such as E3V3M5 instead of just saying GCS = 11. A score of 13 or higher correlates with a mild brain injury, 9–12 is a moderate brain injury, and 8 or less is a severe brain injury.

✦ Mannitol

Typically 0.25-0.5g/kg is given with signs of acutely elevated ICP. Mannitol will expand plasma and ↑cardiac output. It ↓blood viscosity, ↑CBF, and ↑CMRO$_2$. It ↓ICP even before diuresis is produced.

It may precipitate pulmonary oedema and worsen ICP if it leaks through a damaged blood–brain barrier.

Table 7.2 Causes of 'secondary insult' to the brain	
Systemic	**Intracranial**
Hypoxemia	Raised ICP and/or brain shift
Hypotension	Vasospasm
Hyper- and hypocapnia	Seizures
Hyperthermia	Infection
Hyper- and hypoglycaemia	
Hyponatremia	

7.11 Excitation and inhibition in the CNS

Excitatory amino acids

Glutamate and **aspartate** are the main fast excitatory transmitters found within the CNS.

Glutamate is the principal excitatory transmitter of the CNS. Its role as a transmitter begins with its production by the Krebs' cycle, where it is interconverted with α-oxoglutarate. Few drugs interfere specifically with glutamate metabolism. Like many other transmitters, it is stored in vesicles and released in response to Ca^{2+} influx. Following is release, its action is terminated up by neuronal and glial cell uptake.

Aspartate performs a similar, although less important, role.

Excitatory receptors

Ionotropic glutamate excitatory receptors are divided into three subtypes: N-methyl-D-aspartate (NMDA), AMPA, and kainate. There is also a group of metabotropic G-protein-coupled receptors (GPCRs) coupled to either phospholipase C (PLC) or adenylyl cyclase. The structure of the NMDA receptor is shown in Figure 7.34.

AMPA receptors activate fast excitatory synaptic transmission, while NMDA receptors initiate slow elements of excitatory potentials. Modulators affect the function of these two receptors at binding sites distinct from the ligand-binding site. NMDA and metabotropic glutamate receptors:

- Influence synaptic plasticity (important in learning).
- Have a role the development of epilepsy.

The receptors may become targets for drugs affecting Alzheimer's disease. Excitatory receptor antagonism may potentially improve outcome following head injury or stroke, and arrest neurodegenerative decline. Ketamine and phencyclidine antagonize the NMDA receptor by blocking the channel; however, they have other less desirable CNS effects. The few commercially available drugs that antagonize NMDA receptors are associated with the development of hallucinations.

Attempts to antagonize AMPA receptors have been similarly disappointing; the therapeutic window appears to be very narrow and most drugs cause marked respiratory depression.

Inhibitory neurotransmitters

Gamma aminobutyric acid (GABA) and glycine

GABA is found solely within the brain, and is the main inhibitory neurotransmitter. It is released from short interneurons. Virtually all neurons are sensitive to its effects, and it is found at nearly a third of all CNS synapses. Its highest concentrations are found within the basal ganglia.

GABA is formed from glutamate and is transaminated to form α-oxoglutarate. However, its action is terminated by re-uptake rather than by metabolism.

In the brainstem and spinal cord, glycine is the important inhibitory transmitter. It produces inhibitory hyperpolarization if applied to cells of the spinal cord (where it is found in abundance). Interestingly, it also has a role in facilitating stimulation of the NMDA receptor.

Inhibitory receptors

$GABA_A$ receptor

This is a ligand-gated chloride channel. It mediates fast post-synaptic inhibition. It is comprised of α, β, and γ subunits around a central pore. The structure is shown in Figure 7.35. The cortex has the highest concentration of $GABA_A$ receptors.

Benzodiazepines, barbiturates, propofol, and neurosteroids act at the $GABA_A$ receptor. Drugs may act at the binding site, modulatory sites, or the ion channel itself. Benzodiazepines have various actions, but those that selectively potentiate GABA cause sedation by binding to an accessory 'benzodiazepine' site.

$GABA_C$ receptor

This is a ligand-gated chloride channel and is structurally similar to the $GABA_A$ receptor. It is found in particularly high concentrations in the retina. It is not modulated by steroids, barbiturates, baclofen, or benzodiazepines.

$GABA_B$ receptor

This is a G-protein-coupled receptor. It inhibits adenylyl cyclase, and acts both pre- and postsynaptically:

Presynaptically, inhibition of voltage-gated Ca^{2+} channels leads to reduced trasmitter release.

Postsynaptically, it reduces opening of potassium channels, and therefore post-synaptic excitability.

Baclofen is a selective $GABA_B$ agonist, which (unlike GABA) is able to cross the blood–brain barrier. It produces little post-synaptic inhibition. It is used clinically to treat spasticity.

Glycine receptor

The glycine receptor resembles the $GABA_A$ receptor: it is ligand-gated, and its subunits surround a central chloride channel.

Tetanus toxin prevents glycine acting on interneurons. The resulting neuronal hyperexcitability causes muscle spasm ('lockjaw').

Benzodiazepines

Benzodiazepines bind to a specific site on the $GABA_A$ receptor, promoting the fast inhibitory postsynaptic effect. Various $GABA_A$ receptor subtypes are found in different parts of the brain, each with its own specific benzodiazepine sensitivity. Only two of the three γ-subunit types have benzodiazepine receptor activity. Endogenous ligands are as yet unknown.

Antagonists at the $GABA_A$ receptor antagonize the anxiolysis produced by benzodiazepines.

The structure of benzodiazepines allows many modifications to be made without loss of activity. Of the thousands synthesized, more than 20 are currently licensed for use. There are some differences between the receptor interactions of different groups; however, pharmacokinetic differences are the most meaningful clinically.

Clinical effects

Anxiolysis This effect is seen consistently in different animal species. Benzodiazepines also reduce aggression.

Sedation The drugs hasten the onset of sleep and increase its duration. Both effects decline when the drugs taken for more than few weeks. Like all hypnotics, they reduce the duration of REM sleep. This effect is always found in the anxiolytic benzodiazepines.

Reduction of muscle tone Coordination is affected; this is mediated centrally and is independent of sedation.

Anticonvulsant This action is common to all benzodiazepines.

Pharmacokinetics

In general, benzodiazepines show good oral absorption, and strong plasma protein binding with marked lipid solubility.

Duration of action is variable; there are short-, medium- and long-acting varieties. Following metabolism and glucuronidation, they are excreted via the kidney.

Side effects

Tolerance develops with all benzodiazepines. Dependence is also a major problem; sudden cessation after months produces intense anxiety, dizziness, and tremor (especially with short-acting drugs).

Acute overdose is associated with sleep, but relatively little cardio-respiratory depression. However, they potentiate other depressant CNS drugs, including inhibitory effects on respiration. Drowsiness, confusion, amnesia, and incoordination are unwanted effects even at therapeutic doses.

Table 7.3 NMDA receptor (excitatory) properties

	NMDA receptor site	Glycine modulatory site
Endogenous agonists	Glutamate found on NR2 subunit Aspartate	Glycine found on NR1 subunit D-serine
Channel blockers	Phencyclidine, memantidine Ketamine Mg^{2+}	Seem to be prerequisites for NMDA or glutamte receptor activation *in vitro*
Effector mechanism	Ligand-gated cation channel	
Location	Widespread Post-synaptic	
Function	Slow EPSP Synaptic plasticity	

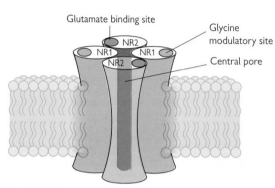

Fig. 7.34 NMDA receptors may consist of either four or five subunits surrounding a central ion pore. The pore gives a high permeability to Ca^{++} and is blocked by Mg^{++}.

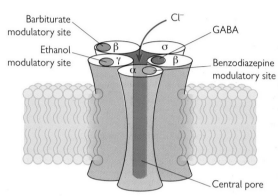

Fig. 7.35 The GABA_A receptor is composed of five sub-units which have 16 known isoforms, each produced by a different gene.

Table 7.4 Inhibitory neurotransmitter receptor properties

	GABA_A			GABA_C	GABA_B	Glycine
	Receptor site	Benzodiazepine site	Other modulatory sites			
Endogenous agonist	GABA	Diazepam binding inhibitor	Steroid metabolites		GABA	Glycine β-alanine
Other agonist	Muscimol	Diazepam	Steroid anaesthetics		Baclofen	
Antagonist	Bicuculline	Flumazenil			Phaclofen	Strychnine
Effector mechanism	Ligand-gated Cl⁻ channel			Ligand-gated Cl⁻ channel	G-protein-coupled	Ligand-gated Cl⁻ channel
Location	Widespread; GABAergic interneurons	Modulating agents induce a change in the protein architecture of the GABA_A complex, which modifies the size of the pore and permeability to Cl⁻. When Cl⁻ enters the neuron, it is hyperpolarized, resulting in an inhibition of neuronal activity and a general anxiolysis. Benzodiazepines reduce anxiety by potentiating the effect of GABA by making the Cl⁻ channel open more frequently. However, modulating molecules have no effect on the neuron's Cl⁻ permeability without GABA present at its receptor.		Retina	Widespread pre- and postsynaptic	Spinal cord and brainstem Postsynaptic
Function	Fast IPSP				↓ calcium entry (presynaptic) ↑ potassium permeability (postsynaptic)	Fast IPSP

Table 7.5 Benzodiazepines, zopiclone and flumazenil

	Name	Diazepam	Lorazepam	Midazolam
Properties	Uses	Short-term anxiety; procedural sedation; co-induction agent for anaesthesia; treatment of seizures, alcohol withdrawal, muscular spasticity.	Short-term anxiety (e.g. pre-medication); treatment of status epilepticus	Co-induction agent for anaesthesia; procedural and intensive care sedation; pre-medication; seizures (unlicenced).
	Chemical	Benzodiazepine	Hydroxybenzodiazepine	Imidazobenzodiazepine
	Presentation	Tablets 2/5/10mg; syrup; rectal solution/suppositories. IV: clear yellow solution or white emulsion 5mg/ml	Tablets 1/2.5mg IV: clear colourless solution 4mg/ml	Buccal liquid 10mg/ml IV: clear, colourless aqueous solution, 1/2/5mg/ml
	Primary actions	Hypnosis, sedation, anxiolysis. Amnesia (anterograde only). Anticonvulsant. Muscular anti-spasmodic.		
	Mode	Binds to the benzodiazepine binding site on the GABA chloride channel complex. This causes allosteric modulation of the GABA complex and potentiates GABAergic activity.		
	Route/dose	PO 2-10 mg tds; PR 0.25-0.5 mg/kg (as solution); 10-30mg (as suppository) IV 2-20mg titrated to effect	PO 1-4mg/day in divided doses. Halve dose in elderly. IV 25-30mcg/kg, repeated if necessary	Buccal 10mg (can use IV solution); IM 0.07 – 0.08mg/kg IV 2mg increased in steps of 1mg, titrated to response. Reduce dose in elderly. Infusion in ITU 30-200mcg/kg/hr
Effects	CVS	Transient small decrease in BP and CO; increased coronary bloodflow; possible decrease in myocardial oxygen consumption.	Cardiostable	SVRI falls by up to 33%; moderate increase in heart rate; small decrease in BP. Obtunds pressor response to laryngoscopy.
	RS	Respiratory depression in large doses	Mild respiratory depression	Minute volume usually unchanged but can cause apnoea in high doses.
	CNS	Anxiolysis, hypnosis, sedation. Anterograde amnesia. Decreased seizure and spinal reflex activity May cause paradoxical excitement	Anxiolysis, hypnosis, sedation. Anterograde amnesia.	Anxiolysis, hypnosis, sedation. Anterograde amnesia. Decreased cerebral oxygen consumption and blood flow.
	GI			Hepatic blood flow reduced
	GU			Renal blood flow reduced
Kinetics	Absorption	Rapid enteral absorption, OBA 86-100%.	OBA 90%	OBA 44%
	Distribution	99% protein-bound; VD 0.8-1.4 L/kg	88-92% protein bound; VD 1L/kg	96% protein bound; VD 0.8-1.5 L/kg
	Metabolism	>99% metabolized. Hepatic; active metabolites including desmethyldiazepam ($t_{1/2}$ 100hr), oxazepam, temazepam; further oxidation/conjugation to soluble products	Hepatic conjugation to an inactive metabolite. Renal disease has no effect on clearance.	Almost completely metabolized in the liver (hydroxylated then conjugated) to active metabolites. Renal disease has minimal effect on clearance
	Excretion	Soluble derivatives excreted in urine. Clearance 0.4ml/kg/min, terminal $t_{1/2}$ 20-40hr.	80% excreted in urine as the soluble metabolite. Clearance 1ml/kg/min, terminal $t_{1/2}$ 8-25h.	Hydroxylated derivatives excreted in urine. Clearance 6-9ml/kg/min. Elimination $t_{1/2}$ 1.5-3.5 hr (longer in critical illness).
	Note	Interaction with cimetidine: clearance of diazepam reduced.	Not affected by co-administration of cimetidine	Some immunosuppressant effects via inhibition of phagocytosis and leucocytes.

	Name	Temazepam	Zopiclone	Flumazenil
Properties	Uses	Anaesthetic pre-medication; hypnotic	Insomnia (short-term use only)	Reversal of benzodiazepine sedation; adjunct to supportive care in benzodiazepine overdose. Has also been used in hepatic encephalopathy and alcohol intoxication.
	Chemical	3-hydroxy benzodiazepine (metabolite of diazepam)	Cyclopyrrolone derivative	Imidazobenzodiazepine structure
	Presentation	Capsules 10/20mg Elixir 2mg/ml	Tablets 3.75/7.5mg. Racemic mixture of 2 stereoisomers, only one of which is active.	Clear, colourless aqueous solution; 100mcg/ml. pH 4.
	Primary actions	Hypnosis, sedation, anxiolysis. Anticonvulsant. Muscular anti-spasmodic.	In addition to benzodiazepine-like properties, zopiclone exhibits barbiturate-type actions.	Benzodiazepine antagonist
	Mode	Binds to the benzodiazepine binding site on the GABA chloride channel complex. This causes allosteric modulation of the GABA complex and potentiates GABAergic activity.	Interacts with GABA-receptor complexes at binding domains close or allosterically coupled to benzodiazepine receptors.	Competitively inhibits activity at the benzodiazepine site on the GABA/benzodiazepine receptor complex
	Route/dose	PO 10-40mg (use lower doses in elderly)	3.75-7.5mg nocte	IV; 100mcg increments titrated to effect. Total adult dose 1mg. Can be infused at 100-400mcg/hr.
Effects	CVS	Insignificant decrease in BP; improves myocardial oxygen supply/demand ratio	Cardiostable	Cardiostable
	RS	Some respiratory depression at high doses	Some respiratory depression at high doses	Nil
	CNS	Anxiolysis, hypnosis, sedation. Anticonvulsant properties.	Hypnosis, anxiolysis, sedation.	May cause seizures in patients on benzodiazepines to control epilepsy, or with severe hepatic impairment or severe cyclic antidepressant overdose. However, flumazenil appears to have minor intrinsic anticonvulsant activity.
	GI		May cause nausea	Nausea and vomiting (11%)

Table 7.5 Continued

	Name	Temazepam	Zopiclone	Flumazenil
Kinetics	Absorption	OBA nearly 100%. May be delayed by antacids.	Rapidly absorbed following oral administration. OBA 67% due to FPM.	Not administered orally.
	Distribution	76% protein-bound, V_D 0.8L/kg	Protein binding 45%. V_D 1.9L/kg.	50% protein-bound; V_D 0.9-101L/kg.
	Metabolism	Congugated to glucuronide in liver. Metabolites inactive.	Hepatic, via decarboxylation, demethylation, and side chain oxidation. Metabolites: N-oxide derivative (12%; weakly active); others inactive.	>99% in liver, by de-ethylation and conjugation. Clearance is hepatic bloodflow-dependent and reduced by 75% in severe hepatic impairment.
	Excretion	80% in urine as glucuronides; 12% in faeces. Clearance 1.5 ml/kg/min,.	75% excreted in urine as metabolites. Terminal $t_{1/2}$ 3.8-6.5hr (prolonged in hepatic insufficiency).	90% - 95% in urine as metabolites; 5% - 10% in faeces. Clearance 15 ml/kg/min.
	Note		Metabolised by CYP3A4; clearance reduced by ketoconazole and clarithromycin (CYP3A4 inhibitors) and increased by rifampicin (a potent inducer)	

→ Isomerism

Isomers are molecules which have the same chemical formula, but different structural formulae – i.e. different spatial arrangements of atoms. There are two main forms of isomerism: structural isomerism, and stereoisomerism.

Structural isomerism

In structural isomerism, the same set of atoms is arranged in different ways. Look at Figure 7.41, and you will see that enflurane is a structural isomer of isoflurane. Types of structural isomerism include *chain isomerism*, where hydrocarbon chains can exist in a number of branched forms; *position isomerism*, where the functional groups occupy different positions on the molecule (isoflurane and enflurane are and example of this specific type of isomerism), and *functional group isomerism*, where the molecules are completely dissimilar – the atoms in the functional groups are split up to give an entirely different molecule.

Tautomerism describes a state where a molecule changes between structural isomers, either spontaneously or in response to changes in the environment (temperaure, pH, and so on). Examples of tautomerism include:

- *Thiopental*. Barbiturates are not easily soluble in water at neutral pH, as they exist in the keto form (so-called after the C=O group in ketones). In the alkaline pH of the ampoule, the keto form changes to the enol form ("ene" for the –C=N– bond, and "ol" for the –SH group). The enol form is water soluble. (The alkaline pH of the ampoule is achieved by the addition of sodium carbonate, which forms alkaline NaOH on the addition of water).

Keto-thiopental
(at low pH; water insoluble)

Enol-thiopental
(at high pH; water soluble)

- At pH 4, *midazolam* forms an open, ionised structure which is water soluble. This aqueous solution is easy to prepare and store. After the aqueous preparation is introduced into the body (at pH 7.4), the structure changes to an unionized ring. This increases lipid solubility, allowing the drug to cross the blood-brain barrier and take effect.

Ionized
(Open; pH 4)

Unionized
(Closed; pH 7.4)

Stereoisomerism

Stereoisomers have the same chemical and structural formulae. The differences between different stereoisomers are in the spatial arrangement of the bonds between the functional groups. There are three types of stereoisomerism: *cis-trans isomerism, conformational isomerism,* and optical isomerism.

Cis-trans isomers possess stiff double or triple bonds between atoms (i.e. the atoms share more than one electron). The functional groups are not free to rotate around double bonds as they are around single bonds. In a compound $R_1R_2C=CR_3R_4$, R_1 and R_3 may be on the same side of the molecule (cis), or opposite sides (trans). The different configurations of the molecule are called *diasteriomers*. *Cis-trans isomerism* tends to impart different physiochemical and pharmacological properties to the different diastereomers.

- Atracurium exists as a mixture of 10 different cis-trans arrangements, as the molecule possesses stiff planar rings which fix its functional groups in position. cis-Atracurium is a single stereoisomer preparation. It is 3-5 times more potent than atracurium, and has a better side effect profile (fewer haemodynamic effects and less histamine release).

Conformational isomerism: this occurs when different 3-D conformations of the molecule exist, even when the functional groups are arranged in the same pattern. It can be thought of as the way molecules and bonds fold. Glucose and other sugars can exist in "boat" and "chair" forms, depending in the folding of the carbon ring. The boat form of glucose is unstable.

Optical isomerism: some molecules possess tetravalent atoms – usually a carbon atom, or ammonium ion (N+) – with four dissimilar groups attached. These structures display "handedness" – i.e. two forms can exist as mirror images of one another but are not superimposable. The mirror image molecules are called enantiomers. Biological molecules produced by enzymes are often produced as a single enantiomer. For example, R(−) lactate is produced during glycolysis.

Enantiomers are optically active, and rotate plane-polarised light to the right (+) or left (−). They are more systematically classified as R or S. If the atom attached to the chiral carbon with the lowest atomic number is imagined pointing away from the observer, the other groups fall into a plane in a triangular arrangement. If the atomic numbers of these three atoms descend in a clockwise direction, the molecule is in its rectus (R) form. If they descend anticlockwise, this is the sinister (S) form. A preparation containing equal proportions of R and S molecules is called a *racemic mixture*, while a preparation containing only one enantiomer is described as *enantiopure*.

Enantiomers tend to possess the same physiochemical properties (boiling point, lipid solubility etc.). However, many pharmacological processes depend on a good fit between a drug and its receptor. In these cases, different enantiomers may have very different pharmacological effects.

- Bupivacaine is presented as a racemic mixture. However, the S enantiomer is less toxic than the R form, and so it is now available as enantiopure S(−) bupivacaine. Ropivacaine is presented as S(−) ropivacaine.

7.12 Other neurotransmitters in the CNS

In the CNS, different types of receptor and transmitter are arranged into intricate systems, producing complex patterns of function.

Noradrenaline

The production, storage, and release of noradrenaline in the CNS is no different from that in the periphery (Section 9.3); and the receptors are identical.

Within the CNS, stimulation of β-receptors generally produces inhibitory responses, and α-receptor stimulation is excitatory.

Noradrenergic neuron cell bodies are found within the pons and medulla. They are thought to be involved in several processes:

- Arousal, alertness and wakefulness.
- Blood pressure regulation.
- Control of mood.
- Functioning of the reward system.

Groups of drugs acting on CNS noradrenergic transmission include antidepressants, cocaine and amphetamines, clonidine, and α-methyldopa.

Serotonin

Less than 1% of serotonin (5-hydroxytryptamine, 5-HT) is found within the CNS. However, serotonergic neurons have a wide distribution with broad-ranging effects, including control of:

- Mood and emotion (SSRIs form an important group of antidepressants).
- Wakefulness.
- Modulation of sensory pathways.
- Body temperature.
- Vomiting.
- Behavioural responses.

Depending on the neuron, 5-HT can exert stimulatory or inhibitory effects, and can act pre- or postsynaptically. There are many receptor subtypes; they operate under the influence of strong local negative feedback.

- **Types 1A, 1B, and 1D** are mainly inhibitory. Antidepressants target the first group. They are G-protein coupled.
- **Type 2** exert an excitatory postsynaptic effect, and are the targets for both LSD and anti-migraine medication. They are G-protein coupled.
- **Type 3** are found in the area postrema (Section 17.10) and are involved in the process of vomiting. They are ligand-gated ion channels.

Synthesis of serotonin is very similar to that of noradrenaline (Section 9.3). The availability of trytophan, which varies with diet, is the rate-limiting step, along with the activity of the first enzyme in the pathway, tryptophan hydroxylase.

The metabolism of 5-HT in the CNS is very similar to that in the periphery. Its re-uptake is similar to that of the catecholamines although the neuronal carrier is different. 5-HT is degraded by monoamine oxidase (MAO). Its final metabolite, 5-HIAA is excreted in the urine; urinary 5-HIAA is a marker of activity.

Acetylcholine

Acetylcholine (ACh) is found abundantly throughout the brain and cord, although it is almost absent from the cerebellum. Both dementia and Parkinsonism are associated with abnormality of ACh pathway function.

Presynaptic muscarinic (mainly M1) receptors are more numerous in the CNS than nicotinic receptors. They affect arousal and learning; the antagonists atropine and hyoscine cause amnesia. Cholinergic drugs that cross the blood–brain barrier (physostigmine) cause EEG evidence of arousal.

Nicotinic receptors are almost exclusively presynaptic and are responsible for the neurostimulatory effects of smoking. They modulate the release of other transmitters such as dopamine.

Acetylcholinesterases are released as neurotransmitters, mainly in the substantia nigra.

Again, storage and metabolism are the same as in the periphery.

Melatonin

Synthesized in the pineal gland, melatonin helps to establish circadian rhythms (although its influence is complex). The diurnal rhythm is controlled by the effect of light on the retina: higher light intensities reduce melatonin secretion. This pathway feeds to the hypothalamus. Melatonin is claimed to be useful in the treatment of jet-lag, although the mechanism is unclear.

Histamine

Sparsely distributed and found only in small amounts within the CNS, histamine may act to produce excitatory or inhibitory effects. Its receptors are type 1, 2, or 3 GPCRs. H_1 receptor blockers cause drowsiness.

Purines

Adenosine and ATP act as transmitters and stimulate a variety of receptors. A_1 receptor agonists are inhibitory whereas A_2 receptors cause arousal and alertness (caffeine is an A_2 agonist).

Nitric oxide (NO)

Neuronal nitric oxide synthetase (NOS) is stimulated to produce nitric oxide (NO) under conditions of raised intracellular Ca^{2+}. This increases cGMP, to produce both inhibitory and excitatory effects. It may play a role in the long-term persistence of depression.

Dopamine

Dopamine synthesis and degradation are similar to that of noradrenaline (for which dopamine is a precursor). Although there are many different types of dopamine receptor (Table 7.6), the known effects are confined to type D_2. This family of receptors may be implicated in schizophrenia, where there is evidence of dopaminergic hyperactivity.

There are three main pathways:

- **Nigrostriatal:** important for motor control. Deficiency of dopaminergic neurons here is associated with Parkinsonism (Figure 7.36). 75% of CNS dopamine is found here.
- **Mesolimbic:** emotion and drug-reward behaviours.
- **Tuberohypophyseal:** regulates pituitary secretions.

Actions of dopamine on the anterior pituitary include:

- Inhibition of prolactin release. Antipsychotic drugs inhibit D_2 receptor function and increase the secretion of prolactin. Bromocriptine, an agonist, suppresses prolactin secretion.
- Stimulation of growth hormone release.

These effects occur in response to ion-channel changes and inhibition of Ca^{2+} mobilization.

Dopamine also acts on the chemoceptor trigger zone to cause vomiting (Section 17.10). Antidopaminergic antipsychotics have antiemetic effects.

Table 7.6 Types of dopamine receptor

Functional role	D_1type		D_2type		
	D_1	D_5	D_2	D_3	D_4
Cortex: arousal, mood	++	–	++	–	–
Limbic: emotion	+++	–	+++	+	+
Basal ganglia: motor control	++	+	+++	+–	+
Pituitary: endocrine	–	–	+++	–	–
Hypothalamus: autonomic	++	+	–	–	–
Agonist: dopamine	Low potency		High potency		
Antagonist: chlorpromazine	+		+++	+++	+
Signal transduction	↑ cAMP		↓ cAMP		
Effect	Postsynaptic inhibition		Pre- and postsynaptic inhibition		

➕ Parkinson's disease (PD)

This degenerative disease occurs frequently in the elderly. It is associated with marked loss of dopamine from the basal ganglia. It has three main symptoms:

- Pill-rolling tremor at rest.
- Cog-wheel muscle rigidity.
- Hypokinesia (poverty of movement).

In the later stages, PD is associated with dementia. It is usually idiopathic but other less common causes of parkinsonism include encephalitis, vascular insufficiency, and chlorpromazine. There is no demonstrable hereditary association.

Symptoms begin when dopamine levels in the substantia nigra fall below 40% of normal; in established cases the level is <10%.

The consequences of damage to the nigrostriatal pathway are:

- ↑ dopamine turnover
- ↑ number of dopamine receptors
- Drug treatments

The aim is to redress the imbalance between dopamine and ACh within the nigrostriatal pathway. Available drugs include:

- Levodopa; replaces dopamine. Used with a peripherally acting dopa-decarboxylase inhibitor such as carbidopa. Loss of effectiveness is probably a result of the natural progression of the disease.
- Bromocriptine: mimics the action of dopamine.
- Selegeline: MAO-B inhibitor; reduces dopamine breakdown.
- Amantadine: possibly increases dopamine release.
- Benztropine: ACh antagonist.

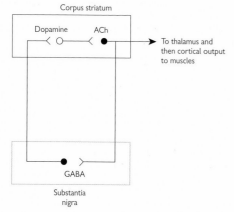

Fig 7.36 The pathway of Parkinson's disease. Neurones from the substantia nigra project to the caudate nucleus and putamen (together termed the corpus striatum), using dopamine as their neurotransmitter. In Parkinsonism, there is profound loss of dopamine in the striatum with cell loss and atrophy in the substantia nigra. Depletion of 80-85% of the dopamine content of the striatum results in Parkinsonism.

➕ Alzheimer's disease

A common age-related dementia without brain infarction. The major pathological features include:

- **Loss of cholinergic neurons** (particularly in the basal forebrain). There is also reduced choline acetyl transferase activity and a reduced density of muscarinic (although not nicotinic) receptors. However, anticholinesterases (e.g. tacrine) have shown only marginal benefit.
- **Amyloid plaques** of precursor protein found in normal neuronal membranes.
- **Neurofibrillary tangles** of highly phosphorylated normal neuronal protein, the significance of which is unknown.

☄ Antipsychotic drugs

These block D_2 receptors; the degree of block is proportional to potency. Predictably, this causes ↑prolactin release and two types of motor disturbance:

- **Tardive dyskinesias:** involuntary movements of the face and limbs that appear after a prolonged period of treatment. Possibly due to a proliferation of D_2 receptors in the corpus striatum. Rarely improve, and difficult to treat.
- **Acute dystonias:** acute onset of Parkinson-like tremor and rigidity. Probably due to blockade of nigrostriatal dopamine receptors. Reversible.

Other common side effects are related to other receptor actions:

- mAChR blockade: dry mouth and blurred vision.
- α-adrenoceptor blockade: hypotension.

Other problems include sedation, weight gain, agranulocytosis and obstructive jaundice.

➕ Malignant neuroleptic syndrome

This is associated with drugs which reduce dopaminergic activity in the hypothalamus, nigrostriatal pathway, and spinal cord. Over 60% of cases occur within the first week of treatment. The incidence is higher in males, especially <40 years of age.

Features include hyperthermia, rigidity, and dysautonomia with delerium or even coma. There are various disturbances:

- **Hypothalamic effects:** elevated temperature set-point and impairment of heat-dissipating mechanisms.
- **Peripheral effects:** ↑calcium release from the sarcoplasmic reticulum, resulting in ↑contractility with hyperthermia, rigidity, and muscle breakdown.
- **Synpatho-adrenal hyperactivity** is due to a reduction in usual tonic inhibition. Blood pressure is typically labile.

Intravenous anaesthetics are primarily used to induce and maintain anaesthesia. Some are also used as sedative agents and in the treatment of epilepsy. Table 7.7 shows the properties of the most commonly used drugs.

Theories of anaesthesia

Many different drugs of variable structure produce anaesthesia, and so it seems unlikely that reaction with one specific receptor is the key. They appear to act on the neuronal membrane. Two main theories of action have developed.

Protein theory

Interaction with ion channels is the currently accepted theory of action. Interactions with the channels themselves or disruption of the molecules that maintain them are both potential mechanisms of action. Voltage gating, ligand gating, and G-protein coupling are all likely to be implicated. All the IV agents except ketamine act on the $GABA_A$ receptor to increase chloride conductance. Ketamine antagonizes NMDA receptors, depressing the sensory relay nuclei and stimulating the limbic system.

Lipid theory

The Meyer–Overton studies examined anaesthetic potency of inhalational agents in tadpoles. By comparing the reciprocal of the molar concentration needed to produce anaesthesia with the olive oil:water partition coefficient of the drug, they demonstrated that potency is related to lipid solubility (Section 7.15). No mechanism was suggested for this relationship at the time, although cell volume expansion and increased membrane fluidity have been proposed since.

This concept has limitations. Alcohols do not exhibit ever-increasing potency with increasing chain length (and lipid solubility); there is a cut-off. This effect could explain the mechanism in greater detail. If the target sites are hydrophobic pockets within membrane proteins, the anaesthetic could bind with greater affinity as it fills more of the pocket. When the molecule becomes too large to fit, the binding affinity will decrease.

Another drawback with theories of non-specific membrane interaction concerns stereoisomers. Agents which exist as stereoisomers can have markedly different anaesthetic potencies, despite identical chemical properties. Isomers have differing effects on both synaptic transmission and ion-channel performance. This is more in keeping with a mechanism of action involving interaction at specific, chiral, protein binding sites.

Ideal IV anaesthetic agents

Of the various agents available, no single one has an ideal set of characteristics. The notion of an ideal agent has relevance to drug development and evaluation. However, different circumstances call for different properties in IV anaesthetics: the hypotension desirable for middle ear surgery is inappropriate for the sick laparotomy, for example.

Below is a classification of characteristics which may be desirable in an IV anaesthetic agent. Many describe the absence of side effects of drugs currently in use.

Physical/pharmaceutical

- Soluble in aqueous medium
- Stable in solution
- Stable in light
- Stable at room temperature
- Long shelf-life
- Inexpensive

Pharmacodynamic

- Analgesic properties
- Anti-emetic properties
- Minimal cardiovascular and respiratory depression
- No excitatory phenomena; non-epileptogenic
- No emergence phenomena
- Does not increase intracranial/intra-ocular pressure
- No pain on injection
- No teratogenicity

Pharmacokinetic

- Rapid onset (within one arm–brain circulation time when given IV)
- Rapid predictable recovery
- Non-cumulative with infusion
- Metabolites inactive and non-toxic
- Elimination not affected by cardiac, hepatic, or renal impairment

Pharmacokinetics of IV agents

Anaesthesia is produced by diffusion of IV agents across the blood–brain barrier (BBB) into the brain. The rate of diffusion into the brain depends on many factors:

- **Extracellular pH** and **pKa** of the agent: these determine the degree of ionization of the drug (Section 7.22). Only the non-ionized fraction of the drug crosses the lipid BBB.
- The **relative solubility** of the IV anaesthetic agent in lipid and water determines the rapidity of transfer from blood to brain. The higher the lipid solubility, the faster the transfer.
- **Protein binding:** only the unbound drug is free to cross the BBB.
- **Potency:** perhaps counter-intuitively, less potent agents tend to have a faster onset of action. The large doses administered result in a greater concentration gradient from plasma to binding site. This leads to faster diffusion to the site of action.

The anaesthetic effects of all IV anaesthetic agents (after a single bolus) are terminated by redistribution to other tissues, notably fat. Triexponential decline is seen.

Classification of IV anaesthetic agents

Anaesthetic agents can be classified according to their structures:

- *Barbiturates*: thiopental, methohexital.
- *Alkyl phenols*: propofol.
- *Imidazole compounds*: etomidate.
- *Phencyclidine derivatives*: ketamine.
- *Steroids*: eltanolone, minaxolone, althesin (a mixture of the two steroids alphaxolone and alphadolone).

Barbituric acid is formed from the condensation reaction between urea and malonic acid. Addition of alkyl groups at the C5 position confers anaesthetic activity, and addition of phenyl groups gives the drugs anticonvulsive properties. Exchanging sulphur for oxygen at C1 increases lipid solubility and speed of onset, and methylating the N1 atom in the ring increases speed of onset but has a pro-convulsant effect. Thiopental and methohexital are the only two barbiturate IV induction agents in use (methohexital is used primarily for electro-convulsive therapy as it is pro-epileptic). Phenobarbital is occasionally used in refractory seizures. Barbiturates cannot be used in patients with porphyria.

Propofol is widely used as an IV induction agent. It is also suitable for total IV anaesthesia (Section 7.14). It is formulated as an emulsion with soya bean oil and egg phosphatide.

Etomidate is relatively cardiostable, but suppresses adrenocortical function. It is painful on injection, and causes excitatory movements, nausea, and vomiting. It is contraindicated in porphyria.

Steroid anaesthetics are no longer available. Althesin was solubilized in cremaphor EL, a compound associated with anaphylactic reactions (although it has been reformulated for veterinary practice).

Table 7.7 Anaesthetics

		Propofol	Thiopental	Etomidate	Ketamine
Properties	Uses	Induction and maintenance of anaesthesia; sedation; status epilepticus	Induction of GA; status epilepticus	Induction of GA	Induction of GA; analgesia; status asthmaticus
	Chemical	2,6-di-isopropylphenol	Thiobarbiturate	Carboxylated imidazole	Phencyclidine derivative
	Presentation	1% or 2% solution in soya bean oil, egg phosphatide, and sodium hydroxide	Hygroscopic yellow powder with 6% sodium carbonate in a nitrogen atmosphere; 2.5% solution has pH 10.8 and pKa 7.6	Clear, colourless solution in 35% propylene glycol and water; pH 8.1	Clear colourless racemic solution
	Action	Hypnotic	Hypnotic and anticonvulsant	Hypnotic	Dissociative anaesthesia
	Mode	Potentiates GABA and glycine	↓postsynaptic sensitivity to neurotransmitters; precise molecular action unknown	Acts on $GABA_A$ (D-isomer only)	Non-competitive antagonism of NMDA receptors at both the Ca^{2+} pore and phencyclidine binding site; modulates mAChR and opioid receptors
	Route	IV; induction dose 1-2mg/kg (but see TIVA) For children, the dose should be ↑ by 50%	IV 2-7mg/kg; may also be administered rectally	IV 0.3mg/kg	IV 1.5-2mg/kg, IM 10mg/kg; also effective orally and epidurally
Effects	CVS	↓BP and SVR 15-25%, without ↑HR. Vasodilatation produced by local release of nitric oxide	Negative inotropic action; ↓CO, SVR, and BP	Relatively CVS stable but when repeated produces ↓CO, ↓SVR, and ↓BP	↑HR, ↑BP, ↑CO due to ↑sympathetic tone; baroreceptor function maintained
	RS	Apnoea; suppression of laryngeal reflexes; ↓V_T and ↑RR with infusion Brochodilatation; hypoxic vasoconstriction is preserved	Apnoea, prolonged respiratory depression; ↓response to CO_2; occasional bronchoconstriction	Transient apnoea, ↓RR, and ↓V_T Coughing and hiccups are common	Stimulation of respiration; preservation of airway reflexes
	CNS	Rapid smooth induction. ↓ICP, ↓CBP, ↓$CMRO_2$; anticonvulsant; intrinsic anti-emetic (D_2 receptor antagonism)	Rapid smooth induction; ↓IOP, ↓ICP, ↓CBP, ↓$CMRO_2$; anticonvulsant Antalgesic effect in low doses	↓IOP, ↓ICP, ↓CBP, and ↓$CMRO_2$ Involuntary muscle movements are common; epileptiform EEG in 20%	↑IOP, ↑ICP,↑ $CMRO_2$; amnesia common; visceral pain poorly obtunded; LA at high doses; causes emergence delirium and hallucinations
	GI		↓ GI activity, splanchnic vasoconstriction	PONV (15%)	PONV common
	Other	Burning, stinging, or cold sensation on injection is common	May transiently ↑K^+ levels		↑Uterine tone; ↑circulating catecholamine levels
Kinetics	Absorption	Only used IV	Good oral and rectal absorption.		Good absorption orally, but only 20% bioavailability because of first-pass metabolism.
	Distribution	97% protein-bound; large V_D (10-20L/kg) due to high lipid solubility	75% protein-bound; V_D 1.96L/kg; rapid onset due to high CBF, lipid solubility, and low state of ionization (40% at pH 7.4)	75% protein-bound; V_D 2-5L/kg.	20-50% protein-bound; V_D 3L/kg
	Metabolism	Liver; via P450, to inactive glucuronide, sulphate, and hydroxide. Some extrahepatic metabolism may occur.	Side-arm oxidation in the liver; 15% metabolized per hour, with 30% remaining in the body at 24hr	Hepatic esterases metabolize etomidate to carboxylates	N-methylation and hydroxylation occur in the liver; some metabolites are active
	Excretion	Metabolites excreted in the urine; clearance ↓ in renal failure	Inactive metabolites excreted in the urine	87% excreted into the urine; only 3% unchanged; the rest is excreted in bile	Conjugates excreted in the urine
	Toxicity	Pain on injection ↓ by use of lidocaine, cooling the drug, and use of a large vein	Use with caution in CVS disease	Potent depressant of steroid synthesis (even after single dose)	Rashes in 15%: emergence delirium can be reduced by benzodiazepine premedication
	Note	Safe in porphyria and MH Solutions support growth of bacteria, fungi	NOT safe in porphyria ↑hypnotic effect in presence of morphine	NOT safe in porphyria	Drug of abuse.

7.14 Total intravenous anaesthesia and pharmacokinetics I

Total intravenous anaesthesia (TIVA) is increasingly popular. Two commonly used drugs in TIVA are propofol (providing hypnosis and anaesthesia) and remifentanil (obtunding the response to surgical stimulation, and as a co-anaesthetic agent). Other agents, such as muscle relaxants and benzodiazepines, are added according to the needs of the anaesthetic and personal preference. The choice and combination of drugs is informed by an understanding of their pharmacokinetic behaviour. Here, we introduce some important principles of pharmacokinetics and look at their practical applications when giving a TIVA anaesthetic. These principles apply to all drugs and should be considered when administering any pharmaceutical agent.

Experimental determination of the pharmacokinetics of propofol and remifentanil has allowed development of population-based target-controlled infusion (TCI) algorithms which incorporate the height, weight, age, and sex of the patient. These algorithms are programmed into syringe pumps. (The algorithms commonly seen are Marsh and Schneider for propofol, and Minto for remifentanil.)

Pharmacokinetic principles

Pharmacokinetic models describe the relationship between dose, plasma concentration, and time and allow numerical analysis of absorption, distribution, metabolism, and excretion. The measurement of drug concentrations in plasma is central to pharmacokinetic analysis.

Single-compartment model
The single compartment model is entirely theoretical, but demonstrates some important pharmacological principles. It describes a system where a dose of drug is administered and distributes instantly and evenly across a volume (the 'compartment') from which it is eliminated. Elimination is (in first order kinetics) an exponential process. (see Figure 7.37)

Pharmacokinetic constants
Volume of distribution

The volume of distribution, V_D, describes the relationship between the total amount of drug in the body, and its plasma concentration. In the single compartment model, where the drug is evenly distributed across the entire volume, the volume of distribution will be equal to the compartment volume. The resulting concentration will be given by the total dose divided by the compartment volume.

When a drug is administered, it may remain as a free drug within the plasma; it may distribute passively between one or more tissue compartments; or it may be sequestered, bound, or actively taken up by specific tissue types. The remaining concentration of drug in plasma will change accordingly. The volume of distribution is **the theoretical volume in which the given dose of drug would have to be distributed to achieve the observed concentration.**

$$V_D = \frac{\text{total dose}}{\text{plasma concentration}}$$

V_D, may be quoted in L/kg to allow comparison between subjects. Although the concept may seem abstract, it can tell us a lot about a drug's distribution in the body. If a drug's V_D is similar to plasma or ECF volume (around 5 or 20 litres respectively), we can infer that the drug remains largely in the plasma or ECF. This may be because it has difficulty crossing cell membranes, or because it is highly bound by plasma proteins. Remifentanil, for example, has a V_D of 0.3 L/kg (much smaller than most opioids) because of its substantial binding to plasma proteins (70%).

If the V_D of a drug is much larger than the plasma or ECF volume, we can infer that it is distributed into tissues. The V_D gives no clue as to where the drug is distributed: it may pass non-specifically into many tissues, or it may be taken up preferentially into specific sites or tissues (e.g. iodine, which is actively transported into thyroid foilicular cells).

Although propofol is one of the most highly protein-bound drugs (98%), it is also extremely lipid soluble. This allows it to redistribute rapidly into all tissues, and its volume of distribution is very large, at 10–20L/kg.

Clearance

The clearance, CL, of a drug refers to **the theoretical amount of blood or plasma from which a drug would have to be completely removed per unit time to account for its observed removal from the body.** Again, this may seem rather abstract, as in reality a smaller proportion of drug is removed from a larger volume per unit time. However, the absolute amount of drug eliminated in unit time is usually not constant, and depends on (among other things) its concentration. If we think of clearance as the rate of elimination of drug (in mg/min) per unit of concentration (in mg/ml), we arrive at a value expressed in ml/min, which is best described by our original statement. Furthermore, this value remains constant for all first-order kinetics (i.e. the vast majority of drugs).

Terminal half-life, rate constant, and time constant

The terminal half-life ($t_{1/2}$) of a drug is **the time required for the plasma concentration to fall by half during the final phase of drug elimination** (see Figure 7.38a). In the single compartment model, concentration falls only as a result of elimination of drug from the compartment (it is not redistributed). $t_{1/2}$ is a constant, related to the ratio of V_D to clearance:

$$t_{1/2} = \ln2\,(V_D/CL) = 0.693\,(V_D/CL)$$

Plotting a graph of the natural logarithm of plasma concentration vs. time (Figure 7.38b) gives a straight line with its y intercept at C_0 (the initial concentration) and slope -k. k is described as the rate constant for the process. It is equal to CL/V_D, and therefore $t_{1/2} = \ln2/k = 0.693/k$.

The time constant, τ (tau) is defined as **the time it would have taken for the concentration to fall to zero, if elimination had continued at the original rate.** The time constant is equal to V_D/CL, and as such is the direct inverse of the rate constant ($\tau = 1/k$). It is equal to the time taken for the concentration to fall to 1/e of its initial value: so in one time contant, the C, falls to C_0/e, or $0.37C_0$. Time constant and half life are related by the equation: $t_{1/2} = \ln2\,\tau = 0.693\,\tau$

Practical application

In theory, just these three simple pharmacokinetic constants can be used to determine the dose regimen, loading dose and infusion rate for any drug. Assuming the bioavailability of the drug is 100% (as in IV dosing):

- The ideal intermittent dose is given by

Target C_P x dose interval x CL

- The ideal dose interval is the half-life of the drug, given by $0.693(V_D/CL)$
- Steady state is achieved within 4–5 half lives. To hasten the onset of action, we can calculate a loading dose, by multiplying the desired plasma concentration, by the volume of distribution

Dose = C_P x V_D

- The infusion rate would be the desired plasma concentration multiplied by the clearance: rate (e.g. in mg/min) = C_P, x CL.

In practice, the single compartment model is too simplistic to be useful. V_D, CL, and $t_{1/2}$ vary between subjects. Furthermore, the model does not account for a number of other active and time-dependent pharmacokinetic processes. Redistribution within tissues, resulting in accumulation outside the central compartment, is the most important of these. It is also important to remember that the single-compartment half-life only describes plasma concentration and may not describe the duration of action of a drug at its effect site.

To account for redistribution and effect site concentrations, more sophisticated multi-compartment constructs are necessary.

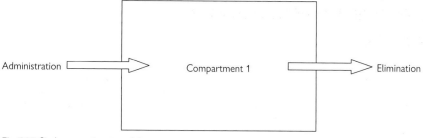

Fig. 7.37 Single compartment model.

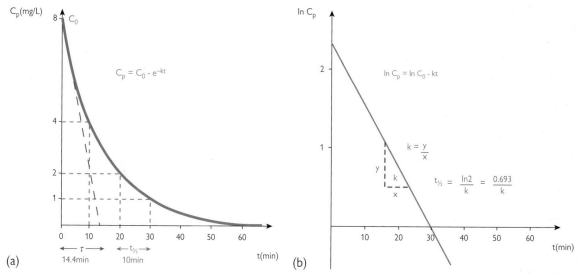

Fig. 7.38 Elimination in the single-compartment model: (a) shows a graph of plasma concentration, C_p, versus time, with an initial plasmA concentration C_0. This curve is described by the equation $C_p = C_0 \cdot e^{+kt}$. The half life, $t_{1/2}$ and time constant, τ, are represented graphically; (b) shows a semi-logarithmic plot of lnC_p versus time. This is a straight line, with y-intercept C_0 and slope $-k$ (k being the rate constant and the inverse of τ).

First order vs. zero order kinetics

The graphs in Figure 7.38 demonstrate first order kinetics. When the rate of elimination, v, follows first order kinetics, the amount of drug eliminated in unit time is related to the concentration of drug present at that time. As the concentration falls, the absolute amount of drug eliminated per unit time falls. What does stay constant is the *proportion* of drug eliminated per window of time: e.g. 50% every 10 minutes (giving a half life of 10 minutes). The clearance remains constant. This is referred to as first order kinetics, because the rate of elimination is proportional to C_p to the power 1 ($C_p^1 = C_p$)

If the drug is elimination at a constant rate from the comparment, regardless of its concentration, its elimination is proportional to C_p^0 ($C_p^0 = 1$). It is said to follow zero order kinetics. Zero order kinetics occur when the elimination mechanism is saturable – it has a maximum work rate which cannot be exceeded. The maximum rate at which a substance can eliminated is denoted v_{max}.

The Michaelis-Menten equation

The Michaelis-Menten equation can be used to predict which type of kinetics a drug will follow.

$$v = \frac{v_{max} \cdot C_p}{k_m + C_p}$$

where k_m is the plasma concentration at which elimination is 50% of v_{max} ($v = 0.5v_{max}$). v_{max} and k_m are constants for any one drug in any given system. It follows that, if $C_p \gg k_m$, then ($k_m + C_p$) will approximate to C_p. v will then approximate to v_{max}, and the system is likely to obey zero order kinetics. The higher the C_p, the more likely that zero order kinetics will supervene. If however $C_p \ll k_m$, then ($C_p + k_m$) will approximate to k_m, v will approximate to v_{max}, C_p/k_m. As v_{max} and k_m are constants, this indicates that v will be proportional to C_p – which defines first order kinetics.

7.15 Total intravenous anaesthesia and pharmacokinetics II

Although the single-compartment model (Section 7.14) is useful for introducing pharmacokinetic concepts, real life requires more complex models to explain the disposition of drugs in the body.

The two-compartment model

The two-compartment model (Figure 7.39) is an extension of the single compartment model which accounts for the observed behaviour of many drugs. Consider a dose of lidocaine injected into a vein in an attempt to reduce the pain of a propofol injection. After such an IV bolus, the lidocaine is first redistributed, and then eliminated. Redistribution, which is not accounted for in the single compartment model, reduces the concentration of the lidocaine in the plasma. However, it does not reduce the total amount of lidocaine present in the body. This removal comes later, primarily by hepatic metabolism.

A semilogarithmic plot of $\ln C_P$ versus time shows a distinctive biexponential decline. A distribution phase, α, is followed by an elimination phase, β. Each of these processes has its own rate constant (and hence its own time constant and half-life).

This biexponential decay can be explained in terms of a two compartment pharmacokinetic model. As well as the central compartment into which drug is given, and from which it is eliminated, there is a second, larger, peripheral compartment. Drug redistributes into this compartment after administration, accounting for the early α phase of the graph. The drug is eliminated from the central compartment and its terminal elimination is described by the β phase of the graph.

The two-compartment model is a theoretical construct and does not have any true physiological or anatomical correlation. However, it can adequately describe the behaviour of many drugs.

TIVA and the three-compartment model

Most anaesthetic drugs fit a three-compartment model (Figure 7.40). In this model, the loading dose is delivered into the central compartment (i.e. the blood) and then distributed into two peripheral compartments (the "fast," vessel-rich tissues e.g. muscle, viscera, and brain; and the "slow," less vascular tissues e.g. fat). This distribution reduces the concentration of the drug in the central compartment, terminating the action of a single IV bolus. Figure 7.37 illustrates this.

A steady central compartment concentration should be maintained: this is best achieved by continuous infusion. However, with a fixed infusion rate, five to six half-lives are needed to reach steady state. To hasten the onset of anaesthesia, a loading dose is used.

Due to tissue loading and slow equilibration between compartments, it is impossible to predict the concentration of anaesthetic agent based on the traditional distribution and elimination half-lives ($t_{\frac{1}{2}\alpha}$ and $t_{\frac{1}{2}\beta}$ respectively). Instead, **context sensitive half time (CSHT)** is used. This is defined as the time for the drug concentration to decline by 50% in the given "context" - the duration that the infusion has been running. Context sensitive half time is not a single number, but changes with infusion duration. A graph showing the context-sensitive half times of fentanyl, propofol, alfentanil, and remifentanil is shown in Figure 7.42. The CSHT increases until all compartments are in equilibrium, when it plateaus at steady state. At this point of full compartment loading, the CSHT is the same as the elimination half-life.

Propofol behaves according to the three compartment model, with its CSHT increasing as described. Remifentanil, on the other hand, is unusual: its CSHT is constant at 3–5min, irrespective of duration of infusion. This is because its rapid elimination by non-specific esterases is too fast to allow tissue loading. Elimination of remifentanil is independent of cardiovascular, renal or hepatic function, and so the CSHT is also independent of co-existing disease.

Delivery of total intravenous anaesthesia (TIVA) is usually achieved with a target controlled infusion (TCI) system.

TCI systems calculate the loading dose and infusion rate based on a real-time pharmacokinetic model. This is designed to achieve a preset target blood concentration. In practice, due to patient variability, the predicted concentration may differ from the measured blood concentration. Many manually controlled infusion algorithms are also available which can deliver broadly comparable levels to those of TCI systems. Remifentanil can be infused at a chosen rate if a purpose built TCI driver is not available. In this case, a syringe driver programmed to deliver in µg/kg/min is easiest to use:

- A starting rate of 0.2 µg/kg/min will take effect within a few minutes. If a therapeutic plasma level is required sooner, a bolus (1.5–2 µg/kg) can be given before starting the infusion.
- If bradycardia occurs, the rate can be dropped to 0.05–0.1 µg/kg/min.

Practical conduct of TIVA

Giving sets

Purpose-built giving sets are available. These have the advantages of fewer connections, and a one-way valve. This increases the reliability of the infusion, greatly reducing the risk of inadvertent awareness.

Starting the anaesthetic

It is best to become familiar with, and use, one particular concentration of each drug. This avoids confusion and reduces risk. 2% propofol (commercially available) and 50µg/ml remifentanil (i.e. 1mg in 20ml) are commonly used. Having said that, for procedures taking less than an hour it is more economical to use 1% propofol and 20µg/ml remifentanil. The following is a guide, which should be adapted to individual patient circumstances and physiological parameters:

- Carry out pre-anaesthetic checks and monitoring according to standard guidelines. Seriously consider depth of anaesthesia monitoring.
- Programme the patient's details (e.g. height, weight age), the concentration of the drug, and the make of syringe into the driver.
- Set the propofol TCI to 4 µg/ml for an elderly patient and 6 µg/ml for others, and the remifentanil to 5ng/ml (or 0.2 µg/kg/min, as described above).
- When cannulating the patient, give 40mg lidocaine IV and wait for 2min before removing the tourniquet. This "mini-Biers block" helps to anaesthetise the vein and reduce pain on injection of propofol (particularly useful when using the 2% preparation). Attach the giving set to the cannula.
- Pre-oxygenate the patient.
- Start the remifentanil infusion.
- Consider a bolus of either midazolam 2mg or propofol 50–80mg to speed up induction (only recommended in young, fit patients).
- Start the propofol infusion. If using only the TCI pump, the induction will tend to be slower than a bolus IV induction.
- Once the patient is anaesthetised, secure the airway. If muscle relaxants are required, give them and ventilate the patient manually until they have had time to take effect.
- It is easiest to adjust the depth of anaesthesia using depth of anaesthesia monitoring (Section 4.9). Adequate depth of anaesthesia usually coincides with a propofol TCI level of 2–4µg/ml.
- It is essential to keep the cannula in sight at all times during TIVA (e.g. by positioning the arm out on a board), as otherwise tissuing or inadvertent disconnection may not become apparent until the patient develops awareness.

Bear in mind that at the end of the anaesthetic, the action of remifentanil will be short-lived. *Additional pain relief (eg. longer acting opioid, regional analgesia) should already have been commenced in expectation of this.*

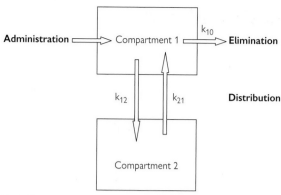

Fig. 7.39

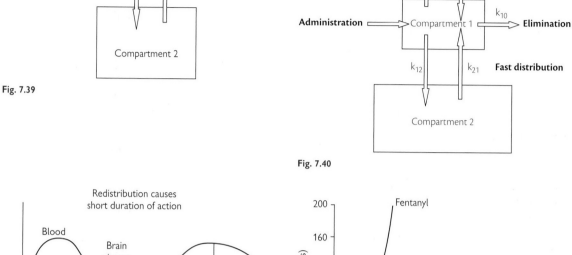

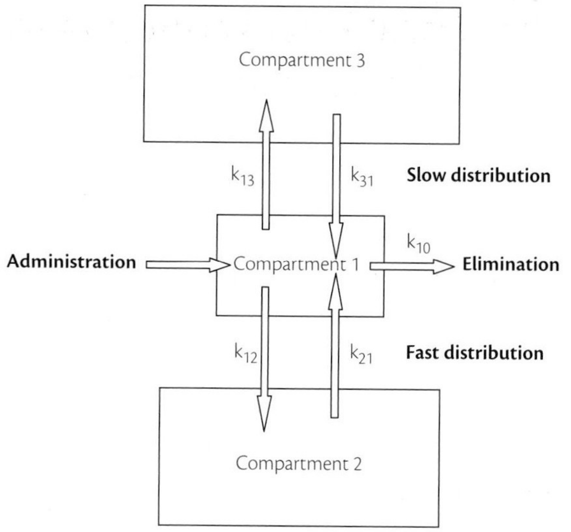

Fig. 7.40

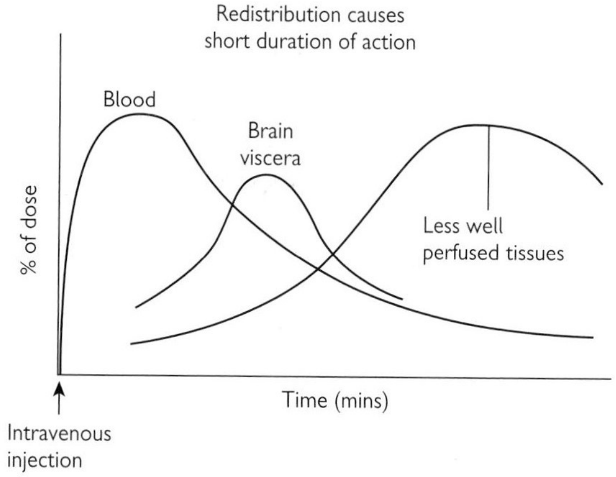

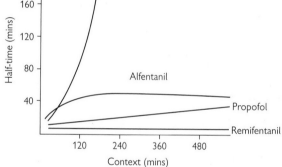

Fig. 7.41 Distribution graph.

Fig. 7.42 Context-sensitive half-time.

Nitrous oxide was synthesized by Priestley in 1772, and first used in anaesthetic practice by Cotton and Wells in 1844. Other inhalational agents introduced since include diethyl ether, chloroform, ethyl chloride, cyclopropane, and trichloroethylene. These agents were either highly flammable, or toxic.

In the 1950s, the idea of fluorinating these hydrocarbons (known to reduce flammability and toxicity) culminated in the manufacture of halothane. Subsequently, it was discovered that substituting a methyl ethyl ether for the alkane group (enflurane, isoflurane) reduced the sensitization of the heart to catecholamines. Sevoflurane and desflurane were subsequently developed as agents halogenated only with fluorine.

Mechanism of action

The exact mechanism of action of inhalational agents is not known. It is unclear whether the anaesthetic action of the volatiles is due to action at a single site, multiple points, or whether different inhalationals act on different targets. Various theories have arisen over time.

Interaction with lipid membranes

In the early 1900s, Meyer and Overton found that agents with greater solubility in oil possess more potent anaesthetic effects. Figure 7.40 shows the Meyer-Overton relationship between oil:gas partition coefficient and potency for a number of inhalational agents. This relationship seemed to indicate a point of action within lipid membranes. However, various anaesthetic substances have been shown to violate this rule.

The critical volume hypothesis was an extension of the lipid solubility theory, and postulated that non-specific expansion of membranes by dissolved agent causes anaesthesia. The number of molecules, rather than the exact agent, was crucial. This view was supported by evidence that anaesthetisia could be reversed in small animals by the use of pressurised containers, which were thought to re-compress the membranes to their original volume. This theory is undermined by findings that membrane expansion can occur with small changes in temperature, without resultant anaesthesia.

Protein interaction

The correlation between potency and lipid solubility suggests a hydrophobic site of action for the volatile agent. The incongruities of purely lipid-based theories led to investigation on specific protein targets. Pre- and post-synaptic effects on neurotransmission have been demonstrated, and various membrane proteins are affected by volatiles. It is not clear whether these effects are due to direct interaction with membrane proteins, or via second messengers, altered neurotransmitter re-uptake, or distortion of ion channels and changes in ion conductance. Possibilities include:

Inhibitory receptors: $GABA_A$ and glycine receptors are agonised by inhalational agents at clinically relevant concentrations. The binding site for inhalational agents is thought to reside on the (subunit; binding here appears to cause allosteric potentiation of GABA. The degree of in-vivo agonism of the receptor and the clinical potency of various isomers of isoflurane show good agreement.

Two-pore-domain potassium (K2P) channels: these are dimeric, non-inactivating potassium channels which are active at all membrane potentials. They are thought to play a role in setting the resting membrane potential in many cells. They are activated by inhalational anaesthetics.

Excitatory receptors: antagonism NMDA, AMPA and kainate receptors may have a role in the action of inhalational agents but this is probably much less significant.

Voltage-gated ion channels: these are affected by inhalational agents only in supra-anaesthetic doses.

5-HT₃ receptors: these are agonised by inhalational agents, but not by propofol. This probably explains the pro-emetic effect of inhalational agents.

Nicotinic ACh receptors: inhalational agents affect these channels, although the clinical significance of this is not clear.

Calcium channels: intracellular calcium release is inhibited by inhalational agents. This may affect neurotransmitter release.

Potency

The Meyer–Overton experiments showed the correlation between the olive oil:gas partition coefficient and potency. Anaesthetic potency increases with lipid solubility (Figure 7.44; note the logarithmic scales).

Minimum alveolar concentration (MAC) is defined as *the minimum concentration of inhalational anaesthetic agent in the alveoli, at equilibrium, at one atmosphere pressure, in 100% oxygen, which produces immobility in 50% of unpremedicated adult subjects when exposed to a standard noxious stimulus*. It is analogous to ED_{50}. MAC is correlated with end-tidal anaesthetic agent concentration, and is used as a guide to the depth of anaesthesia. However, the response to a noxious stimulus is partly mediated at the spinal level, regardless of conscious state. It is more usual in practice to deliver the ED_{95} (the concentration of inhalational agent where 95% of patients will be immobile); this is 1.2–1.4 MAC for most agents (Table 7.8), as the response–concentration curve is very steep.

Studies have shown that the depth of anaesthesia correlates linearly with the bispectral index (BIS); but the BIS value is drug-specific, i.e. equivalent MAC values with different agents will give differing BIS values.

Speed of onset

The rate of uptake of inhaled anaesthetic is classically described by the ratio of alveolar to inspired concentration (F_A/F_I) over time (Figure 7.43). At equilibrium, brain concentration is equal to alveolar concentration, so *the rate of rise of (F_A/F_I) is an index of how quickly anaesthesia is achieved*. Factors which determine how quickly F_A approaches F_I include ventilation, rate of uptake from the alveoli, and concentration of agent delivered.

Ventilation

This can be affected by many factors. During spontaneous ventilation, the uptake of the volatile agent is subject to negative feedback; respiration is depressed by increased depth of anaesthesia (this also serves to limit the adverse cardiorespiratory effects of the agent). During controlled ventilation, this effect is eliminated, and so controlling ventilation can rapidly deepen anaesthesia.

Rate of uptake from the alveoli

This is influenced by the following.

- **Solubility of the agent in blood** (Figure 7.43a) The lower the blood–gas solubility, the faster the increase in alveolar concentration. This is counter-intuitive, as it might be imagined that the higher the content of the agent in the blood, the faster the anaesthetic effect. It is important to remember that it is actually the *partial pressure* of inhalational agent (not the overall blood content) which determines its transfer from blood to brain. Agents which are highly blood-soluble exert a lower partial pressure and so are less available to diffuse across the blood–brain barrier.

- **Pulmonary capillary blood flow**, (Figure 7.43b) which is related to cardiac output. The higher the cardiac output, the faster the removal of agent from the alveolus. This slows its rate of rise and prolongs induction. Conversely, in a shocked patient, gaseous induction is rapid. The effect of cardiac output depends also on the blood:gas solubility of the agents. The more soluble the agent, the greater the influence of cardiac output on its rate of uptake.

- **The partial pressure gradient** between alveoli and pulmonary blood. This is determined by the delivered concentration and tissue uptake of volatile agents, which in turn depends on cardiac output, proportion of vessel-rich tissues to fat, and solubility of the various agents in tissues.

Concentration of agent delivered

If anaesthetic agents were administered at 100% concentration, the uptake would be maximal and constant, as the concentration of agent in the lungs would remain at 100%. This is of course a theoretical situation, since as well as the agent, oxygen must be administered and carbon dioxide will be excreted into the alveolus.

At lower concentrations, each molecule of agent taken up from the alveolus reduces the amount left in the alveolus, and erodes the remaining diffusion gradient. The rate at which the alveolar tension rises to approach the inspired concentration is consequently higher at higher inspired concentrations. See Figure 7.43c.

Second gas effect

See Section 7.16.

Other factors

Pungency: pungent agents can induce breath-holding.

Right-to-left shunts: the effect is to dilute the gas leaving the lungs, slowing induction. This is more marked with less soluble agents.

Age: the behaviour of inhalational agents is influenced by differing ventilation/FRC ratios, tissue water content, proportion of cardiac output distributed to the vessel compared with fatty tissues, and many other factors, all of which change with age.

Elimination of inhalational agents

Most of the factors affecting rate of uptake affect elimination in the same way. The exception is cardiac output: an increased cardiac output will hasten recovery, as there is increased delivery of blood to the alveoli.

Elimination of anaesthetic through metabolism depends on the agent: halothane (20%), sevoflurane (~5%), enflurane (2%), isoflurane (0.2%), desflurane (0.02%), and N_2O (<0.01%). For most agents, the enzyme systems responsible for metabolism are rapidly saturated and contribute little to elimination.

Recovery depends on the duration of anaesthesia, since accumulation occurs in the tissues. An analogy can be drawn with context-sensitive half-time (Section 7.14).

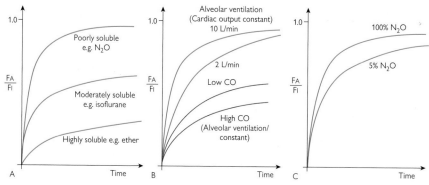

Fig. 7.43 FA/FI vs. time.

Ideal inhalational anaesthetic agent

Physical

- Stable in presence of light and heat; long shelf-life.
- Inert on contact with soda lime, metal and anaesthetic circuit.
- Preservative free.
- Non-flammable, non-explosive.
- Non-irritant, pleasant odour.
- Eco-friendly.
- Economical.

Pharmacodynamic properties

- Smooth rapid induction and emergence.
- Analgesic properties.
- No cardiovascular depression.
- No respiratory depression.
- No effect on blood flow to vital organs .
- No increase in intracranial or intra-ocular pressure.
- Not epileptogenic.
- No effect on uterine tone.
- Non-toxic.
- Does not trigger malignant hyperthermia
- Non-teratogenic, non-carcinogenic.

Biochemical and pharmacokinetic properties

- High oil:gas partition coefficient (potent; low MAC).
- Low blood:gas partition coefficient (rapid induction and emergence).
- Minimal metabolism.

→ Factors affecting MAC

Factors increasing MAC

- Young age (infants/children).
- Hyperthermia.
- Hypernatraemia.
- Elevated CNS catecholamine stores.
- Chronic opioid use.
- Chronic alcohol use.

Factors decreasing MAC

- Increasing age.
- Pregnancy.
- Hypothermia.
- Hyponatraemia.
- Acute alcohol intake.
- Acute intake of CNS depressant drugs: opioids, benzodiazepines, major tranquilizers, TCAs.
- Other drugs: lithium; lidocaine; magnesium.
- Anaemia.
- Hypotension.

Factors not affecting MAC

- Sex.
- Weight/body surface area.
- Duration of anaesthesia.
- Hypo/hyperkalaemia.

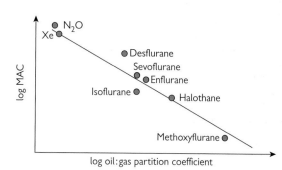

Fig. 7.44 MAC vs. oil:gas partition coefficient.

Table 7.8 Minimum alveolar concentration and ED$_{95}$			
	MAC in oxygen–air (%v/v)	ED$_{95}$	ED$_{95}$:MAC
Halothane	0.75	0.9	1.2
Isoflurane	1.17	1.63	1.4
Sevoflurane	1.8	2.1	1.2
Desflurane	6.6		

A number of different inhalational agents are available for use. All are used for the maintenance (and some for the induction) of general anaesthesia. In addition nitrous oxide is used (in entonox) for analgesia. Halogenated hydrocarbons and methyl ethers are administered with specialised vaporizers (Section 2.8). The pharmacological properties of the inhalational agents are shown opposite. Ether is no longer used but is included for comparison.

Halothane

Structure: halogenated hydrocarbon. It contains bromine, chlorine, and fluorine.

Presentation: clear, colourless liquid. Unstable in light, it contains 0.01% thymol as a preservative and is stored in brown glass bottles. Thymol imparts the characteristic sweet, herbal smell.

Pharmacodynamics:

CNS: general anaesthesia with negligible analgesia; cerebral vasodilatation, increased cerebral blood flow and intracranial pressure; decreases cerebral O2 consumption.

CVS: dose-related myocardial depression with reduction in myocardial oxygen demand. Bradycardia due to vagal stimulation. Hypotension (due to myocardial depression and vasodilatation). Threshold potential and refractory period of myocardium is increased. Halothane sensitizes the myocardium to circulating catecholamines, and doses of adrenaline (e.g. as a local anaesthetic additive) should be limited during halothane anaesthesia.

RS: respiratory depression, with tidal volume predominantly affected (respiratory rate may actually increase).

Other: splanchnic and renal blood flow are reduced, secondary to general circulatory effects. Uterine tone is reduced.

Pharmacokinetics

Halothane is more soluble in blood than most other inhalational agents; when used for inhalational inductions, the onset of anaesthesia is slow. It is very lipid soluble, resulting in significant tissue accumulation – this causes dose- and duration-dependent offset time which is longer than most other agents. Halothane is metabolised to a significant degree (20%) in the liver, and one of its metabolites is probably immunogenic. This is the likely mechanism of halothane hepatitis (see below). The rest is exhaled unchanged.

Adverse effects

Halothane is a potent trigger for **malignant hyperthermia**.

Cardiac dysrhythmias may occur in response to circulating catecholamines.

Halothane hepatotoxicity varies between subclinical liver dysfunction and fulminant hepatic necrosis. It is probably immunologically mediated: trifluoroacetyl chloride, a metabolite, may behave as a hapten (i.e. bind to hepatic proteins and induce antibody formation). Risk factors include: repeated exposure within a short interval, obesity, and perioperative hypoxia. The incidence is lower in children. Mortality is 50-75%. Halothane should be avoided if the patient has been exposed within the last 6 months.

Isoflurane

Structure: halogenated methyl ether containing chlorine, and five fluorine atoms.

Presentation: a clear, colourless liquid. Isoflurane has a strong smell. It is presented in glass bottles with no preservatives.

Pharmacodynamics:

CNS: general anaesthesia with negligible analgesia; cerebral vasodilatation and increased cerebral blood flow at concentrations >1 MAC, but decreased cerebral O2 consumption.

CVS: mild myocardial depression with reduction in systemic vascular resistance, leading to hypotension. However, a reflex tachycardia helps to preserve cardiac output. Threshold potential is increased, and phase IV depolarisation and refractory period are prolonged. Coronary

vasodilation occurs, with a theoretical risk of "steal syndrome" in patients with coronary artery stenosis. However, isoflurane is cardioprotective against ischaemic insults in animal models. Isoflurane is not especially arrhythmogenic.

RS: isoflurane is irritant to the upper respiratory tract and tends to cause coughing, breath-holding, and bronchorrhoea with bronchodilation. It causes respiratory depression, with reduction in tidal volume. The responses to hypoxia and hypercapnia are blunted.

Other: isoflurane reduces the tone of the pregnant uterus.

Pharmacokinetics

Isoflurane has a lower blood:gas partition coefficient than halothane and is less soluble. Equilibration is therefore more rapid. However, its irritant effects make isoflurane impractical for inhalational induction of anaesthesia.

Only 0.2% of the dose is metabolised in the liver (and excreted in the urine). The rest is exhaled unchanged.

Adverse effects

Isoflurane is a trigger for **malignant hyperthermia**, although appears less potent than other inhalational agents. Nevertheless it is absolutely contra-indicated in susceptible patients.

Rarely, hepatic toxicitiy has been reported.

Enflurane

Structure: halogenated methyl ether containing chlorine, and five fluorine atoms. Enflurane is a structural isomer of isoflurane, and as such has similar physical properties (Table 7.9).

Presentation: a clear, colourless liquid with a sweetish smell. It should be protected from light.

Pharmacodynamics:

CNS: general anaesthesia with negligible analgesia; cerebral vasodilatation and increased cerebral blood flow , but decreased cerebral O2 consumption. Enflurane has been associated with tonic-clonic muscle activity and epileptiform EEG changes.

CVS: myocardial depression with reduction in systemic vascular resistance, leading to hypotension. Induces a slight reflex tachycardia. Threshold potential is increased, and phase IV depolarisation and refractory period are prolonged. Coronary vasodilation occurs. Enflurane sensitises the myocardium to the effects of catecholamines, but is not in itself arrhythmogenic.

RS: unlike isoflurane, enflurane is non-irritant to the upper respiratory tract, simply causing bronchodilation. It causes marked respiratory depression, with reduction in tidal volume. The responses to hypoxia and hypercapnia are blunted.

Other: enflurane reduces perfusion to the splanchnic bed and reduces the tone of the pregnant uterus. It may cause hyperglycaemia, and decreases plasma noradrenaline concentrations.

Pharmacokinetics

Enflurane is less soluble in blood than halothane, resulting in a quicker onset of anaesthesia when used during inhalational induction.

2-2.5% of the dose is metabolised in the liver (oxidation and dehalogenation) by the cytochrome P450 system; this results in higher fluoride plasma concentrations than other inhalational anaesthetics. Metabolites are excreted in the urine. Enflurane is also excreted in sweat, faeces, and skin - only 80% of the dose is exhaled unchanged.

Adverse effects

Enflurane is a recognised precipitant of **malignant hyperthermia**, and is absolutely contra-indicated in susceptible patients.

Rarely, **hepatic toxicitiy** has been reported. Due to the relatively large proportion metabolised in liver, plasma fluoride concentrations increase and this presents a theoretical risk of toxicity.

Myocardial dysrhythmias may occur in the presence of sympathetic activity (e.g. hypoxia, light anaesthesia). Doses of adrenaline (e.g. as a local anaesthetic additive) should be limited during enflurane anaesthesia.

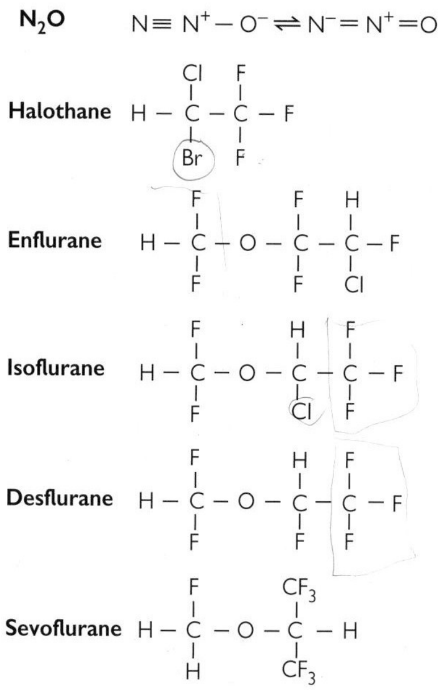

N_2O $N \equiv N^+ - O^- \rightleftharpoons N^- = N^+ = O$

Halothane

$$H - \overset{\overset{\textstyle Cl}{|}}{\underset{\underset{\textstyle Br}{|}}{C}} - \overset{\overset{\textstyle F}{|}}{\underset{\underset{\textstyle F}{|}}{C}} - F$$

Enflurane

$$H - \overset{\overset{\textstyle F}{|}}{\underset{\underset{\textstyle F}{|}}{C}} - O - \overset{\overset{\textstyle F}{|}}{\underset{\underset{\textstyle F}{|}}{C}} - \overset{\overset{\textstyle H}{|}}{\underset{\underset{\textstyle Cl}{|}}{C}} - F$$

Isoflurane

$$H - \overset{\overset{\textstyle F}{|}}{\underset{\underset{\textstyle F}{|}}{C}} - O - \overset{\overset{\textstyle H}{|}}{\underset{\underset{\textstyle Cl}{|}}{C}} - \overset{\overset{\textstyle F}{|}}{\underset{\underset{\textstyle F}{|}}{C}} - F$$

Desflurane

$$H - \overset{\overset{\textstyle F}{|}}{\underset{\underset{\textstyle F}{|}}{C}} - O - \overset{\overset{\textstyle H}{|}}{\underset{\underset{\textstyle F}{|}}{C}} - \overset{\overset{\textstyle F}{|}}{\underset{\underset{\textstyle F}{|}}{C}} - F$$

Sevoflurane

$$H - \overset{\overset{\textstyle F}{|}}{\underset{\underset{\textstyle H}{|}}{C}} - O - \overset{\overset{\textstyle CF_3}{|}}{\underset{\underset{\textstyle CF_3}{|}}{C}} - H$$

Fig. 7.45 Molecular structures of inhalational agents.

Table 7.9 International agents summary

	Halothane	Isoflurane	Sevoflurane	Desflurane	Enflurane	Nitrous (N$_2$O)	Xenon	Ether
MW(Da)	197 Da	184.5 Da	200.1 Da	168 Da	184.5 Da	44 Da	131 Da	74 Da
BP	50.2°C	48.5°C	58.5°C	22.8°C	56.5°C	-88°C	-108°C	35°C
SVP	32.3 kPa	33.2 kPa	22.7 kPa	88.5 kPa	22.9 kPa	5300 kPa (52 bar) - cylinder gauge pressure is 51 bar	Gaseous	7.8 kPa
MAC	0.75%	1.15%	2.00%	6.35%	1.68%	105%	71%	1.90%
B:G	2.4	1.4	0.7	0.42	1.9	0.47	0.12	12.1
O:G	224	98	80	19	98	1.4	1.8	65
% metab	20%	0.20%	3.50%	0.02%	2%	<0.01%	Nil	15%
Metabolites	Trifluoroacetic acid, Cl-, Br-	Trifluoroacetic acid, F-	"Organic + inorganic fluorides Compound A (B,C,D,E)"	Trifluoroacetic acid	Organic and inorganic fluorides	N2		CO2 and water
						T$_{crit}$ 36.5°C		
						P$_{crit}$ 72 bar		

Sevoflurane

Structure: halogenated ether containing seven fluorine atoms (hence the name). It is presented in polythylene naphthalate bottles, since in the presence of glass it can release toxic hydrofluoric acid.

Presentation: a clear, colourless liquid with a reasonably pleasant smell.

Pharmacodynamics:

CNS: general anaesthesia with negligible analgesia; cerebral vasodilatation and increased cerebral blood flow , but decreased cerebral O_2 consumption.

CVS: myocardial depression with some reduction in systemic vascular resistance, leading to hypotension (systolic falls further than diastolic). Does not sensitise the myocardium to catecholamines and does not appear to cause coronary steal syndrome.

RS: sevoflurane is non-irritant to the upper respiratory tract, and is frequently used for inhalational induction of anaesthesia. Reduction in tidal volume is offset by an increase in respiratory rate, so that minute volume is preserved. The responses to hypoxia and hypercapnia are blunted, and hypoxic pulmonary vasoconstriction is inhibited. Sevoflurane causes bronchodilation and is occasionally used in the management of refractory status asthmaticus.

Pharmacokinetics

Sevoflurane has a low blood:gas solubility coefficient of 0.7, resulting in rapid equilibration and a fast onset of anaesthesia when used for inhalational induction.

Around 3.5% of the dose is metabolised in the liver, resulting in increased fluoride plasma concentrations (equivalent to those caused by enflurane). Metabolites are excreted in the urine. The remainder is exhaled unchanged.

Adverse effects

Sevoflurane is a recognised precipitant of **malignant hyperthermia**, and is absolutely contra-indicated in susceptible patients.

Sevoflurane reacts with dry soda lime to produce several compounds, A – E. Concerns about compound A nephrotoxicity remain theoretical: it is nephrotoxic in rats, but thresholds for toxicity are not reached in humans even after prolonged use. Fluoride ions (produced during hepatic metabolism of sevoflurane) are also nephrotoxic, but the amounts produced by sevoflurane metabolism appear not to be sufficient to cause renal damage.

Nitrous oxide (N_2O)

(For the physical properties and storage of anaesthetic gases, see Section 2.2–2.3).

Uses: as an adjuvant to general anaesthesia, as an analgesic, and for cryotherapy. Entonox contains 50% by volume N_2O.

Mechanism of action: the exact mechanism is unclear. It may modulate the effects of CNS encephalins and endorphins, as well as non-competitive antagonism of glutamate at NMDA receptors.

Pharmacodynamics

CNS: N_2O produces CNS depression and analgesia. It decreases the MAC of other inhalational agents when used concomitantly. It increases cerebral blood flow and intracranial pressure.

CVS: N_2O is a mild direct myocardial depressant, but also increases sympathetic activity centrally. Therefore little overall effect is seen in healthy individuals.

RS: N_2O causes a slight decrease in tidal volume and an increase in respiratory rate. Overall there is little change in ventilation.

Pharmacokinetics

N_2O diffuses freely across the alveolar epithelium. Onset and offset of action are fast because of the low blood:gas partition coefficient (0.47). Less than 0.01% is metabolized in humans. It is excreted unchanged via the lungs and skin.

Adverse effects

N_2O is 34 times more soluble than nitrogen and diffuses rapidly through membranes. It tends to expand air-filled cavities as nitrogen diffuses out slowly. Therefore it is contraindicated in pneumothorax and certain types of surgery (e.g. neurosurgery, middle ear procedures). This rapid diffusion gives rise to two related phenomena in the alveoli.

- *Second gas effect:* diffusion of N_2O out of the alveolus is much faster than delivery of nitrogen in. This reduces alveolar volume, increasing the concentration of other alveolar gases (including volatiles). The volatile agent will move faster down this steeper concentration gradient between alveolus and blood, speeding the uptake process. See Figure 7.46. The rapid uptake of N_2O also has the effect of drawing gas from the respiratory bronchiole into the alveolus, effectively increasing ventilation.

- *Diffusion hypoxia (Fink effect):* the reverse of the second gas effect. It occurs at the end of anaesthesia. Oxygen concentration in the alveoli is diluted by rapid movement of N_2O from the blood. This can cause hypoxia if supplemental oxygen is not administered.

Nausea and vomiting are common after N_2O (~15%).

Bone marrow toxicity: N_2O oxidizes the cobalt atom in vitamin B_{12} (cyanocobalamine; a cofactor for methionine synthetase). This leads to inhibition of methionine synthesis, reducing production of methionine tetrahydrofolate and DNA. Exposure to N_2O for a few hours may lead to megaloblastic changes in bone marrow; prolonged exposure may lead to agranulocytosis.

Neurotoxicity: protracted use may lead to peripheral neuropathy.

Management of both bone marrow toxicity and neurotoxicity includes administration of folinic acid, providing an alternate source of tetrahydrofolate.

Teratogenicity: N_2O has been shown to be teratogenic in rats, but evidence in humans is not so strong.

Desflurane

Structure: 2,2,2-trifluro-1-fluoroethyl-difluoromethyl ether.

Presentation: clear colourless solution with no preservatives.

Uses: general anaesthesia.

Mechanism of action: unknown.

Pharmacodynamics

CNS: desflurane produces general anaesthesia. It increases CBF and ICP and decreases CMRO2.

CVS: desflurane causes a dose-dependent decrease in systemic vascular resistance. Myocardial contractility is decreased but sympathetic tone is relatively preserved.

RS: desflurane causes dose-dependent respiratory depression.

Pharmacokinetics

Up to 0.02% of inhaled desflurane undergoes metabolism in the liver by cytochrome P450.

Adverse effects

It is a trigger for malignant hyperthermia. Desflurane is respiratory tract irritant, so cannot be used for inhalational induction.

Xenon

Chemical structure: Xe.

Presentation: inert odourless colourless gas. Manufactured by fractional distillation of air.

Uses: as an adjuvant to general anaesthesia.

Mechanism of action: unknown.

Pharmacodynamics

CNS: xenon produces anaesthetic with significant analgesic properties. It increases CBF and ICP.

CVS: xenon does not alter cardiac contractility but decreases heart rate.

RS: xenon decreases the respiratory rate but increases the tidal volume, thereby maintaining minute volume.

Pharmacokinetics

Xenon is not metabolized in the body. It has a high density and viscosity, which may increase airway resistance. It does not appear to cause diffusion hypoxia.

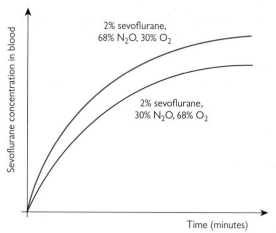

Fig. 7.46 The second gas effect. Uptake of sevoflurane is faster with the higher concentration of N_2O.

Table 7.10 Physical properties of inhalational agents						
	Molecular weight	Boiling point (°C)	SVP at 20°C (kPa)	MAC	Partition coefficient	
					Blood:gas	Oil:gas
N_2O	44	−88	–	105	0.47	1.4
Halothane	197	50	32	0.76	2.4	224
Isoflurane	184.5	48	33	1.28	1.4	95
Enflurane	184.5	56	23	1.68	1.9	95
Desflurane	168	23	89	5–10	0.42	26
Sevoflurane	200	58	22	2.0	0.69	80
Xenon	131	−108	–	71	0.14	1.9

7.19 Epilepsy and anticonvulsants

Epilepsy is a neurological condition characterized by recurrent seizures due to abnormal uncontrolled neuronal activity in the brain. Seizures can be classified into two broad groups:

Generalized seizures

- Tonic–clonic or grand mal
- Tonic
- Atonic
- Myoclonic
- Absence seizures (petit mal)

Partial seizures

- Simple partial seizures
- Complex partial seizures

In some individuals, seizures can be triggered by flashing lights, fever, stress, alcohol, illegal drugs, or changes in hormone levels.

Risk factors for seizures

In most cases, epilepsy is idiopathic. However, it may be secondary to brain injury or disease, when it is referred to as 'symptomatic epilepsy':

- Head injury
- Ischaemic/hypoxic brain injury (e.g. post-cardiac arrest)
- CNS infection
- Drug overdose (e.g. tricyclic antidepressants)
- Pre-existing epilepsy with poor compliance or recent change of treatment
- Electrolyte imbalance (e.g. hyponatraemia, hypocalcaemia, hypomagnesaemia, hypoglycaemia)
- Renal or hepatic failure
- Brain tumour
- Alcoholism.

Epilepsy cannot be cured (except in some instances of symptomatic epilepsy by treatment or resolution of the primary cause). The mainstay of treatment is control of seizures with anticonvulsants and lifestyle changes. In severe epilepsy, neurosurgical options may reduce the frequency and duration of seizures.

Status epilepticus

Status epilepticus is defined as continuous seizure activity for 30min or more, or intermittent seizure activity lasting 30min or more without intervening periods of consciousness.

Status epilepticus affects approximately 14,000 people per annum in the UK and carries an overall mortality of 25% (although much of this results from the underlying condition causing the seizures). When seizures continue beyond 30min, cerebral autoregulation fails, blood flow falls, and ICP rises. Oxygen delivery is inadequate to meet demand, and seizures continue - but clinically they appear to diminish to muscular twitching or even no muscular activity. Cardiovascular, respiratory, and metabolic derangements combine with excitotoxicity to produce neuronal damage. It is vital to terminate seizures rapidly to reduce long term sequelae.

Presentation

Loss of consciousness; tonic–clonic seizures; urinary incontinence. With prolonged seizures, signs may become more subtle, e.g. eyelid twitching.

Clinical management

See status epilepticus algorithm (Section 22.21).

ABC approach: maintain the airway and give 100% oxygen.

Cannulate a vein, take a blood sample for biochemistry and haematology, and check glucose. Treat confirmed hypoglycaemia.

Give IV lorazepam or diazepam (both 0.1mg/kg). Lorazepam is preferred as its duration of action is much longer.

If seizures persist after 10min, give phenytoin (15mg/kg at 50mg/min or less) or fosphenytoin (22.5mg/kg at a rate of up to 225mg/min). Phenytoin carries a risk of hypotension and arrhythmias, and the patient should be monitored. (There is also a reported 6% incidence of a potentially devastating soft tissue reaction with infusion of phenytoin distal to the antecubital fossa: 'purple glove syndrome'.) Fosphenytoin is a water-soluble prodrug which is converted to phenytoin. It can be infused more rapidly, has a lower incidence of cardiovascular side effects, and has no adverse effects on extravasation.

If seizures still persist, furher phenytoin may be given up to a total of 30mg/kg or fosphenytoin up to a total of 45mg/kg.

If the seizures remain refractory, phenobarbital 20mg/kg can be considered. Intubation and ventilation is likely to be necessary at this stage to protect the airway and optimize gas exchange. In any case, general anaesthesia is the definitive treatment for refractory seizures. Propofol or thiopental should be used for induction, with suxamethonium. Longer-acting paralysis should be avoided if possible, as it may mask continuing seizures.

Anaesthesia is maintained with infusions of propofol (2–10mg/kg/hr) or thiopental (3–5mg/kg/hr). There may be significantly delayed recovery after prolonged usage of thiopental. Ideally, either agent should be used in conjunction with continuous EEG monitoring to minimize the dose used to abolish seizures.

Search for an underlying cause (see risk factors).

Treat complications, e.g. hyperthermia, rhabdomyolysis, arrhythmias, pulmonary aspiration.

Arterial blood gases, full blood count, urea and electrolytes, blood glucose, anti-convulsant blood levels.

Consider CT brain.

Where available, EEG.

Anticonvulsants

Anticonvulsants can be classified based on their mechanism of action and their clinical use

Mechanism of action of anticonvulsants

There are three main modes of action for anticonvulsants:

Drugs acting on ion channels

Na^+ channels

- Phenytoin
- Carbemazepine
- Lamotrigine
- Topiramate
- Valproate

Ca^{2+} channels

- Ethosuximide
- Valproate

Drugs enhancing GABA transmission

- Benzodiazepines
- Barbiturates
- Valproate
- Gabapentin
- Vigabatrin
- Felbamate
- Topiramate
- Propofol

Drugs inhibiting excitatory neurotransmitters

- Felbamate
- Topiramate

Drugs acting on sodium channels are useful for treating generalized tonic–clonic or partial seizures. Drugs acting on calcium entry (and clonazepam, a benzodiazepine) are useful for absence seizures. Drugs enhancing GABA transmission are useful for myoclonic seizures as well as for tonic–clonic and partial seizures.

Table 7.11 Anticonvulsants

	Name	Phenytoin	Carbemazapine	Valproate
Properties	Uses	Anticonvulsant Digoxin induced dysrhythmia Trigeminal neuralgia	Epilepsy, especially temporal lobe and tonic–clonic Trigeminal neuralgia Bipolar disorder	Epilepsy, especially petit mal, myoclonic seizures, and infantile spasms Chronic pain
	Chemical	Hydantoin derivative	Iminostilbene derivative (similar to TCAs)	A salt of valproic acid
	Action	Anticonvulsant and anti-dysrhthymic	Anticonvulsant and analgesic	Anticonvulsant
	Mode	Membrane stabilization: slows inward Na and Ca^{2+} flux; delays outward K^+ flux.	Currently unknown	GABAergic inhibition; GABA levels ↑ by reduction of metabolism
	Route	PO 200–600mg/day. IV Load 10-15mg/kg infused slowly, followed by 100mg TDS; dose for dysrhythmia titrated to effect.	PO 100–1600mg/day	PO 600–2500mg/day IV 400–2500mg/day
Effects	CVS	Class I antiarrhythmic; ↑AV nodal conduction; ↓BP and complete heart block may follow too-rapid IV bolusing	Antiarrhythmic; depresses AV conduction	
	CNS	80% epileptics controlled with just this drug; does not raise seizure threshold but stabilizes membrane; primary focus of seizure activity is unaffected	Raises seizure threshold May act as a CNS stimulant	Anticonvulsant; minimal sedation; occasional essential tremor
	Other	↑glucose, ↓Ca^{2+}, alteration in LFTs; suppresses ADH secretion	Antidiuretic effect; potentiates water intoxication	↑ammonium levels
Kinetics	Absorption	Slow PO absorption; 90% bioavailability	Good PO absorption	Rapid and complete absorption
	Distribution	90% protein-bound	75% protein bound; V_d 1L/kg	90% albumin protein bound
	Metabolism	Large genetic variation; hydroxylated and then conjugated with glucuronide in the liver; zero-order kinetics just above the therapeutic range	Hepatic oxidation to active metabolite epoxide; will induce its own metabolism with chronic use	Hepatic oxidation and conjugation with glucuronide to active metabolites
	Excretion	80% actively secreted by renal tubules; <5% excreted unchanged; ↓ dose in hepatic impairment	Urine excretion via unconjugated metabolites	1–3% unchanged in urine
	Toxicity	Acne, gum hyperplasia, hirsuitism and coarsened facies, megaloblastic anaemia, osteomalacia, erythroderma, lymphadenopathy, SLE, hepatotoxicity	Diplopia, nausea, drowsiness, ataxia, rashes; neutropenia common but aplastic anaemia is rare.	GI upset; pancreatitis; liver dysfunction; hair loss; platelet and coagulation disturbances
	Note	Nausea, vomiting, and drowsiness; behavioural disturbance; peripheral neuropathy; potent enzyme inducer; ↓ effect of warfarin and benzodiazepines; phenytoin toxicity produced by metronidazole and isoniazid; ↓ MAC of volatiles and increases LA toxicity	Valproate will increase plasma levels of carbamezepine; regular LFTs and WBC should be performed during chronic therapy	Contraindicated in those with acute liver disease; LFTS should be monitored during chronic therapy; platelet function should be assessed prior to regional anaesthesia

→ Anticonvulsants

Vigabatrin is an analogue of GABA, but it is not a GABA-receptor agonist. It is an irreversible inhibitor of GABA-transaminase, the enzyme that breaks down GABA and increases its synaptic levels.

The [S]-enantiomer of the racemic compound is pharmacologically active.

Lamotrigine possibly inhibits voltage-sensitive sodium channels, stabilizes presynaptic membranes, and modulates transmitter release of excitatory amino acids.

It has relatively few drug interactions although its interaction with valproate is an indication for blood monitoring. Life-threatening skin reactions, including toxic epidermal necrolysis, are a major concern. Rashes may occur in the first 2 months of therapy, or on restarting therapy at the normal dose following a short break.

Gabapentin was synthesized to mimic the chemical structure of GABA, but now is not thought to act on GABA receptors. It is thought to bind to the $\alpha 2\delta$ subunit of CNS voltage-dependent calcium channels.

It is used as second-line drug to control partial seizures and is also used for treating post-herpetic neuralgia and neuropathic pain. It is well tolerated, has relatively few side effects, and is excreted unmetabolized via the kidneys.

7.20 Antidepressants

Around one in ten adults will suffer depression at some stage in their lives; the prevalence is around 5%. Various antidepressant drugs are in use.

Tricyclic antidepressants

Tricyclic antidepressants (TCAs) are named after their original three-ringed structure. However, second-generation TCAs may have different configurations, while retaining the pharmacological properties of their predecessors.

Uses

TCAs are used in the treatment of clinical depression, various chronic pain conditions, and nocturnal enuresis.

Mechanism of action

TCAs prevent the re-uptake of various neurotransmitters (serotonin, noradrenaline, and dopamine) into the nerve terminal.

Side effects

Many of the side effects are antimuscarinic. They include dry mouth, blurred vision, decreased gut motility, constipation, urinary retention and hyperthermia. TCAs can also cause postural hypotension. Amitriptyline in particular has sedative effects, and is usually given at night. TCAs are dangerous in overdose (see opposite).

Interactions

Drugs which inhibit hepatic cytochrome P450 decrease the metabolism of TCAs, leading to higher plasma concentrations.

TCAs increase sensitivity to catecholamines. This can result in hypertension and arrhythmias if sympathomimetics are used. They may enhance the effects of CNS depressants, including alcohol.

Monoamine oxidase inhibitors

Monoamine oxidase inhibitors (MAOIs) are classified according to their pharmacodynamic behaviour. Older MAOIs (such as phenelzine) are non-selective and irreversible, whereas the new generation (e.g. moclobemide) are selective and reversible.

Uses

Used in the treatment of clinical depression. MAOIs are used only when other antidepressants have been tried unsuccessfully.

Mechanism of action

Monoamine oxidase (MAO) catalyses the oxidative deamination of amines. Two types are found:

- **Type A** inactivates noradrenaline and 5-HT.
- **Type B** inactivates tyramine and phenylethylamine.

Both are capable of inactivating dopamine and tyramine.

MAOIs act by inhibiting the metabolism of these neurotransmitters, increasing their concentrations.

Side effects

Common side effects include: dry mouth, insomnia, tachycardia, drowsiness, blurred vision, appetite changes, muscle twitching, restlessness, and impotence.

Interactions

MAOIs can produce an exaggerated hypertensive response with sympathomimetic drugs. This is particularly true of indirectly acting drugs (e.g. ephedrine), which cause endogenous catecholamine release. Indirectly acting sympathomimetics depend on MAO for their metabolism, while the directly acting sympathomimetics can be metabolized by catechol-*O*-methyl transferase (COMT) (Section 9.3).

Pethidine administered in the presence of MAOIs can cause high tachycardia, hypertension, fever, agitation, convulsion, and coma. The mechanism of this reaction is not known, and other opioids are safe alongside MAOIs.

MAOIs react with tyramine-rich foods (hard cheese; soya bean products; aged, preserved, or spoiled meat and fish; Chianti; protein or yeast extracts; ale), leading to 'cheese syndrome'—uncontrolled hypertension with marked postural drop, blurring of vision, and sedation.

MAOIs and anaesthesia

For elective surgery, the traditional advice was to stop MAOIs 2–3 weeks preoperatively. This approach necessitates psychiatric input, as it could put patients at risk of a relapse into depression. However, the newer reversible MAO-A-specific MAOIs are less prone to serious interactions and do not need to be stopped perioperatively. Pethidine and indirectly acting sympathomimetics should still be avoided; if cardiovascular support is indicated, directly acting sympathomimetics can be used with caution.

Selective serotonin re-uptake inhibitors

SSRIs are increasingly being prescribed as they are better tolerated than other classes of antidepressant.

Uses

SSRIs are used in the treatment of clinical depression, anxiety disorders, and premature ejaculation.

Mechanism of action

As the name suggests, SSRIs inhibit the re-uptake of serotonin into presynaptic cells. This increases the amount of serotonin available to the postsynaptic receptors.

Side effects

SSRIs cause fewer side effects than TCAs. GI side effects include nausea, vomiting, and diarrhoea due to the action of serotonin on the GI tract. Cardiovascular side effects include arrhythmias and orthostatic hypotension. SIADH and impaired platelet function have been reported.

Interactions

SSRIs cannot be used concomitantly with MAOIs or TCAs because of the risk of developing serotonin syndrome (tremor, hyperthermia, cardiovascular collapse). Pethidine may also precipitate serotonin syndrome when used with SSRIs.

Lithium

Lithium is commonly used in the form of lithium carbonate salt in the treatment of bipolar depression, mania, and recurrent affective disorder. The precise mechanism of action is unknown. Lithium may mimic sodium, entering excitable cells during depolarization but decreasing neurotransmitter release.

Lithium decreases the seizure threshold in epileptics. It antagonizes ADH, leading to polyuria and polydipsia. Prolonged treatment may damage renal tubules, and cause nephrogenic diabetes insipidus. It can cause thyroid dysfunction. In addition it may increase plasma levels of Na^+, Mg^{2+}, and Ca^{2+}. The therapeutic window is small (plasma level 0.5–1.0 mmol/L). Toxicity occurs at plasma levels >1.5mmol/L; signs include vomiting, ataxia, arrhythmias, confusion, and seizures.

Lithium may reduce anaesthetic requirements because of effects on the brainstem; it prolongs the action of neuromuscular blockers although paradoxically it can often increase generalized muscle tone in awake patients.

Other agents

Other antidepressant drugs include serotonin and noradrenaline re-uptake inhibitors (e.g. venlafaxine, duloxetine), presynaptic α_2-adrenoceptor antagonists (e.g. mianserin, mirtazapine), selective noradrenaline re-uptake inhibitors (SNRIs) (e.g. reboxetine), and others whose mechanism of action is obscure.

→ TCA overdose

TCAs are rapidly absorbed from the gut and undergo first-pass metabolism. Conjugates are renally eliminated. They are lipophilic and highly protein-bound, with a large V_D. Elimination half-life is often >24hr.

The altered pharmacokinetics of overdose reduce excretion and increase toxic effects. Anticholinergic effects delay gastric emptying and acidosis (from respiratory depression and hypotension) reduces protein binding and increases the free active drug.

The toxic effects of TCAs are related to

- Anticholinergic effects
- Direct α-adrenergic blockade
- Inhibition of noradrenaline and serotonin re-uptake
- Blockade of fast sodium channels in myocardial cells, resulting in membrane-stabilizing effects

Anticholinergic effects

Anticholinergic symptoms start within 2hr of ingestion and are typically the first to appear. They include dry mouth, blurred vision, mydriasis, urinary retention, hypoactive or absent bowel sounds, pyrexia, and myoclonic twitching.

Cardiovascular effects

Due to impaired conduction from fast Na^+ channel blockade. This decreases the slope of phase zero depolarization, widens the QRS complex, and prolongs the PR, QRS, and QT intervals. This often leads to heart block and unstable dysrrhythmias. TCAs also depress myocardial contractility, but vasodilatation from direct α-adrenergic blockade is the major cause of hypotension.

Patients with a QRS <100msec are unlikely to develop seizures and arrhythmias, but those with QRS > 160 msec have a 50% chance of developing serious rhythm disturbance.

CNS effects

Include drowsiness, extrapyramidal signs, rigidity, ophthalmoplegia, respiratory depression, delirium, seizure, and coma. Depressed conscious level is due to the antihistamine and anticholinergic effects, while seizures are probably related to increased brain noradrenaline and serotonin levels.

Therapy

Gastric lavage should be performed within 1hr of ingestion; otherwise, it is ineffective.

Clinical deterioration should be anticipated, and early intubation should be considered. Prevention of acidaemia is vital. Serum alkalinization with sodium bicarbonate to pH 7.45–7.55 increases protein binding, decreases the QRS interval, stabilizes arrhythmias, and increases BP.

Class IA, class IC, class II, and class III drugs should be avoided in the treatment of dysrrhythmias.

- Class IA and IC drugs block sodium channels and exacerbate TCA effects on the myocardium.
- Class III drugs prolong the QT interval and increase the risk of a malignant ventricular arrhythmia.
- β-blockers depress myocardial contractility and worsen hypotension.

Class IB anti-arrhythmics increase the rate of phase zero depolarization: phenytoin may correct conduction defects. Magnesium and glucagons may also be useful.

→ SSRI cessation syndrome

SSRI cessation syndrome may occur during or following the interruption, lowering of dose, or discontinuation of regular SSRI or SNRI antidepressant drugs. It usually begins 24 hr to a week after the change in drug dose, depending on its elimination half-life. However, some SSRI medications have a very short half-life with few active metabolites; in these, the brief duration of action means that cessation syndrome may be precipitated by failure to take a single due dose. Some patients have extreme difficulty in discontinuing SSRIs.

SSRIs prevent presynaptic re-uptake of serotonin, resulting in a greater concentration within the synaptic cleft. This causes greater stimulation of pre-synaptic serotonin receptors, leading to reduced serotonin production. Increased synaptic serotonin also leads to downregulation of its post-synaptic receptors. When the SSRI is discontinued, there is neither enough serotonin nor an appropriate number of its receptors to maintain post-synaptic function. Cessation syndrome symptoms may last for up to several weeks.

Symptoms include headache, diarrhoea, nausea, vomiting, chills, dizziness, and fatigue. There are also CNS features including insomnia, agitation, impaired concentration, vivid dreams, depersonalization, irritability, and suicidal thoughts. These symptoms vary in intensity and duration.

→ Serotonin syndrome

A rare but potentially life-threatening side effect, characterized by dangerously high brain levels of serotonin. It occurs when an SSRI interacts with MAOIs which reduce breakdown of the brain amines serotonin and noradrenaline.

It may also occur when SSRIs are taken with St John's wort. Serotonin syndrome requires immediate medical treatment.

Signs and symptoms

- Confusion
- Restlessness
- Hallucinations
- Extreme agitation
- Fluctuations in blood pressure
- Increased heart rate
- Nausea and vomiting
- Fever
- Seizures
- Coma

Treatment of serotonin syndrome is mainly supportive, and the condition usually resolves within 36hr. However, serotonin antagonists such as cyproheptadine (primarily an antihistamine), chlorpromazine, methysergide, and propranolol can be used in some cases.

The motor cortex

The motor area of the brain is anterior to the central sulcus, in the precentral gyrus. It can be divided into three areas.

In the **primary motor cortex** stimulation of nerve bodies produces a set movement.

The **supplementary motor area** (also known as the secondary motor cortex) is found 3cm anterior to the motor cortex, on the superomedial aspect of the hemisphere. The **premotor cortex** is also anterior to the motor cortex, on the lateral surface of the hemisphere. Nerve signals in these two areas produce much more complex patterns of movement than the discrete patterns produced in the primary motor cortex.

Organization of the cortex

The motor cortex is organized topographically. Stimulation of a region will produce stereotyped contraction of a group of muscles. The areas controlling movement of the face, mastication, and swallowing are found near the lateral sulcus. Together with areas for fine hand movements, they dominate the motor cortex.

The areas controlling the face and hands are supplied by the middle cerebral artery. The areas controlling foot movements are dorsomedial, next to the central sulcus, and supplied by anterior cerebral artery. Isolated lesions here result in loss of voluntary movement of the contralateral limb. Speech defects occur if there are lesions within Broca's area.

The corticospinal tracts

Voluntary motor pathways pass from the motor cortex to the cell bodies of the lower motor neurons (Figure 7.47). The fibres pass through the posterior limb of the **internal capsule** (Figure 7.48), where again they are topographically organized.

From the internal capsule the fibres form a compact bundle which occupies the central third of the **cerebral peduncle**. They pass through the **ventral pons**, where they are broken up into smaller bundles.

At the lower end of the pons they coalesce into a single bundle that lies on the ventral medulla, called the **pyramid**. Branches are sent to cranial nerve nuclei. Craniobulbar fibres cross over in the brainstem; some nuclei are bilaterally innervated.

At the lower end of the medulla the majority of pyramidal fibres cross and occupy a central position in the **lateral white column** of the spinal cord. Some fibres remain uncrossed.

Vascular lesions of the motor pathways

The internal capsule is supplied by branches of the middle cerebral artery. Lesions here are associated with complete contralateral hemiplegia and associated sensory loss. The deficit can extend to the optic radiation, giving a contralateral homonymous hemianopia. Fibres of nerve III are often associated, so there are signs of nerve III palsy.

The pons is supplied by the pontine branches of the basilar artery. If the blood supply is compromised, cranial nerves IV and VII are often involved. The result is a contralateral hemiplegia, with ipsilateral lower motor neuron IV and VII nerve lesions.

The medulla is supplied by the anterior spinal branches of the vertebral artery. Vascular defects here often cause bilateral lesions, as the pyramids are close together. The pattern is of tongue paralysis with disturbances of phonation and swallowing.

The spinal cord is supplied by segmental branches of the anterior and posterior spinal arteries.

Extrapyramidal motor pathways

Basal ganglia

The basal ganglia consist of the putamen, caudate nucleus, globus pallidus, and substantia nigra. Their role is indirect control of complex patterns of movement. By projecting to the motor cortex, the premotor cortex, and the supplementary motor area simultaneously, they form part of the corto-basal ganglia motor loop, which is important in

determining how rapidly movement is performed and how large the movement should be.

Lesions in the basal ganglia lead to tremors, athetosis (writhing), chorea (fidgeting), and uncontrolled explosive movements (hemiballismus). Degeneration of dopaminergic neurons within the substantia nigra leads to the development of parkinsonism.

Cerebellum

The cerebellum has a vital role in coordinating the sequence of motor activities. Figure 7.49 is a schematic diagram of the neuronal connections in the cerebellum.

Lesions of the cerebellum lead to disturbances of motor function, e.g. unsteady gait, hypotonia, tremor, nystagmus and dysarthria.

Proprioception and spinal reflexes

Muscle control needs continuous feedback of sensory information from each muscle to the spinal cord. The vital components of this information are the length of muscle, instantaneous tension, and the rates of change of length and tension.

There are two types of specialized sensory receptor.

- **Muscle spindles:** distributed in muscle bellies. These give information on muscle length and its rate of change (Section 8.3).
- **Golgi tendon organs:** located in muscle tendons. These give feedback about tendon tension and its rate of change (Section 8.3).

Spinal cord reflexes which cause muscle spasm

Pain can elicit debilitating reflex muscle spasm. This often occurs where facilitation of the spinal cord is increased by long-standing upper motor lesions.

Children with cerebral palsy often suffer intense muscle spasm, especially exaggerated after painful surgery. Epidural analgesia is often required to control perioperative spasm, especially when benzodiazepines and other drug treatments have proved ineffective. Pertionitis can cause severe abdominal muscle spasm.

The vestibular system and balance

The vestibular system (Figure 7.50) is encased, along with the auditory organ of Corti, within a number of chambers (the labyrinth) in the petrous temporal bone. It comprises the **semicircular canals** (which detect rotational motion), the **utricle**, and the **saccule** (which detect linear displacement).

The system is suspended in a CSF-like fluid called **perilymph**, and contains fluid called **endolymph** (resembling intracellular fluid).

The three semicircular canals are arranged at right angles to each other, reflecting the three-dimensional world. Each canal has a swelling; the ampulla containing hair cells that project from a ridge called the crista into a simple jelly-like substance called the cupula (this is contained in the endolymph; Figure 7.51). During rotational acceleration, endolymph is displaced opposite to the direction of rotation. This bends the hair processes, altering permeability and membrane potential (Figure 7.52). As one semicircular canal is stimulated, its mirror image on the other side is inhibited, amplifying the overall signal reaching the brain. The information transmitted from the semicircular canal is used to:

- predict disequilibrium and produce corrections (e.g. to prevent falling over whilst running)
- enable gaze to remain fixed on an object during head rotation.

The utricle and saccule contain patches of hair cells, the **maculae**. The macula of the utricle lies in the horizontal plane and detects horizontal linear acceleration; the macula of the saccule lies in the vertical plane and detects vertical linear acceleration.

The pathway for the equilibrium reflexes passes from the vestibular nerves to the vestibular nuclei, and then to the cerebellum. There are connections to the reticular system and the spinal cord, and also via the medial longitudinal fasciculus to the oculomotor nuclei. The flocculonodular lobes of the cerebellum are especially concerned with dynamic equilibrium, and lesions here mimic lesions in the semicircular canal.

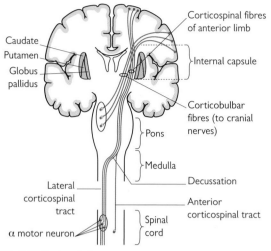

Fig. 7.47 Corticospinal tract.

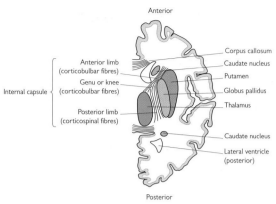

Fig. 7.48 Anatomical relations of the internal capsule.

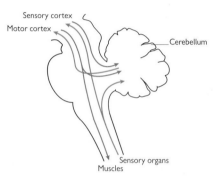

Fig. 7.49 Cerebellum feedback loop.

➕ **Drugs and the vestibular apparatus**

Alcohol diffuses through the christa at a higher rate than through the rest of the semicircular canals, therefore causing a density change compared with the rest of the fluid in the canal. This accounts for the dizziness and nausea that accompany alcohol consumption. Morphine sensitizes the vestibular apparatus, triggering nausea, particularly in patients who are ambulant immediately after surgery.

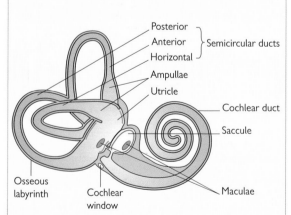

Fig. 7.50 The vestibular apparatus

It provides very precise control over the timing, sequence, and duration of the body's movements. It does so by means of a loop circuit that connects it to the motor cortex thereby modulating by signals that the motor cortex sends to the rest of the body (Figure 7.47). It also plays a role in analysing the visual signals associated with movement. The cerebellum appears to calculate the speed of these movements and adjust the motor commands accordingly. Patients who have suffered injuries to the cerebellum have poor motor control which is thought to be due to errors in such calculations.

➡️ **Hair cells**

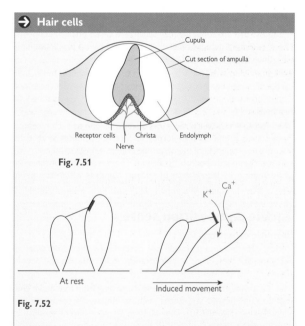

Fig. 7.51

Fig. 7.52

The maculae, christae, and organ of Corti all utilise the same type of sensory receptor—the hair cell. Hair cells possess a number of stiff cilia which can be displaced by movement. In the cochlear, movement occurs as a result of sound waves being transduced by the ossicles and vibrating the basilar membrane in which the hair cell bodies lie. Vestibular hair cells' cilia are bent by movement of the head, which causes displacement of the gelatinous cupula. Cation channels open to depolarise the cell (Figure 7.52). The semicircular canals each respond to rotational or angular acceleration in a specific direction. In contrast, the utricle's hair cells respond to linear acceleration in all directions. The mechanism is so sensitive it can detect rotation of 0.1° per second.

7.22 Somatosensory pathways

There are two main classes of somatosensory information, which are conducted to the brain via two distinct pathways.

- The **dorsal column–medial lemniscus system** carries signals for tactile, vibration, and position sensation from joints, and is described here.
- The **anterolateral system** carries impulses for pain, temperature, itch, and sexual sensation, and is described in Section 7.26.

Sensory receptors

Receptors are formed by the peripheral terminations of the axons of dorsal root ganglion cells.

There are five basic types of receptor: mechanoreceptors, thermoreceptors, nociceptors, chemoreceptors, and electromagnetic receptors. Receptors work by converting sensory stimuli into nerve impulses, a process called transduction. Some of the different varieties of receptor are shown in Figure 7.53.

Sensory transduction

A stimulus alters the membrane permeability of the nerve ending, which in turn produces a depolarization (the 'receptor potential'). If the receptor potential rises above a threshold, an action potential is produced.

Coding for intensity of the stimulus is by means of action potential frequency. The exact relationship varies from receptor to receptor: for example in the Pacinian corpuscle, a mechanoreceptor, the relationship between action potential frequency and the log of the stimulus strength is linear.

Adaptation of receptors

Receptors can vary their response to a stimulus with time. The degree of adaptation varies with receptor.

Receptors that adapt quickly (e.g. touch) are called **phasic receptors**. Phasic receptors detect new stimuli. They also have a predictive function, detecting the rate of change of a stimulus.

Receptors which adapt slowly are called **tonic receptors,** and include carbon dioxide chemoreceptors, muscle spindles, and pain receptors. Tonic receptors provide continuous information for regulating vital functions.

The mechanism by which receptors adapt is unique to each receptor. For instance, in the Pacinian corpuscle, fluid redistributes so that the viscoelastic properties of the corpuscle change: a mechanical event will no longer produce a receptor potential. There is a generic mechanism of adaptation by inactivation of sodium channels within the nerve membrane.

Tactile and position sense

Somatic sensations

Touch, pressure and vibration are detected by the same types of receptor, but these vary in their location within the skin and deeper tissues.

There is a wide array of tactile receptors, ranging from free nerve endings to complicated structures such as Meissner's corpuscle and Merkel's disc (Figure 7.53). They all have slightly different sensitivities and adaptive patterns.

The receptive field

The accuracy with which tactile information can be sensed varies from one region of the body to another, and depends not only on the density of nerve receptors but also on the size of their receptive fields. The receptive field of a somatic sensory neuron is the region of the skin within which a tactile stimulus evokes a sensory response in the cell or its axon. The receptive fields in the finger are smaller than those in the forearm, and so allow more accurate two-point discrimination. Sensory discrimination also depends on input from higher centres; the effects of fatigue, stress, and practice on accurate discrimination of tactile sensation are well reported.

It is becoming clear that somatosensory receptive fields are dynamic, changing according to the history of the stimulus–receptor interaction and according to input from higher centres.

Pathways of mechano-sensory information

The cell bodies of the first-order axons are found in the **dorsal root ganglion** associated with each segmental spinal nerve. As they enter the spinal cord, they divide into ascending and descending branches.

The **descending branches** enter laterally, divide, and terminate on interneurons which further synapse in the anterior and lateral horn of the spinal cord. Some of these connections are responsible for the spinal reflexes (Section 8.3). Others ascend in the spinocerebellar tract and interact with the cerebellum in coordinating movement. Some collaterals are involved in modifying the pain pathways (gate theory, Section 7.27).

The **ascending branches** do not synapse, but climb in the dorsal column tracts all the way to the **medulla** where they synapse in the **gracile** and **cuneate nuclei**. The position of the gracile and cuneate tracts (otherwise known as the dorsal columns) is shown Figure 7.54, along with the positions of the other major spinal cords tracts described elsewhere.

Axons in the dorsal columns are topographically organized, so that sensation from the lower limbs is carried in fibres in the medial part of the dorsal columns (the **gracile tract**). Sensation from the upper limbs, trunk, and neck is carried in the lateral part (the **cuneate tract**). Despite occupying a substantial area of the spinal cord, lesions in the dorsal column tracts have a limited effect on tactile tasks. This may be because some cutaneous mechanoreception is conveyed in anterolateral pathways such as the spinothalamic tract (Section 7.26).

The **second-order neurons** decussate (cross over) to the opposite side of the brainstem and ascend in the **medial lemniscus**. The topographical organization is maintained, but the fibres change position during the crossover. The result is that in the pons and upper midbrain, the upper body is represented in the medial fibres and the lower limbs in the lateral axons. This topographical representation continues all the way to the **venterobasal complex of the thalamus** where the second-order neurons terminate.

In the pons, fibres from the principal nucleus (where the first-order neurons synapse) join the medial leminiscus (part of the trigeminal brainstem complex). These second-order fibres make up the **trigeminal lemniscus**.

Somatosensory cortex

The third-order neurons from the venterobasal thalamus relay to the **somatosensory cortex** which is located just posterior to the central sulcus, and again has a topographical organization. The areas representing the face and hands occupy the lateral areas, and those corresponding to the lower limbs the medial areas. Areas associated with the densest and most complex sensory information (such as the fingertips, lips, and genitalia) occupy a greater proportion of the sensory cortex (Figure 7.56). A representation of the weighting given to different body parts is shown in Figure 7.56. The equivalent representation of the motor cortex is shown in Figure 7.55, for comparison.

The sensory cortex, like other parts of the cortex is organized in units called modules, each involving thousands of nerve cells in repeating patterns. These modules are vertical columns containing six layers of neurons, each layer performing a distinct function (e.g. the second-order neurons from the thalamus relay in layer IV).

Each module detects a different area on the body with a specific sensory modality, e.g. 'light touch from the left little finger'. Different modalities tend to be grouped in discrete areas. For example, sensory information from the proprioreceptors arrives nearest the central sulcus, adjacent to the motor cortex.

In addition, different areas of the sensory cortex are functionally dissimilar. For instance, in the anterior part of the sensory cortex (area 3b), responses tend to be simple (a module might respond to sensation from one finger). More posteriorly (in area 1), a module might respond to stimulation of the whole hand.

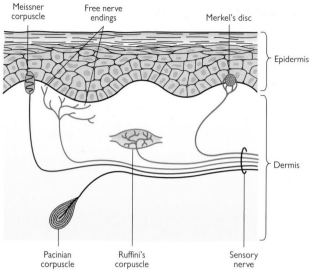

Fig. 7.53 Sensory receptors. Meissner's corpuscles detect light touch; free nerve endings respond to pain and temperature; Ruffini's corpuscles detect skin stretch and joint position; Merckel's discs are sensitive, slowly-adapting mechanoreceptors which are involved in tactile discrimination and texture sense; and Pacinian corpuscles respond to deep touch and vibration.

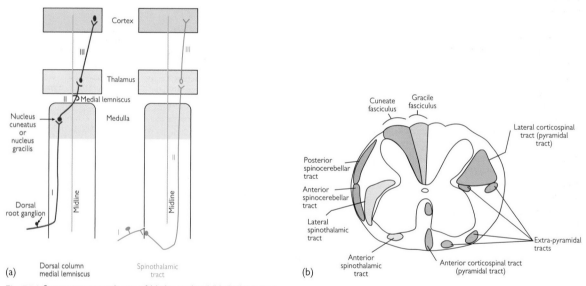

Fig. 7.54 Somatosensory pathways of (a) the cord and (b) the brainstem.

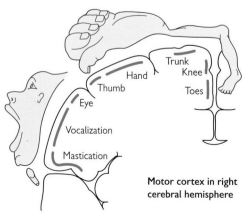

Fig. 7.55 Motor cortex homunculus.

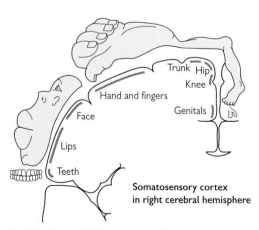

Fig. 7.56 Topographical organization of the sensory cortex: the sensory homunculus.

7.23 Nerve conduction

A membrane potential allows the conduction of an electrical current along and between cells. In this way information is transferred.

Membrane potentials

The **resting membrane potential** (RMP) is a stable 70mV (negative inside the cell). Chemical and electrical gradients tend to move Na^+ into the cell. If it were not for the Na^+–K^+ ATP pump (Figure 7.61), the membrane potential would quickly dissipate.

Local currents are able to alter the membrane potential. If depolarization is sufficient (e.g. a 10–15mV change), the **threshold potential** is reached, and voltage-gated channels open. This allows an inpouring of Na^+ ions. The membrane depolarizes, and actually overshoots to become positive inside the cell. This closes Na^+ voltage-gated channels.

Depolarization opens voltage-gated K^+ channels, allowing K^+ to move along its concentration gradient and out of the cell. This slower sustained process returns the RMP to its resting value. The Na^+–K^+ ATP pump restores the electrochemical gradients.

This process affects the function of adjacent membrane, producing similar changes of depolarization and repolarization. As this is repeated along the axon it produces a wave of change known as an **action potential**. This response has a constant amplitude—'all or nothing.' As a result, communication of stimulus intensity by nerves is by frequency of firing, not the size of the impulse (which cannot vary).

The changes in membrane potential, along with the corresponding ion permeabilities, are shown in Figure 7.59. The positive and negative feedback loops of ion permeability are shown in Figure 7.60.

The refractory period

It is impossible to stimulate a nerve during the period of Na^+ channel opening. This is the **absolute refractory period**.

Following this, there is a 15msec **relative refractory period**, during which the threshold is higher and a larger stimulus is required to produce a response.

The refractory period ensures that impulses are conducted in one direction only. It also limits the maximum frequency of nerve firing.

Compound action potential

Peripheral nerves contain a variety of fibres, each with their respective action potential profiles. Different nerve diameters and the presence of myelin will affect the speed of conduction, represented as a spread of voltage peaks (Figure 7.58).

Classification of nerve fibres

The speed of transmission along nerve fibres depends on myelination and size.

Myelination of nerve fibres

Some nerve fibres are covered by insulating myelin sheaths of Schwann cells. These layers increase the resistance and reduce the capacitance of nerve cells. This allows membrane potential changes only at gaps in the myelin, the nodes of Ranvier. The action potential 'jumps' from one node to the next, a phenomenon known as saltatory conduction (Figure 7.57). This allows the action potential to be transmitted faster in myelinated than in unmyelinated fibres.

The conduction velocities of different nerve fibres are given in Table 7.12

Voltage-gated ion channels

The membrane voltage affects channels that act as specific gateways for Na^+, K^+ and Ca^{2+}.

Sodium channels

Sodium channels are densely packed on the surface of the nerve. Each consists of an internal membrane protein made up of four segments, each containing six α-helices (Figure 7.62). One helix in each segment is positively charged but the negatively charged helices line a central pore that is closed at RMP. With depolarization, the positively charged helix moves outwards, inducing conformational change in each helix and opening of the pore.

During an action potential, the channel opens for 0.7msec. It is selective and allows cations (Na^+, Li^+, K^+) to pass with variable relative permeabilities.

Potassium channels

Potassium channels are 20 times less densely packed on the surface of the nerve than sodium channels. Although potassium channels allow passage of other ions, including thallium, ammonium and rubidium, sodium does not pass. The collection of water molecules that surround a sodium ion makes it too large to cross this pore.

Calcium channels

The sequence of these channels is very similar to that of sodium channels.

The effect of calcium

Low plasma Ca^{2+} affects nerve excitability. Polar phospholipids produce fixed membrane negative charges and these are normally balanced by external calcium ions. When this balance is altered by hypocalcaemia, the fixed negative charges affect the RMP, causing depolarization towards threshold. Smaller, otherwise insignificant, stimuli are more likely to produce an action potential.

Table 7.12 Nerve fibre conduction velocities

	Fibre type	Function	Axon diameter (µm)	Conduction velocity (m/sec)
Myelinated	A_α (I)	Motor a-fibres	9–18	70–120
		Spindle afferents (Ia)		
		Tendon organs (Ib)		
	A_β (II)	Touch and pressure	5–12	30–75
	A_γ (II)	Motor to muscle spindles	3–6	18–36
	A_δ (III)	Pain, pressure, temperature	1–5	4–30
	B (III)	Preganglionic	3/–	3–12
No myelin	C (IV)	Pain, touch, heat	1/–	1–2

Pressure on a nerve affects the larger nerve fibres preferentially, so that touch is affected before pain.

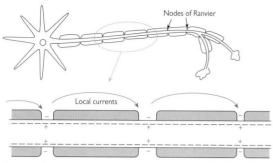

Fig. 7.57 Conduction via the nodes of Ranvier. Saltatory conduction: local reversal of the membrane potenial is detected by surrounding voltage-gated ion channels, which then open themselves.

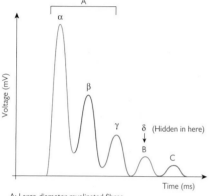

A: Large-diameter myelinated fibres
B: Small myelinated preganglionic antonomic visceral nerves
C: All small diameter unmyelinated motion & sensory fibres

Fig. 7.58 The compound action potential of a mixed peripheral nerve.

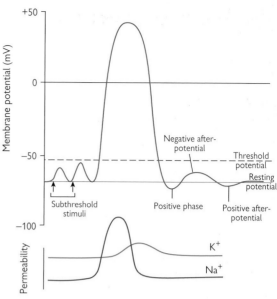

Fig. 7.59 Action potential. The action potential is 'all or nothing' because of the positive feedback of ↑Na+ inflow on membrane depolarization. It is not everlasting because of the effect of ↑K+ permeability, which returns the membrane potential to the resting state.

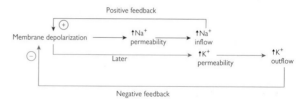

Fig. 7.60 Membrane permeability.

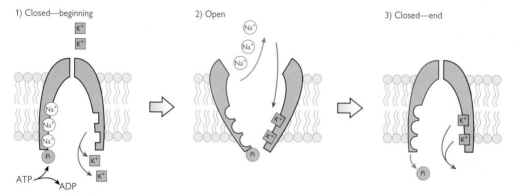

Fig. 7.61 The K+–Na+ pump. Phosphate from ATP binds to the inside of the pump allowing it to open. It discharges Na+ externally. K+ binds to the pump, which closes as the phosphate group dissociates. Thus K+ can enter the cell.

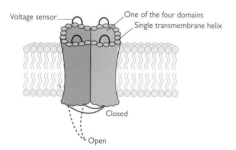

Fig. 7.62 The Na+ channel consists of one α subunit protein consisting of four domains, although there are occasionally additional β1 or β2 subunits. Each domain is made up of six repeating transmembrane α helices. 7000 Na+ ions pass through the channel in the 1msec opening time.

7.24 Local anaesthetics I

Local anaesthetics exert their effects by the blockade of sodium channels. This prevents propagation of nerve action potentials and stops neuronal transmission of nociceptive (and other) impulses.

Uses

For treatment and prevention of pain, local anaesthetics can be used in:
- subarachnoid blocks
- epidural blocks
- regional nerve blocks
- local infiltration
- topical preparations.

Classification

Most local anaesthetics consist of an aromatic ring linked by a carbonyl-containing moiety, through a carbon chain, to a substituted amino group. The two classes are defined by the nature of the carbonyl-containing linkage group (Figure 7.64).
- **Esters** include cocaine, procaine, and amethocaine.
- **Amides** include lidocaine, prilocaine, mepivacaine, and bupivacaine.

Preparations

Local anaesthetics come in various preparations and strengths (see individual drugs). They are formulated as hydrochloride salts to increase water solubility. Various additives are used.
- Preservatives and antifungals to improve shelf life (these can cause arachnoiditis and so preservative-free preparations must be used in subarachnoid blocks)
- Vasoconstrictors to reduce the rate of systemic absorption and increase the duration of anaesthesia. Vasoconstricting preparations should not be used in the region of end-arteries (e.g digital nerve blocks, penile blocks) as there is a risk of ischaemic necrosis.
- Glucose 8% is added to bupivacaine to make it hyperbaric and influence its spread in subarachnoid injections.

Some amide local anaesthetics (bupivacaine and ropivacaine) are presented as enantiopure (Section 7.11) in order to improve their toxicity profile.

Amide local anaesthetics can be sterilized as they are very heat stable. This makes them suitable for subarachnoid and epidural use. Ester local anaesthetics are unstable in solution and cannot be sterilized.

Eutectic mixture of local anaesthetic (EMLA)

Two components which, when mixed, behave with a single set of physical characteristics are said to be eutectic. Although individually crystalline, equal volumes of prilocaine and lidocaine base melt into one another to form an oil. EMLA is 2.5% of each drug in an oil–water emulsion. It provides topical anaesthesia for venepuncture 60–90 min after application under an occlusive dressing.

Because of its prilocaine content, it should be avoided in infants <12 months of age and in patients with methaemoglobinaemia.

Ametop (a cream containing amethocaine) is a good alternative and has a faster duration of action.

Pharmacodynamics

Local anaesthetics block fast voltage-gated sodium channels, which reversibly interrupts the conduction of the action potential. The resting and threshold potentials are not affected. The binding site for the drug is intracellular (Figure 7.63). *In vitro*, local anaesthetics bind preferentially to open sodium channels, so actively firing neurons are blocked first.

Speed of onset

The speed of onset of a local anaesthetic is governed by its rate of diffusion across the neuronal membrane. Like all processes of diffusion, this is governed by **Fick's law**.

Local anaesthetics are weak bases with pKa >7.4. On entering extracellular fluid (at pH 7.4), the B form takes on protons to become the BH^+ form. This charge prevents the drug from crossing the lipid membrane. The further the pKa from 7.4, the greater the extent of ionization.

Because they are less ionized at physiological pH, local anaesthetics with lower pKa (such as lidocaine) enter neurons more readily than those with higher pKa (such as bupivacaine). This increases the speed of onset.

In acidic environments, such as inflamed or infected tissue, penetration can be very slow. In addition, inflammation leads to locally increased blood flow, so the drug is removed from the site of action. For these reasons, local anaesthetics tend to work poorly in inflamed tissues.

Duration of action

The duration of action of is closely related to the degree of protein binding. This is thought to reflect the avidity of binding to the channel, and also to tissue proteins, which may act as local depot.

Potency

Potency of local anaesthetics *in vitro* correlates with lipid solubility. As well as sodium channel blockade, local anaesthetics are thought to have actions arising from non-specific membrane expansion, and distortion of the sodium channel. Note the similarity between this idea and the Meyer–Overton theory of action of anaesthetic vapours (Section 7.13).

The physical properties of some commonly used local anaesthetic agents are given in Table 7.13.

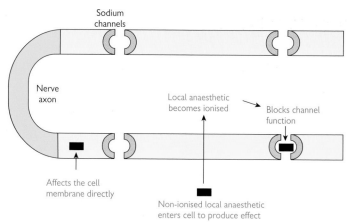

Fig. 7.63 Mechanism of action of local anaesthetics. Local anaesthetic action has two steps. Firstly, the drug enters the neuron by simple diffusion. The rate of entry is governed by Fick's law (see below). Secondly, it becomes protonated (ionized) and interacts with the sodium channel. Local anaesthetics may also affect the lipid membrane directly.

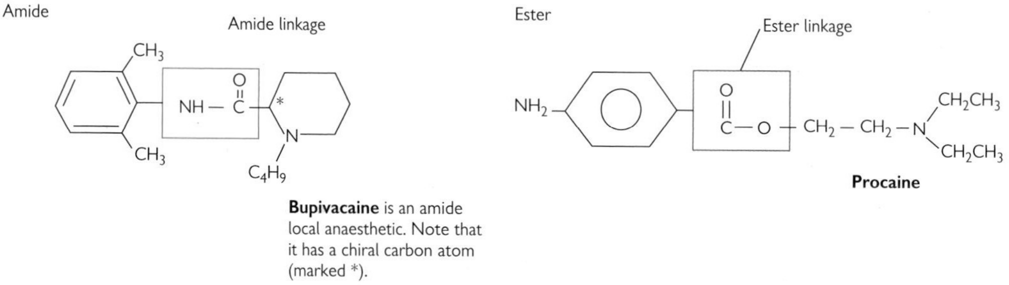

Bupivacaine is an amide local anaesthetic. Note that it has a chiral carbon atom (marked *).

Procaine

Fig. 7.64 Amide and ester structures.

➜ Weak acids, bases, and pKa

A weak acid or base is defined as one which does not completely dissociate in solution. pKa is the negative log of the dissociation constant K_a for a weak acid or base. It is related to pH by the Henderson–Hasselbalch equation:

$$pH = pKa + log\left(\frac{[\text{proton acceptor}]}{[\text{proton donor}]}\right)$$

Acids in solution exist in two forms: AH and A^-. A^- is the ionized form, and is the proton acceptor. Bases exist as BH^+ and B. B is the proton acceptor for a base, and is the non-ionized form.

As pH falls, free protons become available: A^- will tend to acquire protons and become AH (non-ionized), and B will acquire protons to become BH^+ (ionized).

If pH and the pKa are equal, the substance is 50% dissociated: there are equal numbers of molecules in the ionized and non-ionized forms.

At a pH below its pKa, an acid will become predominantly non-ionized and a base will become predominantly ionized. The reverse is true for pH above pKa.

➜ Fick's law

$$\text{Rate of diffusion} = \frac{kA(C_{out} - C_{in})}{D}$$

Fick's law determines the rate of any process of diffusion. Rate is constant for a given system at a given temperature, by an experimentally determined factor k. In the case of local anaesthetics diffusing through cell membranes, k is influenced by molecular weight, lipid solubility, and ionization (which is, in turn, dependent on pKa).

Rate is proportional to:

- The surface area A over which diffusion is taking place. Smaller neurons (C and Aδ, which transmit nociceptive impulses) are blocked faster as they have a greater ratio of surface area to volume and accumulate the drugs more rapidly.
- The concentration gradient ($C_{out} - C_{in}$) across the membrane. Concentrated solutions of local anaesthetic will have a more rapid onset than weak solutions. Increased blood flow to the area of administration (e.g. inflammation) will remove the drug, erode the concentration gradient, and reduce both the speed and duration of action. (When using Fick's law to describe gas diffusion, C is replaced by partial pressure P).

Table 7.13 Properties of local anaesthetics

Drug	Lipid solubility (relative)	Potency (relative)	pKa	Onset	Protein binding (%)	Duration	Plasma $t_{1/2}$ (min)	Toxic plasma concentration (mcg/ml)	Maximum safe dose* (mg/kg)
Lidocaine	150	2	7.9	Fast	70	Medium	120	>5	3 (7 with adrenaline)
Ropivacaine	300	8	8.1	Medium	94	Long	110	>4	3.5
Bupivacaine	1000	8	8.1	Medium	95	Long	180	>1.5	2
Prilocaine	50	2	7.9	Fast	55	Short	120	>5	5 (8 with adrenaline)
Procaine	1	2	8.9	Slow	6	Short	30		12
Amethocaine	200	8	8.5	Slow	75	Long	60		1.5

*To find the dose in a solution of any drug, multiply the volume percent value by 10—this is the number of milligrams per millilitre: 0.5% bupivacaine has 5mg/ml, 8.4% sodium bicarbonate has 84mg/ml, adrenaline 1:1000 = 0.1% (i.e. 1/1000) has 1mg/ml.

7.25 Local anaesthetics II

Pharmacokinetics

Absorption
Because they are lipid-soluble, non-ionized local anaesthetics are well absorbed by most tissues. However, oral lidocaine only has a bioavailability of 25–50% because of first-pass metabolism. Other factors affecting absorption are:

- Volume
- Concentration
- Site and type of block: IV (Bier's block) > intercostal > caudal > epidural > brachial plexus > subcutaneous infiltration.

Distribution
Local anaesthetics can cross the blood–brain barrier and the placenta. As with axonal penetration, pKa is a major determinant of the extent of membrane crossing.

There is variable binding to plasma proteins. Local anaesthetics are basic, and bind α_1 acid glycoprotein with strong affinity. However, albumin represents the bulk of protein binding as it is more abundant in plasma.

Metabolism and excretion
Esters are rapidly metabolized by tissue and plasma esterases (including plasma cholinesterase), except cocaine which is hydrolysed in the liver.

Amides are metabolized in the liver; metabolites are conjugated for excretion in the urine. As they are more stable molecules, metabolism of amides is slower.

Interactions, toxicity, and side effects

Interactions
Hepatic: clearance of local anaesthetics can be reduced by drugs which decrease hepatic blood flow, or inhibit liver enzymes.
Protein binding: verapamil can displace amides from their protein binding sites and increase their free concentrations.

Toxicity
Systemic toxicity can result from an excessive dose, or inadvertent intravascular administration. The 'toxic dose' of the drug must always be considered in the context of the type of block and expected rate of systemic absorption. CNS and cardiovascular effects predominate (Section 25.21).

Other side effects
High or total spinal blockade can complicate subarachnoid and epidural anaesthesia, or other regional techniques close to the spinal column and nerve roots.

Most local anaesthetics have vasomotor effects—generally vasodilator at low concentrations, and vasoconstrictor at high concentrations. Cocaine is an exception: it is a pure vasoconstrictor, increasing local catecholamine concentrations by inhibiting breakdown by MAO and uptake by the uptake 1 mechanism (Section 9.3).

Anaphylactic reactions to local anaesthetics are very rare. Para-aminobenzoate (PABA), a metabolite of ester local anaesthetics, can cause hypersensitivity reactions, and allergy to preservatives has been reported. Prilocaine (e.g. in EMLA cream) can induce methaemoglobinaemia, especially in neonates.

Commonly used local anaesthetics
These can be classified as short- or long-acting agents.

Short-acting agents
Lidocaine is the most commonly used short-acting local anaesthetic in acute pain management. It is primarily a local anaesthetic but is also a Class IB anti-arrhythmic. Once injected, the duration of action is dependent on the site of administration. On average, plain lidocaine 1% will last for 1 hr while the addition of adrenaline will increase this to 1.5–2 hr. Lidocaine is often used with longer-acting agents to produce a combination of rapid onset and long duration of action. Long-term use of lidocaine (e.g. continuous perineural infusions) leads to tachyphylaxis and tolerance. Other short-acting local anaesthetics include prilocaine, procaine, and mepivacaine.

Long-acting agents
The most commonly used are bupivacaine, levobupivacaine, and ropivacaine. These are structurally related amide local anaesthetics. Bupivacaine is a racemic mixture of S- and R-enantiomers; levobupivacaine is the S enantiomer alone (for an explanation of enantiomers, see Section 7.11). Ropivacaine is supplied as a pure S enantiomer. Bupivacaine has a slow onset, and blockade of large nerves may take up to an hour. It has a long duration of action. Epidural bupivacaine lasts for 3–4hr, while blockade of large nerves may last for up to 48hr. Levobupivacaine is clinically similar to bupivacaine. Ropivacaine is similar in structure but is less lipid soluble and so penetrates the myelin sheath less readily. This results in slower onset of action, reduced blockade of motor fibres, and a shorter duration of action.

Why use S-enantiomers?
These S-enantiomers have been shown to exhibit less CVS and CNS toxicity than R-enantiomers or racemic mixtures at equivalent doses with equivalent sensory blockade. Accidental IV injection of bupivacaine in moderate doses results in severe myocardial depression and refractory ventricular fibrillation. Higher doses of levobupivacaine and ropivacaine are required to cause ventricular arrhythmias. Toxicity is ranked:

bupivacaine > levobupivacaine > ropivacaine

Table 7.14 Some properties of local anaesthetics

		Lidocaine	Ropivacaine	Bupivacaine
Properties	Uses	Local anaesthesia (infiltration, nerve blocks, IV regional anaesthesia, topical (as EMLA), epidural), ventricular arrhythmias	Local anaesthesia (NOT for IV regional anaesthesia)	
	Chemical	Aminoacylamide, weak base, pKa 7.7	Amide, weak base, pKa 8.1	Amide, weak base, pKa 8.1
	Presentation	Clear colourless solution 0.5–2% (± adrenaline 1:200,000), spray 10%, aqueous solution 4%, gel, ointment. A component of EMLA cream (with prilocaine)	0.2%, 0.75%, and 2% in 10ml ampoules 2% in 200ml bags for epidural infusion	0.25% and 0.5% in 10ml ampoules (wrapped sterile ampoules available, also with adrenaline 1:200,000) 0.1% and 0.125% for epidural infusion
	Primary actions	Reversible neuronal blockade, type IB anti-arrhythmic.	Reversible neuronal blockade via fast Na^+ channels	
	Mode	Blockade of internal opening of Na^+ channels		
	Route	Infiltration, topical, epidural, intrathecal; IV for cardiac use	Field block, nerve block, epidural	Field block, nerve block, epidural, intrathecal
	Max dose	3mg/kg plain 7mg/kg with adrenaline	3.5mg/kg	2mg/kg
Effects	CNS	CNS effects seen in overdose/toxicity–classically a biphasic response: initial excitatory phenomena (agitation, perioral tingling, audiovisual disturbances, seizures) followed by CNS depression and coma		
	CVS	Prolongs phase 0, raises threshold potential; shortens action potential and refractory period (phase 3 shortened)	Less cardiotoxic than bupivacaine	Produces highly refractory myocardial depression and vasodilatation in toxic doses
Kinetics	Absorption	Depends on site of injection, dose, and presence of vasoconstrictors. OBA 35% due to FPM in liver	Depends on site of injection, dose, and presence of vasoconstrictors.	Depends on site of injection and dose only; vasoconstrictors no effect as highly protein bound in tissues
	Distribution	65% plasma protein bound (α_1 acid glycoprotein); V_D 0.7–1.5L/kg	94% plasma protein bound (α_1 acid glycoprotein), large V_D (60L/kg)	Highly lipid soluble, 95% protein bound, V_D 1L/kg
	Metabolism	70% N-dealkylated in liver, clearance 14ml/kg/min	By cytochrome P-450 system in liver	Hepatic metabolism, rather slow clearance of 9ml/kg/min
	Excretion	Metabolites excreted in urine; elimination $t_{1/2}$ 100min (longer in cardiac or hepatic impairment)	Metabolites mainly excreted in urine, clearance 12mL/kg/min, elimination $t_{1/2}$ 2hr	6% excreted unchanged in urine. Metabolites also renally excreted
	Notes			Potency 4x lidocaine; tissue protein binding accounts for the intransigence of toxic effects; may also bind to Ca^{2+} and K^+ channels.

		Cocaine	Prilocaine	Tetracaine (amethocaine)
Properties	Uses	Topical anaesthesia and vaoconstriction in nasal mucosa	Local infiltration for anaesthesia, peripheral nerve blocks, IV regional anaesthesia. EMLA: topical anaesthesia for venepuncture/split skin graft	Topical anaesthesia of cornea and skin
	Chemical	Ester; naturally occurring plant alkaloid (*Erythroxylon coca*)	Amide, weak base, pKa 7.7 (33% non-ionized at pH 7.4)	Ester
	Presentation	Solution 4–10%, paste 1–4%, Moffatt's solution (2ml 8% cocaine, 2ml 1% sodium bicarbonate, 1ml 1:1000 adrenaline)	Clear colourless solution 0.5–4%; 3% solution with felypressin 0.03IU/ml; as EMLA with lidocaine (section 7.24)	Eye drops 0.5% and 1% Gel 4%
	Primary actions	Reversible neuronal blockade; CNS stimulant effects	Reversible neuronal blockade	
	Mode	Sodium channel blocker, uptake-1 block (i.e. catecholamine re-uptake inhibitor), also inhibits MAO	Sodium channel blocker	
	Route	Topical	Local infiltration, regional blockade, IV with proximal cuff, topical (as EMLA)	Topical
	Max dose	1.5mg/kg recommended, 3mg/kg may cause toxicity	6mg/kg plain 8mg/kg with felypressin	1.5mg/kg
Effects	CNS	Euphoria, mood elevation; can cause agitation, hallucinations, cerebral ischaemia, and haemorrhage in toxic doses. Mydriatic, increases IOP	CNS effects seen in overdose/toxicity–classically a biphasic response. Initial excitation (agitation, perioral tingling, audiovisual disturbances, seizures) followed by CNS depression and coma	Few systemic effects. Causes local vasodilatation and erythema (may assist with venepuncture)
	CVS	Tacyhcardia, hypertension; marked vasoconstriction; can cause arrhythmias (incl. VF), myocardial ischaemia/infarction, and cardiac rupture in overdose	Vasoconstriction at low doses with mild increase in SVR and BP. Vasodilatation and myocardial depression at toxic levels, which can cause cardiovascular collapse	
	Respiratory	Hyperventilation (direct central stimulation); overdose may depress medulla and cause respiratory arrest	Bronchodilator; central respiratory depression may occur in toxicity.	
	Other	Hyperthermia hypertonia/hyperreflexia, nausea and vomiting	A metabolite (o-toluidine) causes methaemoglobinaemia after large doses; fetus/neonate particularly vulnerable as RBCs deficient in methaemoglobin reductase	
Kinetics	Absorption	Well absorbed from mucosal surfaces (intranasal bioavailability 50%)	3× less lipid soluble than lidocaine (although roughly equipotent).	Slow through skin; occlusive dressing required to prolong contact time >30min
	Distribution	98% plasma protein bound, V_D 2L/kg	55% protein bound, V_D 2.7L/kg	75% plasma protein bound, V_D 1L/kg
	Metabolism	Relatively resistant to plasma ChE, metabolized in liver, metabolites may be responsible for some CNS effects.	Phase 1 hydrolysis in liver, kidney, and lung; R(−) more rapidly metabolized and results in higher concentrations of o-toluidine.	By plasma ChE, metabolites include butyl-aminobenzoate
	Excretion	Metabolites excreted in urine, <1% excreted unchanged, clearance 30ml/kg/min, terminal $t_{1/2}$ 48min	Metabolites excreted in urine, clearance 35ml/kg/min, terminal $t_{1/2}$ 100min	Metabolites excreted in urine., very small proportion excreted unchanged, clearance 50ml/kg/min, terminal $t_{1/2}$ 15min
	Notes	Marked abuse potential, overdose treated by ABC approach, benzodiazepines to control agitation ± active cooling. May precipitate arrythmias if used with halothane or cyclopropane	Avoid in anaemia, pre-existing methaemoglobinaemia. IV administration of methylene blue (5mg/kg) is effective in reversing methaemoglobinaemia.	

OBA, oral bioavailability (Section 17.12); FPM, first-pass metabolism (Section 17.12); V_D = volume of distribution (Section 17.14).

Terminology

Pain is a difficult concept to define in all its variety. The International Association for the Study of Pain (IASP) Task Force for Taxonomy define it as *'an unpleasant sensory and emotional experience associated with actual or potential tissue damage, or described in terms of such damage'*. This definition emphasizes that pain is not a simple sensory modality, but a higher conscious process. Pain is subjective. It is defined by the experience of the individual, not by the causative stimulus: 'pain is what the patient says it is'.

Nociception is the process by which the painful stimulus is conveyed by the nervous system to the brain. Nociception can occur without consciousness, whereas pain cannot.

Acute pain is 'pain of recent onset and probable limited duration. It usually has an identifiable temporal and causal relationship to injury or disease'.

Chronic pain 'persists beyond the time of healing of an injury and frequently there may not be any clearly identifiable cause'.

Nociceptive pathway

Nociception is the ability to detect potentially tissue-damaging stimuli. It is an important protective mechanism, initially activating reflex withdrawal. In conscious individuals, nociception usually results in pain; this allows an integrated higher response to the stimulus.

The process involves multiple peripheral and central mechanisms. While nociception is governed by peripheral sensory factors, psychological and environmental factors influence the final experience of pain.

Nociceptors

Innocuous cutaneous sensation is mediated by specific receptors (Section 7.22). **Nociceptors** are preferentially sensitive to noxious stimuli (or those which would become noxious if prolonged). They are naked nerve endings, located in almost all tissues. They activated by different stimuli:

* **Mechanical.**
* **Thermal:** hot (above 45–50°C) or cold.
* **Chemical:** exogenous (e.g. caustic material) or endogenous (e.g. cell membrane damage or inflammation).

Nociceptors can be further classified by their sensitivity to the type of stimulus:

* **Unimodal:** mechanical, thermal; project to A-δ fibres.
* **Polymodal:** mechanical, thermal (hot/cold), chemical, project to C-fibres.

The most abundant type is the *C-fibre polymodal nociceptor*, which responds to a broad range of physical and chemical stimuli. It is activated and sensitized via ionotropic and metabotropic receptors. These respond to mediators produced by tissue damage resulting from infection, inflammation, and ischaemia. This sensitization results in more frequent nerve firing.

Afferent nerve fibres

Sensory fibres are classified into low and high threshold primary afferents:

Low threshold afferents are myelinated fibres with specialized nerve endings that convey innocuous sensation such as light touch, vibration, pressure and proprioception (Section 7.22).

High threshold afferents are medium-diameter lightly myelinated A-δ fibres and small-diameter slow–conducting unmyelinated C-fibres. Their nerve endings are nociceptors. A-δ fibres mediate 'fast' or sharp stabbing types of pain, whilst C-fibres signal 'slow' dull pain. The cell bodies of both types are found in the dorsal root ganglia.

Visceral afferents arise from the internal organs; their fibres travel with the autonomic nervous system. They are relatively spread out, so visceral pain is poorly localized. They converge with cutaneous pathways onto second-order dorsal horn neurons. This is why visceral pain is referred to the body surface in a dermatomal distribution.

Spinal cord laminae

Primary afferents mostly project onto cells in the dorsal horn of the spinal cord (Figure 7.65 inset). The dorsal horn is divided into six laminae (Rexed's laminae), responsible for processing sensory information. The primary inputs are as follows.

* **Lamina I:** large cells and small inhibitory interneurons. Input from A-δ fibres and from C-fibres (indirectly via lamina II interneurons).
* **Lamina II:** substantia gelatinosa. Inhibitory and excitatory interneurons. Input from C-fibres.
* **Laminae III–VI:** input from (mainly) innocuous afferents and low-threshold sensory fibres (A-α and A-β). Lamina V receives input from A-δ fibres onto WDR neurons (see below).

Laminae I and II are known as the *superficial dorsal horn*. They receive input from A-δ and C-fibres. They contain both *nociceptive-specific (NS)* and *wide dynamic range (WDR)* cells. WDR cells respond to both innocuous and noxious stimuli. There are numerous interconnections between laminae; the dorsal horn has an important role in the modulation of pain signals.

Ascending spinal cord pathways

A diagram of the major ascending nociceptive pathways is shown in Figure 7.65.

Spinothalamic tract

A-δ fibres enter lamina I and synapse on small interneurons. These give rise to part of the *spinothalamic tract,* carrying signals to the thalamus and then the somatosensory cortex.

C-fibres synapse with lamina II interneurons. These convey the signals to the cells of the spinothalamic tract in laminae I, IV, and V. The axons of these cells decussate across the spinal cord anterior commissure; the tract then ascends in the anterior quadrant of the contralateral white matter.

The spinothalamic tract transmits information about simple touch, pain, and temperature. It is able to separate 'fast' (localizing) and 'slow' (emotional) components of pain. Fast pain travels directly to the thalamus without synapsing. Slow pain, although travelling in parallel, reaches the thalamus through synapses in the brainstem regions. Slow pain is also transmitted by other pathways, e.g. the spinoreticular tract.

The spinothalamic tract ascends the entire length of the cord, staying in the same location until reaching the brainstem. Fast axons terminate in the ventroposterior nucleus of the thalamus and mediate mainly simple touch and pain. These axons then project to somatic sensory areas. Slow axons innervate the intralaminar nuclei of the thalamus, and the reticular activating system. These form part of the projection to the cortical cingulate gyrus associated with 'emotional' pain.

Spinoreticular tract

The nociceptive input to the spinoreticular tract arises from postsynaptic dorsal horn cells with complex receptive fields including both nociceptive and innocuous afferents. The tract projects to the reticular activating system (Section 7.2).

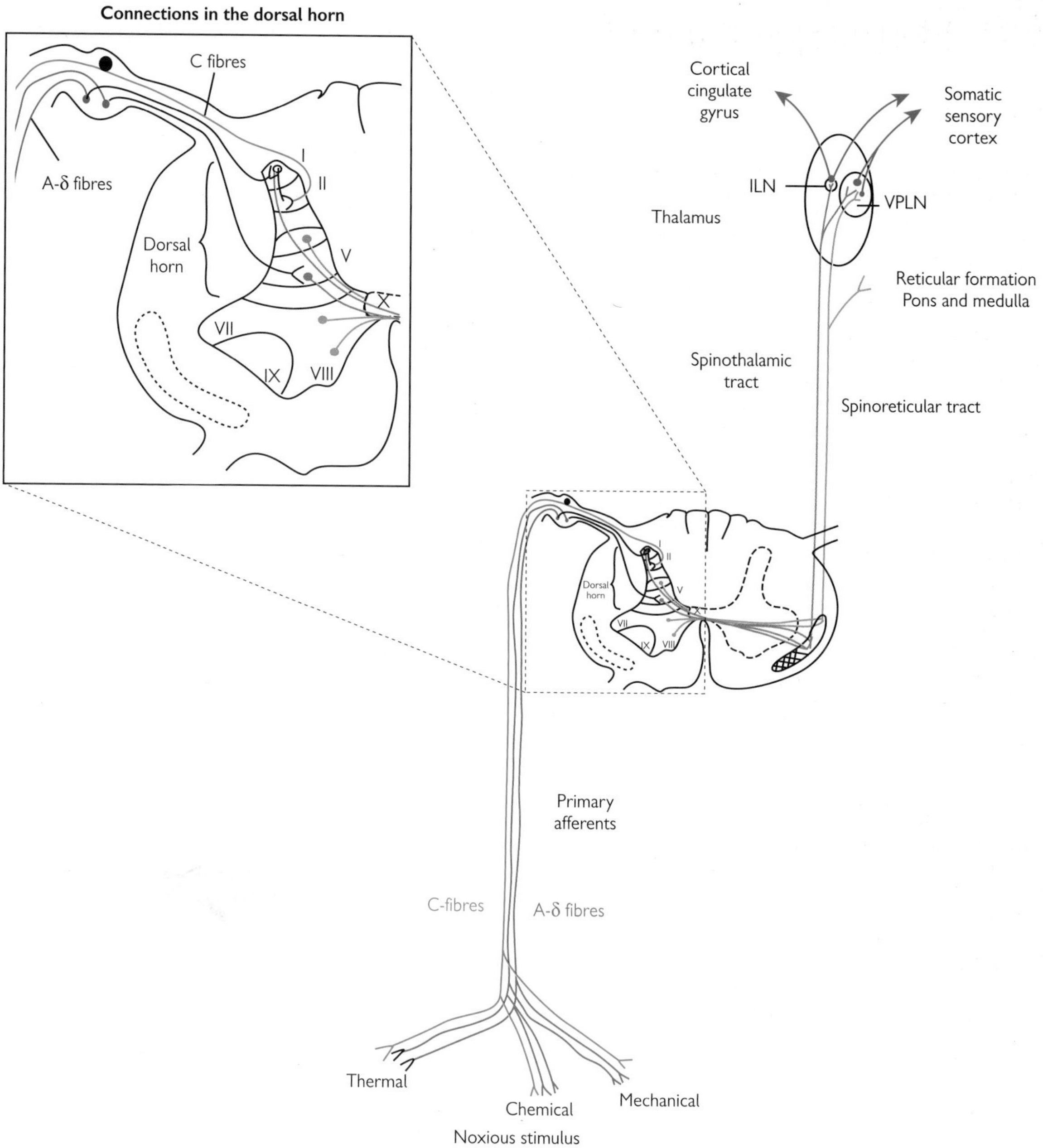

Fig. 7.65 Spinothalamic and spinoreticular tracts conveying nociceptive information within the spinal cord. The **spinothalamic tract** (purple) arises from laminae I, IV, and V. The entire tract decussates and ascends contralaterally. The numerous interneurons within the spinal cord laminae have been omitted for simplicity; but note that slow C-fibre input to lamina II projects onto lamina I, rather than contributing directly to the tract. The **spinoreticular tract** (brown) arises from laminae VII and VIII. Part of this tract does not decussate, but ascends ipsilaterally.

7.27 Physiology of pain II

Neurotransmitters

A large number of neurotransmitters mediate transmission of the sensations of pain in both brain and spinal cord.

- **Excitatory neurotransmitters:** glutamate, tachykinins (substance P, neurokinins A and B).
- **Inhibitory neurotransmitters:** GABA (more than 40% of inhibition in the CNS is GABAergic).
- **Descending pain regulation:** noradrenaline, serotonin, opioid peptides.

Glutamate is released from primary afferent neurons. This activates postsynaptic ionotropic AMPA receptors, rapidly signalling the location and intensity of noxious stimuli. A normal high-intensity stimulus results in brief localized pain, allowing the stimulus response relationship between afferent input and dorsal horn neuron output to be predictable and reproducible.

Peptides including substance P are largely responsible for transmission of slow C-fibre impulses in the dorsal horn.

GABA is widespread in the brain and spinal cord. Together with glycine, it has major inhibitory effects. Interneurons in laminae I, II, and III are GABA-rich, and mediate gate control in the dorsal horn.

Levels of pain modulation

Modulation of afferent pain impulses occurs at numerous levels, from central inhibitory pathways through to the peripheral nerve endings themselves. Figure 7.66 demonstrates the sites of action of the common analgesic modalities.

Therefore there are a large number of sites where analgesics can act: from the central actions of paracetamol and opioids, to spinal cord modulation via local anaesthetics, anticonvulsants, NMDA antagonists, and TENS, to the peripheral effects of anti-inflammatories and nerve blocks.

Descending inhibitory pathways

Descending inhibitory pathways use feedback loops involving various nuclei: the periaqueductal grey (PAG), nucleus raphe magnus (NRM), and locus coeruleus (LC), to name three.

Periaqueductal grey

PAG surrounds the cerebral aqueduct in brain. It is the most important descending pathway; stimulation of PAG results in more profound analgesia than stimulation of the NRM or the LC (see below). Stimulation of the PAG disinhibits GABAergic interneurons, resulting in encephalin-rich neurons exciting the NRM and LC neurons.

Nucleus raphe magnus

Region in medulla. Contains serotoninergic neurons which synapse in lamina II. Stimulation of the NRM results in serotonin release, which appears to activate inhibitory interneurons. Serotonin may also act presynaptically to block C-fibre terminals, preventing the release of glutamate and substance P.

Locus coeruleus

Region in pons. Contains noradrenergic neurons. Descends to exert inhibitory influence on dorsal horn neurons.

These central pathways act at the spinal cord level in two ways:

- **Presynaptic inhibition** of primary afferents. Calcium-channel opening is prevented, inhibiting neurotransmitter release. This prevents synaptic transmission of impulses.
- **Postsynaptic inhibition** of projection cells. This is mediated via the opening of potassium channels, causing hyperpolarization of the membrane.

Pain can also be modulated via the **endogenous opioid system**. Ligands such as endorphins, encephalins and dynorphins act on opioid receptors. They inhibit pain transmission by either hyperpolarizing the cell membrane or closing calcium channels and preventing neurotransmitter release.

Spinal cord

A complex interplay of excitation and inhibition occurs in the spinal cord, which influences the signals transmitted centrally.

With repeated C-fibre stimulation, WDR neurons display 'wind-up'. The post-synaptic membrane becomes progressively more depolarized and a magnesium block is removed from the NMDA receptor. This is mediated by glutamate (acting on ionotropic NMDA receptors and metabotropic glutamate receptors), and also by substance P (acting on neurokinin A receptors). The WDR cell in the dorsal horn progressively increases its output with each stimulus, causing a rapid increase in responsiveness. Such excitatory modulation has a role in the development of chronic pain.

Inhibitory modulation is mediated by non-nociceptive peripheral inputs (gate control, Figure 7.67), descending pathways, higher brain function, and local inhibitory GABAergic neurons.

Peripheral factors

Existing nociceptors can be sensitized, and dormant nociceptors activated, by factors within injured tissues:

- Injured cells release **K$^+$, prostaglandins, and leukotrienes.**
- Platelets release **serotonin.**
- Mast cells release **histamine.**
- Primary afferent nociceptors release **substance P.**

Neuropathic pain

Neuropathic pain is 'initiated or caused by a primary lesion or dysfunction in the nervous system'. Although commonly chronic, neuropathic pain can also be a component of acute pain. Examples include complex regional pain syndrome type I (acute minor trauma) and II (nerve injury), post-stroke pain, trigeminal neuralgia, and painful diabetic neuropathy.

The mechanisms of neuropathic pain differ significantly from nociceptive pain. Neuropathic pain generally occurs because of the following changes subsequent to nerve injury.

- A lowered threshold for activation of injured primary afferents causes ectopic discharges from the injured nerve or the dorsal root ganglion. This is due to changes in the expression of sodium and calcium channels.
- Locally released nerve growth factor results in sprouting of normal axons into the denervated area of skin.
- In the spinal cord the increased peripheral input results in central sensitization (primary hyperalgesia). This is further accentuated by loss of inhibitory mechanisms, reparatory processes in damaged nerves, and reactive changes in adjacent tissues.
- A–β fibres sprout from laminae III and IV into the superficial dorsal horn (laminae I/II), and normally painless sensations are perceived as painful (tactile allodynia).
- Wind-up occurs (increased activity of glutamate in the dorsal horn, increasing the response to C-fibre stimulation).
- There is downregulation of dorsal horn opioid receptors and reduced opioid sensitivity.

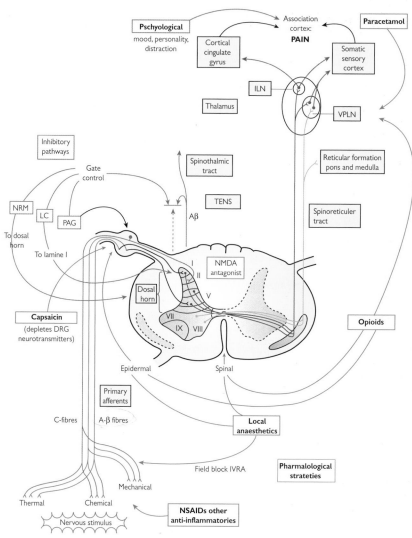

Fig. 7.66 Intervention in pain. The pain pathway is subject to multiple levels of physiological modulation. This figure pinpoints the sites of action of pharmacological interventions.

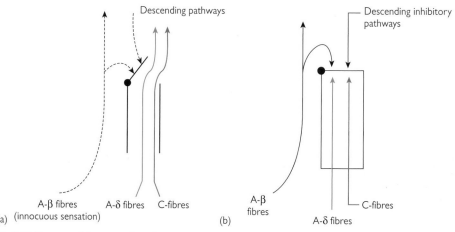

Fig. 7.67 Gate control theory was devised in 1965. It postulates that pain is a function of the balance between the information travelling into the spinal cord through large fibres and small fibres. If there is more activity through the large fibres there should be little or no pain; if there is relatively more activity through the small fibres, pain is conducted centrally. This underlines the fact that transmission of information from primary afferents to secondary neurons in the CNS is subject to modulation (gating). This occurs in the substantia gelatinosa of the spinal cord. A–β and C-fibres coming from the skin give nociceptive input. However, when the stimulus is weak, endogenous encephalinergic interneurons stimulated by A–β fibres inhibit nociceptive transmission. Rubbing a painful area stimulates inhibitory lamina II neurons via innocuous large sensory afferents from the skin, reducing nociceptive transmission and pain.

Paracetamol is a simple analgesic. It can be combined with other drugs, often within the same tablet (these preparations are described as compound analgesics).

It is important to identify which drugs are contained in compound preparations in order to prevent inadvertent overdose. Generic drug name prescribing should help to avoid such errors.

Paracetamol

Paracetamol is a para-aminophenol. It is a potent antipyretic, but has no demonstrable anti-inflammatory action. It is used in the treatment of mild to moderate pain of any cause and fever. It can be given via oral, rectal, and IV routes. Oral paracetamol reduces opioid requirements and duration of PCA morphine use in post-operative patients. Rectal paracetamol does not have the same opioid-sparing effect as it produces suboptimal plasma concentrations. IV paracetamol is as effective as ketorolac as a postoperative analgesic. It is as effective as morphine for dental surgery and is better tolerated.

There is evidence to show that the addition of a NSAID to paracetamol results in superior analgesia.

Mechanism of action

The molecular mechanism of action of paracetamol has not been clearly demonstrated. Paracetamol is an inhibitor of prostaglandin synthesis and is believed to act on COX enzymes within the CNS. Much debate continues as to which specific COX enzyme or enzymes are inhibited. More recently it has been proposed that paracetamol might inhibit COX-3 (a splice variant of COX-1 found in central nervous tissue) (Section 7.29). It has also been suggested that the weak anti-inflammatory activity is due to the reduced ability of paracetamol to inhibit COX in inflamed tissue. It may have an inhibitory action on peripheral bradykinin-sensitive receptors of the afferent nociceptive pathway.

Dose

Adults 1g 4–6 hourly (max 4g in 24hr); children orally initially 20mg/kg, then 15mg/kg (max 90mg/kg in 24 hr). A wide range of preparations are available.

Pharmacokinetics

Absorption

Well absorbed from small bowel (oral bioavailability 80%). Peak plasma levels after 60min of ingestion. 10% protein bound. Variable absorption from rectum (bioavailability is 70–90% of oral route and longer to reach peak plasma concentration)

Metabolism

Conjugated by the liver with glucuronide and sulphate or cysteine. In overdose the glucuronide pathway becomes saturated and P450 CYP2E1 produces the toxic metabolite N-acetyl-p-amino-benzoquinoneimine (NAPQI). This rapidly depletes hepatic glutathione stores.

Interactions, toxicity, and side effects

Side effects: paracetamol has a very low incidence of usage-limiting side effects. Nausea, vomiting and rashes have been described, but are rare with therapeutic doses. Occasionally, methaemoglobinaemia and haemolytic anaemia can develop.

Toxicity: The minimum toxic dose is 150mg/kg taken within 24 hours. NAPQI binds covalently to hepatocyte cell membranes leading to centrilobular necrosis. Features of toxicity can be divided as follows:

- **Early:** nausea and vomiting which may quickly settle
- **Intermediate:** development of right upper quadrant pain suggests hepatic necrosis. Liver function tests become deranged > 18 hours post ingestion (↑ prothrombin time and ↑ bilirubin after 36hr).
- **Late (3–4 days):** signs of severe liver failure (hypoglycaemia, encephalopathy, cerebral oedema, lactic acidosis)
- **Other features** include acute haemolytic anaemia, sweating and erythema.

Overdose is treated with an IV infusion of acetylcysteine or oral methionine (Section 17.13).

Cautions Consider alternative or reduce dose in acute liver disease, alcohol related liver disease and glucose-6-phosphate deficiency.

Compound analgesics

A wide range of simple and compound analgesics are available to the public for over-the-counter use in the community. Many will contain combinations of paracetamol with a weak opioid like codeine and some contain paracetamol with an NSAID such as ibuprofen or aspirin. Several analgesic preparations marketed for cold and flu-like symptoms also contain caffeine. It is useful to question patients about their choice of analgesics used for minor ailments as this may reveal intolerances and undesirable side effects to certain drugs.

Advantages of compound preparations

- Improved patient compliance (fewer tablets to swallow)
- Synergistic action of different drugs. 650mg paracetamol combined with tramadol 75mg has an NNT lower than that for paracetamol 1g alone (Table 7.15).

Disadvantages

- Restricts the titration of the individual components.
- Preparations which contain the full dose of the opioid component may augment analgesic activity but opiate side effects are not avoided.
- Co-proxamol (paracetamol 325mg + detropropoxypheme 32.5mg) was withdrawn from the market due to concerns regarding its safety profile. Mortality from co-proxamol overdose is around 10 times higher compared with other paracetamol–opioid combinations. There is little evidence that it has more analgesic effect than paracetamol alone (NNT 4.4 compared with 3.8 for paracetamol 1g).

Table 7.15 Examples of some commonly available compound analgesics:

	Simple component (mg per tablet)	Opioid component (mg per tablet)
Co-codamol	Paracetamol (500)	Codeine phosphate (8 or 30)
Co-dydramol	Paracetamol (500)	Dihydrocodeine (10, 20, or 30)
Tramacet	Paracetamol (325)	Tramadol (37.5)

Analgesic efficacy

In choosing which analgesic to prescribe, various factors should be considered. The patient's co-existing morbidities (including allergies) should be explored, along with previous experience of analgesics. It then makes sense to choose the most efficacious preparation which is compatible. The Oxford League Table of Analgesic Efficacy is a regularly updated resource which compares randomised controlled trials of analgesics, compared with placebo, and ranks them in order of NNT. Table 7.15 is an abbreviated version; for full details, follow links from www.medicine.ox.ac.uk/bandolier/index.html.

Table 7.16 The 2007 Oxford League Table of Analgesic Efficacy (adapted from www.medicine.ox.ac.uk/bandolier)

	At least 50% pain relief (%)	NNT
Etoricoxib 180/240	77	1.5
Etoricoxib 100/120	70	1.6
Valdecoxib 40	73	1.6
Ibuprofen 600/800	86	1.7
Valdecoxib 20	68	1.7
Ketorolac 20	57	1.8
Ketorolac 60 (intramuscular)	56	1.8
Diclofenac 100	69	1.8
Piroxicam 40	80	1.9
Celecoxib 400	52	2.1
Paracetamol 1000 + Codeine 60	57	2.2
Oxycodone IR 5 + Paracetamol 500	60	2.2
Oxycodone IR 15	73	2.3
Aspirin 1200	61	2.4
Dipyrone 500	73	2.4
Ibuprofen 400	55	2.5
Oxycodone IR 10 + Paracetamol 650	66	2.6
Diclofenence 25	53	2.6
Ketorolac 10	50	2.6
Paracetamol 650 + tramadol 75	43	2.6
Oxycodone IR 10 + Paracetamol 1000	67	2.7
Naproxen 400/440	51	2.7
Piroxicam 20	63	2.7
Naproxen 500/550	52	2.7
Diclofenac 50	57	2.7
Ibuprofen 200	48	2.7
Paracetamol 650 + tramadol 112	60	2.8
Pethidine 100 (intramuscular)	54	2.9
Tramadol 150	48	2.9
Morphine 10 (intramuscular)	50	2.9
Naproxen 200/200	45	3.4
Ketorolac 30 (intramuscular)	53	3.4
Paracetamol 500	61	3.5
Celecoxib 200	40	3.5
Paracetamol 1500	65	3.7
Ibuprofen 100	36	3.7
Oxycodone IR 5 + Paracetamol 1000	55	3.8
Paracetamol 1000	46	3.8
Paracetamol 600/650 + Codeine 60	42	4.2
Aspirin 600/650	38	4.4
Paracetamol 600/650	38	4.6
Ibuprofen 50	32	4.7
Tramadol 100	30	4.8
Tramadol 75	32	5.3
Aspirin 650 + Codeine 60	25	5.3
Oxycodone IR 5 + Paracetamol 325	24	5.5
Ketorolac 10 (intramuscular)	48	5.7
Paracetamol 300 + Codeine 30	26	5.7
Tramadol 50	19	8.3
Codeine 60	15	16.7

Numbers needed to treat are calculated for the proportion of patients with at least 50% pain relief over 4–6 hours compared with placebo in randomized, double-blind, single-dose studies in patients with moderate to severe pain. Drugs were oral, unless specified, and doses are milligrams.

Non-steroidal anti-inflammatory drugs (NSAIDs) are used in mild to moderate inflammatory pain. Postoperatively, they reduce opioid requirements (particularly useful in day surgery).

They are also used for their anti-inflammatory, anti-pyretic, and anti-platelet effects.

Aspirin, although useful in other areas, is not often used for postoperative pain because of its irreversible anti-platelet activity and associated risk of bleeding.

Classification

- Non-specific COX inhibitors:
  - Irreversible (aspirin)
  - Reversible (others).
- Preferential COX-2 inhibitors (oxicams).
- Specific COX-2 inhibitors (coxibs).

Presentations

Oral, rectal, and IV routes are most commonly used. The IM route has declined in popularity because of pain and tissue necrosis with some drugs. Compound preparations also exist.

Mechanism of action

NSAIDs inhibit the enzyme cyclo-oxygenase (COX), which produces prostanoids: prostaglandins ($PGE_{2\alpha}$, PGF_2, and PGD_2), prostacyclin (PGI_2), and thromboxane A_2. The pathways and actions are shown in Figure 7.68. Note that NSAIDs act on COX, preserving and enhancing leukotriene production, whereas steroids act further up the pathway. This accounts for the bronchospastic properties of NSAIDs, in contrast to the bronchodilator effects of steroids.

COX isoforms

There are three forms of the COX enzyme. Traditional NSAIDs exert their actions through COX-1 and COX-2. There is considerable overlap, but broadly speaking:

- COX-1 is the constitutive form, expressed in most tissues. It is involved in maintenance of renal blood flow, haemostasis, and GI mucosal integrity.
- COX-2 is the inducible form, barely detectable unless inflammation triggers its expression. Its products are involved in pain and inflammation.
- COX-3 was described in 2002, and is a splice variant of COX-1. It is present in the CNS and may account for some of the actions of paracetamol.

The interaction with COX is stereospecific: S-enantiomers are biologically active in most cases.

Cox-independent actions of NSAIDs

Analgesic
- Anti-nociceptive at the thalamic level
- Increase levels of plasma β-endorphin

Anti-inflammatory
- Direct inhibition of neutrophil activity
- Reduce heterotopic ossification

Effects of NSAIDs

Neurological Attenuates PG-induced nerve sensitization; analgesic; central anti-pyretic effect.

CVS Can induce heart failure via fluid retention in susceptible individuals.

Renal Reduced renal blood flow can precipitate renal failure (especially in elderly/dehydrated patients or in combination with other nephrotoxic drugs); fluid retention. Aspirin inhibits urate secretion at <2g/day, but is uricosuric at higher doses(>5g/day). Analgesic nephrop-

athy (papillary necrosis and interstitial fibrosis) may occur with prolonged use.

Haematological Anti-platelet effects can increase surgical blood loss to a variable degree (this is not usually significant with NSAIDs other than aspirin). Direct anti-neutrophilic action. Can cause leucopenia and thrombocytopenia with prolonged use. GI bleeding may cause anaemia.

Respiratory Leukotriene production may be increased, causing bronchospasm in sensitive individuals. Around 20% of asthmatics are affected.

GI tract 50% of patients will have dyspepsia, gastritis, or diarrhoea. NSAIDs can cause gastro-duodenal ulceration, perforation, and bleeding (potentiated by antiplatelet effects). The risk is lower with COX-2 inhibitors. Prolonged or high-dose regimens may be hepatotoxic.

Musculoskeletal being weak acids, NSAIDs can accumulate in inflamed joints (ion trapping).

Pharmacokinetics

Absorption NSAIDs are well absorbed orally. Being acidic, they are non-ionized in the stomach, favouring absorption. In practice, however, most absorption occurs in the small intestine because of its much higher surface area.

Distribution NSAIDs are highly plasma protein-bound: 85% (aspirin)–99% (most others). This results in small volumes of distribution, close to plasma volume.

Elimination Most metabolism is hepatic, with excretion via urine and bile. Elimination half-lives are around 2–6hr.

Toxicity, cautions, and interactions

Side effects increase with long-term use and in the elderly. All NSAIDs should be prescribed for the shortest possible duration. NSAIDs can cause allergic reactions. They are irritant when injected (IM or IV).

Cautions Hypersensitivity to aspirin; pregnancy and breastfeeding; coagulopathy; renal, cardiac, or hepatic impairment; heart failure, LV dysfunction, hypertension.

Contraindications Mild to moderate renal impairment; active peptic ulceration (including COX-2 inhibitors); previous history of peptic ulceration (non-selective COX inhibitors); severe heart failure; hypovolaemia/dehydration. Aspirin is contraindicated in children younger than 12 years (risk of Reye's syndrome).

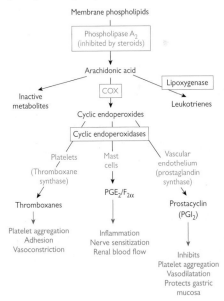

Fig. 7.68 Prostaglandin synthesis.

Because of emerging concerns about cardiovascular safety, selective COX-2 inhibitors should only be used when specifically indicated (increased risk of GI bleeding or perforation). They should be avoided in ischaemic heart disease or cerebrovascular disease.

Interactions NSAIDs are highly protein-bound (mostly to albumin), and can potentiate the effects of other protein-bound drugs (e.g. lithium).

Warfarin is not only displaced from albumin, but many NSAIDs are metabolized by the same enzyme (CYP 2C9). NSAIDs antagonize the effects of antihypertensives, probably by disrupting renal prostaglandin synthesis.

Multiple NSAIDs (e.g. low-dose aspirin plus NSAID) should not be used unless absolutely necessary.

Table 7.17 Common NSAIDs in clinical practice

		Aspirin	Acemetacin	Diclofenac
Properties	Uses	Pain, IHD, cerebrovascular disease, inflammatory/febrile conditions, bone tumours	Inflammatory musculoskeletal disorders, postoperative pain.	
	Chemical	Salicylate	Acetic acid derivative	Phenylacetic acid derivative
	Presentation	Tablets 75–600mg, compound preparations	60mg capsules	Tablets, suppositories, solution for injection (25mg/ml).
	Primary actions	Antiplatelet, analgesic, anti-pyretic, anti-inflammatory.	Analgesic; anti-inflammatory; anti-pyretic	
	Mode	Irreversible non-selective COX inhibition (COX 1 > COX 2)	Weak COX inhibitor; partly a pro-drug for indometacin	Non-selective COX inhibition
	Route and dose	Oral, 75mg o.d. (antiplatelet effect), 300–900mg 4 hourly (max 4g/day) for analgesia	Oral; 60mg bd–tds	Oral/PR/IV; 150mg/day (divided)
Effects	CVS	Antiplatelet activity, ↑blood loss postoperatively, oedema, exacerbation of heart failure	Oedema, exacerbation of heart failure; NSAIDs other than aspirin have variable antiplatelet activity, occasionally of clinical significance	
	RS	Bronchospasm in sensitive patients, ↑O_2 consumption/CO_2 production; hyperventilation + pulmonary oedema in overdose	Bronchospasm in sensitive patients	
	CNS	Analgesic and antipyretic	Analgesia, antipyretic effect; peripheral reduction in nerve desensitization	
	GI	↑risk of GI ulceration and haemorrhage (potentiated by bleeding tendency)	GI upset, ulceration, haemorrhage	
	GU	Proteinuria, haematuria, renal impairment; urate reabsorption at low doses but ↑ excretion at high doses	↑urea; caution in patients with reduced RBF where perfusion may be maintained by PGs (e.g. sepsis, hypotension, atheromatous vascular disease); can cause interstitial nephritis and renal failure	
Kinetics	Absorption	Complete absorption from upper GI tract; some FPM so bioavailability is 70%	Bioavailability 66%; peak plasma concentration 3.5 h after oral dose	Completely absorbed, but bioavailability 50% due to FPM
	Distribution	Hydrolysed rapidly to salicylate; this is 80–90% protein-bound; V_D 0.15L/kg.	Acemetacin 85% protein-bound; indometacin 90%	>99% protein bound; V_D 0.15L/kg
	Metabolism	Hepatic (70%)—zero-order kinetics; other hepatic pathways (15%) and urinary excretion of salicylate (15%) display first-order kinetics.	Hepatic and renal mechanisms	Hepatic, to inactive metabolites; plasma $t_{1/2}$ 2 hr
	Excretion	Renal	Mainly renal	Mainly renal

		Ibuprofen	Ketorolac	Parecoxib
Properties	Uses	Inflammatory musculoskeletal disorders; post-operative pain.	Short-term management of postoperative pain only	
	Chemical	Proprionic acid derivative	Acetic acid derivative	Pyrazole
	Presentation	Tablets 200–600mg, paediatric elixir	Tablets 10mg, injection 10mg/ml	Powder for reconstitution 40mg
	Action	Analgesic, anti-inflammatory, anti-pyretic.		
	Mode	Non-selective COX inhibition		Prodrug for valdecoxib (COX-2 inhibitor)
	Route and dose	PO 20mg/kg/day in divided doses	PO 10mg qds, IM/IV 10–30mg qds (max 90mg/day)	IM/IV 40mg bd
Effects	CVS	Oedema, exacerbation of heart failure; NSAIDs other than aspirin have variable antiplatelet activity, but this is rarely of clinical significance		
	RS	Bronchospasm in sensitive patients		
	CNS	Analgesia, antipyretic effect; peripheral reduction in nerve sensitization.		
	GI	GI upset, ulceration, haemorrhage		
	GU	↑urea; occasionally renal impairment, nephritic syndrome, papillary necrosis can occur; caution in patients with reduced RBF where perfusion may be maintained by PGs (e.g. sepsis, hypotension, atheromatous vascular disease); can cause interstitial nephritis and renal failure.		
	Other	Best side-effect profile.		Avoid in ischaemic heart disease
Kinetics	Absorption	OBA 80%	OBA 85%	
	Distribution	>99% protein bound; V_D 0.15L/kg	>99% protein bound, V_D 0.15 /kg	Apparent V_D of valdecoxib 1.2L/kg as it accumulates in RBCs
	Metabolism	Hepatic, plasma $t_{1/2}$ 2hr	Hepatic phase I and II	Rapid hepatic hydrolysis (CYP 2C9) to valdecoxib; then to various metabolites (one is active).
	Excretion	Mainly renal	Renal; elimination $t_{1/2}$ 5hr	Renal; elimination $t_{1/2}$ 8hr
	Note	S-isomers active		May inhibit other CYP isoforms

OBA, oral bioavailability (Section 17.12); FPM, first-pass metabolism (Section 17.12); V_D = volume of distribution (Section 7.14).

The term 'opioid' describes a substance which interacts with opioid receptors to produce analgesia. 'Opiate' specifically refers to a naturally occuring drug derived from the opium poppy (*Papaver somniferum*).

Uses

Opioids are the mainstay of treatment of severe postoperative pain. The key principle is to titrate the dose to achieve the desired effect, while minimizing unwanted effects.

Other uses include: co-induction agents for general anaesthesia, sedation and endotracheal tube tolerance on ICU, antitussive effects (especially codeine).

Classification

Various classifications are used: structural, pharmacodynamic, or duration of action.

Structural

Opioids can be classified according to chemical structure. Many naturally occurring varieties (including morphine) are phenanthrene derivatives; other synthetic classes are phenylpiperidines, anilinopiperidines, diphenylheptanes, benzomorphanes, and thebaine derivatives. Most opioids are levorotatory isomers, reflecting the configuration of the receptors. Some of the structures of the commonly used opioids are shown in Figure 7.69.

Pharmacodynamic

Opioids can also be classified by their activity at opioid receptors:

- Pure agonist (morphine, fentanyl, pethidine, codeine).
- Partial agonist (nalbuphine, buprenorphine, pentazocine).
- Pure antagonist (naloxone, naltrexone).

Duration of action

- Long-acting: methadone.
- Medium-acting: morphine, diamorphine.
- Short-acting: fentanyl, alfentanil.
- Ultra-short-acting: remifentanil.

Presentations

Virtually all routes can be used for opioid administration, depending on the drug.

Mechanism of action

Initially four receptors were described: mu, delta, kappa, and sigma. Sigma receptors are no longer considered to be opioid receptors (effects are not reversed by naloxone; and the receptor has a high affinity for phencyclidine).

Currently the receptors are classified as OP1 (delta), OP2 (kappa), and OP3 (mu); there are a number of subtypes of each receptor.

Opioid receptors are all G-protein coupled receptors (see Section 9.4). OP1 and OP3 receptors open potassium ion channels. This results in hyperpolarization and a shortened action potential plateau; in turn this reduces calcium-channel influx and neurotransmitter release. OP2 receptors close calcium channels and prevent neurotransmitter release.

Supraspinally, the receptors are found in large numbers in the periaqueductal grey matter. Here they are thought to activate descending inhibitory pain pathways.

In the spinal cord, receptors are found in abundance in the substantia gelatinosa. There are two main locations.

- **Presynaptic terminals of primary afferent sensory neurons.** Presynaptic receptors are responsible for the inhibition of neurotransmitter release.

- **Dendrites of postsynaptic interneurons.** These neurons are responsible for modulation of spinothalamic transmission. The postsynaptic receptors reduce evoked excitatory synaptic potentials.

Peripheral opioid receptors also exist, especially in the GI tract.

Effects of opioids

Opioids produce effects on many systems.

CNS Analgesia (especially for visceral pain). Euphoria, anxiolysis, sedation (OP3 receptors). Dysphoria in high doses (OP2). Nausea (dose-dependent; dopaminergic and 5-HT3 receptors in the chemoreceptor trigger zone (Section 17.10)). Miosis (OP2 and OP3 receptors in the Edinger–Westphal nucleus; responsive to atropine).

CVS Most opioids are relatively cardiostable. Reduction in sympathetic drive causes bradycardia. Histamine release causes vasodilation, contributing to hypotension.

Renal Spasm of the uretero-vesical sphincter and bladder detrusitor muscle; may result in urinary retention.

Respiratory Dose-dependent respiratory depression from stimulation of OP3 (particularly $OP3_2$) receptors. Sensitivity of the respiratory centre to carbon dioxide is reduced; hypoxic drive is less affected. Respiratory rate is reduced more than tidal volume.

Opioids are anti-tussive. Histamine release can cause bronchospasm. At high doses, opioid receptor interaction with CNS. GABAergic interneurons of dopaminergic pathways can cause muscle rigidity, particularly in the chest wall.

GI tract Delayed gastric emptying, decreased peristalsis, and constipation (caused by constriction of sphincters within the GIT). Transient increases in amylase and lipase may occur due to increased tone of the sphincter of Oddi causing reflux of bile into the pancreatic duct.

Endocrine Release of ACTH, prolactin, and gonadotrophic hormones is inhibited (particularly by morphine); increased secretion of ADH results in impaired water excretion and may lead to hyponatraemia.

Other Pruritus is common. Dependence can occur, and is due to suppression of endogenous opioid production.

Table 7.18 Comparative effects of opioid receptors

OP1 (delta)	OP2 (kappa)	OP3 (mu)
Analgesia		
Respiratory depression	Mild respiratory depression	Respiratory depression
Miosis		
Euphoria	Dysphoria	Euphoria
Sedation	Mild Sedation	Sedation
Physical dependence		
↑GI motility	–	↑GI motility
Smooth muscle contraction	–	Smooth muscle contraction
–	Diuresis	–

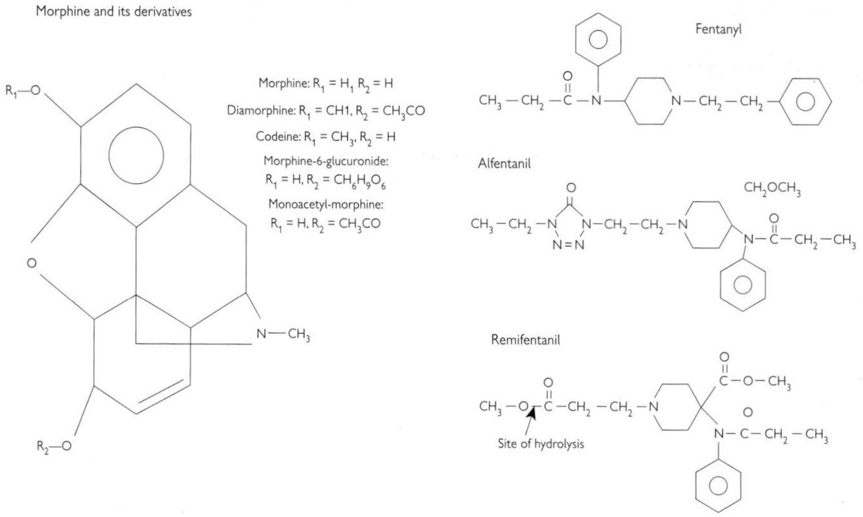

Morphine and its derivatives

Morphine: $R_1 = H$, $R_2 = H$
Diamorphine: $R_1 = CH1$, $R_2 = CH_3CO$
Codeine: $R_1 = CH_3$, $R_2 = H$
Morphine-6-glucuronide:
$R_1 = H$, $R_2 = CH_6H_9O_6$
Monoacetyl-morphine:
$R_1 = H$, $R_2 = CH_3CO$

Fentanyl

Alfentanil

Remifentanil

Site of hydrolysis

Fig. 7.69 Morphine, codeine, diamorphine and their metabolites share a ring structure. Fentanyl, alfentanil and remifentanil possess many structural smilarities. Note the ester link in remifentanil which makes if vulnerable to hydrolysis.

➜ Dose-response relationships

Most drugs exert their effects by occupying receptors in a reversible fashion, with the magnitude of effect being proportional to the fraction of receptors occupied. There are, of course, exceptions to this "rule," such as osmotic diuretics, (no specific receptor), and aspirin (acetylates and permanently inactivates cyclo-oxygenase).

An *agonist* is a drug which combines with a receptor to cause a biological effect: morphine combines with opioid receptors to activate second messenger pathways via G proteins. Association with, and dissociation from, the receptor are subject to random probability. Increasing the concentration of agonist increases the probability that an agonist molecule will find its receptor. A plot of concentration vs. receptor occupancy (Figure 7.70, inset) gives a hyperbola. However, analysis of dose-response relationships is easier if a plot of log concentration vs. receptor occupancy is used (Figure 7.70, main diagram).

At equilibrium, association and dissociation occur at the same rate. The equilibrium dissociation constant, K_D, is the concentration of drug where 50% receptor occupancy occurs. K_D should not be confused with ED_{50}, which is the dose which gives 50% of the maximal response (often this dose corresponds to a plasma concentration of K_D). While the K_D describes the strength of binding between the drug and the receptor (avidity), it says nothing about the magnitude of the response (intrinsic activity, IA). IA takes a value between -1 and +1. A *full agonist* has an IA of 1 (Figure 7.70, line A).

A *partial agonist* is a drug which binds to receptors to give the same type of response as the full agonist, but the response is smaller. The IA is greater than 0 but smaller than 1 (Figure 7.70, line B). Buprenorphine is a partial agonist at opioid receptors. If the partial agonist prevents a full agonist from gaining access to the receptor, it is in effect acting as a partial antagonist at that receptor (Figure 7.70, line A+B).

An antagonist is a drug which combines with a receptor *and has no effect other than to prevent the action of the agonist.* In other words, giving the agonist alone drug should have no effect.

- *Reversible competitive antagonists* (such as naloxone) compete with agonists for access to the receptor. Each can be displaced by sufficient concentrations of the other. Sufficient concentrations of an agonist can completely overcome a reversible competitive antagonist, (Figure 7.70, A + competitive antagonist).
- *Reversible non-competitive antagonists* block the action of an agonist at some point other than its receptor binding site, and therefore are not displaced by increasing concentrations of agonist. In the presence of a non-competitive antagonist, the maximal effect attainable by agonist is reduced (Figure 7.70, A + non-competitive antagonist).

An *inverse agonist* is a drug which combines with a receptor to produce the opposite effect from that of the agonist. Its IA is between -1 and 0. There are few true inverse agonists, but examples include rimonabant, an inverse agonist at CB1 (cannabinoid) receptors (it was used as an anti-obesity drug but has been withdrawn).

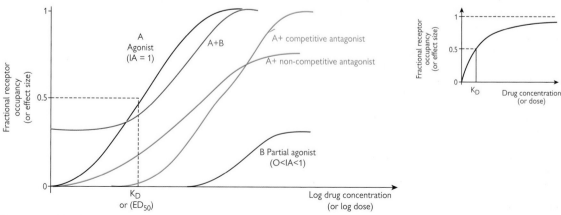

Note: it is assumed that effect size is proportional to receptor occupancy

Fig. 7.70

Pharmacokinetics

The pharmacokinetic behaviour of the opioids is determined by three main factors.

- **Lipid solubility:** this determines the rate of passage into the CNS, and hence the speed of onset.
- **Protein binding:** the extent of protein binding will determine the distribution within body compartments.
- **Ionization:** the degree of ionization depends on the pKa of the drug and the ambient pH. The ionization of the drug contributes to both lipid solubility and protein binding.

Absorption Generally, opioids are well absorbed from the GIT. The majority are weak bases: in the alkaline small intestine they are largely non-ionized and readily absorbed. Despite this, opioids have a relatively low bioavailability because of first-pass metabolism in the intestinal wall and liver (the exception is tramadol, which has an oral bioavailability of 70–100%).

Distribution Distribution within tissues and uptake into the CNS largely depends on lipid solubility. Morphine is distributed gradually, whereas fentanyl (which is 600 times more lipid-soluble) is rapidly absorbed by tissues. The volume of distribution is reduced in the elderly and peak plasma concentrations are higher, giving an increased sensitivity to opioids and their side-effects.

Metabolism Most opioids are largely metabolized in the liver where they are conjugated to active or inactive metabolites. A notable exception is remifentanil, which is hydrolysed by non-specific plasma esterases to an inactive carboxylated metabolite. Metabolites tend to be excreted in the urine, and accumulation occurs in renal failure; active metabolites (e.g. morphine-6-glucuronide, norpethidine) may then cause marked clinical effects.

Intrathecal and epidural opioids

Administration of intrathecal and epidural opioids is widespread. Drugs are administered at lower doses. The opioids once administered via these routes bind to opioid receptors in Rexed's laminae I and II of the spinal cord, influencing pain pathways. Systemic absorption of the drug and spread through the CSF may also contribute to the analgesic effect. The effect of the drug is largely governed by its lipid solubility and molecular size: drugs with high lipid solubility and small molecular size will have a rapid onset of action, but drugs with lower lipid solubility will last much longer. Opioids administered by this route are often co-administered with local anaesthetic drugs, as the two are synergistic.

Intrathecal opioids

There is a risk of delayed respiratory depression with opioids used in this way. Intrathecal opioids may migrate in a cephalad direction into the CSF. Here they may directly depress the respiratory centre, even in the small doses used in spinal analgesia. For this reason, lipid-soluble opioids (fentanyl, diamorphine), which diffuse rapidly into the spinal cord and 'fix' there, are preferred.

Epidural opioids

Because of the termination of the epidural space at the foramen magnum, epidural opioids do not migrate into the CSF around the brainstem. However, during prolonged infusions, systemic absorption of epidural opiates may become sufficient to cause respiratory concentration. Fentanyl is excreted in gastric juice and subsequently reabsorbed by the alkaline small intestine; this enterosystemic cycling may contribute to delayed respiratory depression.

When combining local anaesthetic and opioid in epidural infusions, typical combinations and concentrations include:

- Bupivacaine 0.1–0.2% with fentanyl 2–4mcg/ml
- Bupivacaine 0.1–0.2% with diamorphine 50–100mcg/ml

Toxicity, cautions, and interactions

Side effects In addition to the effects already described, pruritus is common. There is considerable inter-patient variation in the severity of side effects. As well as directly mediated histamine release, opioids can cause true allergic reactions.

Cautions Acute asthma; reduced respiratory reserve; hypovolaemia or hypotension; prostatic hypertrophy. Opioids depress neonatal respiration if given pre-delivery. In head injuries, opioids will affect pupil reflexes and may reduce the GCS. Opioids will exacerbate a paralytic ileus.

Contraindications Acute respiratory depression; acute alcohol intoxication (risk of aspiration or respiratory arrest); IV administration in phaeochromocytoma (histamine-releasing opioids, e.g. morphine, may cause a hypertensive crisis (Section 18.4)).

Interactions Alfentanil and midazolam are metabolized by the same P450 enzyme (CYP3A3/4), so when they are used together, both half-lives are prolonged.

Opioid receptor antagonists

The main clinical use of these drugs is to reverse or limit the effects of opioids:

- Pure antagonists—antagonists at all opioid receptor subtypes.
- Partial agonists—antagonize the effects of pure agonists at receptors without being antagonist themselves.

Partial opioid agonists have been used to try and maintain analgesia whilst reversing the unwanted side effects of other opioids. In practice, however, this is very difficult to do. Some partial opioid agonists are associated with very high incidences of side effects.

Table 7.19 Pharmacodynamics of opioid antagonists and partial agonists

Drug	Type	Agonist at:	Antagonist at:
Naloxone	Ant	–	OP1, 2, 3
Naltrexone	Ant	–	OP1, 2, 3
Pentazocine	Ag/Ant	OP2, sigma	OP3
Nalorphine	Ag/Ant	Partial OP2, sigma	OP3
Buprenorphine	Partial Ag	OP3	–
Ag, agonist; Ant, antagonist			

Table 7.20 Common opioids in clinical practice

		Morphine	Codeine	Diamorphine
Properties	Uses	Moderate/severe pain, palliation, ITU sedation	Mild/moderate pain, cough, diarrhoea	Severe pain, acute MI, pulmonary oedema
	Chemical	Phenanthrene, weak base, pKa 7.9 (76% ionized at pH 7.4)	Phenanthrene (3-methyl morphine), weak base, pKa 8.2	3,6-diacetyl morphine, synthetic
	Presentation	IV clear aqueous solution, tablets, syrup, and suppositories of various strengths	Tablets (15, 50, 60mg), syrup (5mg/ml), clear solution for injection 60mg/ml Compound presentations exist (e.g. co-codamol)	White lyophilized powder for reconstitution (5, 10, 30, 100, 500mg); tablets (10mg)
	Action	See section 7.30	Analgesia, antitussive, reduced GI motility.	Potent analgesia
	Mode	OP3 receptor agonist	Prodrug (10% metabolized to morphine); antitussive effect may be via a separate receptor	Prodrug for morphine; no activity at opioid receptors.
	Route	IV: rescue analgesia 0.05–0.1mg/kg every 5min titrated to pain; continue with IM or SC 0.1–0.2mg/kg 3–4 hourly. IV PCA dose usually 1mg per bolus with a lock-out of 5 min. PO 2-3x parenteral dose.	PO or IM: 30–60 mg qds (children 3mg/kg/day in divided doses)	IV 1–2.5mg; IM/SC 5–10mg; epidural 2.5–5mg; intrathecal 250–500mcg
Effects	For the general effects of opioids, see section 7.28	Effective analgesic but can produce dysphoria at high doses	Pronounced antitussive and constipating effects; fairly low abuse potential	Analgesia, euphoria, and respiratory depression predominate
Kinetics	Absorption	Absorbed in small bowel; FPM so OBA 30%. Peak effect 10–20 min after IV dose	Oral/rectal bioavailability 65%; peak concentration 1hr after oral dose	Well absorbed (lipid solubility 200x morphine) but extensive FPM; OBA 20%
	Distribution	V_D 3.5L/kg (less in the elderly → higher peak concentrations); 35% protein-bound	V_D 5.4L/kg (less after IM route); only 7% protein-bound	Rapidly penetrates tissues; V_D 1L/kg. 40% protein-bound
	Metabolism	Hepatic and renal. 70% to morphine-3-glucuronide; 30% to morphine-6-glucuronide (13x more potent than morphine)	15% to codeine-6-glucuronide; 15% N-demethylated to norcodeine. 10% to morphine by CYP 2D6 (genetic polymorphism can significantly alter the analgesic efficacy)	Plasma $t_{1/2}$ 5min. Rapid ester hydrolysis in plasma, liver, and neural tissue to morphine and 6-monoacetyl morphine (6MAM); both are opioid receptor agonists
	Excretion	Metabolites excreted in urine (NB: accumulation in renal failure); clearance 15mg/kg/min; elimination half-life 3hr	Renal, as free codeine and metabolites; clearance 15ml/kg/min; elimination half-life 3hr	Metabolism as above; then as for morphine
	Notes	The standard agent with which others are compared Not recommended via epidural or subarachnoid routes because of delayed respiratory depression	Dihydrocodeine is similar	Marked abuse potential.

		Fentanyl	Alfentanil	Remifentanil
Properties	Uses	Painful minor surgery (low dose); opioid-based anaesthesia (high dose)	Co-anaesthesia, analgesia, sedation in ICU	Co-anaesthesia, analgesia, sedation, hypotensive anaesthesia
	Chemical	Synthetic phenylpiperidine; weak base, pKa 8.4.	Synthetic anilinopiperidine; weak base, pKa 6.5	Synthetic anilinopiperidine; weak base pKa 7.1.
	Presentation	IV clear colourless solution, 25mcg/ml; also transdermal patches, buccal lozenges/lollipops.	Clear solution for injection, .5 or 5mg/ml	Crystalline white powder: 1, 2, and 5mg vials; includes glycine so not suitable for epidural or spinal use
	Primary actions	Analgesia, sedation	Analgesia, respiratory depression	Potent analgesia, suppression of laryngeal reflexes, hypotension, bradycardia
	Mode	Pure OP3 agonist; potency 100x morphine	Pure OP3 agonist; potency 10–20x morphine	Pure OP3 agonist
	Route	IV: 'low dose' 1–2mcg/kg; 'high dose' 50–100mcg/kg Epidural: 25–100mcg. Intrathecal: 10–25mcg.	IV bolus 10–50/kg; infusion 0.5–1mcg/kg/min.	IV infusion: loading dose 0.5–1mcg/kg over 30sec, then titrate to effect (e.g. 0.05–1mcg/kg/min; less if spontaneous respiration required)
Effects	CNS	Muscle rigidity at high doses	Muscle rigidity; analgesia, some sedation	Potent analgesia but minimal sedation; muscle rigidity common.
	CVS	Bradycardia (vagally mediated). ↓response to laryngoscopy		↓ MAP and heart rate
	Respiratory	Marked respiratory depression; minimal histamine release–bronchospasm uncommon		
Kinetics	Absorption	Extensive FPM, OBA 33%; lipid solubility 600x morphine, rapid onset of action after IV bolus	Peak effect within 90sec of IV bolus; duration 5–10min	–
	Distribution	Rapid; V_D 4L/kg; protein binding 80%; offset of action due to distribution (distribution $t_{1/2}$ 13min)	90% protein bound in plasma; V_D 0.8L/kg	70% bound to plasma proteins; low V_D 0.3L/kg; lipid solubility 20x morphine, but metabolized too rapidly to allow tissue loading
	Metabolism	Hepatic: N-demethylation to norfentanyl, and hydroxylation; metabolites are inactive.	Hepatic: N-demethylation (noralfentanil, inactive) plus other phase I and II pathways	Plasma $t_{1/2}$ 3–10min; rapid hydrolysis to inactive metabolites by non-specific tissue and plasma esterases; offset of action due to metabolism, not distribution
	Excretion	Metabolites excreted in urine; elimination half-life 3hr after single IV bolus	Metabolites excreted in urine; elimination half-life 100min	Metabolites excreted in urine
	Notes	Half-life is highly context sensitive (Section 7.15).	Half-life is context-sensitive	Unaffected by renal/hepatic failure or cholinesterase deficiency; half-life is not context-sensitive

Acute pain in the surgical patient may be due to pre-existing disease; the surgical procedure (with associated IV access, drains, etc.) or a combination of these. Many patients experience avoidable pain in hospital.

Patients at increased risk of inadequate analgesia include:

- Extremes of age (young children and the elderly).
- Critically ill patients.
- Those with communication difficulties—cultural and language barriers, hearing/sight/speech difficulties, cognitive impairment.
- Patients with a history of substance misuse.
- Chronic pain patients already on opioids.

In some patients, untreated acute pain progresses to chronic pain. This is ultimately more complicated to manage, and more disabling.

Adverse effects of pain

Psychological
Distressing, interferes with sleep, distracting. May undermine faith in medical and nursing staff.

Physiological
- **Cardiovascular:** ↑sympathetic drive—hypertension, tachycardia, vasoconstriction; ↑risk of DVT and PE due to immobility.
- **Respiratory:** ↓chest expansion, inability to cough—retained secretions, basal atelectasis, hypoxia, respiratory infection.

Socio-economic
Prolonged hospital stay, delayed return to work, stress on interpersonal relationships.

Planning analgesia

The anaesthetist and patient should agree an analgesic strategy preoperatively. Factors to consider include:

- Anticipated severity of pain: site and size of incision, major versus minor surgery, day case (may want to minimise use of opioids).
- Potential side effects.
- Patient factors: patient expectations and personality.
- Underlying medical conditions, e.g. patients with rheumatoid arthritis, visual impairment, or cognitive deficits may not manage a PCA effectively.

Treatment options
Treatment of acute pain can be divided into non-pharmacological and pharmacological methods. Non-pharmacological techniques include explanation, reassurance, relaxation, and hypnosis. Pharmacological management includes classical analgesics (simple analgesics, NSAIDs, and opioids), local anaesthetics (regional or local blocks), and adjuvant drugs (e.g. ketamine, clonidine, amitryptilline, gabapentin, pregabalin). 'Multimodal analgesia' is the use of more than one drug, each with a different mode of action.

Routes of administration
The oral route is usually preferred. However, it may not always be appropriate because of postoperative nausea and vomiting, or failure of absorption after bowel surgery.

Timing of analgesia
Drugs can be administered at various times:

- **Pre-emptive:** administration of an analgesic prior to an acute pain stimulus, i.e. pre-incisional intervention. There is no good evidence that pre-emptive analgesia has a significant effect on postoperative analgesia.
- **Preventive:** analgesic interventions which 'have an effect on postoperative pain and/or analgesic consumption that exceeds the expected duration of action of the drug' (e.g. NMDA receptor antagonists).
- **Post-incisional:** administration of an analgesic after a skin incision has been made.

Assessment of perioperative pain

History
A thorough pain history is important, even in postoperative patients. Worsening or unexpected patterns of pain may indicate surgical complications or new pathologies.

Scoring systems
Pain severity should be measured in order to monitor efficacy of treatment. As there is enormous variablility between patients, scoring systems are useful.

- *Visual analogue scale:* patient places mark on a line. Distance from the 'pain free' end is measured in millimetres. Avoids ambiguity of words used to describe pain intensity. A pictorial version (e.g. using sad or smiling faces) can be used for children.
- *Verbal rating scale:* e.g. 'none, mild, moderate, severe'. Alternatively, a pain score from 0 to 10.

The Acute Pain Service (APS)
The APS is a multidisciplinary team dedicated to the management of acute pain. Commonly this involves managing patients with opioid PCAs and epidurals. The patient's symptoms, the response to treatment, and the development of any side effects are regularly assessed. The APS is usually lead by a consultant anaesthetist and may include:

- a clinical nurse specialist, responsible for the day-to-day running of the service
- junior doctors
- a pharmacist
- physiotherapists.

The objectives of the APS are as follows.

- Provision of specialist care and advice for difficult acute pain problems (e.g. patients already being treated for chronic pain).
- Communication between different healthcare professionals involved in the patient's care.
- Education and training of staff.
- Patient education.
- Continuing audit of the service.

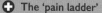 The 'pain ladder'

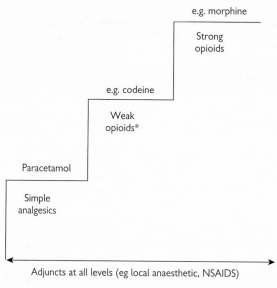

Fig. 7.71 WHO pain ladder.

The World Health Organization pain ladder (Figure 7.71) was originally introduced as a guide to the management of pain in patients with cancer. The three steps are as follows.

- MILD PAIN
  - Non-opioid (regular paracetamol 1g 6 hourly)
  - ± NSAID
  - ± adjuvant
- MODERATE PAIN
  - Weak opioid (e.g. codeine) + paracetamol
  - ± adjuvant
- SEVERE PAIN
  - Strong opioid + paracetamol
  - ± adjuvant

The principles of the pain ladder are that pain relief should be given regularly 'by the clock', not 'as required'. The patient is reassessed at each level. If the pain is not controlled then you should step up the ladder. These principles can be applied to acute pain. However, the anaesthetist usually has to start at the top of the ladder at the time of surgery, with a reduction in analgesic requirements as the patient recovers.

The value of step 2 ('moderate pain') has been questioned, particularly with reference to the variable pharmacokinetic profiles of drugs such as codeine (Section 7.31). It has been suggested that a more appropriate step should involve low-dose strong opioids, whereas step 3 would include higher doses of strong opioids.

Other treatments for pain, such as regional anaesthesia/analgesia, are not included in the pain ladder, and should be considered as appropriate.

Use of patient-controlled analgesia (PCA) and epidural devices mandates the involvement of the acute pain team.

Patient-controlled analgesia

A PCA regime involves the delivery of opioid analgesics via a programmable infusion pump controlled by the patient. Administration is usually IV, but can be as effective subcutaneously. The equipment includes:

- An electronic lockable infusion pump.
- A patient control or 'button'.
- A 'coded' giving set—specific colour or labelled for IV opioids only.
- A non-return valve.
- A supply of opioid (in an infusion bag or syringe, depending on the type of pump in use).

Drugs

The most common choice is morphine, but other opioids can be effectively used: oxycodone, diamorphine, or fentanyl (useful in patients with renal impairment).

Advantages of PCA

- Decreases nursing burden: reduces need for time-consuming checking and administration of opioids.
- Reduces risk of drug administration error (the pump has a safety 'lock-out period').
- Allows patient to feel in control of analgesia.
- Allows pain team to assess opiate requirements.

Disadvantages of PCA

- Inadequate analgesia if settings are inappropriate for the patient (e.g. opioid-tolerant patients).
- The pumps are expensive and may fail.
- Must have dedicated IV cannula.
- Inappropriate for some patients (confused, unable to use button effectively, e.g. rheumatoid hands).

There is no evidence that PCA's provide better efficacy of analgesia, decreased hospital stay, or fewer opioid side effects compared with traditional IM opioid regimes.

Standard parameters for PCA

A standard morphine regime usually involves a 1mg bolus, with a lock-out period (where no further doses can be given) of 5min. Occasionally, a larger bolus or even a continuous background infusion may be beneficial (for paediatric patients, see Section 20.7); a total dose limit for a given period can be programmed if desired. A loading dose should be given before the PCA is initiated; this should be given only by trained staff (and may include opioids administered intraoperatively).

Prescribing for patients with a PCA regime

- Additional opioids or sedatives should not be given.
- Continuous supplemental oxygen should be given to reduce the incidence of hypoxia secondary to respiratory depression.
- Prescribe regular paracetamol ± regular NSAID (if not contraindicated) for their opioid-sparing effects.
- Regular or PRN anti-emetics should be prescribed.

IV naloxone should be prescribed on the 'as-required' side of the prescription chart and should be administered in:

- 100mcg increments for signs of opioid overdose (e.g. respiratory rate <8; patient is difficult to rouse);
- 40mcg increments for troublesome pruritis.

Epidural analgesia

This is the administration of drugs into the epidural space via a catheter. Usually this is done by continuous infusion, but may include patient-controlled top-ups ± a background infusion. The pump is set up with a background rate ± a top-up dose (in millilitres) with a lock-out interval.

Drugs

Usually bupivicaine 0.1–0.25% with fentanyl 2–5mcg/ml or diamorphine 20–50mcg/ml. The usual volume range is a total of 4–15ml/hr, although higher doses may be necessary. A typical lock-out interval for patient boluses is 30min.

Advantages of epidural

- Superior pain relief
- Improved bowel recovery with thoracic epidural in bowel surgery.
- May reduce the incidence of postoperative MI.
- Reduced incidence of postoperative lower respiratory infection.
- Lumbar epidural may help to prevent lower limb graft occlusion in vascular patients.

Disadvantages of epidural

- Complications can be serious. There is a small risk of respiratory depression, hypotension, or even cardiorespiratory arrest if a high block is unnoticed.
- Requires nursing staff trained in the technique.
- Patients require bladder catheterization.

An epidural gives little benefit if an opioid is used as the sole agent. Low-dose local anaesthetic and opioid mixtures provide better pain relief than either drug alone. The addition of adrenaline may improve analgesia and may reduce systemic opioid concentrations.

Monitoring

Because of the risk of respiratory depression and reduced conscious level, patients should have their vital signs and sedation score checked frequently. Observations should also include pain scores and nausea/vomiting assessment. A suggested initial regime for observation is:

- half-hourly for 2hr;
- hourly for 8hr;
- 2 hourly for 8hr;
- then 4 hourly.

For patient-controlled devices, the number of good demands vs. total demands should be assessed regularly. This can indicate whether the pump is programmed appropriately, and illustrate changes in pain control.

For patients with epidurals, motor block should be assessed. The catheter site should be inspected regularly, looking for signs of infection, swelling or leakage of fluid.

All patients with a PCA or epidural should be reviewed daily by the acute pain team.

Junior anaesthetists are often called to review problematic epidurals on the wards. A 'troubleshooting' algorithm is shown in Figure 7.72. This should be used in conjunction with local protocols.

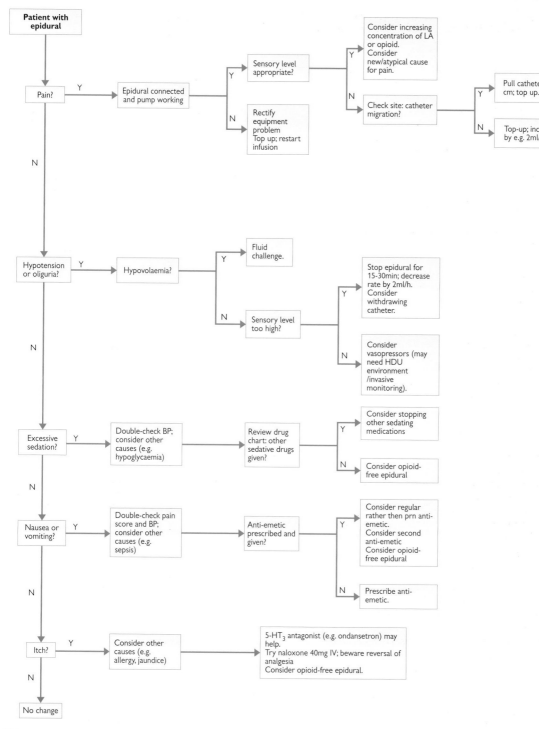

Fig. 7.72 Epidural troubleshooting algorithm.

Notes:
This algorithm assumes the patient is not in extremis. If problems are severe, start with an ABC approach.
If topping up the epidural, observations should be performed every 5 minutes for the first 20 minutes.
After making any change to the epidural, reassess the patient after 15-20min.

Chapter 8

Muscle

209

Topics covered elsewhere

- Malignant hyperpyrexia (Section 25.22)

8.1 The neuromuscular junction

The neuromuscular junction (NMJ) represents the interface between the nervous system and the skeletal muscle. Its transmitter is acetyl choline (ACh).

Skeletal muscle is innervated by A-α motor neurons—large-diameter, myelinated neurons arising from the anterior horns of the spinal cord. At the muscle, the neuronal axon divides into branches, each forming a single junction with a muscle fibre. The group of muscle fibres innervated by a single motor neuron is referred to as a motor unit. Each motor neuron innervates from one to over 2000 muscle fibres; however, each muscle fibre is supplied by only one motor neuron. There are two patterns of innervation:

- *En plaque* **innervation:** the muscle fibre has a single NMJ near its midpoint. The majority of NMJs are like this.
- *En grappe* **innervation:** there are multiple points of innervation on the muscle fibre, giving fine control. The extra-ocular muscles and the intrinsic muscle of the larynx are innervated in this way.

As the fibres approach the muscle termination, they lose their myelination and branch into a number of terminal buttons. The muscle membrane or sarcolemma opposite each button is invaginated to form junctional folds. Nicotinic acetyl choline receptors (NAChRs) are found on the crest of each fold, and anti-cholinesterase enzymes in the trough. The space between the motor end-plate and the terminal button of the motor neuron is called the junctional cleft.

Acetylcholine synthesis and release

The process of acetylcholine synthesis and release is shown in Figure 8.1. Acetylcholine is formed in the cytoplasm from choline and acetyl CoA, under the influence of choline-*O*-acetyltransferase. After formation, 80% is taken up and stored in vesicles. The rest remains within the stroma but cannot be released, forming a stationary store.

The vesicles themselves are formed by the Golgi apparatus of the neuronal cell body (located in the spinal cord). They are transported along the axon to the NMJ. The vesicles also contain ATP, vesiculin, cholesterol, and lipids. After release, the contents are recycled into the terminal.

As the action potential is conducted beyond the last node of Ranvier, local current flow allows an influx of calcium ions (Ca^{2+}) into the presynaptic terminal. The vesicle fuses with the membrane and releases its contents into the junctional cleft, a process known as exocytosis. Calcium-dependent exocytosis involves the formation of a calci-calmodulin complex and assimilation of various structural proteins within the cytoplasm.

The delayed opening of potassium channels later restores the membrane potential.

Nicotinic acetylcholine receptors

Nicotinic acetylcholine receptors (nAChRs) are proteins, each with a molecular weight of 250kDa. They consist of five polypeptide subunits: two identical α, one β, one γ (expressed in the fetus, but replaced by an ε subunit in the adult), and one δ. These combine to form a cylindrical structure surrounding a membrane-spanning ion channel (Figure 8.2). One ACh molecule binds to each α-subunit, displaying positive cooperativity (i.e. occupation of one ACh binding site makes binding at the other one easier; another example of this is the interaction between haemoglobin and oxygen (Section 15.1). The channel opens in response to ACh.

- Channel opening increases the permeability of the sarcolemma to sodium, potassium, magnesium, and ammonium cations.

- This increased conductance (approximately 25pS) allows sodium to flow in and potassium to flow out along their respective electrochemical gradients. The largest flux is of sodium ions.
- Negatively charged amino acid groups at the mouth of the channel repel anions to prevent anion migration.
- The opening of the nicotinic ACh receptors and depolarization of the sarcolemma results in an EPP.
- When this EPP reaches threshold (approximately −55mv), an action potential propagates across the entire sarcolemma.

There are nAChRs on both the pre- and post-junctional membranes. Pre-junctional nAChRs are thought to play a role in mobilizing additional ACh when the muscle is being stimulated. Blockade of these receptors is thought to give rise to the phenomenon of fade, whereby an evoked tetanic contraction is seen to die away in the presence of non-depolarizing muscle relaxants (Section 8.5). Pre-junctional nAChRs are not blocked by α-bungarotoxin.

Motor nerve action potentials

The resting potential of the muscle membrane is about −80 to −90 mV (similar to that in large myelinated nerve fibres). There are two types of depolarizing potential at the motor end-plate, because there are different types of ACh release:

Spontaneous release of acetyl choline

Vesicles in the terminal button of the axon can occasionally randomly and spontaneously fuse with the presynaptic membrane and release ACh molecules into the junctional gap. This only results in small (0.5–1mV) transient electrical changes in the postsynaptic membrane called miniature end-plate potentials (MEPPs). Some drugs and toxins cause an increase in the number and frequency of MEPPs (see opposite).

Evoked release of acetyl choline

The arrival of a nerve impulse releases around 125–200 vesicles, each containing 1200–1500 ACh molecules. The resulting depolarization of the postsynaptic membrane, by 50–75 mV, is an end-plate potential (EPP).

Each nerve impulse releases enough vesicles to activate 10 times the number of receptors required for an end-plate potential. This provides a margin of safety for normal neuromuscular transmission.

Removal of acetylcholine

In order for repolarization to occur, the ACh released into the junctional gap must be removed rapidly. **Acetylcholinesterase** catalyses the hydrolysis of ACh back to choline and acetylCoA.

Mechanisms of neuromuscular blockade

Neuromuscular transmission can be interrupted at any point in its pathway, from ACh synthesis to the ACh receptor. Clinically useful drugs tend to work at the ACh receptor, but many other compounds (mostly toxins and poisons found in nature) interrupt the pathway (see opposite).

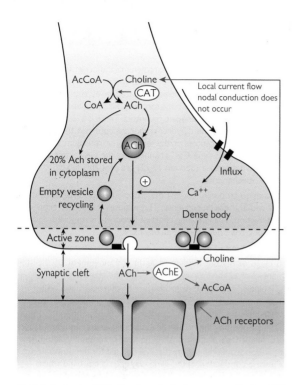

Fig. 8.1 Synthesis of ACh. The dense bodies line up opposite the AChR and are surrounded by vesicles available for immediate release in the active zone. Vesicles behind this active zone form a reserve.

Drugs and mechanisms of neuromuscular blockade

Blockade of ACh synthesis
Hemicholinium

Depletion of ACh stores
Tetanus toxin

Prevention of ACh release
Botulinum toxin, tiger snake venom, β-bungarotoxin
Local anaesthetics
Magnesium ions
Aminoglycoside antibiotics

Blockade of the ACh receptor
Depolarizing blockade
Suxamethonium
Anticholinesterases, e.g. organophosphates
Non-depolarizing blockade
Aminosteroids
Benzylisoquinoliniun esters

Drugs that increase MEPP frequency

Theophylline

Digoxin

Catecholamines

Black widow spider toxin (α-latrotoxin)

These drugs and toxins may increase the rate of MEPP so much that they deplete stores of ACh and lead to failure of neuromuscular transmission.

CHAPTER 8 Muscle

211

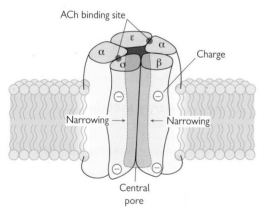

Fig. 8.2 The nicotinic ACh receptors aggregate in clusters on the crests of the sarcolemma. A normal neuromuscular end-plate has, on average, 50 million receptors. Acetylcholinesterase is found in the troughs of the junctional folds, and removes ACh from the junctional cleft, terminating its effect.

8.2 Muscle contraction

Anatomy of striated muscle

Skeletal muscle fibres have diameters of 10–100μm. They are striated, with light and dark bands. This results from the interdigitation of thick and thin filaments, which are organized into cylindrical bundles known as myofibrils. The filaments within each myofibril form a repeating pattern along its length (Figure 8.3). Each subunit is known as a sarcomere.

I Band (isotropic to polarized light)

The light I band lies at the ends of adjacent sarcomeres, and contains the portion of the thin (actin) filaments that do not overlap with thick filaments. The filaments are anchored together across the muscle fibre by Z discs. Each sarcomere contains two sets of thin filaments, the outer ends of which anchor to the Z disc. The inner extremities overlap a portion of the thick filaments and so fall within the A band.

A Band (anisotropic to polarized light)

The thick filaments are arranged in the middle of each sarcomere in an orderly parallel arrangement which produces the wide dark A band. Here, proteins link the central regions of the thick (myosin) forming the M line. The M line maintains the regular array of thick filaments in the middle of each sarcomere.

The **H band,** containing only thick filaments not overlapped by thin filaments, is in the centre of the A band.

Contractile proteins

The proteins which contribute to contraction of muscle are myosin, actin, and the regulatory proteins troponin and tropomyosin. They are shown in Figure 8.4.

Myosin

Thick filaments are composed of myosin, a large, complex protein. It has two globular heads, each of which binds and cleaves ATP. Each head consists of one heavy and two short protein chains. Heads protrude radially from each thick filament, to interact with actin.

The long tail is formed from α helices tightly bound around each other. The tails fuse to form the body of the thick filament, with the heads orientated towards the Z line and the tails towards the M line.

Actin

Six thin filaments surround each myosin strand in hexagonal fashion. The thin filaments are formed by two F-actin chains, wound tightly around one another. The degradation of ATP by the myosin head is potentiated by actin.

Troponin and tropomyosin

Troponin and tropomyosin are the chief regulatory proteins controlling actin and myosin interaction.

Tropomyosin is formed from two α-helical chains. It lies in the channel formed between the two F-actin sequences. Tropomyosin prevents interaction between actin and myosin.

Troponin consists of three subunits:

- Troponin-T binds tropomyosin
- Troponin-C binds calcium
- Troponin-I inhibits the actomyosin ATPase.

Together, they form a globular protein complex found at regular intervals along the filament (every seventh actin monomer).

Excitation–contraction coupling

This is the term used to refer to the sequence of events leading from the action potential in the motor axon to muscle contraction.

Excitation of the muscle

Depolarization of the muscle end-plate via nAChRs generates an end-plate potential (Section 8.1). If this reaches the threshold potential (around 50-55mV), a muscle action potential (AP) results.

This AP is propagated along the sarcolemma and down the T tubules (Figure 8.5) where it activates dihydropyridine receptors (voltage-gated L-type Ca^{2+} channels). Intracellular Ca^{2+} levels rise, and 60 times more calcium is released from the sarcoplasmic reticulum (SR) following opening of adjacent ryanodine receptors. There is a close structural association between the dihydropyridine receptors in the T tubules and the ryanodine receptors on the sarcoplasmic reticulum: a cytoplasmic loop from the L-type Ca^{2+} channel links the two. Some types of malignant hyperpyrexia (Section 22.22) are probably linked to faulty ryanodine mechanisms.

Ca^{2+} binds to troponin, burying the troponin–tropomyosin complex deeper within the actin sequence. This exposes the sites of actin–myosin interaction. The inhibiting effect of troponin-I is removed, and the process of cross-bridge formation begins.

The cross-bridge cycle

Each cycle of myosin binding to actin and movement of the thin filament involves the hydrolysis of one ATP molecule (Figure 8.6).

- ATP binding causes the dissociation of myosin from actin. (After death, without ATP, dissociation cannot occur, resulting in rigor mortis).
- ATP hydrolysis by the myosin head transfers energy to it and causes a conformational shape change—the head becomes angulated. This angulation stores the energy that will be used for the powerstroke of muscle contraction, in the same way as a rubber band stores energy when it is stretched. Angulation of the myosin head lines it up with a new actin binding site. ADP and inorganic phosphate (Pi) remain bound.
- Initial weak binding of myosin and actin releases Pi. The following stronger binding triggers the powerstroke: the myosin head flips back to its low-energy conformation, generating force and pulling the thin filament towards the centre of the sarcomere. ADP is released and ATP binds, allowing dissociation of the myosin and actin. The cycle repeats.

Despite the ratchet-type action, cross-bridges cycle independently of one another, so muscle contraction is smooth rather than staggered.

Relaxation follows a reduction in Ca^{2+} concentration. It is pumped back into the SR by membrane-bound Mg^{2+}-and Ca^{2+}-dependent ATPases. An amount equivalent to that admitted by dihydropyridine receptors is discharged via sarcolemmal Na^+/Ca^{2+} exchange mechanisms. As a result there are fewer available myosin binding sites, fewer cross-bridge interactions, and less muscle tension.

Skeletal muscle energy metabolism

Muscle contraction is accompanied by a large increase in ATP consumption. This ATP can be made via three routes.

- Direct phosphorylation of ADP by creatine phosphate. This has a rapid onset but is limited by the cellular content of creatine phosphate. It lasts until the other two mechanisms can take over.
- Utilization of glycogen stores by glycolysis, i.e. the breakdown of glucose to pyruvate. Does not require oxygen, but only produces small amounts of ATP.
- Oxidative phosphorylation: complete utilization of pyruvate in the mitochondria, requiring oxygen. Supplies most of the ATP requirements during exercise.

Myoglobin

Myoglobin is a haem-containing protein found in skeletal muscle that stores oxygen. It consists of a single globin chain and so cannot exhibit cooperativity of oxygen binding. As a consequence, its oxygen dissociation curve is very different from that of haemoglobin, forming a rectangular hyperbola rather than a sigmoid shape.

It has a P_{50} of approximately 0.3kPa, and is therefore is able not only to load oxygen from haemoglobin but also to load and unload it within the muscle cell as conditions dictate.

Skeletal muscle fibre types

There are two main types of human skeletal muscle fibre. The type depends on whether the myosin isoenzyme is fast or slow with respect to ATPase activity and cycling rate.

Slow fibres

- The most common fibre in human muscle. These fibres respond slowly, requiring repeated stimuli. They have a long duration of contraction.
- Innervation may be either *en grappe* or *en plaque*. They contain many capillaries, much myoglobin, and large numbers of mitochondria. They generate a low peak force of contraction.
- Low in glycolytic and ATPase activity, they use primarily aerobic cellular respiration and have relatively high endurance.

Fast fibres or twitch fibres

These have primarily anaerobic metabolism and relatively low endurance. They are required for infrequent but intense activity. The subclasses of twitch muscle fibres include:

- **Fast fatigue-resistant** (or fast oxidative) contain large amounts of myoglobin and mitochondria. Found in red muscles. They maintain force after a large number of contractions.
- **Fast fatiguable** (or fast glycolytic) are the most powerful, and have high twitch rates of upwards of 120 twitches/sec. They also tire the fastest. The predominant fibre in white muscle, they are used for fine skilled movements. They exhibit a fast onset, and short duration of contraction. Low myoglobin and mitochondria content.

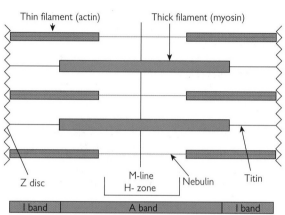

Fig. 8.3 A single sarcomere (2.4μm at rest). A sarcomere is the region between two Z discs. The M line is connected to the Z disc by titin, which limits the length of the sarcomere in tension and contributes to muscle passive tension. Nebulin contributes to the structural integrity of the sarcomere and possibly acts as a template for further sarcomere production.

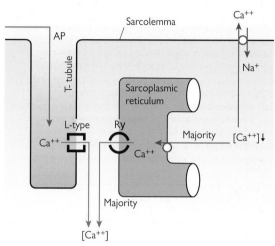

Fig. 8.5 The T-tubules. Invaginations of the muscle membrane occur at regular intervals and are closely related to the SR. Calcium concentrations increase (blue) and are reduced (red).

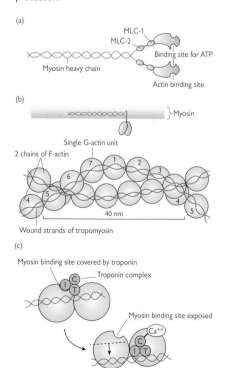

Fig. 8.4 Muscle proteins. (a) The structure of myosin. (b) Actin, myosin and tropomyosin. (c) The binding of Ca²⁺ to troponin induces depression of tropomyosin which reveals binding sites on the thin filament.

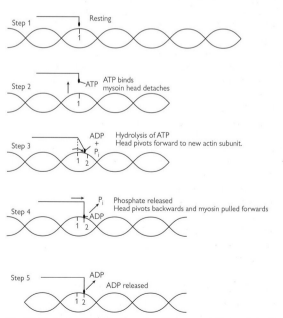

Fig. 8.6 Cycle of cross-bridge formation. Force generation in a skeletal muscle fibre occurs when myosin cross bridges bind to actin filaments, resulting in the relative sliding of thin and thick filaments. This is known as the **sliding filament theory.** It produces muscle shortening with no change in filament length.

Mechanics of muscle contraction

The force exerted on an object by a contracting muscle is known as muscle **tension** and the force exerted on the muscle by the weight of the object is the **load**. In order for muscle fibres to shorten, muscle tension must be greater than the opposing load. Three different types of muscle contraction can occur.

- **Isotonic** Contraction with a constant load but shortening length, e.g. a waiter's biceps as he lifts a tray of drinks.
- **Isometric** Contraction with no change in length: the waiter carefully carrying the drinks in front while walking.
- **Lengthening contraction** Contraction where the external load is greater than the tension developed by the muscle. This causes the muscle to increase in length despite contraction: the waiter lowering the tray onto a table while keeping it supported.

The tension (the amount of force produced) is a function of the proportion of active cross-bridges (Section 8.2). It depends on:

- **Ca^{2+} concentration:** each muscle AP leads to a rise in intracellular Ca^{2+} that is sufficient to bind all troponin molecules and fully expose all of the myosin binding sites on the thin filament.
- The **initial length** of the contracting muscle influences the proportion of active cross-bridges (the length–tension relationship, see below).

Single-fibre contraction

The mechanical response of a single muscle fibre to a single action potential is called a twitch. Following the action potential, there is a latent period before the muscle contraction starts to increase. This period varies between fibre types. Contraction time is the time between the onset of tension development and maximum muscle tension.

Force-velocity relationship (Figure 8.7)

The force generated by a muscle depends on the total number of cross-bridges attached. Cross-bridge attachment takes a finite amount of time. With slower filament velocity more cross-bridges have time to attach, and force increases. If filaments slide past one another more quickly, fewer may become attached and therefore force decreases. The velocity of muscle fibre shortening decreases with increases in load. Maximum muscle velocity occurs at zero load; at very high loads, the fibres will break.

Frequency–tension relationship (Figure 8.8)

Summation is the increase in the mechanical response of a muscle fibre to successive APs occurring during mechanical activity:

- A maintained contraction occurs in response to repetitive stimuli, preventing complete relaxation.
- As the frequency of action potentials increases, the contractions summate to form **tetanus**, and this increases until maximum tension is developed.
- Successive action potentials release Ca^{2+} from the SR before all the previously released Ca^{2+} has been removed. This increases muscle tension.

Length–tension relationship (Figure 8.9)

The tension developed by a muscle fibre varies with changing fibre length prior to contraction. The optimal length (l_o) is that at which the fibre generates the greatest tension. It is explained by the sliding filament theory:

- Overstretching a muscle reduces the amount of overlap between thick and thin filaments, reducing the number of cross bridges formed and therefore the tension.
- Filament overlap is greatest at l_o: at this length the number of cross-bridges formed is greatest, and this produces maximum tension.
- An understretched muscle forms fewer crossbridges due to the spatial arrangement of actin and myosin filaments.

Whole muscle contraction

The tension produced by whole-muscle contractions depends on the number of active fibres in the muscle and the amount of tension developed by each fibre.

Recruitment is the process by which increasing muscle tension is produced by increasing the number of active motor units.

Control of muscle tone and movement

Changes in muscle length are monitored by local motor control mechanisms. The two most important are muscle spindles and the Golgi tendon reflex. Muscle spindles supply the motor system (both locally and centrally) with continuous information about the muscle's length, and its rate of change. In contrast, Golgi tendon organs provide information about the degree of muscle tension. The balance of these two signals allows a fine degree of control of muscle movement.

Muscle spindles (Figure 8.10)

Muscle spindles are small bundles of fibres (intrafusal fibres) 3–10mm long, embedded in parallel with (extrafusal) skeletal muscle fibres. Their central portions act as receptors which sense the length of the muscle (static signal), or the rate of change of length (dynamic signal). Their ends contain contractile elements which alter the length, and therefore the sensitivity, of the fibre. This mechanism is under the control of motor neurones.

There are two types of intrafusal fibre:

- Nuclear bag fibres: so-called because their cell nuclei inhabit a bag-like expansion in the middle of the cell. There are 1–3 per spindle. Bag 1 fibres have low levels of myosin ATPase activity and give rise to a slowly adapting dynamic response. Bag 2 fibres have higher levels of myosin ATPase activity and are quicker to adapt. They are involved with the static response.
- Nuclear chain fibres: these possess nuclei arranged in chains along the fibre. There are 3–9 per spindle.

The sensory innervation of the muscle spindle consists of a single type Ia (primary, fast) and one or two type II (secondary, slower) fibres. Their branches terminate on the middle portions of the intrafusal fibres. The type Ia fibres wrap around them in an annulospiral fashion, whereas the type II fibres exhibit a "flower spray" pattern. The sensory fibres contain stretch-sensitive ion channels; the rate of firing of the afferent nerves increases with increased spindle length.

The primary afferent fibres innervate both the bag and chain fibres. The secondary afferents innervate only the nuclear chain fibres.

Static and dynamic response

During slow muscle stretching, there is an increase in both type Ia and type II afferent signalling. The response is roughly proportional to the absolute length of the muscle. Since the nuclear bag 2 and nuclear chain fibres are innervated by both primary and secondary afferents, they appear to be principally responsible for this static signalling.

During rapid muscle stretching, the primary afferent nerve fibre is stimulated much more powerfully than the secondary fibre. Conversely, during rapid muscle shortening, the Ia signal disappears altogether, before returning to its resting rate when the length of the muscle ceases to change. This suggests that the nuclear bag 1 fibres are primarily concerned with the dynamic response to muscle stretch.

Gamma motor neurones

Gamma motor neurones comprise the motor supply to muscle spindles. By shortening the actin and myosin-containing elements at the ends of the intrafusal fibres, they stretch the central portions of the fibres, increasing the probability that the ion channels on the afferent nerves will open. This increases the sensitivity of the spindle. The γ nerves can be divided into static and dynamic types. The static nerves innervate the nuclear chain fibres, while the dynamic nerves supply the bag fibres. The function of γ motor neurones, the "gamma loop," is described opposite (Figure 8.11).

Function of muscle spindles

Muscle spindles tend to maintain the length of the muscle in status quo. The stretch reflex (Figure 8.12) opposes sudden changes in muscle length. This is important in smoothing out muscular movement; if the innervation of the muscle spindle is severed, movements become jerky. Pre-tensioning of muscles via γ input (which sensitises muscle spindles) tends to stabilise joints and is important in situations of "tense action" – where delicate and exact muscle positioning is necessary (e.g. writing).

Golgi tendon organ

Golgi tendon organs are the main receptors employed in monitoring muscle tension. They are located in the tendons near the junction with the muscle and so are arranged in series with it. They give rise to the tendon reflex:

● Endings of Ib afferent nerve fibres are wrapped around collagen bundles in the tendon. These bundles are slightly bowed in the resting state.

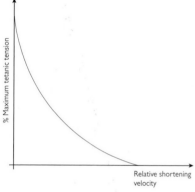

Fig. 8.7 Force–velocity diagram. This demonstrates the dynamic development of cross-bridges between thick and thin filaments.

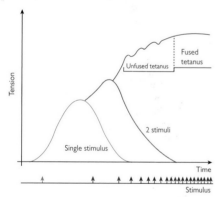

Fig. 8.8 Frequency of stimulation and tension developed, demonstrating summation.

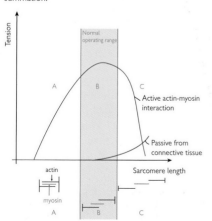

Fig. 8.9 The length–tension relationship demonstrates that generation of isometric tension is a function of overlap between thick and thin filaments.

● Contraction of the muscle pulls on the tendon and this straightens the collagen bundles, distorting the receptor endings.
● A feedback signal is sent to inhibitory neurons in the spinal cord which synapse with the α motor neurons.
● This not only inhibits motor activity and agonist skeletal muscle tone, but also stimulates activity in antagonist muscles.

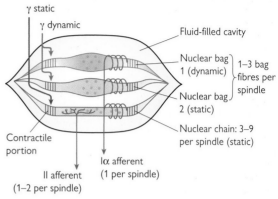

Fig. 8.10 The muscle spindle.

The gamma loop

The cerebellum initiates increased γ fibre activity, causing contraction of the intra-fusal muscle spindle fibres. This results in increased muscle spindle afferent activity, and in turn increased α-motor neuron activity with muscle contraction.

Damage to higher centres alters this pre-tensioning of the muscle spindles. Clinically this manifests as hyper- or hypotonicity of the skeletal musculature.

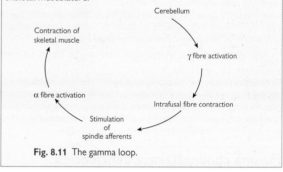

Fig. 8.11 The gamma loop.

The stretch reflex

● Passive stretching of the muscle stretches the muscle spindle as well, stimulating the annulospiral endings in both the nuclear bag and nuclear chain fibres. Both the change and the rate of change of muscle length are important.
● This increases firing of both the Ia and group II afferents.
● These afferents synapse directly with the α motor neurons that stimulate the agonist muscle (monosynaptic reflex). There is a concomitant decrease in antagonist muscle tone via central interneurons (polysynaptic reflex).

With cessation of stretch the Ia sensory output diminishes. There is reduced α-motor neuron activity: the agonist muscle relaxes.

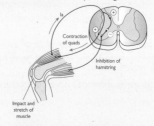

Fig. 8.12 The stretch reflex.

215

8.4 Depolarizing muscle relaxants

Depolarizing muscle relaxants (DMRs) act as agonists at the nicotinic ACh receptors of the NMJ. They produce a persistent depolarization of the NMJ by mimicking the effect of ACh. The only drug of this type in clinical use is suxamethonium.

Mechanism of action
The neuromuscular blocking effect of DMRs is biphasic.

Phase 1 block
- On stimulation, the AChR opens, and there is a high flux of sodium into and potassium out of the cell.
- Depolarization of the end-plate by the relaxant causes the adjacent voltage-gated sodium channels to open.
- A wave of depolarization sweeps along the muscle, characterized by fasciculations or uncoordinated muscular contractions.
- If the depolarizing relaxant is not removed from the cleft, the sodium channels adjacent to the end-plate remain in the inactivated state (see Section 8.1), resulting in muscle paralysis or relaxation.

The depth and duration of blockade is *increased* by the use of anti-cholinesterase drugs (as further accumulation of ACh will add to the agonist activity at the NMJ).

Phase 2 block
Continued use of a DMR can result in the development of phase 2 block, which resembles the block achieved with NDMR. The receptor becomes unresponsive to ACh, an effect that continues for several minutes, even after the drug is gone.

Suxamethonium

Suxamethonium is a short-acting muscle relaxant, which is used when rapid and profound neuromuscular block is required, e.g. as part of rapid-sequence induction. It is also used for modification of the fits of electroconvulsive therapy. One molecule of suxamethonium is basically two ACh molecules joined together (Figure 8.13).

Its side effect profile is troublesome and can be life-threatening (Table 8.2).

Suxamethonium is not susceptible to hydrolysis by acetylcholinesterase and is not eliminated from the junctional cleft easily. Instead, it diffuses away into the plasma, where plasma cholinesterase breaks it down to succinylmonocholine (a weakly active metabolite) and choline. It is further hydrolysed to succinic acid and choline.

Plasma cholinesterase deficiencies

Plasma cholinesterase deficiencies cause suxamethonium apnoea, a syndrome of prolonged duration of action of DMRs. The enzyme is produced in the liver. Cholinesterase deficiencies may be acquired or genetic. Obesity may increase levels of plasma cholinesterase.

Inherited plasma cholinesterase deficiency
The cholinesterase gene is located on an autosomal chromosome (3q26) and several alleles are recognized:
- Usual (U)
- Atypical (A)
- Silent (S)
- Fluoride resistant (F).

There are 10 possible genotypes. The atypical, silent, and fluoride-resistant genes all produce abnormal pseudo-cholinesterase activity.
- 96% of the population is homozygous for the normal pseudo-cholinesterase genotype.
- A normal patient has a dibucaine number of 75–85 (see below).
- Heterozygotes (one normal and one abnormal gene) have a dibucaine number of 40–60.
- Homozygotes (both genes abnormal) have a dibucaine number of <30.

- Silent gene homozygotes have 1–2 hr of apnoea because of the slow speed of suxamethonium hydrolysis (5%/hr).

Dibucaine and fluoride numbers
The dibucaine technique was first described by Kalow and Genest in 1957. Dibucaine is an amide local anaesthetic which inhibits normal plasma cholinesterase. Fluoride has a similar effect. Abnormal variants of plasma cholinesterase are inhibited to a lesser degree than normal plasma cholinesterase.
- A sample of plasma is incubated with butyrylthiocholine and an indicator chemical (5,5'-dithiobis-2-nitrobenzoic acid).
- This produces a coloured product which can be measured: the spectrophotometric absorption is proportional to the pseudocholinesterase activity present.
- The dibucaine and fluoride numbers can be determined by repeating this assay in the presence of standard aliquots of either dibucaine (0.03mmol/L) or fluoride (4mmol/L) in the reaction mixture. This determines the percentage inhibition of enzyme activity caused by these agents, i.e. the dibucaine or fluoride number.
- The dibucaine and fluoride numbers do not measure the concentration of enzyme in the plasma nor the efficiency of the enzyme at metabolizing suxamethonium.

Clinical suspicion of suxamethonium apnoea
Patients with suxamethonium apnoea may remain paralysed for many hours after a standard dose of suxamethonium. They must be kept anaesthetized and ventilated until the suxamethonium is eventually eliminated.

Following recovery, the patient should be screened with estimation of both the dibucaine and fluoride numbers. If the patient's results are abnormal, all blood relatives should be similarly investigated.

Those with evidence of abnormal pseudo-cholinesterase activity should be counselled and advised to wear a MedicAlert bracelet. Determination of the number allows the probability of their genotype to be estimated without resorting to genetic or molecular biology investigations. However, recent evidence suggests that these more expensive investigations remain the gold standard.

Acquired plasma cholinesterase deficiency

Reduced plasma level with pathology
- Renal failure, heart failure, and liver disease
- Malignancy
- Malnutrition
- Burns
- Nephrotic syndrome
- Cardiopulmonary bypass
- Plasmapharesis

Reduced plasma levell without pathology
- Neonates
- Elderly
- Pregnant women (pregnancy may unmask subclinical suxamethonium apnoea)

Reduced activity of plasma cholinesterase
- Anticholinesterases
- Etomidate and ketamine
- Ester local anaesthetics
- Esmolol
- Metoclopramide
- Lithium
- Cytotoxic drugs (e.g. methotrexate)
- Oral contraceptive pill
- Hyperthyroidism

Table 8.1 Characteristics of suxamethonium

	Name	Suxamethonium
Properties	Uses	Profound rapid muscle relaxation
	Chemical	Dicholine ester of succinic acid
	Presentation	Clear aqueous solution; stored at 4°C
	Action	Neuromuscular blockade
	Mode	Causes depolarization before paralysis
	Route	0.5–2.0mg/kg IV; 2.5mg/kg IM
Effects	CVS	↓ HR with repeated doses
	Respiratory	Apnoea with paralysis
	CNS	Fasciculation followed by phase I block. Repeated doses may give rise to phase II block.
	GI	↑intragastric pressures; ↑salivation, ↑gastric secretion
	Other	↑K+ levels
Kinetics	Absorption	IV dosing only
	Distribution	Rapid redistribution
	Metabolism	Hydrolysed rapidly by plasma cholinesterase to succinyl monocholine and subsequently succinic acid plus choline; only 10% of the administered dose reaches the NMJ
	Excretion	2–10% unchanged in the urine; $t_{1/2}$ 2.5–4.5min
	Toxicity	See above

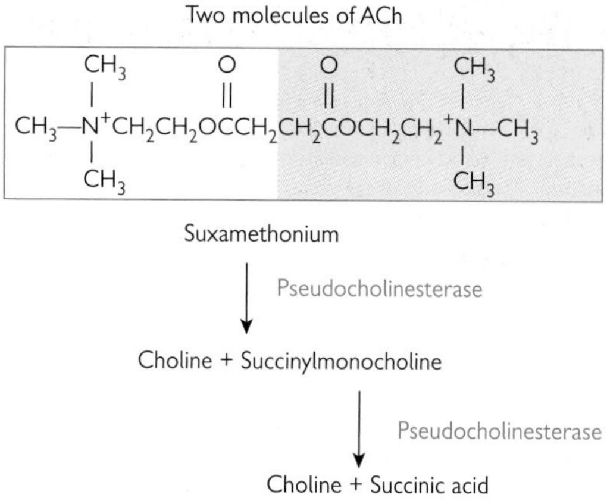

Two molecules of ACh

$$CH_3-N^+CH_2CH_2OCCH_2CH_2COCH_2CH_2^+N-CH_3$$

Suxamethonium

↓ Pseudocholinesterase

Choline + Succinylmonocholine

↓ Pseudocholinesterase

Choline + Succinic acid

Fig. 8.13 Structure and breakdown of suxamethonium. It is virtually all metabolized within 1min.

Table 8.2 Side effects of suxamethonium

Side effect	Mechanism
Bradycardia	Probably via mAChR in the heart; mainly seen in children; opposed by atropine
Myalgia	Most common in young ambulatory female patients; worse in the shoulder and pelvic girdle muscles; caused by muscle damage secondary to fasiculations
Increased intragastric pressure	Thought to be due to abdominal muscle fasiculations; no increased risk of regurgitation as lower oesophageal sphincter tone is also increased (unless this mechanism is altered, e.g. pregnancy)
Increased intracranial and intraocular pressure	Transient rise after injection—of no importance unless there is eye or intracranial pathology: in such cases, the risk–benefit balance should be carefully considered and suxamethonium avoided if possible
Hyperkalaemia	Usually by 0.5mmol/L but higher in certain conditions (see below) when it should be avoided if possible
Hypotension	Caused by muscle relaxation, bradycardia, and histamine release
Tachyphylaxis	Repeated doses may cause a reduced response and lead to a change to phase 2 block (similar to NDMRs); more likely with large doses and infusions (rarely used)
Anaphylaxis	Ranging from minor skin flushing to severe bronchospasm and cardiac arrest
Suxamethonium apnoea	Due to acquired or genetic factors
Malignant hyperpyrexia	Suxamethonium is a potent trigger for malignant hyperthermia

Table 8.3 Characteristics of plasma cholinesterase genotypes

Genotype	Approximate incidence in population (%)	Dibucaine number	Approximate duration of paralysis
U:U	94	75–85	6min
U:S/U:A/U:F	5	40–60	10–20min
F:F	0.0001	65–75	1–2hr
A:A	0.03	15–25	2–4hr
S:S	0.001	0	2–4hr

→ Risk of ↑K+ after suxamethonium use

- Burns
- Spinal injuries and denervating injuries (incuding stroke)
- Critical illness myoneuropathy
- Duchenne muscular dystrophy
- Dystrophia myotonica
- Tetanus
- Renal failure

Mechanism

The increase in serum K+ is usually 0.5mmol/L; however, larger increases (4–9mmol/L) can be seen where there is either damage of the muscle cell membrane (as seen in burns) or formation of nicotinic ACh receptors beyond the NMJ (seen in neurological disease). Patients with renal failure may already have an elevated serum potassium. The additional release caused by the administration of suxamethonium may drive the potassium level high enough to cause clinical effects (Section 11.10)

8.5 Non-depolarizing muscle relaxants

Non-depolarizing muscle relaxants (NDMRs) all contain quaternary amine groups, and act as antagonists of the nAChRs of the neuromuscular junction. Therefore they are generally water soluble, with small volumes of distribution, and follow two-compartment model (Section 7.15). Historically they are related to curare, the generic South American arrow poison containing extracts from the *Chondrodrendon* and *Strychnos* plant species, reported to have first been used in anaesthesia for muscle relaxation in Canada in 1942 by Griffith and Johnson. They can be divided, according to their structure, into two groups: the *benzylisoquiniliniums* and the *aminosteroids*.

NDMRs have similar effects at the NMJ, but differ in their pharmacokinetics, and therefore onset and duration, as well as their excretion, metabolism, and side effects. Different muscles differ in their sensitivity to NDMRs, in the onset as well as the degree of blockade.

Most NDMRs structurally resemble ACh, at least in part. Chain length determines specificity for neuromuscular rather than autonomic receptors: maximum neuromuscular blockade occurs with ten CH_2 groups whereas maximum autonomic effect occurs with six CH_2 groups. Unlike suxamethonium, they are bulky rigid molecules that shield the receptor from ACh.

Characteristics of an ideal NDMR

- Non-depolarizing action with actions confined to the NMJ
- Rapid onset (within one circulation time)
- Short duration, suitable for infusion
- Rapid metabolism to inactive products
- Easily, rapidly, and completely antagonizable
- Not transferred across the placenta or blood–brain barrier
- No local or systemic side effects
- Compatibility with other drugs and solutions
- Long shelf-life without refrigeration
- Cheap and sterilizable

Benzylisoquinolinium compounds

Atracurium
Atracurium was developed in 1974, and was rationally designed to degrade spontaneously at body temperature. This process (Hofmann degradation) yields laudanosine and monoquaternary acrylate. It at least partially avoids the need for clearance by other mechanisms. However, it also undergoes plasma ester hydrolsis to yield monoquaternary acid alcohol. The elimination half-life is around 20min. It is a mixture of 10 stereoisotopes, the *cis–cis* version of which has a more favourable profile.

Cis-atracurium
The *cis-cis* isomer of atracurium. It is said to be approximately four times more potent than atracurium. This carries an associated slower onset of action, since the smaller dose required does not establish such a pronounced diffusion gradient between the plasma and the effect site, and therefore diffusion to the NMJ is slower. It undergoes a greater proportion of Hoffman elimination (77%) and avoids histamine release. Therefore it has a better side-effect profile.

Mivacurium
Structurally related to atracurium, but does not undergo Hoffman elimination. It is a mixture of three isomers:
- *trans-trans* (57%)
- *cis-trans* (36%)
- *cis-cis* (7%).

The *cis-cis* isomer is the least potent, but has the longest duration. The usual dose is 0.1mg/kg. It has a relatively slow onset with little histamine release and a short duration of action: $t_{1/2}$ is approximately 6min, with a single dose lasting approximately 15min. It is metabolized mainly by plasma cholinesterase to inactive metabolites. Although it does not need to be refrigerated, it has a relatively short shelf-life of approximately 18 months.

Aminosteroid compounds

These have two ACh regions at each end of the molecule, although the region on the D ring is the most important for NMJ binding.

Vecuronium and pancuronium
See Table 8.4.

Rocuronium
Rocuronium's name is derived from **r**apid **o**nset **c**urare, as it has the fastest onset of the NDMRs (effective 60sec after an intubating dose). The IV dose is 0.6mg/kg.

Sugammadex

Sugammadex (Org 25969) is a synthetic derivative of cyclodextrin, designed to bind rocuronium selectively. This binding results in a rapid decrease in the free rocuronium concentration in plasma, and subsequently at the motor end-plate, resulting in the restoration of muscle activity.

It benefits from a much more favourable side-effect profile than the anticholinesterases. Although its action is limited to rocuronium, it may become more widespread clinically over the next few years because of the increasing use of rocuronium in the emergency setting.

Key points of NDMR use

- Ensure that you can ventilate the patient with a bag and mask before administering NDMRs.
- Allow enough time for them to work before attempting to intubate the patient. Failure to do so reduces the chance of successful intubation and increases patient morbidity. Nerve stimulator evidence of adequacy of blockade may be useful.
- Ensure that the patient is appropriately anaesthetized once paralysed, as they will not be able to move if they are aware or in pain.
- It is futile trying to reverse the blockade with anticholinesterases too soon. Wait for at least 20min after the last dose.
- Never extubate the patient unless you are certain that paralysis has been adequately reversed. Again, a nerve stimulator may be useful.

Drugs and conditions that affect NDMRs

- *Antibiotics:* aminoglycosides affect both DMRs and NDMRs.
- *CVS drugs:* antiarrhythmic drugs tend to prolong NDMRs.
- *Local anaesthetics* prolong both DMRs and NDMRs.
- *Inhalational agents* all increase duration and degree of block.
- *Electrolyte imbalance:* acute ↓K^+ increases the transmembrane potential at the end-plate with resistance to DMRs and greater sensivity to NDMRs. Hypercalcaemia and hypomagnesaemia increase ACh release from the terminal, producing NDMR resistance.
- *Acid–base imbalance:* acidosis enhances NDMR blockade.
- *Hypothermia:* ↑duration, due to delayed NDMR metabolism.
- *Age:* neonates are more sensitive to NDMRs. The elderly show marked pharmacokinetic variation, with reduced excretion of steroid NDMRs.
- *Disease states:* pancuronium excretion is delayed by liver disease. Other NDMRs tend to be affected more by renal disease.

Table 8.4 Comparison of non-depolarizing muscle relaxants

		Atracurium	Mivacurium	Pancuronium	Vecuronium	Rocuronium
Properties	Uses	Controlled paralysis	Controlled paralysis	Controlled paralysis	Controlled paralysis	Controlled paralysis
	Chemical	Benzylisoquinolinium ester	Benzylisoquinolinium ester	Aminosteroid	Aminosteroid	Aminosteroid
	Presentation	Clear, colourless, 10mg/ml	Clear, pale yellow, 2mg/ml	Clear, colourless, 2mg/ml	Lyophilized powder with citrate and mannitol buffer; diluted in water before use; stable for 24 hr	Clear, colourless, 10mg/ml
	Action	Competetive NDMR	Competitive NDMR	Competitive NDMR	Competitive NDMR	Competitive NDMR
	Mode	Post-junctional nAChR inhibition	Post-junctional nAChR inhibition	Post-junctional nAChR inhibition	Pre- and post-junctional nAChR inhibition	Pre- and post-junctional nAChR inhibition
	Route	IV 0.6mg/kg for intubation	0.1mg/kg for intubation	0.1mg/kg for intubation	0.1mg/kg for intubation	IV 0.6mg/kg for intubation
Effects	CVS	Minimal effects unless histamine release is pronounced	<7% ↑HR and ↓BP	↑HR, ↑BP, ↑CO; no effect on SVR Causes noradrenaline release Vagolytic effect	Only large doses produce ↑CO and ↓SVR; ↑HR with fentanyl	Large doses produce a mild vagolytic effect; ↑HR and ↑MAP
	RS	Apnoea; histamine release provokes bronchospasm	Apnoea; bronchospasm with histamine release	Apnoea; histamine release unlikely	Apnoea; histamine release unlikely	Apnoea; histamine release unlikely
	CNS		No ganglion blockade			
	GI	LOS pressure unaffected			LOS pressure unaffected	
	Other			May reduce APTT and PT	May reduce APTT and PT	
	Distribution	82% protein bound	V_D 0.1–0.03ml/kg; a single dose will last 20min	15–30% protein bound; does not cross BBB; V_D 0.15L/kg	60–90% protein bound; does not cross BBB or placenta	30% protein bound; V_D 0.27 l/kg
	Metabolism	Hoffman degradation and ester hydrolysis	Via plasma cholinesterase	30–45% hepatic breakdown	Liver deacetylation to active metabolites	No metabolites within the urine or plasma
	Excretion	$t_{1/2\beta}$ <20min, unaffected by liver or kidney disease	Metabolites cleared into bile and urine with some unchanged. Renal and liver failure both ↑duration of action	40% excreted unchanged in urine	20% unchanged in urine and 25% unchanged in bile	40% unchanged in bile; 13–31% unchanged in urine; renal failure has little effect on duration of action; hepatic failure does affect it
	Toxicity	Histamine release with predictable clinical effects		Rare reports of anaphylactoid reactions	Rare reports of anaphylactoid reactions	Rare reports of anaphylactoid reactions
	Note	Safe in MH	Safe in MH. Incompatible with barbiturates	Aminosteroid cross-reactivity a possibility	Aminosteroid cross-reactivity a possibility	Aminosteroid cross-reactivity a possibility

There is wide variation in patient sensitivity to neuromuscular blocking agents, so it is always preferable to monitor neuromuscular function. There is increasing evidence that residual neuromuscular blockade is common and may lead to adverse patient outcomes.

As it is difficult to measure the degree of receptor blockade directly, neuromuscular function is indirectly assessed using either clinical assessment or electrical nerve stimulation.

Depolarizing and non-depolarizing blockade give characteristic patterns in response to electrical stimuli (Figures 8.14 and 8.15).

Clinical assessment

Clinical signs of adequate return of neuromuscular function following non-depolarising neuromuscular blockade include:

- Sustained head lift for at least 5 sec
- Generation of a vital capacity of at least 10ml/kg
- Generation of an inspiratory pressure of at least −25cmH$_2$O.

Tidal volume is not a reliable guide to recovery, since normal volumes can be generated with only 20% functional diaphragm muscle receptors.

However, clinical assessment can be influenced by other factors such as residual anaesthesia. It cannot be performed under anaesthesia, and so electrical nerve stimulation is more commonly used.

Electrical nerve stimulation

Measuring the muscle response following an electrical stimulus to a peripheral nerve is the standard assessment of neuromuscular function (Figure 8.15).

The black electrode is negatively charged and depolarizes the membrane, whereas the red electrode is positively charged and hyperpolarizes the membrane. Although stimulation is possible however the electrodes are placed, maximum twitch height is obtained when the negative (black) electrode is closest to the nerve.

The *maximum stimulus* is that which is sufficient to stimulate all the fibres of a motor nerve, producing maximum muscle contraction. The *supramaximal current* is 25% greater than this value, and is used for peripheral nerve stimulation to ensure that a maximum stimulus is achieved.

Single twitch

A single twitch is the simplest mode of stimulation. A square-wave stimulus is applied to a peripheral nerve for a short duration (0.1–0.2ms). This can be used to establish the level at which a supramaximal stimulus is obtained, but is of little use in clinical practice.

Train-of-four stimulation

Train-of-four (TOF) stimulation was developed in 1970 as a clinical tool to assess neuromuscular block in the anaesthetised patient.

Four square-wave stimuli at 2Hz and 50mA are applied to a peripheral nerve, and the resulting muscle action is assessed. This may be by simple observation (which is unreliable), or objectively by measurement of the tension, acceleration, or action potential in the muscle of interest (often the adductor policis). The twitches obtained may be counted, or the relative strength of the last assessed compared with the that of the first assessed.

Train-of-four count

As a neuromuscular block deepens, fewer stimuli traverse the neuromuscular junction. For most general surgery, a block giving less than two twitches is adequate. The TOF count roughly correlates with the number of receptors occupied by NDMR (Table 8.5).

TOF ratio

Presynaptic ACh mobilization is reduced in the presence of NDMRs. Multiple or tetanic stimuli can then deplete ACh in the nerve terminal and cause a reduction in the strength of contraction with each successive twitch, known as *fade*. The degree of non-depolarizing neuromuscular blockade can be described as the ratio of the force generated by the fourth contraction (T4) to that generated by the first contraction (T1). This effect is not seen with DMRs unless a phase 2 block has occurred.

For many years, a TOF ratio of 0.7 was thought to correlate with adequate respiratory function. It was assumed that sustained maximum inspiratory force and minute ventilation indicated safe recovery from neuromuscular blockade.

However, at a TOF ratio of 0.7 there may still be:

- Residual paralysis and laryngeal and pharyngeal muscle function
- Residual paralysis and hypoxic ventilatory control
- Patient discomfort
- A reduced margin of safety of neuromuscular transmission.

These residual effects all disappear with a TOF ratio of at least 0.9. However, when objective monitoring is not available, tetanic stimulation may the most appropriate method to assess residual paralysis.

Tetanic stimulation

This uses a supramaximal stimulus at high frequency (50–200Hz) for a set period of time (normally 5sec).

- Tetanic contraction is seen when less than 75% of receptors are blocked, but in the presence of non-depolarizing muscular blockers (NDMBs) this contraction will show the characteristic fade.
- It is sensitive in eliciting minor degrees of neuromuscular block but the pain of tetanic contraction limits its usefulness to anaesthetized patients only.

Post-tetanic facilitation

Post-tetanic facilitation describes an increased response to a given stimulus following tetanic stimulation. This is due to increased synthesis and mobilization of ACh. This additional ACh is able to compete with NDMRs for receptors (until it is metabolized). Again, the effect is not seen with depolarizing blockade.

Post-tetanic count

The post-tetanic count (PTC) may be useful during deep blockade, when there is no response to single twitch or TOF stimulation. It is mainly used where profound neuromuscular blockade is required, e.g. during retinal surgery. A response will be seen in the early stages of recovery because of post-tetanic facilitation.

- A 5sec tetanic stimulus at 50Hz is applied. If there is no twitch response, it is followed 3sec later by single twitches at 1Hz for 10sec.
- The anaesthetist simply counts how many twitches are visible. When only one or two twitches are visible, the block is deep enough for virtually any surgery. A PTC of 9 correlates with a TOF count of 1.
- PTC should not be repeated within 6min, as the result may be inaccurate.

Double-burst stimulation

Double-burst stimulation (DBS) involves the application of an initial burst of three 0.2ms tetanic impulses at 50Hz, followed by an identical stimulation 750ms later.

- The magnitude of the response generated is about three times greater than the TOF, making it easier to assess the degree of fade present.

Table 8.5		
Receptors occupied	**TOF twitch number**	**Single twitch**
75%	4 is lost	Begins to be reduced
80%	3 and 4 are lost	
90–95%	2, 3, and 4 are lost	Disappears

✚ Which nerve and why?

The chosen nerve must

- have a motor component and be easily accessible
- be close to the skin
- cause a contraction in a muscle group that must either be visible or be available for evoked response monitoring.

Table 8.6 Common sites for neuromuscular monitoring

Nerve	Muscle contraction
Ophthalmic branch, facial nerve	Orbicularis oculi
Ulnar	Adductor pollicis of thumb
Posterior tibial	Plantar flexion of big toe
Peroneal	Dorsiflexion of foot

Different muscle groups have different sensitivities to NDMRs. The reason may be a variation in blood flow, and therefore drug delivery, different muscle fibre types, or variable densities of AChRs.

The diaphragm is the least sensitive, and the muscles of the face and hand the most sensitive. Restoration of facial and hand muscle activity should ensure adequate reversal of respiratory muscle paralysis.

➔ Characteristics of an ideal nerve stimulator

- Portable and battery powered
- Able to generate a pulse stimulus of 0.3ms
- Supramaximal current output to a maximum of 80mA at all frequencies – guarantees that all nerve fibres depolarize
- Monophasic square–wave pulse waveform—maintains a constant current throughout the stimulus
- Action over a range of frequencies, i.e. single twitch (1Hz), TOF (2Hz), and tetanic stimulation (50Hz)
- Displays adequacy of electrical contact on screen
- Indicates polarity of electrodes
- Able to monitor the evoked responses quantatively—assessment of function

✚ Practical points

- TOFC: one twitch or none – intubation may be attempted.
- Reversal agents can be given when the TOF count recovers to 3 or 4.
- TOFC of 1 or 2 increases the risk of inadequate reversal in recovery.
- A TOF should not be repeated for at least 30sec as depletion of ACh will alter the results.
- The time from PTC 1 to TOFC 1 is documented for most relaxants as an index of the duration of action (pancuronium 40min, atracurium 9min).

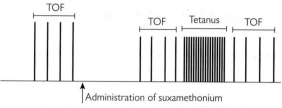

Fig. 8.14 Patterns of evoked muscle responses following administration of depolarizing blockers. Note the absence of fade and the lack of post-tetanic facilitation.

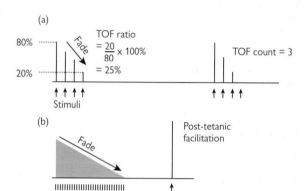

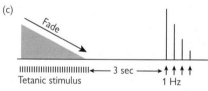

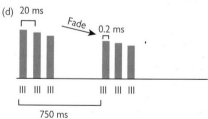

Fig. 8.15 Patterns of evoked muscle responses following administration of non-depolarizing neuromuscular blockers: (a) TOF ratio and count; (b) tetanic stimulation; (c) post-tetanic count; (d) double-burst stimulation.

221

8.7 Acetylcholinesterase inhibitors

Acetylcholinesterase inhibitors are used in anaesthetics in the reversal of NDMBs. They are also used in the diagnosis and treatment of myasthenia gravis (MG), and in the treatment of Alzheimer's dementia. They can augment, or in overdose cause, depolarizing blockade. By preventing the breakdown of acetylcholine, they also result in muscarinic side effects and so are often administered with anti-muscarinic agents.

They act to inhibit the breakdown of acetylcholine by binding to the acetylcholinesterase enzyme. This raises the concentration of acetylcholine at the neuromuscular junction.

Mechanism of action

The acetylcholinesterase enzyme has two binding sites: the anionic binding site, which binds the quaternary amine group of ACh, and the esteratic binding site, which binds the ester group of the ACh molecule. Binding the ester group causes ACh to dissociate, leaving the enzyme itself acetylated. Hydrolysis regenerates the original enzyme. Acetylcholinesterase inhibitors prevent the breakdown of acetylcholine by preventing its binding to the enzyme. They can be divided into two groups according to the type of inhibition.

Reversible
- Edrophonium.
- Carbamate esters (neostigmine, pyridostigmine, physostigmine).

Irreversible
- Organophosphate compounds.

Edrophonium

Edrophonium (Tensilon) is a phenolic quaternary amine. Its quaternary amine group combines reversibly with the anionic site of acetycholinesterase, preventing the access of ACh. It also has direct effects on motor nerves, resulting in increased ACh release. Its quaternary amine group prevents it from crossing the blood–brain barrier.

2–10 mg IV is used in the diagnosis of MG, while 0.5–1.0mg/kg is used in the reversal of non-depolarizing neuromuscular blockade.

Carbamate esters

Carbamate esters contain either a tertiary or a quaternary amine group and a carbamyl group. The amine group binds to the anionic site of acetycholinesterase, while the carbamyl group binds to the esteratic site. The drug then dissociates, leaving the acetylcholinesterase carbamylated (rather than acetylated as occurs with ACh).

This is a similar to the reaction of acetylcholinesterase with ACh. However, the hydrolysis of the carbamylated enzyme is much slower (half-life of minutes) than that of the acetylated enzyme (half-life of microseconds). Therefore the carbamylated enzyme is unavailable for ACh degradation and so ACh concentration increases.

Carbamates may also have direct effects on neuronal transmission, and inhibit the action of plasma cholinesterase.

Neostigmine

Neostigmine is a quaternary amine used for reversal of NDMBs at a dose of 0.05mg/kg IV. Other clinical uses include MG, urinary retention, and paralytic ileus. It is normally available in combination with glycopyrrolate (neostigmine 2.5mg–glycopyrrolate 0.5mg) to prevent the bradycardia caused by muscarinic stimulation. It has a maximum effect approximately 7min after IV administration and a terminal half-life of approximately 30min. A single dose has a duration of action of approximately 50min. The duration of action of glycopyrrolate mirrors that of neostigmine, as shown in Figure 8.18.

Oral bioavailability is low because of first pass metabolism. It is mainly metabolized by plasma esterases, although there is some metabolism in the liver with excretion in the bile, and some elimination of the unchanged drug in the urine.

Pyridostigmine

Also a quaternary amine, pyridostigmine is used in the treatment of MG and is given orally at a dose of 30–120mg 4–12 hourly. It is more potent than neostigmine, with better oral bioavailability, a slower onset, and a longer duration of action.

It has fewer muscarinic side effects. Its metabolism is similar to that of neostigmine: it is mainly metabolized by plasma esterases, although there is some metabolism in the liver with excretion in the bile, and some non-metabolized elimination in the urine.

Physostigmine

Physostigmine is a tertiary amine and is therefore well absorbed from the gut, and able to cross the BBB and placenta.

It was formerly a treatment for central anticholinergic syndrome and used topically in narrow angle glaucoma. It is no longer available in the UK.

Organophosphates

Organophosphorus compounds were shown to inhibit acetycholinesterase in 1937, and have subsequently been used as insecticides and chemical weapons. They can be absorbed enterally, via the lungs or skin, and are rapidly distributed to all tissues. They cause inhibition of acetycholinesterase by phosphorylation of the esteratic site, resulting in a stable enzyme complex that is resistant to hydrolysis and reactivation. For this reason, they are considered to be irreversible inhibitors of acetylcholinesterase.

The majority of these chemicals have similar effects on plasma cholinesterase. Symptoms of organophosphorous poisoning are classically described by the acronym SLUD: Salivation, Lacrimation, Urination, and Diarrhoea.

Other symptoms include muscle weakness and fasciculation, and CNS excitation with tremor and convulsions. CNS depression with coma and apnoea may also occur.

Treatment is with acetylcholinesterase reactivators such as pralidoxime. In addition, atropine 2mg IV every 30min until full atropinization should be given for up to 3 days. Anticonvulsants, sedation, and ventilation may also be necessary.

Sarin

Sarin (Figure 8.17) is a nerve agent classified as a weapon of mass destruction. It has an activity profile similar to that of malathion and other insecticides.

At room temperature it is colourless and odourless. Its low saturated vapour pressure (0.4kPa) would seem to make it a relatively inefficient terrorist agent. However, sarin is efficiently absorbed across any membrane, including the skin. It is fatal in even minute amounts, being 500 times more toxic than cyanide.

In 1995, the outlawed group Aum Shinrikyo carried out its second sarin attack, killing 12 people on the Tokyo underground system. This demonstrated a powerful new terrorist technique with devastating potential.

Ecothiopate

This is a quaternary amine organophosphorous compound, now withdrawn from the UK. It was previously used as a miotic agent in narrow-angle glaucoma. Its use was associated with prolonged apnoea after suxamethonium administration because of the inhibition of acetylcholinesterase and plasma cholinesterase.

Table 8.7 Comparison of acetylcholinesterase inhibitors

Name		Neostigmine	Pyridostigmine	Edrophonium
Properties	Uses	For reversal of NDMRs; MG therapy	Main use in MG; Can be used to reverse NDMR block	Tensilon test. Reversal of NDMRs
	Chemical	Quaternary amine	Pyridine analogue of neostigmine	Synthetic quaternary ammonium compound
	Presentation	Clear colourless solution for IV injection	Clear colourless solution for IV injection 5mg/ml	Clear colourless solution, 10mg/mL
	Action	Cholinergic	Cholinergic; fewer muscarinic effects than neostigmine	Cholinergic
	Mode	Reversible acid-transferring cholinesterase inhibitor; binds to the esteratic site	Reversible acid-transferring cholinesterase inhibitor; binds to the esteratic site	Competes with ACh at the anionic site of cholinesterase; some pre-junctional action
	Route	MG dose: 15–50mg 2–4hrly Reversal: 0.05mg/kg, with anticholinergic agent	IV, IM, or PO for MG; 60mg tablets; dose titrated to effect	IV administration; more rapid onset and briefer duration than neostigmine
Effects	CVS	↓HR and ↓CO, ↑conduction time, ↓ refractory period.	Slower onset ↓HR and ↓CO; ↑conduction time and ↓refractory period	↓HR, ↓CO; ↑conduction time
	RS	↑secretion, bronchoconstriction	↑secretion, bronchoconstriction	↑secretion, bronchoconstriction
	CNS	High doses: causes neuromuscular blockade by direct receptor effects and accumulation of ACh	High doses: causes blockade by direct effect and accumulation of ACh	Agitation, miosis; weakness and fasciculation in normal subjects
	GI	↑salivation, ↑gastric secretions, ↑motility	↑salivation, ↑gastric secretions, ↑motility	↑salivation, ↑GI motility, ↑gastric acid secretions
	Other	↑ureteric peristalsis	↑ureteric peristalsis	↑ureteric peristalsis
Kinetics	Absorption	Poor oral absorption; 1–2% oral bioavailability	<10% oral bioavailability	
	Distribution	Highly ionized; 6–10% protein bound		V_D 0.9–1.3L/kg
	Metabolism	Metabolized to quaternary alcohol by plasma esterases; some biliary excretion	<25% metabolized and subsequently glucuronidated	Uncertain; it is not hydrolysed by esterases
	Excretion	66% excreted in the urine; renal failure leads to accumulation	Renal excretion accounts for 75% of clearance	Unknown
	Notes	Prolongs action of suxamethonium	Longer to peak effect than neostgmine	Cardiac arrest has been reported

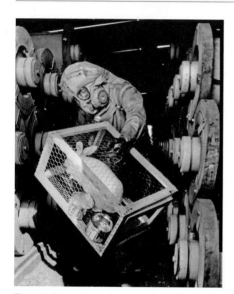

Fig. 8.16 Storage facility for sarin in the 1950s. Rabbits were used as an early warning system in the detection of leaks.

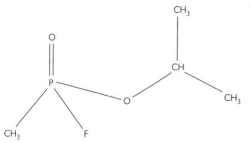

Fig. 8.17 Structure of sarin.

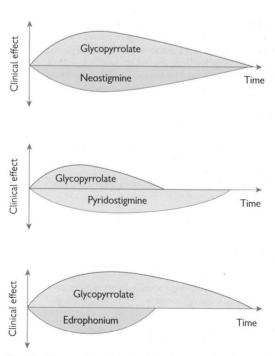

Fig. 8.18 Diagram of the clinical profiles of glycopyrrolate vs. some common acetylcholinesterase inhibitors. Glycopyrrolate is often used to antagonise the cholinergic side effects of acetylcholinesterase inhibitors. The degree and duration of antagonism is best matched to neostigmine (top). The effects of pyridostigmine are longer-lasting than those of glycopyrrolate (middle), and so late cholinergic effects (bradycardia, bronchoconstriction) may supervene. Conversely, if used to antagonise edrophonium, the anticholinergic effects of glycopyrrolate itself may be undesirably long-lived (bottom).

Myasthenia gravis

Myaesthenia gravis (MG) is an autoimmune condition, with a prevalence of around 4:100,000 and peak incidence at 30 years of age. It is twice as common in women than in men. It is due to IgG auto-antibodies against the ACh receptor, detectable in over 90% of cases.

Associations

- Thymic hyperplasia in 70% under 40 years of age with MG.
- Thymic tumours in 10% of patients (Figure 8.19).
- Other autoimmune diseases.
- HLA B8 and DR3 genotypes.

Clinical signs

- The major symptom is weakness, which improves with rest. This may affect ocular muscles (resulting in ptosis and diplopia), bulbar muscles (dysarthria, aspiration), and limb and respiratory muscles.
- Most hospital admissions present with an established diagnosis, with an exacerbation of disease due to another pathology.

Myasthenic crisis

Generally due to insufficient medication. Such crises may also be provoked by infection, stress, pregnancy, or use of other drugs (see opposite).

Cholinergic crisis

Results from an excess of cholinesterase inhibitors, and resembles organophosphate poisoning (Section 8.7).

Myasthenic and cholinergic crises are difficult to distinguish clinically, since both cause bronchospasm, bronchorrhoea, respiratory failure, diaphoresis, and cyanosis.

Diagnosis

- Made by Tensilon test, in which edrophonium 2mg and then 8mg is administered IV.
- A brief improvement in muscle strength confirms the diagnosis.
- The test can also be used to differentiate a cholinergic from a myasthenic crisis (the latter will be improved).
- EMG studies can be used to demonstrate the marked fatiguability of muscle. ACh antibodies may be present in the blood.

Therapy

Treatment with acetylcholinesterase inhibitors such as pyridostigmine (30–120mg 6 hourly) or neostigmine (15–30mg 4 hourly) can be successful but often causes muscarinic side effects and may cause a cholinergic crisis. Concurrent anti-muscarinic therapy can prevent predictable abdominal pain, diarrhoea, and salivation.

Immunosuppressive drugs, such as steroids, azothiaprine, cyclosporine, and cyclophosphamide, modify the immune system and improve outcome

Thymectomy improves symptoms in over 50% of patients, especially those with thymomas and thymic hyperplasia. It can result in a cure for some, but the effects can take from weeks to 5 years to become apparent.

Gradual failure of ventilation and poor secretion clearance are the main causes of admission to ICU for ventilation. Regular spirometry helps determine when respiratory support is necessary. As FVC approaches tidal volume, patients will not be able to cough.

Anaesthetic implications

Myasthenia gravis has several important anaesthetic implications.

- It may be associated with poor respiratory and bulbar function.
- Patients undergoing a general anaesthetic will almost always require assisted ventilation.
- Patients show resistance to DMRs, with an increased risk of dual block development.
- There is greatly increased sensitivity to NDMRs; 90% dose reduction is necessary together with careful monitoring of neuromuscular blockade.
- Many commonly used drugs, such as antibiotics and local anaesthetics, increase weakness in MG.

Dystrophia myotonica

Myotonias are characterized by continued involuntary muscle contraction after cessation of voluntary effort. The most common is dystrophia myotonica, with a prevalence of 5 in 100,000. It is inherited in an autosomal dominant fashion, and caused by a trinucleotide (CTG) repeat in the DM1 protein kinase gene on chromosome 19q13.3. The age of onset of symptoms is inversely proportional to the length of the CTG repeat.

Clinical signs

Many patients have characteristic facies (Figure 8.20).

There is myotonia, with progressive distal muscle weakness and ptosis, and weakness of the facial muscles and sternocleidomastoid muscles.

Associated abnormalities include mitral valve prolapse in 20%, cardiomyopathies, and cardiac conduction abnormalities. Other signs include cataracts, cognitive impairment, male-pattern baldness, poor bulbar function, hypogonadism, and poor respiratory function.

Therapies

There is no specific treatment for the weakness and wasting, although the myotonia is sometimes treated with phenytoin.

Anaesthetic implications

- Patients with myotonia have an increased sensitivity to anaesthetic agents and opiates.
- They have poor cardiac and respiratory reserve, and an increased risk of aspiration due to poor bulbar function.
- They show an increased sensitivity to NDMRs.
- Suxamethonium, acetylcholinesterase inhibitors, and nerve stimulators can all stimulate dystonia.
- The patient must be kept warm, since both cooling and shivering will precipitate dystonia.

Duchenne's muscular dystrophy

This X-linked recessive disorder has an incidence of approximately 1 in 3000 males. Presentation usually occurs by the age of 4, with death in the early twenties. The mutation results in the absence of dystrophin, a rod-shaped muscle cytoskeletal protein.

Clinical signs

Symptoms include proximal limb weakness, which may present with Gower's sign (the patient appears to 'climb up' himself when rising from a squatting position), and calf pseudohypertrophy. In the later stages of the disease, limb contractures can occur.

Myocardial disease may cause dilated cardiomyopathy, mitral valve prolapse, and ECG abnormalities.

Investigations

Muscle biopsy reveals muscle fibre necrosis with fat replacement, and the absence of dystrophin. EMG shows a myopathic tracing.

There is often a raised serum creatinine.

Anaesthetic implications

- Patients often present for muscle biopsy or orthopaedic procedures.
- Poor bulbar, respiratory, and cardiac function with kyphoscoliosis and delayed gastric emptying present significant anaesthetic risks.
- Suxamethonium and volatile anaesthetic agents can provoke rhabdomyolysis, with associated hyperkalaemia and myoglobinuria.
- Non-depolarizing NDMRs can be used with reduced doses and neuromuscular monitoring.

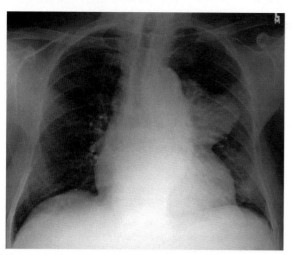

Fig. 8.19 CXR demonstrating a thymoma in a patient with myaesthenia gravis.

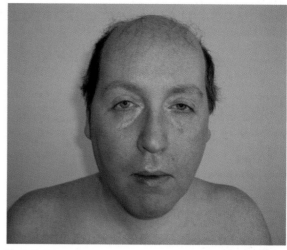

Fig. 8.20 Facial features of dystrophia myotonica.

➔ **Risk factors increasing the need for postoperative ventilation in MG**

- Disease history greater than 6 years
- Coexisting respiratory disease
- Preoperative vital capacity of <2.9L
- Pyridostigmine dose requirements >750mg/day

Drugs which worsen symptoms of MG

Antibiotics
Macrolides, fluoroquinolones, aminoglycosides, tetracycline, and chloroquine

Antiarrhythmics
β-blockers, calcium-channel blockers, quinidine, lidocaine, procainamide, and trimethaphan

Miscellaneous
Diphenylhydantoin, lithium, chlorpromazine, muscle relaxants, levothyroxine, adrenocorticotropic hormone (ACTH), and (paradoxically) corticosteroids

➔ **Eaton–Lambert syndrome**

This is a rare autoimmune condition where production of IgG autoantibodies against voltage-dependent Ca^{2+} channels results in reduced ACh release. It is usually a non-metastatic manifestation of malignancy (usually small cell bronchial carcinoma) but it may occur on its own as an autoimmune disorder.

The main symptom is proximal muscle weakness which improves with exercise. The reduced reflexes are reduced or absent and improve similarly. Autonomic involvement may result in dry mouth and urinary hesitance. The treatment mainstays are immunosupression and therapy for the underlying cause. Patients show an increased sensitivity to DMBs and NDMBs, and so doses for each should be reduced.

Exercise produces great demands on the cardiovascular, respiratory, and metabolic systems. Physiological change is directed towards allowing the muscles to work at their maximum potential and the responses are dependent on whether the exercise is unusual or part of a training programme. In general, exercise-related changes in women are the same as for men except for quantitative differences caused by differences in levels of testosterone, body size, and body composition. The integrated response to exercise can broadly be divided into different components:

Neurological phase

Anticipation of exercise leads to activation of sympathetic and inhibition of parasympathetic outflow. Passive movement of limbs induces a similar response. There is an increase in ventilation that precedes actual exercise: it is unclear whether this anticipatory response is learned or innate. It does not result from altered blood gases since a mild respiratory alkalosis is produced.

Metabolic phase

O_2 uptake and CO_2 production change in linear fashion, yet blood gas levels remain unchanged; the mechanism for this remains unexplained. Minute volume is able to increase to $20\times$ normal, possibly in response to feedback from metaboreceptors in muscles detecting the local build up of products of exercise.

Afferent input from muscle chemo- and mechanoreceptors influences the medullary cardiovascular centre and facilitates the impact on autonomic neurons from higher brain centres.

Finally, arterial baroreceptors play a role, further inhibiting parasympathetic outflow and increasing sympathetic discharge.

Compensatory phase

As exercise proceeds, oxygen intake is matched by the production of CO_2. At increased intensity, this relationship changes and the amount of CO_2 produced relative to oxygen taken up increases proportionally. This is called the anaerobic threshold (AT) (Section 1.7) .

Anaerobic metabolism of glucose produces lactate, which is buffered by bicarbonate to form CO_2. The AT is the point at which lactate production begins in significant amounts. The Cori cycle (Figure 8.23) describes the movement of lactate produced by anaerobic glycolysis to the liver, where glucose is regenerated. This circulates back to the muscles to re-enter the glycolytic pathway.

Respiratory changes

With increased exercise, more ventilation becomes necessary. Initially, this is achieved by larger tidal volumes which still lie on the steep part of the compliance curve, representing energy cost efficiency.

Further increases in minute volume are due to increased respiratory rate. As tidal volume becomes maximal (on the flat upper part of the compliance curve) energy costs are higher; a rate rise is more energy efficient.

During exercise, there is an increase in surface area for diffusion and oxygen-diffusing capacity increases. This is due to the following.
- Increased pulmonary blood flow and capillary perfusion. The proportion of dead space per tidal breath is reduced.
- Recruitment of pulmonary capillaries secondary to increased CO. The downside is that faster RBC transit within the pulmonary capillary means that there is less time available for gas diffusion. Those with lung disease might demonstrate diffusion limitation (Section 13.11).
- Increased A–a gradient. The hyperventilation of the anticipatory stage raises P_AO_2 and the increased peripheral oxygen extraction of this stage results in lower mixed venous O_2 saturation. The two combine to increase the gradient for diffusion.

Maximal breathing capacity is about 50% greater than the actual total pulmonary ventilation of maximal exercise. This provides a buffer for athletes that can be called on in conditions such as high altitude and excessive heat. It also means that in health, pulmonary function does not act as the limiter of exercise performance.

Cardiovascular changes

During exercise, the cardiac output can increase from a resting value of 5L/min to a maximal value of 35L/min (in athletes). Most of the increase goes to the exercising muscles, but there are also increases in flow to the skin (dissipation of heat) and the heart (for the additional work of pumping and increased output). The increased flow through these three areas is the result of arteriolar vasodilation mediated by local metabolic factors (muscle and heart) and sympathetic tone (skin).

The change in cardiac output is due initially to an increase in stroke volume (around 50%) and, later, heart rate (around 270%). Increase in stroke volume reaches its maximum by the time the cardiac output has increased only 50% of its maximum. These changes represent the greatest energy efficiency for the heart: at low levels of exercise; increased SV impacts less on myocardial O_2 delivery.

As muscles vasodilate, there is greater venous return and therefore preload, and this will increase SV. Preload will also increase because of the effect of circulating catecholamines.

Mean arterial blood pressure increases by a small amount as the rise in cardiac output is greater than the decrease in peripheral resistance. Pulse pressure increases markedly due to the reduced SVR. Muscle vasodilatation facilitates the increased speed of stroke volume ejection.

Sympathetic stimulation causes peripheral arteriolar vasoconstriction and reduced flow to internal organs. Although this also affects muscle blood flow, local production of vasodilatory substances increases flow and is the stronger effect.

Limiters

Once SV has been maximally increased, CO is raised by increasing HR. The first sign of embarrassment is the development of a metabolic acidosis, demonstrating a failure of adequate O_2 supply.

Respiratory function is not the exercise limiter; this is the gradual failure of the CVS and muscles to deliver, and use O_2 in sufficient quantity.

Training

Training affects the level of onset of the anaerobic threshold. It improves the following.
- Oxygen delivery to the tissues. This is determined by the oxygen uptake of the lungs, the transport of O_2 by the CVS, and the blood oxygen content.
- The ability of the tissues to extract and use oxygen. This is a function of the capillary density (and therefore ease of diffusion of oxygen from the blood to the muscle tissues), the number of mitochondria, and the quantity of enzymes that support aerobic metabolism.

Muscles functioning under no load will increase little in strength, whereas muscles contracting at >50% of their maximal contractile force will rapidly increase in strength due to muscle hypertrophy. Not only do skeletal muscles hypertrophy during training but the myocardium may be similarly affected. Heart enlargement and increased pumping capacity only occur through endurance training of appropriate duration, frequency, and intensity.

Oxygen consumption in an athletically trained male may increase to around 4000ml/min from a baseline of 250ml/min. The abbreviation for the rate of oxygen usage under maximal aerobic metabolism is $VO_{2\,max}$.
- Athletic training has a progressive effect on increasing $VO_{2\,max}$ although there is a strong genetic influence.
- Athletes tend to have a higher stroke volume than non-athletes, but have a normal cardiac output at rest because of a decreased resting heart rate.

→ Creatine

A muscle cell needs energy more quickly than it can be supplied: an extra storage source is needed. Muscle cells use phosphorylated creatine to store and transport energy within the cell.

The phosphate group can be quickly transferred to ADP to regenerate the ATP necessary for muscle contraction (Figure 8.21). Hydrolysis of creatine phosphate to creatine releases 10.3kcal/mole.

Advantages of this system:

● Phosphorylated creatine represents a buffer stock of energy, which can be provided very quickly.

● It is small, which increases the speed of energy transfer.

It is metabolically inert and is particularly suitable for the loss-free transport of energy. This is in contrast to ATP and ADP, which interact with many enzymes and structural proteins.

The contribution of the various systems of energy production in muscle over time is shown in Figure 8.22. At the onset of exercise, available stores of ATP are used within a couple of seconds. For the fastest conversion of ADP back to ATP, the phosphate group from phosphocreatine is moved onto ADP. The resulting ATP is immediately available for muscular work.

There is enough phosphocreatine to keep ATP levels up for several more seconds, allowing almost 10sec of energy for the muscles (ATP + creatine).

The body can recharge creatine back to phosphocreatine in less than 60sec. This ATP + creatine system (shown schematically in Figure 8.21) makes up the fastest component of the anaerobic system, and is most used by power athletes.

Endurance athletes rely on the production of energy from the aerobic system of FA metabolism, a slower process that can produce vast quantities of energy for prolonged periods (Figure 8.24).

Creatine comes from two sources:

● Dietary (animal flesh).

● Internally manufactured by the liver and kidneys from glycine, arginine, and methionine.

A 70kg adult has 120g of creatine in the muscles, with a daily turnover of 2g. 50% of this is replaced by the diet and the rest is synthesized. The endogenous production of creatine is negatively influenced by exogenous intake.

Creatine is eliminated from the body by the kidneys as either creatine or creatinine, which is formed from the non-enzymatic degradation of creatine.

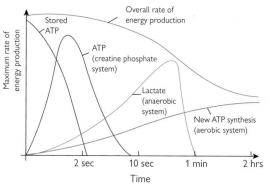

Fig. 8.22 Rate of energy production.

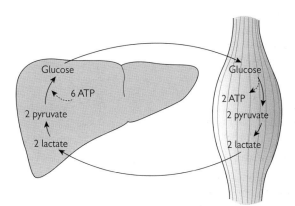

Fig. 8.23 The Cori cycle.

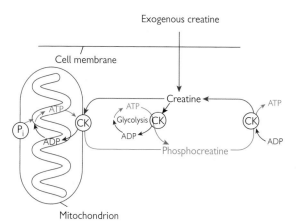

Fig. 8.21 Cellular shuttle of creatine phosphate–ATP: CK, creatine kinase; Pi, phosphate

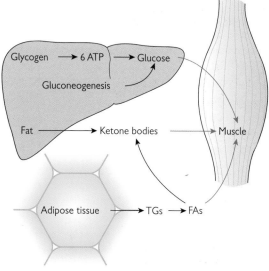

Fig. 8.24 Effect of exercise on metabolism. Energy from fatty acid metabolism requires oxygen since fatty acids enter the tricarboxylic acid (Krebs) cycle as acetyl CoA.

Chapter 9

Autonomic nervous system

Topics covered elsewhere

- The adrenal glands (Section 18.3)
- Disorders of the adrenal glands (Section 18.4)

9.1 The autonomic nervous system

Other than innervation of the skeletal muscle, the autonomic nervous system conveys all output from the CNS. There are three components:

- The sympathetic system
- The parasympathetic system
- The enteric nervous system.

The enteric system is able to function independently of the CNS, but the other two cannot function without it. A schematic diagram of the parasympathetic and sympathetic nervous systems is shown in Figure 9.1. The effects and receptor types are given in Table 9.6.

Sympathetic system

Pre-ganglionic cell bodies lie in the lateral horn of the grey matter of the thoracic and lumbar spinal cord. On leaving the cord, they may follow different routes.

- Most synapse in the para-vertebral sympathetic chain.
- A few synapse in the unpaired pre-vertebral ganglia within the peritoneum, eventually innervating the abdominal and pelvic viscera.
- Fewer still do not synapse at all and innervate the adrenal medulla. This is modified post-ganglionic tissue.

Each pre-ganglionic fibre branches and makes connections at several different ganglia. The post-ganglionic fibres of the sympathetic chain rejoin the spinal nerves, travelling along this route until they reach their destination.

Parasympathetic

The cranial outflow

This consists of pre-ganglionic fibres of cranial nerves III, VII, IX, and X. The ganglia lie adjacent to the target organ and the post-ganglionic fibres are very short.

The sacral outflow

Fibres leave the cord in a bundle of nerves known as the nervi erigentes. They synapse in the pelvis at a number of ganglia that also carry sympathetic fibres. The two systems are anatomically indistinct at this point.

Enteric system

There are probably more cells in this system than there are in the spinal cord. It consists of neurons within the intramural plexuses of the gastrointestinal tract. It is pharmacologically complex and involves many different transmitters and neuropeptides.

It receives input from both the sympathetic and the parasympathetic systems. Some neurons provide local reflex pathways that control function independently of this supply.

It controls the secretory and the motor functions of the gut.

Function

Although there is a specific role for the sympathetic system during emergencies, minute-to-minute, the whole system controls many varied local functions.

In some places the two systems produce opposing effects:

- Heart.
- Gut smooth muscle.
- Bladder smooth muscle.

In some places, only one system operates:

- Blood vessels (sympathetic)
- Sweat glands (sympathetic)
- Ciliary muscle (parasympathetic).

In some places the situation is more complex:

- Bronchial smooth muscle has only parasympathetic innervation but it is very sensitive to circulating catecholamines
- Resistance arterioles only have sympathetic innervation; but sympathetic function is opposed by nitric oxide.

Transmitters

Acetyl choline and noradrenaline have well-defined, traditional roles as neurotransmitters. They are released at synapses, cross the synaptic cleft and act on post-synaptic receptors to elicit intracellular effects. However, there are additional mechanisms that need to be considered. Pre- and postsynaptic effects are often referred to as neuromodulation: a mediator changes the action of another neurotransmitter.

Presynaptic modulation

The process of synthesis and release of the neurotransmitter is affected by the transmitter, and other substances, produced locally:

- Homotropic: the transmitter binds to presynaptic receptors and affects the terminal from which it is released.
- Heterotropic: one neurotransmitter affects the release of another.

Presynaptic receptors affect release of neurotransmitter by regulating the entry of calcium into the cell. Action potential arrival opens voltage-gated N-type Ca^{2+} channels, allowing calcium into the cell.

- Adenylyl cyclase (GPCR regulation) facilitates Ca^{2+} entry.
- Phospholipase C (GPCR regulation) inhibits Ca^{2+} entry.

Postsynaptic modulation

This appears to be due to changes in Ca^{2+} and K^+ channel function, mediated by a second messenger.

Co-transmission

ACh and noradrenaline are not the only ANS neurotransmitters. Many individual autonomic neurons contain several different effector molecules and release more than one transmitter. These effector molecules are often active at both pre- and postsynaptic receptors, affecting both transmitter release and the effect produced.

The proportions of transmitters released may be influenced by other factors. Neuropeptide Y (NPY) and noradrenaline are stored in different vesicles, but the former is released at high frequencies of stimulation and has been shown to reduce the release of noradrenaline in the rat vas deferens.

A combination of effectors will produce different results. Potentially, summation produces a rapid onset *and* prolonged duration.

For example, in the sympathetic system:

- ACh produces a rapid response
- Nitric oxide produces an intermediate response
- Vasoactive intestinal polypeptide (VIP) produces a slow response.

In the parasympathetic system:

- ATP produces a rapid response
- Noradrenaline produces an intermediate response
- NPY produces a slow response.

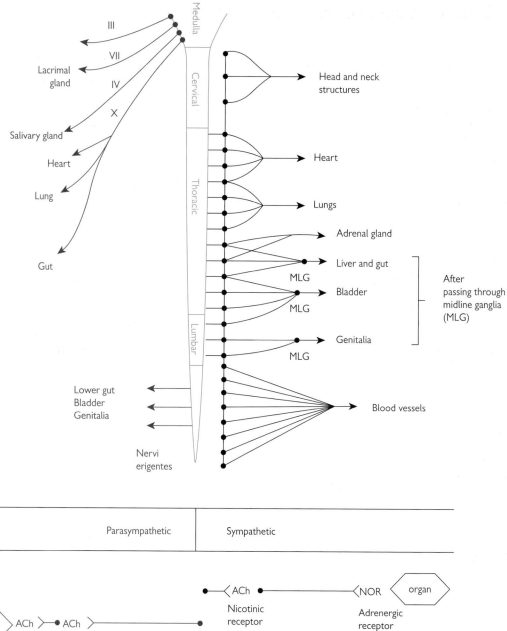

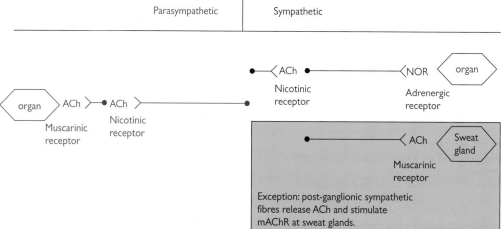

Fig. 9.1 Anatomy of the autonomic nervous system.

9.2 Parasympathetic transmission

ACh can assume three-dimensional structures that are similar to muscarine and nicotine. It can interact with these quite different receptor proteins because of its molecular flexibility. ACh is an agonist at both nicotinic and muscarinic receptors but is more potent at the latter.

The neurotransmitter at both sympathetic and parasympathetic ganglia is ACh. The main receptors at the autonomic ganglia are nicotinic.

Nicotinic receptors

Nicotine: alkaloid extract from *Nicotiana tobacum*.

Nicotinic acetyl choline receptors (nAChRs) are ligand-gated ion channels. In muscle, there is a strict pentameric structure, but within the ganglia and brain there are many receptor subtypes that have different subunit compositions, and different pharmacological and biophysical properties. 17 subunits have been identified, including nine different α and four different β types. The molecular weight of each is 40–58kDa.

Broadly, each of the subunits contains four transmembrane α helices, and one from each subunit (the M2 helix) lines the transmembrane pore. The M2 helix contains a single residue which determines whether the pore is cation-selective (excitatory) or anion-selective (inhibitory, as in the case of GABA receptors).

There is a physical constriction within the pore formed by angulation of each of the lining α helices. The ACh binding sites lie at each α subunit N-terminal, and both need to be occupied in order to open the pore. ACh binding induces a conformational change at the constriction and opens the channel.

There are two types of nAChR. They are structurally similar but differ in their subunit composition. Although pharmacologically distinct, both are ionotropic receptors:

- **Nicotinic muscle (Nm):** found at the NMJ.
- **Nicotinic neuronal (Nn):** found in the CNS and in the parasympathetic ganglia.

They are diverse in structure. The Nn subunits have been divided into four subfamilies (I–IV) based on similarities in protein sequence. In addition, subfamily III has been further divided into three tribes.

The receptor subtypes can be further subdivided:

- **Homomeric:** formed of only one type of subunit eg α7-α9.
- **Heteromeric:** formed from α and β subunits.

Muscarinic receptors

Muscarine is the poisonous ingredient of the fungus *Amanita muscarina*.

There are five types of muscarinic receptors and they are all G-protein coupled (metabotropic). They are all blocked by atropine.

- M1, M2, and M3 are well characterized. Their features are summarised in Table 9.1.
- M4 and M5 are less well understood.

The different types are classified according to which agonists and antagonists react with them.

- M1, M3, and M5 couple to Gq/11 and act via the inositol phosphate pathway.
- M2 and M4 couple to Gi/o and act by inhibiting adenylate cyclase.

The overall effects of muscarinic agonists and antagonists are shown in Table 9.2.

Postganglionic parasympathetic fibre ACh release

M2 receptors autoinhibit release of ACh in a similar manner to the action of presynaptic α_2 receptors in the adrenergic neuron.

Unlike the NMJ, there is no obvious synaptic cleft. ACh has to diffuse a great distance to muscarinic receptors.

ACh release at autonomic ganglia

ACh is synthesized, stored, and released in a similar manner to that of the neuromuscular junction (Section 8.1).

Some ACh is hydrolysed within the cleft before receptor interaction. At the receptor, the ACh is hydrolysed within 1ms.

The amount of ACh released and the number of AChR activated is 100x less than at the NMJ: muscle cells are much larger than neurons and require a larger synaptic current for activation of an AP.

Initial stimulation of the nicotinic receptors (nAChR) produces a fast EPSP or an EPP, followed by:

- Slow IPSP. 2-5 secs duration. Hyperpolarising: K^+ conductance increases. M2 receptor mediated, although dopamine and adenosine assist.
- Slow EPSP. 10 secs duration. M1 mediated K^+ channels closure.
- A late slow EPSP. 1-2 minutes duration. K^+ conductance reduction mediated by peptide co-transmitters such as substance P.

Ganglion stimulants

Nicotinic receptor agonists may affect both ganglia and the motor end plate but some are selective. See Table 9.3.

Ganglion blocking drugs

These may act in several different ways.

- Prevention of ACh release e.g. botulinum, Mg^{2+} and hemicholinium.
- Prolonged depolarization: Nicotine
- Post-synaptic interference by blocking nAChR or ion channels.

Clinical effects

Arteriolar vasodilatation and hypotension result from blockade of sympathetic ganglia. There is blockade of the cardiovascular reflexes. This produces postural hypotension and post-exercise hypotension. Other signs include:

- Skin: warm and dry
- Dry mouth and throat
- Bladder: retention of urine and impotence
- Gut: poor gastric motility with constipation
- Eye: failure of accommodation with mydriasis. Absence of tears
- Temperature control: marked heat loss and tendency to hypothermia.

Anaesthetic implications

Their many side effects have rendered this class of drugs obsolete. Trimetophan was formerly used for hypotensive anaesthesia.

Tubocurarine causes some blockade at the autonomic ganglia and was formerly used as part of a hypotensive anaesthetic technique.

Table 9.1 Important features of M1, M2 and M3 receptors

M1 'Neural'	Found in CNS and PNS, and in gastric parietal cells	Act via inositol phosphate pathway Exert excitatory effects $\downarrow K^+$ conductance, causing membrane depolarization.	Deficiency of this receptor possibly associated with dementia
M2 'Cardiac'	Found in cardiac atria and conducting tissue, and in presynaptic terminals	Inhibit adenylate cyclase Exert inhibitory effects $\uparrow K^+$ conductance and inhibit Ca^{2+} channels	Slow the heart and reduce the force of contraction
M3 'Glandular'	Found in smooth muscle, vascular endothelium, and glandular tissue	Act via inositol phosphate pathway Exert excitatory effects	Stimulation of glandular secretion and contraction of visceral smooth muscle May also cause vasodilatation via NO

Table 9.2 Clinical effects of muscarinic agonists and antagonists

Muscarinic agonist (e.g. ACh, muscarine, carbachol, pilocarpine)	System	Muscarinic antagonist (e.g. atropine, hyoscine, ipatropium, pirenzepine)
Reduced HR Reduced CO Mainly due to a reduced force of atrial contraction: the ventricles have few muscarinic receptors and little parasympathetic innervation	**CVS**	Increased HR HR response to exercise is unchanged BP unchanged Resistance vessels have little parasympathetic innervation
Contraction	**Bronchial smooth muscle**	Relaxation
Increased peristalsis	**GI smooth muscle**	Reduced motility. Large doses are required
Contraction	**Bladder smooth muscle**	Relaxation
Increased	**Sweating** **Lacrimation** **Salivation** **Bronchial secretion**	Reduced
Pupillary constriction Accommodation	**Eye**	Pupilary dilatation Cycloplegia
	CNS	Excitation, restlessness, agitation

Table 9.3 Parasympathetic receptor agonists and antagonists

Agonists	Methacholine		Dimethylphenylpiperazinium	Suxamethonium
	Muscarine		Nicotine	
	Carbamylcholine			
	Acetylcholine			
Receptor	M1 Neural	M2 Cardiac	M3 Glandular	Nn Nicotinic neuronal-type	Nm Nicotinic muscle-type
Antagonist	Atropine			Nicotine	
	Pirenzipine	AF-DX 116	Tiotropium	Hexamethonium/trimetaphan	Tubocurarine

Lobeline: a tobacco plant extract and partial nicotine agonist, which has been used in commercial preparations to help stop smoking. There is no evidence that it works.

Noradrenergic cell bodies lie within sympathetic ganglia. The cells' axons are long and branched. The branches have numerous varicosities, each of which houses a large number of noradrenaline-containing vesicles.

Noradrenaline synthesis

The synthetic pathway is illustrated in Figure 9.2

Phenylethanolamine N-methyltransferase (PNMT) catalyses the methylation of noradrenaline to adrenaline. It is found in the brain and also in the adrenal medulla, in cells that liberate adrenaline. PNMT is not present at birth but develops in response to steroid influence.

Drugs affecting noradrenaline synthesis

Methyldopa

Used today mainly in the treatment of hypertension of late pregnancy. It is taken up, decarboxylated, and hydroxylated to form the false transmitter α-methylnoradrenaline. It displaces noradrenaline from the vesicles.

It accumulates because it is not metabolized by MAO. On release it acts (weakly) on α_1 receptors and (more strongly) on α_2 receptors. In this way it produces its action: the α_2 stimulation effects significant auto-inhibition.

It has a central and peripheral action. Side effects include immune haemolytic reactions, liver toxicity, and sedation.

Noradrenaline storage

Each vesicle contains between 1500 and 15000 molecules of noradrenaline; little is found free within the cytoplasm. A specific transporter that uses the transvesical proton gradient as its driving force maintains this concentration difference. Noradrenaline forms a complex with ATP and chromogranin A and this helps limit the amount that diffuses out into the cytoplasm.

ATP has a transmitter function: it produces the fast EPSP at smooth muscle cells.

Drugs affecting noradrenaline storage

Reserpine

Reserpine binds to the transport protein and blocks the uptake of noradrenaline into terminal vesicles. Noradrenaline is degraded by MOA in the cytoplasm, and levels fall sufficiently to effectively block adrenergic transmission.

Reserpine also depletes 5-HT stores and dopamine, resulting in depression.

Noradrenaline release

The arrival of an action potential stimulates release of vesicular noradrenaline in the same manner as at any other synapse. However, there are some important differences between the adrenergic neuron and the focused anatomical relationships of the NMJ.

- An impulse will only discharge a few hundred vesicles although there are thousands of varicosities.
- The vast majority of adrenergic varicosities remain inactive when an action potential arrives.

Presynaptic modulation is an important control mechanism for noradrenaline release and many different substances exert this effect. An overview of the process is shown in Figure 9.3.

Drugs affecting noradrenaline release

Noradrenergic-blocking drugs: guanethidine

Guanethidine is used today for the treatment of complex regional pain syndrome.

It is taken up into vesicles in the same way as noradrenaline. The catecholamine is displaced and undergoes cytosolic metabolism by MAO. The overall effect is similar to that of reserpine. Since it enters the terminal via uptake-1, inhibitors of this route will affect its function.

Additionally, it may interfere with initiation of exocytosis. Long-term use produces structural changes within the neuron.

Indirectly acting sympathomimetic amines

Ephedrine, amphetamine, and tyramine.

Structurally related to noradrenaline, they enter the neuron under the influence of uptake 1. They then inhibit this uptake mechanism. Again in common with reserpine, they displace noradrenaline from the vesicle, some of which is oxidized by MAO in the cytosol. The rest escapes via uptake 1 to act on α_1 receptors. The inhibited uptake 1 mechanism prevents termination, increasing the action of noradrenaline at the receptors. They have weak direct adrenoceptor actions:

Substances that modify adrenergic transmission significantly affect the action of indirectly acting sympathomimetic amines:

- Reserpine depletes the terminal of noradrenaline and abolishes its effects.
- MAO inhibitors dangerously potentiate their effects by preventing the breakdown of cytosolic transmitter, which is then able to escape. This is of special importance for tyramine, which is itself a substrate for MAO. Foods rich in tyramine, such as cheese, can provoke sudden hypertensive crises.

Termination of effect

Re-uptake (uptake 1) is the mechanism responsible for terminating the effect of noradrenaline. Once taken up it is degraded.

Adrenaline is more dependent on uptake 2. It similarly then undergoes degradation.

Uptake 1

- Neuronal.
- High affinity, selective for noradrenaline.
- Low maximum rate of uptake.
- The mechanism co-transports noradrenaline, Na^+, and Cl^-. Changes in the Na^+ gradient can alter the uptake direction.

Uptake 2

- Extra-neuronal.
- Low affinity; route of removal for adrenaline and isoprenaline.
- High maximum rate of uptake.

Degradation

MAO and COMT are the two main enzymes responsible for the degradation of catecholamines, including noradrenaline.

Monoamine oxidase (MAO)

MAO is cytosolic, bound to the mitochondrial surface membrane. It is abundant in noradrenergic nerve terminals but is also found in the liver and the gut epithelium. It can also oxidize other monamines including dopamine.

Catechol-O-methyl transferase (COMT)

COMT is widespread, and is found in many different tissues. It further metabolizes catecholamines and their deaminated products.

Inhibitors of uptake 1

TCAs, cocaine, and amphetamine. The effect of noradrenaline is potentiated.

Amphetamine, guanethidine, and phenoxybenzamine share structural similarities with noradrenaline binding sites. They also act at other points of the sympathetic transmission pathway.

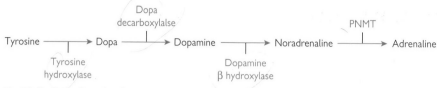

Fig. 9.2 Synthesis of noradrenaline.

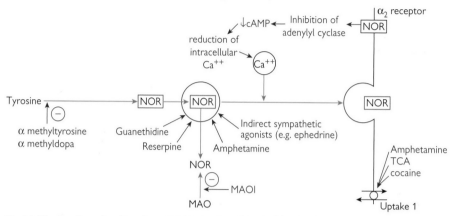

Fig. 9.3 Diagram of noradrenaline release. Inhibition by drugs (blue labels) and the effect of α_2 negative feedback are shown.

→ Anatomy of the sympathetic system and cervical ganglia

Sympathetic outflow only occurs from pre-ganglionic cell bodies in the lateral horns of T1–L2. However, the chains extend the whole length of the column.

- Fibres exit the cord via the ventral ramus and enter the sympathetic chain through the white ramus.

Cervical (Figure 9.4, top)

- On entering the ganglion, the fibres have three options:
  - Ascend or descend to synapse in a ganglion at another level.
  - Synapse at that level, rejoining the spinal nerve via the grey ramus.
  - Carry on through the ganglion to synapse within a plexus (cardiac or cardiac).
- The inferior cervical ganglion is fused with that of T1, forming the stellate ganglion.
- The three cervical ganglia have additional vascular branches which distribute sympathetic fibres to major vessels and structures within the skull. This arrangement allows a more complete innervation than would be possible with the somatic and visceral branches alone.
- Cardiac supply: T1–T5. All fibres are post-ganglionic.
- There are cardiac branches from each of the cervical ganglia.

Lumbar (Figure 9.4, bottom)

- L1 and L2 have white rami communicans.
- Lumbar and splanchnic plexus fibres are all pre-ganglionic.

The sympathetic chain T_1–L_2 each segment receives input directly from the cord

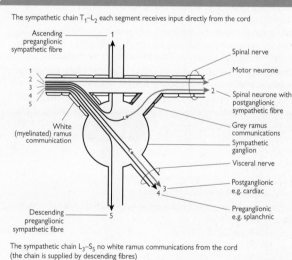

The sympathetic chain L_3–S_5 no white ramus communications from the cord (the chain is supplied by descending fibres)

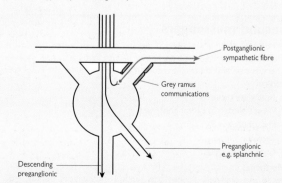

Fig. 9.4 Anatomy of sympathetic system ganglia.

9.4 Adrenergic transduction

Adrenergic receptors are members of the G-protein coupled family. They transduce a signal (such as noradrenaline) into a cellular response with the help of a second messenger.

G proteins

So called because of their interaction with the guanine nucleotides GDP and GTP. G proteins are hetero-trimeric structures with subunits α, β, and γ anchored to the membrane via a fatty acid residue. The various combinations of these subunits produce over 1500 different G proteins: each one demonstrates selectivity for both receptor and effector. The function of G proteins is shown in Figure 9.5.

G-protein coupled receptors (GPCRs)

G protein-coupled receptors (GPRCs) comprise the largest family of receptors with over 1000 different types. They respond to a wide range of extracellular signals and not just catecholamines. These signals include hormones, amines, and even light.

There are several distinct groups of GPCRs:

- Group 1—adrenergic/rhodopsin activated
- Group 2—secretin activated
- Group 3—glutamate and GABA activated
- Group 4—fungal mating pheromone receptors
- Group 5—cyclic AMP receptors
- Group 6—frizzled/smoothened.

Not surprisingly, GPCRs produce their effects by acting with G proteins. Each receptor has an extracellular domain specific for its ligand and an intra-cellular portion between transmembrane proteins 3 and 4 specific to its G protein (Figure 9.6). The specific receptor–G protein coupling will determine which second-messenger system is activated. Some ligands will activate more than one receptor type and the response produced will depend on the downstream effects of the receptor.

Similarly, some GPCRs activate multiple G proteins with the overall response a summation of second messenger actions.

This convoluted process conveys several advantages. There is amplification of the signal and a few thousand receptors can produce millions of second-messenger molecules. It allows integration of input from several stimuli (convergence), and regulation of more than one effector (divergence).

ACh activates five muscarinic receptor subtypes:

- M1, M3, and M5 subtypes couple to Gq/11
- M2 and M4 subtypes couple to Gi/o

Epinephrine (adrenaline) and norepinephrine (noradrenaline) activate three classes of GPCR:

- α_1 couple to Gq/11
- α_2 couple to Gi/o
- β couple to Gs.

Second messengers

When the cellular signalling molecule does not enter the cell it may initiate a defined cascade, known as a second-messenger system. There are several important second messengers, each with its specific control:

- Adenylate cyclase/cAMP
- Phospholipase C/inisitol phosphate
- Phospholipase A_2
- Tyrosine kinase
- Guanylate cyclase.

Hormones usually exert their effect via intracellular receptors. Ligand-gated ion channels do not use second messengers but may be influenced by them.

Control by G protein

Adenylate cyclase, phospholipase C, and phospholipase A_2 are controlled by G proteins.

Adenylate cyclase/cAMP

Cyclic AMP controls many cellular functions and a variety drugs, hormones and neurotransmitters affect its concentration. It is produced continuously by adenylate cyclase and hydrolysed by phosphodiesterases to 5'AMP. G proteins control the function of adenylate cyclase.

Adenylate cyclase is activated by the hormones glucagon and adrenaline and inhibited by adenosine. The activation varies betweeen tissues: liver adenylate cyclase responds more strongly to glucagon, but in muscle adrenaline exerts the stronger effect. In this way, sympathetic stimulation will mobilize glucose for its use in muscles.

Cyclic AMP activates protein kinases (often PKA) that catalyse the phosphorylation of cytoplasmic serine and threonine residues. The target enzyme may be activated or inhibited. Examples include:

- Myosin light chain kinase. This is inactivated by cAMP-dependent protein kinase and produces smooth muscle relaxation. In this way, β-adrenergic stimulation of bronchial smooth muscle will provide relief for asthmatics.
- Conversely, phosphorylation of voltage-activated Ca^{2+} channels in heart muscle increases calcium entry, increasing contractility. This is, again, a product of β stimulation.

G_i inhibits adenylate cyclase and the reduced cAMP concentration is the mechanism of action of M2ACh, α_2, and opioid receptors.

There are tissue-specific phosphodiesterase isoenzymes responsible for the degradation of cAMP. Inhibition of the form expressed in genital blood vessels is the basis of action of sildenafil (Viagra).

Forskolin directly stimulates adenylate cyclase, increasing the concentration of cAMP. It is not used clinically.

Phospholipase C

Different G proteins administer this second-messenger system. Phospholipase C_β splits PIP_2 into IP_3 and DAG, both of which are active.

Inositol phosphate and intracellular calcium

Calcium is actively scavenged and sequestered from the cytoplasm in order to keep its concentration low.

IP3 releases Ca^{2+} and raises its concentration 100-fold. It achieves this by acting on specific receptors on the endoplasmic reticulum, releasing calcium from its vesicular stores within.

Diacylglycerol (DAG) and protein kinase C (PKC)

DAG remains within the membrane (it is lipophilic).

- The raised Ca^{2+} produced by the action of IP_3 on the endoplasmic reticulum is essential for the migration to, and activation of, PKC by DAG.
- PKC is then able to promote phosphorylation of a number of intracellular proteins by acting on their serine and threonine residues.

PKC has a piovotal role of in mediating cellular responses to extracellular stimuli. PKC is not a single enzyme but a family of at least 10 isoforms, classified by their activation requirements.

Phospholipase A_2

Phospholipase A_2 activation occurs in a very similar fashion to activation of phospholipase C_β. It produces arachadonic acid and its metabolites have been shown to influence potassium channel function and also to have a paracrine role:

- Ion channel regulation
- Division of α and $\beta\gamma$ into active moieties.

➔ Types of receptor

Receptors may be integral membrane or intracellular proteins. There are four main superfamilies of membrane receptor.

- **Channel-linked (ionotropic)** These mediate fast responses and affect membrane potential.
- **G-protein coupled receptors (metabotropic)** These mediate slower transmission and affect metabolic processes.
- **Kinase-linked**
- **Receptors containing intrinsic enzyme activity** Gene transcription takes place at intracellular receptors.

Both ionotropic and metabotropic receptors are found in the autonomic nervous system.

➔ Signal transduction

Signal transduction is the conversion of a signal into another stimulus. Diabetes, heart disease and cancer are thought to arise from defects in signal transduction pathways.

Most receptors will respond to only one specific ligand. These are synthesized, stored, and secreted prior to transport to the target cell. Recognition of the ligand by the receptor results produces a conformational change and defined chemical reactions within the cell. These steps amplify the process of response before the ligand is removed from the receptor.

➔ The α subunits

These can be divided into four families based on sequence homology.

G_s family

Permanently stimulates adenylate cyclase. This is the mechanism of the fatal effects of infection with *Vibrio cholerae*. Also used in taste and smell.

G_i family.

Produce inhibition of adenylate cyclase. React with the effector phospholipase.

The pertussis toxin can inhibit most G_i proteins. G_t and G_g proteins have similar sequences and are often included in this group.

G_t protein (transducin) is a component of the light-recognition pathway of retinal cells.

G_g protein is a component of taste recognition for bitter.

G_q family.

Use phospholipase C as effector.

G_{12} family.

Activated by thromboxane and thrombin receptors.

Stimulate p115 RhoGEF, a guanine nucleotide exchange factor for the monomeric G protein RhoA.

They may play a role in cancer metastasis.

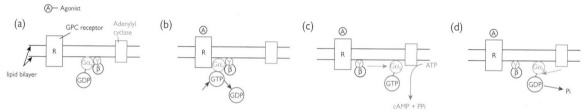

Fig. 9.5 Function of G protein-coupled receptors and G proteins.
(a) When the agonist binds to the GPCR, a conformational change increases its affinity for its G protein. (b) The G protein, with attached GDP molecule, associates with the receptor. Once attached, the G protein releases GDP and binds GTP. (c) This activates the G protein and causes dissociation of the Gα subunit, which activates its second messenger system (in this case, the $Gα_s$ subunit activates adenylyl cyclase). (d) This leads to hydrolysis of the GTP to GDP, in turn causing release of the Gα subunit from the second messenger apparatus and re-association with its β and γ subunits.

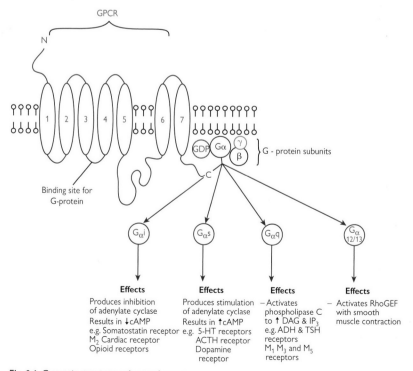

Fig. 9.6 G protein structure and second messengers.

9.5 Adrenergic receptor agonists and antagonists

The sympathetic system orchestrates its effects through the activity of adrenergic neurons and the actions of circulating catecholamines. A table of the autonomic receptor types and their effects is given in Table 9.6. Here we discuss the various drugs which interact with α and β adrenoceptors. A summary of adrenergic receptors is given in Table 9.4; and adrenaline, noradrenaline, and dobutamine are considered in more detail in Table 9.5.

α-adrenergic receptor agonists

Specific α-adrenergic agonists
α_1: Phenylephrine, metaraminol

α_2: Clonidine

Non-specific α-adrenergic agonists
Adrenaline and noradrenaline. Both also have actions at β-adrenergic receptors.

α-adrenergic receptor antagonists

Clinical uses
α blockade causes peripheral vasodilatation and a fall in blood pressure. It is associated with an increase in sympathetic cardiac activity. Concomitant α_2 blockade worsens the reflex tachycardia.

Non-selective α agonists
Phenoxybenzamine has a long duration of action because it binds covalently to the receptor. It also antagonizes at ACh, histamine, and 5-HT receptors. Used as a preoperative treatment for phaeochromocytoma.

Phentolamine binds reversibly and so has a shorter duration of action.

Selective α_1 antagonists
Doxazosin causes less reflex tachycardia than non-selective α agonists, because there is still scope for α_2-mediated reduction of noradrenaline release.

Tamsulosin is used for its ability to relax the smooth muscle of the bladder neck for patients with benign prostatic hypertrophy.

Selective α_2 antagonists
Yohombine is not in clinical use. It causes vasoconstriction, and is used socially as an aphrodisiac.

β-adrenoceptor agonists

Dobutamine (selective β_1 agonist) increases both heart rate and force of contraction, and increases oxygen consumption. Excessive stimulation of β_1 receptors can precipitate, dysrhythmia. β-induced vasodilatation is mediated via endothelial secretion of NO and is a feature of dobutamine use, which reduces SVR via its effect on the muscle vascular bed.

Carbohydrate metabolism is affected by β_1 stimulation: glycogen synthase is inhibited and phosphorylase is enhanced, resulting in increased production of glucose by the liver, and increased G6P (for cellular fuel) in muscle.

Broadly, β stimulation results in relaxation of most types of smooth muscle through the action of cAMP and the inactivation of myosin light chain kinase. β stimulation also results in lower intracellular Ca^{2+} levels, further reducing contraction force. Selective β_2 agonists (e.g. salbutamol) bronchodilate through this mechanism. This group is also used to reduce uterine tension and end premature labour.

β_2 agonists also increase skeletal white (fast) muscle twitch tension through an action on the contractile proteins rather than the muscle membrane. They are on the International Olympic Committee (IOC) of list of banned substances because of their effects on twitch tension, even though red muscle twitch tension is reduced. They also commonly produce tremor.

β-adrenergic receptor antagonists

Heart failure
β-blockers reduce heart rate, prolong diastolic filling and lengthen coronary perfusion time, and lower the myocardial energy expenditure.

They also improve the ejection fraction. In heart failure β-blockers reduce the absolute risk of death by 4.5% over 12 months.

Post MI
β-blockers reduce the incidence of sudden death for at least 25 months following MI. For maximum effectiveness, they should be started within 2 weeks of infarction. MI-associated heart failure is not a contraindication.

Hypertension
β-blockers are no longer considered first-line anti-hytpertensives; they have been shown to increase the incidence of diabetes when used in combination with thiazide diuretics.

They may be used in hypertensive emergencies, e.g. control of BP during aortic root dissection.

Other uses include the treatment of:
- Glaucoma: a more favourable side-effect profile compared with anticholinesterase drugs or muscarinic agonists
- Thyrotoxicosis
- Anxiety states
- Reduction of portal pressure in variceal bleeding
- Migraine prophylaxis
- Benign essential tremor.

Pharmacology
The performance of each drug is related to the following properties.

Degree of receptor specificity: receptor specificity is important in that β_1 agonists are less likely to provoke bronchoconstriction.

Intrinsic sympathomimetic activity: drugs with ISA exert low-level agonist activity whilst also acting as an antagonist. They stimulate β-receptors when levels of catecholamines are low. This is important in those that are excessively bradycardic with β-blockade. They have no benefit post MI and are not useful in angina or for the control of tachycardia.

Membrane-stabilizing activity: some block membrane Na^+ channels, which, at toxic levels, causes prolongation of the QRS complex and impairment of conduction. This group also has a higher incidence of seizure activity.

Lipid solubility: β-blockers that cross the BBB produce nightmares and hallucinations. Lipophilic β-blockers are primarily metabolized by the liver, whereas hydrophilic β-blockers are eliminated more or less unchanged by the kidneys and may be removed by renal replacement therapies.

Class III anti-dysrhythmic activity: sotolol is unique in that it has this activity and might potentiate QT interval lengthening and torsades de pointes.

Complications of B-blockers
- Bronchoconstriction: a problem of non-specific agents.
- Cardiac failure: despite evidence that some patients benefit from β-blockade, others suffer worsening heart function.
- Bradycardia
- Hypoglycaemia: this is of little consequence in the healthy, but in diabetics β-blockers impair recognition of the signs of hypoglycaemia (e.g. ↑HR) and reduce the generation of glucose by the liver.
- Worsening of peripheral vascular disease (PVD). Those with mild to moderate PVD may similarly be given β-blockers safely, but patients with severe PVD (pain at rest, ischaemic ulcers) should probably not receive β-blockers.
- Fatigue: probably associated with an insufficient cardiac output during exercise.
- Cold extremities.
- Bad dreams: the result of penetration of the CNS by lipid-soluble drugs (e.g. propranolol).

Table 9.4 Adrenergic receptor summary

	α₁ Vascular	α Presynaptic	β₁ Heart	β₂ Smooth	β₃ Fat
Agonist	Phenylephrine	Clonidine			
	Methoxamine	α-methyl noradrenaline			
			Dobutamine	Terbutaline	
	Noradrenaline			Salbutamol	Noradrenaline
	Adrenaline				
			Isoprenaline		
Receptors	**α₁** Vascular	**α** Presynaptic	**β₁** Heart	**β₂** Smooth	**β₃** Fat
Antagonists	Labetolol			Labetolol	CGP20712A
	Phentolamine		Propranolol		
	Phenoxybenzamine		Atenolol	Butoxamine	
	Prazosin	Yohombine	Metoprolol		
Potencies	A = NA » Iso	A = NA » Iso	Iso > A = NA	Iso > A » NA	Iso = NA > A

A, adrenaline; NA, noradrenaline; Iso, isoprenaline.

Table 9.5 Characteristics of some adrenergic receptor agonists

	Name	Noradrenaline	Adrenaline	Dobutamine
Properties	Uses	Refractory hypotension	Anaphylactoid and anaphylactic shock Cardiac arrest Low cardiac output states ↑duration of action of LAs Reduction of IOP in glaucoma	Used to aid cardiac performance in shock states, cardiomyopathy Dobutamine stress testing of the heart
	Chemical	Catecholamine	Catecholamine	Synthetic isoprenaline derivative
	Presentation	Clear colourless solution	Clear colourless solution	Clear colourless solution
	Action	↑SVR	Sympathomimetic	Positive inotrope, mild peripheral vasodilatation
	Mode	Indirect and direct sympathomimetic active at α > β	Direct α and β agonist	Direct β₁ agonist
	Route	IV infusion	IV bolus and infusion; inhaled	IV infusion
Effects	CVS	↑ SVR with ↑BP; reflex ↓HR; ↑renal blood flow in shock states	↑inotrope and chronotrope ↑SVR, ↑BP, ↑HR	↑contractility; ↑SAN automaticity; ↑rate of AV conduction; β₂ vasodilatation causes ↓SVR
	RS	↑MV and mild bronchodilation	↑RR and ↑Vₜ, bronchodilator	
	CNS	Weakly mydriatic; ↑CBF proportional to ↑BP	Excitatory effect; weakly mydriatic	Stimulation only at high dose
	GI	↓hepatic & splanchnic blood flow		↑urine OP secondary to ↑CO
	Other	↓insulin secretion, ↑glucagon, ↑glycogenolysis and so ↑[glucose] ↑contractility of the pregnant uterus leading to fetal asphyxia	↓insulin secretion, ↑glucagon, ↑glycogenolysis and so ↑[glucose] ↑plasma renin ↑FFA concentration ↑BMR and ↑temperature	↓glucose; ↑FFA concentration
Kinetics	Absorption	Very high first-pass metabolism	Slower SC/IM absorption	
	Metabolism	Metabolism by both MAO and COMT resulting in urinary excretion of VMA	Mainly uptake 2 and COMT metabolism, although some uptake 1 and MAO metabolism	COMT deactivation followed by glucuronidation
	Excretion			Excreted in urine
	Toxicity		CNS excitation, CVS ischaemia and dysrhythmia	
	Notes	Co-administration of MAOIs or TCAs results in marked hypertension	Limit the dose with inhalational agents (especially halothane) in order to prevent serious ventricular dysrhythmias	Tachyphylaxis

Table 9.6 Receptor effects within the sympathetic and parasympathetic systems

	Receptor type	Parasympathetic	Organ	Sympathetic	Receptor type
Heart	M2	↓ rate	**SA node**	↑ rate	β_1
	M2	↓ force	**Atrial muscle**	↑ force	β_1
	M2	↓ conduction velocity	**AV node**	↑ automaticity	β_1
	M2	No effect	**Ventricular muscle**	↑ automaticity and force	β_1
Blood vessels	–	No effect	**Veins**	Dilatation	β_2
	–	No effect	**Veins**	Constriction	α
	–	No effect	**Coronary arterioles**	Constriction	α
	–	No effect	**Muscle arterioles**	Dilatation	β_2
	–	No effect	**Viscera arterioles**	Constriction	α
	–	No effect	**Skin arterioles**	Constriction	α
	–	No effect	**Brain arterioles**	Constriction	α
	–	No effect	**Salivaryglands arterioles**	Constriction	α
	M3	Dilatation	**Erectile tissue arterioles**	Constriction	α
Viscera	M3	Erection	**Sex organs**	Ejaculation	α
	M3	Constriction	**Bronchi smooth muscle**	No sympathetic innervation	β_2
	M3	Secretion	**Bronchi glands**	No effect	
	M3	↑ motility	**GI smooth muscle**	↓ motility	$\alpha_1, \alpha_2, \beta_2$
	M3	Dilatation	**GI sphincters**	Constriction	α_2, β_2
	M3	Secretion	**GI glands**	No effect	
	M1	Secretion	**Stomach glands**	No effect	
	–	Variable	**Uterus pregnant**	Constriction	α
	–	Variable	**Uterus non-pregnant**	Relaxation	β_2
Eye	M3	Constriction	**Pupil**	Dilatation	α
	M3	Contraction	**Ciliary muscle**	Relaxation	β
Other	–	No effect	**Sweat secretion**	Secretion (cholinergic fibres)	α
	–	No effect	**Pilomotor**	Piloerection	α
	M3	Secretion	**Salivary secretion**	Secretion	α, β
	M3	Secretion	**Lacrimal secretion**	No effect	
	–	No effect	**Kidney**	Renin secretion	β_2
	–	No effect	**Liver**	Glycogenolysis	α, β_2
	–	No effect	**Liver**	Gluconeogenesis	α, β_2

Chapter 10

Cardiovascular system

10.1 The heart

The circulation rapidly transports oxygen, nutrients, hormones, heat, and waste products around the body.

The circulation can be considered in two parts: the low-pressure pulmonary system and the high-pressure systemic circulation. The energy needed to pump blood around these two systems is derived from contraction of the heart.

Gross anatomy

The heart is a hollow muscular organ consisting of four chambers: the right atrium and ventricle collect blood from the great veins and pump it into the pulmonary circulation. The left atrium collects oxygenated blood from the pulmonary veins and the ventricle pumps it into the systemic circulation.

Blood vessels

The **right coronary artery** (RCA) arises from the anterior aortic sinus. It passes forwards between the right atrium and pulmonary trunk and descends along the atrioventricular groove to the inferior border of the heart where it turns round to the posterior surface and anastomoses with the left coronary artery at the posterior interventricular groove.

The right coronary artery supplies:

- the sinoatrial node in 60% of individuals
- the atrioventricular node in 85% of individuals
- the posterior and inferior parts of the left ventricle.

In 80% of cases, the RCA terminates as the posterior interventricular branch, which supplies the interventricular septum. Conduction abnormalities are commonly associated with occlusion of the right coronary artery.

The **left coronary artery** arises from the posterior aortic sinus. It passes forward behind the pulmonary trunk and then divides in the space between the aorta and the pulmonary artery into the left anterior descending artery and the circumflex branch. The left anterior descending artery passes along the anterior interventricular groove towards the apex, turns round the lower border, and anastomoses with the posterior interventricular artery

The **circumflex artery** passes around the left border of the heart to reach the posterior interventricular groove. It supplies

- The sinoatrial node in 40% of individuals
- The lateral wall of the ventricle via the marginal arteries.

The blood vessels of the heart are demonstrated in Figure 10.1.

Myocardial blood supply

Basal blood flow in the myocardium is 70–80ml/100g/min. The maximum is 300–400ml/100g/min.

The blood supply to the myocardium flows from the left and right coronary arteries. Because of the high intramural pressure during systole, most of the flow takes place during diastole. While these arteries anastomose with each other, this is insufficient to maintain a collateral circulation. They are functional end arteries.

The coronary perfusion pressure is the difference between aortic root diastolic pressure and left ventricular end diastolic (LVEDP) pressure. In effect myocardial capillaries function as a Starling resistor. In systole, driving pressure and LV pressure are the same, so flow to the left ventricle will cease. In the right ventricle, pressures are lower so some flow will take place during systole. (Figure 10.3)

Systolic pressure is not transmitted equally to all parts of the ventricular wall; the epicardial arteries are slightly removed from this intraventricular pressure. This may further impact on flow.

Systemic vasoactive agents (e.g. adrenaline, AVP) may influence the tone of large and small coronary vessels. Platelets (serotonin, ADP) also release substances that affect vascular tone.

Coronary blood flow and autoregulation

At rest the heart extracts 70–80% of the oxygen delivered to it. Myocardial metabolism can only significantly increase with increased coronary blood flow and oxygen supply. Marked reactive hyperaemia is seen when coronary blood flow is interrupted for as little as 1sec.

The coronary circulation shows considerable autoregulation. The calibre of the vessels (and hence blood flow) is influenced by pressure changes in the aorta, and also by chemical and neural factors.

Chemical factors

The close relationship between coronary blood flow and myocardial oxygen consumption implies that products of metabolism cause coronary vasodilatation. The leading suspects are oxygen deficiency and increased local concentrations of CO_2, H^+, K^+, lactate, prostaglandins, adenine nucleotides, and adenosine. More than one of these vasodilator metabolites may be involved.

Asphyxia, hypoxia and intracoronary injections of cyanide all increase coronary blood flow by 200–300% in both denervated and intact hearts. Myocardial tissue hypoxia is common to these three stimuli.

During exercise, coronary flow increases 4–5 times: metabolic autoregulation counteracts sympathetically mediated vasoconstriction.

Neural factors

The coronary arterioles contain:

- α-adrenoceptors, which mediate vasoconstriction.
- β-adrenoceptors, which mediate vasodilation.

Stimulation of noradrenergic nerves to the heart and injections of noradrenaline cause vasodilation. However, both simultaneously increase heart rate and the force of cardiac contraction: the vasodilation is due to production of vasodilator metabolites in the myocardium secondary to the increase in its activity. When the inotropic and chronotropic effects of noradrenaline discharge are blocked by β-adrenergic blocking drugs in unanaesthetized animals, stimulation of the noradrenergic nerves or injection of noradrenaline elicits coronary vasoconstriction. Thus the *direct* effect of noradrenergic stimulation is constriction rather than dilation of the coronary vessels.

Stimulation of myocardial vagal fibres dilates the coronaries.

Special features of the coronary circulation

- Smaller muscle fibres with high capillary density so a shorter diffusion distance.
- High basal oxygen extraction (>60%); this can increase to >90% during exercise.
- Well-developed autoregulation
- Metabolic vasodilation dominates regulation (possibly adenosine, K^+, and acidosis).
- β-adrenoceptors ensure that sympathetic activity causes vasodilation

Venous drainage

Almost all (95%) of the myocardial venous blood drains via the coronary sinus into the right atrium. This is a continuation of the great cardiac vein and enters the right atrium near the orifice of the inferior vena cava. Its PO_2 is very low (3kPa). The remaining veins drain directly into the left ventricle and constitute a fixed shunt:

- The thebesian vein.
- The anterior sinusoidal vein.
- The anterior luminal veins.

Pericardium

The heart is separated from the rest of the thoracic viscera by the pericardium. The myocardium is covered by the fibrous epicardium. The pericardial sac normally contains 5–30ml of clear fluid, which lubricates and allows contraction with minimal friction.

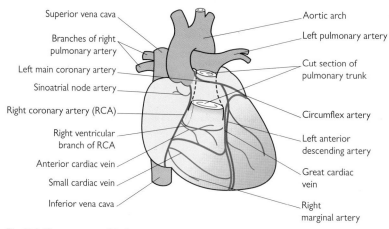

Superior vena cava

Branches of right
pulmonary artery

Left main coronary artery

Sinoatrial node artery

Right coronary artery (RCA)

Right ventricular
branch of RCA

Anterior cardiac vein

Small cardiac vein

Inferior vena cava

Aortic arch

Left pulmonary artery

Cut section of
pulmonary trunk

Circumflex artery

Left anterior
descending artery

Great cardiac
vein

Right
marginal artery

Fig. 10.1 Gross anatomy of the heart.

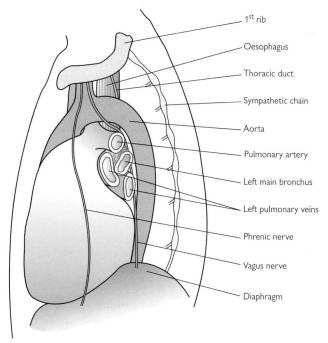

1st rib

Oesophagus

Thoracic duct

Sympathetic chain

Aorta

Pulmonary artery

Left main bronchus

Left pulmonary veins

Phrenic nerve

Vagus nerve

Diaphragm

Fig. 10.2 View of the mediastinum from the left pleural space.

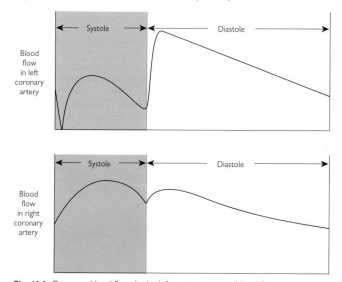

Systole

Diastole

Blood
flow
in left
coronary
artery

Systole

Diastole

Blood
flow
in right
coronary
artery

Fig. 10.3 Coronary blood flow. In the left coronary artery, blood flow occurs predominantly during diastole. In the lower-pressure right heart, blood flow occurs throughout the cardiac cycle.

When the heart contracts, blood is ejected into the vessels of the systemic and pulmonary circulations. These vessels vary depending on the blood pressure and function they perform.

Structure

The systemic vessels comprise:

- Arteries, which supply blood to organs at high pressure
- Arterioles, which are smaller vessels with muscular walls that directly control flow through each capillary bed
- Capillaries which consist of a single layer of endothelial cells; their thin walls allow exchange of nutrients between blood and tissue
- Veins return blood from the capillary beds to the heart. They act as a reservoir, and venous tone is important in maintaining the return of blood to the heart. In severe haemorrhage, sympathetic stimulation causes venoconstriction, with less pooling and more centripetal flow.

All blood vessels except capillaries are made up of three layers: the tunica intima, the tunica media, and the tunica adventitia. The proportion of each layer varies, depending on the function of the vessel and the intraluminal pressure (Figure 10.4).

Arteries

Elastic arteries exit from the heart (e.g. aorta, pulmonary trunk). The aorta is expanded during systole when only a third of the ejected blood volume enters the peripheral circulation, the rest distending the aorta. In diastole the competent aortic valve prevents the return of blood into the LV and the stored potential energy in the wall of the vessel is converted into kinetic energy, propelling the blood forward in a more continuous fashion. Thus the elastic wall of the aorta acts as a second pump, an effect known as hydraulic filtration.

This effect reduces with age. Peripheral vasodilatation with increased run-off causes systemic flow to become more intermittent.

Muscular arteries are low-resistance low-volume high-pressure conduits. They also perform hydraulic filtration.

They have a thinner tunica media than elastic arteries but the internal elastic lamina is prominent and clearly separates the intima from the media. Smooth muscle cells predominate in their tunica media.

The systolic stretching of the wall marches along the vessel (at speeds in the order of metres per second) much quicker than the flow of blood (centimetres per second). It is this pressure wave that is palpated peripherally as the pulse.

Arterioles are the smallest arteries (diameter 0.3 μm or less) (Section 10.3).

Capillaries

Capillary endothelia are surrounded by an underlying basal lamina and occasional pericytes. They have a small radius and so, from Laplace's law, they have a low wall tension and do not need supporting connective tissue.

Pericytes contain actin, myosin, and tropomyocin, suggesting a contractile function for these cells in regulating blood flow through the capillary. There is also evidence that these cells are stimulated to proliferate and differentiate into endothelial and smooth muscle cells following injury.

Three types of capillaries can be distinguished on the basis of their structures and functions.

Continuous capillaries

Found in muscle, brain and connective tissue, they are characterized as a continuous sheet of endothelial cells and joined by tight junctions. Water, O_2, CO_2 and small hydrophilic molecules can diffuse or be transported across the endothelial plasma membrane, but large molecules are transported by transcytosis.

Fenestrated capillaries

Typical of intestines and kidneys. They contain numerous pores 60–80nm in diameter that allow the rapid exchange of water and small molecules.

Sinusoidal capillaries

Found in the liver, bone marrow, and some endocrine glands. They are irregular channels of up to 40μm in diameter that allow the slow circulation of blood. Both the endothelium and the basal laminae of sinusoidal capillaries are discontinuous.

Pressure pulse contours

The pressure waveform varies with progression distally along the arterial tree. Diastolic and mean pressures fall and the systolic pressure wave becomes narrowed. The incisura is lost and the dicrotic notch becomes prominent.

The elderly have stiffer and less compliant vessels, and these changes are not so pronounced. Additionally, the elderly have an impaired upstroke due to reduced myocardial contractility and a higher peak pressure due to reduced aortic compliance.

MAP is the average arterial pressure and approximates to

$$\text{diastolic pressure} + \left(\frac{\text{pulse pressure}}{3} \right)$$

- The pulse pressure (systolic pressure – diastolic pressure) is determined by the stroke volume and the elastance of the arterial system.
- An ↑SV increases SBP but DBP less so, and so pulse pressure will increase.
- Increased elastance (stiffness) means that for the same SV, SBP will rise.

Blood flow

The flow of a Newtonian fluid through a rigid, unbranching cylinder or tube is laminar and governed by Poiseuille's equation, where

$$\text{Flow} = \frac{\pi r^4 \Delta P}{8 \eta l}$$

Where r = radius of the vessel, ΔP = pressure gradient along the tube, η (eta) = fluid viscosity, and l = tube length.

Although this equation is often said to govern blood flow, there are several important deviations from it.

- Blood flow is pulsatile and it is not until the capillary that flow becomes almost continuous.
- Vascular structure: vessels are distensible and are not rigid. The variable compliances offer different pressure–flow relationships.
- Blood viscosity is not constant at a given temperature and changes according to ambient temperature at the skin: cool air encourages stasis and increases viscosity. Increasing the haematocrit from 0.45 to 0.60 doubles viscosity.
- Viscosity also falls with reducing vessel diameter such that the flow of whole blood through capillaries matches that of plasma. In these small vessels, RBCs move to the centre of the vessel, occupying the axial stream. This effect is also seen at high flow rates, where it is known as shear thinning.
- Turbulent flow does not move in discrete laminae but in a disorganized fashion. The flow rate is proportional to the square root of the driving pressure and more energy is required for a given flow rate. The Reynolds number is used to predict when flow will become turbulent (Section 2.7).

However, although the formula is not strictly applicable, small changes in radius will result in large changes in flow rate. This is especially evident in muscular arterioles.

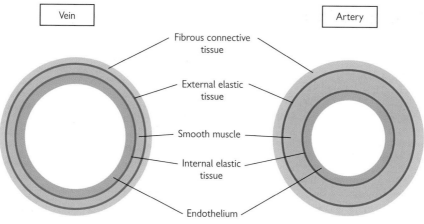

Fig. 10.4 Veins contain 75% of the circulating blood volume, in contrast to the 20% found in the arterial system. Changes in the morphological characteristics of arteries accompany this gradual progression in vessel size.

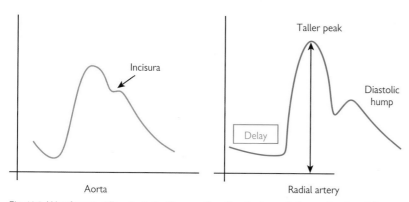

Fig. 10.5 Waveforms in different arteries. The sensation of a pulse is merely the continuation of the pressure wave. It is worth remembering that the pressure wave travels much faster than blood can flow. Its presence indicates that the heart is pumping; it does not mean that blood is flowing within that vessel.

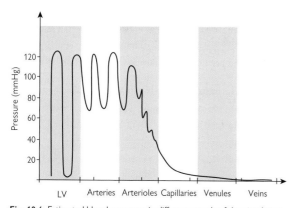

Fig. 10.6 Estimated blood pressures in different vessels of the circulation.

10.3 The circulation II

Arterioles

Arterioles consist of a scant adventitial layer, with one to six layers of smooth muscle surrounding a thin endothelium. They have a number of important clinical effects.

- Control of local blood flow. The diameter of capillaries in different tissue beds varies with organ activity.
- Arterioles affect systemic vascular resistance and blood pressure. They are the major influence on SVR, and since BP = CO × SVR arterioles have a major effect on BP. The sympathetic system, in turn, has a major influence on their resting tone.
- The arterioles of an individual organ bed can change calibre independently of any other vascular bed. The relative vasodilatation of the vascular bed determines the proportion of cardiac output that it will receive.
- Capillary hydrostatic pressure is affected by arteriolar tone. Vasoconstriction reduces downstream hydrostatic pressure, which results in movement of interstitial fluid into the circulation (Section 11.5).
- Arterioles affect distal capillary hydrostatic pressure. Vasoconstriction reduces hydrostatic pressure downstream and increases the flow of fluid from the interstitium to the vascular compartment.

Regulation of local blood flow

Almost all arteriolar beds exhibit autoregulation. The uterine and hepatic portal circulations are maximally vasodilated and are notable exceptions.

Autoregulation allows organs to determine their own flow. There are two major mechanisms for this.

Myogenic

Smooth muscle fibres contract in response to increased pressure: local resistance increases and the flow to the organ remains constant. The reverse happens with a fall in perfusion pressure. This is the most influential mechanism in the arteriolar beds of the brain and kidney.

Metabolic

A number of chemical substances, such as norepinephrine, angiotensin II, vasopressin, endothelin-1, and thromboxane A_2, can cause contraction. Each of these substances binds to specific receptors on the vascular smooth muscle (VSM) cells (or to receptors on the endothelium adjacent to the VSM), which then leads to VSM contraction. The mechanism of contraction involves different signal transduction pathways, all of which converge to increase intracellular calcium. This is of importance in the heart, skeletal muscle, and brain.

In addition to autoregulation, other mechanisms also influence the flow of blood within tissues.

- *Local vasoactive control* Local release of bradykinin by intestinal glands increases blood flow to the gut. The local release of NO synthesized by endothelial cells results in local vasodilatation. Similarly, endothelins and thromboxane A_2 cause vasoconstriction.
- *Sympathetic supply* Arterioles receive rich sympathetic innervation, and this exerts a significant basal tone. α stimulation results in constriction in most vascular beds although $β_2$ stimulation of vessels in skeletal muscle causes vasodilatation. This is important in the skin, kidneys, and gut.
- *Parasympathetic* This is unimportant in humans; only the genitalia have a significant parasympathetic vasodilatatory supply.
- *Hormones*. Adrenaline is released from the adrenal medulla in response to increased sympathetic outflow. It causes either vasoconstriction or vasodilatation depending on the relative proportions of α and β receptors present in the arterioles.

The constancy of supply pressure allows tissues to control their blood flow by adjusting local vascular resistance. The sympathetic nervous system is the major influence maintaining a constant blood pressure. The brain, heart, and kidneys have relatively poor neurogenic control and so their blood flow will not be adversely affected by sympathetically mediated vasoconstriction.

Vascular smooth muscle

The contractile characteristics and the mechanisms that cause contraction of VSM are very different from those in cardiac muscle. VSM undergoes slow sustained tonic contractions, whereas cardiac muscle contractions are rapid and of relatively short duration (a few hundred milliseconds). Although VSM contains actin and myosin, it is not organized into distinct bands. Neither does it have the regulatory protein troponin.

Although not striated, VSM is highly organized and well suited for its role in maintaining tonic contractions and reducing blood vessel lumen diameter (Figure 10.8). As blood flow is proportional to the fourth power of the vessel radius, small changes in VSM tone have large effects on blood pressure and flow.

Different types of stimulus initiate contraction of VSM.

- *Mechanical:* passive stretching of VSM can cause contraction that originates from the smooth muscle itself and therefore is termed a myogenic response
- *Electrical:* depolarization of the VSM cell membrane also elicits contraction. This is most likely due to opening of voltage-dependent L-type Ca^{2+} channels, which cause an increase in the intracellular concentration of calcium.

The terminal ends of arterioles empty into the capillaries, which form a branching and anastamosing network of endothelial tubes (8–10μm in diameter) between arterioles and venules.

Smooth muscle does not contain troponin. Various agents increase intracellular Ca^{2+} through depolarization of the sarcolemma and entry via L-type calcium channels and from release from the sarcoplasmic reticulum. Ryanodine receptors and inisitol triphosphate (ITP) receptor channels, control sarcoplasmic release.

Calcium and calmodulin combine and activate myosin light-chain kinase (MLCK), which results in the phosphorylation of myosin and shortening of the muscle cell. Although calcium levels fall within a few minutes, the force of contraction does not fall immediately. This is possibly because of the persistence of a number of dephosphorylated cross-bridges.

Figure 10.7 is a schematic diagram of excitation-contraction coupling in smooth muscle.

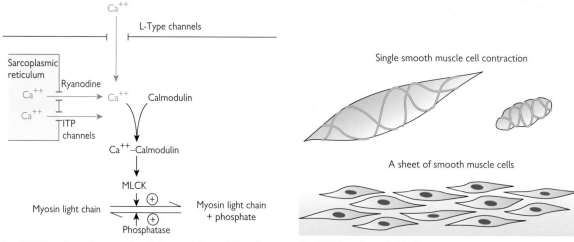

Fig. 10.7 Smooth muscle contraction: An increase in intracellular calcium causes MLCK to phosphorylate myosin, causing muscle shortening.

Fig. 10.8 Smooth muscle histology.

Table 10.1 **The differences between skeletal, smooth, and cardiac muscle**			
	Skeletal muscle	Smooth muscle	Cardiac muscle
Control	Voluntary and involuntary	Involuntary	Involuntary
Stimulation of contraction	Contraction is initiated with nerve AP at each NMJ and then to each muscle cell. Duration of depolarization 5–10msec	Receptor stimulation on the smooth muscle itself or on cells a short distance away; SM is also sensitive to chemical agent stimulation; contraction often appears spontaneous	Pacemaker cells stimulate contraction AP spread by specialized conducting cells; AP also conducted between cells
Muscle spindle	Yes	No	No
Major source of Ca^{2+}	Some entry from the ECF but mostly from the sarcoplasmic reticulum; the dihydropyridine receptor triggers the release of Ca^{2+} from the SR by opening its channels	Regardless of stimulation, signal transduction leads to an increase in Ca^{2+}; this is mostly from the ECF, entering via voltage-gated Ca^{2+} channels	Similar to skeletal muscle
Ca^{2+} binding	Ca^{2+} binds to troponin C; this induces movement of troponin I and reduces its inhibition, allowing exposure of the myosin binding sites.	Ca^{2+} binds to calmodulin upon entry to the cell; the Ca^{2+}–calmodulin complex activates myosin light-chain kinase	Similar to skeletal muscle
Activation of myosin ATPase	Does not need phosphorylation	Active myosin light-chain kinase is required to phosphorylate myosin ATPase; this allows cross-head formation and the process of contraction	Similar to skeletal muscle
Contraction	Usually short-lived and under an element of voluntary control 7.5–100msec but depends on the type of fibre	Typically tonic contractions of long duration; Ca^{2+} is pumped externally by ATP-dependent Ca^{2+} pumps or the Na^+–Ca^{2+} exchanger.	300msec in the ventricles
Resting membrane potential	Stable RMP	No RMP	RMP changes with time (until the threshold potential is reached); this change is under the influence of various factors (Section 10.5)

Veins

Veins function as a low-pressure collection system for the return of blood from the capillary beds to the heart. They are typically classified on the basis of size and, in general, have thinner walls and larger lumens than their companion arteries. Although veins generally conform to the three-layered system already described, the adventitial layer is their thickest tunica.

- **Post-capillary venules** receive blood draining from the capillary bed and have a diameter of 15–20μm. They are similar in appearance to capillary vessels and consist of an endothelium surrounded by a basal lamina with associated pericytes.
- Many **medium-sized veins** contain valves that enable blood to flow in only one direction. Venous return of blood is facilitated by contraction of skeletal muscles which compress the veins within them.
- The **vena cavae** are the largest veins in the body, which empty into the heart. Their thin walls are characterized by longitudinally arranged adventitial smooth muscle.

Venous reservoirs

Generally, the whole venous system can be considered a reservoir, but functionally the most important organs are the lungs, liver, gut, and skin. The spleen has only a minor role.

On standing, there is reflex sympathetic venoconstriction of the veins of the legs, which aims to maintain venous return and cardiac output. In this way leg veins serve a reservoir function. The reflex is mediated via the low-pressure baroreceptors of the veno-atrial junction.

Venous distensibility

Veins have low elastance and so can accommodate large volumes with relatively little change in pressure. At low pressures, veins collapse and their resistance rises, but with larger volumes of blood they distend and thus can be described as being able to buffer blood volume.

In view of the high compliance of veins, posture and hydrostatic pressure significantly influence their diameter.

Venous return

The major factors affecting venous return are as follows.

Venous valves

These allow only unidirectional blood flow.

Respiratory pump

At the onset of inspiration, the combination of the negative intra-thoracic and positive intra-abdominal pressures increases the flow of blood back to the right atrium. Thoracic blood volume increases by 250ml and right ventricular stroke volume increases by 20ml. This change in pressure adversely affects the return of blood to the LV and reduces its SV. During expiration the pressure gradients favour reduced venous return and a 5% increase in left ventricular stroke volume.

In vigorous exercise, subdiaphragmatic IVC partially collapses during inspiration due to increased intra-abdominal pressure. This results in a moderate flow limitation and so the increase in blood flow through the right heart is not as great as might be expected.

Skeletal muscle pump

The rhythmic contraction of skeletal muscles compresses veins and expels blood. The venous valves ensure that this blood is returned to the heart.

Venomotor tone

Sympathetic stimulation reduces the compliance and increases venous return to the heart in response to hypovolaemia and exercise.

The effect of the cardiac cycle

During the early rapid ventricular filling of diastole, atrial pressure falls, facilitating the return of blood from the systemic and pulmonary veins. Similarly, during contraction the fibrous atrioventricular ring is pulled towards the apex, increasing atrial volume, reducing atrial pressure, and increasing venous return (the x-descent; Section 4.6).

The pressure gradient for venous return

The mean systemic filling pressure (MSFP) is an assessment of the hydrostatic filling of the CVS. It is the static pressure in the system following cardiac arrest and equilibration between the veins and the arteries. In this somewhat artificial setting, the arterial pressure falls more than the venous pressure rises, largely because of the difference in compliance between the two systems.

In the intact person, the MSFP approximates to the mean venous pressure. The pressure gradient across the venous system is the major determinant of blood flow back to the heart where

$$\text{venous return} = \frac{(\text{MSFP} - \text{RAP})}{\text{resistance to venous return}}$$

Systemic vascular resistance (SVR) determines the resistance to venous return. For example, during exercise there is skeletal muscle vasodilatation, an increased venous return, and increased CO.

For any given right atrial pressure (RAP) and SVR, MSFP will govern venous return. It can also be seen that with the higher right heart pressures of heart failure, venous return suffers as a result of the reduced pressure gradient for return (the distensibility of the venous system allows blood to pool).

Cardiac output and venous return

Although there is minor variability with phase of ventilation, CO must equal VR within a short period of time.

Curves can be drawn for both CO and VR against RAP. The point at which these curves intersect is the equilibrium point, and is the RAP at which the CO and VR are equal. This is the operating point for the circulation at that circulating volume and level of sympathetic stimulation. If either circulating volume or level of sympathetic stimulation change, the equilibrium point will also change.

Two mechanisms are important in equilibrating cardiac output with venous return.

Heterometric autoregulation

As predicted by Starling's law, increased venous return will increase ventricular end-diastolic volume and produce a greater force of contraction and stroke volume. Similarly stretching of the sinoatrial node fibres will also increase heart rate, albeit modestly.

This is important in keeping left and right outputs matched and is a very rapid response to change in venous return.

Homeometric autoregulation

There are also autoregulatory changes that result from an increase in intracellular Ca^{2+} availability. This causes an increase in contractility which is independent of both pre- and afterload.

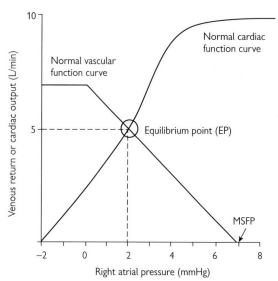

Fig. 10.9 MFSP is the point where RAP is so high that VR ceases. The plateau of venous return develops as RAP becomes more negative. Extrathoracic veins collapse at −4mmHg pressure and act as Starling resistors. This is the major limiting factor for venous return.

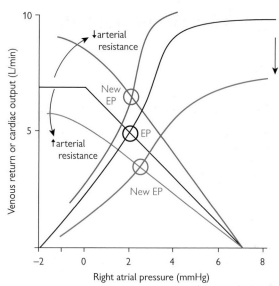

Fig. 10.11 Resistance and MSFP. 2% of blood is contained within the arterioles. Vasoconstriction reduces venous return and CO and rotates the curve anticlockwise. Vasodilatation has the opposite effect. Increased arterial resistance (one cause of an increased afterload) will also cause depression of the cardiac function curve and a new equilibrium point.

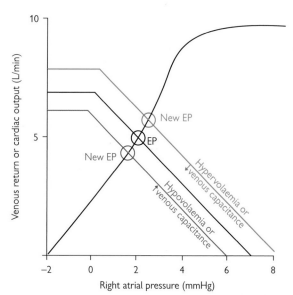

Fig. 10.10 Volume and MSFP Changes in venous tone and blood volume do not affect the position of the cardiac function curve. However, they do affect the vascular function curve and so the equilibrium point is changed. Reduced venous capacitance (e.g. as with vasoconstrictor administration or sympathetic stimulation) has an identical effect to that of hypervolaemia. Increased capacitance approximates to hypovolaemia.

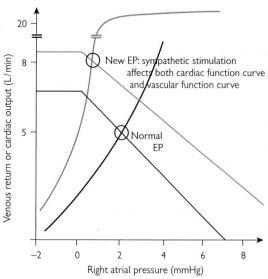

Fig. 10.12 Effect of sympathetic stimulation. A significant amount of the increased CO is related to the venoconstriction and elevation of the MSFP curve. The new CO increases as a result of changes in HR, SV, and the peripheral circulation that alters venous return. High sympathetic blockade produces opposite changes: the cardiac function curve moves to the right and the vascular function curve moves to the left. The equilibrium point is reduced.

10.5 Control of heart rate

Rhythmicity of the heart

Although almost all cardiac tissue has intrinsic pacemaker activity, the sinoatrial (SA) node fires at the fastest rate, suppressing automatic impulses from the rest of the myocardium. The sinoatrial action potential spreads via gap junctions between the fibres sufficiently quickly to allow simultaneous contraction in both atria. The impulse is conducted to the left atrium via Bachmann's bundle, a special sinoatrial pathway.

Cardiac action potentials

There are two types of cardiac action potential: the slow action potential of pacemaker cells, and the fast action potential of the rest of the myocardium.

SA node: slow response

All cardiac cells produce spontaneous action potentials but the SA node produces them the most rapidly. Therefore it functions as the pacemaker. It measures 2mm × 8mm and is located at the junction of the right atrium and the SVC. The resting discharge rate is 100/min without ANS influence. It is made up of two types of cell:

- Long elongated cells
- Small round cells that probably act as the pacemakers.

The membrane potentials of cells in the SA node differ from those of other cardiac cells. There are only three phases (Figure 10.13):

- *Phase 4* There is a fall in K$^+$ permeability (reduced potassium conductance, gK$^+$) and an increase in inward Na$^+$ slow current: the 'funny' potential (I_f). T channels open and increase Ca^{2+} permeability (I_{Ca-T}); this inward movement of calcium drives the electrogenic calcium sodium exchange mechanism.
- *Phase 0* When the membrane potential reaches a critical threshold potential of about –40mV, L-type calcium channels open, resulting in depolarization. *Thus, in contrast with other cardiac cells, the depolarization phase of the action potential in the SA node cells results mainly from the increase in calcium ion permeability.* Because the movement of calcium is not rapid, the slope (rate of depolarization) is not steep. Involvement of the fast sodium channel is negligible and T-channel activity is similarly terminated.
- *Phase 3* Similar to that in non-pacemaker cells, although the absolute refractory period in pacemaker cells is longer. Produced by the outward movement of K$^+$ following an increase in its permeability. L-type Ca^{2+} channels close.

Atrioventricular (AV) node

This lies at the base of the RA near the coronary sinus. It contains fewer round cells and is the only conduction pathway between the atria and the ventricles. It has three zones:

- AN: transitional, between atria and AVN
- N: nodal
- NH: the origin of the bundle of His.

The transitional and node zones are responsible for the 0.1sec delay in the action potential between the atria and the ventricles. It is this that allows the atria to finish filling the ventricles before ventricular systole.

The action potential of cells in the AV node also depends on slow calcium channels rather than fast sodium channels. This acts to slow conduction through the AV node, allowing sufficient delay between atrial and ventricular contraction.

Phase 4 is slower than that of the SA node, which means that the SA node will act as pacemaker.

Ventricular conduction

1cm beyond the AV ring the bundle of His splits into the left and right bundles. These further divide, ultimately supplying the Purkinje fibres that innervate the ventricular cells. Purkinje fibres exhibit very fast conduction and this allows rapid ventricular activation. They have a long refractory period and this helps to block abnormal atrial impulses. Like all cardiac tissue, they have innate rhythmicity.

The endocardial surfaces depolarize first and the wave then spreads to the epicardial surface: the outside of the thinner right ventricle depolarizes before the left. Both apices contract before the body and this makes the contraction efficient.

Myocardium: fast response

- *Phase 0*. When the cell depolarizes, sodium channels in the membrane open and greatly increase the permeability to sodium. Sodium then enters the cell, making the interior positive.
- *Phase 1* Almost as soon as the fast sodium channels have opened, they start to close and sodium permeability returns to the resting state.
- *Phase 2* As the potential of the cell membrane becomes more positive voltage-gated calcium channels open. This allows calcium to enter the cell, initiating crossbridge formation and muscle contraction. The slow calcium channels remain open for approximately 300–400msec giving the myocardial action potential its characteristic plateau phase.

The long plateau is important for two reasons. During this phase the heart is refractory and cannot respond to a further stimulus. As a result the heart contracts as a single unit and, under normal circumstances, cannot undergo a tetanic contraction.

The long plateau also allows calcium to enter the cell and so increases the force of contraction. During contraction calcium is also released from stores within the sarcoplasmic reticulum.

- *Phase 3* Following depolarization the slow calcium channels close and calcium is removed from the cell by a passive sodium–calcium exchange mechanism and an active calcium pump. Free intracellular calcium is also reduced by re-uptake into the sarcoplasmic reticulum. As the free intracellular calcium concentration falls, contraction is terminated. As the permeabilities for sodium, calcium, and potassium return to normal, the cells repolarize.
- *Phase 4* Like all excitable tissue the cardiac myocyte has a resting membrane potential. This potential is formed from the chemical and electrical balance between the ions on both sides of the cell membrane, and is about –80mV. The concentrations of sodium and potassium are maintained by the membrane sodium–potassium pumps. The resting cell membrane is relatively more permeable to potassium, and as potassium leaks out of the cell down its concentration gradient it changes the resting membrane potential, tending to make it depolarize.

Cardiac output and heart rate

The heart acts as a demand pump in that it supplies blood in response to changes in the tissues, which demonstrate metabolic autoregulation. As tissue activity increases, there is vasodilatation and increased venous return, which increases cardiac output according to the mechanism of Starling's law.

Primary changes in either HR or SV have little effect on cardiac output in the absence of increased venous return. Without more blood entering from peripheral tissues, large vein transmural pressure would fall, resulting in collapse of the veins that supply the heart. Increasing the heart rate alone would only result in a reduced SV.

This can be demonstrated by measuring cardiac output in response to a changing heart rate by administering atropine or overpacing the subject.

Table 10.2 Types of ion channel involved in the myocardial AP process*

	Channel	Features
Sodium channels	Fast Na+	Phase 0 depolarization of non-pacemaker cardiac action potentials
	Slow Na$^+$	The 'funny' pacemaker current (I_f) in cardiac SAN tissue
Potassium channels	Inward rectifier (I_{ir} or I_{K1})	Maintains phase 4 negative potential in myocardial cells
	Transient outward (I_{to})	Contributes to phase 1 of non-pacemaker cardiac action potentials
	Delayed rectifier (I_{Kr})	Phase 3 repolarization of cardiac action potentials
Potassium channels (not part of the myocardial AP process)*	ATP-sensitive ($I_{K, ATP}$)	K_{ATP} channels; inhibited by ATP; therefore, open when ATP decreases during hypoxia; in vascular smooth muscle, adenosine removes the ATP inhibition and opens these channels, producing vasodilation
	Acetylcholine-activated ($I_{K, ACh}$)	Activated by acetylcholine; Gi-protein coupled
	Calcium-activated ($I_{K, Ca}$ or BK_{Ca})	Open in response to Ca^{2+} influx in vascular smooth muscle
Calcium Channels	L-type (I_{Ca-L})	Slow inward long-lasting current; phase 2 non-pacemaker cardiac action potentials, and phases 4 and 0 of SA and AV nodal cells; important in vascular smooth muscle contraction
	T-type (I_{Ca-T})	Transient current that contributes to phase 4 pacemaker currents in SA and AV nodal cells

*For completeness, other potassium channels are included.

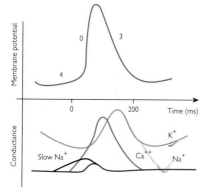

Fig. 10.13 Action potentials and conductance changes at the SAN.

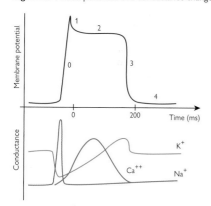

Fig. 10.14 Action potentials and conductance changes at the ventricular myocardium.

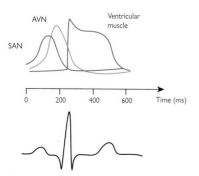

Fig. 10.15 Different action potentials within the heart.

➔ Regulation of heart rate

This occurs through the pacemaker cells within the SA node. Electrophysiological alteration of heart rate can occur in one of three ways:

- Altering the rate of phase 4 depolarization
- Altering the threshold potential
- Altering the resting membrane potential.

Many factors influence SA node activity; in particular, the SA node has an extensive autonomic innervation.

Vagal stimulation results in slowing of the heart rate. ACh released from vagal nerve endings has two effects:

- It increases the permeability of the cell membrane to potassium, increasing the leak of positively charged potassium ions from the cell and thereby increasing the negative cell resting potential.
- It reduces the cell membrane permeability to calcium ions, reducing the slope of phase 4 depolarization.

Sympathetic nerve stimulation and circulating catecholamines increase the heart rate by:

- Increasing the rate of phase 4 depolarization (by increasing calcium ion permeability)
- Lowering the threshold potential.

➔ Refractory period

While the resting membrane potential remains more positive than about −45mV, the cardiac muscle cell is insensitive to further stimulation (absolute refractory period).

Following this, the cell shows reduced sensitivity to additional stimulation (relative refractory period).

Contraction of the muscle cell begins soon after the onset of the action potential and peaks towards the end of the plateau phase. Therefore contraction occurs entirely within the refractory period and consequently heart muscle cannot be tetanized.

10.6 Cardiac cycle

The cardiac cycle refers to the mechanical and electrical events during a single cycle of contraction and relaxation. It describes both the patterns of change observed in individual measurements of mechanical and electrical function and how the timing of events in different chambers of the heart relate to each other.

Atrial pressure

There are three peaks in atrial pressure, known as 'a', 'c', and 'v' waves. Throughout ventricular diastole there is a pressure gradient favouring blood flow through the open AV valve into the ventricle.

- The **a wave:** atrial pressure remains at about 1mmHg until atrial systole, where it peaks at 6mmHg. The atrium then relaxes and ventricular pressure starts to reverse the pressure gradient, closing the AV valve. This is magnified (*giant a wave*) in tricuspid stenosis or pulmonary hypertension (usually in combination with a raised JVP). Intermittent *cannon waves*, where the atrium contracts against a closed tricuspid valve, may be seen in complete heart block.

- The back-pressure on the valve cusps during isovolumic ventricular contraction, causes a secondary rise in atrial pressure, the **c wave**.

- The **x descent** results from atrial lengthening accompanying ventricular contraction. It is not seen in atrial fibrillation (AF).

- Blood continues to enter the atria from the venous system; since the AV valves are closed, there is a steady increase in atrial pressure, the **v wave**. This becomes a very dominant wave in tricuspid regurgitation (accompanied by peripheral oedema and a pulsatile liver).

- The **y descent**: the AV valves reopen as the rapidly falling pressure in the relaxing ventricle drops below that in the atrium. In tricuspid stenosis, this is slow to fall.

Ventricular pressure

This is the simplest of the three relevant pressure waves. During most of ventricular diastole, intraventricular pressure is <1mmHg. Atrial systole raises it to 5mmHg at the end of diastole.

As the atrium relaxes, the pressure falls but ventricular systole, or contraction, then commences and pressure rises rapidly, reaching a peak of about 120mmHg in the left ventricle.

The waveform in the right ventricle is identical in shape to the left but the peak pressure during systole is only 25mmHg. Again, the pressure falls back to its original low value as the ventricle relaxes in diastole.

As heart rate increases, diastole shortens and cardiac pumping becomes inefficient due to inadequate ventricular filling.

Aortic pressure

During ventricular diastole, there is a gradual decline in aortic pressure to a minimum of about 80mmHg. Throughout this period, aortic pressure is higher than left ventricular pressure and so the aortic valve remains closed.

During systole, the ventricular pressure rises above aortic pressure, opening the valve and allowing blood to be ejected into the aorta. Aortic pressure follows ventricular pressure closely during systole, peaking at about 120mmHg, but as the pressure in the ventricles start to decline there is a much slower drop in aortic pressure. This reflects the elasticity of the aorta, which is stretched by the rapid inflow of blood during ventricular systole. The stored elastic energy is then released during diastole as the walls of the aorta passively recoil, thus maintaining aortic pressure.

As a result, the aortic and ventricular pressure waves cross once more and the aortic valve closes. This halts the backflow of blood towards the ventricle and the force generated as the momentum of this blood is dissipated shows up as a brief increase in aortic pressure—the dicrotic notch.

Pressures in the pulmonary trunk follow a similar pattern but are much lower at 25/10mHg compared with 120/80mmHg for the aorta. This reflects the lower resistance of the pulmonary circulation; pulmonary and systemic blood flow is almost equal.

Ventricular performance

In systole, the atria and then the ventricles contract, ejecting blood into both the pulmonary and systemic circulations. Following systole, the four chambers relax sequentially.

The pressure–volume area represents the total external work performed by the heart and its heat generated during contraction. It is a reflection of the amount of oxygen comsumed during each systole.

The pressure increase of isovolumic contraction is converted into heat energy since no external work is done. The potential energy available during contraction agrees closely with the heat released during systole.

Myocardial oxygen consumption

Myocardial work is measured as the product of pressure and volume, but the oxygen cost depends on how that work is performed. For the same cardiac output (product), the cost is greater when higher pressures are involved, rather than higher volumes.

The major determinants of myocardial oxygen consumption are:

- Ventricular wall tension
- Contractility
- Heart rate.

Other factors that have a lesser effect include:

- Basal energy metabolism. Although this is 25% of the total, it is relatively constant.
- Energy for electrical activation. This is less than 1% of the total.
- External work performed has been shown experimentally to correlate poorly with cardiac oxygen consumption.

Clinical estimation of myocardial oxygen consumption requires measurement of both arterial and venous content (with sampling from the both the aortic root and the coronary sinus) and estimation of the total coronary flow. This application of the Fick technique is clearly impractical.

The tension time index is the area under the LV pressure–time curve during systole. It has been shown to reflect myocardial oxygen consumption when contractility is held constant.

Other myocardial substrates

Substrate utilization is determined by availability: the amount used is proportional to its supply concentration. The myocardium takes up glucose under the influence of insulin, and metabolism of this carbohydrate produces 40% of the heart's energy. Fatty acids supply the other 60%, although ketones may be used when conditions dictate.

Myocardial blood flow and oxygen consumption are tightly coupled. The coronary circulation has a very high oxygen extraction ratio and blood returning via the coronary sinus has PO_2 <3kPa. The heart relies heavily on aerobic metabolism.

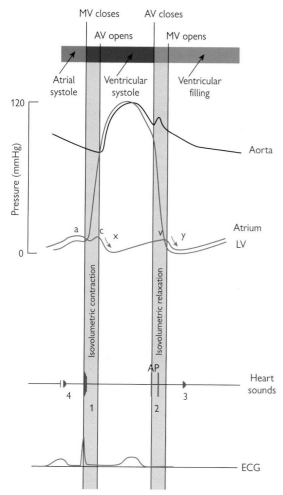

Fig. 10.16 Pressure changes within the chambers of the heart, and their correlation with heart sounds and the ECG. The cardiac output (CO) is the product of heart rate (HR) and the volume of blood ejected per cycle, stroke volume (SV):

$$CO = HR \times SV.$$

→ **Left ventricular pressure–volume loop**

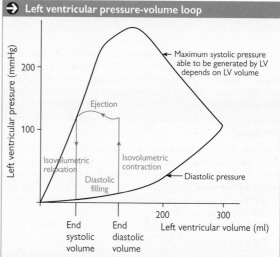

Fig. 10.17 Pressure–volume loop for the left ventricle The maximum systolic pressure is the sum of pressure developed during systole and diastolic pressure.

- Opening of the mitral valve indicates the start of ventricular filling.
- Closure of the mitral valve at the start of systole, the isovolumic contraction phase.
- Opening of the aortic valve at the start of ventricular ejection.
- Closure of the aortic valve at the start of the isovolumetric relaxation phase
- Closure of the aortic valve at the start of the isovolumetric relaxation phase.

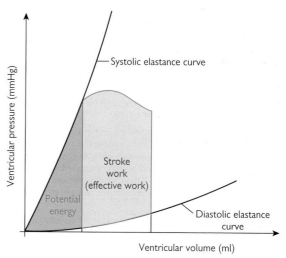

Fig. 10.18 Left ventricle pressure–volume relationship of diastole, and stroke work and potential energy. The effective work (EW) performed by the ventricle in raising the pressure and ejecting the SV is the area of the loop. The total work of the ventricle is EW plus the potential energy (PE).

The quantity of blood ejected from the ventricle is known as the stroke volume (SV). The SV does not stay constant, but changes from minute to minute (and indeed from beat to beat), under the influence of various factors, including preload, afterload, cardiac contractility, and ventricular function.

Preload

Stretching the muscle fibres prior to contraction enhances their subsequent contractile energy (illustrated in Figure 10.22). This is Starling's law of the heart (the force–length relationship). Stretching increases the force of contraction by:

- Changing the geometry of the actin and myosin so allowing more cross-bridges to form
- Increasing sensitivity to intracellular calcium
- Promoting sarcoplasmic Ca^{2+} release.

The greater the force of contraction, the greater the ejected stroke volume will be. Figure 10.19a shows the relationship between preload (as indicated by increased LVEDV) and stroke volume.

In the intact heart the LVED volume is an index of preload. This is difficult to measure, so the LVED pressure is used instead, although ventricular elastance must be considered.

Clinically, right heart preload is estimated from the mean CVP. Left ventricular preload is assessed using the pulmonary artery occlusion pressure (PAOP). When the pulmonary artery catheter is in place and the balloon is inflated, there is a continuous column of blood between its tip and the left atrium. This column is uninterrupted, is of low resistance, and is at the same horizontal level. Left atrial pressure is almost the same as the LVED pressure and so the PAOP can be used as an estimation of preload.

This relationship fails when there is a significant difference in the pressure between the tip of the catheter and the left ventricle (e.g. mitral stenosis or COPD).

Using CVP to determine intravascular filling

Many factors affect the pressure of the central venous compartment, including circulating blood volume, right heart function, pulmonary vascular pressure, degree of sympathetic stimulation, intrathoracic pressure, lung volume, and the presence of pleural fluid or gas. Many of these factors change with time. Therefore, single CVP readings are of limited use in steering fluid management; observation of trends gives a better guide.

When measuring the CVP, one is really trying to make an inference about volume: the elastance equation relates the two parameters, where elastance is the change in pressure per unit change in volume (the inverse of compliance). The CVP should rise, and remain elevated, in response to intravascular filling. If the CVP falls, remains unchanged, or rises and then falls, the venous compartment (at least) still has room for more fluid.

What fluid should be used? Any that stays within the vascular compartment is acceptable, but remember that the volume of isotonic crystalloid will be distributed across the entire ECF, unlike colloid which initially, at least, will remain in the vascular space. For the reasons described above, CVP is likely to change with time and so the response to filling should be checked regularly.

Afterload

This is the force opposing shortening of the muscle fibres during contraction. It can also be described as the tension that develops in the muscle during contraction which approximates to Laplace's law:

$$T = \frac{P \times R}{2W}$$

where T is the tension in the ventricular muscle wall, P is the pressure in the ventricle, R is the radius of the ventricle, and W is the wall thickness.

Increasing the pressure in the ventricle, increasing the diameter of the ventricle, and reducing ventricular wall thickness will all increase the wall tension and hence afterload.

A reduction in pressure and ventricular diameter together with an increase in wall thickness will all reduce afterload.

Afterload changes *during* ejection because of the changing geometry of the ventricle and pressure gradients within the ventricular cavity. In the normal heart wall, thickness and ventricular diameter vary only with the cardiac cycle; hence the cavity pressure, which is related to blood pressure, is the major variable determining afterload.

Increases in afterload will decrease stroke volume (Figure 10.19b). Arterial vasodilation will reduce the pressure in the ventricle, reducing afterload and so increasing stroke volume.

Contractility

This is a change in the contractile energy of the heart not related to changes in fibre length or afterload.

Contractility generally changes with factors external to the myocyte, such as extracellular calcium levels and the degree of sympathetic stimulation.

For a given muscle fibre with a constant preload, if the contractility is increased (positive inotropic state), then the force and rate of contraction will increase together with the stroke volume (Figure 10.19c). An estimate of contractility can be made by measuring the maximum rate of pressure increase in the ventricle during the isovolumetric contraction; this is known as dP/dt_{max}.

A problem with this estimation is that it is not independent of myocardial loading factors (pre- and afterload). Technically, it is difficult to measure accurately and so it is not routinely used.

Ventricular systolic function

Normal areas of the myocardium contract concentrically. Myocardium damaged by ischaemia is usually akinetic or shows abnormal movement. These dyskinetic areas paradoxically move outward during systole and often contain very little active myocardium. Wall motion abnormalities usually indicate local coronary artery disease. Normal myocardium compensates for areas of damage (provided that they are not too extensive) by increased muscle shortening.

Ventricular diastolic function

The major determinants of diastolic performance are:

- Myocardial recoil and relaxation
- Ventricular compliance
- Atrial function
- Heart rate.

The maximum negative dP/dt during the isovolumetric relaxation phase gives a measure of the heart's ability to relax. Relaxation can be slowed by both pressure and volume overload which primarily prolong contraction. Drugs, such as some catecholamines and phosphodiesterase inhibitors, which enhance the rate and extent of relaxation are known as positive lusiotropes.

Ventricular elastance (stiffness) is the change in pressure per unit change in volume and is the mathematical inverse of compliance (distensibility). Diastolic elastance changes with LV volume and its value is the gradient at any point on the volume–pressure curve (Figure 10.21).

Stiffness increases with conditions that increase the bulk of the LV, such as hypertension, aortic stenosis, and HOCM. It will also worsen with restrictive cardiomyopathy and amyloid infiltration.

Pericardial effusions increase the pressure for any given diastolic ventricular volume. This causes an upshift of the elastance curve.

Abnormalities of diastolic function are illustrated in Figure 10.20.

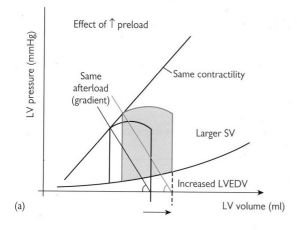

(a)

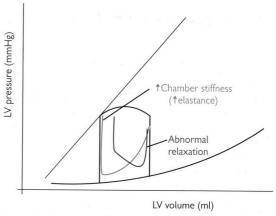

Fig. 10.20 Abnormalities of pressure–volume loops.

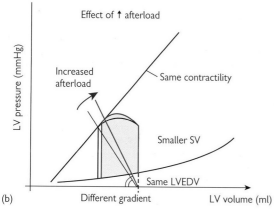

(b)

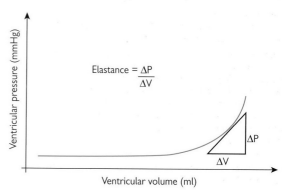

Fig. 10.21 Elastance. The flat part of the curve demonstrates that the ventricle is very easy to fill. The stiffer ventricle is harder to overfill, and because the sarcomere length is not increased much beyond its optimal, the force of contraction will not be too badly affected.

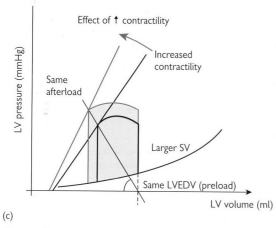

(c)

Fig. 10.19 Pressure–volume loops. The black lines represent normal baseline function.

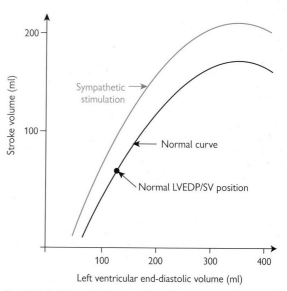

Fig. 10.22 Starling curve. The normal heart lies on the ascending part of the curve.

10.8 CNS control of the cardiovascular system

Many centres within the CNS influence the performance of the cardio-vascular system:

- Medullary premotor sympathetic cells
- Medullary premotor parasympathetic cells
- Cerebral cortex
- Hypothalamus
- Cerebellum
- Periaqueductal grey matter.

The medulla integrates the afferent information and alters autonomic activity accordingly.

Central sympathetic cells

The cells of the rostral ventrolateral medulla (RVLM) moderate blood pressure by integrating inputs from many different sources. They are tonically active and send information via the intermediolateral column of the spinal cord to increase cardiac output and vascular resistance. The tonic activity is inhibited by the baroreceptor reflex. The RVLM cells are able to affect different tissue circulations specifically.

Cells of the caudal ventrolateral medulla (CVLM) influence the activity of the RVLM and act as a cardiovascular depressant. Like the RVLM, the CVLM receives a variety of influences before producing an integrated response.

Central parasympathetic cells

The nucleus ambiguus of the ventrolateral medulla and the dorsal vagal nucleus are the sources of pre-ganglionic parasympathetic fibres. They discharge synchronously with the cardiac cycle because of baroreceptor input from the nucleus tractus solitarius (NTS). Medullary inspiratory neurons directly inhibit parasympathetic firing to cause the tachycardia of inspiration: sinus arrhythmia.

Nucleus tractus solitarius

The NTS is the main site of termination not only for the glossopharyngeal and vagus nerves but also for second-order afferents from other receptors. Therefore the NTS plays an important role in the response to baroreceptor information. Hypertension will lead to:

- An increased parasympathetic output.
- A simultaneous stimulation of CVLM cells which in turn inhibit RVLM activity and sympathetic output.

The NTS also receives input from other parts of the brain, including the higher centres and the RLVM. These afferents probably moderate the information relayed from the baroreceptors, altering the sensitivity of the system.

Ablation of the NTS induces sustained hypertension.

Other CNS influences over CVS responses

Cerebellum

Spinocerebellar pathways send information about joint position and proprioception from muscles and skin. The cerebellum mediates the CVS response at the onset of exercise and in preparation for flight.

Periaqueductal gray matter

Stimulation produces the features of a defence reaction and different PAG regions supply specific cells of the RVLM to induce changes in specific vascular beds.

Hypothalamus

The defence area of the hypothalamus inhibits the baroreceptor response at the NTS.

The depressor area is quite different and enhances the baroreceptor reflex.

Reduced input from the baroreceptors via the NTS will increase production of ADH in the supra-optic nucleus.

Limbic system

Stimulation of one of the components of the limbic system, the amygdala, produces rage and fear and activates the hypothalamic defence area.

Cerebral cortex

This may be important for the onset of responses required at the beginning of exercise.

Receptors

Baroreceptors

Baroreceptors are spray-like nerve endings found in the walls of the carotid sinus and the transverse arch of the aorta. They fire in response to stretch of the vessel: the tunica media of the carotid sinus is thin and relatively more compliant than adjacent arterial wall.

The threshold for firing of the whole group is approximately 60mmHg. Individual receptor nerves have their own narrow thresholds, and these vary: it is the combination of these that provides the baroreceptors with such an effective range of response.

Baroreceptors demonstrate dynamic sensitivity by firing in response to a rapid change in vessel stretch. Their rate of firing varies even within the cardiac cycle, an effect amplified because those that respond to higher pressures are recruited during systole. They demonstrate accommodation where the range of response is reset. This occurs in response to actual blood pressure change, but may also be caused by central mechanisms.

They are responsible for the short-term control of blood pressure only.

Cardiopulmonary receptors

Myelinated vagal veno-atrial stretch receptors send information from the junction of the large veins and the atria about the circulating volume. Both A and B types sense overfilling and produce the Bainbridge reflex:

- Reflex tachycardia due to sympathetic SAN stimulation.
- Water and salt excretion via ANP and reduced ADH secretion.

Unmyelinated vagal and sympathetic mechanoceptors form a network within the atria, especially the LV. They fire during ventricular and, to a lesser extent, atrial systole. They have a role in preventing sustained hypertension

Vagal and sympathetic chemoceptors respond to substances produced by ischaemic cells.

Chemoreceptors

Peripheral chemoeceptors respond to the hypoxia and acidaemia of marked hypotension. They increase sympathetic output at pressures significantly below 60mmHg.

Other reflexes and responses

Other reflexes transiently influence the cardiovascular system. For example, the diving reflex slows the heart and vasoconstricts in response to the application of cold water to the face.

Effectors

- Heart
- Vessels
- Kidneys and water balance

The efferent pathways affect the CVS via the parasympathetic and sympathetic systems and include a number of hormones. Their effects will be considered in more detail later.

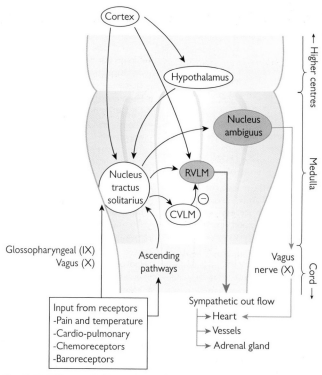

Fig. 10.23 CNS control of the cardiovascular system. Areas that affect the RVLM: input excitation—glutamate; input inhibition—GABA.

➔ **Defence reaction or 'fight or flight' response**

↑Heart rate

↑Cardiac output

↑Blood pressure

Dilatation of skeletal muscle blood vessels

Vasoconstriction of GI and renal blood vessels

➔ **Control of cardiac output**

- The supply of a constant perfusion pressure allows different tissues to determine their own blood flows. This is the responsibility of the nervous system and its reflexes.
- Metabolic activity and autoregulation change the resistance to blood flow within individual organs. This will ultimately affect the systemic vascular resistance.
- If BP remains constant, the tissues control CO as a consequence of their own metabolic activity and autoregulation.
- CNS activity to maintain perfusion pressure causes vasoconstriction in some tissues but the important ones (heart, brain and kidney) remain unaffected by this sympathetic effect.

10.9 Other CVS influences

Exercise

The systemic cardiovascular response to exercise depends on whether muscle contractions are primarily isometric or isotonic with the performance of external work.

Isometric muscle contraction

Heart rate rises with just the thought of performing a muscle contraction: this is probably the result of psychic stimuli acting on the medulla oblongata. The increase is largely due to decreased vagal tone, although there is increased sympathetic discharge.

Within a few seconds of the onset of an isometric muscle contraction, systolic and diastolic blood pressures rise sharply. Stroke volume changes relatively little and blood flow to the steadily contracting muscles is reduced as a result of compression of blood vessels.

Isotonic muscle contraction

Again, there is a prompt increase in heart rate but also a marked increase in stroke volume. In addition, there is a net fall in total peripheral resistance due to vasodilation in exercising muscles. Consequently, systolic blood pressure rises only moderately, whereas diastolic pressure usually remains unchanged or falls.

This difference in response occurs because, unlike isotonic exercise, in isometric activity the muscles are tonically contracted and consequently contribute to increased total peripheral resistance.

During isotonic exercise cardiac output is increased to values that may exceed 35L/min, the amount being proportional to the increase in oxygen consumption. The maximum heart rate achieved during exercise decreases with age.

There is a large increase in venous return, although this is not the primary cause of the increase in cardiac output. Venous return is increased by:

- The large increase in the activity of the muscle and thoracic pumps
- Mobilization of blood from the viscera
- Increased pressure transmitted through the dilated arterioles to the veins
- Noradrenergically-mediated venoconstriction, which decreases the volume of blood in the veins.

The amount of blood mobilized from the splanchnic area and other reservoirs may increase the blood in the arterial portion of the circulation by as much as 30% during strenuous exercise.

After exercise, the blood pressure may transiently drop to subnormal levels, presumably because accumulated metabolites keep the muscle vessels dilated for a short period. However, the blood pressure soon returns to the pre-exercise level. The heart rate returns to normal more slowly.

Blood loss

When blood volume is reduced and venous return is decreased, the arterial and venous baroreceptors are stretched less and sympathetic output is increased. This causes the following (Figure 10.27):

- Reflex tachycardia. With ongoing haemorrhage the heart rate rises even further.
- Increased contractility.
- Venoconstriction.
- Vasoconstriction: This is generalized, sparing only the vessels of the brain and the heart. Vasoconstriction is most marked in the skin, where it accounts for coolness and pallor, and in the kidneys and viscera. The intense vasoconstriction of the splanchnic vessels shifts blood from the visceral reservoir into the systemic circulation.

- Glomerular filtration rate is decreased but renal plasma flow is decreased to a greater extent, so that the filtration fraction increases.
- Haemorrhage is a potent stimulus to adrenal medullary secretion. Circulating noradrenaline is also increased.
- Plasma renin activity is increased, leading to increased circulating angiotensin II. This is followed by increased aldosterone secretion. The increased levels of aldosterone cause retention of Na^+ and water, which helps to re-expand the blood volume. However, aldosterone takes about 30min to exert its effect.
- The CNS ischaemic response is the most potent cause of sympathetic outflow stimulation, caused by a reduction in medullary blood flow and local acid accumulation. It is a last ditch attempt to maintain blood flow to the brain.

ADH release is stimulated by a 20% reduction in blood volume and is sensed in the high-pressure baroreceptors of the arch and sinus. Hypovolaemia is a much more potent stimulus to release than change in osmolality. It causes:

- Vasoconstriction
- Conservation of water at the kidney.

The change in Starling's forces at the capillary moves fluid from the interstitium to the circulating compartment. This is an efficient process and up to 1L/hr is moved in this way.

Increased ACTH levels are found following trauma, and cortisol increases the responsiveness of vessels to catecholamine stimulation.

Haemorrhage reduces oxygen delivery to the carotid and aortic bodies. Anaemia, stagnant hypoxia, and acidosis stimulate these chemoreceptors and are probably the main cause of the respiratory stimulation of shock.

Standing up

The tendency is for blood to pool in the legs, with a resulting fall in both cardiac output and blood pressure. The carotid baroreceptors stimulate a sympathetic response that produces peripheral vasoconstriction (more) and venoconstriction (less), increased heart rate, and increased contractility. These combine to increase blood pressure and maintain cerebral perfusion.

On standing, hydrostatic pressure changes reduce cerebral perfusion, although brisk walking and the ensuing effect of the muscle pump soon restore this deficit.

In the elderly, these responses are less pronounced and are worsened by comorbidity and medication (e.g. ACE inhibitors and β-blockers).

Anaesthesia

All the volatile anaesthetic agents are myocardial depressants. The extent of this depression varies with the particular agent. Systemic hypotension occurs predominantly as a result of a reduction in systemic vascular resistance. A reflex tachycardia suggests that the carotid sinus reflex is preserved.

The heart is not sensitized to catecholamines with the commonly used volatile agents except for halothane, which is now infrequently used in the UK.

There is a dose-dependent reduction in cardiac output and blood pressure with intravenous anaesthetics, except for ketamine which increases cardiac output. Etomidate causes only slight cardiovascular depression.

→ The Valsalva manoeuvre

The Valsalva manoeuvre (Figure 10.24) is a simple test of the baroreceptor reflex. The patient tries to breathe out forcefully against a closed larynx (straining), resulting in an increased intrathoracic pressure.

Phase 1

Brief period where increased intrathoracic pressure increases return of blood to the left heart. Starling's law increases SV and BP also rises because of the increased intrathoracic pressure itself. The baroreceptor reflex reduces heart rate.

Phase 2

Blood pressure falls with failure of venous return. Sympathetic stimulation causes ↑HR and vasoconstriction. The aim is to maintain BP but organ perfusion suffers.

Phase 3

After release of straining, the BP and CO fall for several beats since venous return to the left heart falls as the reduced pressure allows pulmonary vessels to dilate. HR is unchanged.

Phase 4

CO is restored as venous return to the left heart returns but the peripheries are still vasoconstricted so ↑BP results. Baroreceptors sense the BP overshoot and ↓HR.

HR responses are less obvious in the elderly.

The square wave response of congestive cardiac failure (Figure 10.25)

↑BP during phase 2 and no ↑BP when the strain is released. The abnormal response is probably due to the increased reservoir of blood within the pulmonary vasculature.

Absent overshoot (Figure 10.26)

This is a feature of autonomic dysfunction.

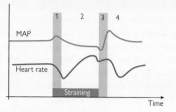

Fig. 10.24 The Valsalva manoeuvre.

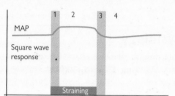

Fig. 10.25 Square-wave response

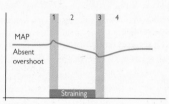

Fig. 10.26 Absent overshoot

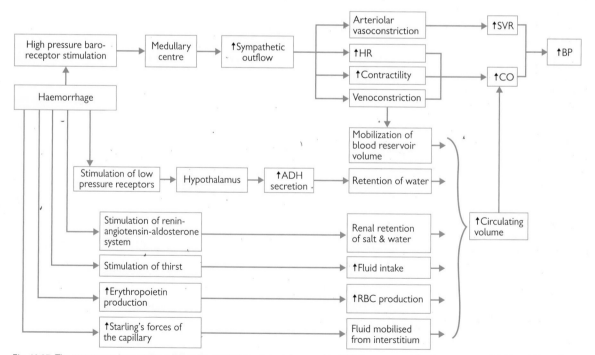

Fig. 10.27 The response to haemorrhage. When the circulating volume is increased by 20%, the reverse of the above sequence is initiated. The only way to return CO and BP to normal is to excrete excess fluid.

Myocardial ischaemia can occur as a result of increased myocardial oxygen demand, reduced myocardial oxygen supply, or both. With incomplete coronary obstruction, an increase in myocardial oxygen requirement caused by exercise, tachycardia, or emotion leads to a transitory imbalance known as demand ischaemia. This is responsible for most episodes of chronic stable angina.

Supply ischaemia, is responsible for myocardial infarction (MI) and most episodes of unstable angina (UA), and is caused by occlusion of the coronary vessels.

Pathophysiology

Ischaemic heart disease (IHD) is characterized by the presence of coronary artery stenoses. Plaques increase resistance: the longer the lesion, the greater the resistance. Two parallel stenoses compound the problem.

In addition to physical obstruction, there are a number of important endothelial effects that determine disease evolution and the progression of angina to an acute coronary syndrome.

Endothelial vasodilatation

Nitric oxide (NO) secretion in epicardial arteries causes vasodilatation. Substances which act similarly include serotonin, histamine, bradykinin, and substance P. The response to these substances is markedly impaired in patients with atherosclerosis. This loss of response occurs even prior to detection of atherosclerosis by angiography. This loss of NO bioavailability is related to risk factors for atherosclerosis and is caused by both reduced synthesis and accelerated breakdown of NO.

Endothelial function is impaired in atherosclerosis, and risk factors for atherosclerosis play an important role in the development of acute coronary syndromes. In the presence of coronary artery stenosis, loss of endothelium-dependent dilation puts even stable angina patients at risk of myocardial ischaemia. Epicardial arteries need to dilate during exercise; however, paradoxical vasoconstriction often occurs at the site of coronary stenoses.

Serotonin and other products of platelet aggregation and thrombosis cause paradoxical coronary artery constriction in the presence of plaque fissuring or rupture, a hallmark of unstable angina and MI. Indeed, patients with unstable coronary syndromes have augmented release of serotonin into the coronary circulation.

NO is an important anti-atherogenic and plaque-stabilizing substance. Reduced levels of NO not only enhance vasoconstriction at sites of disrupted atherosclerotic plaques but also destabilize these plaques.

Endothelial hyperpolarization

Endothelium-derived hyperpolarization factor (EDHF) has been proposed as a mediator of endothelium-dependent vasodilation. It produces hyperpolarization of the underlying smooth muscle through activation of Ca^{2+}-activated K^+ channels in vascular smooth muscle cells. EDHF is upregulated as NO levels fall, helping to maintain coronary artery vasodilatation.

Endothelial vasoconstriction

The endothelium is also a source of vasoconstrictor factors, characterized by endothelins (e.g. ET-1). Plasma concentrations of ET-1 are raised in a variety of CVS diseases including hypercholesterolaemia, hypertension, atherosclerosis, acute MI, and congestive heart failure. Macrophages and activated smooth muscle cells also produce ET-1, and are found in high numbers in vulnerable or ruptured plaques.

Plaque evolution

Plaque formation starts relatively early in life (Figure 10.28). Macrophages accumulate at future plaque sites and incorporate cholesterol to become 'foam cells'. A lipid-rich core develops with further cell accumulation and, over this sits a fibrous cap. The plaque grows outwards at first and this is accompanied by compensatory vessel enlargement (known as positive vessel remodelling). Initially it does not impact on vessel patency. Later, the more advanced plaque becomes calcified.

Endovascular plaques eventually thicken and rupture, exposing a thrombogenic surface upon which platelets aggregate with formation of thrombus. The excessive mortality rate of coronary heart disease is primarily due to rupture and thrombosis of the atherosclerotic plaque. Patients with STEMI usually have vessels occluded by thrombus, with angiographic evidence seen in more than 90% of patients.

Local inflammation causes plaque destabilization, and systemic inflammatory, thrombotic, and haemodynamic factors lead to clot formation. The role of the platelet is central: it contributes to both plaque inflammation and thrombosis.

Coronary artery inflammation

Arterial inflammation may be caused by or related to infection or precipitated by extrinsic causes such as fever, tachycardia, thyrotoxicosis, hypotension, anaemia, or hypoxaemia. Cocaine-related coronary artery dissection is an unusual cause of acute coronary syndrome (ACS). Other rare causes include Marfan's syndrome; Kawasaki disease; Takayasu arteritis, and dissection of coronary aneurysms.

Clinical features of IHD

When myocardial oxygen demand increases, coronary artery narrowing becomes clinically significant and results in angina.

Angina is usually described as a sensation of chest pressure or heaviness, which is reproduced by activities or conditions that increase myocardial oxygen demand. Some present with only neck, jaw, ear, arm, or epigastric discomfort. Associated symptoms include exertional dyspnoea that resolves with pain or rest, decreased exercise tolerance, nausea from vagal stimulation. and diaphoresis from sympathetic discharge.

Elderly persons and those with diabetes may have particularly subtle presentations and present with non-specific symptoms.

As many as half of cases of ACS are clinically silent in that they do not cause the classic symptoms described above and consequently go unrecognized by the patient.

Stable angina

- Episodic pain lasting 5–15min
- Provoked by exertion and relieved by rest or nitroglycerin.

Variant angina (Prinzmetal angina)

Occurs primarily at rest and is thought to be due to coronary vasospasm, triggered by smoking. It is frequently seen in connective tissue disease.

Unstable angina

A change in pattern or severity of symptoms, e.g. increasing frequency or duration or refractory to nitroglycerin or angina at rest. Patients have increased risk for adverse cardiac events, such as MI or death.

Myocardial damage

The clinical findings are similar to angina but last longer and are frequently associated with ventricular complications and signs of shock.

Examination findings

The patient will usually lie quietly in bed and may appear anxious, sweaty, and pale. Hypertension may precipitate angina or reflect sympathetic activity. Hypotension indicates poor ventricular performance or acute valvular dysfunction. Cardiogenic shock is associated with signs of organ insufficiency.

Dyslipidaemia (elevated LDL, cholesterol, triglyceride, and low HDL)

Hypertension

Diabetes mellitus

Cigarette smoking

Family history of coronary artery disease (CAD)

Ageing

Menopause

Mutations in the enzyme nitric oxide synthetase (NOS)

Hyperhomocystinaemia

➕ **Treatment options for angina**

- Treatment for the underlying risk factors
- *β-blockers:* reduce myocardial VO_2 by reducing HR and inotropy
- *Calcium-channel antagonists:* inhibit calcium ions from entering slow channels and voltage-sensitive areas of vascular smooth muscle and myocardium. Decrease myocardial oxygen demand by reducing peripheral vascular resistance, reducing heart rate by slowing conduction through SA and AV nodes, and reducing ventricular inotropy
- *Long-acting nitrates:* Relax vascular smooth muscle by stimulating intracellular cGMP. Decrease LV pressure (preload) and arterial resistance (afterload), reducing cardiac oxygen demand.
- *Short-acting nitrates* for relief of acute symptoms.
- *Antiplatelet therapy* at the development of ACS.
- *Percutaneous interventions* at the development of ACS.

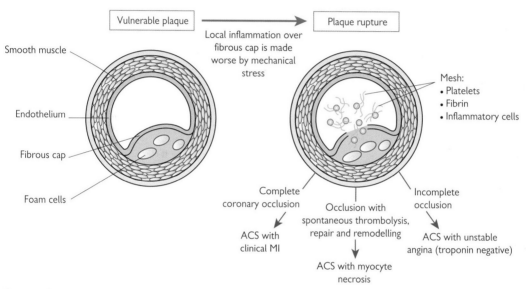

Fig. 10.28 Evolution of plaque rupture and coronary artery occlusion. Foam cells are mononuclear cells which migrate into the intima and phagocytose LDL. Their activation leads to secretion of growth factors and cytokines that both develop the plaque and promote its inflammation and rupture

Table 10.3

The often confusing array of definitions for ACS. British Cardiac Society (BCS) definitions are those now used in the UK. The Myocardial Infarction Audit Project (MINAP) began in late 1998 when a broadly based steering group developed a dataset for acute myocardial infarction (AMI). This allowed clinicians to examine the management of myocardial infarction within their hospitals against targets specified by the National Service Framework for Coronary Heart Disease (NSF) (www.rcplondon.ac.uk).

	• History consistent with diagnosis • ST segment and other ECG changes consistent with MI • Troponin raised	• History consistent with diagnosis • ECG changes consistent with MI • **NO** ST changes • Troponin raised	• Rapid resolution of ST elevation (usually following rapid reperfusion therapies) • Small troponin rise	• Dynamic ECG changes consistent with fluctuating ischaemia • Small troponin rise	• NO troponin rise • Dynamic ECG changes consistent with fluctuating ischaemia
Troponin level	≥1.0	≥1.0	≥0.01 and <1.0	≥0.01 and <1.0	<0.01
BCS terminology	ACS with clinical MI	ACS with clinical MI	ACS with myocardial necrosis	ACS with myocyte necrosis	ACS with unstable angina
MINAP dataset definitions	STEMI	Non-STEMI	MI aborted	Unstable angina (troponin positive)	Unstable angina (troponin negative)
AKA			Threatened MI	ACS troponin positive	ACS troponin negative

The stratification of treatment of myocardial damage depends on

- The changes seen on ECG.
- The results of troponin investigation.

Investigations

Troponin studies

Troponin is a protein that only takes part in the contractile process and therefore is usually absent from the plasma. It is detectable within 3–6hr of MI, remaining elevated for 14 days.

Cardiac and skeletal troponin T and I are encoded by different genes and so are distinctly different from one another. Highly specific assays for cardiac troponins T and I mean that elevated blood levels reliably, albeit with some exceptions, predict cardiac damage.

Troponin I is the preferred diagnostic marker for myocardial necrosis, rising with greater sensitivity and specificity than CK-MB. It has prognostic value: size of infarct, risk of future CVS complications, and risk of death are determined by the degree of troponin elevation and amount of muscle injury. Its biochemical profile makes it particularly useful for those who have coexisting skeletal muscle damage, e.g. following chest trauma.

Troponin T has similar release kinetics to troponin I. Similar to troponin I, levels of troponin T remain elevated for 14 days and also identify those at risk of further cardiac events.

Other causes of troponin levels without other evidence of ACS include:

- Supraventricular tachycardia
- Myocarditis
- Pulmonary embolism
- Sepsis syndrome
- Inflammatory muscle disease
- Renal failure
- Endurance athletes.

Other tests

CK-MB levels begin to rise within 4hr after MI, peak at 18–24hr, and subside over 3–4 days. A level within the reference range does not exclude myocardial necrosis. Serial tests for CK-MB over a 24hr period are required in order to attain a sensitivity near 100% and a specificity of 98%. Small infarcts would be missed if CK-MB alone were used.

Myoglobin is also released from infarcted myocardium and may be detected as early as 2hr after MI. Myoglobin levels are highly sensitive but not cardiac specific.

Cardiac markers should be used at regular intervals in the evaluation of patients with episodes of ischaemic pain, with new changes on ECG, or in those in whom the diagnosis of ACS is being considered.

ECG changes of infarction

See Figure 10.29.

Relevance to anaesthesia

The aims of anaesthesia for the patient with IHD are to maintain adequate oxygen balance and avoid demand ischaemia. This translates as avoiding tachycardia and extremes of blood pressure.

Premedication

Premedication may relieve anxiety and reduce tachycardia, therefore improving myocardial oxygen balance. Studies with preoperative administration of both β-blockers and clonidine have not consistently shown benefit for patients with IHD undergoing non-cardiac surgery.

Induction

Most IV anaesthetic agents are direct myocardial depressants and often further reduce MAP by causing peripheral vasodilatation. These effects are more profound in the hypovolaemic patient, where compensatory tachycardia worsens coronary blood flow. Judicious administration is required.

Ketamine poses a different risk: its indirect sympathetic stimulation increases myocardial work by increasing both afterload and heart rate, neither of which is helpful in this patient group.

Laryngoscopy is a powerful stressor, and should be avoided unless the type of surgery or clinical risk demands it. Fentanyl at 2μg/kg attenuates but does not abolish the response to laryngoscopy.

Standard monitoring allows the anaesthetist to detect potential problems such as increased heart rate and signs of ischaemia (e.g. ST segment changes).

5% of patients over the age of 35 years have asymptomatic ischaemic heart disease. Until recently, anaesthesia and surgery within 3 months of MI carried a 40% risk of perioperative re-infarction. This rate decreases to 15% at 3–6 months and 5% thereafter.

Research findings suggest that, with intensive perioperative monitoring, much lower rates of re-infarction can be achieved (at less than 3 months and at 3–6 months). Mortality from postoperative infarction is 40–60%.

Elective surgery should generally be postponed until 6 months after infarction. Unstable angina is particularly associated with an increased risk of perioperative myocardial infarction.

Maintenance

Volatile agents have variable CVS effects. Although they broadly preserve cardiac output, they cause vasodilation, and isoflurane has been implicated in the 'coronary steal' syndrome. Halothane increases dysrhythmias, especially in the presence of high levels of catecholamine.

High doses of opioids reduce the stressor response to surgery.

Recovery

Reversal of muscle relaxation with a neostigmine and glycopyrrolate causes tachycardia, and extubation in itself is a stressor.
Tachycardia, pain, hypothermia, shivering, hypoxia, and anaemia all worsen oxygen balance. The use of supplemental oxygen in the postoperative period is one of the most effective means of preventing myocardial ischaemia. It should be continued for 3 days postoperatively whilst the patient is still in hospital.

Regional anaesthesia

This has the theoretical advantage of ablating tachycardia and reducing afterload. However, these advantages are outweighed by the hypotension, with attendant reduction in coronary blood flow, that these techniques can produce. Volume loading is essential.

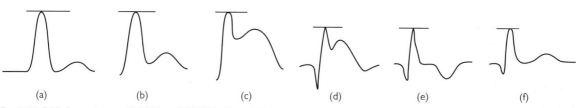

Fig. 10.29 ECG changes in acute MI. (a) Normal. (b) Within hours: ST elevation. (c) Within hours: worsening ST elevation. (d) Within days: reduced R-wave voltage and Q waves. Less ST elevation. (e) Within a week: T-wave inversion develops. (f) Months later: abnormal Q waves and reduced R amplitude persist. T waves return to normal.

263

Table 10.4 **Treatment options for ischaemic heart disease**				
Treatment options	**ACS with clinical MI STEMI**	**ACS with clinical MI NON STEMI**	**ACS with myocyte necrosis**	**ACS with unstable angina**
Aspirin	300mg immediately, continued long term	300mg immediately	300mg immediately	300mg immediately
Clopidogrel	300mg immediately, continued for 4 weeks	300mg immediately, continued for 3 months	300mg immediately	300mg immediately
Glycoprotein IIb/IIIa receptor antagonist	No	Yes	Yes	Yes
LMW heparin	Yes	Yes	Yes	Yes
Fondaparinux	Yes, if not undergoing reperfusion therapy			
Oral β-blocker	Yes, if no CCF or bradycardia, continued long term	Yes, if no CCF or bradycardia, continued long term	Yes, if no CCF or bradycardia, continued long term	Yes, if no CCF or bradycardia, continued long term
24hr tight glycaemic control	Yes, if diabetic	Yes, if diabetic		
Primary percutaneous coronary reperfusion	Yes			
Thrombolytic therapy	Yes, if angioplasty not available within 90min. Fibrin-specific agent, e.g. tissue plasminogen activator			
Rescue percutaneous coronary intervention	Yes, if fail to re-perfuse with thrombolysis, within 6hr of onset of symptoms			
Statins	Yes, prior to discharge, continued long term	Yes, prior to discharge, continued long term	Yes, prior to discharge, continued long term	Yes, prior to discharge, continued long term
ACE inhibitor	Yes, to start within 36 hr, continued long-term.	Yes, to start within 36 hr, continued long-term.	Yes, continued long term	Yes, continued long term
Aldosterone receptor antagonist	Yes, if EF <40%	Yes, if EF <40%		
Non-invasive ventilation	Yes, if cardiogenic pulmonary oedema	Yes, if cardiogenic pulmonary oedema	Yes, if cardiogenic pulmonary oedema	Yes, if cardiogenic pulmonary oedema
Balloon pump support	Yes, if ACS with cardiogenic shock or VSD or papillary muscle rupture with a plan for immediate coronary revascularization	Yes, if ACS with cardiogenic shock or VSD or papillary muscle rupture with a plan for immediate coronary revascularization	Yes, if ACS with cardiogenic shock or VSD or papillary muscle rupture with a plan for immediate coronary revascularization	Yes, if ACS with cardiogenic shock or VSD or papillary muscle rupture with a plan for immediate coronary revascularization
Cardiac surgery	If VSD or papillary rupture within 48hr	If VSD or papillary rupture within 48hr	If VSD or papillary rupture within 48hr	If VSD or papillary rupture within 48hr

Heart failure is seen in 10% of the >75-year-old age group, and is associated with increased mortality following anaesthesia. The most common cause is ischaemic heart disease, but other causes include hypertension, valvular heart disease, and cardiomyopathy. Mortality increases with worsening systolic function: 30% of untreated patients with an ejection fraction of <40% will die within a year.

Heart failure is a multisystem disorder characterized by abnormalities of cardiac muscle, skeletal muscle, and renal function, stimulation of the sympathetic nervous system, and a complex pattern of neurohumoral changes.

Myocardial diastolic dysfunction

This occurs when the ventricle becomes less compliant, which impairs ventricular filling. Both systolic and diastolic dysfunction cause higher ventricular end-diastolic pressure. The Frank–Starling mechanism is recruited to augment stroke volume. (Similarly, with dilated cardiomyopathy, the ventricle dilates as preload pressures increase in an attempt to maintain normal stroke volumes.)

Myocardial systolic dysfunction

The primary abnormality in non-valvular heart failure is impairment in left ventricular function with a fall in cardiac output. Contractility is reduced as a result of alterations in the cell transduction pathways responsible for regulating inotropy. The fall in cardiac output leads to activation of several neurohormonal compensatory mechanisms aimed at improving the mechanical environment of the heart.

Sympathetic system activation maintains cardiac output with an increase in heart rate, increased myocardial contractility, and venoconstriction. Activation of the RAAS results in vasoconstriction (angiotensin) and an increase in blood volume, with retention of salt and water (aldosterone). Concentrations of vasopressin and natriuretic peptides increase. With time, there is progressive cardiac dilatation and remodelling.

The cardiac function curve of heart failure in shown in Figure 10.31.

Neurohormonal activation

Although these compensatory neurohormonal mechanisms of chronic heart failure provide valuable support for the heart in normal physiological circumstances, they also have a fundamental role in the development and subsequent progression of chronic heart failure.

Renin–angiotensin–aldosterone system (RAAS)

Stimulation of the RAAS in heart failure leads to increased concentrations of renin, plasma angiotensin II, and aldosterone. Angiotensin II is a potent vasoconstrictor of the renal (efferent arterioles) and systemic circulations, where it stimulates release of noradrenaline from sympathetic nerve terminals, inhibits vagal tone, and promotes the release of aldosterone. This leads to the retention of sodium and water and the increased excretion of potassium.

In addition, angiotensin II has important effects on cardiac myocytes and may contribute to the endothelial dysfunction that is observed in chronic heart failure.

Sympathetic nervous system

The sympathetic nervous system stimulates increased inotropic and chronotropic activity. However, chronic sympathetic activation has deleterious effects on cardiac function.

The earliest increase in sympathetic activity is detected in the heart, and this seems to precede the increase in sympathetic outflow to skeletal muscle and the kidneys that is present in advanced heart failure.

Sustained sympathetic stimulation activates the RAAS and other neurohormones, leading to increased venous and arterial tone (and greater preload and afterload, respectively), increased plasma noradrenaline concentrations, progressive retention of salt and water, and oedema.

Excessive sympathetic activity is also associated with cardiac myocyte apoptosis, hypertrophy, and focal myocardial necrosis. Longer term, it produces downregulation of α-receptors and baroreceptor dysfunction, both of which further worsen cardiovascular performance.

Natriuretic peptides

There are three natriuretic peptides, with similar structures, which exert a wide range of effects on the heart, kidneys, and CNS.

- Atrial natriuretic peptide (ANP) is released from the atria in response to stretch, leading to natriuresis and vasodilatation.
- In humans, brain natriuretic peptide (BNP) is also released from the heart, predominantly from the ventricles, and its actions are similar to those of ANP. It is released from stretched ventricular wall. BNP, particularly the N-terminal portion of pro-BNP, is a sensitive marker of CCF and a predictor of outcome.
- C-type natriuretic peptide is limited to the vascular endothelium and CNS and has only limited effects on natriuresis and vasodilatation.

ANP and BNP increase in response to volume expansion and pressure overload of the heart and act as physiological antagonists to the effects of angiotensin II on vascular tone, aldosterone secretion, and renal-tubule sodium reabsorption. There is currently interest in the diagnostic and therapeutic potential of these peptides.

Antidiuretic hormone

Antidiuretic hormone (vasopressin) concentrations are also increased in severe chronic heart failure. High concentrations of vasopressin are common in patients receiving diuretic treatment, contributing to the development of hyponatraemia.

Endothelins

Endothelin is secreted by vascular endothelial cells and is a potent vasoconstrictor peptide with pronounced effects on the renal vasculature, promoting the retention of sodium. Importantly, the plasma concentration of endothelin-1 is of prognostic significance: it is increased in proportion to the symptomatic and haemodynamic severity of heart failure, need for admission to hospital, and death.

Relevance to anaesthesia

Anaesthesia and surgery in patients with cardiac failure carry an increased risk of morbidity and mortality. The cause of the heart failure should be elucidated and treatment instituted before elective surgery (see Table 10.5).

When surgery is unavoidable, senior help is advisable and invasive cardiovascular monitoring essential. Early consultation with ICU is useful since these patients often need cardiorespiratory support postoperatively. Minimal doses of induction agent should be used. A balanced technique is usually appropriate and it is extremely important to maintain oxygen saturation and an adequate MAP. Contractility should be maintained and an inotrope infusion may be required.

Depending on the site of surgery, a low subarachnoid or epidural block may be useful in some patients with cardiac failure since afterload is reduced and cardiac output is preserved. Caution needs to be observed as the sympathetic block produces venodilation and a reduction in preload. Excessive hypotension is counter-productive and a high block should be avoided.

Preoperative left ventricular failure should be treated with diuretics, ACE inhibitors, and nitrates. Anaemia should be corrected to a haematocrit of 30%.

The demands of anaesthetic management are similar to those which apply to the hypertensive patient: close monitoring, avoidance of tachycardia and bradycardia, maintenance of normotension, and careful choice of anaesthetic agent.

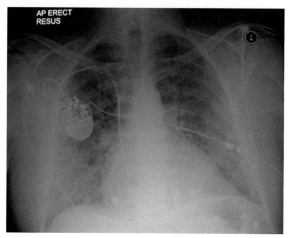

Fig. 10.30 The CXR findings of heart failure

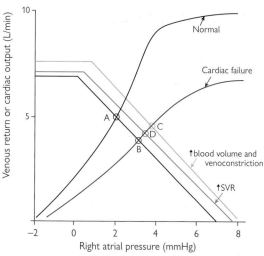

Fig. 10.31 Cardiac function curve of heart failure. Both systolic and diastolic heart failure cause changes in SVR, blood volume, and venous pressure. A, normal point of operation; B, the decrease in cardiac performance causes a downward shift in the slope of the cardiac function curve; C, the increase in blood volume and venoconstriction causes a parallel shift to the right of the systemic vascular function curve; D, systemic vascular resistance also increases, and the slope of the vascular function curve shifts downwards.

➜ Classification of heart failure (NYHA grading)

Class I (Mild)

No limitation of physical activity. Ordinary physical activity does not cause undue fatigue, palpitation, or dyspnoea (shortness of breath).

Class II (Mild)

Slight limitation of physical activity. Comfortable at rest, but ordinary physical activity results in fatigue, palpitation, or dyspnoea.

Class III (Moderate)

Marked limitation of physical activity. Comfortable at rest, but less than ordinary activity causes fatigue, palpitation, or dyspnoea.

Class IV (Severe)

Unable to carry out any physical activity without discomfort. Symptoms of cardiac insufficiency at rest. If any physical activity is undertaken, discomfort is increased.

Table 10.5 Clinical features and treatment options for heart failure

	Symptoms	Investigation findings	Treatments
Left ventricular systolic dysfunction	Fatigue Exertional dyspnoea Orthopnoea PND Pulmonary oedema Crackles, rhonci Chronic non-productive cough S3, gallop rhythm Exercise intolerance Confusion or decreased level of consciousness Nocturia	Abnormal CXR findings ECG evidence of IHD Echo evidence of systolic and/or diastolic dysfunction	Diuretics Vasodilators ACE inhibitors β-blockers
Diastolic dysfunction	Similar clinical features to systolic dysfunction (above) Possible S4 due to atrial ejection into stiff ventricles	Abnormal CXR findings ECG evidence of IHD Echo evidence of systolic and/or diastolic dysfunction	Diuretics Calcium-channel blockers β-blockers ACE inhibitors
Right ventricular systolic dysfunction	Fatigue JVD Hepatojugular reflex (>1cm) Ascites Peripheral oedema (may extend into thighs and abdomen) Nausea/vomiting Anorexia Right upper quadrant pain (hepatomegaly) Venous stasis	Abnormal liver enzymes Prolongation of coagulation studies	Diuretics Sodium/fluid restriction Paracentesis Anticoagulation (atrial dysrhythmia prophylaxis)

Angiotensin-converting enzyme inhibitors

These drugs are used in all grades of heart failure in patients with MI with left ventricular dysfunction, where prognosis is improved. They are also used in hypertension, and in insulin-dependent diabetics with nephropathy. However, hypertension is relatively resistant to ACE inhibition in the black population where concurrent diuretic therapy may be required.

Their mechanism of action involves the inhibition of the angiotensin-converting enzyme (ACE), reducing the production of the potent vasoconstrictor angiotensia II. This leads to various common effects:

- A decrease in both preload and afterload, afterload being reduced more. Caution needs to be exercised, with starting dose hypotension being common.
- A decrease in renal perfusion pressure. Bilateral renal artery stenosis or unilateral renal artery stenosis to the single functioning kidney are contraindications to treatment.
- Aldosterone levels may fall and renin, potassium, urea, and creatinine may be increased.
- A persistent cough may result from a rise in bradykinin level, caused by the lack of ACE which breaks down bradykinin.

ACE inhibitors should not be used with potassium-sparing diuretics since hyperkalaemia can result. The potential for precipitating renal failure is high if used concurrently with NSAIDs.

Angiotensin II receptor antagonists

Angiotensin II receptor antagonists are used in the treatment of hypertension. As the name suggests they block a subtype angiotensin II receptor AT_1. They block the negative feedback of angiotensin II on renin secretion, and although both renin and angiotensin II levels increase, this has little impact because of comprehensive AT_1 receptor blockade.

Like the ACE inhibitors, AT_1 receptor antagonists are contraindicated in bilateral renal artery stenosis.

Calcium-channel antagonists

These drugs are all effective in specifically blocking the entry of Ca^{2+} through L-type channels, while leaving T-, N-, and P-type Ca^{2+} channels unaffected. The L-type channel is widespread in the cardiovascular system and is responsible for the plateau phase (slow inward current) of the cardiac action potential. It triggers the internal release of Ca^{2+}. There are three classes of calcium-channel antagonist.

Class I (e.g. verapamil)

Used in the treatment of certain supraventricular arrhythmias and angina. It slows conduction of the action potential at the SA node and the AV node, slowing the heart rate. It also has a mild negative inotropic effect and vasodilates peripheral vasculature.

Class II (e.g. amlodipine, nifedipine)

Used in the prophylaxis and treatment of angina and hypertension. They reduce tone in peripheral and coronary arteries, resulting in a fall in blood pressure associated with a reflex increase in heart rate and contractility.

Nimodipine has the ability to cross the blood–brain barrier and is specifically used in the prevention and treatment of cerebral vasospasm following subarachnoid haemorrhage.

Class III (e.g. diltiazem)

Used in the prophylaxis and treatment of angina and hypertension. Prolongs AV conduction, reduces contractility, and reduces the systemic vascular resistance. BP is reduced without a reflex tachycardia.

Diuretics

Diuretics are widely used in the treatment of mild heart failure and hypertension, alone or in combination with other drugs. There are many groups of diuretics drugs, all of which increase urine production. The different groups, of diuretics include the thiazides, the loop diuretics, potassium-sparing diuretics aldosterone antagonists, osmotic diuretics and carbonic anhydrase inhibitors. They work at different sites within the kidney and have differing mechanisms of action. Diuretics are discussed in more detail in Section 12.6, but the two most commonly used in heart failure will briefly be considered here.

The thiazides are moderately potent and act mainly on the early segment of the distal convoluted tubule by inhibiting Na^+ and Cl^- reabsorption. This leads to increased Na^+ and Cl^- excretion and therefore increased water excretion. In addition, thiazides reduce systemic vascular resistance and reduce carbonic anhydrase activity, resulting in increased bicarbonate excretion. Side effects include hypokalaemia, hypochloraemic alkalosis, hyponatraemia, increased urate (precipitating gout), and hyperglycaemia.

The loop diuretics are used in severe heart failure to reduce peripheral and pulmonary oedema. They inhibit Na^+ and Cl^- reabsorption in the thick ascending limb of the loop of Henle, and to a lesser extent in the early part of the distal tubule. This impairs the action of the counter-current multiplier system and reduces the hypertonicity of the medulla, which reduces reabsorption of water in the collecting system. The thick ascending limb of the loop of Henle has a large capacity for NaCl reabsorption, so when ion reabsorption is blocked the effects are marked. Loop diuretics also produce arteriolar vasodilation, reducing systemic vascular resistance. The preload is also reduced before diuresis is seen.

Potassium-channel activators

Nicorandil is a potassium-channel activator with a nitrate moiety. It is used as prophylaxis for and treatment of hypertension, angina, and heart failure. ATP-sensitive K^+ channels are closed during the normal cardiac cycle but are open (activated) during periods of ischaemia when intracellular levels of ATP fall. In the open state K^+ passes down its concentration gradient out of the cell, resulting in hyperpolarization. This closes Ca^{2+} channels, resulting in less Ca^{2+} for myocardial infarction. Nicorandil activates the ATP-sensitive K^+ channels within the heart and the arterioles.

The cardiovascular effects are venodilation and arteriolar vasodilation, resulting in reduced pre-and afterload. Cardiac output is increased and coronary blood flow is improved, and nicorandil is effective at suppressing torsade de pointes associated with a prolonged QT interval. Contractility and AV conduction are not affected.

Centrally acting agents

Methyldopa

Methyldopa is an antihypertensive agent with two modes of action. It is a DOPA decarboxylase inhibitor, reducing peripheral and central levels of dopamine, adrenaline, and noradrenaline. In addition, it is metabolised to α-methylnoradrenaline, an α_2-adrenergic agonist with a similar action to clonidine (below).

Although methyldopa has been superseded by other antihypertensives in most clinical settings, it retains a role in the management of hypertensive disease in pregnancy. It is relatively safe for the fetus compared with other antihypertensive drugs.

Clonidine

Clonidine is an α_2-agonist with an affinity for α_2 receptors 200 times that for α_1 receptors. It stimulates the α_2 receptors in the lateral reticular nucleus, resulting in reduced central sympathetic outflow, and in the spinal cord, where they augment endogenous opiate release and modulate the descending noradrenergic pathways involved in spinal nociceptive processing. Initially a rise in blood pressure may be seen, which is mediated by peripheral α_1 stimulation. This is followed by a more sustained fall in blood pressure.

Clonidine also has sedative properties and can reduce the MAC of volatile anaesthetic agents by up to 50%.

β- and α-blocking agents

β-blockers are no longer recommended for control of hypertension because they are less effective at reducing CVS events such as stroke. When compared with ACE inhibitors and calcium-channel blockers, they are less effective at preventing diabetes.

Table 10.6 Characteristics of cardiovascular drugs

	Name	Ramipril	Losartan	Amlodipine
Properties	Uses	Anti-hypertensive Treatment of CCF, especially following MI Used to delay diabetic renal disease	Anti-hypertensive Used to delay diabetic renal disease	Anti-hypertensive Anti-anginal
	Chemical			Dihydropyridine
	Action	A pro-drug; ester of ramiprilat	Anti-hypertensive	Anti-hypertensive
	Mode	Lowers production of angiotensin II	Angiotensin II type 1 receptor antagonist	Ca^{2+} channel blocker
	Route	Oral 1.25–10mg daily	Oral 25–100mg/day	Oral 5–10 mg daily
Effects	CVS	↓ SVR; small reflex; ↑HR; CO unchanged	Peripheral vasodilatation and lower MAP	Relaxation of smooth muscle, ↓SVR, ↓BP
	CNS			
	Other	↑RBF but little ↑GFR; ↑renin secretion	↑renin secretion (↓feedback inhibition)	
Kinetics	Absorption	28% bioavailability	32% bioavailability	60–90% bioavailability
	Distribution	Protein-binding 56% ramiprilat		
	Metabolism	Hepatic, to ramiprilat; half-life 2–4hr	Mainly hepatic with active metabolite	Mainly hepatic to inactive metabolites; half-life 30–50hr
	Excretion	Renal 60%, faecal 40%	60% biliary with 25% renal; 6% unchanged in urine.	Renal
	Toxicity			May cause peripheral oedema in 10%
	Note	Not to be used in renal artery stenosis May worsen hypoglycaemic effect of other drugs		Not to be used in cardiogenic shock

	Name	Bendrofluazide	Nicorandil	Methyldopa
Properties	Uses	Anti-hypertensive Diabetes insipidus Renal tubular acidosis	Anti-anginal	Anti-hypertensive
	Chemical	Thiazide	Ethyl nitrate	Phenylalanine
	Action	Diuretic and anti-hypertensive	Vasodilator	Anti-hypertensive
	Mode	Inhibits Na^+ and Cl^- co-transport in the DCT with ↑water, Na^+, and K^+ loss	K^+ channel activation and NO stimulation of GMP	Metabolized to α-methyl-noradrenaline, which exerts central action via α_2 agonism
	Route	2.5–10mg daily	Oral up to 30mg daily	
Effects	CVS	↓plasma volume, slight ↓CO, and mild vasodilatation	Arterial and venous dilatation. No effect on contractility or conduction	↓SVR but HR and CO unchanged
	CNS	CNS depression at toxic dose		
	Other	↑urinary Ca^{2+} loss; slight ↓RBF and GFR		No effect on GFR, RBF, or placental blood flow ↓renin activity
Kinetics	Absorption	Completely absorbed	75%	Markedly variable absorption
	Distribution	95% protein bound	Protein-binding 25%	50% protein-bound
	Metabolism	Some metabolites are active	Hepatic.	Hepatic metabolism
	Excretion	Mainly urinary	Renal	Variable amount excreted via kidneys
	Toxicity	↓K^+ and ↑Ca^{2+} precipitate dysrrhythmia under GA	Hypovolaemia worsens hypotensive effect	
	Note	Glucose due to ↑synthesis and ↓insulin secretion. ↑TGs and cholesterol		Effects prolonged in liver and renal failure; associated with nasal congestion

Most patients with essential hypertension have a normal cardiac output but a raised peripheral resistance. Prolonged smooth muscle constriction in small arterioles induces structural changes, thickening of vessel walls, and an irreversible rise in peripheral resistance.

The pathophysiology of hypertension is still uncertain. Many factors contribute to its development and the relative importance of these probably varies between individuals.

The control of peripheral vascular resistance

Vascular endothelial cells play a key role in cardiovascular regulation by producing a number of potent local vasoactive agents including NO and the vasoconstrictor peptide endothelin. Dysfunction of the endothelium has been implicated in human essential hypertension. Modulation of endothelial function is an attractive therapeutic option.

Clinically effective antihypertensive therapy appears to restore impaired production of NO, but does not seem to restore the impaired endothelium-dependent vascular relaxation or vascular response to endothelial agonists. This indicates that such endothelial dysfunction is primary and becomes irreversible once the hypertensive process has become established.

Vasoactive substances

Many other vasoactive systems and mechanisms affecting sodium transport and vascular tone are involved in the maintenance of a normal blood pressure.

- Bradykinin is a potent vasodilator inactivated by ACE. Consequently, ACE inhibitors may exert some of their effect by blocking bradykinin inactivation.
- Endothelin is a powerful endothelial vasoconstrictor which may produce a salt-sensitive rise in blood pressure. It activates local renin–angiotensin systems.
- Nitric oxide is produced by arterial and venous endothelia and diffuses through the vessel wall into the smooth muscle causing vasodilatation.
- Atrial natriuretic peptide is secreted from the atria in response to increased blood volume. It increases sodium and water excretion from the kidney, and a defective secretion cause fluid retention and hypertension.

Hypercoagulability

Patients with hypertension demonstrate abnormalities with prothrombosis:

- *The vessel wall:* endothelial dysfunction or damage.
- *Blood constituents:* abnormal levels of haemostatic factors, platelet activation, and fibrinolysis.
- *Blood flow:* abnormal rheology, viscosity, and flow reserve.

These abnormalities are related to target organ damage and long-term prognosis, and may be altered by antihypertensive treatment.

Renin–angiotensin system

The renin–angiotensin system may be the most important of the endocrine systems that affect blood pressure. Renin is secreted from the juxtaglomerular apparatus of the kidney in response to glomerular underperfusion or reduced delivery of sodium to the distal nephron. It is also released in response to stimulation from the sympathetic nervous system.

Autonomic nervous system

Adrenaline and noradrenaline do not have a clear role in the aetiology of hypertension. Nevertheless, drugs that block the sympathetic nervous system do lower blood pressure and have a well-established therapeutic role.

General considerations

For hypertensive patients, it is important to consider the following questions preoperatively.

- Is the patient known to be hypertensive and, if so, are they on antihypertensive medication? Are they compliant? Does therapy need alteration before surgery?
- If this is presentation of their hypertension, does the patient have a treatable cause?
- Should surgery be postponed until blood pressure is controlled?

Relevance to anaesthesia

Preoperative drug optimization may improve outcome. Undertreated hypertensives are at risk of blood pressure lability and increased CVS morbidity and mortality. However, isolated hypertension is not universally accepted as a risk factor for many types of surgery. Deferring surgery is recommended by some authorities for those with diastolic pressures >110–115mmHg, or systolic pressures of >180–200mmHg. Others emphasize the importance of maintaining haemodynamic near-normality (pressures of within 20% of usual values), and optimization of organ perfusion with adequate fluid and oxygen administration.

Organ autoregulation curves of hypertensives are shifted to the right and higher perfusion pressures may be required.

Abrupt and marked reductions in blood pressure may occur on induction of anaesthesia. Short-acting opioids such as fentanyl may diminish stimulatory effects although the dose required is high.

High concentrations of volatile agents can cause hypotension by decreasing the systemic vascular resistance and depressing the myocardium. Volume loading reduces this risk. Nitrous oxide can be used safely.

Light anaesthesia, pain, hypoxia, and hypercarbia potentiate hypertension with increased myocardial work and oxygen demand, subendocardial ischaemia, or infarction. Regional anaesthesia may provoke significant hypotension, necessitating fluid and vasopressor resuscitation. Intra-arterial monitoring improves BP monitoring, allowing early pharmacological intervention.

In the recovery room, patients may develop hypertension due to pain, bladder distension, confusion, disorientation, or anxiety. It is important that is remains a calm environment with staff trained to anticipate and treat these problems.

Adequate warming is essential: shivering and tachycardia promote hypoxia and increase myocardial oxygen consumption and risk.

Antihypertensive drugs and anaesthesia

Elective surgical cases should be given their regular antihypertensive medications on the morning of surgery with caution. All anaesthetic agents may cause vasodilation and cardiac depression, with cumulative hypotensive results.

Perioperative continuation of ACE inhibitors potentiates hypotension, especially in the presence of marked blood loss or regional anaesthesia. Renal function should be carefully monitored in those patients taking ACE inhibitors and NSAIDs concomitantly, since this combination can precipitate acute renal failure.

Anaesthetic agents such as ketamine (inhibits re-uptake of noradrenaline) and pancuronium should be avoided because of their cardiovascular stimulatory properties.

Regular antihypertensive medication should be re-started postoperatively

Drug action and side effects

β-blockers reduce the degree of any induced tachycardia. However they may precipitate bradycardia; if severe, this can be treated with anticholinergics.

Perioperative β-blockade reduces the risk of in-hospital death in high-risk, but not low-risk, patients with CVS disease undergoing major non-cardiac surgery.

➕ Treatment of hypertension

UK NICE guidelines (June 2006)

Suggest that drug therapy should be offered to patients with:

- Persistent high blood pressure of 160/100 mmHg or more
- Persistent blood pressure above 140/90mmHg and raised cardiovascular risk (10-year risk of cardiovascular disease of at least 20%, existing cardiovascular disease or target organ damage).

The aim of treatment is to reduce blood pressure to 140/90mmHg or less, adding more drugs as needed.

Lifestyle changes

Exercise regularly.

Reduce caffeine intake.

Reduce salt intake.

Cessation of smoking.

Initiation of social support to encourage all the above.

➔ Classification of hypertension

	Systolic (mmHg)	Diastolic (mmHg)
Normal	<130	<85
High normal	130–139	85–89
Hypertension		
Stage 1 (mild)	140–159	90–99
Stage 2 (moderate)	160–179	100–109
Stage 3 (severe)	180–209	110–119
Stage 4 (very severe)	>210	120

➔ Why hypertension is important

It is a risk factor for other CVS disease.

It causes end-organ damage.

Investigation may reveal an important secondary cause.

It adversely affects anaesthetic outcome.

➔ Preoperative causes

Primary or essential hypertension

Secondary (10%) including:

- Renal—chronic pyelonephritis, renal artery stenosis, polycystic kidneys
- Endocrine—phaeochromocytoma, Cushing's syndrome, Conn's disease
- Pregnancy associated
- Coarctation of the aorta.

➔ Perioperative causes

Pain.

Light anaesthesia.

Hypoxia.

Hypercarbia.

Fluid overload.

Drug interactions/vasopressors given.

Surgical effects.

Malignant hyperthermia.

Measurement error.

➔ Hypertensive crises

The manifestations of are those of end-organ dysfunction:

- Hypertensive encephalopathy.
- Acute aortic dissection.
- Acute myocardial infarction.
- Acute cerebral vascular accident.
- Acute hypertensive renal injury.
- Acute congestive heart failure.

The absolute level of BP may not be as important as the rate of increase. Patients with long-standing hypertension may tolerate systolic BPs of 200mmHg or diastolic BPs of up to 150mmHg without developing hypertensive encephalopathy, while children or pregnant women may develop encephalopathy with diastolic BPs of 100mmHg.

Malignant hypertension: DBP >140mmHg and signs of papilloedema

Treatment of malignant hypertension: MAP should be reduced by 25% within the first 24–48hr. IABP monitoring might be appropriate.

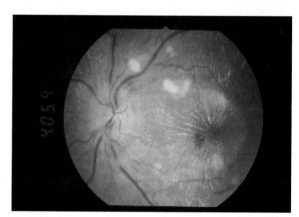

Fig. 10.32 Hypertensive retinopathy: grade 0, no changes; grade 1, minimal arteriolar narrowing; grade 2, obvious arteriolar narrowing with focal irregularities; grade 3, grade 2 + retinal haemorrhages and/or exudate; grade 4, grade 3 + swollen optic nerve (malignant hypertension). This figure demonstrates grade 4.

➔ Surgery associated with increased risk for hypertensives

- Asymptomatic patients with mild to moderate hypertension (DBP≤110mmHg) are not at increased risk and can be anaesthetised safely.
- The presence of severe end-organ damage (LVH, CRF, CVA, CAD, LVF) increases the risk significantly.
- Isolated systolic hypertension <200mmHg should not defer surgery unless for aortic surgery, carotid endarterectomy, CABG, craniotomies (aneurysm clipping), AVM, posterior fossa surgery. (increased risk).

10.15 Cardiac imaging

New cardiac imaging methods such as cardiac magnetic resonance imaging (MRI) and cardiac computed tomography (CT) are providing more information about the dynamic function of the heart in a less invasive manner.

Transthoracic echocardigraphy

Transthoracic echocardiography (TTE) uses ultrasound to visualize cardiac structures. The medical imaging portion of the sound spectrum begins in the megahertz range, well above the maximum audible frequency of 15kHz. In the 2–7MHz range used by ultrasound imaging, the wavelengths of the acoustic pulses are <1mm and therefore are capable of resolving fine anatomic structures.

One of the main advantages of acoustic medical imaging is its minimal disturbance of normal tissue physiology and function. This allows ready and repeated use of this technique for assessing tissues and organs. However, acoustic imaging has limitations because it works best with soft tissues and is very adversely affected by interposed bone or air (e.g. ribs or lungs!).

The short-axis view is obtained with the transducer along the left parasternal border between the rib spaces, giving a cross-sectional view of the left ventricular cavity. The normal left ventricular myocardium is approximately circular with the exception of the two papillary muscles. The interventricular septum tends to contract in a circular manner towards the high pressure left ventricular cavity. The apical four-chamber view (Figure 10.33) is achieved by placing the probe in the region of the maximal apical impulse.

TTE is better than Transoesophageal echocardiography (TOE) at visualization of minor valvular regurgitation, quantification of stenotic lesions, mitral valve prolapse, and assessment in the presence of non-tisssue heart valves.

Transoesophageal echocardigraphy

TOE is performed using a miniature high-frequency (5MHz) ultrasound transducer mounted on the tip of a directable gastroscope-like tube about 12mm in diameter. Using topical oral anesthesia and a little sedative, most individuals can swallow the probe without difficulty. Because the transducer lies in the lower oesophagus in close direct fluid contact with the posterior of the heart, the images are superb and there is no interference from lung tissue.

Knobs at the operator end of the probe allow different views of the heart to be obtained. TOE is particularly good at providing evidence of intracardiac infection, clot, and shunt, investigation of intra- or paracardiac masses, and aortic dissection, and detection of air embolism.

Contraindications to this technique include cervical instability, oephageal varices, recent upper GI surgery, and an uncooperative patient.

Cardiac MRI

MRI uses large magnets and radiofrequency waves to produce high-quality still and moving pictures of the body's internal structures. The scan monitors energy changes in tissues reacting to magnetic forces. A computer analyses these changes and creates a composite image of the tissues. The images can be shown in two or three spatial dimensions in either static or dynamic cine mode and and can show abnormal patterns of blood flow in the heart and great vessels.

MRI displays abnormalities in cardiac chamber contraction and can identify heart muscle that does not receive an adequate blood supply from the coronary arteries. With the aid of the non-iodine-based enhancing agent gadolinium–DTPA, it can also clearly identify areas of muscle that have become damaged as a result of infarction.

Cardiac CT

A traditional CT scan is an X-ray procedure which, with the aid of a computer, combines many X-ray images to generate cross-sectional views of the body. Cardiac CT uses advanced CT technology with or without intravenous iodine-based contrast to visualize cardiac anatomy, including the coronary arteries and great arteries and veins. With multidetector scanning, it is possible to acquire high-resolution three-dimensional images of the heart and great vessels.

Cardiac CT is especially useful in evaluating the myocardium, coronary arteries, pulmonary veins, thoracic aorta, pericardium, and cardiac masses such as thrombus of the left atrial appendage.

High-speed helical non-contrast enhanced cardiac CT scans are being used more frequently to detect calcium deposits found in atherosclerotic plaque in the coronary arteries before symptoms develop (Calcium-Score Screening Heart Scan). Although the predictive value of coronary calcium score screening is not fully defined, more coronary calcium indicates more atherosclerosis, and a greater likelihood of arterial narrowing and future cardiovascular events.

Coronary angiography

Coronary angiography is the radiographic visualization of the coronary vessels after injection of radio-opaque contrast media. It is most commonly performed with specialized intravascular catheters. The procedure is usually included as part of cardiac catheterization, which may also involve angiography of other vascular structures, such as the aorta and left ventricle.

The purpose of coronary angiography is to define the coronary anatomy and the degree of luminal obstruction of the coronary arteries. It is most commonly used to determine the presence and extent of obstructive coronary artery disease and to assess the feasibility and appropriateness of various forms of therapy, such as revascularization by percutaneous or surgical interventions. It is also used when the diagnosis of coronary disease is uncertain and cannot reasonably be excluded by non-invasive techniques.

The risk of major complications is <2%, but factors such as the presence of shock, acute renal insufficiency, and cardiomyopathy significantly increase risk. A number of relative contraindications to the procedure have been reported. Of these, pre-existing renal impairment, particularly in a patient with diabetes, and a history of prior anaphylactic reaction to contrast medium require special attention before coronary angiography to reduce the risk of subsequent complications.

The angiogram in Figure 10.34 shows the left coronary circulation. The distal left main coronary artery (LMCA) divides into its main branches:

* the left circumflex artery (LCX);
* the left anterior descending (LAD) artery,

The LAD has two large diagonal branches.

⊕ Congenital heart defects

The four most common congenital heart defects are: atrial septal defect; ventricular septal defect; patent ductus arteriosus; and tetralogy of Fallot.

Atrial septal defect (including patent foramen ovale)

Patients are often asymptomatic. The ASD usually results in a left-to-right shunt. In patients in whom the defect has not been closed, one must be careful of paradoxical emboli.

The more severe form, atrioventricular septal defect (AVSD), is associated with Down´s syndrome and results in severe pulmonary hypertension if not treated in infancy.

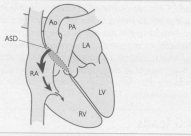

Ventricular septal defect

This is the most common form of congenital heart disease. Clinical effects depend on how many are present and their size. A small single VSD may be asymptomatic with a small left-to-right shunt. In patients who have not had corrective surgery, it is important to prevent air emboli and fluid overload and to remember antibiotic prophylaxis.

Patients with a moderate-sized single VSD often present with mild heart failure. The have markedly increased pulmonary blood flow. If the lesion is not recognized, these patients are at risk of pulmonary hypertension and shunt reversal. Avoid hyperventilation and high inspired oxygen levels.

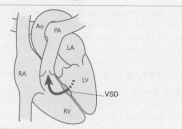

Patent ductus arteriosus

Patients with PDA may have a moderate left-to-right shunt which can result in an elevated pulmonary vascular resistance rather like a moderately sized VSD.

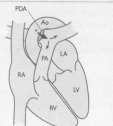

Tetralogy of Fallot

These patients have:
- Pulmonary stenosis
- VSD
- Over-riding aorta
- Right ventricular hypertrophy.

Total repair is usually undertaken between the ages of 3 and 8 months. Prior to definitive surgery the ratio of systemic vascular resistance (SVR) to pulmonary vascular resistance (PVR) determines both the systemic blood flow and blood oxygen saturation.

If these patients require surgery prior to their repair they should be intubated and ventilated in order to maintain a low PVR. Cyanosis should be treated with hyperventilation, intravenous fluid and systemic vasopressors (e.g. phenylephrine).

Eisenmenger's syndrome has a markedly increased morbidity and mortality. Patients have an abnormal and irreversible elevation in PVR resulting in cyanosis and right-to-left shunting. The degree of shunting depends on the PVR-to-SVR ratio. Increasing SVR or decreasing PVR leads to better blood oxygen saturation.

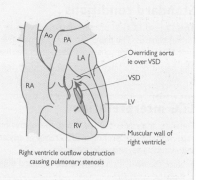

Right ventricle outflow obstruction causing pulmonary stenosis

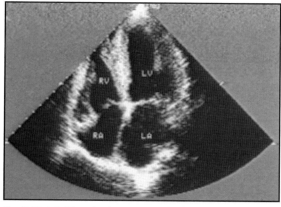

Fig. 10.33 Apical four-chamber view, transthoracic echo.

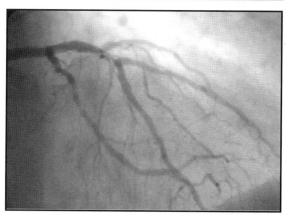

Fig. 10.34 Coronary angiogram.

The ECG is a representation of electrical activity in the myocardium. It provides valuable information about heart rate, rhythm, and conduction disturbances. It can also indicate myocardial disease (ischaemia, inflammation), and give clues to structural abnormalities (e.g. hypertrophy, valvular disease). Inferences can be drawn about other conditions such as changes in electrolyte balance (especially K^+), hypothermia, pulmonary disorders, and drug effects or toxicity. It gives no indication of cardiac output.

ECG leads

The heart is represented as a series of ECG leads, each displaying the potential detected at a particular point around the heart. The principles of vectors apply when interpreting these signals: a positive (upward) deflection represents a depolarization wave moving towards the electrode (or a repolarization wave moving away). If the electrical current is at right angles to the lead, no deflection will occur.

Limb leads

The limb leads show a view of the heart in the frontal (coronal) plane. The 'standard' bipolar leads I, II, and III each record a difference between two surface electrodes, e.g. lead I is the potential difference between the right and left arm leads. Augmented leads AVR, AVL, and AVF are unipolar, as they show a potential at the electrode contact point, relative to a calculated null point. Two schematic representations of the limb leads are shown in Figure 10.35.

Chest leads

The unipolar leads V1–6 view the heart in an approximately transverse plane (Figure 10.36). Each displays the potential at its own point on the chest wall, relative to a calculated null or 'zero' point in the middle of the heart.

Standard conditions

The 12-lead ECG is printed on paper with large (5mm) and small (1mm) squares. The paper scrolls at 25mm/s: five large squares represent 1sec, one large square is 0.2sec, and one small square is 0.04sec.

The height of the trace is also standardized: 1cm (two large squares) is 1mV.

ECG interpretation

Detailed analysis is beyond the scope of this book. Remember that reporting and interpreting an ECG requires a systematic approach. The following is a suggested framework:

* Note the patient's name, and the date and time
* Rate
* Rhythm
* Cardiac axis
* Conduction intervals
* QRS segments
* ST segments
* T waves.

Interpret the ECG first and foremost as 'normal' or 'abnormal'. Then detail the abnormalities systematically. Conclude with a differential diagnosis and a plan of action.

Features of the normal 12-lead ECG

Rate

60–100bpm. Calculate by 300/R–R interval in large squares.

Rhythm

Sinus If each P wave is followed by a QRS at a constant interval, then sinus rhythm is present (see arrhythmias, Section 10.17).

Cardiac axis

−30° to +90° Formally assessed by adding the vectors of leads I and AVF. As a rule of thumb, it is normal if I and II are both positive. If I is positive and II is negative, then **L**eft axis deviation is present. If I is negative and II is positive (**R**eaching toward one another), **R**ight axis deviation is present.

Conduction intervals

PR 0.12–0.2sec (3–5 small squares). Represents mainly AV node conduction.

QRS <0.12sec (3 small squares). Represents ventricular depolarization from the bundle of His.

QT <0.44sec for males, <0.46sec for females (corrected for rates other than 60bpm: $QTc = QT/\sqrt{R-R}$ interval in seconds). Represents ventricular repolarization.

QRS segments

Right ventricular leads (V1 +/- V2): S wave > R wave.

Left ventricular leads (V5 and 6): R wave <25mm height and Q waves <2mm deep and 1mm wide. (These small Q waves are septal in origin and are the only non-pathological Q waves).

ST segments

These should always be isoelectric. Elevation or depression indicates that abnormal currents (injury currents) are occurring within the myocardium, suggesting damage. Patterns may be consistent with a particular coronary artery territory, suggesting ischaemia or infarction; or global, suggesting a more widespread process such as myocarditis. In young fit individuals, 'high take-off' may be mistaken for ST elevation.

T waves

The T wave should be upright except in III, VR, and V1. Afro-Caribbeans may have inverted T waves in V2 and V3.

ECG monitoring in theatre

Although an ECG trace can be obtained with the electrodes attached in a variety of positions, conventionally they are placed in a standard position each time so that abnormalities are easier to detect. Most monitors have three leads and are connected as follows:

* Red—right arm
  (or second intercostal space on the right of the sternum).
* Yellow—left arm
  (or second intercostal space on the left of the sternum).
* Green (or black)—left leg
  (or more often in the region of the apex beat).

A good electrical connection between the patient and the electrodes is required to minimize the resistance of the skin.

Most monitors can only show one lead at a time and therefore the lead that gives as much information as possible should be chosen. Lead II, a bipolar lead with electrodes on the right arm and left leg, is most commonly used. It is the most useful lead for detecting cardiac arrhythmias as it lies close to the cardiac axis and allows the best view of P and R waves.

The CM5 lead is useful for detection of myocardial ischaemia. This is a bipolar lead with the right arm electrode placed on the manubrium and the left arm electrode placed at the surface marking of the V5 position (just above the fifth interspace in the anterior axillary line). The left leg lead acts as a neutral and may be placed anywhere. To select the CM5 lead on the monitor, turn the selector dial to 'lead I'. This position allows detection of up to 80% of left ventricular episodes of ischaemia, and as it also displays arrhythmias it can be recommended for use in most patients.

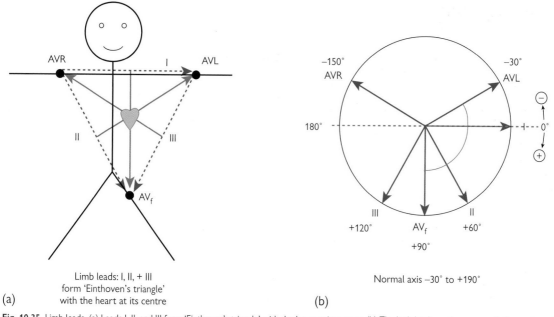

Fig. 10.35 Limb leads. (a) Leads I, II, and III form 'Einthoven's triangle' with the heart at its centre. (b) The limb leads can be represented as vectors. The cardiac axis is the overall vector of depolarisation and is normally in the range −30° to +90°.

The heart as viewed by the chest leads V1–6 major conduction pathways are shown in red

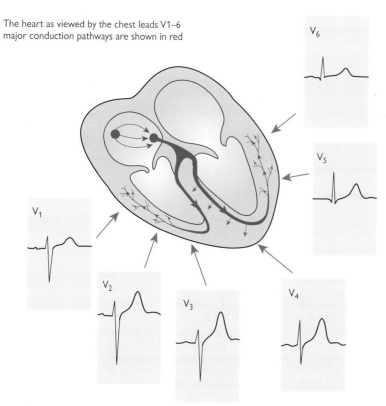

Fig. 10.36 The heart as viewed by the chest leads V1-6. Major conduction pathways are shown in red.

Abnormal electrical activity in the heart may result in changes in heart rate, rhythm, or conduction. Management depends on evaluation of the rhythm, its cause, its effect on cardiac function, and the risk of progression to a more malignant arrhythmia.

For rapid recognition and management, arrhythmias can be divided into narrow complex and broad complex.

Narrow complex arrhythmias arise above the bifurcation of the bundle of His, and are therefore 'supraventricular'. QRS duration is less than 0.12s (three small squares).

Arrhythmias originating from the SAN

Sinus arrhythmia

This is a baroreceptor-mediated change in heart rate with respiration, and is normal in children and athletes. It is markedly attenuated by general anaesthesia and IPPV.

Sinus tachycardia

In sinus tachycardia, the SA node discharges at a rate >100bpm; the ECG is otherwise unremarkable. Sinus tachycardia is a normal response to a variety of physiological states: anxiety, pain, hypovolaemia, anaemia, sepsis, fever, and pregnancy. Other causes include drugs (cyclizine, sympathomimetics, vagolytics, caffeine), light anaesthesia, hypercapnia, thyrotoxicosis, PE, and heart failure.

The cause should be sought and corrected. If it is poorly tolerated and the cause is not immediately remediable (e.g. thyrotoxicosis), β-blockers can be considered.

Sinus bradycardia

This describes a heart rate of <60bpm, with otherwise normal conduction. Rates of 40–60bpm may be well tolerated but if <40bpm, there is a risk of sinus pause or, in extreme cases, asystole.

Bradycardia is often produced by surgical vagal stimulation. Stimuli include cervical and peritoneal stretch, or the oculocardiac reflex. It is more common in children because the sympathetic innervation of the heart is immature and vagal tone predominates. Generally the heart rate improves when the surgical stimulus is removed. If not, atropine or glycopyrrolate can be given. Refractory cases may require isoprenaline or adrenaline, or even CPR. Bradycardia caused by β-blocker overdose is treated with glucagon.

In most people, the right coronary artery supplies the SAN: bradycardia can complicate right coronary artery disease. In the elderly, sick sinus syndrome may be heralded by episodes of sinus bradycardia. These can progress to sinus pauses, sinus arrest, or alternating bradycardia/tachycardias.

Atrial arrhythmias

Atrial fibrillation

Atrial fibrillation (AF) is seen on the ECG as an absence of p-waves and an irregular baseline (the atrial fibrillation trace). QRS complexes are narrow, but irregularly irregular. The heart rate may be slow, normal, or fast. A cause for new AF should always be sought; precipitants include electrolyte disturbances, hypovolaemia, sepsis, and myocardial ischaemia. It is common during thoracic surgery.

After correcting any precipants, drugs such as β-blockers, digoxin, or amiodarone, may be necessary to control the ventricular rate. Immediate DC cardioversion is indicated if there is a clinically significant reduction in cardiac output.

Atrial flutter, atrial tachycardia.

Ectopic atrial activity in the atria may outpace the SAN. Typically the rate is >150bpm. The rhythm may be paroxysmal or sustained. In atrial flutter, the baseline has a characteristic jagged appearance. In atrial tachycardia, deflections resembling P waves occur but their morphology is unusual.

In anaesthetized patients, synchronized DC cardioversion is the first-line treatment and is almost always successful. Anti-arrhythmics may restore sinus rhythm, or AV nodal blocking agents (e.g. β-blockers, verapamil) can be used to control the rate.

Atrial ectopics

Atrial ectopics are occasional early beats with bizarre P waves. They are usually benign, but occasionally herald the onset of other atrial arrhythmias.

Junctional arrhythmias

Junctional or AV nodal tachycardia

Previously and confusingly termed supraventricular tachycardia (SVT), these rhythms are now separated into AV node re-entry tachycardia (AVNRT), AV re-entry tachycardia (AVRT), and His bundle tachycardia. They involve re-entrant circuits arising in or near the AV node (AVNRT), or occasionally via fast accessory pathways conducting between the atria and ventricles (AVRT or pre-excitation). Because of the fast ventricular rate, P waves are often buried within the QRS complexes or T waves, and the rhythm can be mistaken for fast AF or flutter. However, the ventricular rate is regular, and non-conducted P waves can be seen in some complexes. Again, the rhythm may be paroxysmal and self-terminating, or sustained. Vagal manoeuvres may be effective; administration of adenosine will reveal normal atrial activity, and in many cases terminate the arrhythmia. Failing this, verapamil or β-blockers can slow the re-entrant current and control the rate. If cardiac output is compromised, synchronized DC cardioversion is indicated.

Wolff–Parkinson–White (WPW) syndrome

This pre-excitation syndrome is caused by an accessory conduction pathway between atria and ventricles. This pathway lacks the inbuilt delay of the AV node, and causes the slurred QRS upstroke (delta wave) on the ECG. If the ventricles depolarize from the normal His bundle pathways, the QRS complex will be relatively normal. However, if the accessory pathway depolarizes the ventricles, the QRS complex becomes distorted and prolonged. Diagnosis requires two ECG criteria, plus a clinical criterion:

- A short PR interval (<0.2sec in the presence of sinus rhythm).
- Widened QRS complex (>0.12sec) with a delta wave.
- Episodes of paroxysmal tachycardia.

AV node blockers such as verapamil and digoxin should not be used as they tend to direct the action potential along the abnormal pathway. The ensuing abnormal ventricular conduction can degenerate into VF.

Heart block

Heart block occurs when a defect in the conducting system of the heart causes electrical signals travelling from the AV node to the ventricles to become slowed or even stopped. The major risk from heart block is bradycardia, which can cause dizziness, syncope, or even asystole. Heart block usually occurs as a result of degeneration of the conducting system with age. Other causes include myocardial infarction, valvular disease or surgery, or cardiomyopathy. When treatment is indicated, a permanent pacemaker is the first-line choice. The classification of heart block is shown on p 276.

Bundle branch blocks

Bundle branch blocks occur when there is a conduction delay below the bifurcation of the bundle of His. The portion of the myocardium beyond the block depolarizes late and irregularly, giving rise to a widened bizarre QRS complex. The leads in which the late portion of the complex is seen indicate the site of the block.

Right bundle branch block (RBBB)

There is a second late depolarization wave, which is positive in the right ventricular precordial lead V_1 and negative in the left ventricular leads (V_{4-6}). This gives an RsR' pattern in V_1 with a deep slurred S wave in V_{4-6}, AVF, and I.

Left bundle branch block (LBBB)

This gives opposite changes to RBBB: the late positive portion of the QRS complex is in the left ventricular leads V4–6, giving an M-shaped appearance. The septum also depolarizes abnormally (R→L instead of L→R), and so leads V2 and V3 are affected, with loss of septal Q waves.

Left anterior hemiblock

This represents blockade in the anterior fascicle of the left bundle. This fascicle has a single end-arterial supply and so is vulnerable to damage. The features are: left axis deviation, a small Q wave in V_1, and a small R wave in V_3, with a normal QRS width.

Left posterior hemiblock

This is less common, and features right axis deviation, a small R wave in V_1, and a small Q wave in V_3. The QRS width is normal.

Bifascicular and trifascicular blocks

Bifascicular block occurs when RBBB is combined with a left hemiblock.. Trifascicular block is bifascicular block with a prolonged PR interval (first-degree heart block).

◎ How do arrhythmias occur?

Arrhythmias occur when the normal conducting system in the heart becomes unstable. The three main arrhythmogenic mechanisms are: re-entry circuits, enhanced automaticity, and triggered activity (caused by early or late after-depolarizations).

Re-entry circuits

Re-entry circuits occur when a loop of cardiac tissue possesses a limb with a prolonged refractory period. The action potential is conducted normally down one limb, but more slowly down the other. By the time the limbs re-join, the fast limb has repolarized, its refractory period is over, and the AP from the slow limb can then be conducted retrogradely as well as onward through the remaining conduction pathway. This not only re-activates the slow limb at the beginning of the loop, but blocks normal action potential impulses from reaching it.

Re-entry loops can occur between the junctions of normal and ischaemic cardiac tissue. They are also a problem in WPW tachycardias, where the normal AV nodal delay provides the slow limb of the loop.

Enhanced automaticity

The principles of automaticity in the SAN apply to all other areas of the myocardium with inbuilt pacemaker activity. The rate of firing can be increased by increasing the resting membrane potential, lowering the depolarization threshold, or increasing the rate of rise of phase 4 of the action potential. This can occur in the context of increased sympathetic stimulation, digoxin toxicity, or ischaemia. Under some circumstances, the rate of discharge can become inappropriately rapid and create an ectopic pacemaker.

Triggered activity

Some arrhythmias appear to be triggered by random fluctuations in membrane potential which, under circumstances of enhanced excitability, can trigger full action potentials. There are two main types of trigger.

- **Early after-depolarizations** These are small depolarizing impulses occurring during the plateau phase of the cardiac action potential. They are more frequent with bradycardia, hypomagnesaemia, and hypokalaemia, and drugs that increase the plateau period (e.g. class IA and III anti-arrhythmics and tricyclic antidepressants). Their overall effect is to prolong the QT interval, which may lead to the R-on-T phenomenon and induce torsade de pointes.

- **Late after-depolarizations** These occur after repolarization is complete. They are more common at increased heart rates, and with increased intracellular calcium. They may summate to cause full-blown action potentials, and may be the mechanism behind some sustained tachycardias, including digoxin-induced arrhythmias.

⊕ Classification of heart block

First-degree block

PR interval >0.2sec (one large box); each P is followed by a QRS. PR interval is measured from the beginning of the P wave to the beginning of the QRS.

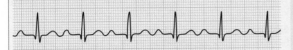

Fig. 10.37 First-degree block. PR interval is approximately 0.28sec.

Second-degree block—Möbitz type 1

Also called 'Wenkebach'. PR interval becomes progressively longer each beat until finally a QRS is 'dropped' (missing).

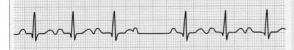

Fig. 10.38 Second-degree block type 1. Note the increasing PR interval before the QRS is dropped. Then the cycle is repeated.

Second-degree block—Möbitz type 2

Look out! This is a more serious conduction problem than Möbitz type 1. PR intervals are constant and a QRS is 'dropped' intermittently. The block is further described by the ratio of P waves to QRS complexes, e.g. 2:1 or 3:1 block. Blocks of 2:1 or worse are high-grade arrhythmias with a significant risk of progression to complete heart block and asystole.

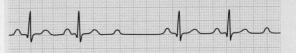

Fig. 10.39 Second-degree block type 2. Note the dropped QRS after the third P waves.

Third-degree (complete) block

In third-degree block the AV node does not conduct impulses from the atria to the ventricles. The heart rate is maintained by a ventricular escape rhythm, typically around 40 bpm. The atrial rate is completely independent of the ventricular rate and so the PR interval is random. The QRS complex is wide and bizarre unless it originates before the bifurcation of the bundle of His. Not only is the ventricular rate often insufficient to maintain an acceptable cardiac output, but there is a high risk of progression to asystole.

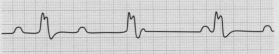

Fig. 10.40 Third-degree block. Note that the P waves and QRS waves are independent of one another.

Broad complex arrhythmias usually arise from the ventricles. Less commonly, they are conducted aberrantly from a site above the ventricles. The QRS duration is >0.12sec.

Ventricular ectopics

These are due to an episode of enhanced automaticity in ventricular muscle (Section 10.5). A wide unusual QRS complex appears prematurely on the ECG, followed by a compensatory pause as the next sinus impulse encounters refractory muscle. These can occur in normal hearts, but may also be caused by hypoxia, hypercapnia, anti-arrhythmic drugs, catecholamines, electrolyte disturbances (especially hypokalaemia), fever, and acid–base imbalances. If they persist at >5/min despite correction of the cause, or occur in runs of >3, or if they fall on the upstroke or apex of the T wave (R-on-T), they should be treated: lidocaine (1–1.5mg/kg over 2min at 5min intervals, maximum 200mg; then an infusion of 2–4mg/min) is the first-line therapy.

Ventricular escape rhythms

These occur in the presence of severe bradycardia or complete heart block, when a ventricular pacemaker emerges. QRS complexes are widened and bizarre, the axis may be markedly deviated, and P waves, if seen, are unrelated to the QRS complexes. The rate is usually slow (40bpm), and the pacemaker may be unreliable. After treating causes of bradycardia (Section 10.17), temporary pacing is indicated. If an underlying heart block persists for more than 2 weeks, a permanent pacemaker is the treatment of choice.

Ventricular tachycardia (VT)

VT arises from single (monomorphic) or multiple (polymorphic) foci in the ventricles. It is defined as run of at least three consecutive ventricular ectopic beats at a rate of >120bpm (but usually 130–250 bpm). There may be occasional normal (or near-normal) **capture beats**, or **fusion beats** where a normally conducted beat meets an ectopic beat travelling in the opposite direction. Occasionally an SVT with aberrant conduction may be mistaken for VT. Features which suggest VT rather than SVT include:

- Concordance between leads (all complexes either negative or positive).
- Marked left axis deviation.
- Capture and fusion beats.
- AV dissociation (although P waves are often hidden).
- Failure to respond to IV. adenosine.

Treatment depends on whether there is a pulse (for pulseless VT, see management of cardiac arrest (Section 25.15)). If a pulse is present, consider whether there are adverse features. These include chest pain, confusion, hypoxia, heart failre, marked hypotension (SBP <90mmHg).

If adverse signs are present, immediate synchronized DC cardioversion is needed. This should be followed by an infusion of amiodarone (see below) to prevent recurrence.

If the patient is stable, the first priority is to identify and correct the cause (causes are as for ventriular ectopics). Failing that, amiodarone 300mg over 20–60 min, followed by 900mg over 23hr, is the first-line therapy.

Torsade de pointes is a specific type of VT. It resembles VF, but can be distinguished by its characteristic twisting axis. The outline of the ECG resembles two opposing sine waves. It is most usually precipitated in the presence of a long QT interval by the R-on-T phenomenon. Treat by stopping any QT-prolonging drugs, and administering magnesium 8mmol/15min. Overdrive pacing can also be used.

SVT + aberrant conduction

Any narrow-complex tachycardia can combine with abnormal ventricular conduction to produce a rhythm which mimics VT on the ECG. Features which favour the diagnosis of VT are discussed above. However, it must be remembered that AV-blocking drugs, such as verapamil or β-blockers, reduce the activity of normal AV conduction pathways and may make VT more difficult to treat. In addition, VT is the more common of the two scenarios. *If in doubt, treat as VT.*

Accelerated idioventricular rhythm

This resembles VT, arising from an ectopic ventricular pacemaker, but the rate is <120bpm. There is usually an adequate cardiac output. The rhythm is most often seen during reperfusion following treatment for MI, and may actually be a good prognostic sign. It requires careful monitoring.

Ventricular fibrillation (VF)

VF is seen on the ECG as random chaotic activity with no discernible QRS complexes. It is incompatible with a cardiac output and requires immediate implementation of the Advanced Life Support protocol (Section 25.2). If the arrest is witnessed or monitored, a precordial thump may be of value (acting as a low-energy shock). The prognosis depends upon prompt delivery of a DC shock, which should not be delayed by intubation, IV access, etc.

VF usually begins as 'coarse,' with an amplitude of around 1cm on ECG (1mV). Without treatment, tt gradually deteriorates into fine VF and then asystole.

Many cardiac diseases will progress to VF if cardiac output is severely compromised for a significant period. It may also be caused by electric shock, electrolyte disturbances (particularly hyperkalaemia), or degeneration of other arrhythmias. An **R-on-T phenomenon**, where a ventricular impulse coincides with the upstroke or peak of a T wave, can precipitate VF: the presence of both depolarized and repolarized cells in the myocardium gives rise to multiple disorganized re-entry circuits.

→ **Anti-arrhythmic drugs**

Various schemes exist for classifying anti-arrhythmic drugs. The Vaughan Williams classification (Table 10.7) was developed in 1970 and categorizes drugs according to their actions on channels and receptors. However, not all drugs are included and some occupy more than one category. The 'Sicilian gambit' of 1991 is a more complex pharmacodynamic classification, and describes drug action on channels, receptors, and pumps within the myocardium.

A more user-friendly classification describes the uses of anti-arrhythmic drugs in the clinical setting, but leaves the individual to learn their pharmacology:

Drugs used for supraventricular tachyarrhythmias

These include adenosine, digoxin, verapamil, β-blockers, and quinidine.

Drugs used for ventricular tachyarrhythmias

These include lidocaine and mexiletine.

Drugs used for both supraventricular and ventricular arrhythmias

These include amiodarone, flecainide, procainamide, disopyramide, propafenone, and sotalol.

Drugs used for bradyarrhythmias

These include atropine, glycopyrrolate, isoprenaline, and adrenaline.

Table 10.7 The Vaughan-Williams classification of anti-arrhythmics

Class	Mode of action	Drugs
I	Na$^+$-channel blockade	
	(a) prolongs action potential	Quinidine, procainamide, disopyramide
	(b) shortens action potential	Lidocaine, mexiletine
	(c) no effect on action potential	Flecainide, encainide, propafenone
II	β-blockade: antagonize catecholamines	β-blockers Bretylium
III	K$^+$-channel blockade: prolong action potential	Amiodarone Sotalol Bretylium
IV	Ca$^+$-channel blockade	Verapamil Diltiazem

Table 10.8 Characteristics of anti-arrhythmics

	Name	Adenosine	Amiodarone	Atropine
Properties	Uses	Suspected AVNRT; reveals atrial ECG trace in narrow complex tachycardia	Pre-excited tachycardia; other refractory tachycardias	Bradycardia and asystole; anti-sialagogue premedication
	Chemical	Endogenous nucleoside (adenine + D-ribose)	Iodinated benzofuran derivative	Naturally occurring tropane alkaloid (from *Atropa belladonna*)
	Presentation	Colourless solution in saline, 3mg/ml; 2ml glass vials	Colourless solution for dilution in 5% dextrose; 150mg ampoules; tablets (100 or 200mg)	Racemic mixture; colourless solution 600mcg/ml; minijet 500mcg in 5ml
	Action	Blocks conduction at the AV node	Increases duration of action potential and refractory period	Anti-muscarinic: vagolytic action causes tachycardi
	Mode	A_1 receptors (Gi-protein coupled)	Potent K^+ channel blocker; moderate α- and β-blockade; some Na^+ and Ca^{2+} channel block.	Muscarinic acetyl choline receptor blockade (minimal nicotinic blockade at therapeutic dose)
	Route and dose	IV bolus, 6 mg initially followed by 12 mg if not effective	IV: e.g. 150–300mg loading dose over 1h, then 900mg over 23h; central vein. Oral 200mg tds for 1/52, bd for 1/52, then od	IV/IM/SC: max 20mg/kg (for treatment of bradycardia 5–10mg/kg boluses titrated to effect). (Bradycardic PEA or asystole: 3mg single dose IV).
Effects	CVS	Transient atrioventricular block; chest pain or cardiac 'thump'; vasodilatation.	Cardioversion of narrow and broad complex tachyarrhythmias; negative ino- and chronotropy	Early bradycardia (due to initial muscarinic agonist effect); then tachycardia
	RS	Bronchospasm	Pneumonitis, pleuritis, or pulmonary fibrosis, expecially with high FiO_2 in critical illness.	Bronchodilation and increased dead space; reduction in bronchial secretions
	CNS	Dizziness, syncope.	Corneal deposits: 'haloes' or blurred vision	Mydriasis, anti-emesis, amnesia, sedation
	GI		Minor GI upset, metallic taste. Jaundice, hepatitis, and cirrhosis can occur (monitor LFTs)	↓lower oesophageal sphincter tone and gastric secretions
	Other		Thyroid dysfunction (↑ or ↓): baseline thyroid tests prior to starting; skin discoloration and photosensitivity.	Loss of sweating may cause pyrexia (especially in paediatric patients).
Kinetics	Absorption	Transient effects: plasma $t\frac{1}{2}$ is only 8-10sec because of cellular uptake	Oral bioavailability 60%	Rapid but variable absorption from intestine.
	Distribution		Highly protein-bound, accumulates in muscle and fat; V_D varies from 2–70L/kg	Cosses cell membranes readily including BBB. 50% plasma protein bound.
	Metabolism		Hepatic: metabolites have some activity.	Hepatic esterases.
	Excretion		Biliary, skin, tears; elimination $t_{\frac{1}{2}}$ 7 weeks.	Urine; elimination $t_{\frac{1}{2}}$ 2.5h
	Note		Multiple interactions: potentiate protein-bound drugs, digoxin, AV blockers. Avoid with QT interval-prolonging drugs	Large doses may cause central anticholinergice syndrome

Table 10.8 Continued

	Name	Bretylium	Digoxin	Flecainide
Properties	Uses	Life-threatening ventricular tachyarrhythmias	Atrial fibrillation/flutter; heart failure (positive inotropic effect)	Ventricular tachyarrhythmias, pre-excited re-entry tachycardias
	Chemical	Bromobenzyl quaternary ammonium derivative	Glycoside	Amide local anaesthetic
	Presentation	Colourless solution 50mg/ml; 10ml glass ampoule	Colourless solution for injection 25mcg/ml; tablets 625-250mcg	10mg/ml solution for injection; 50 + 100mg tablets
	Action	Suppression of ventricular arrhythmias	Slowing of pacemaker rate and AV conduction; positive inotropy	Suppression of ectopic discharge and accessory pathway conduction
	Mode	Blockade of K^+ channels; some β-blockade; accumulates in sympathetic ganglia to ↓NAdr release	Inhibits Na^+/K^+ cell membrane pump; increased intracellular sodium then causes displacement of intracellular calcium, leading to pacemaker slowing; AV conduction delay and increased AV refractory period; is also positive inotropy and enhanced ventricular automaticity	Class Ic: blockade of sodium channels with no change to action potential duration; maximum rate of depolarization is reduced, especially in accessory pathways
	Route	Refractory VF or pulseless VT: 5mg/kg rapid IV 1–2mg/min by IV infusion IM route also used	Loading dose IV/PO: 10–20mcg/kg 6–12 hourly until effective; maintenance dose 10–20mcg/kg/day, adjusted according to response and plasma concentration	IV infusion: 2mg/kg loading dose over 10min; then 1.5mg/kg/hr for 1hr, then 0.25mg/kg/hr
Effects	CVS	Initial NAdr release, then hypotension (keep patient supine).	Slowing of ventricular rate; ECG shows increased PR interval, shortened QT interval, and 'reverse-tick' ST depression with T-wave flattening. In toxicity, digoxin can cause arrhythmias (especially bradyarrhythmias and bigeminy)	May be negatively inotropic, but relatively cardiostable in most cases
	RS	Possible neuromuscular blockade → ventilatory impairment		
	CNS	Nausea and vomiting; confusion	In toxicity: drowsiness, confusion, visual disturbance (green-yellow haloes), weakness, coma	May cause visual disturbances, headaches, paraesthesiae, and dizziness
	GI	Diarrhoea	In toxicity: anorexia, nausea, vomiting, diarrhoea in toxic doses	Reversible liver damage
	GU		Mild diuretic effect	
Kinetics	Absorption	Oral bioavailability poor (20%)	Variable; oral bioavailability 60–90%	Rapid absorption; oral bioavailability 90%
	Distribution	Protein-binding 1–6; large V_D (8L/kg). Appears to accumulate in cardiac tissue.	25% protein-bound in plasma; large V_D (5–11L/kg). Accumulates in cardiac tissue.	Approximately 50% protein-bound; V_D 6–10 L/kg
	Metabolism	Excreted in urine; clearance approx. 6 x GFR.	Only 10% metabolized (phase I reactions in liver)	Hepatic; two major metabolites. 50-90% metabolized
	Excretion		Mostly (60%) unchanged in urine; accumulates in renal impairment (increase dose interval)	Unmetabolized fraction and metabolites excreted in urine; clearance 10ml/kg/min; elimination $t_{1/2}$ 11hr (IV dose) or 20hr (PO dose)
	Toxicity		Digoxin-specific antibodies can be used in toxicity. Not significantly removed by dialysis. Likelihood of toxicity increased by hypokalaemia and hypomagnesaemia, hypernatraemia and hypercalcaemia, hypoxaemia, renal failure, and acid–base imbalance	Flecainide increases plasma digoxin levels. Not removed by dialysis.
	Note	Can cause hyperthermia	Therapeutic plasma concentration 1–2ng/ml	

	Name	Glycopyrrolate	Magnesium	Sotalol
Properties	**Uses**	Bradyarrhythmias; to counteract the muscarinic effects of anticholinesterases; anti-sialogogue	Hypomagnesaemia; pre-eclampsia; torsade de pointes and other ventricular tachyarrhythmias; asthma; cerebral oedema; acute myocardial infarction; tetanus	Ventricular tachycardia; prophylaxis of AVNRT and AVNT; also controls ventricular rate in AF
	Chemical	Quaternary amine	Ion, formulated as the inorganic sulphate	Substituted isopropylphenylethylamine
	Presentation	Clear solution for injection (0.2mg/ml); fixed-dose combination with neostigmine	Colourless solution for injection (2.03mmol/ml ionic magnesium)	Racemic mixture Clear solution for injection, 10mg/ml in 4 ml ampoule Tablets 40–200mg
	Action	Anticholinergic (especially anti-secretory).	Smooth muscle relaxation; cofactor in many enzyme systems; essential for nucleic acid production and protein function	Suppresses ventricular arrhythmias, slows ventricular rate
	Mode	Competitive ACh antagonism at peripheral muscarinic receptors	Mechanism(s) of action unknown; presynaptic inhibition of ACh release at the NMJ	Non-selective β-blocker; also some class III activity
	Route	IV or IM: 0.2–0.4mg (paediatric 4–10mcg/kg)	IV or IM; regimes vary, e.g. pre-eclampsia 16 mmol over 20min, then 4–8mmol/hr.	IV: 50–100mg over 20min (monitor ECG)PO: 80–160mg bd
Effects	**CVS**	Increased heart rate, reduction in bradycardic response to vagal stimulus; BP largely unaffected	Vasodilatation and decreased SVR, can cause hypotension; slows SA node pacemaker discharge, prolongs SA node action potential, PR interval, and AV node refractory period	Catecholamine antagonism: reduced HR; prolongs cardiac action potential; not a myocardial depressant; may cause long QT and torsade de pointes, exacerbated by hypokalaemia
	RS	Bronchodilatation, increased dead space; reduces secretions.	Bronchodilatation; attenuates hypoxic pulmonary vasoconstriction	Can cause bronchospasm in sensitive individuals
	CNS	Does not cross BBB but can cause headache and sleepiness; pupils unaffected	Anticonvulsant properties; inhibition of sympathetic discharge at high doses	Dizziness, lethargy, headache may occur
	GI	Antisialogogue (5× more potent than atropine); reduced gastric volume and motility; reduces LOS tone		
	GU	Difficulty in micturition can occur	Renal vasodilatation, diuretic effect; tocolytic and may improve placental perfusion; may cause neonatal hypotonia and respiratory depression	
Kinetics	**Absorption**	Poor oral bioavailability (5%)	Oral absorption and bioavailability variable	Well absorbed; oral bioavailability almost 100%
	Distribution	Rapid redistribution; V_D 0.5L/kg: can cross the placenta and cause fetal tachycardia	30% protein-bound in plasma	No significant protein binding; V_D 1.3L/kg
	Metabolism	Little biotransformation in humans		Not metabolized
	Excretion	Urine 85%, bile 15%; mostly (80%) unchanged	Excreted in urine	90% in urine, 10% in bile
	Note	May cause pyrexia through loss of sweating	Serum levels should be monitored; loss of deep tendon reflexes indicates impending toxicity	L- and D-isomers have class III activity; β-blockade is from the L-isomer

Table 10.8 Continued

Cardiac output is an extremely useful measurement to make during anaesthesia and critical care. Many methods exist to measure and monitor cardiac output. They vary in accuracy, ease of use, expense, and degree of invasiveness.

Pulmonary artery flotation catheter

The pulmonary artery flotation catheter (PAFC), while mainly superseded by other monitoring devices, provides a great deal of information about the cardiovascular system. The balloon-tipped fluid-filled catheter is generally 'floated' into position from a central vein such that the tip lies in a large pulmonary artery. Various parameters can then be measured.

Modern catheters are fitted with a distal heated filament, which allows automatic thermodilution measurement via heating the blood and measuring the resultant thermodilution trace. This provides near-continuous cardiac output monitoring. The PAC is used in assessment of haemodynamic status and direct intracardiac and pulmonary artery pressures. The distal (pulmonary artery) port allows sampling of mixed venous blood for the assessment of oxygen transport and the calculation of derived parameters such as oxygen consumption, oxygen utilization coefficient, and intrapulmonary shunt fraction.

The PAC is tipped with a balloon which can be inflated to occlude the pulmonary artery; the subsequent back pressure is a reflection of the left atrial filling pressure and until recently was considered a good indicator of preload.

Other derived values can be calculated from measured values such as:

CI	CO/body surface area	2.4–4L/min/m^2
SV	CO/heart rate	40–70ml/beat
SVR	MAP – CVP/CO	900–1200dyn/s/cm^{-5}
PVR	MPAP – PAOP/CO	100–200dyn/s/cm^{-5}

The pressure trace obtained from the distal lumen during insertion of a PAFC is shown in Figure 10.41.

The pulmonary artery wedge pressure (or pulmonary artery occlusion pressure PAOP) has been superseded by more reliable techniques such as intrathoracic blood volume or stroke volume variation as indicators of volume status. The PAC has fallen out of common use as clinicians favour less invasive and less hazardous technologies for monitoring haemodynamic status. Considerable controversy exists over whether the PAC increases mortality; recent studies suggest that it neither increases nor improves mortality. Complications such as cardiac tamponade, pulmonary artery rupture, and air emboli are a danger.

Ultrasound and Doppler methods

Blood flow is increasingly being assessed by Doppler techniques, which are very convenient because they are non-invasive (or minimally invasive). These machines transmit an ultrasonic vibration into the body and record the change in the frequency of the signal that is reflected from the red blood cells. Doppler techniques measure velocity, not flow; the flow can be obtained by integrating the signal over the cross-sectional area of the vessel.

The Doppler equation

The oesophageal Doppler technique is based on measurement of blood flow velocity in the descending aorta by means of a Doppler transducer (4MHz continuous or 5MHz pulsed wave, according to the type of device) at the tip of a flexible probe. The probe can be introduced orally in anaesthetized mechanically ventilated patients. Following its introduction, it is advanced gently until the tip is located approximately at the mid-thoracic level; it is then rotated so that the transducer faces the aorta and a characteristic aortic velocity signal is obtained. Probe position is optimized by slow rotation in the long axis and alteration of the depth of insertion to generate a clear signal with the highest possible peak velocity. Gain setting is adjusted to obtain the best outline of the aortic velocity waveform.

Measurement of stroke volume using oesophageal Doppler is derived from the well-established principles of stroke volume measurement in the left ventricular outflow tract using transthoracic echo and Doppler. Several assumptions are required for transposition of this algorithm from the left ventricular outflow tract to the descending aorta: accurate measurement of descending aortic blood flow velocity; a 'flat' velocity profile in the descending aorta; an estimated aortic cross-sectional area close to the mean value during systole; a constant division of blood flow between the descending aorta (70%) and the brachiocephalic and coronary arteries (30%); and, finally, a negligible diastolic flow in the descending aorta.

Accurate velocity measurement requires good alignment between the Doppler beam and blood flow, and knowledge of the angle at which the blood flow is insonated. Alignment is optimal where the signal is brightest on the spectral representation (CardioQ, Deltex Medical Ltd, Chichester, UK; Waki, Atys Medical, Soucieu en Jarrest, France) or when the aortic walls are well defined on M-mode echocardiography (HemoSonic, Arrow International, Reading, PA, USA), and when peak velocity is maximum (all devices). The angle between the Doppler beam and the flow is presumed to be the same as that between the transducer and the probe (45° or 60°, depending on the device), because the oesophagus and aorta are usually parallel in the thorax. The discrepancy between the true and theoretical angles is more problematic when the inclination of the transducer is 60°. Indeed, a discrepancy of 10° will result in an error ranging between +28% and –32% for a 60° transducer (5MHz) but only +16% to –19% for a 45° transducer (4MHz).

The assumption regarding the velocity profile is that all red blood cells are moving at approximately the same speed.

Finally, some manufacturers of oesophageal Doppler devices provide measures of systemic cardiac output rather than descending aortic blood flow. They calculate the systemic values by assuming a constant partition of blood between cephalic (30%) and caudal (70%) territories. Although this may be valid in healthy resting persons, the partition may vary depending on haemodynamic conditions, reflex activation, or metabolic activity within different organs. Therefore the assumed constant ratio between cephalic and caudal territories may become inaccurate under a variety of pathophysiological conditions.

Doppler systems may utilize a continuous or pulsed ultrasound technique

Continuous Doppler system

This can measure high velocities but averages the frequency shifts along the whole length of the ascending aorta so that the exact point at which the velocity is measured is unknown. Therefore it is difficult to know where to measure the aortic diameter.

The pulsed Doppler system

This uses the same transducer to generate and receive the ultrasound but produces short pulses instead of a continuous stream of ultrasound. The great advantage of this system is that the beam can be focused so that the operator knows the precise depth at which the measurement is being made. However, there is a limit to the velocity of blood flow which can be measured since high velocities lead to a large Doppler shift. Increasing the pulse repetition frequency extends the range of velocity measurement, but decreases the possible depth of measurement since the signals must have time to return to the transducer before the next pulse is emitted.

Table 10.9 Normal values for cardiovascular parameters

Measured values		Value
CVP	Central venous pressure (Reflects right atrial pressure)	1–6mm Hg
PAP	Mean pulmonary artery pressure	Systolic 15–30mmHg Diastolic 6–12mm Hg
PAOP	Pulmonary artery occlusion pressure (Estimates left atrial heart pressure and left ventricular end diasolic pressure)	6–12mmHg
CO	Cardiac output	3.5–7.5 L/min
P_vO_2	Mixed venous partial pressure of oxygen Drawn from end of pulmonary artery catheter. Used to calculate how well oxygen is extracted by the tissue	70–75%
RVEDV	Right ventricular end-diastolic volume	
RVESV	Right ventricular end-systolic volume	

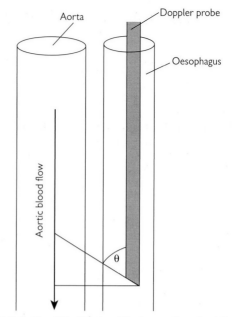

Fig. 10.42 Position of the Doppler within the oesophagus in relation to blood flow through the adjacent aorta.

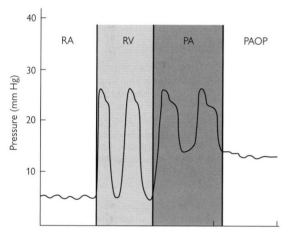

Fig. 10.41 Pressure recorded from the tip of the PAC as it advances through the various chambers prior to arrival in the pulmonary artery. Pressure waveforms: RA, right atrium; RV, right ventricle; PA, pulmonary artery; PAOP, pulmonary artery occlusion pressure.

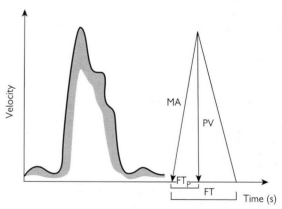

Fig. 10.43 Velocity–time Doppler waveform segments and measurements made: MA, mean acceleration; PV, peak velocity; FT, flow time; FTp, flow time to peak velocity.

➔ Doppler shift

$$F_d = 2F_t V\cos\theta/C$$

where F_d is Doppler shift, F_t is the transmitted Doppler frequency, V is the speed of blood flow, $\cos\theta$ is the cosine of the angle between blood flow and beam, and C is the speed of sound in tissue.

Table 10.10 Construction of oesophageal Doppler cardiac index

Stroke distance	Flow time × peak velocity
Minute distance	Stroke distance × heart rate
Stroke volume	Stroke distance/cross-sectional area of the aorta
Cardiac output	Stroke volume × heart rate
Cardiac index	Cardiac output/body surface area

Dilution methods

Dilution methods measure how fast flowing blood can dilute an indicator substance introduced to the circulatory system, usually using a pulmonary artery catheter. Early methods used a dye; the cardiac output is inversely proportional to the concentration of dye sampled downstream. More specifically, the cardiac output is equal to the quantity of indicator dye injected divided by the area under the dilution curve measured downstream (Stewart–Hamilton equation) (Figure 10.44).

The indicator generally used now is a known volume of cold 5% glucose solution and the change in temperature is measured downstream. Cardiac output can be affected by the phase of respiration, especially under mechanical ventilation, and therefore should be measured at a defined phase of the respiratory cycle (typically end-expiratory).

Cardiac output is inversely proportional to the area under the thermodilution curve.

Arterial pulse contour analysis

This is a technique combining transpulmonary thermodilution and arterial pulse contour analysis. Estimation of cardiac output based on pulse contour analysis is an indirect method, since cardiac output is not measured directly but is computed from a pressure pulsation on the basis of a criterion or model. The origin of the pulse contour method for estimation of beat-to-beat stroke volume is based on the Windkessel model described by Otto Frank in 1899. Most pulse contour methods are explicitly or implicitly based on this mode. They relate an arterial pressure or pressure difference to a flow or volume change. Nowadays, three pulse contour methods are available: PiCCO, PulseCO, and Modelflow. All three pulse contour methods use an invasively measured arterial blood pressure and need to be calibrated.

PiCCO is calibrated by transpulmonary thermodilution, PulseCO by transpulmonary lithium dilution, and Modelflow by the mean of three or four conventional thermodilution measurements equally spread over the ventilatory cycle. The output of these pulse contour systems is calculated on a beat-to-beat basis, but presentation of the data is typically within a 30sec window.

PiCCO

Transpulmonary thermodilution using the Stewart–Hamilton principle is used as the independent calibrating technique. This measures the change in temperature at a femoral arterial line following three episodes of bolus injection of cold saline through a central venous line. Calibration of the arterial pulse contour analysis is derived from this cold-saline thermodilution.

The PiCCO algorithm uses mathematical analysis of the pulse contour waveform to calculate continuous cardiac output. Since the thermodilution fluid passes through the right heart, the pulmonary circulation, and the left heart, further mathematical analysis allows approximation of cardiac filling volumes, intrathoracic blood volume, and extravascular lung water.

Additional information generated includes stroke volume variation (SVV) and pulse pressure variation (PPV), which can be used to estimate response to volume replacement in mechanically ventilated patients.

LiDCO

The PulseCO algorithm used by LiDCO is based on pulse power derivation and does not depend on waveform morphology. Once again, independent calibration is required and although this utilizes the Stewart–Hamilton principle, this time it is performed using lithium chloride. This is injected and the resulting arterial lithium concentration–time curve is recorded by withdrawing blood past a lithium sensor attached to the patient's existing arterial line.

This has the advantage of not requiring central venous access; it is usable with a peripheral vein and a peripheral arterial line. However, it does not provide information about heart volumes or extravascular lung water. Other disadvantages include error in the presence of certain muscle relaxants and the fact that dilution measurements cannot be performed too frequently.

FloTrac and PRAM (pressure recording analytical method) technology

More recent developments are the FloTrac and PRAM systems which can derive cardiac output from the arterial waveform without the need for an independent method of calibration. The cardiac output is derived from an estimation of stroke volume which is calculated from the pulse pressure. Continuous cardiac output can then be displayed directly from a conventional arterial line. The methodology has yet to be extensively evaluated, but early studies suggest that it may be accurate.

Impedance cardiography

Impedance cardiography (ICG) is an advanced technique which was developed for the space industry. It calculates cardiac output based on the measurement of changes in impedance in the chest over the cardiac cycle (changes in blood volume). The rate of change of impedance is a reflection of cardiac output. It is thought to be useful in estimating changes but not for absolute measurements. This technique has progressed clinically and allows low-cost non-invasive estimations of cardiac output and total peripheral resistance, using only four paired skin electrodes (Figure 10.45).

- An alternating current is transmitted through the chest.
- The current seeks the path of least resistance: the blood filled aorta.
- Baseline impedance to current is measured.
- Blood volume and velocity in aorta change with each heartbeat.
- Corresponding changes in impedance are used with ECG to provide haemodynamic parameters.

Limitations

Contraction of the heart produces a cyclical change in transthoracic impedance of about 0.5%, unfortunately giving a rather low signal-to-noise ratio. Although the method has been reported to give accurate results in normal subjects, several studies show some inaccuracy in critically ill patients.

Aortovelography

This is use of a continuous wave Doppler ultrasound probe in the suprasternal notch to measure blood velocity and acceleration in the ascending aorta. The role of the USCOM device (USCOM Ltd) in haemodynamic monitoring is evolving. It should be noted that the USCOM monitor is limited to cardiac output measurement and gives no indication of other haemodynamic variables, such as pressure measurements, vascular resistance, or stroke work calculations. In addition, it does not provide the means of measuring mixed venous oxygenation. Thus the USCOM monitor does not completely replace the pulmonary artery catheter. However, in situations where cardiac output measurement is most pertinent to patient management, the USCOM monitor is superior in speed, safety, and cost. It has potential applications in intensive care, anaesthesia, cardiology, and research.

The portable unit can be used on adult and paediatric patients, whether they are awake, intubated, or unconscious. USCOM can detect low or high cardiac output states in sepsis, confirm normal circulatory function with no risk to the patient, and assess haemodynamic response to fluid, inotropes, and vasoactive therapy.

Potentially the machine has a role in the worldwide adoption of Early Goal Directed Therapy and the Surviving Sepsis Campaign. The greatest benefit of the device is that it really provides cardiac output in real time at the bedside and has the ability to bring a critical care approach to all clinical areas.

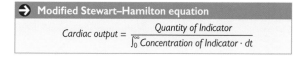

Modified Stewart–Hamilton equation

$$Cardiac\ output = \frac{Quantity\ of\ Indicator}{\int_0^\infty Concentration\ of\ Indicator \cdot dt}$$

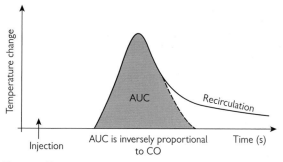

Fig. 10.44 Temperature change measured at the distal arterial sensor, following bolus injection of cold saline.

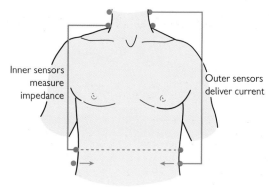

Fig. 10.45 Electrode set-up for impedance cardiography.

Chapter 11

Body compartments and fluid balance

11.1 Body compartments

Body water

Total body water (TBW) accounts for approximately 60% of body mass. This varies with fat and muscle content, so the value is lower for females (50%), may be lower for the elderly, and is higher for infants (70%).

Body water is contained within two main compartments:

- Extracellular fluid (ECF)
- Intracellular fluid (ICF).

The two compartments are separated by the cell membrane.

In real terms, approximately 55% of body water (23L) is in the ICF and 45% (19L) is in the ECF. However, the ECF water of bone and dense connective tissue is kinetically a very slow compartment, so for functional purposes the ratio of ICF to ECF is considered to be 2:1. This is the ratio to use for determining the distribution of infused fluids. It is consistent with the common clinically accepted distribution in a 70kg man (Figure 11.1):

- TBW = 42L (70kg × 60%)
- ICF = 28L
- ECF = 14L, of which 11L are interstitial fluid and 3L are plasma fluid (note that the total circulating volume is 5L; red cells make up 2L if the haematocrit is 40%).

The ECF is in turn subdivided into several smaller compartments: interstitial fluid (ISF), intravascular fluid, water held within dense connective tissue and bone, and transcellular fluids.

Transcellular fluids are formed from the transport activities of cells and are found in epithelia-lined spaces. They include CSF, joint fluid, bile, and aqueous humour.

Normally only small amounts of fluid are found in the peritoneal and pleural cavities. However, significant accumulations can occur with ascites and pleural effusions. These are ultrafiltrates of plasma with variable amounts of albumin, and count towards the ECF volume.

Similarly, oedema is an accumulation of an ultrafiltrate of plasma in the interstitial space and is usually found in dependent areas.

Measurement of compartment volumes

Compartment volumes are usually measured by administering a known amount of a 'tracer' substance (Table 11.1). This distributes within a compartment, and its concentration is measured after mixing. For example, deuterium or tritium oxide can be used to measure total body water. The volume of the compartment is calculated from the formula:

$$\text{volume} = \frac{\text{mass administered}}{\text{concentration}}$$

An ideal tracer substance should:

- Be confined to the compartment being measured
- Not alter fluid distribution
- Rapidly and uniformly distribute throughout the compartment
- Be non-toxic
- Not be metabolized or excreted (allowance for metabolism or excretion can be included in the calculation; for example, the amount excreted might be measured, or a plot of concentration vs. time can be extrapolated back to time zero to allow for metabolism).

ECF tracers

All tracers differ in some aspects from ideal. Isotope tracers (e.g. $^{35}SO_4$ and chloride isotopes) often enter cells to some extent, overestimating ECF volume. Crystalloid tracers (e.g. inulin and mannitol), which are larger molecules, do not diffuse equally throughout the whole of the ECF, so ECF volume can be underestimated. The results obtained may vary with the time allowed for distribution since the different components of the ECF have different kinetic characteristics.

Blood and plasma tracers

Blood volume can be determined from measurement of the plasma volume and the haematocrit. The plasma volume can be calculated using tracers such as Evans blue or radio-iodine, both of which bind to serum albumin. However, since some albumin is lost to the interstitial space, causing an exponential decline in tracer concentration in the plasma, multiple samples are taken. A graph of concentration vs. time is extrapolated back to time zero. This provides the tracer concentration immediately after the mixing phase.

Once the plasma volume has been determined, blood volume can be calculated from the formula:

$$\text{blood volume} = (\text{plasma volume} \times 100)/(100 - \text{Hct})$$

where Hct is the haematocrit (per cent).

Again, this step can introduce error. Haematocrit varies between the venous and arterial circulations as red cells swell in the veins with chloride shift (carbon dioxide transport results in an increase in the number of particles inside the cell; Section 13.12).

^{51}Cr can be used to label red cells. The whole-blood volume can be determined if the tracer concentration in whole blood is measured. Alternatively, the red cell volume can be determined if tracer concentration in a known volume of red cells is quantified.

Using both ^{131}I and ^{51}Cr allows simultaneous measurement of both red cell mass and plasma volume so that the blood volume can be determined without using the haematocrit.

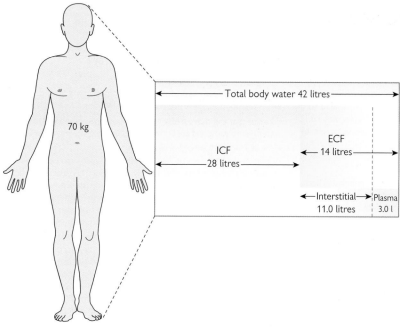

Fig. 11.1 Graphical representation of body compartments in a 70kg man.

Table 11.1 **Tracers used to measure body compartments**				
	Total body water	**Extracellular fluid**	**Whole blood**	**Plasma**
Tracer	Isotopically labelled water: deuterium (^{2}H), tritium (^{3}H)	Thiosulphate Inulin Mannitol Radiochloride Radiosodium	Labelled red cells: ^{51}Cr	Labelled albumin: radio-iodine or Evans blue dye.

11.2 Movement of water across cell membranes

Osmosis and osmotic pressure

Water crosses cell membranes readily along osmotic gradients, i.e. until the osmolality (particle/water ratio) is the same on both sides.

When solutes are added to water, intermolecular forces lead to a reduction in the random movement of the water molecules i.e. a reduction in activity. Where different compartments are separated by a semipermeable membrane (i.e. a membrane permeable to water but not to solute), water will move from areas of high activity to those of low activity until equilibrium is reached.

This movement of water is called osmosis. A solution containing particles exerts osmotic pressure: this is the hydrostatic pressure that would need to be exerted to oppose the osmotic movement of water (Figure 11. 2).

Osmotic pressure is one of the colligative properties of a solution (see opposite). The osmotic pressure of a solution can be calculated using the van't Hoff equation:

$$\text{osmotic pressure} = n \times (c/M) \times RT$$

where n is the number of particles into which the substance dissociates (e.g. glucose counts as one particle, whereas salt (NaCl) dissociates into sodium and chloride, and therefore counts as two particles), c is the concentration (g/L), M is the molecular weight of the molecules, R is the universal gas constant and T is the absolute temperature (K).

Osmolality

The osmolality of a solution is the **number of osmoles of solute per kilogram of solvent**. One osmole contains Avogadro's number (6.02 $\times 10^{23}$) of particles. The osmolality of body fluids is determined by particles in milimolar concentrations, so the units used are **mosm/kg**. An osmometer measures the osmolality of the specimen (e.g. by depression of freezing point.)

Osmolarity

The osmolarity of a solution is **the number of osmoles of solute per litre of solution**. (NB: the volume of a solution changes with temperature.) The osmolarity of body fluids can be estimated by adding the concentrations of those substances present in millimolar concentrations according to the formula (the units are **mosm/L**):

$$\text{osmolarity} = 2([Na^+] + [K^+]) + [\text{urea}] + [\text{glucose}].$$

Note that the sodium and potassium contribution is doubled, because each cation of Na^+ or K^+ will have an associated anion (mainly chloride).

There is a difference between measured osmolality and calculated osmolarity as the calculation does not include particles present in low concentrations (e.g. calcium, magnesium, and their accompanying anions). This difference is known as the osmolar gap and should be no more than 10:

measured osmolality – calculated osmolarity = osmolar gap.

A raised osmolar gap is due to the presence of other unmeasured particles in milimolar concentrations (e.g. ingested alcohols).

Tonicity (effective osmolality)

Tonicity is the **osmolality due to effective osmoles.**

Only particles restricted to one of the compartments will determine water distribution; these are termed effective osmoles.

Particles that can move freely across the cell membrane will not effect water distribution, and are known as ineffective osmoles. These include urea, glucose (see below), and alcohol.

Administered glucose is usually an ineffective osmole, since in the presence of insulin it enters cells readily. Thus 5% dextrose, while being isosmolar, is effectively hypotonic as the administered water distributes throughout the body. It contains no effective osmoles to restrict water to any specific compartment. All pure dextrose solutions are hypotonic, although their osmolarities will vary with the actual dextrose concentration used.

In diabetics, lack of insulin inhibits glucose entry into muscle and fat cells. Glucose concentrations can then rise and glucose will act as an effective osmole (Figure 11.3). Therefore water will move out of these cells, leading to a fall in $[Na^+]$. $[Na^+]$ falls by approximately 1.5mmol/L for every 5.5 mmol/L rise in [glucose] from normal (Table 11.2). In contrast, liver cells do not need insulin and have a glucose concentration equal to the ECF so the hyperglycaemia *per se* has no influence on water shifts in the liver. However the fall in $[Na^+]$ caused by water movement out of muscle cells will cause water to enter hepatocytes and they will swell.

Effective osmoles (tonicity) determine water movement. The number of effective osmoles in each compartment determines the volume of that compartment.

ICF effective osmoles

The major intracellular particles are large macromolecular anions and K^+. Since these macromolecules are largely proteins and organic phosphate esters (ATP, RNA, DNA, creatine phosphate, phospholipids), which are essential for cell function, only small net changes in their content occur. The total number of ICF particles is therefore relatively constant in number.

Therefore changes in ICF tonicity are due to changes in cellular water content (see Section 11.4). *Tonicity reflects cell volume.*

ECF effective osmoles

The major effective osmoles in the ECF are Na^+ and its accompanying anions, and so the *tonicity* of the ECF is largely determined by the sodium *concentration* $[Na^+]$, while the *volume* of the ECF is determined by the total number of Na^+ particles, i.e. the Na^+ *content*.

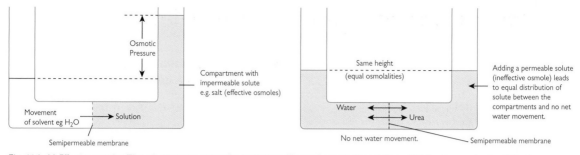

Fig. 11.2 (a) Effective osmoles. The solvent moves across the semipermeable membrane to the solution, which has lower solvent activity. As a consequence, the hydrostatic pressure rises. At equilibrium, the hydrostatic pressure will equal the osmotic pressure and solvent will not move. (b) Ineffective osmoles. No net water movement, with equal osmolarity and osmotic pressure either side of the semipermeable membrane.

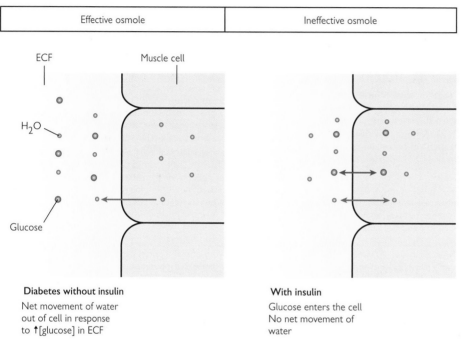

Fig. 11.3 Clinical example of effective and ineffective osmoles:

Plasma tonicity = $2([Na^+] + [K^+]) + [glucose]$.

Plasma osmolarity = $2([Na^+] + [K^+]) + [glucose] + [urea]$.

NB: In most individuals, [glucose] is kept constant but in diabetics this may change significantly. Table 11.2 illlustrates this.

Table 11.2 **Effects of hyperglycaemia on plasma sodium and tonicity**			
	[Na⁺] (mmol/L)	**[glucose] (mmol/L)**	**Tonicity**
Normal	140	5	Normal
Hyperglycaemia (DKA, no insulin)	128	49	↑, despite hyponatraemia
As a guide, [Na⁺] falls by 1.5mmol for every 5.5mmol rise in [glucose]. When the glucose is removed, water will flow back into cells and [Na⁺] will rise.			

➜ **Colligative properties of solutions**

Colligative properties are the properties of solutions containing non-volatile solutes, which depend on the concentration of the solute (number of particles). The four colligative properties are:

• **Solvent vapour pressure (Section 2.8):** decreases as solute concentration increases (Raoult's law).
• **Freezing point:** depression as solute concentration increases (this property is exploited in osmometry).
• **Boiling point:** elevation as solute concentration increases.
• **Osmotic pressure:** increases with solute concentration.

11.3 Tonicity and sodium concentration

Effects of changes in tonicity

Hypotonicity causes cell swelling, and hypertonicity causes cellular dehydration. The organ most readily affected is the brain, contained within the rigid skull (Monro–Kellie doctrine, Section 7.10).

Therefore the symptoms of tonicity changes are largely neurological. Swelling may result in raised intracranial pressure, diminished blood supply, and ultimately herniation and death. Shrinkage, on the other hand, may stretch vascular connections (leading to intracranial haemorrhage) or cause venous sinus thrombosis.

Plasma sodium concentration and tonicity

Since water moves freely, ICF and ECF tonicity are equal. Cellular volume (i.e. water content) can be determined simply by measuring ECF tonicity. **[Na$^+$] is used as a marker for this.**

Hypernatraemia

In adults, the most common clinical manifestation of hypernatraemia (hypertonicity and therefore cellular dehydration) is altered mental state and a decreasing level of consciousness. In small children, alternating periods of lethargy and irritability may be seen. Tachypnoea, nausea and vomiting are also common. Seizures may occur.

Hypernatraemia *always* means hypertonicity and intracellular dehydration. The patient requires free water to replenish intracellular volume, irrespective of any ECF volume changes. ECF volume may be increased, normal, or reduced.

Hyponatraemia

Symptoms that appear with a slow reduction in [Na$^+$] include headache, nausea, vomiting, muscle cramps, lethargy, and irritability. Large or rapid declines in [Na$^+$] can lead to serious complications, including seizures, coma, brainstem herniation, respiratory arrest, and death.

Hyponatraemia *usually* means hypotonicity and cell swelling, but sometimes other particles can act as effective ECF osmoles so that tonicity is normal or even increased. Such particles include glucose *in the absence of insulin* (i.e. diabetes, Section 11.2), mannitol, and glycine. The presence of extra unmeasured particles can be discovered by comparing the calculated osmolarity with the measured osmolality. An increased **osmolar gap** demonstrates the presence of unmeasured particles, but does not tell you what they are, or whether or not they are effective osmoles. For example, consider a patient with:

- [Na$^+$] 120mmol/L
- normal [urea]
- normal [glucose]
- normal measured osmolality.

Clearly some unmeasured particle is contributing to the serum osmolality (Table 11.3). Consider the different effects which would be seen if the particles were alcohol or mannitol molecules.

- *Alcohol:* the patient's ECF will be hypotonic (and cell water content increased) as alcohol molecules pass freely into cells (ineffective osmoles) and do not alter tonicity.
- *Mannitol:* the patient's ECF will still be isotonic as mannitol is an effective osmolar substance. Cell water content will be normal.

The clinical setting provides the clues to the identity of the particles. For example, during transurethral prostate resection, irrigation fluids containing particles such as mannitol or glycine are used which may be absorbed into the circulation. Both these particles act as effective osmoles, holding water in the ECF. Glycine distributes only slowly into muscle cells and almost not at all into the CNS. The absorption of these solutions will lead to a fall in [Na$^+$]. However, in order to define the real tonicity change, the serum osmolality must be measured. Simple inspection of [Na$^+$] will be misleading.

Regulation of tonicity

Changes in tonicity (and therefore cell volume) can be life-threatening. The body has sensors to detect this and effector mechanisms to restore normality. These are very sensitive, responding to swings of just 1–2%.

Osmoreceptors might more appropriately be called tonicity receptors. Located in the hypothalamus, they swell or shrink in response to changes in tonicity.

- Hypertonicity activates thirst and secretion of ADH. This causes renal free water retention (see below).
- Hypotonicity switches off thirst and inhibits the secretion of ADH. In the absence of ADH, dilute urine is excreted. (This inhibition of ADH release may be overridden by non-osmotic stimuli for ADH; see below).

Antidiuretic hormone (ADH)

ADH (also called arginine vasopressin (AVP)) has been characterized as a nine amino acid peptide. It is synthesized in specialized (magnocellular) neural cells in two areas of the hypothalamus: the supra-optic and paraventricular nuclei (Figure 11.4). The peptide is enzymatically cleaved from a pro-hormone and transported to the posterior pituitary where it is stored within neurosecretory granules. Specific stimuli, such as osmoreceptor signals, cause secretion into the bloodstream.

For water to cross a lipid membrane, a channel is required. In the distal nephron; this channel is called aquaporin-2 (AQP-2). When ADH binds to AVP V$_2$ receptors on the basolateral aspect of the distal nephron (collecting tubule) cells, cAMP is formed (Figure 11.5). This activates protein kinase A, in turn causing phosphorylation of AQP-2. AQP-2 is located in vesicles in the cytosol. When ADH acts on the kidney these vesicles fuse to the cell membrane, increasing the number of pores, and water transport is enhanced.

Water moves out of the nephron because of differences in tonicity across the membrane. A hypertonic medulla (generated by the loop of Henle) provides this gradient (Section 12.4). In conditions where this is impaired (e.g. recovery from acute tubular necrosis) the kidney cannot concentrate the urine, and patients will be polyuric. This can result in inappropriate water loss and hypertonicity if water excretion is not matched with intake.

ADH also increases the permeability of the medullary collecting duct to urea (the hypertonicity of the medulla 'pulling' water out of the nephron is generated by high concentrations of NaCl and urea).

This is a finely tuned regulatory system which adjusts the rate of free water excretion accurately to the ambient plasma tonicity via changes in ADH secretion. The rapid response of ADH secretion to tonicity changes, coupled with the short half-life (10–20min) of ADH enables this system to adjust renal water excretion to changes in tonicity on a minute-by-minute basis.

ADH is also secreted in response to non-osmotic stimuli, which has important clinical implications. ADH levels rise in response to hypovolaemia, hypotension, and situations of impaired arterial circulation. Information from baroreceptors is relayed to the nucleus tractus solitarius of the brain stem and ultimately to the hypothalamus. Higher levels of ADH stimulate V$_1$ receptors on blood vessels to increase vascular resistance and maintain blood pressure.

Nausea (with or without vomiting) is the most potent stimulus for ADH secretion. The reason for this is unknown. A variety of drugs also stimulate ADH secretion.

Therefore it can readily be appreciated that a number of potential stimuli for ADH secretion exist in the perioperative setting, potentially resulting in water retention, hypotonicity and cell swelling.

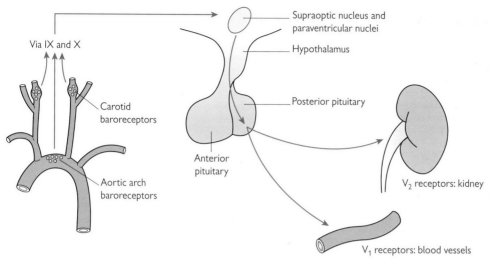

Fig. 11.4 Stimuli for the production of ADH. Osmoreceptors in the supra-optic nucleus respond to tonicity changes. Cells begin to synthesize and secrete ADH at an effective osmolality of 280mosm/kg. Maximum water retention occurs at a P_{osm} of 290mosm/kg. Urea is an ineffective osmole. A 10% reduction in blood pressure results in less baroreceptor stretch and ultimately in increased ADH secretion. This information is conveyed by cranial nerves IX and X.

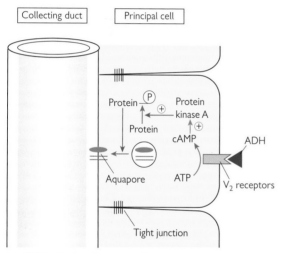

Fig. 11.5 Production of aquaporins. V_2 receptors on the basolateral membrane of principal cells are GPCRs that stimulate production of cAMP. Stimulation leads to insertion of aquaporin channels into the apical membrane.

> ➡ **Aquaporins**
>
> Aquaporins are water channels that mediate transcellular water transport within the nephron. Currently 11 discrete types have been identified.
> - Aquaporin 1: apical and basolateral membranes of the proximal tubule and descending thin limb of the loop of Henle.
> - Aquaporin 2: apical plasma membrane of principle cells in the collecting duct. AVP regulated.
> - Aquaporin 3 and 4: basolateral membrane of CD cells in the collecting duct.

Table 11.3 The influence of ineffective and effective osmoles on tonicity and osmolality in the presence of hyponatraemia

Additional molecules	Nil	Alcohol ingestion	Mannitol
Na⁺	120	120	120
K⁺	5	5	5
Urea	5	5	5
Glucose	5	5	5
Calculated osmolality	260	260	260
Measured osmolality	270	310	310
Osmolar gap	≤10	>45	>45
Significance	No additional unmeasured particles	Additional particles present	Additional particles present
Tonicity	Hypotonic	Hypotonic: **ineffective osmoles**	Hypertonic: **effective osmoles**
Cell size	Swollen	Swollen	Shrunken

ECF fluid balance

In contrast with ICF particles (Section 11.2), the total number of ECF particles (mostly sodium and accompanying anions) can change significantly. Tonicity changes in the ECF can be due to changes in sodium content, water content, or both. Therefore Na *concentration (tonicity)* tells you nothing about the *amount* of sodium in the body (and consequently the ECF volume). This must be determined by clinical examination: ECF overload is characterized by raised JVP or CVP and oedema (systemic or pulmonary), while depletion can be seen as low venous pressures, cool peripheries, hypotension, tachycardia, and reduced skin turgor.

Since sodium content determines ECF volume, the regulation of ECF volume is essentially the regulation of sodium balance. Sensor and effector mechanisms exist to control this. However, apart from venous volume receptors, these receptors detect changes in the 'effective arterial circulation' rather than the actual volume of ECF. This has important clinical consequences.

The promotion of Na retention

When the central venous volume is high, atrial natriuretic peptide (ANP) is released from the right atrium. This decreases vascular resistance and promotes NaCl excretion. It also diminishes the release of aldosterone from the zona glomerulosa. When venous volume is low, ANP release is in inhibited.

Sodium retention is promoted by receptors in the arterial circulation. Low blood pressure is detected by baroreceptors in the aortic arch, and increased sympathetic activity promotes increased sodium reabsorption by the proximal convoluted tubular (PCT) cells of the kidney and stimulates renin release from the juxtaglomerular apparatus. A low renal perfusion pressure also causes renin release.

Renin acts on angiotensinogen to produce angiotensin I, which is converted to angiotensin II by ACE in the lung. Angiotensin II causes vasoconstriction, promotes reabsorption of Na^+ by the PCT, and stimulates aldosterone release. It also stimulates thirst.

Increased Na^+ absorption by the PCT is accompanied by passive water absorption to maintain isotonicity.

Aldosterone promotes Na^+ reabsorption by the distal tubule in exchange for K^+ or H^+.

Conditions resulting in impaired arterial circulation (e.g. heart failure) or impaired renal perfusion (e.g. renal artery stenosis) lead to activation of Na^+-retaining mechanisms, and expansion of the ECF. Although this will lead to increased ANP secretion, Na^+ retention predominates (GFR will be reduced in these situations, and so ANP becomes less effective).

Non-osmotic ADH release

In conditions of reduced effective arterial circulation, ADH secretion is promoted, resulting in water retention (Section 11.3). Even if this leads to hypotonicity, ADH release will continue if non-osmotic stimuli remain (ECF volume maintenance takes priority over tonicity).

Therefore the administration of significant volumes of hypotonic fluids in situations where ADH has been released will result in hyponatraemia, hypotonicity, and cell swelling. If this occurs quickly enough, it may be fatal, and cases continue to be reported in both adults and children inappropriately prescribed hypotonic fluids, such as one-fifth normal saline in dextrose or dextrose solutions, in the perioperative period.

Defence of brain cell volume

The total number of particles in the ICF in most cells rarely changes, but changes do occur in brain cells during *chronic* shrinking or swelling. This is advantageous since the consequences of brain swelling or shrinkage can be devastating. Cell swelling can cause increased intracranial pressure, leading to cerebral ischaemia, infarction, or even coning; conversely, neuronal shrinkage can lead to traction on meninges and vessels, and in some instances, intracranial haemorrhage. In order to return swollen cells to normal, intracellular electrolytes (K^+ and Cl^-) and amino acids or small peptides are extruded. In contrast, the mechanism to gain ICF volume in states of cellular dehydration involves an influx of small particles, probably Na^+. The particles that change within the ICF of the brain in response to volume changes have been termed 'idiogenic osmoles'.

This explains why patients may be asymptomatic despite marked changes in tonicity [Na^+]. In this situation it is important not to try to correct [Na^+]

too quickly. Returning [Na^+] to normal in an individual with chronic hyponatraemia will result in shrunken cells unless it is done slowly enough for the cells to regain the particles that they have previously extruded. Too-rapid correction of hyponatraemia has resulted in the development of osmotic demyelination syndromes such as central pontine myelinolysis, which can result in an irreversible quadriparesis with bulbar involvement.

In chronic hyponatraemia the rise in [Na^+] should be limited to <8mmol/day.

Symptomatic changes in [Na^+] need to be treated acutely to stop the symptoms. Once asymptomatic, further correction can be achieved more slowly.

Hyponatraemia

The most common setting for acute and potentially life-threatening hyponatraemia is in the perioperative period.

Excess water intake is usually excreted rapidly. For hyponatraemia to occur there must be excess water intake *and* inhibition of the normal excretory mechanisms. Removal of the excess requires glomerular filtration and subsequent excretion. Therefore retention will occur if there is loss of filtration (uncommon) or inhibition of excretion, i.e. ADH secretion (common).

In cases of hyponatraemia, there will always be water intake (e.g. IV fluids) and, and in the absence of filtration failure, ADH secretion, which may be appropriate or inappropriate. Appropriate ADH secretion occurs in the perioperative period and is usually due to an ECF deficit.

In these cases, restoring the ECF volume with isotonic fluids will turn off the ADH, excess water will be excreted, and [Na^+] will rise. On the other hand, administering hypotonic fluids (such as one-fifth normal saline in dextrose) will cause a further decrease in [Na^+] *before* an adequate amount of salt has been given to replete the ECF deficit. The resulting brain swelling can be fatal, with the patient progressing quickly from feeling unwell to developing seizures, respiratory arrest, and brainstem death.

In cases where ADH has been secreted in response to non-osmotic stimuli, and the ECF volume is normal, simple restriction of water to less than obligatory losses will allow the excess water to be lost slowly and cell volume will return to normal with restoration of a normal [Na^+].

If the patient is symptomatic, [Na^+] must be raised more quickly, at least initially (although beware too-rapid changes). Increasing [Na^+] by a few mmol/L is usually enough to stop symptoms. The options for doing this include giving Na^+-containing infusions that are of a higher concentration than the patient's serum. Occasionally hypertonic saline is needed: 3ml/kg of 3% saline is usually enough to raise [Na^+] and stop immediate symptoms; further rises can be attained more slowly. The scope for giving saline infusions may be restricted if the patient already has ECF expansion and there is concern that pulmonary oedema may occur.

Free-water excretion can be promoted using a loop diuretic. By interfering with the loop of Henle, the generation of a hypertonic renal medulla is impaired. This in turn impairs the ability of ADH to cause water retention (since this depends on the hypertonic medulla). Although the diuretic causes sodium loss, the water loss is usually greater and so [Na^+] tends to rise.

Use of a loop diuretic can be combined with saline infusion to increase the rate of rise of [Na^+].

Note that distal tubular diuretics, such as thiazides, impair Na^+ reabsorption but leave water-retaining mechanisms intact. Thus their use may *cause* hyponatraemia.

Table 11.4 shows the relative changes in sodium and water which must occur to cause hyponatraemia, while Table 11.5 summarises the approach to management.

Hypernatraemia

Free water administration (nasogastric water or IV infusions of hypotonic fluids) is required to replenish cell volume.

Management of the ECF volume depends on clinical examination. If there is an ECF deficit, this requires repletion and isotonic saline is appropriate despite the hypernatraemia. If the ECF is normal or expanded, salt should be avoided. With ECF expansion, a diuretic might be indicated to promote excretion of the excess salt. Figure 11.7 demonstrates that ECF volume changes are not reflected by plasma sodium concentration: oedema (ECF, and therefore total body sodium *content*) may or may not be associated with derangements in [Na^+].

→ Principles of management of hypo- and hypernatraemia

The key principles of ICF and ECF volume and tonicity should always be rigorously applied to management of sodium derangements.

- Always consider ECF volume (Na^+ balance/content) and intracellular volume (tonicity/water balance) separately.
- Hypernatraemia *always* means hypertonicity and ICF water depletion. The patient requires free water for intracellular rehydration.
- Hyponatraemia *often* means hypotonicity, but the osmolar gap and clinical history may indicate normal or even increased tonicity.
- Sodium *concentration* **tells us nothing** about *total sodium balance* and *ECF volume*. Clinical examination is required to gauge the ECF volume status of the patient.
- Chronic changes are better tolerated than acute changes. As a rule of thumb, derangements should be corrected at the rate they occurred.

Table 11.4 Hyponatraemia (and therefore swollen cells) may result from these changes to water and Na content

Hyponatraemia			
↑water	↑↑ water	Normal water	↓ water
Normal Na	↑ Na	↓ Na	↓↓ Na

Table 11.5 Principles of management of hyponatraemia*

Options	Indications	Notes	Notes
Restrict free water to less than obligatory losses	As sole management only for asymptomatic patients with normal or expanded ECF	[Na^+] will rise slowly	Avoid hypotonic fluids unless trying to prevent too-rapid a rise in [Na^+]
Give saline solutions of higher [Na^+] than patient	For patients with depleted ECF	Usually normal saline will suffice	Occasionally in symptomatic patients, hypertonic saline is indicated, e.g. 3ml/kg 3% saline to raise [Na^+] by a few mmol/L, then slow down rate of rise
Promote free water loss using a loop diuretic	For patients with normal or expanded ECF	If normal ECF then replace urinary losses with normal saline to avoid ECF depletion	Combining a loop diuretic with saline infusion will increase the rate of rise of [Na^+]

*Which option you choose depends on the urgency of treatment and the patient's ECF volume and consequent ability to tolerate a Na^+ load and consequent ECF expansion.

→ ADH secretion may be:

Appropriate Vascular baroreceptors sense reduced circulatory volume, as seen with plasma volume depletion, CCF, cirrhosis, and nephrotic syndrome. Hypovolaemia will stimulate secretion of ADH and override osmotic influence at the hypothalamus, causing hyponatremia.

Inappropriate This occurs when there is dysregulation of cells synthesizing and secreting ADH. The posterior pituitary is not always the source of ADH secretion. Different types of tumour, drugs, and various CNS and lung disorders are associated with inappropriate secretion of ADH.

The keys to diagnosis of SIADH are:

- Hyponatraemia
- Inappropriately elevated urine osmolality (>300mOsm/kg) with decreased serum osmolality
- Excessive urine sodium excretion (U_{Na} >30mEq/L).

The diagnosis can only be made in those who are Na^+ replete, and therefore without stimulus for **appropriate** ADH secretion. They should not be receiving diuretic therapy and should have normal cardiac, renal, adrenal, hepatic, and thyroid function.

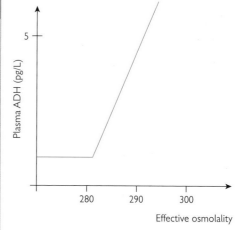

Fig. 11.6 The secretion of ADH.

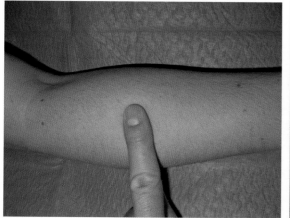

A

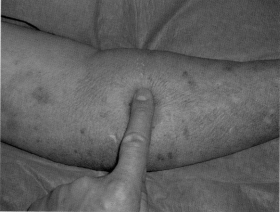

B

Fig. 11.7 (a) Normal arm: plasma [Na^+] = 140mmol/L. (b) Oedematous arm: plasma [Na^+] = 140mmol/L. ECF volume is determined by sodium *content*. This cannot be deduced from the plasma *concentration*.

Starling forces

Movement of fluid across the capillary wall involves hydrostatic and osmotic forces. Intravascular hydrostatic pressure comes from the work of the heart. Only large molecules such as plasma proteins can be effective osmoles across the capillary wall; small ions and glucose are ineffective, as the capillary is permeable to them.

The osmotic pressure due to plasma proteins is called **colloid osmotic pressure** or **oncotic pressure.**

Overall, forces tending to move an ultrafiltrate out of the capillary are capillary hydrostatic pressure and tissue oncotic pressure. Forces tending to push fluid into the capillary are tissue hydrostatic pressure and plasma oncotic pressure. Net movement is due to:

- The balance of these forces
- The surface area available for fluid transfer
- The permeability of the capillary membrane to fluid and small molecules
- The permeability to proteins.

This relationship is expressed by Starling's law (Figure 11.8).

Capillary hydrostatic pressure

Capillary hydrostatic pressure, and therefore the rate of capillary filtration, can be held relatively constant despite changes in blood pressure. This is termed autoregulation, and is largely under local control, e.g. by metabolic factors, vessel wall stretch receptors, humoral and neural factors.

Factors determining capillary hydrostatic pressure are arterial pressure, the resistance at the pre-capillary sphincter, and post-capillary resistance in the venules and veins. Alterations in pre-capillary sphincter tone help maintain capillary hydrostatic pressure. Resistance at the venous end is less well regulated, so changes in venous pressure tend to produce parallel changes in capillary hydrostatic pressure.

Capillaries in different organs have different haemodynamic and permeability characteristics. For example, alveolar capillaries have both a lower hydrostatic pressure and a lower transcapillary oncotic pressure gradient than skeletal muscle capillaries. As a result, hypoalbuminaemia is less likely to cause oedema here than in other capillary beds. On the other hand, glomerular capillaries differ in that they have a much higher hydrostatic pressure gradient with a high permeability, allowing a high rate of filtration.

Determinants of oncotic pressure

From van't Hoff's equation (Section 11.2) the oncotic pressure should be a linear function of protein concentration. However, the oncotic pressure measured is greater than that predicted. This difference is due in part to the **Gibbs–Donnan equilibrium.** This applies when one compartment contains non-diffusible ions (in this case, negatively-charged plasma proteins), and states that the product of the diffusible ions in each compartment is equal. Assuming for simplicity that the only diffusible ions in plasma and interstitial fluid are Na^+ and Cl^-, the equilibrium is satisfied by the equation:

plasma $[Na^+]$ x plasma $[Cl^-]$ = interstitial $[Na^+]$ x interstitial $[Cl^-]$

The $[Na^+]$ and $[Cl^-]$ in the interstitial fluid are equal. However, for electrical equilibrium, plasma $[Na^+]$ would need to be approximately 15mmol/L higher than $[Cl^-]$ to balance the negative charge on the plasma proteins.

Satisfying both the Gibbs–Donnan equation and the need for electrical neutrality, and assuming an interstitial $[Na^+]$ and $[Cl^-]$ of 145mmol/L each, we can calculate plasma concentrations of sodium and chloride: $[Na^+]$, 152.7mmol/L; $[Cl^-]$ 137.7mmol/L.

Therefore the total number of Na and Cl particles in the plasma is 290.4mmol/L, compared with 290mmol/L in the interstitium; therefore 0.4mosm/L oncotic pressure comes from the sodium and chloride ions themselves. As normal plasma protein concentration is approximately 0.9mmol/L, the total osmotic effect is 1.3 mosm/L. Since 1mosm/L generates an osmotic pressure of 19.3mmHg, this effect increases the capillary oncotic pressure from 17.4mmHg (0.9 × 19.3) to 25.09mmHg (1.3 × 19.3). Other poorly understood factors may also be involved.

Given the above, it might be expected that small decreases in plasma oncotic pressure, or increases in capillary hydrostatic pressure, would lead to interstitial oedema. In fact, relatively large changes are required. This is due to protective mechanisms, including:

- Increased lymphatic flow removing excess filtrate
- Falling interstitial oncotic pressure due to dilution and removal by the lymphatics (see below)
- Increasing interstitial fluid volume resulting in an increased interstitial hydrostatic pressure.

A falling albumin concentration leads to reduced entry of albumin into the interstitium and a parallel decline in interstitial protein concentration. This helps to maintain the *transcapillary* oncotic pressure gradient near normal and minimize fluid loss out of the capillary.

Oedema secondary to hypoalbuminaemia is only likely where it is acute, leaving little time for the interstitial oncotic pressure to fall (e.g. crystalloid resuscitation for massive bleeding), or where the plasma albumin concentration is less than 10g/L, when the transcapillary oncotic gradient cannot be maintained as the interstitial concentration cannot fall any further.

Lymph and lymphatics

The lymphatic system consists of capillaries located in virtually all tissues. Exceptions include the central nervous system, bone, and cartilage. These drain via lymph nodes, returning fluid to the venous system via the thoracic duct (at the junction of the left subclavian and internal jugular veins) and the much smaller right lymphatic duct. Lymph vessels usually travel with arteries and veins. Lymph nodes contain sinusoids lined by macrophages (part of the reticuloendothelial system), which filter and phagocytose bacteria and debris. Lymphocytes are also present in the nodes, proliferating on exposure to specific antigens. Lymph capillaries are blind-ending with flap valves, allowing interstitial fluid to enter but not to return to the interstitium. Larger vessels have smooth muscle in their walls. Flow is promoted by compression from surrounding structures, e.g. muscle contraction and nearby arterial pulsation. Valves prevent reflux.

Lymphatics return protein and excess fluid to the circulation, and transport fat as chylomicrons from the small intestine. Lymph from the small intestine is milky in appearance after a meal. Protein removal keeps the interstitial protein concentration low (approximately 20g/L), helping to prevent oedema formation.

Lymph generally reflects interstitial fluid in its composition. Since hepatic sinusoids are very permeable to proteins, the protein concentration in hepatic lymph is higher (60g/L), which gives rise to a thoracic duct lymph protein concentration of about 50g/L.

Net filtration at the arterial end of capillaries is about 20ml/min, with 18ml/min returning to the circulation at the venous end. The net lymph production is therefore about 2ml/min, i.e. 10% of fluid filtered in the capillaries returns to the circulation as lymph. The majority (approximately 100ml/hr at rest) returns via the thoracic duct. Lymph production can increase markedly with exercise.

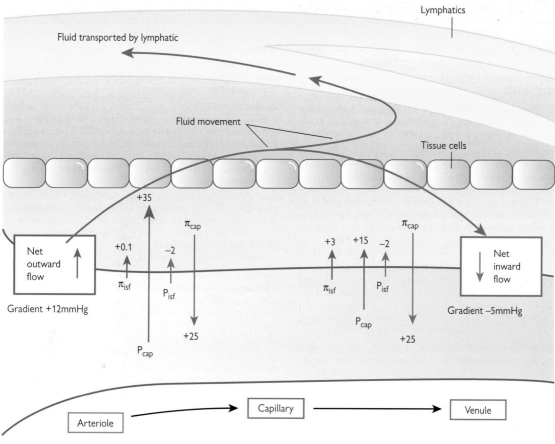

Fig. 11.8 Starling's forces. Typical numerical values are shown (these vary between different tissues):

$$\text{net filtration} = L_pS \left[(P_{cap} - P_{isf}) - s(\Pi_{cap} - \Pi_{isf}) \right]$$

where L_p is the unit permeability (or porosity) of the capillary wall, S is the surface area available for fluid movement, P_{cap} and P_{isf} are the capillary and interstitial fluid hydraulic pressures, respectively, Π_{cap} and Π_{isf} are the capillary and interstitial fluid oncotic pressures, respectively, and s is the reflection coefficient of proteins across the capillary wall (values range from 0 (completely permeable) to 1 (completely impermeable)). The capillary hydrostatic pressure falls along its length. This results in net fluid flow out of the capillary at first but by the end there is a smaller net flow back into the vessel. The fluid that does not drain back into the capillary is transported back to the circulation by the lymphatics.

11.6 Crystalloids and colloids

Available fluids are traditionally divided into crystalloids and colloids, but they should be also considered in terms of tonicity.

Crystalloids

Crystalloids provide water, electrolytes, and glucose in varying composition according to the specific formulation of individual fluids. Therefore their osmolarity and tonicity vary.

5% dextrose

This has an osmolarity of 278mosm/L, but since glucose is normally an ineffective osmole its tonicity is zero. Giving pure dextrose solutions is equivalent to giving pure water which will distribute throughout the body in a $^2/_3:^1/_3$ ratio across the ICF and ECF respectively (Figure 11.9). Excessive administration of such dextrose solutions will lead to hypotonicity and cell swelling, indicated by a falling [Na$^+$], unless the excess water is excreted.

Normal saline

This contains 154mmol/L of NaCl and therefore is expected to have an osmolarity of 308mosm/L. Since Na$^+$ and Cl$^-$ are effective osmoles restricted to the ECF, the tonicity and osmolarity are identical and close to normal body tonicity. Therefore it is isotonic. Since it is restricted to the ECF, it will distribute throughout that compartment (approximately 25% intravascular and 75% interstitial).

One-fifth normal saline in 4% dextrose

The tonicity is one-fifth normal, so that giving a 1000ml infusion would effectively be the same as giving 200 ml of normal saline and 800 ml of dextrose.

Lactated Ringer's solution (Hartmann's solution)

Hartmann's solution is more physiological than saline in terms of electrolyte composition and is approximately isotonic, so it is commonly used for ECF replacement. The lactate is metabolized as the whole lactate molecule rather than the lactate ion, consuming H$^+$ and leaving net bicarbonate in its place (the H$^+$ comes from carbonic acid). Use of this fluid for ECF expansion does not result in the acidosis seen with large-volume saline infusions (Section 11.13).

Excessive administration of isotonic fluids will lead to ECF expansion with oedema and increased vascular pressures. Crystalloid solutions are cheaper than colloids, and are non-allergenic.

Colloids

Colloids contain larger particles which cross the capillary membrane less easily and therefore exert a similar oncotic effect to plasma proteins. This results in a slower loss of the infused fluid from the circulation compared with isotonic crystalloids. Use of colloids to replace blood loss results in less total ECF expansion, and therefore less oedema and weight gain, compared with isotonic crystalloids.

The controversy as to whether isotonic crystalloids or colloids are better for volume resuscitation remains ongoing. Colloids are more expensive and, depending on the specific solution, vary in their physical and chemical properties and potential side effects.

The main colloids currently available are gelatins, starches, dextrans, and albumin. Synthetic colloids are polydisperse molecules of variable size and they generally exhibit similar effectiveness in maintaining colloid oncotic pressure, but there are differences in their side-effect profiles. Selection of a specific colloid has often been based predominantly on cost and availability and therefore colloid use varies between countries (gelatins are unavailable in the USA).

Colloid preparations are generally suspended in normal saline, although preparations suspended in a more physiological 'balanced' solution do exist. Perceived benefits of these include reduced changes in electrolyte and acid–base status compared with a large saline load.

Gelatins

These are polypeptides formed from degradation products of animal collagen. The gelatins are either succinylated or linked to urea and are usually suspended in normal saline.

Starches

Hydroxyethyl starch (HES) is synthesized by partial hydrolysis of amylopectin plant starch and hydroxylation at the C2, C3, and C6 positions of the constituent glucose molecules. Starch preparations are generally suspended in normal saline. HES is clinically available in a number of formulations differing in both average molecular weight and extent of molar substitution.

In the USA, only high molecular weight (450kDa) of 0.7 molar substitution (HES 450/0.7) is used routinely. In Europe, HES products of varying molecular weight and/or molar substitution have been introduced on the basis that adverse effects are primarily attributable to less easily cleared preparations of higher molecular weight and greater molar substitution. However, this remains to be proven.

Dextrans

These are naturally occurring linear polysaccharide molecules synthesized by *Leuconostoc mesenteroides* bacteria growing in sucrose-containing media. They may be suspended in normal saline or 5% dextrose.

Albumin

This is a 69kDa protein purified from human plasma. It is available in 5% and 25% preparations and the incidence of adverse events is low. It is more expensive than the artificial preparations and its use has declined.

Reported side effects of colloids

Anaphylactoid reactions

These are relatively infrequent, occurring most commonly with gelatins and least commonly with albumin, dextrans, and starch.

Pruritus

This is largely confined to HES (although there have been occasional reports of occurrence in dextrans). It appears to be dose-dependent (more common with repeated doses) and typically delayed in onset, ranges from mild to severe, and is generally unresponsive to treatment. It has occurred in patients receiving less than the maximum recommended dose.

Coagulopathy

HES administration can lead to reduction in the levels of circulating factor VIII and von Willebrand factor, impairment of platelet function, prolongation of partial thromboplastin time and activated partial thromboplastin time, and increased bleeding complications. Manufacturers provide recommendations on dosage. Excessive administration of any colloid may cause dilution of clotting factors and platelets.

Renal failure

All three artificial colloids have been associated with renal impairment, although the highest incidence appears to be with HES.

Tissue deposition

HES is deposited in a variety of tissues including skin, liver, muscle, spleen, intestine, trophoblast, and placental stroma. Deposition has been associated with pruritus. Deposits may persist for years.

Rheology

Alterations in plasma viscosity are complex and depend on a number of factors including molecular weight of colloid, speed, and degree of degradation, and size of particle produced, as well as the effect of cumulative doses. Low molecular weight dextrans are often used to improve the microvascular circulation by decreasing blood viscosity. They also reduce platelet and red blood cell aggregation by coating endothelial cells; however, this may predispose to bleeding.

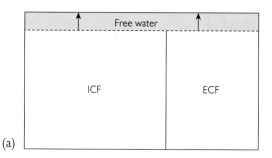

Addition of free water (i.e. water without effective osmoles) causes proportional expansion of all compartments. Reduced [Na$^+$] indicates the changed tonicity

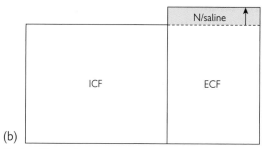

Addition of isotonic fluids (e.g. saline) expands the ECF compartment. This is detected by clinical examination. If [Na$^+$] remains unchanged, tonicity will be unchanged and ICF volume will remain the same.

Fig. 11.9 The distribution of (a) free water and (b) isotonic crystalloid across the intra- and extracellular compartments.

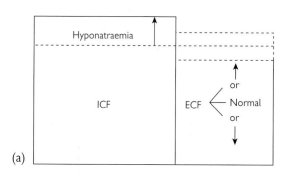

Hyponatraemia will usually mean hypotonicity. ICF volume is increased and cells become swollen.
The ECF volume may be reduced, normal or increased.

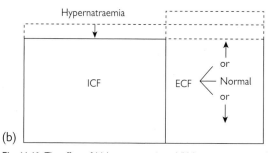

Hypernatraemia means hypertonicity and shrunken cells.
The ECF volume may be reduced, normal or increased.

Fig. 11.10 The effect of (a) hyponatraemia and (b) hypernatraemia on ICF volume.

There is no universal regimen for fluid prescription that can be applied to every patient. Prescribing will require fine-tuning as predicted losses and requirements will vary under the influence of both hormonal and inflammatory responses and underlying renal and cardiovascular function. Abnormal losses will also require consideration, e.g. drainage following major surgery.

When there is a perceived deficit the fluid prescribed should be appropriate to that deficit, i.e. intracellular, intravascular, or interstitial. Therefore 'replacement' regimes should be tailored to the compartment to be filled and not by simply increasing 'maintenance' regimes.

The best approach requires:

- An understanding of the underlying principles
- A willingness regularly to examine the patient to determine ECF volume changes
- Regular examination of blood results to determine tonicity and electrolyte changes.

Salt balance and water balance must be considered separately, and clinicians should regularly review the patient for signs of water retention, or loss and/or sodium retention or loss. Table 11.6 gives some clinical scenarios of fluid balance derangements.

Salt balance

Since Na^+ and its accompanying anions are the major effective osmoles of the ECF, ECF volume is determined by the total amount of sodium present. Too much salt leads to expansion of the ECF and too little salt leads to depletion. The volume of the ECF is assessed by clinical examination.

Having examined a patient, you should be able to state whether or not you consider their interstitial space to be obviously expanded, apparently euvolaemic, or obviously depleted. The vascular compartment should be similarly examined and its volume inferred. Only then are you in a position to decide what you need to do about the ECF, i.e. should salt be given or restricted?

Clinical examination cannot detect subtle changes, and so volume changes ≤15% will be missed. Clues suggesting possible ECF volume change can be gained from the patient's history and knowledge of the normal physiological responses. For example, with ECF deficit (in the absence of renal disease or recent diuretics) the urinary $[Na^+]$ should be low (< 10mmol/L) because of the action of aldosterone. Plasma [urea] tends to rise more than [creatinine], and so the urea-to-creatinine ratio is elevated. With ECF volume contraction, there is not only a reduced GFR but also enhanced reabsorption of urea from the renal tubule. Urate similarly undergoes increased tubular reabsorption.

Salt deficit

ECF contraction results in proportional fluid loss from both the interstitial fluid volume (IFV) and the circulating volume (CV). Many of the physical signs associated with ECF contraction are the signs of circulatory changes, and (with the exception of the JVP) reflect circulatory efficacy rather than volume *per se*. Abnormalities in circulatory efficacy may also be caused by cardiac dysfunction or changes in the peripheral vasculature. **They are not pathognomonic of volume deficits**.

ECF contraction is rectified by treatment with isotonic solutions.

Salt excess

Cases of total ECF excess are more complex as the two main compartments (IFV and CV) do not always change proportionately, or even in the same direction.

Oedema requires interstitial expansion of at least a few extra litres before it can be detected clinically. Its presence always denotes a total increase in ECF volume. However, while this may be accompanied by a proportional increase in circulating volume, (e.g. in cases of renal failure), at other times it may be accompanied by a decrease in circulating volume, (e.g. capillary leak syndromes such as sepsis and burns).

Management of ECF expansion depends on the circulating volume.

- Where this is also increased the patient will need to lose salt.
- If the CV is depleted, the patient will require further salt (despite the expanded interstitial space) and should be given isotonic fluids. Further oedema will inevitably occur. Development of oedema may be reduced with the use of colloids, but there is no definitive evidence that this results in better outcome.

Water balance

Cell volume is determined by water balance:

- Too much water causes cell swelling and hypotonicity as indicated by ↓$[Na^+]$
- Too little water causes cell shrinkage and hypertonicity (↑$[Na^+]$).

Therefore patients with high $[Na^+]$ require free water (i.e. water without effective osmoles) and those with low $[Na^+]$ should have free water restricted, irrespective of what is required for the ECF.

Maintenance fluids

The baseline for fluid prescription is usually prescription of 'normal maintenance requirements', with extra added to cover abnormal losses. The standard 'maintenance' regime for adults reflects a 'normal' intake of approximately 3L of water and up to 154mmol of Na^+ daily (e.g. 1L 0.9% saline and 2L 5% dextrose). However it is essential to appreciate the difference between obligatory requirements and so-called 'normal' maintenance.

Obligatory requirements are those that replace obligatory losses and are the minimum that must be provided. Obligatory requirements are usually significantly less than normal maintenance volumes; administration of the latter relies on excretion of the excess Na^+ and water. This may not be possible in those with inadequate renal or cardiovascular function. Conversely, others may have increased obligatory losses, e.g. from drains, stomas or urine (e.g. in polyuric states), and require more than standard maintenance regimens.

Furthermore, postoperative secretion of aldosterone and ADH will cause retention of both salt and water, exacerbated by excessive IV fluids. Some authorities now advocate giving ≤2L/day for baseline maintenance postoperatively, although these lower volumes may prove inadequate for some patients.

Administration of 3L/day over several days may result in excess sodium or water retention in a number of patients.

Administration of hypotonic fluids in the presence of ADH secretion or hyponatraemia increases mortality and morbidity from encephalopathy. Children and young women are most at risk. Unfortunately, despite the causes being well known and documented, cases are still occurring perioperatively and as a consequence the National Patient Safety Agency (NPSA) in the UK has made recommendations for the administration of IV fluids to children (Section 20.3).

Desalination

Simply prescribing only isotonic fluids does not remove the risk of hypotonicity completely: the Na and Cl of the infused fluid may be excreted but the water retained through the action of ADH.

For example, if 2L of N-saline are infused but only 1L of urine is produced, with $[Na^+]$ and $[Cl^-]$ concentrations of 308mmol each, effectively 1L of free water would have been retained. Assuming a normal ECF volume in this example, urinary excretion of a high concentration of NaCl is appropriate. If the plasma $[Na^+]$ is low, the stimulus for ADH secretion must then be non-osmotic. Management should simply be to restrict/stop all fluids and allow loss of the excess water.

Cerebral salt-wasting

Rarely, excessive renal sodium excretion may be the result of a centrally mediated process with intracranial disease, termed cerebral salt wasting (CSW). This is characterized by excessive Na^+ loss, possibly due to impaired Na^+ reabsorption in the proximal tubule. These patients have signs of ECF volume contraction with inappropriately high $[Na^+]$ in the urine. It may be caused by one or both of:

- Disruption of sympathetic input to the kidneys.
- Production of a circulating natriuretic factor (probably brain natriuretic peptide).

In these situations, ADH secretion is appropriate because of the decreased ECF volume secondary to the renal Na^+ loss. Treatment mandates Na^+ administration in excess of losses, e.g. with hypertonic saline. When the tonicity of input fluid exceeds that of the urine, it allows plasma tonicity to return to normal.

→ **Diuretics and urine output**

Diuretics should not be prescribed simply to increase urine output. The primary indication for a diuretic is to remove excess salt and water. They do not increase GFR, so even if they result in an increased flow of urine they will not have altered underlying renal perfusion or function in any way except by impairment of sodium reabsorption. Indeed, in the patient who is oliguric because of decreased renal blood flow, a diuretic is only going to make things worse.

→ **Dehydration**

Non-specific terms such as 'dehydration' are best avoided, as they are often used inappropriately. Dehydration refers to water balance (and therefore tonicity), but is often used interchangeably with ECF depletion. This causes confusion, as the management of these conditions requires different fluids.

Since the different body compartments may change in different directions with regard to volume, it is essential to think about them independently rather than using single terms for the whole body such as 'wet' and 'dry'.

The terms hypervolaemia and hypovolaemia typically refer to the circulating volume.

Table 11.6 Clinical fluid management scenarios

History	[Na⁺] (mmol/L)	ECF examination	Interpretation	Principles of management
Confused, history of URTI, ↑temperature, ↓oral intake	165	Normal	Hypertonicity, i.e. water deficit Na⁺ balance clinically normal	Replace water deficit: NG water or IV dextrose, usually over 24–48hr to avoid rapid osmotic changes
Renal failure	Normal	Expanded Oedema + ↑JVP, ↑BP, good circulation	Expansion of all ECF compartments Normal tonicity	Remove salt to reduce ECF volumes (diuretics or renal replacement therapy).
Sepsis Bowel anastomotic leak ↑temperature ↑WBC IV infusion of 5% dextrose in progress	130	↓JVP, ↓BP, ↓urine Oedema ++	Total ECF expansion but circulatory inadequacy with hypovolaemic component Hypotonicity due to non-osmotic stimulus for ADH plus water administration	Isotonic fluid to replete CV despite total ECF expansion; avoid hypotonic fluids Other measures (e.g. inotropes/vasopressors) may be required to support circulation further.
Hepatic failure	125	Expanded Oedema ++ Ascites ++ ↑↑JVP, ↓BP, ↓urine	Total ECF expansion, but circulatory inadequacy despite hypervolaemia Hypotonicity due to non-osmotic stimulus for ADH ± water administration (e.g. IV fluids)	Restrict all fluids Other measures (e.g. inotropes/vasopressors) may be required to support circulation further
Diarrhoea ++ Weight loss, drinking fluids Dizzy on standing	120	Depleted ↓JVP, ↓BP, ↓UO, ↑HR, ↓skin turgor	Total ECF deficit, depleted CV and ISV Hypotonicity due to non-osmotic stimulus for ADH plus water intake --(drinking)	Isotonic fluids to replete ECF volume. This will turn off ADH and excess water (hypotonicity) will be excreted. Avoid hypotonic fluids.

Until recently, clinical practice has been influenced by the concept of 'third-space' losses where internal redistribution of ECF fluids following surgery was considered to reduce the functionally available extracellular volume. This functional extracellular deficit was replaced with isotonic fluids, and replacement volumes of up to 15ml/kg/hr were recommended for laparotomies, often leading to postoperative weight gains of 3–7kg.

More recently the existence of a 'third space' has been questioned and concerns expressed over the consequences of excessive fluid administration, including increased morbidity and mortality.

Improved postoperative outcomes in large bowel surgery have been reported using a more restrictive fluid practice, both intraoperatively (e.g. 1500ml total isotonic + 500ml colloid fluid administration with additional fluids only if blood loss >500ml) and postoperatively. The aim of this practice is to limit fluids to maintenance plus replacement of actual losses without also filling a putative third space, resulting in minimal postoperative weight gain. Restrictive practices have also been advocated in thoracic surgery to limit the potential for pulmonary dysfunction.

Traditionally the need for fluid has been based on cardiovascular monitoring and urine output. However, many of the parameters used are affected by variables other than absolute volume, e.g. anaesthetic drugs, concomitant medication, effects of neuraxial blockade. Many of these effects are transient, and treatment with fluids risks volume overload when the effects wear off.

Oesophageal Doppler monitoring has been advocated as a better guide to intraoperative fluid management used to optimize haemodynamics. This approach has shortened hospital stay for both orthopaedic and colorectal surgical patients. Interestingly, in one study, there were no differences in the overall amounts of fluid given to the two groups (which were in keeping with restricted regimens) but the Doppler group received more fluid in the first quarter of the operating time, suggesting that the timing of fluid intervention may be important.

Other invasive methods for guiding fluid management are sometimes used without evidence of effect on outcome. CVP (and, less frequently, PAOP) has commonly been used to guide fluid management, particularly where significant changes are expected or where the patients' comorbidities suggest they are more at risk of complications. However, there is not a linear relationship between pressure and volume; there is a wide 'normal range' and the numbers generated need to be interpreted together with other clinical indications of circulatory adequacy and the response to fluid challenges (Section 4.6).

As yet there is no universally accepted approach to the management of perioperative fluids. While evidence is accumulating, the overall quality is poor and difficult to interpret for the following reasons:

- The number of studies is small
- Different definitions of standard and restricted regimens have been used
- The quality of the studies varies from observational to randomized controlled trials
- Different anaesthetic techniques have been used which may influence the results, e.g. the use of epidurals with their attendant haemodynamic effects.

⊕ Clearly, too much or too little fluid may result in morbidity. The perioperative physician should look for the following signs.

- ECF volume expansion or contraction.
   Is there oedema? What is the circulating volume?
- Hypotonicity or hypertonicity.
   What is the plasma [Na$^+$]?

In hypovolaemia, administration of hypotonic fluid is extremely dangerous as ADH will be secreted in response to ECF deficit. Water will be retained at the expense of tonicity, leading to cell swelling. The severity of associated neurological symptoms depends on the rate and extent of the decline in plasma sodium. Signs may appear suddenly

when plasma [Na$^+$] falls abruptly to only moderately low levels (e.g. 128mmol/L), as may be the case postoperatively.

Tonicity problems will come to light with regular review of plasma [Na$^+$]. Changes in tonicity should be managed by administering or restricting free water as appropriate.

Intraoperative fluid prescription

Patients should arrive in the anaesthetic room euvolaemic, but frequently do not, especially for emergency surgery or following bowel prep. Deficiency of ECF necessitates replacement prior to induction.

Crystalloid solutions are normally given during surgery (in addition to blood when appropriate) to maintain ECF volume and therefore cardiovascular stability and urine output. However, the volume and composition of fluid used remains the subject of debate.

Patients undergoing minor surgery do not need IV fluids as they usually resume oral intake soon after the procedure. However, there is evidence that 1L of IV fluid reduces minor postoperative morbidity.

Those undergoing more major surgery are usually managed with isotonic crystalloids (e.g. Hartmann's) for maintenance with or without colloids used to maintain haemodynamic stability or replace blood loss (on a volume-to-volume basis). When colloids are used, the volumes of fluid infused are significantly less than when crystalloids alone are used. Isotonic crystalloid is distributed throughout the ECF and so approximately three times the volume of blood lost is required when crystalloids alone are used as replacement. Transfusion should be performed if the patient's haemoglobin falls, or is likely to fall, to inadequate levels.

Postoperative fluid prescription

Postoperatively, maintenance regimes are usually crystalloid-based with volumes of 2–3L per day. Additional isotonic fluid should be prescribed for extra losses, e.g. from drains or stomas. However, maintenance regimes need to be altered in response to clinical examination (including weight changes) and measurement of plasma electrolytes.

Potassium supplementation will be required in most patients and is usually prescribed at an initial rate of 60mmol/day, adjusted to individual clinical circumstances. Potassium loss in the urine will be accentuated in the presence of hypovolaemia with concomitant aldosterone secretion.

Postoperative volume deficits may occur despite well-managed intraoperative fluid administration. This may be due to losses from drains, haemorrhage, or internal fluid shifts. Signs suggestive of possible ECF volume deficit include CVS dysfunction and inadequate urine output. Replacement fluid should be isotonic, reflecting the osmolarity of the ECF, and should be given as a bolus, i.e. 250–500ml, repeated as necessary to achieve resolution of the clinical signs.

Measurement of CVP may be helpful when the patient's volume status is difficult to determine, particularly if volume overload is a risk. Vasopressors or inotropes may be indicated if the patient remains hypotensive despite adequate filling.

Points of note

- Isotonic fluids may potentiate sodium excess and ECF expansion.
- Hypotonic fluids may cause hypotonicity with consequent cell swelling, especially if they are speeded up for the treatment of hypotension.

Urine output

To stay in a steady state the body needs to excrete the waste products of metabolism. The minimum volume of urine required to do this depends on the:

- excretory load
- renal concentrating ability.

For example, if an individual has an excretory load of 600mosmol (approximately that of a 70kg man on a standard Western diet) and can concentrate their urine to 1200mosm/L they will need to produce 0.5L of urine, i.e. a urine output of approximately 21ml/hr. On the other hand, an individual with impaired renal concentrating ability, e.g. maximum concentration of 300mosm/L, will need to produce 2L of urine daily, i.e. approximately 83ml/hr.

Thus the standard recommendation of a urine output of 0.5ml/kg/hr does not guarantee adequate excretion in all, and indeed is more than is required in some.

Oliguria raises the possibility of a pre-renal deficit. However, there are other reasons for oliguria including a stress hormone response causing water and sodium retention.

Clinical evidence of an ECF deficit associated with oliguria is an indication for isotonic fluid administration. However, in the presence of a 'good' circulation (i.e. adequate mean arterial pressure and peripheral perfusion), slavish administration of fluid to achieve an arbitrary urine output may be associated with excess fluid retention and complications of fluid overload.

Polyuria

This can *usually* be taken as an indication of a good circulation and renal function, with appropriate excretion of excess salt and water. However, other causes of polyuria (see below) should always be excluded before accepting this. If the patient does have an appropriate high-volume diuresis, consideration should be given as to whether they are receiving too much fluid.

Polyuria may be inappropriate, leading to excessive water and salt loss with attendant tonicity problems and ECF volume deficit. It can occur secondary to an osmotic diuresis, e.g. with hyperglycaemia or in the recovery phase of acute tubular necrosis (ATN). In the latter condition, the kidney initially has recovering filtration without normal tubular function and therefore has impaired renal concentrating ability. Furthermore, as filtration improves there will be an osmotic diuresis secondary to filtration of the particles that accumulated during the oliguric period of ATN. Therefore polyuria is to be expected with a relatively greater water than sodium loss.

If the patient is euvolaemic to start with, they will need to be given increased volumes of water until their concentrating ability is restored. However, if they have accumulated salt and water before the onset of the polyuric phase they can be allowed to excrete the excess with a careful eye kept on their ECF volume (regular clinical exam) and tonicity (regular review of [Na$^+$]).

It should be noted that in such a patient with a urine output of 100ml/hr, a drop to 30–40ml/hr may actually be an indication of decreasing renal blood flow and glomerular filtration, despite the apparently 'normal' urine output.

Other causes of polyuria include mannitol administration and diabetes insipidus.

⊘ How not to do it

History, management, and fatal outcome

A fit healthy 30-year-old 49kg female underwent an apparently uneventful hysterectomy with minimal blood loss. She had received Hartmann's solution intraoperatively. A postoperative fluid prescription of dextrose saline (one-fifth normal saline in 4 % dextrose) had been prescribed 6 hourly over 24 hours. This was speeded up up because of nausea and oliguria. A total of 5L was administered over 16hr. The patient subsequently fitted, and became brain dead with a [Na$^+$] of 124mmol/L.

Pathophysiology

For this degree of hypotonicity and brain swelling, ADH must be secreted and free water given. The water in this case was provided by medical staff as hypotonic IV fluid. ADH was secreted due to non-osmotic stimuli, including ECF volume depletion (as evidenced by oliguria) and nausea.

Mistakes

1. The type of additional IV fluid administered should have been tailored to the compartment that needed to be filled. In the treatment of oliguria, potential ECF deficit needs to be addressed; isotonic fluids should have been given.

2. The dangers of excess hypotonic fluid administration to patients who are likely to secrete ADH were not appreciated.

Assuming a [Na$^+$] of 138mmol/L at the end of the operation, what would be the effect of giving 5L of dextrose saline (assuming all the water and Na$^+$ was retained)?

- 5L dextrose saline is the same as 4L 5% dextrose + 1L normal saline.
- TBW=55% of 49kg = 27L; ECF (before fluid) = 9L.
- Normal saline distributes only within the ECF. Water will fill all compartments in the ratio of their volumes.
- ECF (following fluid) = 9 + 1(normal saline)+ 1.3(1/3 of dextrose saline) = 11.3L.
- Na content (before fluid) = 9 × 138mmol = 1242mmol.
- Na content (after fluid) = (9L × 138)+(154 in 1L normal saline) = 1396mmol.
- [Na$^+$] after fluid = (1392/11.3) = 123mmol/L.

⊕ Summary of approach to fluid prescribing

Consider fluids in terms of tonicity, and the compartment you wish to influence. Crystalloid is a non-specific term that covers a range of fluids of varying tonicity. Administration of the wrong crystalloid can have devastating effects. Colloids are typically isotonic as they are suspended in normal saline.

The starting point of an assessment of a patient's ECF volume is examination, not simply an inspection of the fluid balance chart. The latter tells you nothing about the current volume state but simply the apparent (often inaccurate) relative change over 24hr. Fluid balance charts can be useful where losses are increased (e.g. via drains), to help plan replacement. Short-term weight variation reflects fluid balance changes.

Think of salt balance and water balance separately:

- To determine the ECF volume, examine the patient regularly. This will determine the requirement for Na$^+$ restriction or administration of isotonic solutions.
- To determine the ICF volume look at [Na$^+$] to determine tonicity (i.e. water balance) and the likelihood of cell swelling or contraction.

Where there are clear signs of excess of either salt or water, be prepared to restrict as appropriate. This may mean giving nothing. All too often fluids are prescribed on the simple but wrong premise that 'everyone needs maintenance fluids'. If patients have too much salt or water do not give more; simply let them excrete the excess or help them to do so with diuretics if appropriate.

In those with normal clinical examination and normal [Na$^+$] it is appropriate to continue with your maintenance regime. However, where deviations are detected, the prescription must be altered accordingly.

11.9 Potassium

Almost all (98%) potassium ions (K^+) are in cells (40–50mmol/kg body weight, i.e. close to 4000mmol in a 70kg adult).

Intracellular [K^+] has a concentration of 150mmol/L. It is the primary intracellular cation and is balanced electrically by macromolecular anions (mainly organic phosphates).

Total K^+ content in the ECF is <1mmol/kg body weight (i.e. close to 60mmol in a 70kg adult) with a normal range of ECF [K^+] of 3.6–4.8mmol/L, and it has a key role in generating the resting membrane potential (RMP). The ICF:ECF [K^+] ratio is 30–40:1 and passive diffusion of K^+ out of cells is responsible for the majority of the RMP.

Hyper- or hypokalaemia may predispose the patient to cardiac dysrthymias.

The initial defence against a K^+ load is its entry into cells. A typical Western diet containing 70mmol leads to only a 0.1mmol/L rise in plasma [K^+] in normal individuals. K^+ intake varies with different cultures, ranging from 10–400mmol/day.

K^+ balance is maintained by increasing or decreasing K^+ excretion in the urine and virtually all regulation occurs in the cortical collecting duct (CCD). On a typical Western diet approximately 1mmol/kg per day needs to be excreted (Figure 11.11).

Obligatory potassium loss

Non-renal

Sweat contains 10mmol/L; however, the volume varies greatly between 0.2 and 12L/day. Stool loss is normally about 10mmol/day; however, with diarrhea the K^+ concentration is close to 40–50mmol/day. In cholera, 6L of water containing 750mmol of Na^+ and 100mmol K^+ can be lost in 24hr.

Renal

A normal person with a K^+ deficit should excrete a minimum of 10mmol/day (and with K^+ surplus up to 400mmol/day).

Hyperkalaemia stimulates aldosterone release. Aldosterone enters the principal cell (segment-specific cell of the collecting duct) via the basolateral membrane and binds to a specific cytosolic receptor. The hormone receptor complex enters the nucleus and causes the synthesis of new proteins. Early action is opening of luminal Na^+ channels and later actions include insertion of more Na^+/K^+ATPase units into the basolateral membrane and K^+ channels into the luminal membrane. This promotes Na^+ reabsorption which may be *with* Cl^- or in *exchange* for K^+ or H^+ depending on clinical conditions. K^+ secretion is by the principal cells.

Aldosterone also acts on the colon to promote faecal K^+ loss, but this is only quantitatively important in patients with chronic renal failure. It also promotes K^+ loss in sweat, which may be relevant in athletes training in a hot environment.

K^+ shift across cell membranes

Factors causing intracellular shifts lead to a fall of <1mmol/L when acting individually, but a larger fall may occur if factors act together.

Hormones

Insulin shifts K^+ into cells.

Clinically this is important, as insulin can be used to treat hyperkalaemia. Also, care must be taken not to cause hypokalaemia when treating diabetic ketoacidosis (DKA) with insulin. Insulin also leads to an increase in the content of intracellular anions (e.g. phosphate esters such as RNA) requiring intracellular uptake of K^+.

Catecholamines

β_2 agonists stimulate the movement of K^+ into cells.

With the usual dose of β_2 agonist for bronchospasm, the plasma [K^+] usually falls by only 0.2–0.3mmol/L, but with massive overdose this reduction may be 1.5–2.0mmol/L. The plasma [K^+] rises by only around 0.3mmol in normal subjects on β-blockers.

Drugs

Some drugs can promote transcellular K^+ shifts. These include drugs promoting or antagonizing the hormonal effects discussed above.

β_1 agonists promote renal renin secretion, leading to increased aldosterone levels and increased K^+ excretion in the urine.

α agonists cause K^+ to shift out of cells and inhibit insulin release (which further affects K^+ uptake in its own right).

Cardiac glycoside toxicity can cause serious hyperkalaemia.

Acid–base changes

Acidosis causes a shift of K^+ out of cells. This is most marked with hyperchloraemic acidosis where H^+ enters cells and K^+ moves out. With organic acids such as lactic acid and ketoacids, the organic anions can enter cells with protons; therefore there is no shift in K^+. The primary cause for hyperkalaemia in DKA is insulin deficiency.

Similarly, there are only small changes in plasma [K^+] with respiratory acid–base disorders. Retained CO_2 diffuses into cells where it first forms carbonic acid, which dissociates into protons and bicarbonate. There is no change in electrical charge across the membrane and so K^+ will not leave the cell.

Metabolic alkalosis causes a shift of potassium into cells.

Catabolic and anabolic states

Catabolic states cause a loss of intracellular anions (mainly organic phosphates) with a parallel loss of K^+.

Anabolism (e.g. recovery from DKA, or when malnourished individuals are re-fed) causes cellular K^+ uptake.

Cell damage and necrosis

Cell necrosis causes K^+ loss into the ECF. Hyperkalaemia from cell damage may be seen where there is acute organ necrosis or trauma, or following cytotoxic treatment for neoplasms.

Rhabdomyolysis can release large amounts of K^+ from damaged cells, but if renal function is normal this is usually rapidly cleared. Reperfusion of ischaemic tissues releases K^+ into the systemic circulation.

Lysis of red blood cells on blood sampling can lead to a falsely elevated [K^+]. In these cases, the plasma is pigmented due to Hb. More rarely, leukaemia cells may be unduly fragile and similarly falsely elevate the [K^+] following sampling damage.

Stored blood has a high [K^+] because of K^+ loss from the inactive cells.

Cell depolarization

Widespread cellular depolarization, e.g. with succinylcholine, causes a rise in K^+, usually of the order of <1mmol/L. However, it can be much more pronounced and life-threatening with certain disease states. Normally, K^+ release on depolarization of muscle cells is into the T-tubules, and not the general pool of interstitial fluid. However, in certain patients (e.g. where there has been muscle wasting) disturbed muscle architecture may allow a greater loss of K^+ to the interstitial fluid. Levels >11mmol/L have been seen in ICU patients following succinylcholine for intubation.

Excessive fist clenching before blood sampling may elevate the measured [K^+].

Exercise

Plasma [K^+] may rise by several mmol/L (e.g. up to 8mmol/L) following exhausting exercise. This may be a combination of muscle cell depolarization and cell damage (mechanical rupture of muscle and red blood cells). Its duration is short-lived (half-life 25sec) and it is well tolerated by normal subjects.

Inherited disorders

Inherited disorders include hyper- and hypokalaemic periodic paralysis. Both these disorders result in periodic paralysis associated with [K^+] changes thought to be secondary to alterations in ion channels responsible for membrane excitability.

➜ Milli-equivalents	
1mmol K^+	1mEq
1mmol Ca^{2+}	2mEq
2mmol Mg^{2+}	4mEq
3mmol Fe^{3+}	9mEq

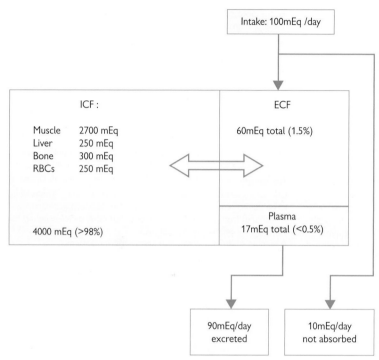

Fig. 11.11 Potassium balance: intra- and extracellular [K^+] change very little day by day.

Hypokalaemia

Dangers of hypokalaemia

- Cardiac dysrthymias, especially in presence of digitalis
- Muscle weakness and fatiguability. This is common.
- May worsen hepatic encephalopathy.
- Produces a renal concentrating defect (reduced aquaporin-2 in the luminal membrane of the medullary collecting duct), causing polyuria and nocturia.
- Ileus (smooth muscle weakness) and constipation.
- Rhabdomyolysis (with extreme K^+ depletion).

ECG changes correlate poorly with plasma $[K^+]$; they usually start with T-wave flattening or inversion. ST segments become depressed and U waves may appear. Dysrthymias and conduction defects may occur. These abnormalities are exaggerated by hypercalcaemia.

Aetiology

Most clinical problems are due to increased loss. However, K^+ intake and shift into cells must also be considered.

Chronic hypokalaemia is rarely due to inadequate intake, as renal excretion of K^+ falls to very low levels (10–15mmol/day) in K^+ depletion. However, poor people on a diet low in meat or vegetables, or those living in parts of the world where diet mostly consists of polished rice, are at risk.

Hypokalaemia is usually due to K^+ loss associated with GI tract fluid loss or renal losses (e.g. diuretics). Note that even with GI tract fluid losses (including vomiting, NG suction, and diarrhoea), the major route of K^+ loss is renal, as aldosterone is secreted secondary to ECF volume depletion, promoting K^+ loss in the urine. However, loss of colonic contents can lead directly to hypokalaemia, particularly with a villous adenoma.

Other causes include primary increases in renin or aldosterone and intracellular K^+ shifts (see above).

Hypothermia causes a transient drop in serum K^+ that usually resolves during rewarming. Lethal cases of hypothermia can cause a paradoxical hyperkalaemia due to cell death.

Magnesium depletion impairs renal reabsorption of K^+ and causes refractory hypokalaemia unless treated.

Management of hypokalaemia

Unless $[K^+]$ is <3mmol/L, few symptoms should be attributed to hypokalaemia. Indeed, there is a lack of proof that treating modest hypokalaemia (3–3.5mmol/L) really does reduce the incidence of cardiac dysrthymias. However, hypokalaemia may enhance the proarrhythmic effects of other conditions such as myocardial ischaemia, magnesium depletion, and digitalis treatment. The ECG changes seen in hypokalaemia are shown in Figure 11.12(a).

Several hundred millimoles of K^+ are usually required to correct severe hypokalaemia. However, it is difficult to predict the total body deficit accurately from the plasma $[K^+]$. A fall from 4 to 3 mmol/L is usually associated with a total body K^+ deficit of 100–400mmol. To lower the plasma $[K^+]$ further by 1mmol/L requires a much larger deficit.

The safest route for K^+ replacement is orally, and intake can be increased with:

- foods rich in K^+ (fresh fruits, juices, and meats);
- K^+ supplements (liquid or solid preparations).

However, if there are GI tract problems or severe hypokalaemia with respiratory muscle weakness and cardiac arrhythmias, or an anticipated intracellular shift of K^+ (e.g. as seen with treatment of DKA), the IV route should be used.

A chloride deficit is usually associated with potassium depletion and so KCl is the rational replacement fluid. The $[K^+]$ concentration of the replacement fluid should be <60mmol/L if infused peripherally. For more urgent replacement, a central vein should be used since potassium solutions are hyperosmotic, cause pain on injection, and damage veins. Typical practice is to give 20mmol of K^+ in 100ml of normal saline and infuse at a maximum rate of 20mmol/hr.

If the K^+ deficit is associated with loss of intracellular anion (phosphate), potassium phosphate should be used. Clinically, this is most relevant in anabolic states, e.g. growth, total parenteral nutrition, and recovery from DKA (where close to half the K^+ deficit is due to the loss of K^+ with phosphate).

Hyperkalaemia

Dangers of hyperkalaemia

- Hyperkalaemia predisposes the patient to potentially lethal cardiac dysrthymias. It can also cause severe weakness.
- Serious effects may occur when the plasma $[K^+]$ is >6mmol/L; however, the correlation between plasma $[K^+]$ is not perfect, and the rate of development is as important as the degree of rise.

Aetiology

Chronic hyperkalaemia suggests impaired excretion of K^+. This is likely to be due to renal failure/dysfunction or low aldosterone bioactivity. K^+ can shift from cells in the presence of hormone deficiencies, acidosis, drugs, or cell damage (see above).

A number of drugs may cause or aggravate hyperkalaemia.

Treatment of hyperkalaemia

Management should be aimed at the underlying cause. However, at times it is necessary to reduce $[K^+]$ to avoid life-threatening complications, especially cardiac dysrrthymias, in the presence of ECG changes (Figure 11.12b). The options for management are as follows.

- Stop any further K^+ intake and drugs that impair K^+ excretion. K^+-sparing diuretics and aldosterone antagonists such as spironolactone or triamterene should be stopped.
- Discontinue any drugs that cause cell lysis. This prevents further shifts of K^+ from the ICF to the ECF.
- Physiologically antagonize the effects of hyperkalaemia by giving IV Ca^{2+} salts. These decrease membrane excitability within minutes but the effect is relatively short-lived (20–30min). However, it provides time for other strategies to work. The usual dose is 10ml 10% calcium gluconate given IV over 3min which can be repeated after 5–10min if ECG changes persist.

If there are signs of circulatory compromise, calcium chloride may be preferred. 10ml of 10% calcium chloride contains three times more elemental calcium (27g vs. 9g) and this may be better at maintaining peripheral vascular tone. Calcium chloride is hypertonic (2000mosmol/L) and ideally should be given through a central vein. Extravasation into tissues will cause tissue damage. As calcium potentiates digitalis cardiotoxicity, it must be given cautiously to those receiving this drug. If the hyperkalaemia is a manifestation of digitalis toxicity, calcium is contraindicated.

- Shift K^+ into cells by using insulin. Although simply giving a bolus of glucose will stimulate endogenous insulin release, most sources recommend adding insulin. For the diabetic, a bolus of insulin *must* be given with the glucose. A typical regimen is to give a bolus of 50ml of 50% glucose containing soluble insulin (5–10 units) over 5–10min. This can be repeated if necessary.
- Shift K^+ into cells by using $NaHCO_3$. If the patient has a metabolic acidosis, the acidaemia may shift K^+ from the ICF; $NaHCO_3$ will counteract this. Even in patients with a normal blood pH, $NaHCO_3$ may lower the $[K^+]$. HCO_3^- delivered to the cortical collecting duct promotes K^+ excretion in the presence of aldosterone. The mechanism is unknown, but may be due to an inhibition of the reabsorption of Na^+ with Cl^-, therefore promoting exchange for K^+. Typically, 50mmol is given over 5–10min, repeated 30min later if necessary.

Both insulin and $NaHCO_3$ strategies are effective within 1 hr.

- Increase K+ loss from the ECF by either increased urinary or GI tract losses. Urinary K+ loss can be promoted by increasing sodium delivery to the CCD where it can be exchanged for K+. These measures should have an effect within 1–4hr.

  If the ECF is expanded a loop diuretic may be given. If contracted, isotonic NaCl or NaHCO₃ may be given.

  Those patients with a low aldosterone level can be given mineralocorticoid replacement as 9-α fludrocortisone (100mcg).

- GI tract K+ loss can be promoted by using K+ binding exchange resins. Rectally administered resins work more rapidly as the rate of secretion of K+ in the colon exceeds that in the proximal GI tract. However, these enemas are poorly tolerated by patients (and nurses). Orally administered resins take more than 6hr to have an effect.

- Insufficient renal function for K+ excretion is an indication for renal replacement therapy. Haemodialysis or haemofiltration is more efficient at removing K+ than peritoneal dialysis. The preceding therapies buy time for replacement therapy to be started. Once instituted, its effect is extremely rapid.

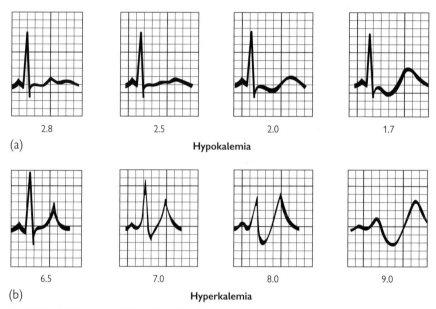

| 2.8 | 2.5 | 2.0 | 1.7 |

(a)   **Hypokalemia**

| 6.5 | 7.0 | 8.0 | 9.0 |

(b)   **Hyperkalemia**

Fig. 11.12 ECG changes with (a) hypokalaemia and (b) hyperkalaemia.

The normal ECF $[H^+]$ can be expressed directly, as $[H^+]$ (in nmol/L), or indirectly, as pH (the negative logarithm to base 10 of the hydrogen ion concentration).

The term p denotes negative logarithm. A negative logarithm is the same as the logarithm of the reciprocal:

$$\text{negative log } [H^+] = \frac{\log 1}{[H^+]}.$$

Therefore pH is a doubly non-linear transformation of $[H^+]$. Starting with the variable $[H^+]$, we take its reciprocal (a non-linear process) and then take the logarithm of the result (another non-linear process). Therefore it is difficult to appreciate quantitatively what is happening when pH values are cited.

The numerical value of the pH logarithm goes from plus infinity, through zero, to minus infinity as $[H^+]$ goes from 0 through 1 to plus infinity (NB: log 0 = 1).

As $[H^+]$ increases from zero to 1M/L, pH decreases from plus infinity to zero. Any solution that does not contain H^+ has pH of plus infinity. pH continues to decrease from zero towards minus infinity as $[H^+]$ increases above 1M/L.

It is very difficult to get $[H^+]$ in aqueous solutions below $\sim 10^{-15}$M/L, so the practical limits on a pH scale are −1.2 and 15. pH meters are usually arbitrarily scaled from 0 to 14.

- pH 7 = 10^{-7}, i.e 100nmol/L $(1/10^{-7})$.
- pH 8 = 10^{-8}, i.e. 10nmol/L $(1/10^{-8})$.

The normal ECF pH of 7.4 reflects a $[H^+]$ of 40nmol/L. Intracellular H^+ is more acidic at 80–100nmol/L. The range of $[H^+]$ in the blood that is compatible with human life is approximately 16–126nmol/L, i.e. pH 6.9–7.8

Traditional approach to acid–base physiology

According to Bronsted's definition:

- Acids are compounds that are capable of donating H^+.
- Bases are compounds that are capable of accepting H^+.

When an acid (HA) dissociates it yields H^+ and its conjugate base (anion A^-):

$$\text{HA} \leftrightarrow \text{H}^+ + \text{A}^- \qquad \text{(e.g. lactic acid} \leftrightarrow \text{H}^+ + \text{lactate}^-).$$

An acid–base reaction always involves a conjugate acid–base pair, made up of the proton donor (HA) and corresponding proton acceptor (A^-). Each acid has a characteristic affinity for its proton. Those with a high affinity are weak acids and dissociate only slightly; those with low affinity are strong acids and readily lose H^+ ions. The tendency of any given acid to dissociate is given by its dissociation constant Ka.

The pKa is the negative logarithm of Ka and bears the same inverse relationship to Ka, as pH does to $[H^+]$.

Strong acids have a high Ka, and therefore low pKa, and strong bases have a low Ka and high pKa values.

For an acid HA at a given temperature is:

$$Ka = \frac{[H^+][A^-]}{[HA]}.$$

Solving for $[H^+]$:

$$[H^+] = \frac{Ka[HA]}{[A^-]}$$

which is the Henderson equation. Changing to logarithms (base 10):

$$\log [H^+] = \log Ka + \log \frac{[HA]}{[A^-]}.$$

Changing to negative logarithms

$$-\log [H^+] = \log Ka + \log \frac{[HA]}{[A^-]}.$$

Since pH and pK are the negative logarithms of $[H^+]$ and K respectively

$$pH = pKa - \log \frac{[HA]}{[A^-]}.$$

Since

$$-\log \frac{[HA]}{[A^-]} = \log \frac{[A^-]}{[HA]}$$

this can be rewritten as

$$pH = pKa + \log \frac{[A^-]}{[HA]}$$

This is the Henderson–Hasselbalch equation, which can be expressed in a more general form as

$$pH = pKa + \log \frac{[\text{proton acceptor}]}{[\text{proton donor}]}$$

Solving the Henderson–Hasselbalch equation provides an estimate of the magnitude of an acidosis, but not the cause (see anion gap, Section 11.12).

When the concentrations of proton donor and acceptor are the same, their ratio equals 1. Since the log 1 = 0), the pKa is equal to the pH when $[A^-]$ = $[HA]$, i.e. $[A^-]/[HA]$ = 1. The acid at this point is 50% dissociated.

Buffers

A conjugate acid–base pair can act as a buffer and resist changes in pH. Its capacity to do so is greatest when pH = pKa, as at this point $[A^-]$ = $[HA]$ and there are equal numbers of proton donors and acceptors. To be effective, there also needs to be a high enough concentration of both the H^+ donor and acceptor in solution. *Thus a buffer is best placed when the environmental pH is equal to the buffer system's pKa, and when the buffer exists in sufficient concentration to deal with the likely magnitude of changes in [H⁺]* (Figure 11.13). 'Closed' buffer systems possess fixed quantities of buffer. The addition of sufficient acid or alkali can overwhelm the system and allow the pH to change once buffers have been consumed. Conversely, 'open' buffer systems can adapt to the prevailing conditions by changing the quantity of acid or conjugate base. The bicarbonate buffer system (BBS) is an example of such an open system, where rapid changes in CO_2, and later changes in HCO_3^-, can preserve buffering capacity in the face of changing acid-base conditions (Figure 11.14). Failure of ventilation or of renal function can convert this open system to a closed system, allowing much larger acid-base derangements to occur (Table 11.7).

The free $[H^+]$ in the ECF is very small (40nmol/L) despite a large amount of daily acid production (see below).

Such control is important, as H^+ ions may affect cellular function, particularly through alterations in hydrogen bonding and protein structure.

The maintenance of a low $[H^+]$ despite a large daily production depends initially on buffers, and then on excretion of the acids. Buffers act only as a temporary measure.

The two major buffer systems are the BBS, with pKa 6.1, and the protein buffer system (largely via the imidazole group in histidines), with an average pKa of 6.8.

The BBS is the initial buffer for a H^+ load (except H_2CO_3, since it cannot buffer itself) and is the major buffer in the ECF. Plasma proteins contribute to ECF buffering (ECF phosphate exists in too low a concentration to contribute).

The BBS is also important in the ICF, although here the HCO_3^- concentration is approximately half that found in the ECF. Intracellular proteins (especially Hb) and, to a lesser extent, phosphates contribute to ICF buffering.

In chronic disorders, bone also acts as an extracellular buffer. Na^+ and K^+ ions on the surface of the bone may exchange with protons, or bone mineral may be dissolved, and this leads to buffer release into the ECF.

Phosphate is an important urinary buffer where pH is lower and phosphate concentration higher.

Close to 1000mmol of H^+ can be buffered: approximately 350mmol by ECF HCO_3^-, 330mmol by ICF HCO_3^-, and 400mmol by ICF proteins.

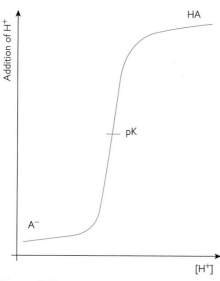

Fig. 11.13 Buffer activity and pH change. As acid is added to a buffered solution operating at a pH near its pKa, the overall $[H^+]$ will not change significiantly.

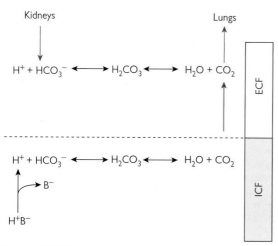

Fig. 11.14 The BBS: an open buffer system. Increased ventilation removes CO_2 and moves the equation to the right. This allows further buffering to take place. At first sight, the BBS is a weak buffer system in that its pKa (6.1) is dissimilar to the pH at which the system operates. However, a major strength of the BBS is that it is an open system, where both CO_2 and HCO_3^- may be independently changed.

Table 11.7 **Metabolic acidaemia ($\downarrow HCO_3^-$) with pH change produced by open and closed systems***									
	With appropriate hyperventilation (example of open system)			Without hyperventilation (example of a closed system)			Without hyperventilation (higher PCO_2)		
HCO_3^-	PCO_2 (kPa)	$[H^+]$	pH	PCO_2 (kPa)	$[H^+]$	pH	PCO_2 (kPa)	$[H^+]$	pH
20	4.66	42	7.38	5.33	48	7.32	8	72	7.14
15	4	50	7.30	5.33	64	7.19	8	96	7.02
10	3.33	60	7.20	5.33	96	7.02	8	143	6.85
5	2.67	96	7.02	5.33	191	6.72	8	287	6.54

*A closed situation could occur when a patient is placed on a mechanical ventilator: control of PCO_2 by the patient is not possible. In these examples, the ventilator is maintaining the PCO_2 at 5.33kPa and 8kPa. The pH is significantly lower in the latter.

11.12 Acid production

Net acid production by the body can be divided into:

- Respiratory (volatile)
- Metabolic (non-volatile) acids.

Organic metabolic acids (e.g. lactic acid) turn over on a day-to-day basis: they are produced and metabolized, but do not contribute to net acid production unless their rates of production or removal are altered.

Respiratory acid (volatile acid)

Carbon dioxide, the major end-product of oxidative metabolism, constitutes respiratory acid. Normal metabolism results in the production of 10mmol/min of CO_2 at rest, which is excreted via the lungs. Thus more than 14,000mmol of CO_2 are produced daily at rest. CO_2 dissolves in water to form carbonic acid, which dissociates into equimolar amounts of H^+ and the anion HCO_3^- (conjugate base).

Therefore a rise in CO_2 causes a respiratory acidosis, and a fall in CO_2 causes a respiratory alkalosis. The degree of change is quantified by the change in PCO_2, as $[H_2CO_3]$ is a function of PCO_2:

$$[H_2CO_3] = PCO_2 \text{ (kPa)} \times 0.234.$$

Chronic changes in CO_2 are accompanied by compensatory metabolic changes that return the pH towards normal. These mechanisms include renal retention of HCO_3^- in chronic respiratory acidosis and excretion of HCO_3^- in respiratory alkalosis (the strong ion theory, discussed in Section 11.13, explains these compensatory mechanisms through renal excretion or retention of Cl^-, respectively, thereby altering the strong ion difference).

CO_2 is transported in the blood from the tissues and is excreted through the lungs. The BBS cannot buffer itself, so the CO_2 added by the tissues is buffered mainly by haemoglobin (Hb).

CO_2 produced in tissues diffuses rapidly into the interstitial fluid and blood. It does not form carbonic acid in the plasma to any significant extent because the hydration reaction is slow. Dissolved CO_2 passes into the red cells. Here, under the influence of carbonic anhydrase, hydration occurs readily, producing carbonic acid. This undergoes dissociation into H^+ and HCO_3^- and the process is enhanced by the interaction of H^+ with Hb (Section 13.12).

Ultimately 70–75% of the CO_2 transported for excretion is carried as HCO_3^- (most of the remainder is carried as carbamino compounds).

Net metabolic (non-volatile) acid

The majority of net metabolic acid production is from protein breakdown (e.g. sulphuric acid from sulphur-containing amino acids) and organic phosphate metabolism. With a standard Western diet, a net metabolic acid load of approximately 1mmol/kg is produced daily. Acids are also produced if there is insufficient oxygen (lactic acid) or insulin (ketoacids). They can also be produced from the metabolism of potentially toxic compounds such as alcohols.

When an acid (e.g. lactic acid) is added to the ECF, it is initially buffered by bicarbonate. This reaction results in a fall in the bicarbonate concentration and a rise in the acid anion (e.g. lactate) concentration:

$$H^+An^- \text{ (acid)} + Na^+ + HCO_3^- \text{ (ECF)} \rightarrow Na^+ + An^- + H_2CO_3$$

$$H_2CO_3 \rightarrow H_2O + CO_2 \text{ (excreted via lungs).}$$

From the Henderson-Hasselbalch equation we know that

$$pH = 6.1 + \log \frac{[HCO_3^-]}{[H_2CO_3]}.$$

With the low pKa, this would not appear to be a good buffer system at physiological pH. However, as we have already seen, its effectiveness is enhanced because it is not a closed system: the body can alter the ratio of $[HCO_3^-]$ to $[H_2CO_3]$ by altering ventilation to change the concentration of H_2CO_3 or via renal mechanisms to retain or excrete HCO_3^-

Anion gap

Calculating the anion gap (AG) helps characterize the mechanism of an acid–base derangement.

The AG is the difference between the concentration of the major cation (Na^+) and the routinely measured anions (Cl^- and HCO_3^-). A normal AG is <12mmol/L. Most of the AG is accounted for by negatively charged proteins such as albumin, and so the AG is reduced by hypoalbuminaemia (this is important in critically ill patients who often have a reduced albumin concentration).

A rise in AG implies that an acidosis is due to acid accumulation, with HCO_3^- being replaced by the unmeasured anion. The common causes are lactic acidosis, diabetic ketoacidosis, the acidosis of renal failure, and metabolism of alcohols.

Alternatively, when HCO_3^- is lost from the body (e.g. in diarrhoea), it is lost with sodium. Therefore there is no change in the anion gap. Therefore a normal AG acidosis implies bicarbonate loss due to either GI loss or renal dysfunction. In the latter there may be either:

- Actual urinary HCO_3^- loss from failure to reabsorb filtered HCO_3^- (proximal renal tubular acidosis), or
- 'Indirect' renal loss, where HCO_3^- is not excreted in the urine. This occurs when the distal tubule either fails to secrete H^+ or fails to produce NH_3 for buffering (both forms of distal renal tubular acidosis). Acid anions are then not excreted with H^+ or NH_4^+ but instead with Na^+. Failure of these processes means that the HCO_3^- originally consumed by buffering the acids as they were added to the ECF is not regenerated.

Base excess and deficit

Since the $[HCO_3^-]$ concentration changes with both respiratory and metabolic acid–base changes, and coexisting metabolic and respiratory changes are to be expected as a consequence of compensatory mechanisms, simple inspection of $[HCO_3^-]$ is insufficient to quantify the degree of metabolic disturbance. A number of methods for assessing the metabolic contribution to a disorder have been devised. These include the 'standard bicarbonate' and 'base excess'.

The standard bicarbonate is the value of $[HCO_3^-]$ once PCO_2 is standardized to 40mmHg.

The base excess (BE) is defined as the concentration of titratable H^+ required to return the pH to 7.4 while the PCO_2 is maintained at 40 mmHg (5.3 kPa). Many blood gas machines now calculate BE from equations involving the variables pH, $[HCO_3^-]$, and [Hb]. The normal range for BE is +2 to −2 with a positive BE denoting a metabolic alkalosis and a negative BE (base deficit) a metabolic acidosis.

The BE represents the net change due to metabolic disturbances; therefore it can be normal if metabolic acidosis and alkalosis coexist.

In this case, an increased AG provides a clue to the presence of an acidosis: a normal pH with a normal PCO_2 means that a concomitant alkalosis must be present.

Anaesthesia in acidaemic patients

Metabolic acidosis should stimulate hyperventilation, a lower P_aCO_2, and ultimately a reduced rise in $[H^+]$ (respiratory compensation). It is important for anaesthetists to bear this in mind, as when they induce anaesthesia and impose IPPV, they remove the patient's ability to control ventilation and compensate. This results in a marked rise in $[H^+]$.

Alternatively, trying to match the patient's compensating minute volume with IPPV may cause significant cardiovascular impairment, especially in the presence of hypovolaemia. With induction of anaesthesia, sympathetic nervous system support of the circulation is often abolished. Anaesthetic drugs may also adversely affect the CVS. Therefore the scene is set for circulatory collapse when inducing anaesthesia in sick acidaemic patients.

→ Regeneration of HCO₃⁻ consumed in buffering

Progressive acidaemia is prevented by:

- The removal of acid anions produced from metabolism
- Repletion of the HCO_3^- consumed in buffering that acid.

Organic acids such as lactate are metabolized (mainly in the liver and kidney), and bicarbonate is generated in the process, thus there is no net effect as long as the metabolism of lactate keeps pace with its production.

Non-volatile acids that cannot be metabolized are excreted by the kidney. The kidney filters large volumes of plasma and in order to maintain homeostasis it must reabsorb filtered $NaHCO_3$. This is done in the proximal convoluted tubule (PCT) and involves secretion of H^+ by the PCT cells. These secreted H^+ are not excreted in the urine but are consumed in the "indirect" reabsorption of HCO_3^-.

The remaining filtered acid anions (eg sulphate) with accompanying cations (eg Na^+) then pass through the kidney to distal tubular sites. Here, H^+ is secreted by the distal tubular cells (DTC) and Na^+ is reabsorbed. H^+ secreted by the DTC is excreted in the urine. Whenever H^+ is excreted by the kidney, as either free H^+ or in combination with phosphate or ammonia, HCO_3^- is added to the ECF: i.e. HCO_3^- is regenerated (Figure 11.15).

The lowest urinary pH that the kidney can generate is 4 (a free $[H^+]$ of 0.1 mmol/L, or 100,000 nmol/L). Since on average we need to excrete a net load of 70 mmol non-volatile acid per day, that would require 700 litres of urine. However, the large proton excretion is achieved with smaller volumes with the aid of urinary buffers. These are

- Mono-hydrogen phosphate (HPO_4^{2-}) which combines with H^+ to form $H_2PO_4^-$ and
- Ammonia (NH_3), which combines with H^+ to form NH_4^+.

The amount of phosphate that can be excreted is limited, so in times of increased acid load the kidney increases its excretion of NH_4^+ (the NH_3 required comes from glutamine metabolism). Free H^+ and $H_2PO_4^-$ in the urine are known as titratable acids, and NH_4^+ as non-titratable.

As long as non-volatile acid excretion keeps pace with acid production there will be no change in $[H^+]$ or $[HCO_3^-]$. However, when acid production exceeds the body's ability to excrete or metabolize acid, the $[HCO_3^-]$ falls and the acid anion concentration rises. This can be detected as a rise in the anion gap.

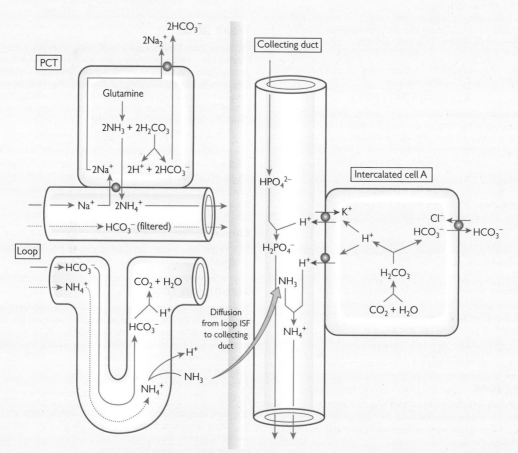

Fig. 11.15 Bicarbonate regeneration. This is a different process from reabsorption (Section 12.2). NH_4^+ is liberated from glutamine and exchanged for sodium in the PCT. In the loop of Henle, this dissociates into ammonia which, following absorption, diffuses across the interstitium into the collecting duct. Here, it combines with H^+ that has been actively secreted into the lumen by two mechanisms: the aldosterone-sensitive H^+ pump and the K^+/H^+ATPase counter-transport. Overall, there is net regeneration of bicarbonate.

11.13 Strong ion difference

Stewart has proposed that the $[H^+]$ concentration in aqueous solutions is determined by the ionization of water and has examined the physicochemical factors that influence this. Different definitions of acids and bases are used in this analysis.

- An acid is a substance that increases hydrogen ion (and decreases hydroxyl ion) concentration when added to an aqueous solution.
- A base is a substance that decreases hydrogen ion (and increases hydroxyl ion) concentration when added to an aqueous solution.

Therefore pure water is always neutral, although its $[H^+]$ concentration and therefore pH is temperature dependent (see below).

Physical chemistry of water

Water is a highly ionizing solvent, and salts dissolved in it separate into ionic components. Strong ions are completely dissociated at physiological pH. Thus NaCl added to water is completely ionized and exists only as dissolved Na^+ and Cl^-; there are no dissolved NaCl molecules. Weak ions are only partially dissociated (e.g. H_2CO_3) and molecules of dissolved H_2CO_3 will coexist with the dissolved products of dissociation: H^+ and HCO_3^- ions.

Water is itself slightly ionized, forming a negatively charged hydroxylated ion (OH^-) and a positively charged protonated ion (HnO^+). For simplicity, these are referred to as OH^- and H^+ ions (protons), respectively.

The degree of dissociation of a substance is given by its dissociation constant K. For water, the relationship is:

$$K_w \times [H_2O] = [H^+] \times [OH^-].$$

The dissociation constant for water (K_w) is very small and therefore self-ionization of water is miniscule. Since the dissociation is very small and the water concentration ($[H_2O]$) is >55mol/L, dissociation has little effect on the water concentration. Therefore $[H_2O]$ can be considered constant and combined with K_w into a new constant K'_w called the ion product for water:

$$K'_w = K_w \times [H_2O].$$

Therefore $K'_w = [H^+] \times [OH^-]$.

In aqueous solutions $[H^+] \times [OH^-]$ must always equal K'_w.

In pure water $[H^+] = [OH^-]$.

Dissociation constants are temperature dependent, and therefore so is the ionic product for water.

In pure water at 25°C, $K_w = 1 \times 10^{-14}$ (mol/L), i.e. the $[H^+]$ and $[OH^-]$ concentrations are both 10^{-7}mol/L (= 100nmol/L, pH 7).

At higher temperatures dissociation is increased and at lower temperatures it is decreased such that:

- at 0°C, $[H^+] = 3.4 \times 10^{-8}$mol/L (pH 7.5);
- at 100°C, $[H^+] = 8.8 \times 10^{-7}$mol/L (pH 6.1);
- at 37°C, the pH of pure water is 6.8.

Strong ions

These ions are completely dissociated (e.g. Na^+ and Cl^-). Since the system must maintain electrical neutrality, any change in the charge difference in strong ions must be balanced by alterations in the dissociation of weaker ions.

Consider a solution containing only strong ions and water. Because strong electrolytes are completely dissociated, the only equilibrium to keep track of is water dissociation.

If specified amounts of NaOH and HCl are added to water, the resulting simple solution would contain only Na^+, Cl^-, OH^-, and H^+.

Electrical neutrality requires that $[Na^+] - [Cl^-] + [H^+] - [OH^-] = 0$.

If there is a difference in $[Na^+]$ and $[Cl^-]$ this is termed the strong ion difference (SID). It must be balanced by an opposite difference in $[H^+]$ and $[OH^-]$.

However, water dissociation still requires that $[H^+] \times [OH^-] = K'_w$. If sodium ions outnumber chloride ions by 1mmol/L ($[Na^+] - [Cl^-] = $ 1mmol/L) and $K'_w = 10^{-14}$, then $[OH^-]$ must be just greater than 1mmol/L (i.e. close to 10^{-3}mol/L) to balance the excess positive charge of Na^+ and the very small positive charge of H^+.

$[H^+]$ would be just less than 10^{-11}mol/L since $[OH^-] \times [H^+] = 10^{-14}$. The solution would be very alkaline, with pH just over 11.

Conversely, a solution containing $[Cl^-] > [Na^+]$ would require $[H^+] > [OH^-]$ and the solution would be acidic. In order to conserve electrical neutrality, any strong ion difference must be associated with differences in $[H^+]$ and $[OH^-]$ in aqueous solutions.

Where $[Na^+] = [Cl^-]$ with no SID, $[H^+]$ must equal $[OH^-]$ and the solution will be neutral.

From any values of $[Na^+]$ and $[Cl^-]$ in solution we can calculate the respective values of $[H^+]$ and $[OH^-]$. The difference between total strong cation and total strong anion concentrations is positive in body fluids, and therefore the net positive electrical charge must be counterbalanced by the net negative charge supplied by anions including OH^-. The specific identities of the strong ions do not matter.

Weak acids

Of course body fluids do not consist solely of strong ions in water. Most of the weaker electrolytes are weak acids, including proteins (largely albumin in the ECF) and phosphate. Since they are weak acids, they are only partially dissociated at physiological pH and the degree of dissociation varies with physiological and pathophysiological changes. In body fluids these weak acids can all be expressed by the general term HA and dissociation is expressed by:

$$HA \leftrightarrow H^+ + A^- \text{ (with a single dissociation constant } K_a\text{)}.$$

The presence of a weak acid solution changes the $[H^+]$ (and pH) of the solution at any SID value to more acid. The degree of change depends on the amount of weak acid present and its level of dissociation.

Consider the solution of sodium chloride in water with a positive SID described previously. The presence of a weak acid now adds acid anions (A^-) and H^+ to the solution, making it more acidic.

Carbon dioxide

CO_2 reacts with water chemically so that its solution behaves like a weak acid. It is found in significant amounts in all body fluids.

Strong ion theory

Stewart's strong ion theory states that three independent variables determine the $[H^+]$ in biological aqueous solutions and any change in $[H^+]$ (or any other dependent variable, including HCO_3^-) is always due to a primary change in one or more of these three independent variables. The three independent variables are:

- strong ion difference;
- total concentration of weak acids (A_{tot});
- PCO_2.

The most abundant strong ions in the extracellular space are Na^+ and Cl^-. Other important strong ions are K^+, SO_4^{2-}, Mg^{2+}, and Ca^{2+}. The charge difference between strong cations and strong anions is calculated by (concentrations in mEq/L):

$$SID = ([Na^+] + [K^+] + [Ca^{2+}] + [Mg^{2+}]) - ([Cl^-] + [\text{other strong anions, e.g. lactate: } A^-])$$

$$= 40\text{–}44\text{mEq of charge}.$$

SID is always positive and is balanced by equal amounts of acid anion (also known as 'buffer base'), chiefly phosphate, albumin and bicarbonate ($[OH^-]$ is very small).

Thus an increase in SID, other factors remaining constant, will be associated with a higher $[OH^-]$ and lower $[H^+]$ and will cause alkalosis. Conversely, a decrease in SID causes acidosis.

Since the strong ion theory states that all changes in acid–base are secondary to changes in the independent variables, and as the total concentration of weak acids is normally constant, it follows that renal mechanisms to maintain homeostasis including compensatory responses to respiratory disturbances must be through strong ion balance. Further, since Na^+ content maintains ECF volume and $[Na^+]$ is a major determinant of the tonicity of body fluids, it follows that alterations in SID balance are best achieved by changes in $[Cl^-]$, i.e. renal Cl^- retention or excretion. This will not affect sodium content (ECF volume) or concentration (tonicity).

> ➲ The strong ion difference in any solution is defined as (the sum of all the strong base cation concentrations) minus (the sum of all the strong acid anion concentrations) expressed in mEq/L.

Metabolic acidosis caused by IV saline

IV administration of large volumes of 0.9% NaCl alters two of the three independent variables: SID and the total concentration of weak acids (A_{tot}). The decrease in A_{tot} will tend to cause an alkalosis. However, the effect on SID, which causes an acidosis, is stronger.

Consider a solution of volume 1L containing 140mmol Na^+ and 110mmol Cl^- with SID = 30. Add 1L of NaCl containing 154mmol of each ion. There is now a 2L solution containing 294mmol Na^+ and 264mmol Cl^-. The ion concentrations are now 147mmol/L Na^+ and 132mmol/L Cl^-. SID is now 15, and therefore the solution is more acidic (Figure 11.16).

The effect of colloid solutions is also determined by their SID, and since most colloids are suspended in normal saline, they will be acidifying.

The traditional and strong ion approaches to acid–base

The traditional approach to acid–base described previously is based on the Henderson–Hasselbalch (HH) equation. Although this equation correctly describes an equilibrium that must exist, it does not say anything about cause and effect. However, the implication is that primary changes in $[HCO_3^-]$ lead directly to changes in $[H^+]$, but mechanistically this may not be correct (see below).

Furthermore, the Bronsted definitions of acids and bases lead to consideration of acids and bases in terms of proton donors or acceptors. This causes confusion when considering why administration of NaCl to patients causes an acidosis.

The strong ion theory proposes a different mechanism for acid–base changes. According to this theory, both HCO_3^- and H^+ are dependent variables within the system and any change in either of their concentrations will always be due to changes in one or more independent variables (although the equilibrium relationship described by the HH equation is of course correct).

While the traditional approach remains the most widely used in clinical practice, strong ion theory is being more frequently referred to in anaesthetic and critical care literature.

Important considerations

- A normal pH does not exclude acid–base disorders. However, it may signal a chronic stable condition.
- An abnormal pH always signifies an acute component to an acid–base disturbance.
- A worsening acidosis is always a cause for concern and may be due to a life-threatening process. Treating the underlying cause should be the focus of management.
- The acidosis due solely to renal failure develops slowly (the base excess changes only a few mmol/24 hr). A metabolic acidosis developing more quickly than this always has another contributory cause.

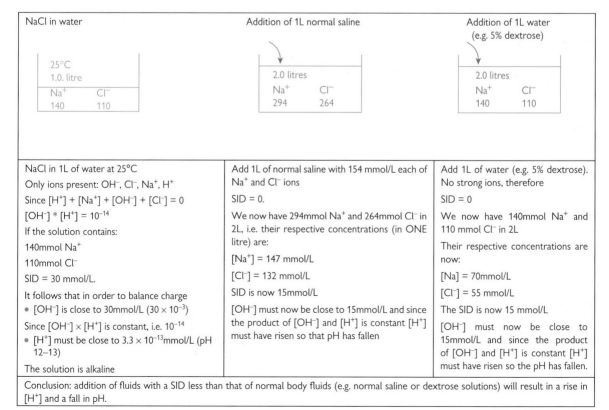

NaCl in water	Addition of 1L normal saline	Addition of 1L water (e.g. 5% dextrose)
25°C 1.0. litre	2.0 litres	2.0 litres
Na⁺ 140 Cl⁻ 110	Na⁺ 294 Cl⁻ 264	Na⁺ 140 Cl⁻ 110
NaCl in 1L of water at 25°C Only ions present: OH^-, Cl^-, Na^+, H^+ Since $[H^+] + [Na^+] + [OH^-] + [Cl^-] = 0$ $[OH^-] * [H^+] = 10^{-14}$ If the solution contains: 140mmol Na^+ 110mmol Cl^- SID = 30 mmol/L. It follows that in order to balance charge • $[OH^-]$ is close to 30mmol/L (30×10^{-3}) Since $[OH^-] \times [H^+]$ is constant, i.e. 10^{-14} • $[H^+]$ must be close to 3.3×10^{-13}mmol/L (pH 12–13) The solution is alkaline	Add 1L of normal saline with 154 mmol/L each of Na^+ and Cl^- ions SID = 0. We now have 294mmol Na^+ and 264mmol Cl^- in 2L, i.e. their respective concentrations (in ONE litre) are: $[Na^+]$ = 147 mmol/L $[Cl^-]$ = 132 mmol/L SID is now 15mmol/L $[OH^-]$ must now be close to 15mmol/L and since the product of $[OH^-]$ and $[H^+]$ is constant $[H^+]$ must have risen so that pH has fallen	Add 1L of water (e.g. 5% dextrose). No strong ions, therefore SID = 0 We now have 140mmol Na^+ and 110 mmol Cl^- in 2L Their respective concentrations are now: $[Na]$ = 70mmol/L $[Cl^-]$ = 55 mmol/L The SID is now 15 mmol/L $[OH^-]$ must now be close to 15mmol/L and since the product of $[OH^-]$ and $[H^+]$ is constant $[H^+]$ must have risen so the pH has fallen.

Conclusion: addition of fluids with a SID less than that of normal body fluids (e.g. normal saline or dextrose solutions) will result in a rise in $[H^+]$ and a fall in pH.

Fig. 11.16 SID and the addition of fluid

Chapter 12

Renal system

12.1 Renal physiology

The kidneys have four main functions.

Two are related to the formation of urine:

- Elimination of solute waste and drugs
- Control of electrolyte and water balance.

Two are hormonal (see Section 18):

- Vitamin D metabolism
- Erythropoiesis.

It is essential for the anaesthetist or critical care specialist to have a good working knowledge of the normal structure and function of the kidneys. It is also vital to develop an understanding of the changes that take place in disease states, affecting the body as a whole, and the kidneys and renal tract in particular.

General features

The normal adult has two functioning kidneys (the incidence of congenital absence of one kidney is 0.3%) that weigh approx 250g each.

The most notable feature of the kidneys is their very large blood supply given their size: 20–30% of cardiac output. The number of renal arteries is variable, with two or even more to each kidney being a common feature (26%).

In order for a normal adult in the UK to remain in steady state, it is essential to be able to excrete the daily load of water and solute waste that is presented to the body. In western society the normal adult solute load is of the order of 600 mOsm/day and is made up of the following:

- **Sodium:** may vary between 50mmol (salt free diet) and 100mmol (no added salt) to upwards of 200mmol where a high-salt diet is consumed.
- **Protein:** intake may vary from 40g/day to more than 100g/day, resulting in the production of variable quantities of urea.
- **Potassium:** intake tends to follow the quantity of protein intake although certain foods contain high potassium levels e.g. bananas.
- **Water:** intake varies from less than one to several litres per day.
- **Non-volatile hydrogen ions:** production associated with non-metabolized anion is of the order of 80mmol/day.

In the diseased state this excretory load may vary widely in relation to tissue injury, fluid administration or fluid loss. Kidney function therefore has to be able to respond to a wide variety of situations and yet maintain steady state.

Understanding the function of the kidney is best approached by consideration of the individual nephron. Each kidney contains approximately a million nephrons, which are present from birth. This number of nephrons can only decrease during life.

At birth, tubular function is relatively immature with limitations in both maximal solute and water conservation. However, by the age of 3 years, tubular function approaches adult levels. In premature babies tubular function is even less developed and commonly causes major problems with solute and water balance and waste excretion.

It had long been considered that glomerular filtration rate (GFR) always falls as one enters the eighth decade of life. However, longtitudinal studies have not supported this inevitability and it is now clear that this cannot be assumed for all individuals. It is the common morbidities of increasing age that reduce renal function and affect GFR.

Nephron structure and function

The nephron can be divided initially into 2 major components:

- The renal corpuscle (containing the glomerulus)
- The renal tubule.

The role of the glomerulus in the production of urine is the generation of a large volume of filtrate. The filtrate is then modified by the tubular system, which may be considered as three sections, each with a distinct action (Figures 12.1 and 12.2):

- **The proximal tubule**, which reabsorbs the bulk of filtered sodium, water and electrolytes essential for normal physiological function.
- **The loop of Henle**, which creates a concentration and dilution mechanism and provides the conditions that allow control of water balance.
- **The distal nephron** (including distal tubule, conducting tubule and collecting duct) where fine control of sodium, potassium, non-volatile hydrogen ion and water balance is exercised.

All the tubular epithelial cells other than the intercalated cells in the distal nephron possess a single non-motile cilium, which protrudes from the luminal membrane into the tubular space. The cilium functions as a tubular flow rate sensor and chemoreceptor, detecting changes in content and flow and causing activation of calcium-dependent pathways which control cell function, differentiation, proliferation, and apoptosis.

The glomerulus

The glomeruli are situated in the cortex and act as plasma filters, producing the initial large filtrate volume of approximately 180L/day in the adult. Waste solutes are present in low concentrations in the plasma, so large-volume filtration allows enough into the tubular system to achieve adequate clearance from the body and maintenance of steady state.

The glomerulus (Figure 12.3) is composed of a tuft of two to five capillary loops invaginated into a dilated portion of the tubule (Bowman's capsule). This is supported by the mesangium and basement membrane, and is supplied by an afferent (pre-glomerular) arteriole and drained by the efferent (post-glomerular) arteriole. The pressure within the capillaries is relatively high ($\approx$50mmHg) and is almost constant throughout their length.

The pressure drop occurs at the efferent arteriole and this allows sufficient driving pressure to achieve the glomerular filtration rate of approximately 125mls/min/1.73m^2 (on average slightly higher in men and lower in women, but with a significant individual variation).

The endothelial cells of the capillaries are extremely thin and have fenestrations that allow direct contact of blood with the basement membrane. The podocytes (epithelial cells) lining the outer surface of the glomerular capillary basement membrane have interdigitating podia with slit pores through which glomerular filtrate passes. These features explain the very high hydraulic permeability of the glomerular capillary, which, together with the high driving pressure and the lack of pressure drop within the capillary, produce the high GFR.

The axial mesangium has a contractile structure that controls the surface area available for filtration in response to circulatory and tubular stimuli. Under normal circumstances, the basement membrane of the capillaries prevents the filtration of solute with an effective radius of >4nm. Because the basement membrane and slit pores are highly negatively charged, molecules <4nm, but with marked negative charge are prevented from passage through the glomerular capillary (Figure 12.4). The most notable example of this is albumin, which has a radius of 3.5nm but undergoes no significant passage in normal health. Inflammation within the glomerulus (e.g. glomerulonephritis) damages the charged structure of the basement membrane and slit pores. Under these circumstances, large quantities of albumin may pass into the filtrate, and hence into the final urine.

It is essential to understand that the energy consumption to create glomerular filtrate takes place within the heart and the muscular arterial resistance vessels, not the kidney. *Kidney function is totally dependent upon the circulation to provide adequate renal perfusion pressure and blood flow to enable the production of glomerular filtrate.*

→ Renal statistics	
Renal blood flow	1.25 l/min (20–30% cardiac output)
Renal plasma flow	625 ml/min
Glomerular filtration rate	125 ml/min
Filtration fraction	0.2 (GFR/RPF)

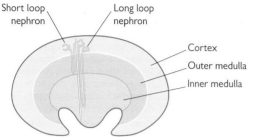

Fig. 12.1 A cross section through the kidney, showing the arrangement of nephrons.

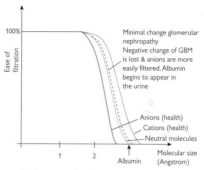

With 100% ease of filtration, the concentrations in the glomerular capillary and Bowman's space are equal.

Fig. 12.4 The effect of molecular size and charge on passage across the glomerular membrane. With 100% ease of filtration, the concentrations in the glomerular capillary and Bowman's capsule are equal. In minimal change glomerular nephropathy, the negative charge of the basement membrane is lost and anions are more easily filtered. Albumin begins to appear in the urine.

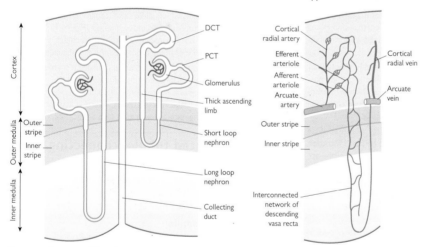

Fig. 12.2 Anatomy of the tubules

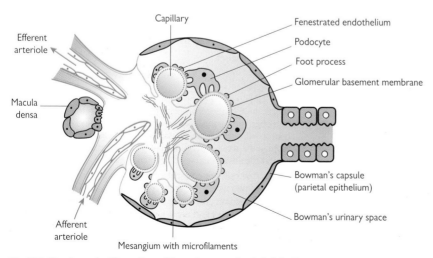

Fig. 12.3 The glomerulus. The surfaces of the podocytes and endothelial cells are covered by a negatively charged glycocalix. This affects the passage of molecules into Bowman's space.

Proximal tubule

Glomerular filtrate passes from the Bowman's capsular space into the proximal tubule. Here, the tubular epithelial cells have a luminal brush border of microvilli providing a large surface area to allow bulk reabsorption. In normal circulatory states, some 60-65% of the glomerular filtrate is reabsorbed here (Figures 12.5 and 12.6). This occurs as follows:

- Non-energy-dependent passive diffusion down the electrochemical gradient, through both cellular and paracellular pathways (the tight junctions between the epithelial cells here are particularly 'leaky').
- Non-energy-dependent facilitated (or carrier-dependent) diffusion e.g. sodium and glucose or amino acid co-transport (both enter the cell) or sodium and hydrogen ion counter-transport (sodium enters and H^+ leaves the cell).
- The ubiquitous energy-dependent active transport $3Na^+/2K^+$ ATP exchange pump provides the driving energy for all these mechanisms. It is present on the anti-luminal baso-lateral cell border.
- Hydraulic conductivity: the luminal membrane has a high density of aquaporin-1 and this allows easy passage of water.

In this fashion, sodium plus accompanying anions and coupled co-transport compounds move from lumen to cell to peri-tubular capillaries; the last transfer is effected by active transport.

Tubular cells have numerous mitochondria, and the tubular cell mass (both proximal and distal) accounts for 8-10% of total body oxygen consumption. This predominantly occurs within the cortical and outer medullary area of the kidney, with blood supply from the efferent arterioles of the glomeruli.

The small quantities of protein filtered by the glomerulus (40mg/L or around 7 g/day) are reabsorbed by endocytosis, either intact or partially degraded. Normally all protein is reabsorbed, but this mechanism is close to saturation under normal conditions and therefore abnormal rises in protein filtration produce detectable proteinuria.

Organic anions and cations (endogenous by-products of metabolism and exogenous compounds e.g. drugs) are excreted by both filtration and efficient secretion within the proximal tubule. Organic anions are actively secreted against their concentration gradients in exchange for α-ketoglutarate. Organic cations are transported into PCT cells and excreted into the lumen via a hydrogen ion-linked antiporter.

By the time tubular fluid enters the descending limb of the Loop of Henle, over 90% of potassium and bicarbonate, all amino acids, glucose and the small quantities of filtered protein have been reabsorbed, in addition to 65% of filtered sodium and water (see Figure 12.8).

Proximal reabsorption of bicarbonate

The majority of filtered bicarbonate must be reabsorbed, otherwise the bicarbonate buffer system would quickly fail. H^+ is secreted into the lumen via:

- The Na^+/H^+ exchanger
- An H^+ antiporter.

Carbonic anhydrase catalyses the breakdown of bicarbonate into CO_2 and OH^-, which combines with H^+ to form water. CO_2 diffuses into the cell where carbonic anhydrase catalyses the reaction in the opposite direction, leading to the formation of protons and bicarbonate.

The process is completed with the secretion of protons, as described above, and the carrier mediated transport of $Na^+/HCO_3^-/CO_3^{2-}$ across the basolateral membrane (Figure 12.9).

Loop of Henle

Having passed through the outer medulla and the proximal tubule, the remaining tubular fluid enters the descending limb of the loop of Henle, within the inner medulla. This section of the nephron is lined with thin epithelial cells and is freely permeable to water due to the high density of aquaporin-1. However, it is not permeable to sodium. The thin limbs are permeable to urea (particularly the ascending thin limb) but thereafter urea is not freely permeable across the luminal membrane until the inner medullary collecting duct where AVP-controlled urea transporters are present. This allows urea recycling to provide a high solute concentration in the medulla, and maximum concentrating conditions.

Water leaves the lumen as the loop descends into the hypertonic medulla, with the osmolarity of the tubular fluid rising *pari passu*. Within the papillae of the medulla of the kidney, the loop makes a hairpin bend and the ascending limb is formed. From this point on, the nephron is impermeable to the passage of water other than in the presence of membrane aquaporin-2 in the distal tubule and collecting duct, under the influence of arginine vasopressin (AVP) (see Section 12.4).

As the ascending limb reaches the outer medulla, the lining cells become cuboidal in shape with sparse microvilli and mitochondria supplying the $3Na^+/2K^+$ ATP exchange pump at the basolateral border. This is the thick ascending limb (TAL) of the loop of Henle, and in this section the luminal surface co-transporter of $Na^+/K^+/2Cl^-$ promotes the reabsorption of sodium and chloride while the passage of water is prevented (Figure 12.7). There is also significant calcium and magnesium reabsorption, mainly via the para-cellular route.

The osmolarity of the tubular fluid falls as it proceeds toward the distal nephron. The reabsorbed solute enters the descending vasa recta capillaries arising from the efferent arterioles and lying parallel to the loops of Henle. They carry the solute into the inner medulla, creating the counter-current multiplier, which allows the formation of a gradient of increasing osmolarity from outer to inner medulla (Figure 12.11). Flow through the vasa recta is mediated by pericytes, which are influenced by the paracrine influence of many agents (e.g. NO, PGE_2, adenosine).

As the tubular fluid leaves the TAL and enters the distal segment of the nephron, the osmolarity is approximately 100 mOsm/kgH₂O. The total sodium and fluid volume will have been reduced by a further 20-30%. At the end of the TAL is the macula densa, which is attached to the hilum of the tubule's originating glomerulus (see Section 12.5).

Distal convoluted tubule, connecting tubule and collecting duct

By this level of the nephron the reduction of the tubular fluid volume and solute content allows fine control of sodium, potassium, non-volatile hydrogen ion, bicarbonate and water balance.

Distal convoluted tubule

Here, the epithelium has microvilli and a dense network of mitochondria. The luminal thiazide sensitive Na^+/Cl^- co-transporter allows further dilution of the tubular fluid to a minimum of 50mOsm/Kg H_2O (Figure 12.7).

Connecting tubule

This contains specific connecting tubular (CNT) cells.

Collecting duct

This is lined by collecting duct (CD) or principal cells and intercalated cells.

Both CNT cells and principal cells are responsive to AVP via aquaporin-2. Mineralocorticoid receptors on both the CNT and CD cells open luminal sodium channels, which can be blocked by amiloride (glucocorticoids activate the same receptors but normally are inactivated in the distal nephron by 11-OH dehydrogenase. In high dosage glucocorticoids will activate potassium secretion).

Intercalated cells are essential for non-volatile hydrogen ion control. There are two types:

- Type A secretes protons via an H^+-ATPase on the luminal border
- Type B secretes bicarbonate by having the H^+-ATPase on the basolateral membrane.

Within the inner medullary collecting duct, the CD cells express the AVP-sensitive urea transporter.

Even with the relatively high sodium intake of a Western diet, normally no more than 200 mmol/day has to be excreted in order to remain in steady state. Given that the tubular system is presented with 180L/day of plasma filtrate containing roughly 25,000mmol of sodium, it can be appreciated that mechanisms for sodium reabsorption are remarkably efficient.

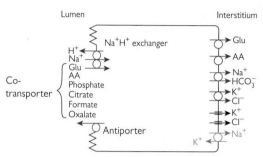

Fig. 12.5 Proximal convoluted tubule: showing carrier-mediated transport mechanisms (green) and active transport (red).

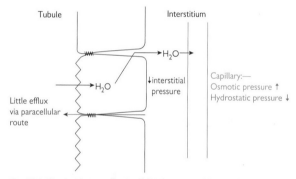

Fig. 12.6 Physical factors affecting PCT absorption. Uptake of fluid by the peritubular capillaries depends on the balance of oncotic and hydrostatic pressures across their endothelium. This usually favours reabsorption of fluid. When the intra-capillary hydrostatic pressure increases or the oncotic pressure is reduced, less fluid is taken up. Interstitial pressure rises and paracellular efflux back into the tubule increases.

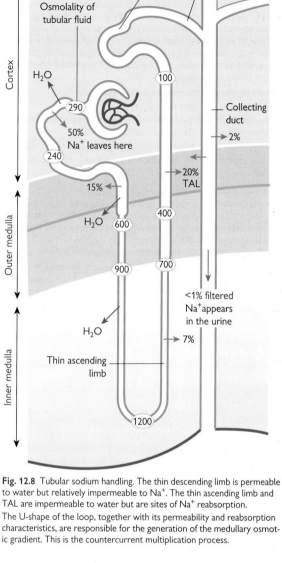

Fig. 12.8 Tubular sodium handling. The thin descending limb is permeable to water but relatively impermeable to Na^+. The thin ascending limb and TAL are impermeable to water but are sites of Na^+ reabsorption.

The U-shape of the loop, together with its permeability and reabsorption characteristics, are responsible for the generation of the medullary osmotic gradient. This is the countercurrent multiplication process.

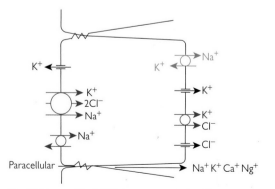

Fig. 12.7 Loop of Henle TAL transport mechanisms The cotransporter is the major route of entry of ions into the cell. Trans-epithelial potential difference drives paracellular ion movement.

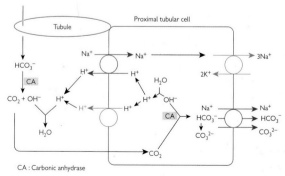

Fig. 12.9 Reabsorption of bicarbonate.

Renal circulation

The structure and response of the renal circulation is of critical importance to the function of the kidney. As previously stated, the high blood flow is essential for the production of the large volume of ultrafiltrate to allow efficient waste solute excretion. This high blood flow is associated with a low overall oxygen extraction. The arterial blood supply is delivered to the glomeruli in the cortex of the kidney (there is no arterial supply to the medulla).

Blood from the efferent arteriole is distributed to:

- The peritubular capillaries.
- The vasa recta (depending on the position of the glomerulus, these may be cortical or juxtamedullary).

The outer and mid-cortical efferent arterioles supply the cortical peritubular capillaries. The medulla is supplied by the juxtamedullary glomerular efferent blood (Figure 12.2).

The vasa recta

The vasa recta have a specific distribution and enter the medulla in discrete vascular bundles: vessels entering the hypertonic inner medulla do not have contact with the tubules of the outer medulla. Ascending vasa recta also leave the inner medulla in bundles and traverse the inner stripe of the outer medulla before supplying its outer stripe.

Together, the vasa recta and the loop of Henle form a countercurrent exchanger of solute (Figure 12.11) The supply of the outer stripe tubules with ascending vasa recta blood is thought to prevent the loss of solute from the medulla.

Flow through the vasa recta is under the control of mediators acting upon the pericytes (e.g. angiotensin II endothelin, adenosine, NO and prostaglandins) ultimately producing fine control of blood flow within the medulla and hence the efficiency of the concentrating mechanism of the kidney.

These long capillaries run parallel to the nephron loop. Blood flow is in the opposite direction to that of the filtrate.

The vasa recta are freely permeable to salt and water. As they descend into the medulla, parallel to the ascending limb of the loop of Henle, solutes diffuse down their concentration gradient from the ISF into the blood vessels. Water flows in the opposite direction, from the dilute blood to the concentrated medullary ISF. The plasma concentration in the vasa recta will parallel that of the nephron and ISF.

As the vasa recta ascend, solutes diffuse out of them and into the ISF, where they promptly diffuse back into the descending limb and are carried back down into the medulla. The concentrated blood gains water from the progressively less concentrated ISF.

Blood flow through the vasa recta is extremely slow, allowing time for equilibration of the steep concentration gradients. The hairpin construction of the vasa recta, coupled with their very slow flow rate, allows blood to pass through the medulla with minimal disturbance to the medullary osmotic gradient. If the blood vessels of this region were similar to those found in the cortex, they would carry away the salt transported out of the ascending limb of the loop, and prevent the development of the countercurrent gradient.

Simply put, the vasa recta trap solutes in the medulla, helping to maintain the high solute concentration of its ISF (Figure 12.15).

Autoregulation of renal blood flow

In health, renal blood flow (RBF) is maintained across a wide range of mean arterial pressures (Figure 12.9). This mechanism is important for two reasons:

- It protects the glomerular capillary from excessive pressure increases.
- It preserves renal perfusion pressure in situations of hypovolaemic or vasodilatory stress.

- This is effected by:
- Myogenic responses in response to distending pressure and shear forces in the glomerular arterioles, effected by calcium dependent mechanisms.
- Tubuloglomerular feedback (see Section 12.4).

Factors that influence renal blood flow

The chronically hypertensive

In the hypertensive patient, the autoregulation relationship is shifted to the right. Autoregulation is not perfect and a sudden increase in arterial blood pressure will cause a pressure natriuresis both by the increase in renal plasma flow and GFR, and the rise in interstitial hydrostatic pressure. This latter response appears to be mediated through NO production. Since renal perfusion is adequate, the macula densa tubuloglomerular feedback response to the increased distal delivery of NaCl will be minimal (Section 12.4). Again, this is mediated via NO production within the cells of the macula densa.

The sympathetic nervous system

This affects RBF via afferent signals generated by the central arterial baroreceptors and central vein/atrial volume receptors.

The afferent and efferent arterioles are supplied with sympathetic nerves, which are triggered when low arterial pressure or diminished central venous return occurs. The sympathetic system also directly stimulates the production of angiotensin by the juxtaglomerular apparatus.

The renin-angiotensin-aldosterone system

The renin-angiotensin-aldosterone (RAA) system is also activated directly by receptors within the afferent arteriole, which detect the reduced vessel stretch that accompanies diminished perfusion pressure. This releases renin from specialised afferent arteriolar cells leading to local angiotensin production. In turn this effects contraction of the mesangium and allows reduction in filtration in the cortical glomeruli by reduction of the surface area available for filtration.

Local angiotensin production also produces contraction of both the afferent and efferent arterioles: the efferent arteriolar contraction is more pronounced. This allows for maximal maintenance of GFR as renal plasma flow (RPF) falls (until perfusion pressure falls to a point where filtration ceases).

Eicosanoids

These metabolites of arachidonic acid have significant effects upon intra-renal blood flow. They are produced by:

- The cyclo-oxygenase (COX) system. Isoforms COX-1 and COX-2 are both expressed within the kidney, producing primarily PGE_2 and PGI_2. Both PGE_2 and PGI_2 are vasodilators and act to balance the vasoconstrictor effects of angiotensin and the sympathetic mediator norepinephrine. PGE_2 also has major effects on both the control of vasa recta blood flow by its dilator effects upon the pericytes, and inhibition of distal sodium reabsorption. Thus, it provides a protective mechanism to ensure adequate oxygen delivery to the medulla.
- Cytochrome P450 metabolites (e.g. 20-hydoxyeicostetranoic acid).

ANF

Atrial natriuretic peptide (ANP) and brain natriuretic peptide (BNP) secretion is stimulated by a rise in blood pressure and an increase in ECF volume. ANP is released from the atria and ventricles of the heart and acts on the medullary collecting duct to inhibit salt and water reabsorption. AVP release is also inhibited by both these hormones. Action is via cell membrane guanyl cyclase receptors in the CD cells.

Urodilatin is similar in structure and action to ANP but is produced locally within the distal tubule in response to blood pressure rise and ECF volume increase. It is more potent than ANP/BNP

Pathology

Autoregulation may be impaired by the presence of vasoactive drugs or pathological processes such as systemic inflammatory response syndrome.

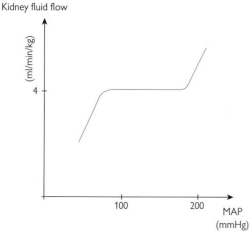

Kidney fluid flow

Fig. 12.10 Autoregulation: between MAP 80mmHg and 180mmHg renal blood flow is constant.

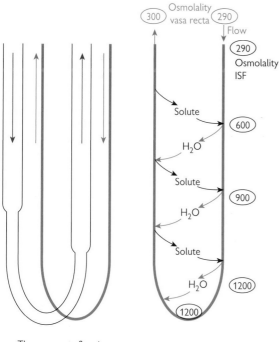

The vasa recta flow is opposite to that of tubular fluid.

Fig. 12.11 Countercurrent exchanger

Plasma enters the descending limb of the vasa recta at 285-290 mosmol/kgH$_2$O. It comes into contact with the high Na$^+$, Cl$^-$ and osmotic concentrations of the medullary ISF through the capillary wall. Water flows out of the descending limb following the osmotic gradient, and Na$^+$ and Cl$^-$ diffuse in, resulting in increasing plasma osmolarity as the fluid approaches the tip of the papilla.

As this concentrated fluid flows into the ascending limb of the vasa recta and back toward the cortex, the gradient is reversed. Water then flows down the osmotic gradient into the ascending vasa recta and Na$^+$ and Cl$^-$ diffuse out.

The volume and osmotic concentration of plasma leaving the vasa recta exceed that of entering plasma

• Trapping of solute is not complete: the rate at which solute is carried out by the vasa recta exceeds that carried in.

• Water is reabsorbed from the descending limb of the loop and from the collecting tubule and is carried out by the vasa recta.

Medullary osmotic concentration reaches steady state when the rate of solute transport out of the thick ascending limb is balanced by the rate of solute leakage into the exiting plasma of the ascending vasa recta.

Tubuloglomerular feedback

Tubuloglomerular feedback represents signalling between different nephron segments. At the hilum of the glomerulus in the cleft between the afferent and efferent arterioles there is close association between a specialised section of the distal nephron (the macula densa) and the mesangium (juxtaglomerular apparatus, JGA) (Figure 12.16). The macula densa senses the flow of solute into the distal nephron and the JGA senses the circulatory supply to the nephron.

In the presence of hypovolaemia, if sodium delivery to the distal nephron is felt to be excessive then GFR is diminished by the JGA to prevent inappropriate loss of solute with further compromise of the circulation. The mediators responsible for this effect are thought to be adenosine and nitric oxide.

Formation of a hypertonic medulla: urea trapping

The counter-current system concentrates urea in the ISF and tubular fluid (Figure 12.15). A reduction in available urea reduces countercurrent effectiveness and decreases the maximal concentration of solute in the final urine.

Vasa recta

Urea diffuses into the vasa recta flowing into the medulla. It is trapped by the counter-current exchange mechanism. Urea trapping of depends ultimately upon active salt transport by the thick ascending limb. This establishes the gradient for water reabsorption and so the gradient for urea diffusion out of the inner medullary collecting duct.

Urea trapping adds to the osmotic gradient forcing water from the descending limb of the loop of Henle and from the collecting tubule.

- Inner medullary CD urea concentration is very high due to the relatively higher water reabsorption proximally. Urea diffuses from the ISF into the vasa recta.
- As it descends in the vasa recta, urea concentration exceeds that of the surrounding ISF and it diffuses out into the ISF.
- Urea concentration in adjacent descending vasa recta is less than that of the ISF. Hence urea diffuses back in to become trapped.

Production of dilute urine

The first requirements for the kidney to be able to excrete a water load are: that there is no stimulus for sodium retention, and there is normal delivery of adequate tubular volume to the distal nephron.

As previously stated, in the situation of sodium retention (e.g. ECF volume depletion or cardiac failure) the percentage of the filtered salt and water reabsorbed proximally rises with a marked reduction of distal delivery of tubular volume. Release of AVP is also stimulated by central volume receptors, causing continued water reabsorption of what little fluid reaches the distal nephron, regardless of the plasma osmolarity. Therefore, the urine will have a high osmolarity regardless of plasma osmolarity. Under these circumstances administration of free water either orally or intravenously will result in water retention and the development of progressive hyponatraemia.

It follows that the syndrome of inappropriate antidiuretic hormone (AVP) secretion (SIADH) cannot be diagnosed unless it has been shown that the patient is not in a salt retaining state. This requires the performance of accurate Na$^+$ balance studies.

Under euvolaemic conditions the structure and function of the loop of Henle, the accompanying vasa recta, and the distal nephron and collecting ducts produce a balanced system that can be modulated to retain or lose free water (non solute-containing) dependent upon the plasma osmolarity under the influence of the central osmoreceptors (Figure 12.18).

Excretion of free water

Fluid leaving the distal nephron in the absence of AVP secretion has an osmolarity of around 50mOsm/KgH$_2$O. In a water-losing state or in the pathological absence of AVP this dilute urine passes directly to the bladder with only a small amount of salt urea and water being reabsorbed within the medullary collecting duct.

Potentially 18L/day of low osmolarity urine can be excreted provided adequate intake can be maintained to prevent a fall in circulating volume and consequent increased proximal fluid reabsorption (e.g. diabetes insipidus).

Requirements for production of dilute urine

- Adequate delivery of solute to the diluting sites
  - Normal GFR
  - Normal proximal salt and water reabsorption
- Distal tubular impermeability to water
- Normal solute transport in diluting site

Production of concentrated urine

When water retention is required, AVP released from the posterior pituitary under the influence of the hypothalamus concentrates the final urine to an osmolarity well in excess of the plasma. By early adulthood this may reach a maximum of 1500mOsm/KgH$_2$O. This maximum declines with age and with increasing renal failure (higher solute load per nephron, with a relative osmotic diuresis).

In the presence of AVP, maximum carriage of water passes via cell membrane aquaporins (Section 11.3). This occurs immediately beyond the DCT through to the collecting ducts in the medulla. The reabsorbed water is returned to the body via the ascending vasa recta (Figure 12.18).

Requirements for production of concentrated urine

- Adequate delivery of solute to distal sites
  - Normal GFR
  - Normal proximal salt and water reabsorption
- Development of a hypertonic medulla
- ADH must be present
- The kidney must respond normally to ADH

Chronic renal failure

In chronic renal failure there is permanent loss of nephrons.

At birth there are approximately 2 million nephrons within the two kidneys. In steady state the normal solute load of approximately 600mosmol/day in the adult is cleared with a relatively modest load of solute per nephron. This provides a significant compensatory reserve and explains the ability of the kidney to adapt to a variety of solute and water conditions in both health and disease.

As nephrons are lost, the solute and volume load per nephron rises and produces the equivalent of an osmotic diuresis with a progressive loss of ability to conserve salt and water. Therefore the concentrating and diluting ability of the kidney diminishes as the nephron number falls.

By the time GFR has diminished to less than 30mls/min, the ability of the kidneys to concentrate urine will be poor and there will be an obligatory loss of water and solute. In fact, concentration will only occur once renal blood flow and glomerular filtration have fallen secondary to ECF volume loss, and this will further compromise renal function. This is the reason that patients with chronic renal failure should not be fasted without providing adequate parenteral fluid to compensate for the obligatory urinary loss of water and solute. Preoperative total starvation regimes for patients with chronic renal failure are particularly dangerous.

The last function that is lost in terminal chronic renal failure is the ability to dilute the urine, by which time renal replacement therapy should ideally have been instituted.

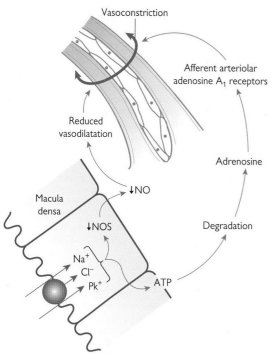

Fig. 12.12 Tubuloglomerular feedback. The luminal surface co-transporter of $Na^+/K^+/2Cl^-$ takes up solute at the macula densa. The subsequent response is mediated by adenosine (acting on A1 receptors on the afferent arteriole) and possibly by ATP, and is modulated by NO and Angiotensin II.

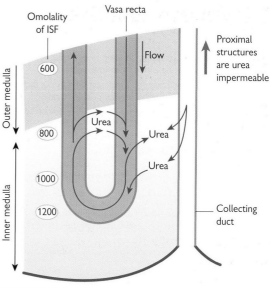

Fig. 12.13 Urea trapping

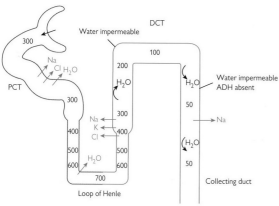

Fig. 12.14 Production of dilute urine

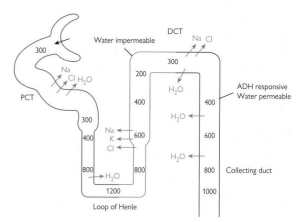

Fig. 12.15 Production of concentrated urine.

As the preservation of circulating volume is essential for human survival, it is very efficiently defended by several mechanisms.

Initially, the response is an attempt to maintain GFR in the face of a falling renal plasma flow (RPF) with a resultant rise in filtration fraction (FF). This is achieved by the release of renin, and the local production of angiotensin II. The efferent arteriole is much more sensitive to angiotensin II than the proximal arteriole, and therefore the pressure within the glomerular capillaries is maintained in the face of falling renal perfusion.

As GFR falls, a higher proportion of filtered fluid is reabsorbed from the proximal tubule. This is due to:
- Active transport
- The effect of the increased solvent drag caused by the higher than normal oncotic pressure in the peritubular capillaries, itself a result of the increase in filtration fraction.
- Direct stimulation of sodium reabsorption by sympathetic nerve stimulation in the proximal tubule.

The concentrating mechanisms in the loop of Henle and the distal nephron work with maximum efficiency due to:
- Slowed tubular fluid flow distal to the PCT.
- The increased levels of AVP that follow from central volume receptor stimulation.

Any distal delivery of sodium that does occur will be reabsorbed, stimulated by:
- Diminished distal delivery of Na^+
- Direct sympathetic nerve stimulation of the TAL of the loop of Henle
- Increased aldosterone production caused by the activation of the renin-angiotensin system.

Very little fluid will be delivered to the distal nephron; and what little fluid leaves this segment will have minimal sodium content. The volume delivered may not allow for significant excretion of potassium, non-volatile hydrogen ion, or water. Urine volume is diminished to a very low level with a very low concentration of sodium and a high osmolarity (provided that no diuretic has been administered).

Within the kidney, as circulating volume decreases, cortical blood flow is diverted from the outer cortical nephrons to the juxta-medullary glomeruli. This preserves the blood supply to the oxygen-dependent outer medulla where most of the major metabolic activity of the kidney resides. The reduction in solute delivery also allows for a reduction in oxygen consumption within the kidney as renal blood flow falls. This pattern of blood flow and oxygen extraction is very different from most other organs in the body. It was demonstrated by the work of Schlichtig and coworkers, who compared the oxygen consumption of the kidney with that of the other organs of the body, as the circulating volume was decreased in dogs.

These adaptive mechanisms are produced by the release of many different mediator systems (e.g. renin-angiotensin, adenosine, autonomic nerves, prostaglandin E, and nitric oxide) and it is obvious that any drug that interferes with these systems will impair the ability of the kidney to defend the body maximally against the effects of circulatory impairment. Such drugs include ACE inhibitors, NSAIDs, β-blockers, and calcium channel blockers.

Many of these drugs are used as anti-hypertensives. This explains why those taking common antihypertensives are so vulnerable to early onset renal dysfunction in situations of salt and water loss, bleeding or loss of normal autoregulation following prolonged severe hypotension, sepsis or systemic inflammatory response syndrome.

Acute renal failure

Acute renal failure (ARF) is normally reversible and occurs when there is a sudden deterioration of renal function that is not immediately remediable by correcting the cause (or, more commonly, multiple causes). Certain overwhelming insults will cause acute renal failure on their own:
- Prolonged loss of renal perfusion: usually >30-40 minutes of total absence of renal perfusion (e.g. abdominal aortic occlusion/dissection/thrombosis, severe prolonged haemorrhagic shock)
- Severe direct tubular toxicity (e.g. paracetamol, mercuric chloride, platinum salts, carbon tetrachloride)
- Severe aggressive glomerular disease (e.g. rapidly progressive glomerulonephritis, vasculitis).

However, ARF usually ensues following exposure to an insult when an individual's kidneys are already stressed, with the normal compensatory mechanisms activated or compromised. This has been found in the developed experimental models, where it is difficult to produce ARF unless the experimental animal is rendered salt and water depleted prior to the administration of the specific insult that results in acute renal failure.

Compensatory mechanisms may be activated by situations where effective renal perfusion is impaired, including effective circulating volume depletion, chronic cardiac failure, cirrhosis, and diuretic administration.

Compensatory mechanisms may be compromised by the following:
- Medication that interferes with intra-renal haemodynamics, autoregulation, and the normal responses to physiological stress (e.g. ACE inhibitors, angiotensin II receptor blockers, COX inhibitors, β-blockers)
- Pathological conditions that interfere with the normal responses of the renal vasculature to stress (e.g. systemic inflammatory response of whatever cause, with loss of autoregulation and inducible NO production, or diabetes mellitus with impaired endothelial NO production).

The effects of the combined insults are to severely compromise the perfusion of the outer medulla of the kidney, with damage to the highly metabolically active cells of both the proximal and distal nephron. This ultimately results in the reduction of GFR by reducing the filtration coefficient (K_f, Section 12.1) of the glomeruli, and the programmed death of tubular cells. These cells then regrow and once the tubule is re-populated, cell signalling via the JGA/Macula densa permits the resumption of filtration.

Management of acute renal failure

ARF may occur following:
- Volume depletion and/or hypotension
- Cytotoxic, ischaemic, or inflammatory insults to the kidney
- Obstruction to the passage of urine
- Any combination of the above.

An ABCDE assessment will help determine the clinical imperative. Failure of opiate clearance might affect airway control, pulmonary oedema will impair oxygenation, and the effects of hypovolaemia might affect cerebral perfusion.

Early, aggressive treatment is aimed at preservation of the remaining functional renal mass, since a large proportion is damaged before any biochemical evidence of renal dysfunction is appreciated. The relationship between the GFR and the serum creatinine level is not linear: a graph of GFR vs. serum creatinine follows a rectangular hyperbola. It follows that, at lower serum creatinine levels, a small increase in serum creatinine signifies a large deterioration in GFR. Conversely, when renal function is poor or end-stage, a small drop in GFR can cause a large increase in measured creatinine.

Identification of the underlying cause and institution of the appropriate therapy may reverse some of the renal damage.

Maintenance of volume and pressure homeostasis should be urgently achieved, since the majority of cases of ARF are due to these eminently treatable causes.

All nephrotoxic agents should be avoided and all medications cleared by renal excretion should have their doses adjusted appropriately.

Table 12.1 Causes and management of ARF

	Diagnostic pointers and therapy
Pre-renal Haemorrhage, sepsis, GI losses from vomiting or diarrhoea	If the signs of intravascular depletion are difficult to interpret, invasive monitoring (e.g. CVP or cardiac output monitoring) might be indicated. Renal ultrasound examination will be normal, i.e. no obstruction, normal sized kidneys. *Therapy* Treat the underlying condition. Try a volume challenge e.g. 250 ml bolus of isotonic fluid. Look for signs of improved vascular compartment filling. Repeat the fluid challenge until the vascular compartment remains well-filled. Once intra-vascular filling is deemed adequate, perfusion should be increased with the aid of vasopressors or inotropes. If the hypotensive patient has an adequate cardiac output, α-adrenergic vasoconstriction with vasopressors (e.g. noradrenaline) may be used to increase MAP and renal blood flow. Positive inotropes such as dobutamine can improve poor CO and therefore renal blood flow.
Intra-renal *Vascular* (e.g. TTP, HUS) *Glomerular* (e.g. Wegener's) *Tubular* (e.g. tumour lysis syndrome or contrast nephropathy) *Interstitial* (e.g. sarcoid, SLE, penicillin's)	Clinical signs of the underlying disease. Renal ultrasound examination will be normal (see above). Early nephrologist input is essential for this group of disorders. A renal biopsy can be useful in establishing the diagnosis and is often performed when renal function does not return for a prolonged period. A diagnosis may aid long-term management. It is occasionally performed prior to the initiation of immunosuppressive medication. *Therapy* Treat the underlying condition, e.g. immunosuppresion for vasculitis. Consider renal replacement therapy (see below).
Post-renal Prostatic disease, bladder carcinoma, ureteric ligation or calculus obstruction	Renal ultrasound examination allows estimation of kidney size, assessment of obstruction of the urinary collecting system and review of pre-existing disease. For example, small kidneys suggest chronic renal failure. The degree of hydronephrosis changes with time and its presence does not confirm complete obstruction. Obtaining good quality renal images may be difficult in the obese or in those with ascites, gas, or a collection of fluid in the retroperitoneal space. Further CT imaging should be performed in these patients. *Therapy* An obstructed urinary system should be drained (e.g. by percutaneous nephrostomy): failure to do so will impair renal function. Drainage of a renal empyema is a urological emergency, essential in the treatment of urinary sepsis. Plans should be made for treatment of the underlying disease.

327

✚ Obstuctive uropathy

In animal models, following acute ureteric obstruction there is a rise in tubular pressure and dilatation of the afferent glomerular arteriole. This can only offset part of the decrease in hydrostatic gradient, to restore GFR to approximately 75% of normal. Within 5hr of the obstruction RBF proximal tubular pressure falls. The fall in RBF is due to the constriction of the afferent arterioles. This is caused by a rise in angiotensin II and thromboxane, and a fall in NO production. An inflammatory infiltrate of the interstitium then commences and ultimately results in the permanent changes that are seen if obstruction is not rapidly relieved. The degree of permanent damage (nephron loss) is related to the time to relief of the obstruction. This probably begins as early as 72 hours.

Distal tubular functional change is marked after obstruction. Concentrating ability is severely impaired (max 400mosmol/Kg). In addition to damage to the juxtamedullary nephrons, there is no response to AVP due to loss of aquaporin-2. There are also distal sodium, potassium and hydrogen ion handling defects that may result in salt loss, hyper or hypokalaemia, and metabolic acidaemia. These may be permanent and recovery is slow. Care must be taken to manage these defects carefully following release of obstruction.

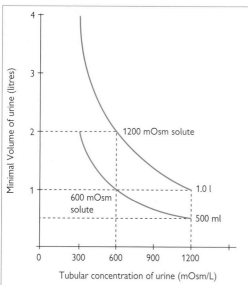

Fig. 12.16 Relationship between minimum volume of urine to concentrating ability and solute load.

If tublular function is sufficient to concentrate urine to 1200mOsm/L, only 500ml/day urine will be required for a daily solute load of 600mOsm/L (or 1000ml for a daily solute load of 1200mOsm/L).

If tubular function will only concentrate to 300mosmol/L, the daily minimal volume of urine required to maintain steady state is vastly different: for a load of 600mosmol it will be 2000ml, and for a load of 1200 mosmol, 4000ml of urine will need to be produced.

Indications for renal replacement therapy
Control of:
- Hyperkalaemia
- Volume (e.g. for control of pulmonary oedema)
- Acid (e.g. for control of metabolic acidaemia)
- Solute (e.g. for control of symptomatic uraemia)
- Specific removal of a drug or toxin (e.g. aspirin, lithium)

12.6 Diuretics

The inhibition of Na^+ reabsorption is the common mode of action by which all diuretics act. They also affect handling of water and a number of other solutes, either directly or as a consequence of their natriuretic effects.

Changing the total body Na^+ content will naturally affect the ECF volume.

Diuretic effect

Several factors are important in determining the diuretic effect.

Sites of action (Figure 12.17)

- Osmotic diuretics act at the PCT and the thin descending limb.
- Carbonic anhydrase inhibitors act at the PCT.
- Loop diuretics act at the TAL of the loop of Henle.
- Thiazides act at the early diluting part of the DCT.
- Potassium sparing diuretics act at the late part of the DCT and the initial part of the CCD.

Response of other nephron segments

The reduced absorption of Na^+ at a proximal site increases Na^+ delivery to the distal nephron. The ability of these more distal sites to handle the increased delivery of Na^+ determines the overall effect of the diuretic's action.

Delivery to their site of action

With the exception of aldosterone antagonists, most diuretics act from within the lumen. They are either freely filtered at the glomerulus, or actively secreted at the PCT via organic anion and cation secretory systems. Manipulation of such systems allows alteration of effect.

ECF volume

ECF volume depletion and low cardiac output states reduce GFR and the filtered load of sodium. This enhances the reabsorption of sodium at the PCT. Distally acting diuretics on their own, would be less effective, since less sodium is delivered to the DCT compared with normal.

Mechanisms of action

Osmotic diuretics (e.g. mannitol)

These increase the osmolarity within the nephron lumen, thereby reducing water reabsorption. They do not affect a specific membrane transport protein.

They are freely filtered at the glomerulus and remain within the lumen. They affect the segments with high permeability to water and so are active at the PCT and the descending limb of the loop of Henle. Both NaCl and water reabsorption are reduced by the increased luminal Osmolality.

Since 60% of solute is reabsorbed at these sites, they may have a powerful diuretic effect, although some of this is offset by increased Na^+ reabsorption at distal sites.

Osmotic diuretics are also associated with an increase in medullary blood flow, which dissipates the osmotic gradient of the medullary ISF. This impairs water reabsorption from the collecting duct and urea trapping (see Section 12.4).

Carbonic anhydrase inhibitors (e.g. acetazolamide)

Inhibition of carbonic anhydrase causes diuresis because >30% of PCT Na^+ reabsorption occurs in exchange for H^+ through the PCT Na^+/H^+ antiporter. Without functioning carbonic anhydrase, there will be fewer protons to exchange for Na^+ (see Section 12.2).

Despite the significant effect on Na^+ reabsorption, the overall diuretic effect is modest since the distal sites are able to compensate and reabsorb more Na^+ than usual. Na^+ excretion rates are only 5-10% of the filtered load.

Predictably, carbonic anhydrase inhibition also leads to reduced bicarbonate reabsorption at the PCT and development of a mild degree of metabolic acidosis.

Loop diuretics (e.g. furosemide)

These are secreted into the lumen by the anion secretory pathways of the PCT, but they work by inhibiting the $K^+/Na^+/2Cl^-$ symporter on the apical surface of the TAL cells. The natriuresis disrupts the countercurrent multiplication process and reduces the osmolality of the ISF of the medulla. Without this, the distal tubules and collecting ducts cannot concentrate urine. In addition, water is not reabsorbed from the descending limb of the loop due to the reduced medullary ISF osmolality, resulting in even greater water loss.

Na^+ excretion may reach 25% of the filtered load, and because distal segments have a limited ability to reabsorb the excess, the result is an impressive diuresis. This may have significant circulatory effects.

Thiazides (e.g. chlorothiazide)

These organic anions are plasma protein-bound, and are secreted into the proximal tubule like loop diuretics. They act through inhibition of Na^+ reabsorption in the early part of the DCT by blocking the apical membrane Na^+/Cl^- symporter. This is the site where urine is diluted; while these agents are natriuretic, they can also prevent excretion of a free water load.

Their action is cortical and not medullary, and so they do not affect the ability of the kidney to concentrate urine. Na^+ loss is 5-10% of the filtered load.

Like loop diuretics, they are weak inhibitors of carbonic anhydrase and this may contribute to the action of diuresis.

Potassium-sparing diuretics

These drugs act on the latter part of the DCT and the CCD. There are two types:

- Some act by antagonizing the effect of aldosterone (e.g. spironolactone) at the principal cell: both Na^+ reabsorption and K^+ secretion are impaired.
- Some block entry of Na^+ into principal cells through the Na^+-selective channels of the apical membrane (e.g. amiloride). With reduced Na^+ uptake, there is less Na^+ extrusion across the basolateral membrane and concomitantly less cellular K^+ uptake. The Na^+ changes also alter voltage differences across these cells, further reducing K^+ loss into the lumen. Triamterene and amiloride are secreted by active mechanisms of the PCT.

The natriuresis is only 3-5% of the filtered load.

It is worth noting that aldosterone antagonism with ACE inhibition, in combination with loop diuretics, reduces morbidity from CCF. Aldosterone causes myocardial fibrosis and the mortality benefit of ACE inhibition appears to be independent of the renal effects.

Aquaretics

ADH V_2 receptor antagonists have been developed, and their action results in excretion of dilute urine. They might prove useful where excretion of water is required in the presence of non-osmotic, non-haemodynamic stimulation of ADH secretion (SIADH).

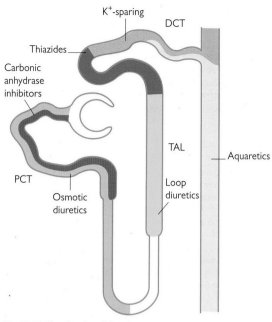

Fig. 12.17 Site of action of diuretics

Table 12.2 Actions of diuretics

	Na⁺ excretion (%)	K⁺ excretion	Bicarb excretion	Ca²⁺ excretion	Free water excretion
Osmotic	10	↑	↑	↑	↑
CAI	5–10	↑	↑	↑	↑
Loop	25	↑	↓	↓	↓
Thiazide	5–10	↑	↓	↓	↓
Potassium-sparing	3–5	↓	↑	NA	NA
Aquaretic	0	NA	NA	NA	↑

➜ **Aldosterone (see Section 18.3)**

Aldosterone acts as a steroid hormone at principal cells. It binds to a cytoplasmic receptor and is transported to the nucleus where the complex binds to DNA elements. Na^+/K^+-ATPase and Na^+ channel synthesis are enhanced, allowing increased Na^+ reabsorption in exchange for K^+.

It also stimulates luminal H^+ secretion by type A intercalated cells.

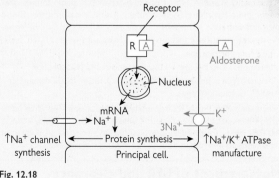

Fig. 12.18

12.7 Assessment of renal function

Urine volume

Urine volume is the crudest method of assessment.

If the quantity of urine falls below the minimum volume that the daily solute load can be concentrated into, then the patient has renal failure. However, the fact that urine volume is greater than this minimum volume does not mean that renal function is normal, since this depends totally upon the ability of the nephrons to concentrate.

If there is a fall in the total nephron mass, each nephron will have to process an increased number of solute molecules. Concentration is then impaired by:

- The increased tubular fluid flow rate.
- An osmotic diuresis for the diminished number of nephrons.

An increase in solute load (e.g. after a major surgical procedure or trauma) produces similar conditions and once again, there is an increased nephron solute load that acts as an osmotic diuretic. Figure 12.19 shows the relationship of minimum urine volume to concentrating ability and solute load.

The fractional excretion of sodium

Urinary electrolytes are used as indicators of functioning renal tubules. The fractional excretion of sodium (FE$_{Na}$) is a commonly used indicator but interpretation of results from patients, with glomerulonephritis, and under the influence of diuretics should be viewed with caution.

$$EF_{Na} = \frac{(U_{Na}/P_{Na})}{(U_{Cr}/P_{Cr})} \times 100$$

Normally, FE$_{Na}$ is less than 1%: around 25,000mmol/day are filtered, yet only 200mmol/day appears in the urine. Similarly in pre-renal disease, the FE$_{Na}$ is less than 1% since with poor renal perfusion, it is expected that the kidney should retain sodium.

In acute tubular necrosis (ATN), the FE$_{Na}$ is usually greater than 1% although the fractional excretion of sodium of ATN caused by contrast media, burns, acute glomerulonephritis, and rhabdomyolysis may be less.

Urea and creatinine

Traditionally available as part of the biochemistry panel of measurements, these have been used to reflect overall renal function. Blood urea concentration is, however, significantly influenced by the degree of urea reabsorption within the kidney. This varies with

- Daily urea production
- Situations of AVP release which maximise urea reabsorption
- Any changes in protein intake or load (e.g. major tissue damage or upper GI haemorrhage).

Creatinine suffers much less from variation in production, which is related to the skeletal muscle mass, and whose level more closely reflects the GFR more closely. Rhabdomyolysis will increase the production of creatinine and may impair its use as an indicator of renal function.

Measurement of GFR and clearance

In humans GFR measurement can only be performed indirectly and is done by using the clearance of a substance excreted solely via filtration. The ideal marker is freely filtered and is neither secreted into nor re-absorbed from the tubular system.

Clearance (C) is the virtual volume of plasma that is completely cleared of a substance per unit time. It can be expressed for the marker substance as $C = A/P$, where A is the amount of substance removed from the plasma and P is the average plasma concentration. C is expressed as units of volume per unit time.

Inulin

In experimental situations, the classical substance that satisfies the ideal criteria is the polymerised sugar inulin (5200 Da, no charge).

It is not metabolised and is non-toxic, but it is necessary to infuse the substance to achieve a steady state. The following are important:

- All urine is collected over a fixed period of time & the concentration of inulin (U) and volume (V) are measured
- Measuring plasma inulin concentration (P) at the mid point of the collection.

$$C = \frac{\text{Urinary concentration} \times \text{Volume}}{P}$$

This method is cumbersome to perform and in clinical practice endogenous markers are used. Traditionally, creatinine (113Da) has been used due to its ease of measurement and relatively constant release into the circulation from phosphocreatine metabolism in skeletal muscle (and to a small extent from meat in the diet). However there are several factors that affect the accuracy of creatinine as a marker for calculating GFR:

- Patient not in steady state (e.g. rapidly changing renal function), as creatinine concentration lags behind the GFR change.
- Creatinine is secreted by the tubules, and so GFR is overestimated. This secretion is also competitively blocked by drugs such as trimethoprim and cimetidine, thus suggesting a fall in GFR. As GFR is reduced these effects become proportionally greater.
- Creatinine in gut secretions is degraded by gut bacteria and this form of clearance is also increased as creatinine levels rise.
- Technical factors in the collection of the urine sample (e.g. spillage, missed volume, blood sample taken outside the collection period) will compromise the assessment of GFR.

Because of the inconvenience and potential for errors in measuring clearance formulae have been developed to provide estimates of GFR based on age, sex, bodyweight, ethnicity and creatinine (e.g. the Cockcroft-Gault and Modification of Diet in Renal Disease MDRD formulae).

These are affected by rapidly changing renal function and also by variation in the method of creatinine measurement when comparing results from different laboratories.

Cystatin C

This low molecular weight (130Da) protein is produced at a steady rate by all nucleated human cells. Production is constant (between 1 and 50 years of age) and unaffected by diet, body mass or sex. Higher levels are found in infants and the elderly.

Cystatin C is freely filtered by the glomerulus, but is both reabsorbed and metabolised within tubular cells. Assays are not yet calibrated between laboratories and so it is not ready for widespread assessment of urinary clearance.

Measurement of renal plasma flow (RPF)

Using the same principles of clearance, para-amino hippurate (PAH), an organic acid that is both filtered and actively secreted in the proximal tubule can be used to measure RPF. PAH is almost completely cleared from the plasma in a single pass, provided the concentration is less than 10mg%.

$$RPF = \frac{(U_{PAH} \times V)}{P_{PAH}} = \text{PAH clearance}$$

Where U_{PAH} and P_{PAH} are concentrations of PAH in the urine and plasma.

$$\text{Renal Blood Flow} = \left(\frac{RPF}{100\text{-haematocrit}}\right) \times 100$$

Limitations:

- If the level is greater than 10mg%, clearance is not complete and RPF is underestimated.
- Interference can occur with drugs that are organic acids and in disease states associated with an increase in toxins or metabolites that are weak organic acids.

Radionuclide techniques

For these investigations, the patient is given a small IV injection of radionuclide before gamma camera imaging several hours later.

Renogram (DTPA scan)

Diethylene triamine pentaacetic acid (DTPA) is a polyamino carboxylic acid chelated with technetium. This technique assesses blood flow to the kidneys, particularly if renal artery stenosis as a cause of hypertension is suspected. A small dose of ACE inhibitor makes this enquiry more sensitive.

DTPA scanning also demonstrates relative left and right function and may be used to demonstrate obstruction to urine flow. As such it is useful in assessing the function of renal transplant grafts.

Static renal scan (DMSA scan)

Tc-99m dimercaptosuccinic acid (DMSA) is used to assess the function of viable tissue within the kidney. It gives information about size, shape and position and the appearance of the kidneys following infection. It is useful for the assessment of active reflux disease of childhood, and pyelonephritis.

Chapter 13

Respiration

13.1 Control of ventilation

The major function of the lungs is the exchange of oxygen and carbon dioxide between alveoli and blood. Despite massively variable metabolic demands, PaO_2 and $PaCO_2$ vary very little. This is testament to the exquisite integration of responses between the sensors, controllers, and effectors of the respiratory system.

Brain stem control

The **medullary respiratory centre** drives the effectors of ventilation and is itself modulated by various feedback mechanisms (Figure 13.1). Its major output is to the phrenic nerves.

The centre is a poorly defined collection of cells found in the floor of the fourth ventricle, rather than an obvious anatomical structure. There are two identifiable areas.

Dorsal respiratory group

The dorsal respiratory group (DRG) is mainly associated with inspiration. It processes the afferent signals from a variety of peripheral receptors. It lies near the nucleus of the tractus solitarius, the termination of input from both the glossopharyngeal and vagus nerves.

When all other inputs have been abolished, these cells fire repetitively to act as the pacemaker for the muscles of inspiration. However, the view that these cells are wholly responsible for the rhythmic nature of inspiration is not completely accepted.

Ventral respiratory group

The ventral respiratory group (VRG) is mainly associated with expiration. Quiet expiration is passive, and so this group is quiescent until exercise when forceful expiration is required.

Six different types of nerve cell have been identified within these two groups. The rate of firing of each group has been linked to a phase in the respiratory cyle: early inspiratory, inspiratory ramp, late onset inspiratory, early expiratory, early peak whole expiratory, and expiratory ramp. Overall, there are three phases (Figure 13.2).

- **Inspiration:** there is ramped (progressively increasing) activity of the inspiratory neurons (and muscles).
- **Early expiration:** there is a decrease and then a second peak in activity of the inspiratory neurons.
- **Late expiration:** inspiratory neurons are inactive. With increasing ventilatory effort, the normally quiescent expiratory neurons become progressively more active.

Apneustic centre

The apneustic centre is found in the lower pons. Its name is derived from the apneuses or inspiratory gasps that result from sectioning above this area. Its role in humans is unclear, although its activity is associated with the prolongation of the ramp inspiratory potentials of the dorsal respiratory group.

Pneumotaxic centre

The pneumotaxic centre is found within the upper pons. It turns off the inspiratory ramp, allowing the inspiratory group neurons to re-initiate activity immediately. This manifests as reduced tidal volume and increased respiratory rate. A normal respiratory ramp can exist following destruction of the pneumotaxic centre.

Other brain influences

Cerebral cortex

The cortex is able to coordinate breathing for speech and swallowing, and a limited amount of hyperventilation is also possible. Pain and anxiety increase respiratory rate, sometimes as an effort to reduce tidal volume and the discomfort associated with deep breathing.

Hypoventilation and breath-holding are quite different, and very difficult to control. Duration of breath-holding is influenced by PaO_2 and $PaCO_2$.

Limbic system and hypothalamus

Rage and fear influence the pattern of breathing.

Other receptors

The central control areas do not act in isolation, but receive input from a variety of other sources. Many of these are mechanoreceptors. They include:

- Nasal and pharyngeal receptors
- Stretch receptors in the lung
- Joint and muscle receptors
- Baroreceptors
- Temperature and pain receptors and pathways
- Chemoreceptors.

The nose and pharynx

Receptors here appear to respond to changes in rates of flow. However, they are more likely to be reacting to changes in the temperature of the gas in the upper airway.

Receptors in the pharynx sense swallowing, and are associated with the cessation of breathing. This reduces the risk of aspiration whilst eating.

The lung

The lung contains two types of myelinated receptor. These are categorized based on the speed of their response to changes in lung volume.

- *Slowly adapting stretch receptors (SARs)* are found among the smooth muscle cells of the airway wall, and fire at different rates according to lung volume. They may aid the termination of inspiration as tidal volume increases sharply.
- *Rapidly adapting stretch receptors (RARs)* are found in association with the epithelial cells of the larger airways, especially at the carina. They increase their firing in response to the rate of change in lung volume; once the lung volume becomes constant, they assume a basal rate of firing (Figure 13.3). They also respond to chemical stimuli, and were formerly known as irritant receptors because of their response to cigarette smoke. Cough, bronchospasm, and mucorrhoea occur in response to such stimulation.

C-fibre (unmyelinated) receptors detect various changes in the pulmonary circulation and interstitial space, and carry information to the brain in the vagus nerve. There are several types:

- *J receptors* are found in juxtaposition with the pulmonary capillaries and are activated in response to higher capillary pressures.
- *Other C-fibre receptors* arise within smaller bronchi, and respond to a range of stimuli including smoke, histamine, prostaglandins, and other inflammatory mediators.

Chest wall

Both muscle spindles and Golgi tendon organs (Section 8.3) monitor and report changes in lung volume. They are able to assess the muscle load and provide feedback about the work being performed by the muscle pump. In effect, this integrates intended with actual lung expansion.

Other receptors

Extreme hypotension stimulates an increased respiratory rate, an effect produced via baroreceptor input to the medullary centres. Reflex hypoventilation is produced by hypertension.

Impulses from moving limbs stimulate respiratory rate.

Heating of the skin increases ventilation.

Pain causes an initial period of apnoea, followed by hyperventilation.

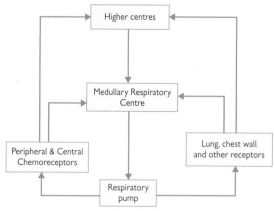

Fig. 13.1 Feedback loop of the medullary respiratory centre.

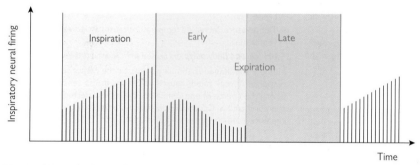

Fig. 13.2 The summed output from the various inspiratory groups. Activity increases rapidly during inspiration and is turned off by the action of inhibitory neurons. During early expiration there is a second burst of inspiratory neuron activity which is thought to cause a lengthening contraction, slowing the expiratory flow rate and allowing smooth breathing.

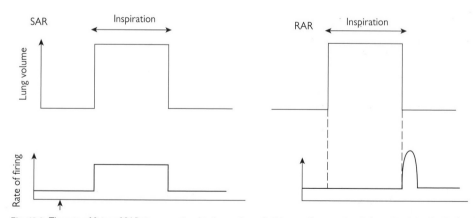

Fig. 13.3 The rate of firing of SARs is proportional to lung volume. In this way, the receptors help to signal that inspiration should cease. The rate of firing of RARs changes with rapid rates of change in lung volume during expiration. This signals that the next breath may be delivered.

Chemoreceptors occur within both the central nervous system and the periphery, and have a key role in maintenance of respiratory homeostasis.

Central chemoreceptors

The central chemoreceptors are quite separate from the medullary respiratory centre previously described (Section 13.1). Nerves that respond to changes in $PaCO_2$ are found on the ventral surface of the medulla (near the exit of the glossopharyngeal and vagus nerves), and on its dorsal surface.

Chemoreceptor cells are sensitive to their immediate milieu, the ECF. ECF composition is governed by CSF, local blood flow, and metabolism. The BBB is relatively impermeable to protons, but CO_2 will diffuse across it freely. On entering the CSF, CO_2 dissociates and ultimately liberates H^+. It is these CO_2-derived protons which influence the central chemoceptors: increased H^+ concentration increases ventilation (Figure 13.4).

Respiratory acidaemia

Normal CSF pH is 7.32, but because it contains relatively little protein buffer, any increase in CO_2 produces a proportionally greater pH change in the CSF than in the blood.

In order to compensate for prolonged hypercapnia, the kidneys regenerate bicarbonate; eventually the concentration of bicarbonate in the CSF also rises. This buffers the increased CSF CO_2, blunting its effect on respiratory drive.

Metabolic acidaemia

Although the central chemoreceptors respond to changes in proton concentration, *in vivo* they have little role in the response to metabolic acidaemia. Protons are slow to diffuse across the BBB and act centrally, whereas they produce a swift response at peripheral chemocreceptors.

Peripheral chemoreceptors

Peripheral chemoreceptors respond to both oxygen and carbon dioxide pressure. They also respond to temperature and pH.

Both the carotid and aortic bodies contain chemoreceptors, although in humans, only the carotid bodies seem to respond to oxygen tension. The two structures are similar anatomically: they possess dense capillary networks and command a high blood flow for their size. Although their metabolic rate is very high, the arteriovenous oxygen difference is small; they are sensitive to changes in arterial rather than venous oxygen pressure. In this way, they are able to sense and respond to whole-body oxygen requirements. Varying oxygen content (by varying Hb concentration), as opposed to partial pressure, does not affect their response.

The carotid and aortic bodies are composed of two cell types.

- *Type 1 (glomus cells)* contain large amounts of dopamine and other neurotransmitters. They are intimately positioned close to nerve endings (the carotid sinus nerve supplies the carotid bodies, and the vagus nerve supplies the aortic bodies).
- *Type 2 (sustentacular cells)* resemble glia, and form supporting structures.

Mechanism of action

The peripheral chemoreceptors are electrically excitable: stimulation blocks potassium currents and causes membrane depolarization. Voltage-gated Ca^{2+} channels open, and the influx of calcium provokes exocytosis of neurotransmitters from storage vesicles. These substances (acetyl choline, noradrenaline, dopamine, substance P, and met-enkephalin) stimulate the nerve endings to produce action potentials.

Peripheral chemoreceptors respond to the following.

- *Hypoxia:* only peripheral sites detect hypoxaemia. Bilateral carotid surgery has been shown to abolish hypoxic ventilatory drive. The response to PaO_2 is non-linear, and although firing starts at a PaO_2 of 67kPa, it dramatically increases below 7.5kPa (Figure 13.7). The mechanism of detection of PaO_2 is not well understood.
- *Carbon dioxide:* when CO_2 diffuses into the cell and liberates protons it changes intracellular pH. The protons alter potassium currents, causing opening of the voltage-gated channels. Although they produce a smaller response to hypercarbia than the central chemoreceptors, they are quicker to respond. The combined central-peripheral response to carbon dioxide is illustrated in Figure 13.6.
- *Temperature:* increased temperature causes an increase in ventilation.
- *pH (carotid body only):* decreased pH causes increased ventilation.

Multiple simultaneous stimuli potentiate the response. The rate of response is very rapid; natural variations in gas tension occurring during the course of one ventilatory cycle are detected by peripheral chemoreceptors. Central conduction and processing of the peripheral chemoreceptor response is illustrated in Figure 13.5.

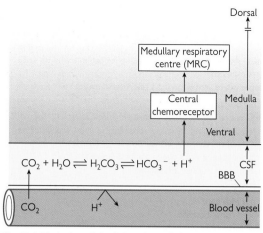

Fig. 13.4 Mechanism of stimulation of central chemoreceptors.

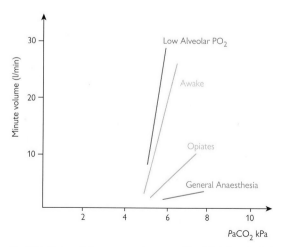

Fig. 13.5 Peripheral chemoreceptors and their pathways of conduction to the medullary respiratory centre.

NTS nucleus tractus solitarius
NA   nucleus ambiguus
MRC medullary respiratory centre

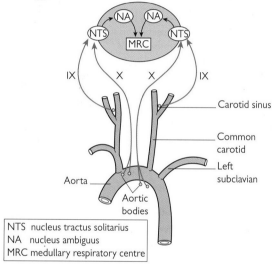

Fig. 13.6 The ventilatory response to oxygen. Blood $PaCO_2$ varies by less than 0.5kPa/day and is the most important factor controlling ventilation. For each 0.13kPa rise in $PaCO_2$, ventilation will increase by 2–5L/min.

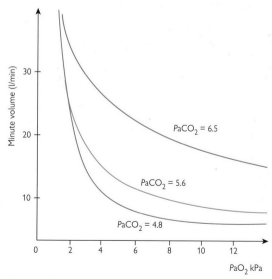

Fig. 13.7 The ventilatory response to O_2. This is purely peripherally driven, since hypoxia will itself depress the medulla. The ventilatory response is amplified by hypercarbia.

Obstructive sleep apnoea

Definition

Obstructive sleep apnoea–hypopnoea syndrome (OSAHS) is defined as the coexistence of excessive daytime sleepiness with irregular breathing at night. It occurs because the upper airway collapses intermittently during sleep. Airway collapse can be:

- Complete, with total obstruction of the lumen and no respiratory airflow for more than 10sec (apnoea), or
- Partial, with reduction in the cross-sectional area of the upper airway lumen, causing hypoventilation by more than 50% of baseline (hypopnoea).

Clinical features

- Excessive daytime sleepiness
- Impaired concentration
- Irritability/personality change
- Decreased libido
- Snoring
- Unrefreshing restless sleep
- Choking episodes during sleep
- Witnessed apnoeas
- Nocturia

Predisposing factors include male sex, age, obesity, and sedating drugs. There is a prevalence of 1–2% in middle-aged males, many of whom remain undiagnosed.

Diagnosis

The diagnosis is made when the sleep study demonstrates periods of apnoea with associated physiological disturbance. This investigation involves measurement of oximetry, heart rate, airflow, and chest wall movement (Figure 13.8).

Management

Weight loss is crucial, and can be curative. Nasal CPAP at night is a very effective therapy for reducing daytime somnolence.

Sleep nasendoscopy helps to determine whether surgery (palatoplasty) will be useful. Mandibular advancement splints can be used in milder cases, but are much less effective.

Clinical implications

- Patients with untreated sleep apnoea are at risk of suffering fatal vehicle accidents and have increased risk of cardiovascular complications, including pulmonary hypertension, and death.
- Because of their physiognomy, many patients with sleep apnoea are difficult to intubate.
- Many have coexistent obesity-related hypoventilation (Pickwickian syndrome), with type 2 respiratory failure.
- OSA patients are at greater risk of opioid-induced respiratory depression and may require postoperative care in a HDU where facilities for NIV or CPAP are available.

Central hypoventilation syndrome

In some patients, hypoventilation and apnoea occur during non-REM sleep, despite relatively normal ventilatory responses in the wakeful state. This is known as central hypoventilation syndrome, or Ondine's curse*. This is thought to be due to brainstem abnormalities leading to failure of chemoreceptor input.

Non-invasive ventilatory support

Indications (BTS Guidelines 2002)

Non-invasive ventilation (NIV) can be used in hospital given the following minimum facilities:

- A consultant committed to developing an NIV service
- Nurses on a respiratory ward, HDU, or ICU who are trained in NIV techniques
- An ICU that is able to provide back-up for patients who do not improve on NIV
- A non-invasive ventilator and a selection of masks.

NIV is particularly indicated in:

- COPD with a respiratory acidaemia pH 7.25–7.35 (H+ 45–56nmol/L).
- Hypercapnic respiratory failure secondary to chest wall deformity (scoliosis, thoracoplasty) or neuromuscular diseases.
- Cardiogenic pulmonary oedema unresponsive to CPAP.
- Weaning from tracheal intubation.
- Decompensated OHAHS

NIV is not indicated in:

- Impaired consciousness.
- Severe hypoxaemia.
- Patients with copious respiratory secretions.

These patients require intubation and ventilation.

The benefits of an acute NIV service

It is probable that fewer patients will be referred to ICU for intubation and ventilation, with concomitant shorter stays.

Absolute contraindications to NIV

- Facial trauma/burns.
- Recent facial, upper airway, or upper GI tract surgery.
- Fixed obstruction of the upper airway.
- Vomiting.

Relative contraindications

- Inability to protect airway
- Haemodynamic instability
- Severe comorbidity
- Confusion/agitation.
- Bowel obstruction
- Focal consolidation on chest radiograph
- Undrained pneumothorax

NIV can be used to avoid invasive ventilation, despite the presence of these relative contraindications, if it is to be the 'ceiling' of treatment or if treatments are to be limited.

When to use non-invasive ventilation

There should be potential for recovery to a quality of life acceptable to the patient. Treatment should be in accordance with the patient's wishes.

Clinical state

The patient should be able to protect their airway. They should be conscious, cooperative, and haemodynamically stable with few comorbidities and respiratory secretions. NIV is not appropriate for patients who appear moribund.

Blood gases

NIV is appropriate in cases of respiratory acidaemia ($PaCO_2$ >6.0 kPa, pH <7.35) that persists despite maximum medical treatment and appropriate controlled oxygen therapy. Patients with pH <7.25 respond less well and should be managed in an HDU/ICU, where more advanced modes of ventilation are available.

Patients with a high A–a oxygen gradient (i.e. severe life-threatening hypoxaemia) may be more appropriately managed by tracheal intubation and ventilation.

---

*Legend tells of Ondine, a water nymph, who cursed her husband after finding him asleep in the arms of another woman. As he had pledged his love to her 'with every waking breath', he would breathe only while awake; sleep would mean certain death.

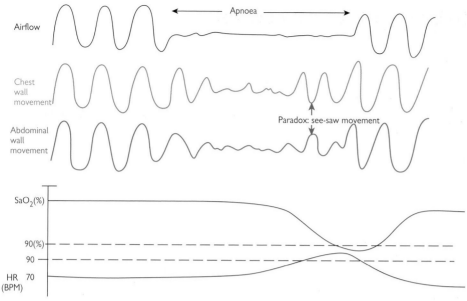

Fig. 13.8 Sleep study demonstrating apnoea due to obstruction. Chest wall and abdominal wall efforts continue during the period of apnoea, eventually becoming paradoxical. Such efforts resolve after a period of arousal, as would be seen on the subject's EEG (not shown).

339

➔ Oxygen sensitivity in type 2 respiratory failure

When additional oxygen is administered to some patients with COPD or kyphoscoliosis, their $PaCO_2$ rises and there is a danger that they will become apnoeic. This is said to be evidence that they rely on hypoxia for the maintenance of respiratory drive. This is at best a curious statement.

The explanation often given is that with hypercarbia there is renal bicarbonate generation. CSF bicarbonate also subsequently rises, and it is this that blunts respiratory response to carbon dioxide. However, this does not explain why a further rise in $PaCO_2$ would not once again stimulate ventilation. A more likely explanation is that chronic hypercarbia alters the response of the central control mechanism in some other way: the body accepts that the energy cost of maintaining a normal $PaCO_2$ is too high.

Administration of oxygen will always increase the $PaCO_2$. There are three reasons.

- Administration of oxygen will reduce minute ventilation and this will increase $PaCO_2$. This is a small effect.
- The Haldane effect (Section 13.12) means that at higher PaO_2, less CO_2 will be carried by Hb, causing an increase in $PaCO_2$.
- Reversal of hypoxic pulmonary vasoconstriction as supplemental oxygen diffuses into poorly ventilated alveoli: more blood enters units that remain poorly ventilated and so $PaCO_2$ must rise.

By increasing the $PaCO2$, the administration of oxygen and increase in $PaO2$ may not actually reduce minute ventilation. However, if the rise in $PaCO2$ is high enough, it can produce CNS depression in its own right.

Clinical recommendations
- ALL patients need enough oxygen, and this will vary with both the individual and the disease process.
- Simple exacerbations of COPD are likely to be controlled with small increases in FiO_2
- More significant exacerbations (e.g. pneumonia) will need more oxygen. Start with enough to ensure SaO_2 >90%, and reduce the FiO_2 to the lowest level that maintains this.
- Patients with documented oxygen sensitivity should be highlighted with an alert system

➔ Chronic oxygen therapy

Oxygen is used to relieve dyspnoea and/or improve prognosis. The use of long-term oxygen therapy (LTOT) has been shown to extend survival in patients with chronic hypoxaemia due to COPD, pulmonary fibrosis, and congestive cardiac failure. Patients are advised to use oxygen for at least 16hr/day. Supply is via an oxygen concentrator, with cylinders for back-up.

Indications
- PaO_2 <7.3kPa in the stable state measured on two occasions
- PaO_2 <8.0kPa in the stable state measured on two separate occasions with pulmonary hypertension or cor pulmonale

Other indications for home oxygen therapy
- Nocturnal oxygen for documented nocturnal desaturation despite normal daytime blood gases (e.g. COPD, obesity)
- Palliative, for relief of dyspnoea in malignancy or end-stage organ failure
- Ambulatory oxygen therapy with small portable cylinders for documented desaturation with exercise

Short-burst oxygen via cylinder for relief of dyspnoea in patients without chronic hypoxaemia should be avoided, as there is poor evidence of efficacy.

➔ Classification of respiratory failure

Type 1 respiratory failure
PaO_2 <8kPa $PaCO_2$ normal or low

Type 2 respiratory failure
PaO_2 <8kPa $PaCO_2$ >6.7kPa

➔ Features of Pickwickian syndrome

Type II respiratory failure and alveolar hypoventilation secondary to obesity. Features of breathlessness, somnolence, and headache.

Therapy
Lose weight, oxygen as required, NIV.

The human respiratory system provides not only the mechanisms of gas exchange, but also important homeostatic, endocrine, and immune functions. Diseases of the respiratory system are common, and may impact greatly on an individual's health or ability to tolerate medical interventions.

The branching structure of the airways ideally suits them to distributing air throughout the lungs, warming and moistening the air, and removing inhaled particulates and pathogens. It is an efficient system: a 2cm water pressure gradient is enough to produce a gas flow rate of 1L/sec.

Functional anatomy of the lung

The trachea divides into progressively smaller generations, 23 in all. Two distinct zones are identifiable.

- **The conducting zone** This comprises airways without alveoli and extends to the terminal bronchioles of the 16th generation. Cartilage is absent from the 11th generation onwards and at this point, lung volume determines the calibre of the airway (Figure 13.10). As the conducting airways do not participate in gas exchange, this region creates an anatomical dead space of around 150ml in a normal adult.

- **The respiratory zone** Alveoli begin to appear in the 17th generation, the respiratory bronchioles. The alveolar ducts at division 20 give rise to the alveolar sacs of terminal division 23. Alveolar histology is shown in Fig. 13.9. The majority of lung volume resides here (approximately 3L). It is the site of gas exchange. The distance from the terminal bronchiole to the most distal alveolus is small (only a few millimetres).

During inspiration, air is drawn down to the terminal bronchioles. Beyond this point, bulk flow gives way to diffusion, with very small rates of forward gas flow. This is a function of the massive increase in the cross-sectional area of the airways beyond the terminal bronchioles. Because of the significant decrease in gas flow, this region is where particles tend to settle.

Dead space

There are different definitions of dead space. For the clinical implications, see Section 13.15.

Anatomical dead space

This is the volume of gas that is contained within the conducting airways without any possibility of performing gas exchange. It amounts to approximately 150ml per tidal breath.

Anatomical dead space is not completely fixed, but depends on a number of other factors.

- **Ventilatory rate** For a set minute volume, a high respiratory rate with small tidal volumes will give a higher proportion of dead space than the same minute volume delivered in fewer larger tidal volumes.
- **Very large tidal volumes** will also increase dead space because of the pull on bronchi by the surrounding lung tissue which increases their internal volume.
- **Posture.** On head-down positioning, the pressure of the abdominal contents will compress the conducting airways, reducing dead space.

The volume of the anatomical dead space can be measured by Fowler's method (Figure 13.12). This measures the volume of the conducting airways to the interface between inspired gas and that gas remaining in the lungs.

Physiological dead space

The alveolar dead space is that volume of alveoli that are ventilated but not perfused. These alveoli do not take part in gas exchange. The sum of anatomical and alveolar dead space is termed the physiological dead space. It is approximately 170ml in an adult male.

Anatomical dead space + alveolar dead space = physiological dead space

Bohr's method (see opposite) estimates the physiological dead space, determining the volume of lung that does not excrete CO_2.

In health, the anatomical and the physiological dead-space values are 150ml and 170ml, respectively. However, with disease, the latter may increase considerably as V/Q mismatch becomes apparent.

Measurement of alveolar ventilation

Alveolar ventilation (V_A) can be summarized as equal to the total expired minute volume (V_E) minus the dead-space ventilation (V_D):

$$V_A = V_E - V_D.$$

No gas exchange occurs in dead space; only alveolar gas provides CO_2.

$$\dot{V}_{CO_2} = \dot{V}_A \times \frac{\%CO_2}{100}$$

$\dot{V}$ is volume per unit time

$\dot{V}_{CO_2}$ is volume of CO_2 produced per unit time

$\dot{V}_A$ is volume of alveolar gas exhaled per unit time.

$[\frac{\%CO_2}{100}]$ is the fractional concentratiion of CO_2, F_{CO_2}

$$\dot{V}_A = \frac{\dot{V}_{CO_2}}{F_{CO_2}}$$

Since partial pressure is proportional to fractional concentration (by Dalton's law of partial pressures):

$$PCO_2 = F_{CO_2} \times K \text{ (where k is a constant)}$$

Therefore,

$$\dot{V}_A = \frac{\dot{V}_{CO_2}}{PCO_2} \times K$$

From this relationship, we can see that $PaCO_2$ is inversely proportional to alveolar ventilation. $PaCO_2$ depends only on the rate of CO_2 production, $\dot{V}_{CO_2}$ (which may vary with exercise or basal metabolic rate), and alveolar ventilation, $\dot{V}_A$.

Non-respiratory functions of the lung

The lung has a number of important non-respiratory functions.

- **Host protection** The lungs have a surface area of almost 100m²; this is a large interface with the environment, which demands protection. The nose filters larger pieces of debris. Clearance of smaller particles is performed by the mucociliary escalator; the beating cilia of epithelial cells move debris towards the larger airways, where it is subsequently coughed out. Mucus is secreted by goblet cells, which line the bronchioles. Within the alveoli, IgA provides an initial defence, and particles coated with these antibodies are ingested by macrophages.
- **Metabolic functions** These include inactivation of bradykinin, removal of proteases (e.g. removal of trypsin by α_1-antitrypsin), and conversion of angiotensin I to angiontensin II. 5-HT is taken up by lung tissue. Proteins and surfactant are synthesized by specialized pulmonary cells.
- **Blood reservoir** There is usually 450ml of blood in the lungs. This volume can be increased by recruitment and distension of pulmonary vessels. It can also be ejected to compensate for hypovolaemia, when the volume remaining in the pulmonary vasculature may be as little as 250ml.

Blood filtration

- **Heat regulation** The warming and humidification of gas by the large airways requires energy (latent heat of vaporization). This accounts for 12% of basal heat loss.
- **Speech** The lungs support the production of speech by generating airflow across the vocal cords.

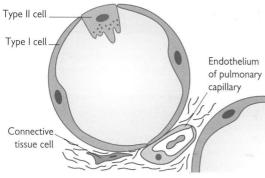

Type II cell

Type I cell

Connective tissue cell

Endothelium of pulmonary capillary

Fig. 13.9 Cells of the alveolus.

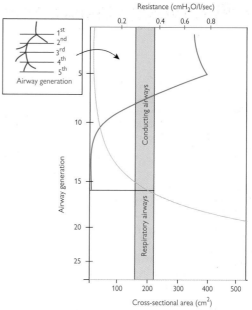

Fig. 13.10 Airway divisions and resistance. Most of the pressure drop occurs in the first seven airway divisions. The massive increase in airway numbers, and therefore the cross-sectional area, accounts for the small contribution of the peripheral airways to resistance. It also explains why a significant amount of small airways disease can be present before it becomes detectable.

341

Bohr equation and estimation of physiological dead space

All expired CO_2 comes from alveolar ventilation. P_ECO_2 is the PCO_2 of mixed expired gas. $PaCO_2$ is assumed to be identical to $PACO_2$. Fractional concentration (F) is proportional to partial pressure. P_ECO_2 is the partial pressure of CO_2 in mixed exhaled ges.

$$V_T \times F_E = V_A \times F_A$$

$$V_T = V_A + V_D$$

$$V_A = V_T - V_D$$

$$V_T \times F_E = (V_T - V_D) \times F_A$$

$$\frac{V_D}{V_T} = \frac{(F_A - F_E)}{F_A}$$

$$\frac{V_D}{V_T} = \frac{(PaCO_2 - P_ECO_2)}{PaCO_2}$$

See Section 13.15 for an explanation of how the Bohr equation and the shunt equation are related.

Fowler's method of estimating the anatomical dead space

This measures the volume of gas contained within the conducting bronchioles down to the midpoint of the transition to alveolar gas.

The subject inhales a single breath of 100% O_2, and exhales through a continuous nitrogen analyser. The graph below is obtained. The first portion of gas exhaled is that of the dead space; since it takes no part in gas exchange, it contains no nitrogen.

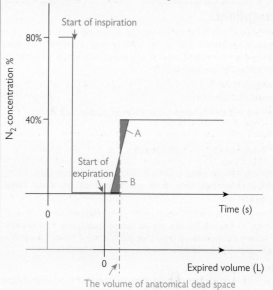

The volume of anatomical dead space

Fig. 13.11 When area A equals area B, the expired volume is an estimate of the anatomical dead space, the mid-point of the transition from conduction to gas exchange.

Ventilation

Alveolar gas exchange relies upon a pressure gradient of respiratory gases being maintained across the alveolar membrane. Constant ventilation of the alveoli is required to replace oxygen and remove CO_2. Creation of a pressure gradient between the alveoli and the proximal airway moves air in and out of the chest. Thoracic volume increases in all three planes and is an active process, whereas expiration is passive during quiet breathing.

In a healthy adult, tidal volumes of 500ml and a respiratory rate of 12 breaths/min generate a minute volume of 6L. The alveoli receive smaller tidal volumes since a proportion of air remains within the dead space, which does not contribute to gas exchange.

The inspiratory muscles

The phrenic nerve (C3,4,5) supplies the diaphragm, which descends 2cm during quiet and 10cm during forceful inspiration. This single muscle is responsible for 70% of the tidal volume. The external intercostals move the ribs, increasing both the anteroposterior and lateral diameters of the thoracic cage (Figure 13.12). The scalene muscles raise the rib cage along the AP axis (although the sternocleidomastoid performs the same task, it is only active during forced breathing).

The increased intrathoracic volume of inspiration reduces pleural pressure from −5 to −8cmH$_2$O (Figure 13.15).

The expiratory muscles

Expiration, although passive during tidal breathing, does require energy. It is driven by elastic recoil of the lung (70% due to surface tension, 30% due to elastic fibres). It is opposed by the chest wall, which has a tendency to expand.

Muscular activity accompanies this process only when respiratory effort is increased. The muscles of the abdominal wall increase intra-abdominal pressure, aiding elevation of the diaphragm. The internal intercostals move the ribs down and in, reducing intra-thoracic volume.

Compliance

Compliance is defined as the change in volume per unit change in pressure across the wall of the subject structure (the transmural pressure*). The compliance of the chest as a whole reflects the compliances of its components:

- lung compliance;
- chest wall compliance

The lung and chest wall compliances are in parallel, and so

$$\frac{1}{Compliance_{total}} = \frac{1}{Compliance_{chest\ wall}} + \frac{1}{Compliance_{lung}}$$

The lung and the chest wall compliance are about the same: 200ml/cmH$_2$O. Therefore total chest compliance will be about 100ml/cmH$_2$O.

Chest compliance increases with lung volume up to a point (Figure 13.14) and so the whole compliance curve is non-linear. However, convention dictates that compliance is reported between the FRC and 1L above FRC, and this part of the curve is straight.

Static lung compliance

This is measured from consecutive measurements of oesophageal pressure (which equates to intrapleural pressure) and mouth pressure

at a number of lung volumes throughout inspiration and expiration. With an open glottis and no gas flow, alveolar pressure equals mouth (i.e. atmospheric) pressure.

Muscular activity of the chest wall does not influence the measurement of lung compliance.

Dynamic compliance

Dynamic compliance differs in that the measurement is made during tidal breathing, with values taken at points of momentary cessation of gas flow (at the beginning and end of the breath).

Static compliance exceeds dynamic compliance: in the latter, a greater pressure gradient is required for the same change in volume because the resistive forces will need to be overcome quickly. This also explains why compliance is frequency dependent, with higher respiratory rates reducing dynamic compliance.

Specific compliance

Specific compliance (total compliance divided by FRC) removes the influence of lung size, allowing comparison of different sizes of patient. The typical value (0.05/cmH$_2$O) is the same for both adults and neonates.

Clinical considerations

Lung compliance

Reduced lung compliance occurs with loss of connective tissue elasticity and alveolar surface tension, and is found in interstitial lung disease, pulmonary oedema, and pleural thickening. Increased lung compliance, indicating loss of elastic recoil, is seen with increasing age, especially in emphysema (Figure 13.16). However, at larger lung volumes, gas trapping reduces compliance and increases the work of breathing.

Chest wall compliance

Just as in the lungs, chest wall compliance is influenced by disease, posture, and position. Ossification of the costal cartilages, scars resulting from burns of the chest, and severe spinal deformities reduce compliance. The diaphragm passively transmits intra-abdominal pressure (increased in obesity and pregnancy). With postural changes, this mechanism reduces total static compliance by up to 60%.

Alteration of lung or chest wall compliance alters work of breathing.

Total compliance

This depends on factors that affect the chest wall and lung, including the phase of ventilation.

Application of lung compliance measurement

In practice, although compliance can be measured in awake non-ventilated subjects, it has little clinical application. In ventilated patients, both static and dynamic measurements of compliance guide the use of PEEP (Section 22.4).

Differences between base and apex

The pressure–volume relationship is sigmoid (Figure 13.14), and this explains the marked variation in ventilation between base and apex. At FRC in the erect position, the weight of the lung in the thorax gives rise to a less negative pressure at the base than the apex.

- The base is subject to less negative intrapleural pressure. The lung is relatively compressed, but it is also able to expand significantly with inspiration since it lies on the steep part of the pressure–volume curve: it has greater compliance.
- The apex is subject to a more negative intrapleural pressure. Although it is held more open at rest, it is on a flatter part of the pressure–volume curve, and so does not ventilate as well as the base.

During forced expiration (with lung volumes below FRC) there are further differences in compliance. Now, intrapleural pressure around the base is higher than atmospheric pressure and is sufficient to cause basal alveoli to close. Apical lung remains patent, and so is now relatively better ventilated.

---

*Transmural pressure is the difference in pressure across the wall of any object. It is denoted as positive if it tends to distend the object. Because there is no reliable method of estimating alveolar pressure, transpulmonary pressure is preferred (Figure 13.13).

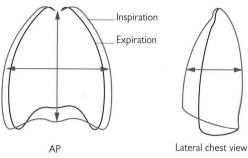

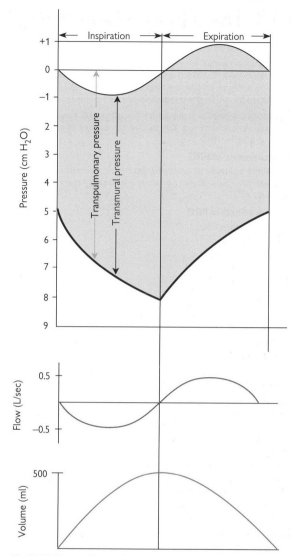

Fig. 13.12 Chest volume. The action of respiratory muscles leading to increased AP, vertical, and coronal diameters and therefore greater chest volume.

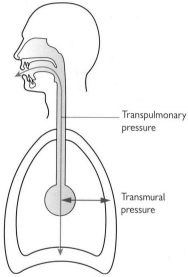

Fig. 13.13 Transmural pressure.

Fig. 13.15 Pressure, flow, and volume curves.
Transmural pressure = alveolar pressure − intrapleural pressure.
Transpulmonary pressure = mouth pressure − intrapleural pressure.
Mouth pressure is atmospheric and taken as zero.

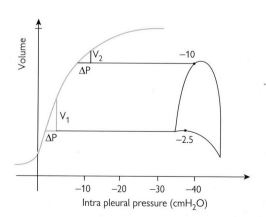

Fig. 13.14 Differences in compliance between the base and apex. For a given change in pressure (ΔP) the change in volume at the base (V_1) is much greater than the change in volume at the apex (V_2). The curve flattens at the top, demonstrating the reduction in compliance at maximal lung volume.

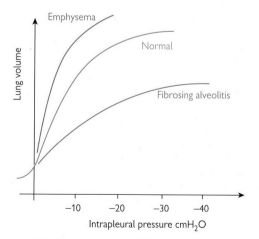

Fig. 13.16 Compliance curves of different conditions. Emphysema: increased compliance with larger TLC. Fibrosing alveolitis: reduced compliance and TLC but greater intrapleural pressures.

13.6 Functional residual capacity

The functional residual capacity (FRC) is the point at end-expiration where the forces acting to spring the chest wall outwards are balanced by the forces acting to collapse the lungs inwards (Figure 13.17 and 13.18). It is affected by various physical, pathological, and therapeutic factors.

Less compliant lungs (e.g. pulmonary fibrosis) result in a lower FRC. Increased distensibility (e.g. due to alveolar damage in emphysema) results in a higher FRC.

Measurement of FRC

FRC cannot be measured directly by spirometry, and must be calculated using either helium dilution or body plethysmography techniques (Section 1.4).

Factors affecting FRC

Factors increasing FRC

- ↑ Height of patient
- Erect posture
- ↓ Lung elastic recoil

Factors decreasing FRC

- Obesity
- Pregnancy
- Supine position
- ↑ Elastic recoil of the lungs (e.g. pulmonary fibrosis)
- Pregnancy
- Anaesthesia

From the diagram of lung volumes (Section 1.4) it can be seen that

$$FRC = ERV + RV.$$

In healthy children and adults FRC is approximately 30ml/kg in the supine position. It does not decrease with age, unless other pathologies develop.

Physiological features of the FRC

- The FRC allows oxygen storage. The store buffers the intermittent delivery of oxygen to the lungs during normal breathing, and maintains a steady P_AO_2 during tidal ventilation. The store of oxygen is enhanced with pre-oxygenation.
- The FRC prevents airway collapse and atelectasis by keeping the lungs partially inflated at all times. The closing volume encroaches progressively upon the expiratory reserve volume (ERV) with age, and may eventually be reached during normal tidal ventilation.
- Pulmonary vascular resistance is minimized at FRC.
- Airways resistances are kept low when airways are kept open.
- Compared with extremes of lung volume, at FRC the lungs have increased compliance and low resistance, and so work of breathing (WOB) is reduced.

Surface tension

A molecule in the middle of a liquid is subject to forces of attraction in all directions from the molecules surrounding it. Because of the symmetry of these forces, there is no resulting molecular movement.

A molecule on the surface of a liquid is subject to similar forces in all directions apart from the air–fluid interface where the intermolecular forces are weaker. The net forces direct the surface molecule towards the centre of the fluid and the surface contracts (Figure 13.19). The strength of this contraction is the surface tension, defined as:

- The force with which a surface contracts per unit length of surface (units, dyn/cm^2).

The result of these forces is that the fluid will reduce its surface area to a minimum. A fluid will assume the shape of a sphere under the conditions of zero gravity.

Surfactant

The air–liquid interface at the alveolus generates surface tension which impacts upon lung compliance and hence WOB. It is estimated that this surface tension is responsible for 70% of the elastic recoil of the lung.

Type II pneumocytes produce both surfactant and the type I cells that line the alveoli. The surface tension of alveoli is reduced by the presence of pulmonary surfactant. This is composed of (by volume):

- 80% dipalmitoyl phosphatidyl choline. This is amphipathic: the hydrophilic choline head and the hydrophobic palmitoyl tail orientate the molecule within the alveolus.
- 10% neutral lipid.
- 4% plasma proteins.
- 2% carbohydrate.
- 4% surfactant protein (SP) subunits A–D. These molecules have hydrophobic and hydrophilic poles. They align on the alveolar surface, reducing the force of attraction between adjacent water molecules. The effects are proportional to the concentration of surfactant and so are greater in alveoli of small radius. This is beneficial in counteracting the high pressures found in small alveoli, a problem predicted by Laplace's law (Section 10.7). SP-B and SP-C are hydrophobic, and are responsible for the spread of surfactant. SP-A and SP-D are hydrophilic and regulate surfactant turnover and composition and entry of plasma proteins into the alveolar fluid.

Surfactant molecules move between the alveolus and type II pneumocytes with the phase of ventilation. During inspiration, molecules of surfactant are drawn from their cells, or sub-alveolar fluid layer micelles, into the fluid lining the alveolus. During deflation, some of the molecules are degraded but others are extruded to form collections of micelles beneath the alveolar fluid layer. These micelles are available for use during the next inhalation. The density of surfactant is constant during the second half of exhalation.

Regular deep breaths are required to distribute surfactant uniformly throughout the lung. In patients who cannot inhale deeply, inadequate surfactant function can result in atelectasis and increased WOB. Surfactant also reduces the tendency to form pulmonary oedema; otherwise alveolar surface tension would tend to draw fluid from the capillary.

Neonates born prematurely may develop infant respiratory distress syndrome. Here the lack of pulmonary surfactant and immature lungs results in the development of atelectasis and pulmonary oedema.

Hysteresis

As can be seen from Figure 13.20, the pressure–volume curves for inflation and deflation of an air-filled lung are different. This is known as hysteresis, and is mainly due to changes in surface tension within the alveoli during the ventilatory cycle.

Inflation

The flat initial part of the inflation curve demonstrates low compliance because surface tension is high. As surfactant is recruited into the alveolar lining, surface tension reduces and compliance increases, and the gradient becomes steeper. At high lung volumes, surfactant density is unchanged and the major determinant of lung compliance is tissue elasticity. The lung is stretched and its compliance is reduced.

Exhalation

The density of surfactant rapidly increases and reduces surface tension. The initial portion of the curve is flat. During mid-exhalation the compliance is constant because some surfactant is extruded and so its density remains the same. At lower lung volumes, surfactant density is higher than during inspiration.

Minor influences on hysteresis

- Recruitment of collapsed alveoli: this contributes to the flat lower part of the inspiratory curve.
- Stress relaxation: elastic recoil diminishes when larger lung volumes are sustained. It plays a very small part in the flat upper part of the deflation curve.

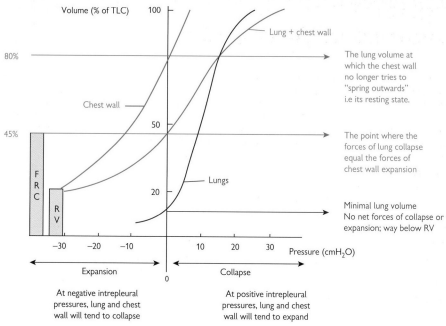

Fig. 13.17 The relaxation pressure–volume curves for chest wall and lung. Static measurements made with a spirometer.

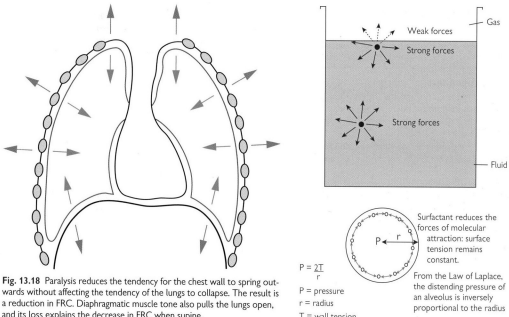

Fig. 13.18 Paralysis reduces the tendency for the chest wall to spring outwards without affecting the tendency of the lungs to collapse. The result is a reduction in FRC. Diaphragmatic muscle tone also pulls the lungs open, and its loss explains the decrease in FRC when supine.

$P = \dfrac{2T}{r}$

P = pressure
r = radius
T = wall tension

Surfactant reduces the forces of molecular attraction: surface tension remains constant.

From the Law of Laplace, the distending pressure of an alveolus is inversely proportional to the radius

Fig. 13.19 The effects of surface tension.

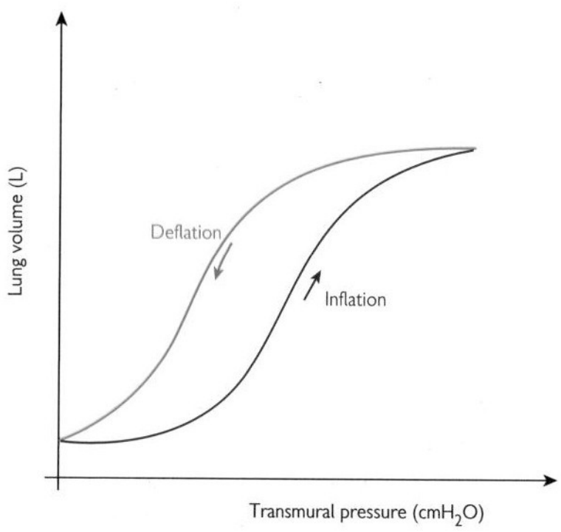

Fig. 13.20 Hysteresis. Higher expanding pressures are required to maintain lung volume during inspiration when compared with expiration. The delay in movement of surfactant from deeper layers during inspiration accounts for the reduced compliance of inflation. Surfactant has a greater effect during expiration than inspiration.

13.7 Closing capacity

Closing capacity (CC) is the volume of the lung when small airways begin to collapse during expiration. It is the sum of the residual volume (RV) and the closing volume (CV):

$$CC = RV + CV$$

In health, closing capacity is significantly less than the FRC and approximates to the residual volume. If closing volume encroaches further into the ERV or even the FRC, airway closure may eventually occur during normal expiration. This prevents ventilation of areas distal to the closure, worsening the ventilation/perfusion relationship (V/Q).

Closing volume slowly increases with age, smoking, and lung disease. Lung elasticity is lost, reducing the radial traction forces that maintain airway patency. The impact of airway closure is one of the main causes of a progressive fall in PaO_2 with advancing age.

In the supine position, closing capacity exceeds FRC by the mid-forties, and in the erect position by age 60 years. The reduced FRC seen during general anaesthesia may fall below closing capacity, so even young patients may have an increased V/Q mismatch.

The lungs are subject to the effects of gravity, and the pleural pressure is less negative at the base. This less negative pressure is transmitted to the alveoli, reducing basal lung volume. This explains why the dependent areas close first. Closed airways shift down to the flat part of the pressure–volume curve. A larger pressure must be generated to move a small amount of air.

 Airway closure above residual volume increases the work of breathing.

The single-breath nitrogen test

This is a test that determines the closing volume (Figure 13.21). 100% O_2 is inspired from residual volume to TLC. This volume is slowly exhaled and the N_2 content measured with a rapid N_2 analyser and plotted against lung volume.

- With inspiration from RV, the upper alveoli initially expand and receive the dead-space gas that contains a high N_2 (i.e. air) concentration.
- These apical alveoli are larger and expand less than basal alveoli during inspiration of the vital capacity breath.
- Basal units expand later and relatively more, drawing in a higher concentration of oxygen.
- With exhalation, N_2 concentration plateaus at a low concentration as the alveoli are emptied.
- As basal units close, the proportion of apical units emptying increases and the N_2 content rises. The lung volume at which this occurs is the CV.

Time constants

The time constant tau (τ) expresses how quickly a lung compartment can react to an alteration of pressure and gives an indication of its filling or emptying velocity. It is a measure of how well alveoli fill and empty. Filling a lung unit will be 95% complete after three time constants. For normal lung, with a time constant of 0.2sec, this takes 0.6sec (Figure 13.22).

The lung consists of a large number of compartments with variable time constants. This heterogeneity is often exaggerated with lung disease (e.g. pneumonia, pulmonary fibrosis). The more non-homogeneous the lung ventilation, the wider the variation in regional time constants. This causes variation in the filling and emptying periods, and the filling volumes, for individual compartments.

The time constant of a lung compartment is a function of its resistance and compliance. At a given pressure, a compartment with high resistance and good compliance fills slowly with a resulting large volume (e.g. asthma). Conversely, a compartment with poor compliance and low resistance fills quickly, but with a smaller volume (e.g. pulmonary fibrosis).

In a lung whose different units have varying time constants, dynamic compliance is frequency dependent. It decreases as frequency increases.

Work of breathing

Work of breathing (WOB) is the work required to move the chest wall and lungs during inspiration and expiration. In this context, it is most convenient to measure work as the product of pressure and volume. This can be explained by considering the dynamic pressure–volume relationship in quiet inspiration and quiet expiration (Figure 13.23). In spontaneous respiration, the WOB involves the work necessary to overcome:

- The elastic forces of surface tension and the elasticity of the lung tissue. This is stored as potential energy during inspiration.
- Non-elastic forces or the flow resistance of the airways. This is dissipated as heat.

Clinical implications

In health at rest, the normal oxygen consumption of the muscles of respiration is 3ml/min (or 0.5ml/min/L minute volume). This increases with increased respiratory effort (both rate and tidal volume) and disease.

In obstructive ventilatory disorders, more work is needed to overome flow resistance, particularly if positive intrapleural pressures are generated in expiration. In restrictive disorders, more elastic respiratory work is required during inspiration.

In the ICU, respiratory work is increased in intubated patients because of the increased flow resistance of the tracheal tube and ventilator tubing.

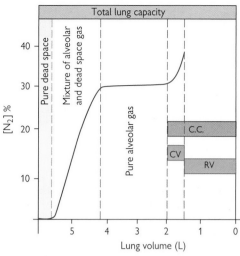

Fig. 13.21 Closing volume: the single-breath nitrogen test.

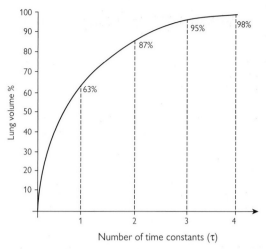

Fig. 13.22 Time constants: 95% of a lung will fill within three time constants (usually 0.6sec). This is a simple exponential process.

→ **Work of breathing**

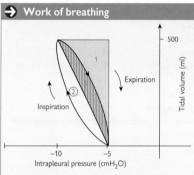

Fig. 13.23 Work performed during ventilation.

Work done from FRC: tidal volume 500ml and intrapleural pressure −5cmH$_2$O.

Elastin fibres are stored in the alveoli and lung tissue. Surface tension is responsible for 70% of the elastic recoil of the lung.

Area 1: potential energy stored in elastic tissues during inspiration.

Area 2: work versus frictional forces of inspiration.

Area 3: work versus frictional forces of expiration.

With tidal breathing in health, stored elastic energy accounts for passive exhalation, i.e. area 1 > area 3.

Tachypnoea or increased airway resistance increases areas 2 and 3.

In these cases, stored elastic energy might be insufficient, necessitating use of the muscles of exhalation, i.e. area 3 > area 1.

It is natural to deduce from Poiseuille's law (Section 2.7) that the chief site of resistance in the bronchial tree must be the smallest airways. In fact, direct measurement confirms that the major culprits are the medium-sized bronchioles proximal to the seventh generation. The distal airways dramatically increase in number and so the cross sectional area also increases enormously. This reduces their effect on resistance to less than 20% of the total.

Small peripheral airways are difficult to assess clinically; significant disease progression can occur before it becomes apparent.

Factors affecting resistance

- Lung volume: as the lung expands, radial traction opens the airways and resistance falls. This is shown graphically below: the relationship is hyperbolic (note that conductance is the reciprocal of resistance).
- Bronchial smooth muscle.
- Properties of the inspired gas.

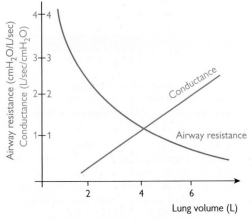

Fig. 13.24 Work performed during ventilation.

Asthma

Definition

Asthma is a chronic inflammatory disorder of the airways. It is characterized by:

- Widespread but variable airflow obstruction (which is reversible spontaneously or with treatment
- An increased airway response to a variety of stimuli.

Pathology

There is infiltration of the bronchial epithelium and submucosa with eosinophils, T lymphocytes, and mast cells. There is also epithelial disruption, mucus gland hypersecretion and thickening of the basement membrane. Acute attacks involve airway oedema and mucous plugging.

Clinical features

A typical history is of wheeze, dyspnoea, and/or cough. The symptoms are intermittent, worse at night, and provoked by triggers. Diagnosis depends upon documenting the presence of polyphonic wheeze or variable airways obstruction by spirometry or PEFR, with exclusion of other causes of airways obstruction.

Asthma phenotypes

- Infantile post-viral wheeze
- Classical atopic asthma
- Aspirin-sensitive asthma (with nasal polyps, forms Samter's triad)
- Occupational asthma
- Exercise-induced asthma
- Adult-onset non-atopic asthma
- Asthma-plus syndromes (allergic bronchopulmonary aspergillosis, Churg–Strauss syndrome)

Lung function tests

See Section 1.4.

Practical points

Most asthmatics are well controlled with modern inhaled therapies, and few are locked into the cycle of repeated acute admissions. The key to effective management is education about compliance and inhaler technique, regular inhaled steroids, and avoidance of trigger factors, including smoking. The British Thoracic Society's guidelines for the management of acute severe asthma in adults are shown opposite.

Risk factors for poor outcomes (hospitalization, ICU admission, death) include disease severity, poor compliance, psychosocial problems, and inadequate initial treatment.

General anaesthesia poses few problems for most asthmatics, provided that their asthma is well controlled with a stable prescription regime. It is worth noting preoperatively whether the asthmatic patient is able to take NSAIDs. This class of drugs should be used with caution but are NOT contraindicated in asthma. Only one in five asthmatics displays NSAID sensitivity.

CHAPTER 13 Respiration

349

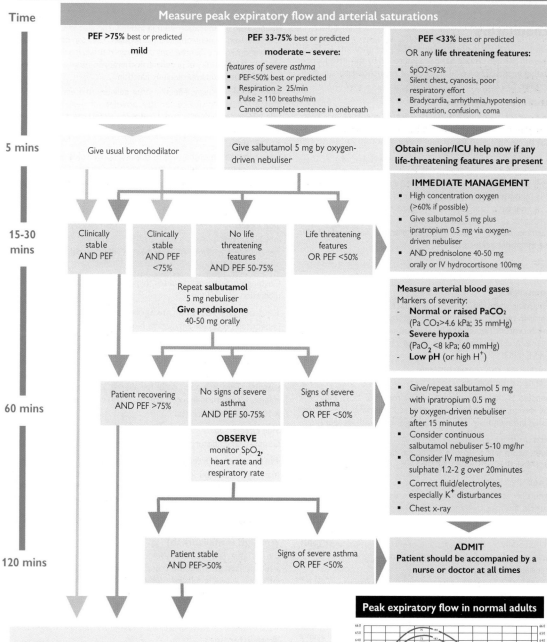

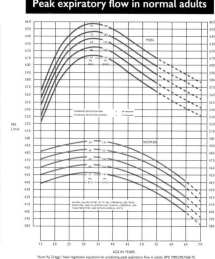

Fig. 13.25 British Thoracic Society Asthma Guidelines. (Reproduced with permission).

Bronchodilators

Bronchodilators are used in obstructive disorders (e.g. asthma, COPD). Effectiveness in chronic disease has been improved by the introduction of long-acting agents. The cellular action of bronchodilators is illustrated in Figure 13.27.

β₂-adrenoreceptor agonists

Circulating catecholamines act on β_2-adrenoreceptors in airway smooth muscle to cause bronchodilation. This effect is mirrored by inhaled β_2 agonists, and these agents are indicated for acute and chronic management of asthma and COPD.

- Short-acting, e.g. salbutamol, terbutaline
- Long-acting e.g. salmeterol, formoterol

Delivery is by metered dose inhaler, which is particularly effective if used with a volumatic (spacer) device (Figure 13.26). Nebulized delivery allows higher doses in acute situations. IV salbutamol can be used in acute asthma, although there is no clear evidence for benefit, and it may cause metabolic acidosis.

Side effects

Tachycardia, tremor, cramps, hypokalaemia.

Anticholinergics

Parasympathetic vagal fibres provide bronchoconstrictor tone for airway smooth muscle. Anticholinergic muscarinic antagonists block muscarinic receptors, notably the M_3 subtype, causing bronchodilation. These agents are indicated for acute and chronic management of asthma and COPD.

- Short-acting, e.g. ipratropium bromide
- Long-acting e.g. tiotropium

As for inhaled β_2 agonists, delivery is by metered dose inhaler ± volumatic device, or by nebulizer in the acute setting. These drugs are not used intravenously. They act synergistically with β_2 agonists.

Side effects

Dry mouth, acute angle closure glaucoma, tachycardia, paradoxical bronchoconstriction.

Xanthines

These agents act as bronchodilators, but are also mildly anti-inflammatory, diuretic, and positively inotropic. The mechanism of action is unclear, but is thought to involve inhibition of phosphodiesterase, leading to increased intracellular cAMP concentrations in airway smooth muscle. Used orally for the management of chronic asthma and COPD, and intravenously for acute brochoconstriction.

- Theophylline, aminophylline.
- Newer PDE-4 inhibitors (available soon) may offer an improved side-effect profile.

There is a wide variability in pharmacokinetics, and a narrow therapeutic window. These factors limit the use of xanthines in stable airways disease. They are now largely superseded by long-acting inhaled agents. IV aminophylline is used in acute asthma and COPD, although there is limited evidence for benefit.

Side effects

Nausea and vomiting, tachycardia, cardiac arrhythmia, convulsions, abdominal pain.

Anti-inflammatory agents

Corticosteroids

Corticosteroids are highly effective at downregulating multiple pathways in airway inflammation. They affect nuclear transcription factors for pro-inflammatory genes. They are particularly effective against the eosinophilic inflammation seen in asthma, and also in COPD which is characterized by neutrophilic inflammation. They can be used orally or intravenously for exacerbations of airways disease. Inhaled corticosteroids are the mainstay of prophylactic therapy to reduce symptoms and exacerbations, and improve lung function.

With inhaled therapy, effective drug delivery (metered dose inhaler plus a volumatic device, or dry powder inhaler) is crucial, and side effects are generally rare. Long-term use of oral steroids is associated with serious side effects and should be limited to only the most severe cases.

Long-term (>3 months) use of oral corticosteroids leads to risk of adrenal suppression with trauma, surgery, or serious illness.

For major surgery, give the usual oral steroid dose on the morning of surgery, followed by hydrocortisone 25–50 mg IV at induction, then 25–50 mg IV TDS for 24–72hr.

Side effects

Inhaled steroids

Adrenal suppression in children, hoarse voice, candidiasis.

Oral steroids

Cushingoid features, diabetes, hypertension, osteoporosis, peptic ulceration.

Leukotriene receptor antagonists

Leukotriene receptor antagonists block the effects of cysteinyl leukotrienes in the airway, reducing both airway inflammation and smooth muscle contraction. They are less potent than corticosteroids because they affect only one pathway, with a considerable heterogeneity of response. They are effective as an add-on therapy for those on inhaled steroids. They are also useful for allergic asthma with concomitant rhinitis, for exercise-induced asthma, and in children. Used orally only.

- Montelukast, Zafirlukast

Side-effects

GI upset, sleep disturbance, rash.

Mast cell stabilizers

Mast cell stabilizers inhibit the release of mediators from sensitized mast cells. Because of their relatively weak effect and short duration of action, their use has largely been superseded by inhaled steroids, except in children.

- Sodium chromoglycate, nedocromil sodium

Anti-IgE (omalizumab)

Omalizumab is a recently developed monoclonal antibody against IgE, which is used as an add-on therapy in allergic asthma uncontrolled on currently available inhaled therapies. Administered by subcutaneous injection every 2–4 weeks.

Side effects

Flu-like symptoms, rash.

Antihistamines

Antihistamines act on H_1 histamine receptors. Older agents are generally of shorter duration of action and cause sedation due to CNS penetration. Second-generation antihistamines can be taken once daily (orally) and cause less (or no) sedation. They are useful for a variety of allergic conditions, including allergic rhinitis and urticaria. However, they are generally ineffective in asthma.

- Short-acting: chlorpheniramine, acravistine
- Non-sedating: fexofenadine, loratadine, cetirizine

Side effects

Sedation, anticholinergic effects.

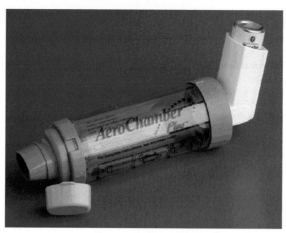

Fig. 13.26 Metered dose inhaler and volumatic spacer.

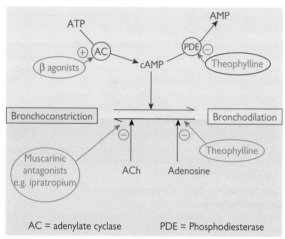

AC = adenylate cyclase   PDE = Phosphodiesterase

Fig. 13.27 Cellular action of bronchodilators.

Other respiratory drugs

Respiratory stimulants

Doxapram

A central stimulant, acting on carotid chemoreceptors and brainstem respiratory centres. Used traditionally in hypercapnic respiratory failure in COPD exacerbations, although it has largely been superseded by NIPPV. Can be used in patients in whom NIPPV is contraindicated, or in those too drowsy for NIPPV (and not for intubation). Given as IV infusion 1.5-4mg/min.

Side effects

Agitation, confusion, fasciculations.

Mucolytics

Carbocysteine, mecysteine

Related to *N*-acetyl cysteine, these agents facilitate expectoration by reducing sputum viscosity. Indicated in bronchiectasis and COPD/chronic bronchitis, with excess sputum production and frequent exacerbations. Studies show a modest effect on exacerbation rates. Used orally. These drugs cause minimal side-effects.

Dornase alpha

Human DNAase, used to reduce sputum viscosity by cleavage of neutrophilic nuclear material. Used to improve pulmonary function in cystic fibrosis only. Administered via nebulizer.

Side effects

Pharyngitis, voice change

Antitussives

The only clinically effective cough suppressant agents are opioids such as codeine and morphine, which can be used in low doses for persistent cough in malignant disease or idiopathic chronic cough.

Definition

Chronic obstructive pulmonary disease (COPD) is a progressive, generally irreversible, airways obstruction caused by a combination of airway and parenchymal damage due to chronic inflammation, predominantly as a result of tobacco smoking.

This term includes patients labelled as chronic bronchitis, emphysema or chronic airflow limitation (CAL). Airflow obstruction is defined as FEV_1 <80% of predicted and FEV_1/FVC ratio <70% of predicted.

Pathology

Inflammation leads to damage due to protease–antiprotease imbalance and oxidative stress, causing acinar destruction in the parenchyma with development of emphysema and bullae.

In the bronchi, inflammation causes goblet cell hyperplasia, smooth muscle hyperplasia, and fibrosis, leading to chronic sputum production and fixed airflow limitation. The airflow limitation is also influenced by loss of elasticity in the parenchyma.

Clinical features

Patients with COPD experience progressive symptomatic deterioration which mirrors the gradual decline in lung function. After an initial asymptomatic period there is progressive exertional dyspnoea. Patients may also develop a productive cough, wheeze, and weight loss, depending on the relative contribution of the different components: chronic bronchitis, emphysema, and fixed airflow limitation.

Important physical signs include chest hyperexpansion, quiet breath and heart sounds, wheeze, pursed-lip breathing, and use of the accessory muscles of ventilation.

Exacerbations are a characteristic feature, with increased symptoms and complications such as respiratory failure. They are usually triggered by viral or bacterial infections, and are a leading cause of hospital admission and mortality.

In the later stages of COPD, patients often develop chronic hypoxia, cor pulmonale, polycythaemia, and type 2 respiratory failure.

Investigation

Lung function testing aids the diagnosis of COPD (Section 1.4).

Management

Treatments are directed at the following potentially reversible components of the disease:

- Bronchial smooth muscle contraction
- Bronchial mucosal congestion and edema
- Airway inflammation
- Increased airway secretion.

Pharmacological

Some patients respond objectively to inhaled or oral steroids, and this therapy reduces the rate of further deterioration. Inhaled β_2 agonists often produce symptomatic relief, but objectively show less benefit compared with asthma. There is similar relief with inhaled anticholinergic agents.

Xanthines are used less commonly because of their narrow therapeutic window. Mucolytics have no place in regular therapy, and antibiotics should be reserved for infective exacerbations.

Pulmonary rehabilitation

A structured training programme improves exercise performance.

Smoking cessation

Community outreach teams

The outreach team approach has been shown to prevent admission and readmission, reduce the length of hospital stay, and reduce the COPD complication rates.

Non-invasive ventilation

This is used for both acute exacerbations, and for those with chronic type 2 respiratory failure.

Practical points

Nihilistic approaches to COPD patients are no longer appropriate. Modern treatments, including better inhaled therapies, pulmonary rehabilitation, and outreach teams, are able to reduce exacerbation rates and improve quality of life.

- Smoking cessation and long-term oxygen therapy (LTOT) are the two interventions that affect long-term prognosis.
- Use of non-invasive ventilation has improved outcomes for severe exacerbations.
- Outcome of ICU admission with intubation in carefully selected patients (based on their functional ability) is surprisingly good.
- COPD patients represent increased but not excessive operative risk. Minimal abnormality on spirometric testing, walking distance, and blood gases represents lower perioperative risk.

Flow–volume loop

Expiratory flow–volume curves allow the identification of large and small airways airflow obstruction (Figure 13.28)

Initiation of expiration is effort-dependent, and the shape of the curve identifies poor effort or technique. However, after only a fraction of expiration, the curve becomes effort-independent, with flow determined by airway resistance and elastic recoil.

Small airways disease (COPD, chronic asthma, bronchiolitis obliterans) is characterized by reduced mid-expiratory flow rates. In emphysema, flow-dependent collapse of small airways leads to a 'scooped-out' appearance of the curve and a reduced maximum mid-expiratory flow.

The inspiratory flow–volume curve is usually symmetrical. Flattening of the curve may be seen in extrapulmonary airway obstruction (e.g. retrosternal goitre).

Flow limitation, dynamic pressure points, and gas trapping

During expiration, positive pleural pressure is transmitted to the alveoli. Since this is higher than mouth pressure, exhalation ensues. Flow reaches a maximum that cannot be exceeded even if expiratory effort is increased. This is the effect of dynamic airways compression (Figure 13.30).

During expiration, positive pleural pressures and elastic recoil of the lung are opposed by positive pressure within the airway. As expiratory flow begins, the resistance of the airway dictates that there will be a pressure drop along its length. The point at which the opposing pressures are matched is termed the equal pressure point (EPP), and at this point airway transmural pressure is zero. Effectively, the pressures that compress the alveoli also compress the airways, forcing them to collapse just proximal to the EPP (Figure 13.29).

The lung unit functions as a Starling resistor, where flow is determined by the pressure gradient across the airway wall rather than the difference between the alveoli and the mouth. Increased effort increases alveolar pressure but also increases airway compression and therefore will not increase flow.

Factors that determine the site of the EPP are important in determining maximum flow rates and the ability of the lungs to limit gas trapping at higher ventilatory rates.

- In emphysema, loss of elastic tissue support promotes airway collapse.
- There is reduced radial traction on airways at low lung volumes.
- Increased airway resistance means that pressure falls more rapidly, moving the EPP towards alveoli. These airways are more easily compressed.

The above factors produce expiratory flow limitation, gas trapping, hyperexpansion, and greater work of breathing. The use of PEEP during ventilatory support counteracts airway collapse and can improve tidal volumes and reduce gas trapping (Section 22.4).

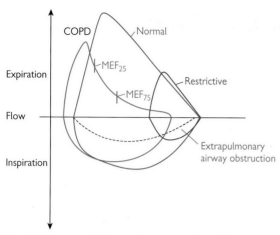

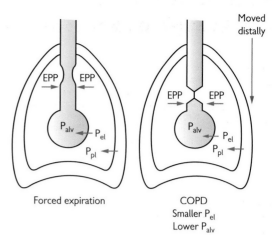

Fig. 13.28 Diagram of F–V loop with superimposed pathologies. Inhalation from RV to TLC is followed by forced expiration. Expiratory flow depends only on lung volume. The COPD curve demonstrates dynamic airway compression. MMEF (maximum mid-expiratory flow) approximates to the average flow between 25% and 75% of TLC. A low average correlates with small airways disease.

Fig. 13.29 Equal pressure point:

alveolar pressure (P_{alv}) = **elastic recoil pressure (P_{el})** + **pleural pressure (P_{pl}).**

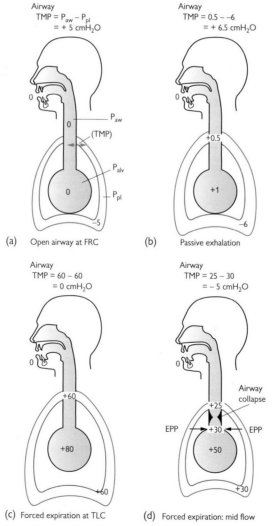

Airway
TMP = $P_{aw} - P_{pl}$
= + 5 cmH$_2$O

Airway
TMP = 0.5 – –6
= + 6.5 cmH$_2$O

(a) Open airway at FRC

(b) Passive exhalation

Airway
TMP = 60 – 60
= 0 cmH$_2$O

Airway
TMP = 25 – 30
= – 5 cmH$_2$O

(c) Forced expiration at TLC

(d) Forced expiration: mid flow

Fig. 13.30 Dynamic airways compression. (a) and (b) show the transmural pressures of the open airway at FRC and during passive exhalation, respectively. (c) shows forced expiration from TLC; the EPP is in the large airways and cartilage in their walls prevents collapse. (d) shows forced expiration at mid-flow. Lung volume and airway calibre are smaller; but with greater resistance and pressure drop along the airway length. Palv reduces with lung volume; transmural pressure soon becomes negative and this forces airway collapse. At the EPP (which has moved distally; arrows), transmural pressure is zero.

13.11 Gas exchange

The key respiratory units of the lung are the alveoli, which are closely associated with the pulmonary circulation. The total surface area of the 300–500 million alveoli in the healthy adult lung is very large—up to 100m^2. Their diameter varies with lung volume; at FRC it is 0.2mm. Gas exchange takes place across the alveolar walls, which form septae between adjacent alveoli. The septae are flat, and so the alveolus is not spherical but more polyhedral in shape.

The walls are lined by thin type I cells. Type II cells are also present and are responsible for the formation of surfactant and the generation of further type I cells. The space between adjacent alveoli contains pulmonary capillaries. The fragile nature of this anatomy makes it vulnerable to damage (Section 13.4).

Diffusion

All gases move across the alveolar membrane by passive diffusion at a rate predicted by Fick's law (Section 7.24). The diffusion constant D is gas specific: it is proportional to the solubility of the gas and inversely proportional to the square root of its molecular weight:

$$V \propto (A/T) \times D \times (P_1 - P_2)$$

$$D = \frac{(solubility)}{\sqrt{(molecular\ weight)}}$$

Where A is the area available for diffusion, T is the thickness of the membrane, and $P_1 - P_2$ is the partial pressure gradient driving diffusion.

CO_2 diffuses 20 times more quickly than oxygen because of its superior solubility despite its similar molecular weight.

In clinical practice, is not possible to measure the lung surface area A or its membrane thickness T. Instead, the diffusing capacity D_L is approximated:

$$V_{gas} = D_L \times (P_1 - P_2).$$

Carbon monoxide is usually used to measure D_L. Its partial pressure in capillary blood is so small that it can be ignored, so

$$D_L = V_{gas}/PACO$$

The diffusing capacity is the volume of CO that diffuses across the lung membrane per minute per kPa alveolar partial pressure.

Rates of gas exchange

When breathing air with a minute volume of 5L/min, only 4L/min will reach the alveoli. Of this, only 840ml will be oxygen. 250ml oxygen enters and 200 ml CO_2 leaves the circulation (giving rise to a respiratory quotient of 0.8). Most inhaled oxygen leaves the lungs without reaching the bloodstream.

The composition of alveolar gas

There is rapid equilibration of oxygen and carbon dioxide between the alveolus and the blood as it passes through the pulmonary capillaries. The primary factors affecting alveolar gas pressures are:

- The composition of inspired gas.
- Alveolar ventilation: this supplies O_2 and removes CO_2.
- The rate of removal of O_2 and addition of CO_2 by pulmonary blood flow. Increased oxygen demand reduces PvO_2 and increased CO_2 production increases $PaCO_2$.

Oxygenation

Uptake from the capillary

Oxygen moves along its partial pressure gradient (not, as is often stated, along its concentration gradient).

Perfusion limitation

In health, at rest, RBCs are within the pulmonary capillary for 0.75sec. Oxygen combines with Hb within the RBC, and PaO_2 begins to rise from its baseline partial pressure in mixed venous blood. Within 0.25sec, Hb is fully saturated and PaO_2 is virtually equal to PAO_2. Further transfer of oxygen can be described as **perfusion limited**: it requires more perfusion with blood of a low PO_2.

This perfusion-limited uptake also occurs with nitrous oxide, which does not combine with Hb (Figure 13.32). Its blood partial pressure rises very quickly, reducing the gradient for diffusion. More can cross into the blood only when more blood (with a lower partial pressure of nitrous oxide) arrives.

Diffusion limitation

When the alveolar membrane is thickened (e.g. after fibrosis), PaO_2 does not equilibrate with PAO_2, and so transfer of oxygen is now **diffusion limited**.

This concept is also applicable, for different reasons, when considering CO. CO moves rapidly across the membrane to combine avidly with Hb. The tight bonding process occurs within the cell and, as a consequence, the partial pressure of CO hardly rises at all, allowing the diffusion gradient to be maintained. Since equilibration of partial pressures across the membrane does not occur, this transfer is also diffusion limited.

Abnormal diffusion

Exercise and membrane thickening

In health, diffusion reserves are enormous. With exercise, the RBC is in the capillary for only 0.25sec but this is still long enough for adequate oxygenation to take place.

However, thickening of the alveolar membrane impedes the movement of oxygen, and PaO_2 may not reach PAO_2 within the shortened time-frame imposed by exercise, resulting in hypoxia (Figure 13.33).

Altitude

Although the partial pressures of both inhaled and mixed venous oxygen are lower at high altitude, the inhaled PO_2 is reduced more. The gradient for diffusion across the alveolar membrane is reduced, and the passage of oxygen will be slower. At rest, this should present little problem, as there is still ample time for diffusion to occur. However, with reduced time in the capillary during exercise and slower diffusion of oxygen, this will result in hypoxia.

The oxygen cascade

Oxygen moves passively throughout the body. For this to occur, a partial pressure gradient must exist at every point where oxygen is transferred: from the atmosphere to the alveoli (where the pressure gradient occurs as a result of the mechanical work of breathing); and to the capillaries, tissues, and mitochondria (where the gradient is ultimately maintained by the consumption of oxygen in oxidative phosphorylation). The oxygen cascade describes these sequential falls in oxygen partial pressure (Figure 13.31).

The CO_2 content of alveolar gas

The alveolar CO_2 concentration depends on:

- CO_2 output which in turn depends on metabolic rate and transfer of CO_2 to the lungs;
- alveolar ventilation

The percentage of alveolar CO_2 is equal to CO_2 output divided by alveolar ventilation:

$$\%\ alveolar\ CO_2 = CO_2\ output/V_A$$

CO_2 diffuses 20 times more quickly than oxygen because of its greater solubility. However, thickening of the alveolar membrane can still impair release of CO_2.

The alveolar gas equation

$$PAO_2 = PIO_2 - (PACO_2/R)$$

This is used to work out the PAO_2 of the ideal alveolus. The equation produces a small error: the inspired and expired gas volumes do not quite match. A more accurate version of this equation adds a correction factor (See opposite).

CO_2 rapidly diffuses out of the vessel and equilibrates within the alveolus, and so arterial and alveolar CO_2 are assumed to be the same: Therefore $PaCO_2$ can be taken from the arterial blood gas. Knowledge of $PaCO_2$ and FiO_2 allows calculation of PAO_2. Comparison of PAO_2 with PaO_2 allows calculation of the A–a gradient.

→ **Diffusion constant: the single-breath method of assessment**

A single vital capacity breath (of dilute CO mixture) is held for 10sec and the rate of disappearance of CO is determined using IR gas analysis on exhalation. Helium is also added to the mixture to allow for determination of lung volume.

The CO transfer coefficient (K_{CO}) is equivalent to D_L/V_A (alveolar volume). It estimates the gas transfer per litre of lung volume and adjusts for a reduction in accessible lung volume.

- $D_L CO$ and K_{CO} will be low in emphysema (reduced alveolar capillary membrane) and fibrosing alveolitis (both have poor V/Q matching and reduced gas diffusion) and pulmonary vascular disease.
- K_{CO} will be normal and $D_L CO$ will be reduced with small lung volumes (pleural effusion, muscle weakness, and consolidation).

Alveolar haemorrhage provides more blood for reaction with CO and so will cause to be overestimated. Anaemia will underestimate it.

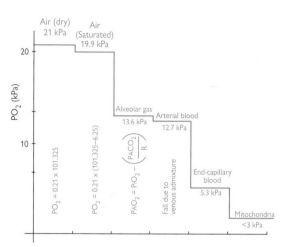

Fig. 13.31 The oxygen cascade. The partial pressure of oxygen falls at successive points along its journey to the mitochondrion. Diffusion deficit does not affect PO_2 at rest, but may become apparent at altitude or with exercise.

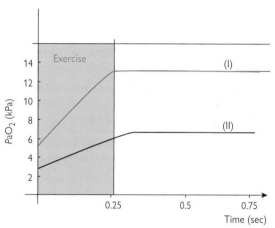

Fig. 13.33 Uptake from the capillary: (I) during exercise there is enough time to load the RBC with O_2; (II) abnormally slow oxygenation when PaO_2 is low (altitude) because of the reduced diffusion gradient. Exercise will be poorly tolerated.

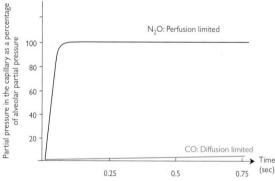

Fig. 13.32 Perfusion- versus diffusion-limited uptake of gases from the alveolus. The partial pressure of N_2O rapidly equilibrates across the alveolar membrane; the only way of maintaining the diffusion gradient is for new blood (without N_2O) to enter the capillary. This is perfusion limitation. Carbon monoxide hardly equilibrates at all across the membrane, and so is diffusion limited.

→ **Complex form of alveolar gas equation**

$$PAO_2 = FiO_2 \times (P_B - P_{H_2O}) - PACO_2 \times \frac{FiO_2 + (1 - FiO_2)}{R}$$

When $FiO_2 = 1.0$, RQ is irrelevant. When $FiO_2 < 1.0$, the correction factor is more accurate when $RQ \neq 1$. At $RQ = 1$, the volume of oxygen removed equals the volume of CO_2 added.

Each minute, 250ml oxygen is taken up into the blood, equal to the volume consumed in the body. The amount delivered to the tissues each minute is known as the oxygen flux, and is normally 1000ml/min.

Oxygen transport

Oxygen is carried in the blood both bound to haemoglobin (Hb) and dissolved in the plasma. The vast majority is carried by haemoglobin.

Haemoglobin

Normal adult haemoglobin consists of four polypeptide chains, 2α and 2β, and an iron-porphyrin compound. Oxygen binds reversibly with the ferrous compound to form oxyhaemoglobin and reaction with each of the four subunits facilitates reaction with the next. Each stage has successively faster kinetics, which means that although fewer binding sites are available, the speed of reaction at the last site is not slower. These reactions account for the S-shaped oxygen dissociation curve (ODC; Figure 13.34).

The significance of the oxygen dissociation curve

PaO_2 can fall significantly, and yet Hb will remain well saturated. The steep part of the curve demonstrates that a lot of oxygen can be removed from Hb with minimal effect on its partial pressure. Therefore the oxygen diffusion partial pressure gradient from the RBC to the cell is maintained.

Binding with haemoglobin

The binding of O_2 to Hb is rapid and takes 0.2sec. The reaction can be considered to be the sum of two stages:

- Diffusion through the alveolar wall, RBC wall, and cell interior.
- Reaction with Hb. This amount of Hb available for oxygen carriage can be severely affected by carbon monoxide poisoning; the effect of carbon monoxide on the ODC and oxygen content of blood is shown in Figure 13.35.

In practice, both parts offer approximately equal resistances.

Transfer to peripheral capillaries

20ml O_2 per 100ml of blood is delivered to the tissues, where 5ml O_2 per 100ml of blood is transferred. In doing so, the mixed venous PO_2 falls to 5kPa.

O_2 diffuses down its partial pressure gradient from the RBC to peripheral tissues. O_2 oxygen released from Hb as the blood PO_2 falls, maintaining delivery to the tissues.

The Bohr effect

Increases in CO_2, proton concentration, and temperature (such as are found in metabolically active tissues) shift the ODC to the right, and this promotes oxygen liberation from Hb and transfer to peripheral tissues. The reverse occurs in the pulmonary circulation, where CO_2 is offloaded and its partial pressure falls.

2,3-diphosphoglycerate (2,3-DPG)

2,3-DPG is made primarily during glucose metabolism (Embden–Meyerhof pathway, Section 17.6). It binds only to deoxygenated β-chains by forming bridges with lysine and histidine in the periphery of the deoxy pocket. As it does so, it alters the shape of the molecule to make release of oxygen more likely.

Production increases with conditions of reduced peripheral O_2 delivery: hypoxia, anaemia, CCF, and COPD. Raised levels shift the ODC to the right, again favouring oxygen offloading in the tissues.

Dissolved oxygen

The amount of O_2 dissolved is proportional to its partial pressure (Henry's law). Although very little oxygen is transported in this way, it is the dissolved portion that diffuses into the tissues. (The obvious analogy here is with protein-bound drugs: although most of the drug present in the plasma is in combination with protein, only the unbound portion is free to act.)

Flux equation

$$\text{Oxygen flux} = CO \times [(\text{Hb } O_2 \text{ carriage}) + (O_2 \text{ dissolved})]$$
$$= CO \times [([\text{Hb}] \times SaO_2 \times K)] + (PaO_2 \times 0.0225)]$$

where [Hb] is the concentration of Hb (g/dl). $K = 1.34\text{ml } O_2/\text{g}$ is Hufner's number, which is the amount of O_2 that combines with and fully saturates 1g Hb at 37°C. The factor 0.0225 is the number of millilitres of O_2 dissolved in 1 decilitre of blood per kPa PO_2. It is roughly equivalent to 0.3ml dissolved O_2 in 100ml blood with $PO_2 = 13.3\text{kPa}$. CO is cardiac output. It is essential to ensure that CO is expressed as decilitres per minute, since oxygen content is given per decilitre.

A typical example: CO = 50dL/min, Hb = 15, oxygen saturation = 98%, and PaO_2 = 100kPa. Then:

$$\text{Oxygen flux} = 50 \times [15 \times [(98/100) \times [1.34] + [100 \times 0.0225]$$
$$\approx 1000\text{ml/min.}$$

Carriage of carbon dioxide

Cellular metabolism produces CO_2, which moves down its partial pressure gradient into the blood where it is found in three forms.

- **Dissolved:** CO_2 is much more soluble than O_2. 10% of CO_2 output is carried to the lungs in the dissolved form.
- **Bicarbonate:** carbonic anhydrase in the endothelium and in RBCs catalyses the otherwise slow combination of CO_2 and water. The subsequent degradation of carbonic acid into bicarbonate and protons is fast.
- **Carbamino compounds** are formed when CO_2 reacts with terminal amine groups of proteins, and the amine groups of lysine and arginine side chains.

Haemoglobin is the most important source of carbamino compounds, since it is abundant and it is a tetramer with four amino terminals for reaction. Additionally, formation increases significantly as haemoglobin becomes deoxygenated (See below).

There is 48ml CO_2 per 100ml arterial blood, and 52 ml CO_2 per 100ml venous blood (Figure 13.37). The higher content in the venous system is due to peripheral generation of CO_2 and its addition to the circulation. There is significantly more CO_2 content than O_2 content in blood.

The chloride shift

Following oxygen unloading, deoxygenated Hb is a better buffer of protons produced by the action of carbonic anhydrase and the dissociation of carbamino compounds (Figure 13.36). Intracellular bicarbonate concentration rises following degradation of carbonic acid, and it diffuses out of the RBC in exchange for chloride. The capnophorin transporter found in the RBC membrane ensures that this is an efficient process. Without the chloride shift to maintain electrochemical neutrality, bicarbonate could not move freely in and out of the RBC, inhibiting further formation of bicarbonate.

Although carbamino compounds carry CO_2, they are completely dissociated at physiological pH and so place a greater proton buffering strain on Hb within the RBC.

Haldane effect

Once Hb offloads oxygen, it can carry more CO_2. The CO_2 dissociation curve demonstrates this phenomenon, known as the Haldane effect. This is because:

- Carbamino compounds are formed, and this increases once O_2 is offloaded. This accounts for 70% of the Haldane effect.
- Deoxyhaemoglobin is more basic than the oxygenated form, and mops up more of the protons released from the degradation of carbonic acid. This allows more degradation of carbonic acid.

Transfer of CO_2 within the lungs

The pulmonary capillary PCO_2 is higher than that of the alveolus, and this induces movement out of the blood. By the end of the pulmonary capillary, the partial pressure is almost identical to that of the alveolus.

The diffusion gradient of partial pressures can be traced from the point of production in the mitochondria all the way to the alveolus.

In the pulmonary capillaries $PaCO_2$ and [H$^+$] fall, and this favours loading with oxygen. By reviewing the Bohr effect, we can see that in the presence of lower CO_2 pressure, more oxygen can be carried by haemoglobin.

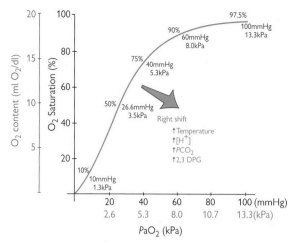

Fig. 13.34 Oxygen dissociation curve. Oxygen content, rather than oxygen saturation, can be shown by changing the y-axis. This curve is for Hb 15g/dl. Clearly, Hb concentration impacts on O_2 content.

Mixed venous point

This is an anomaly. The mixed venous point will not lie on the arterial dissociation curve because of its different CO_2 content and pH (Bohr effect).

P_{50}

This is the point at which Hb is 50% saturated, and is the index of shift for the dissociation curve (affinity for oxygen). It is on the steepest part of the curve, and so is very sensitive at detecting change with different conditions.

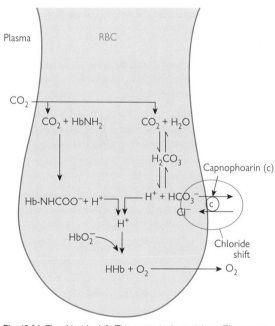

Fig. 13.36 The chloride shift. This occurs in the periphery. The reverse happens in the lungs, when O_2 is loaded and CO_2 lost. Carbamino compounds are formed from the reaction of CO_2 with the terminal amine groups of proteins and the amino groups of amino acid side chains. Hb is an important source because it is the most prevalent protein and it is a tetramer (with four terminal amine groups). Carbaminohaemoglobin is almost completely dissociated at pH 7.4; the protons are buffered by Hb's histidine residues.

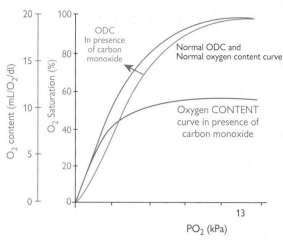

Fig. 13.35 The effect of carbon monoxide on the ODC. The curves shown are for Hb 15g/dl in the presence of carbon monoxide (HbCO 7.5g/dl). Only 50% of the Hb is available for oxygen carriage. Carbon monoxide will significantly alter the O_2 content: the curve is both left-shifted and markedly reduced in size. It will also shift the ODC to the left because of the conformational change induced in Hb that increases its affinity for O_2.

Table 13.1 Carriage of CO_2 in the blood

	Total carriage	Contribution to A–V difference
Dissolved CO_2	5%	10%
Bicarbonate	90%	60%
Carbamino compounds	5%	30%

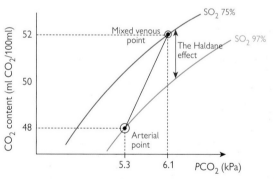

Fig. 13.37 CO_2 dissociation curve. Different CO_2 content curves exist for different levels of oxygenation because of the Haldane effect. In health, oscillation occurs between the arterial and the mixed venous points. The straight CO_2 curve means that any perfused alveoli will increase CO_2 excretion in response to an increased minute volume. This occurs in all V/Q ratios other than **dead space** and **shunt**. This is unlike the ODC, where the flat upper part means that there is not much additional oxygen that can be added by hyperventilation.

In the periphery, the $PaCO_2$ rises only slightly despite a significant increase in blood CO_2 *content*; this is due to the enhanced ability of Hb to carry CO_2 once it has offloaded oxygen.

The lungs have two distinct circulations.

- The **bronchial circulation** provides oxygenated blood at systemic blood pressure to the airways of the lung. It receives 1% of the cardiac output. A significant proportion of it drains into the pulmonary veins, and constitutes a shunt.
- The **pulmonary circulation**, whose physiological characteristics differ in a number of aspects from the systemic circulation. The major role of the pulmonary circulation is to facilitate gas exchange at the site of the alveolar capillaries.

From the right ventricle, divisions of the pulmonary artery follow those of the airways as far as the terminal bronchioles. They then divide to form the capillaries that line the alveoli, an arrangement that results in a sheet of blood surrounding the air spaces. After coalescing to form the pulmonary venules and veins, vessels carry blood back to the left heart.

Pulmonary vessels are usually maximally vasodilated, and so although they are innervated by the autonomic system, the significance of this remains unclear. Experimentally, vasoconstriction is produced by stimulation of either α-adrenoceptors or muscarinic receptors, whereas β-adrenoceptor stimulation causes vasodilatation.

Anatomical differences

The pressure in the aorta is six times that in the pulmonary artery, and the pressure gradient across the systemic circulation is 10 times more than that across the pulmonary vascular system. In keeping with these low pressures, the walls of the pulmonary vessels are thin.

Unlike the systemic circulation, the vascular bed accepts the whole cardiac output. The vessel wall musculature is poorly developed compared with the systemic circulation, since major changes in blood distribution in response to pulmonary metabolic activity are not required: the lungs behave as one organ. The right ventricle develops pulmonary artery pressures just high enough to allow blood to flow to the lung apices.

Pulmonary capillaries act as Starling resistors (Figure 13.40); they are subject to the effects of transmural pressure. They are surrounded by alveolar gas, whose pressure influences the diameter of the vessel. If alveolar pressure rises above capillary pressure, blood flow will cease as the vessel collapses. The rest of the vascular tree is subject to other forces. The elastic forces of the lung cause radial traction and so vessel diameter increases with increasing lung volume.

Vascular resistance

With the same blood flow through the pulmonary circulation as through the systemic, but one-tenth of the pressure drop along its length, the vascular resistance is low (~100dyn sec/cm^{-5}). This resistance can vary in response to changing requirements (Figure 13.38). The mechanisms are as follows.

- *Distension:* at even higher pressures, vessel calibre increases and the cross-sectional area becomes circular rather than flattened. This is the predominant mechanism of action.
- *Recruitment:* as either arterial or venous pressure rises, vessels that are closed become open, allowing blood to flow through them. The mechanism is unclear.

Lung volume also influences pulmonary vascular resistance (PVR) (Figure 13.39). Drugs influencing the smooth muscle of the extra-alveolar vessels affects PVR, particularly at low lung volume. The autonomic system exerts weak control over PVR, and acidaemia seems to increase pulmonary vascular tone, especially in the presence of alveolar hypoxia.

Hypoxic pulmonary vasoconstriction

When the PO_2 of alveolar gas is reduced, there is contraction of smooth muscle in the walls of the vessels supplying the hypoxic lung unit. The response only occurs in response to alveolar gas composition: if the PO_2 of the arteriolar blood is reduced, the effect is not replicated.

The mechanism of action remains obscure, despite the sequence of events being so well described. It occurs in isolated preparations but, even so, the presumed vasoactive trigger has yet to be identified. The intra-cellular events of vascular smooth muscle contraction seem to occur in standard fashion (Section 10.13).

Distribution of blood flow

In the erect human there is a steady decrease in blood flow from the base to the apex of the lung. Basal flow does not change when the person lies down, although in the supine position apical flow increases as does flow to the more dependent posterior regions. It has long been assumed that the causes of blood flow variation are purely gravitational. This is a gross simplification, since imaging techniques have shown heterogeneity even in the horizontal plane. Nevertheless, the concepts are presented as zones of variable flow (Figure 13.40).

There is significantly better blood vessel conductance in the posterior chest. Also, local chemical (NO and prostacyclin) production alters vessel calibre and blood flow, and mediators synthesized elsewhere in the body (such as serotonin and bradykinin) may also affect vessels similarly. Additional influences on blood flow include lung volume: at low volumes, extra-alveolar vessels collapse and blood flow ceases. This is seen at the bases where the parenchyma is poorly expanded.

Pulmonary hypertension

Definition

Normal pulmonary artery pressure has a mean value of 12–16mmHg. The pulmonary circulation has low resistance but high flow, and can accommodate large increases in cardiac output. Pulmonary hypertension is defined as a mean pressure of 20mmHg, or systolic pressure of 30mmHg. A large number of pulmonary and systemic disorders cause pulmonary hypertension. Primary pulmonary hypertension is defined by raised pulmonary artery pressure in the absence of a known cause.

Cor pulmonale is a term used to describe dilatation and failure of the right ventricle secondary to pulmonary hypertension. It is usually due to chronic hypoxic lung disease (e.g. COPD).

As we have already seen, alveolar hypoxia causes localized vasoconstriction, diverting blood away from the region and reducing the V/Q mismatch. General hypoxia, as seen in severe lung disease, results in generalized vasoconstriction. This in turn causes pulmonary hypertension.

Management

Management of secondary pulmonary hypertension should be directed at the underlying cause. Therapy should be started as early as possible in order to prevent progression to cor pulmonale. General supportive therapy, which also applies to primary pulmonary hypertension, includes:

- Correction of chronic hypoxia with long term oxygen therapy.
- Diuretics
- Anticoagulants
- Calcium antagonists
- Prostacyclin analogues
- Endothelin antagonists, e.g. bosentan
- Sildenafil.

Thrombo-endartectomy can be used for chronic thrombotic disease. Severe disease in younger patients is an indication for lung or heart–lung transplantation.

Anaesthetic implications

Laryngoscopy has been shown to increase pulmonary artery pressure and resistance, worsening right heart performance. IPPV, especially with application of PEEP, reduces venous return: this is potentially disastrous since elevated filling pressures must be maintained otherwise right heart output deteriorates.

Table 13.2 Pulmonary and systemic vascular pressures

	Pressure (mmHg)		Pressure (mmHg)
RA	2	LA	5
RV	25/0	LV	120/0
PA	25/8	Aorta	120/75
Arteriole	12	Arteriole	30
Capillary		Capillary	20
Vein	8	Vein	10

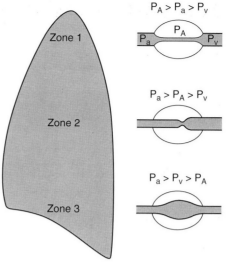

$P_A > P_a > P_v$

Fig. 13.40 Zones of blood flow:
Zone 1

$$P_A > P_a > P_V.$$

Flow is impossible because the vessels are closed flat
Zone 2

$$P_a > P_A > P_V.$$

Flow is related to the pressure difference between the artery and the alveolus. This is the behaviour of a Starling resistor.
Zone 2

$$P_a > P_V > P_A.$$

The usual arterio-venous pressure difference determines blood flow.
The concept of regional blood flow being determined by these pressure gradients is an oversimplification. However, it does illustrate the effects of variations in blood flow on alveolar dead space and appropriate V/Q matching.

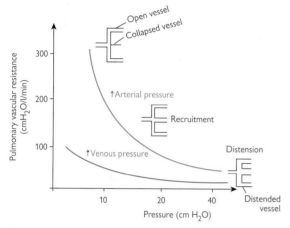

Fig. 13.38 Pulmonary vascular resistance and changing pressure. With increasing arterial pressure (venous pressure held constant) the resistance falls as vessels are recruited. At higher vascular pressures for both systems, distension is the major reason for the fall in resistance.

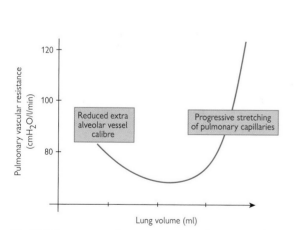

Fig. 13.39 Pulmonary vascular resistance vs. lung volume. At very low volumes, extra-alveolar vascular elastic tissue causes the vessels to reduce calibre or collapse. Vascular resistance is higher at these lower lung volumes. At higher lung volumes the extra-alveolar vessels are stretched open but the capillaries are stretched tightly shut.

→ Hypoxic pulmonary vasoconstriction and anaesthesia

Hypoxic pulmonary vasoconstriction (HPV) is an adaptive mechanism that allows redirection of blood flow to alveoli with higher oxygen pressure, thereby reducing ventilation/perfusion mismatch. The oxygen pressure of pulmonary artery blood has no influence over distribution of flow.

With prolonged hypoxia, this mechanism promotes development of chronic hypoxic pulmonary hypertension. Potassium channels are downregulated, reducing the inward potassium current. The resulting depolarization of the pulmonary artery smooth muscle opens the L-type voltage-dependent Ca^{2+} channels which raise intracellular calcium and cause smooth muscle contraction.

The usual balance between vasoconstrictor molecules (e.g. endothelin-1, thromboxane) and vasodilators (e.g. NO, prostacyclin) is altered by hypoxia.

Inhalational agents block this mechanism, allowing blood to flow to areas of low PaO_2. This results in increased V/Q mismatch and worsening PaO_2.

359

The V/Q ratio determines the partial pressures of all gases in each lung unit. V/Q ratio abnormalities will affect **both** oxygen intake and carbon dioxide excretion.

Figure 13.41 explains how the partial pressures of oxygen and carbon dioxide are affected. For optimal gas exchange, alveolar ventilation (V) and perfusion (Q) should be matched (i.e. a V/Q ratio of 1).

Regional gas exchange

Figure 13.42 demonstrates that, from top to bottom, both ventilation and perfusion increase. However, perfusion increases proportionally much more. The V/Q ratio falls from over 3.0 at the apex to less than 0.7 at the base.

At the apex, lung units function as zone 1, the V/Q ratio is high, and the composition of alveolar gas is that of inspired gas (effectively dead space). At the base the converse is true and here the lung units are predominantly zone 3 (close to shunt). The partial pressures of basal alveolar gas are now more akin to that of the blood returning to the lungs.

V/Q mismatch

It is important to understand that perfusion and ventilation perform as a *ratio*.

- For a given cardiac output, a change in minute volume will change the V/Q ratio of all lung units.
- For a given minute volume, a change in cardiac output will change the V/Q ratio.

This has important implications in the evolution of blood gas abnormalities with respiratory disease.

Dead-space ventilation

In dead space, there is an infinite V/Q ratio (V/Q = ∞). For a constant minute volume, as alveolar dead space increases, alveolar ventilation will fall. $PaCO_2$ is inversely proportional to alveolar ventilation, so it will rise. (Remember that alveolar ventilation is ventilation of lungs units that are able to excrete CO_2, because they are perfused.)

Subsequent stimulation of the chemoreceptors causes an increase in minute and alveolar ventilation, and, since the CO_2 dissociation curve is linear, all perfused lung units are able to increase excretion in response to hyperventilation. Therefore $PaCO_2$ can only remain unchanged at the expense of increased respiratory effort.

Causes

- Compared with spontaneous ventilation, IPPV distributes gas towards the apex and reduces cardiac output, both of which may contribute to greater dead space.
- PEEP may similarly worsen lung perfusion, especially when perfusion pressure is already poor (e.g. shock states).
- Reduced cardiac output such as with hypovolaemia or pulmonary embolus.

Clinically, these patients have a minute volume much greater than expected for their $PaCO_2$. This is difficult to assess in ward patients and is more readily seen in patients ventilated on ICU where MV is measured by the ventilator. This may be an early sign of a reduced cardiac output.

Shunt

In an area of shunt, the V/Q ratio is zero (V/Q = 0). The Thebesian veins of the heart and the A–V shunts within the lung are true anatomical shunts. Shunted blood is poorly oxygenated, and this depresses the PO_2 of post-pulmonary capillary blood significantly (Figure 13.41).

A shunt is an extreme form of V/Q mismatch, and deserves to be mentioned specifically. Simply increasing FiO_2 cannot reverse hypoxaemia due to shunt.

Causes of shunt

Pathological causes of shunt block the ventilation of alveoli whilst still allowing them to be perfused. The airway or bronchial tree may be obstructed, or the alveoli may be filled with pus, blood, fluid, or cells. Clinical shunts include pneumonia, alveolar haemorrhage of Goodpasture's syndrome, pulmonary oedema, and advanced alveolar cell carcinoma.

Clinical relevance

Mismatching of ventilation and perfusion in disease adversely affect both oxygen intake and carbon dioxide excretion. Perfusion of alveoli that are inadequately ventilated (e.g. pneumonia) results in alveolar shunting and hypoxia. Although the blood flow to such alveoli might be expected to diminish due to hypoxic vasoconstriction, the disease process sometimes maintains vascular patency.

The hallmark of shunting is the development of hypoxia with a normal or low $PaCO_2$. Shunting would tend to increase $PaCO_2$ (Figure 13.41), but this in turn increases ventilatory drive. With an increase in minute volume, all perfused alveoli are able to excrete CO_2, a function of the linear CO_2 dissociation curve.

As disease progresses, further reduction in PaO_2 stimulates peripheral chemoreceptors, causing further increases in ventilation and a fall in $PaCO_2$. Disease processes may also specifically affect oxygen and carbon dioxide levels via other sensors, e.g. mechanoreceptors in the chest and cortical input secondary to anxiety of illness.

What happens with a 50% shunt?

Shunted lung units are not able to take up O_2 or excrete CO_2. Any tendency for CO_2 to increase stimulates the chemoreceptors (as does significant reduction in PaO_2). This results in hyperventilation. Since the dissociation curve for CO_2 is linear, hyperventilated and perfused lung units will be able to increase CO_2 excretion, lowering their $PaCO_2$ and the $PaCO_2$ of the blood draining them. This increased excretion of CO_2 may more than compensate for the decreased excretion through the shunt, provided that hyperventilation can be maintained.

While hyperventilated lung units will increase their PaO_2, and therefore the PaO_2 of blood draining them, they add little to the O_2 content of that blood, since capillary Hb is already almost fully saturated. Therefore hyperventilation is unable to compensate for the effects of the shunt on oxygenation. This mixed effect is seen in Table 13.3.

Table 13.3 The effect of high V/Q ratio and shunted lung units on mixed blood oxygen and CO_2 content				
	Normal	High V/Q ratio units (50% flow)	Shunt units (50% flow)	Final arterial blood
PaO_2 (kPa)	13.3	16	5.3	6.7
O_2 content (ml/100ml blood)	20	20.5	15	17.75
SaO_2 (%)	97	99	75	80
$PaCO_2$ (kPa)	5.3	2.67	6.1	4
CO_2 content (ml/100ml blood)	48	38	54	46

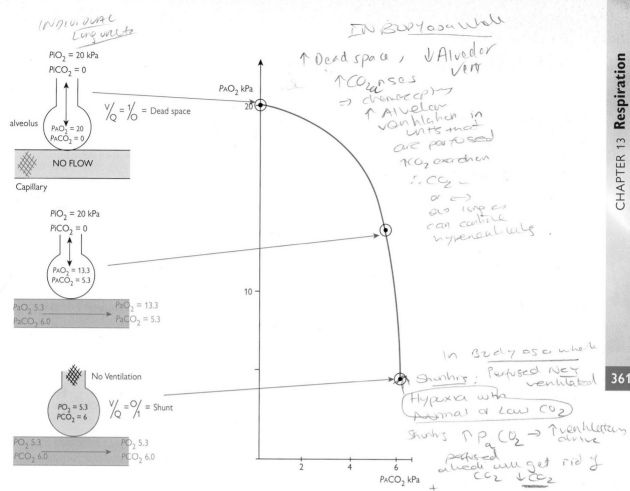

Handwritten annotations:

INDIVIDUAL Lung units

$PiO_2 = 20$ kPa
$PiCO_2 = 0$

$V/Q = 1/0$ = Dead space

alveolus
$PAO_2 = 20$
$PACO_2 = 0$

NO FLOW

Capillary

$PiO_2 = 20$ kPa
$PiCO_2 = 0$

$PAO_2 = 13.3$
$PACO_2 = 5.3$

PaO_2 5.3 → $PaO_2 = 13.3$
$PaCO_2$ 6.0 → $PaCO_2 = 5.3$

No Ventilation

$PO_2 = 5.3$
$PCO_2 = 6$

$V/Q = 0/1$ = Shunt

PO_2 5.3 → PO_2 5.3
PCO_2 6.0 → PCO_2 6.0

PAO_2 kPa
20
10

$PACO_2$ kPa
2 4 6

IN BODY as a Whole
↑ Dead space, ↓ Alveolar Ven
↑CO_2 rises
⇒ chemoreceptors
↑ Alveolar ventilation in units that are perfused
↑CO_2 excretion
∴ CO_2 ↓
or (→)
as long as can continue hyperventilate.

In Body as a whole
Shunting: Perfused NOT ventilated
Hypoxia with Normal or Low CO_2
Shunts ↑P_aCO_2 → ↑ ventilation drive
perfused alveoli will get rid of CO_2
↓CO_2

Fig. 13.41 Diagram of alveoli and PaO_2 and $PaCO_2$ in capillaries. As the V/Q ratio varies, alveolar PO_2 and PCO_2 will change. The extremes of dead space and shunt are shown. This graph reflects the PO_2 and PCO_2 of alveoli and their capillaries for different V/Q ratios. For a gas of known composition (in this case $PiO_2 = 20$kPa and $PiCO_2 = 0$kPa) and mixed venous blood of known composition (in this case $P\bar{v}O_2 = 5.5$kPa and $P\bar{v}CO_2 = 6.0$kPa) lung units of all V/Q ratios must lie on the purple line. Altering either the composition of the blood or the gas alters the position of the line and therefore gas pressures within the alveoli or capillary blood.

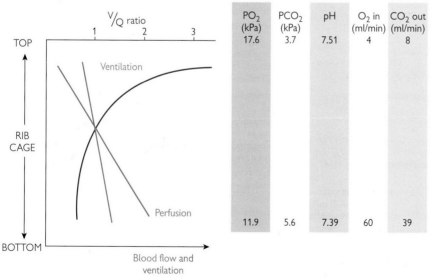

	PO₂ (kPa) 17.6	PCO₂ (kPa) 3.7	pH 7.51	O₂ in (ml/min) 4	CO₂ out (ml/min) 8
	11.9	5.6	7.39	60	39

V/Q ratio

TOP
Ventilation
RIB CAGE
Perfusion
BOTTOM
Blood flow and ventilation

Fig. 13.42 V/Q ratios vs. height of ribs.

Common causes of V/Q mismatch include pulmonary embolus and respiratory infection.

Pulmonary embolus

This is usually caused by embolized thrombus obstructing the pulmonary arteries. It usually originates in the deep veins of the leg, although it may also originate in the central veins and right atrium. Other causes of embolus include:

- Tumour (malignant invasion of great veins).
- Air (after surgery or instrumentation).
- Fat (after fracture) and amniotic fluid. These cause most of their clinical effects from initiation of the inflammatory cascade rather than from obstruction of blood flow.

Affected lung units will be ventilated but not perfused, constituting dead-space ventilation. Subsequent changes, such as pulmonary infarction, inflammation or superimposed infection, may also cause development of low V/Q areas, further contributing to gas exchange abnormalities.

Risk factors

- Recent surgery (abdominal, orthopaedic).
- Obstetric (late pregnancy, puerperium).
- Malignancy.
- Immobility.
- Thrombophilia (e.g. factor V Leiden, antiphospholipid syndrome).
- Exogenous oestrogens (oral contraceptive pill, hormone replacement therapy).
- Previous thromboembolism.
- Varicose veins.
- Coexisting comorbidity (cardiac failure, COPD, neurological disorder).
- Obesity.
- Long-distance travel.

Clinical features

Symptoms: The patient might be asymptomatic, although dyspnoea, pleuritic chest pain, and haemoptysis are common. Some present in extreme shock.

Signs: Tachypnoea, tachycardia, cyanosis, hypotension, raised JVP, right heart strain. Several patterns of presentation are seen:

- Sudden death.
- Cardiac arrest/peri-arrest.
- Acute hypoxia/hypotension.
- Pulmonary infarction (pleuritic chest pain, haemoptysis).
- Sudden deterioration of chronic cardiorespiratory disorder.
- Chronic multiple PE (dyspnoea, pulmonary hypertension).

Diagnosis

A negative D-dimer test reliably excludes PE in patients with intermediate or low clinical probability. Many conditions cause raised D-dimers, so this should not be used to justify imaging for PE without other clinical criteria.

Abnormalities on routine investigations, such as CXR (oligaemia with wedge-shaped infarcts) and ECG (RBBB, right heart strain, P pulmonale), can suggest, but not confirm, the diagnosis. In the presence of a normal CXR, isotope scanning may still be preferred to computed tomographic pulmonary angiography (CTPA) in some centres. The presence of perfusion defects is taken as evidence of emboli.

CTPA is superior to ventilation/perfusion scanning for the diagnosis of PE, and has a better probability of providing the correct diagnosis if PE is in fact absent.

Management

- High-flow oxygen.
- IV fluids and circulatory support.
- Low molecular weight heparin (LMWH) adjusted for weight (enoxaparin 1.5 mg/kg daily subcutaneously).

- Oral warfarin therapy: duration determined by risk factors.
- Thrombolysis (alteplase 100mg IV over 90min) may be used in the peri-arrest patient or in the presence of cardiovascular compromise. Echocardiography may aid assessment if it is rapidly available, but if clinical suspicion is high, thrombolysis is indicated.

Prophylaxis

Up to 50% of pulmonary emboli occur in patients already in hospital or long-term care. These are preventable with appropriate strategies for thromboprophylaxis (usually with LMWH) for high-risk medical and surgical patients.

Pneumonia

Definition

Pneumonia is an acute illness characterized by:

- Lower respiratory tract symptoms (cough, dyspnoea).
- Fever and evidence of systemic inflammation.
- New lung consolidation, visible on CXR.

Many of the consolidated lung units will be perfused but not ventilated (shunt), or poorly ventilated with low V/Q ratios.

Severity assessment

In-hospital outcome is related to organ dysfunction and derangement of physiology. Ward physicians often use 'at risk' scoring systems to assess a patient's likely need for ICU support. Other clinical features associated with poor outcome include severe hypoxia and bilateral infiltrates on CXR.

Management

Antibiotic choice will depend upon clinical subtype and local antibiotic policy. For instance, a penicillin plus macrolide combination is often used for uncomplicated community-acquired pneumonia. Antibiotics should be given intravenously, without delay and with accurate dose intervals. Correction of physiological upset is crucial to outcome in pneumonia. High-flow oxygen and fluids are needed in patients with severe disease, with close attention to correction of hypoxaemia, hypotension, and metabolic acidosis.

Practical points

Non-specific symptoms, such as malaise, headache, vomiting are common at presentation.

The term 'atypical pneumonia' is misleading and should be avoided.

Streptococcus pneumoniae is easily the most common pathogen in community-acquired pneumonia (CAP). Blood cultures are routinely required. However, extensive microbiological investigations such as PCR or antigen testing are only needed for severe disease.

Anaesthetic relevance

With pneumonia, complication rates increase under anaesthesia. It is best to avoid anaesthesia for elective surgery until all the symptoms, signs, and investigations have returned to normal. For the patient with pneumonia who requires emergency surgery, a number of problems may be predicted.

Pneumonia may cause hypoxia via a number of different mechanisms, including worsening dead space, V/Q mismatch, and low mixed venous oxygen content.

Exhaustion results in hypercapnia and the need for IPPV. Untreated hypovolaemia further affects venous return, exacerbating reductions in cardiac output and blood pressure.

Induction and intubation may provoke significant CVS instability, in the septic hypotensive patient. Vasopressor agents may be required pre-induction.

Signs of sepsis are frequently associated with metabolic acidaemia, whilst the respiratory effects of pneumonia are often complicated by respiratory acidaemia.

→ Diagnosis of pulmonary embolism

Diagnosis of pulmonary embolus is difficult, and cannot be confirmed with simple bedside assessment. Because of the high mortality if left untreated, a high index of suspicion is needed, especially in patients with unexplained dyspnoea. Scoring systems such as the Wells score help with risk stratification:

Suspected DVT	3 points
Alternative diagnosis less likely than PE	3 points
Heart rate > 100/min	1.5 points
Immobilization/surgery within 4 weeks	1.5 points
Previous DVT/PE	1.5 points
Haemoptysis	1 point
Malignancy	1 point

Total score: <2 indicates a low probability of PE (mean probability 3.6%); 2–6 indicates a moderate probability of PE (20.5%); >6 indicates a high probability of PE (66.7%).

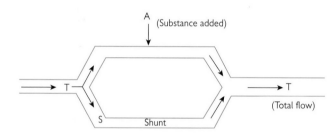

The ratio of flow through S to total flow = $\dfrac{\text{Actual dilution of added substance due to bypass flow}}{\text{Maximum possible dilution of added substance if all flow through the bypass channel}}$

SHUNT EQUATION

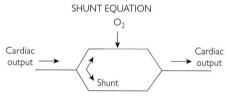

$$\frac{Q_S}{Q_T} = \frac{\text{Actual dilution of } O_2 \text{ by shunt}}{\text{Max possible dilution if all flow through shunt}}$$

$$= \frac{\text{Max possible } [O_2] - \text{Actual } [O_2]}{\text{Max possible } [O_2] - \text{minimum possible } [O_2]}$$

$$= \frac{\text{Capillary } [O_2] - \text{Actual } [O_2]}{\text{Capillary } [O_2] - \text{Mixed venous } [O_2]}$$

If ALL flow through shunt $\dfrac{Q_S}{Q_T} = \dfrac{1}{1} = 1$

If NO flow through shunt $\dfrac{Q_S}{Q_T} = \dfrac{0}{1} = 0$

BOHR EQUATION

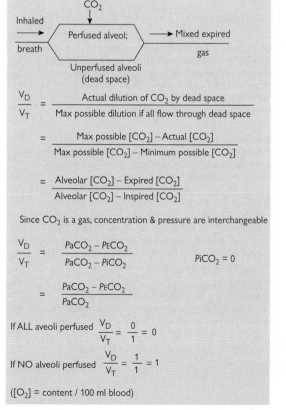

$$\frac{V_D}{V_T} = \frac{\text{Actual dilution of } CO_2 \text{ by dead space}}{\text{Max possible dilution if all flow through dead space}}$$

$$= \frac{\text{Max possible } [CO_2] - \text{Actual } [CO_2]}{\text{Max possible } [CO_2] - \text{Minimum possible } [CO_2]}$$

$$= \frac{\text{Alveolar } [CO_2] - \text{Expired } [CO_2]}{\text{Alveolar } [CO_2] - \text{Inspired } [CO_2]}$$

Since CO_2 is a gas, concentration & pressure are interchangeable

$$\frac{V_D}{V_T} = \frac{PaCO_2 - PeCO_2}{PaCO_2 - PiCO_2} \qquad PiCO_2 = 0$$

$$= \frac{PaCO_2 - PeCO_2}{PaCO_2}$$

If ALL aveoli perfused $\dfrac{V_D}{V_T} = \dfrac{0}{1} = 0$

If NO alveoli perfused $\dfrac{V_D}{V_T} = \dfrac{1}{1} = 1$

([O_2] = content / 100 ml blood)

Fig. 13.43 The shunt and Bohr equations are constructed on the same principles. [O_2] = content / 100ml blood.

Causes of tissue hypoxia

As seen with the oxygen cascade, PO_2 falls in a stepwise manner from the atmosphere to the mitochondria (Section 13.11).

The PO_2 of alveolar gas is only 66% of dry air at sea level. As we have already seen, this is because alveolar PO_2 represents a balance between oxygen removal and replenishment. Consumption varies little at rest, so PaO_2 is affected mainly by alveolar ventilation and FiO_2.

V/Q mismatch and shunts further reduce arterial PO_2 and by the end capillary, PO_2 will have fallen to approximately 5kPa as a result of diffusion into cells. Diffusion deficits do not affect the transfer of oxygen into the blood in health.

With a mitochondrial PO_2 of <1kPa, any upstream problem will cause significant cellular effects. These upstream problems include:

- Hypoxic hypoxia: low Hb saturation (see below)
- Anaemic hypoxia: reduction in functioning Hb
- Stagnant hypoxia: failure of sufficient blood to reach the tissues
- Histotoxic hypoxia: inability of the tissues to utilize oxygen.

Hypoxic hypoxia

- Reduced FiO_2
- Hypoventilation
- V/Q mismatch (including shunt; Figure 13.44)
- Diffusion abnormalities
- Low mixed venous oxygen content.

Interruption of the integrity of the process of ventilation may occur at any point and involve the sensors, effectors, or controllers.

Hypoventilation and apnoea

Hypoventilation will cause both hypoxia and hypercarbia (Section 13.2). Increasing FiO_2 will improve this hypoxia. These changes are described by the alveolar gas equation:

$$PaO_2 = PiO_2 - \left(\frac{PaCO_2}{R}\right)$$

During marked hypoventilation, the diffusion gradient from blood to alveolus is quickly lost and CO_2 accumulates at the rate of 0.5kPa/min with a concomitant respiratory acidosis. There is inter-individual variation in the rate of Hb desaturation with hypoventilation. Once desaturation starts, the descent is steep, especially with reduced FRC, inadequate pre-oxygenation, or increased oxygen consumption.

Apnoea

At the onset of apnoea, the balance of gas exchange alters radically. The massive reserves of CO_2 rest in solution within the body, unable to leave because the alveolar PCO_2 no longer provides a diffusion gradient. Only a few millilitres per minute enter the alveoli.

Alveolar oxygen is removed constantly from the alveoli at its usual rate (250ml/min) during apnoea. Provided that the airway remains patent, gas applied at the mouth is drawn passively into the lungs to replace oxygen lost to the blood. Thus, application, via a mask, of 100% O_2 will increase the duration of apnoea tolerated. An added advantage is that the supplied oxygen will only be drawn to perfused alveoli.

With an obstructed airway, hypoxia develops due to:

- Lack of passive inhalation.
- Thoracic depressurization: gas is continually removed from the alveoli, but if there is nothing to replace it, intra-alveolar pressure must decrease (absorption atelectasis). This will affect PaO_2 and the diffusion gradient into the blood.

Other clinical considerations of apnoea include the following.

- High FiO_2 is associated with absorption atelectasis: this risk is increased with anaesthesia, when the FRC is less than in the awake state.
- Inhalational anaesthesia cannot be maintained during apnoea.
- Exhaled gas monitoring is impossible.
- If the airway appears obstructed and the patient is desaturating, remember to apply 100% O_2 via mask whilst attempting to re-establish airway patency. There may be some diffusion to the alveoli.

Diffusion abnormalities

There is a very small difference in PO_2 between the alveolus and the pulmonary capillary. This is almost unmeasurable in health, but becomes apparent during exercise or with illness (Section 13.11).

The effect of pre-oxygenation

Inhaling 100% O_2 prior to induction will replace the nitrogen removed from the alveoli with oxygen. Additionally, if hyperventilation occurs during pre-oxygenation, PaO_2 will be increased (this is a small effect).

The FRC (breathing air) contains approximately 250ml O_2 at rest, enough for 1min of O_2 consumption. With pre-oxygenation, the volume of oxygen within the lungs rises to over 1.8L. Pre-oxygenation produces no significant increase in the oxygen content of any other tissue, including blood.

Usually patients are asked to breathe 100% O_2 via a tight-fitting face mask for at least 3min, with normal respiratory rate and volume. Eight vital capacity breaths have been shown to be equivalent in efficacy. Infants may be pre-oxygenated more rapidly (within 1min) because of their greater ratio of minute volume to FRC.

The adequacy of pre-oxygenation can only be objectively assessed by analysis of expired gas. The aim is to increase the ETO_2 to ≥90%. Estimation of haemoglobin saturation is not a guide to efficacy of pre-oxygenation, as full saturation will be achieved long before the lungs have adequately de-nitrogenated.

Respiratory equations

The A–a gradient

The alveolar–arterial (A–a) gradient is the difference in PO_2 between alveolar and arterial blood:

$$\text{A–a gradient} = PaO_2 - PaO_2.$$

It is mainly affected by V/Q mismatch (including shunting). Rarely, it may be affected by diffusion abnormality, e.g. fibrosing alveolitis.

In healthy young adults in the erect posture, the A–a gradient is usually <1kPa. It is due to the normal scatter of V/Q abnormalities plus true anatomical shunts.

The shunt equation

The shunt equation accurately describes how much *true* shunt would be required to account for the observed degree of oxygenation defect. In real life, lung units of high and low V/Q ratio all affect oxygenation: the calculated degree of true shunt is unlikely to be actually present, since V/Q spread mimics the effect.

The Bohr equation (Section 13.4)

This demonstrates how much dead space would be required to explain the reduction in mixed CO_2 content of expired gas, compared with alveolar gas.

Although the lungs contain many different V/Q ratio units, $PaCO_2$ will be equal to $PACO_2$ as CO_2 is so diffusible. The spread of V/Q ratios will not affect the accuracy of the Bohr equation's estimate of physiological dead space.

Table 13.4 Causes and treatment of hypoxia: all physiological abnormalities should be considered

Potential causes	Physiological problem	Treatment strategies
↓ alveolar O_2	• ↓ FiO_2, e.g. altitude • Hypoventilation	• ↑ FiO_2, ↑ ventilation
Intrinsic lung disease	• V/Q mismatching • Shunting • Diffusion problems	• ↑ FiO_2 • PEEP, CPAP • Prone positioning • Treatment of underlying problem, e.g. pulmonary oedema drainage of pleural fluid or gas • Optimization of CO
↓ mixed venous O_2 content	• ↓ O_2 delivery due to • Low cardiac output (this magnifies the effects of low V/Q ratio and shunt) • Low Hb • ↑ O_2 consumption	• ↑ FiO_2 • Optimization of [Hb] • Optimization of CO • ↓ O_2 consumption, e.g. paralysis

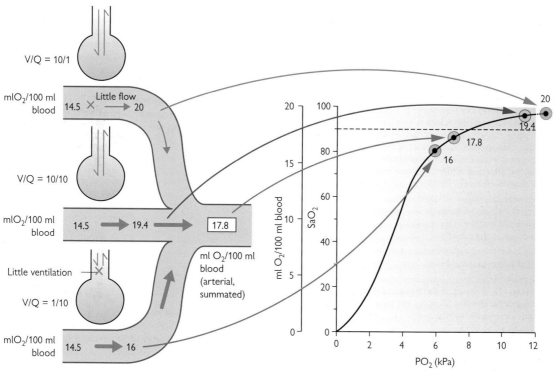

Fig. 13.44 The effect of increasing FiO_2 on the PO_2 of blood leaving lung units with different V/Q ratios: high V/Q (10/1); equal V/Q (10/10); low V/Q (1/10). Shunts will not increase oxygen levels and their capillary blood will continue to resemble mixed venous. Very low V/Q ratio units will increase O_2 content in post-pulmonary capillary blood. Units with a high V/Q ratio will increase O_2 content slightly, mainly as dissolved O_2. Administering oxygen cannot increase the O_2 content of unventilated units; hence hypoxia due to shunt will not imporve simply by increasing FiO_2.

Diving physiology

Pressure increases by 1atm for every 10m of descent. Gases follow Boyle's law and are compressible. With increasing depth and total pressure, the partial pressure increases (Dalton's Law) and with it, the amount of gas dissolved in the blood (Henry's Law).

Diving reflex

This reflex follows immersion: HR slows, there is selective vasoconstriction, and the subject becomes temporarily apnoeic.

Immersion alters the external hydrostatic pressure gradient across vessels of the peripheries, resulting in less peripheral pooling of blood. The increased venous return increases SV and CO and causes stimulation of both low- and high-pressure baroreceptors. Diuresis results from a reduction in ADH secretion and increased ANP secretion.

Hyperbaric effects on the respiratory system

Whilst treading water, breathing normally through the mouth, residual volume and FRC are reduced and work of breathing is increased. Alveolar pressure approximates to atmospheric pressure and the hydrostatic effects of the water oppose the outward movement of the chest wall. This effect is more pronounced with a snorkel, which is only safe to use when less than 1m long (i.e. breathing at atmospheric pressure at a depth of less than 1m). Beyond this, dead space also becomes excessive.

At greater depth and pressure the volume of a fixed mass of gas within the lungs will reduce in accordance with Boyle's law. Excessive reduction of alveolar volume may result in pulmonary oedema or haemorrhage. Problems may also develop during ascent from a dive breathing compressed gases. With the reducing pressure of ascent, lung gas (and volume) expands and failure to exhale this increased volume would cause alveolar rupture.

Breathing compressed gases at depth increases the density and turbulence of the gases, increases airway resistance, and results in increased work of breathing. This is partially offset by using helium, which is less dense, as the carrier gas.

During a dive, the resulting high P_AN_2 increases the pressure gradient governing its diffusion into the blood. Some tissues (e.g. fat) have a large storage capacity for N_2.

At high pressures, N_2 dissolved in the tissues adversely affects membrane and ion-channel function. Clinically, the diver is seen to become less dexterous with reduced mental agility.

Decompression sickness

With rapid ascent, the removal of N_2 from the lungs is insufficient and bubbles form in the tissues, causing significant morbidity. CNS bubble formation produces neurological defects such as blindness and deafness, and gaseous distention of joint tissues causes abnormal posture, known as the bends. The formation of large gas bubbles in the pulmonary circulation is known as the 'chokes'.

Oxygen toxicity

Pulmonary oedema and haemorrhage are associated with breathing very high PiO_2 and occur more quickly with increasing oxygen tension. Symptoms develop within 5hr of breathing a PiO_2 of 200kPa.

Sinus and middle ear pain

Air-filled cavities are subject to the effects of increased pressure at depth. If the pressure is not equalized across the cavity boundary, tissue tension will cause pain for the diver. Raising intra-pharyngeal pressure by swallowing or nose blowing helps reduce pain.

Other effects of diving

Communication is difficult, with low levels of natural light and attenuation of hearing. Hypothermia rapidly develops as water temperature drops and heat conduction from the body is rapid.

Altitude medicine

Ambient pressure falls exponentially with increasing altitude: the ambient pressure at 5800m is half that at the Earth's surface. PiO_2 falls similarly as the O_2 concentration remains constant. A number of physiological responses help humans acclimatize to altitude.

CVS effects

Increased sympathetic activity increases HR and SV very soon (hours) after ascent. However, within a few days, SV falls and CO returns to pre-ascent levels. This reduction in SV reduces the maximum CO attained during exercise.

Hyperventilation

The sensitivity of the carotid bodies increases with altitude and hypoxia stimulates peripheral chemoreceptors to induce an increase in minute volume. This is maximum by 600m, where MV is 160% of that at sea level.

Hyperventilation causes a metabolic alkalosis, which would tend to reduce MV. This effect is lessened by movement of HCO_3^- out of the CSF, which returns its pH to normal. Renal excretion of HCO_3^- further returns the pH to normal.

Hyperventilation reduces $PaCO_2$ and the alveolar gas equation predicts that PaO_2 will rise.

Hypoxic pulmonary vasoconstriction

This occurs in response to alveolar hypoxia but it is not beneficial: it results in pulmonary hypertension and increased cardiac work. Prolonged exposure to high altitude results in right ventricular hypertrophy.

Polycythaemia

Hypoxia stimulates increased renal secretion of erythropoietin, which leads to a greater red cell mass and increased oxygen-carrying capacity and tissue delivery. The downside to this is that the viscosity of the blood is also increased, leading to worsening peripheral blood flow and oxygenation.

2,3-DPG

Levels increase with metabolic alkalosis, shifting the ODC to the right with better unloading of oxygen at peripheral tissues.

Hormonal changes

There will be variable increases in secretion of catecholamines, ADH, glucocorticoids, and thyroid hormones. Circulating volume tends to increase initially, although within a week levels of ADH and aldosterone are reduced as a consequence of the increased RBC mass.

Anaesthetic considerations

- During anaesthesia, the abilty to hyperventilate is reduced with deleterious effects on PaO_2 and CSF pH.
- At altitudes above 1500m nitrous oxide provides very little anaesthetic benefit. Its MAC is very high and at altitude its partial pressure would have to be low in order to accommodate a necessarily higher FiO_2.
- Excretion of bicarbonate reduces its buffering capacity.

The actual output of the vaporizer at high altitude is

$$\text{concentration (\%)} \times P_{\text{sea level}}/P_{\text{altitude}}$$

By replacing the terms, a vaporizer set to 1% at sea level would deliver (at an ambient pressure of 630mmHg)

$$(1/100) \times 760/630 = 1.2\%$$

However, it is the vapour partial pressure and not its concentration that is important in determining the depth of anaesthetic. 1% of isoflurane at sea level translates to 7.6mmHg. 1.2% of isoflurane at 630mmHg altitude is 7.56mmHg. Regardless of altitude, the clinical effect is not changed

- Flowmeters are calibrated for sea level and gas density is altered by changes in ambient pressure.

→ The effects of breathing compressed gases at ↑depth

30 msw	Euphoria, reduced mental agility
50 msw	Loss of concentration, reduced coordination
90 msw	Loss of consciousness, nausea, dizziness

(msw = metres sea water depth)

→ Adaptation to living permanently at high altitude

- Hyperventilation is 20% less than that of an acclimatized low-level person. The advantage of this is lower energy consumption.
- The carotid bodies are hypertrophied and the response to hypoxia is blunted.
- Lung diffusing capacity is 20% greater, largely because of a greater alveolar surface area and larger pulmonary blood volume.
- Lung volumes are larger for a given size of person.
- Cardiac output at rest and during exercise is no different from someone living at sea level.
- ↑ 2,3-DPG shifts the ODC to the right.
- Exercise produces higher PA pressures, probably because of an exaggerated hypoxic pulmonary vasoconstriction response.
- Thyroid hormones and glucocorticoid levels are higher.

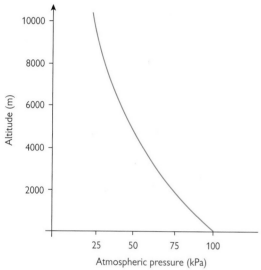

Fig. 13.45 Pressure change with altitude.

→ Acute mountain sickness

Acute mountain sickness (AMS) is the mild end of a spectrum of diseases and is defined as headache plus other symptoms including:

- gastrointestinal (anorexia, nausea or vomiting)
- fatigue or weakness
- dizziness or lightheadedness
- difficulty sleeping.

Contributing factors include the rate of ascent, the altitude attained, the amount of physical activity at high altitude, and individual susceptibility.

High-altitude cerebral oedema (HACE)

This is a severe and fatal form of cerebral oedema. It may progress rapidly and can be fatal within hours of onset.

The exact process is unknown. The hypoxia-induced cerebral vasodilatation probably causes the headache, which itself may be responsible for nausea and malaise (features of mild AMS). Alternatively, acute mountain sickness may be due to mild cerebral oedema.

The results of imaging studies suggest that all people who ascend develop cerebral oedema, although the aetiology remains obscure. Potential reasons include hypoxic alteration of the integrity of the BBB, altered autoregulation, sustained vasodilatation and elevated cerebral capillary pressure. If raised intracranial pressure is at fault, those with a greater range of compensation (e.g. greater CSF volume) should be more resistant to the development of HACE.

High-altitude pulmonary oedema (HAPE)

HAPE generally occurs within 4 days of rapid ascent to at least 2500m (8000ft). Hypoxia is the important element, causing non-cardiogenic pulmonary oedema associated with pulmonary hypertension and elevated capillary pressure. Oedema develops due to circulatory shear stress following pulmonary arterial vasoconstriction and is also associated with increased ADH secretion.

Predisposing factors include cold weather, physical exertion at high altitude, young age, and acclimatized individuals returning to high altitude following a short spell at a lower level.

The earliest signs and symptoms include decreased exercise tolerance and slow recovery, weakness, and dyspnoea on exertion. They may be tachycardic and tachypnoeic at rest, with signs of pulmonary oedema.

Other common features include low-grade fever, persistent respiratory alkalosis, and leukocytosis. The condition typically worsens at night and periodic breathing during sleep is common.

Prevention of AMS

(in those with a history of AMS)

- Avoid heavy exertion at high altitude.
- Slow ascent.
- Avoid abrupt ascent to sleeping elevations over 3000m.
- Avoid alcohol and sedatives.

Treatment

Includes rest, administration of oxygen, and descent to a lower altitude if symptoms are severe. If diagnosed early, recovery may be achieved with a descent of only 500–1000m.

A portable hyperbaric chamber or administration of supplemental oxygen reduces pulmonary artery pressure, heart rate, respiratory rate, and symptoms. Medication (e.g. nifedipine to reduce PA pressure) is only required if descent is impossible or supplemental oxygen is unavailable.

Chapter 14

Immunology

Basic cells of the immune system

Myeloid cells

Myeloid cells are derived from a common myeloid progenitor cell in bone marrow.

Neutrophils

100 billion neutrophils are produced per day by bone marrow at rest. Each is only in circulation for 6–10hr. They are activated by signals from the innate (non-adaptive) immune system.

The neutrophil is a primary phagocytic cell which envelops pathogens, and kills them within vacuoles using proteases and altered local charge conditions (which disrupt bacterial membranes).

Neutrophils also perform essential 'debris clearance' after tissue damage.

Macrophages

Macrophages (called monocytes when in the circulation) are larger, longer-lived, and more complex than neutrophils, but share their phagocytic duties.

They form a link between innate and adaptive immunity by presenting processed antigens from phagocytosed micro-organisms to lymphocytes in order to generate specific responses and memory.

Macrophages produce many protein messengers (cytokines) that activate or suppress the wider immune response.

Dendritic cells

Dendritic cells are tissue cells with complex function. They are phagocytes when immature, but antigen-presenting cells in lymph nodes when mature.

Eosinophils

Relatively few in number, eosinophils release granule contents in response to parasites that have first been coated in antibody.

Mast cells

Mast cells are present in tissue. They possess granules which contain multiple vasoactive compounds, including histamine. Granules are released in response to IgE. IgE is involved in response to parasitic infection, and acute anaphylaxis.

Basophils

These cells have an uncertain function, but share some behaviours with mast cells.

Lymphoid cells

Lymphoid cells are derived from a common lymphoid progenitor cell in bone marrow.

B lymphocytes (B cells)

B cells differentiate in **b**one marrow. They pass between the circulation and lymph nodes/spleen. After meeting specific antigen, they mature into antibody-producing *plasma cells*. The process is shown in Figure 14.2

T lymphocytes (T cells)

T cells differentiate in the **t**hymus. They circulate in a similar way to B cells. They react to specific antigen after presentation by macrophages or dendritic cells. They mature into activated *effector T cells* with a variety of possible functions depending on the amount and type of antigen, and local cytokine concentrations.

Natural killer cells (NK cells)

NK cells are activated by innate immune system, and are involved in killing virally infected cells by non-antigen-specific mechanisms.

Other immune components

Antibody

An antibody (immunoglobulin) is a specialized protein that binds to a particular target molecule, its antigen (Figure 14.1). All antibodies have a common general structure, but the antigen binding site is subject to great variation. Antibodies bind to pathogens and prime them for interaction with other cells (e.g. for phagocytosis).

Antibodies are divided into groups according to the type of heavy chain they contain. The heavy chain, in turn, determines their function.

- IgA: α heavy chains. Secreted onto mucosal surfaces.
- IgD: β heavy chains, function uncertain.
- IgE: ε heavy chains, involved in allergic and anaphylactic reactions.
- IgG: γ heavy chains, majority of plasma immunoglobulins.
- IgM: μ heavy chains, early response during acute infection.

Antigen

An antigen is any molecule that can bind specifically to an antibody (the name stems from **anti**body **gen**eration).

Antigen presenting cells

Antigen presenting cells (APCs) are specialized cells that process antigens and display peptide fragments on the cell surface, along with co-stimulatory molecules.

Cytokines

Cytokines are protein messengers released by cells, which affect the behaviour of other cells by binding to specific receptors.

A subset of cytokines that are made by lymphocytes are called lymphokines, or more commonly interleukins. A further subset involved in limiting viral replication are called interferons. Other examples include tumour necrosis factor (TNF), and granulocyte colony-stimulating factor (GCSF).

Cytokines may induce activation, suppression, differentiation, cell death, or other changes in target cells.

Chemokines

Chemokines (from **chemo**tactic cyto**kines**) form a subset of cytokine protein messengers; released by cells, that attract other cells carrying chemokine receptors. Examples include interleukin-8 and C5a.

Phagocytosis

Phagocytosis refers to the ingestion of particulate matter, predominantly by neutrophils and macrophages. Bacteria are ingested in this way, initially into a vesicle called a phagosome. The phagosome then fuses with other intracellular vesicles containing proteases and other substances that destroy its contents.

Inflammation

Inflammation describes a non-specific response to injury or infection characterized by swelling, redness, heat, and pain at the site of injury.

Major histocompatibility complex

The major histocompatibility complex (MHC) is a cluster of genes on chromosome 6 coding for cell surface glycoproteins (MHC molecules). Class 1 and 2 molecules are the sites of presentation of antigen on APCs (Figure 14.3). The system is known as HLA (human lymphocyte antigen) in humans.

- MHC class I contains three genes called HLA-A, HLA-B, and HLA-C. Proteins from these genes are expressed on all nucleated cells.
- MHC class II genes are called HLA-DR, HLA-DQ, and HLA-DP. MHC class II genes are expressed on B cells, APCs, and macrophages. They present different types of antigen to lymphocytes, and stimulate different components of the adaptive immune response.

The function of the MHC system of glycoproteins is to present fragments of antigens to T cells. T-cell receptors (TCRs) can only recognize antigen fragments in complex with MHC proteins.

T-cell receptor

The T-cell recepter (TCR) is an antigen-specific molecule on the surface of a T lymphocyte which recognizes specific peptides presented to it in combination with MHC class I or II molecules. If co-stimulatory molecules are also present, the lymphocyte will become activated. T cells are sometimes characterized by the subtypes of chains in the TCR: α:β or γ:δ.

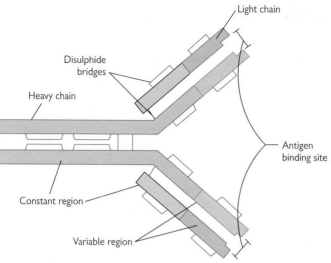

Fig. 14.1 Antibody structure demonstrating the relationship between light and heavy chains, and the antigen binding site.

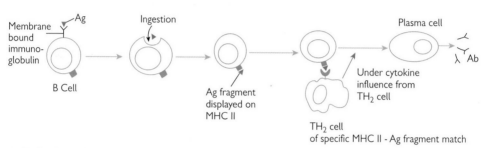

Fig. 14.2 A naive B cell with membrane-bound immunoglobulin which matches its antigen (Ag). The Ag is ingested by the cell, following which fragments are displayed on the cell surface via MHC II molecules. When this complex binds with its specific matching TH-2 cell, the latter releases cytokines that induce maturation of the B cell into a plasma cell. This produces the antibody that matches the original antigen; the resulting Ab–Ag complexes are cleared by the spleen and liver.

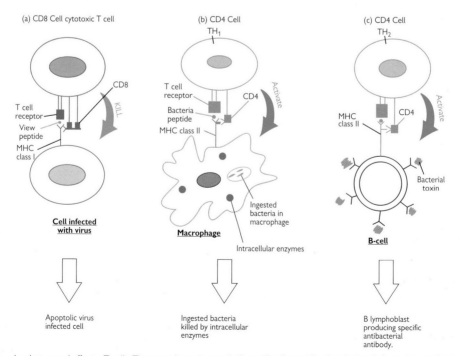

Fig. 14.3 MHC molecule type and effector T-cells. There are three classes of effector T cell, specialized to deal with three classes of pathogen. (a) CD8 (cytotoxic) cells kill target cells that display peptide fragments of cytosolic pathogens, notably viruses, bound to MHC class I molecules at the cell surface. CD4 cells are T 'helper' cells which may be (b) TH$_1$ or (c) TH$_2$. Both express the CD4 co-receptor and recognize fragments of antigens degraded within intracellular vesicles, displayed at the cell surface by MHC class II molecules. TH$_1$ cells activate macrophages, enabling them to destroy intracellular micro-organisms more efficiently. TH$_2$ cells drive B cells to differentiate and produce immunoglobulins.

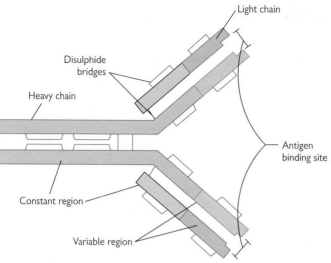

The immune system is extraordinarily complex, but is essentially a mechanism for recognizing 'self' from 'non-self' and trying to mount an appropriate response. Here 'self' means the host or patient, and 'non-self' means anything else: bacteria, viruses, fungi, or other foreign material.

The innate immune system

The innate immune system is the first line of defence against micro-organisms once physical barriers (e.g. skin) are breached. It is present from birth, and provides a response that is not specific to a particular pathogen.

The innate immune system developed very early in evolution and exists even in very simple organisms. The key concept in innate immunity is the recognition of 'danger signals'—patterns of molecules that are typically found in pathogenic micro-organisms (pathogen-associated molecular patterns (PAMPs)). When these are found, prompt killing mechanisms are activated.

The molecular basis for the innate immune system is being increasingly understood. For example, the process by which the 'danger signal' of Gram-negative endotoxin is recognized by multiple cell types (via Toll-like receptor 4) has recently been elucidated.

Complement cascade

The complement cascade is an example of an innate immune pathway (Figure 14.5). Three pathways (the classical, alternative and lecitin pathways) are able to activate this system. Each results in the formation of a protein complex (the 'membrane attack complex' (MAC)) on the surface of micro-organisms, and production of potent signals of inflammation and phagocyte recruitment (chemokines) and molecules that prime for phagocytosis (opsonins). The MAC causes micro-organism lysis and cell death, and the attracted phagocytes assist in this process and clear up the cellular debris.

The three pathways differ in the activation steps.
- The classical pathway requires antibody.
- The alternative and lectin pathways are activated directly by the presence of different PAMPs.

Once activation has occurred there is a common pathway centred on the activation of complement protein 3 (C3) and the MAC, formed from complement proteins 5–9.

Mannose-binding lectin

Mannose-binding lectin (MBL) is a liver-derived plasma protein that recognizes repeating sugar arrays on the surface of many micro-organisms, and activates complement in an antibody-independent fashion. It is important in the response to many common infections.

Plasma levels are determined to a large degree by very common structural gene (and promoter) polymorphism mutations. About a third of the UK population are deficient in MBL, with 10% having a profound deficiency. This is important because children and adults with low MBL levels are at increased risk of systemic inflammation and sepsis, and may have an increased risk of death in intensive care.

The adaptive immune system

The adaptive immune system is responsible for the specific responses to an individual pathogen and the generation of targeted immunological memory. This is the vital process utilized by immunizations, by which subsequent exposure to the same pathogen is more readily handled by the immune system. Adaptive immunity involves the generation of both specific antibodies and specific lymphocytes against pathogens following immunization or infection, so that the contribution of adaptive immunity to protection of the host increases with time and 'immunological experience'.

Linkage of the two systems

While adaptive and innate immunity are typically considered separately, there are numerous points at which they link.

For example, the early destruction of pathogens via the innate response is a stage towards the essential initiating step for adaptive immunity of controlled processing and display of bacterial or viral proteins called 'antigen presentation'. Dendritic cells become activated and phagocytose micro-organisms in inflamed tissues as part of the innate response. They subsequently migrate to local lymph nodes, where they present antigen to lymphocytes and provide stimuli for antigen-specific lymphocyte activation.

Local inflammation also provides signals that recruit macrophages and neutrophils. Once these macrophages are activated, they in turn produce cytokines that accelerate the recruitment to the tissues of the activated antigen-specific lymphocytes produced in response to the antigen presentation.

The separation between innate and adaptive immunity has become even less distinct recently as populations of T-cells that can recognize antigen directly, termed γ:T-cells, have been recognized.

The CD4 subset of T-lymphocytes are activated in this way and differentiate into one of two forms known as TH_1 or TH_2 cells. The choice between TH_1 and TH_2 is determined by many factors, including the type of antigen being attacked and also the relative concentrations of different cytokines produced by the antigen presenting cells.

This distinction is important because TH_1 cells are predominantly involved in causing further macrophage activation and lymphocyte-mediated killing of (particularly virally) infected cells (the cytotoxic response).

In contrast, TH_2 responses are predominantly responsible for accelerating the production of antibody from B cells (also termed the humoral response). A balanced response involving both TH_1 and TH_2 cells may be optimal, and excessive skewing of the adaptive response to either TH_1 or TH_2 is associated with disease processes. Autoimmune diseases such as multiple sclerosis and psoriasis are now thought to reflect, in part, an excess of TH_1 responses over TH_2 responses, while others, including systemic lupus erythematosus, may be associated with an excessive TH_2 response.

Generation of diversity

One of the great achievements of the adaptive immune system is the seemingly impossible state of having specific antibodies and T cells 'waiting in the wings' (lymph nodes) that are directed against antigens that the host has not yet encountered. The number of antibody specificities that can be generated by an individual is estimated at 10^{11} or greater. This is far greater than the number of genes in the human genome ($3-5 \times 10^5$). This is achieved by:
- Combinatorial diversity
- Junctional diversity
- Somatic hypermutation.

These processes occur in the developing B or T lymphocytes in production of the proteins that form the various chains of antibody or T-cell receptor.

In summary, genes for the antigen binding sites of antibodies (or TCRs) exist in groups, and only one of each group is randomly chosen in the process of creating a product from that germline DNA. For example, the immunoglobulin heavy chains have 40 functional gene elements to choose from in the variable (V) region, 25 in the diversity (D) region, and six in the smaller joining region. Any one of these three is chosen. This 'gene rearrangement' is one component of the combinational diversity.

Junctional diversity is an additional process whereby the joints between these recombinations have nucleotides added or subtracted. Further combinatorial diversity is generated by the various pairs of chains required to complete an antibody molecule. Finally, the vulnerability of the 'variable' regions of these genes to point mutuations, especially in activated B-lymphocytes, may further refine antigen binding. This final stage is called somatic hypermutation.

T-cell receptor diversity is less than that of antibodies, because their gene sequences do not undergo somatic hypermutation.

> ### ➜ Features of innate and adaptive immunity
>
> #### Innate immune system
> * Older phylogenetically—present in all multicellular organisms
> * Present from birth
> * Immediate, non-specific response
> * No memory
> * Cellular components—phagocytic system (monocytes, macrophages, dendritic cells) and natural killer cells
>
> #### Adaptive immune system
> * Evolved later—present only in vertebrates
> * Learned responses with exposure to antigens
> * Slower but pathogen- and antigen-specific response
> * Memory specific to antigen
> * Cellular components—T and B lymphocytes

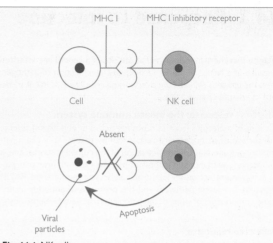

Fig. 14.4 NK cells.

NK cells are cytotoxic lymphocytes derived from the lymphoid stem cell. They are an important component of the innate immune system. After releasing perforins and granzymes, the cells die from apoptosis. Recent advances suggest that these cells require activation prior to their killing (Figure 14.7).

NK cells also have a role in humoral immunity: antibody-coated cells are targeted for destruction via Fc receptors on the NK surface.

Another important action is the destruction of cells with poor expression of MHC class I proteins. Tumours cells and cells that contain microbes classically downregulate MHC class I protein expression, thus reducing the ability of CD4 and CD8 cells to attack. NK cells counter this (Figure 14.9).

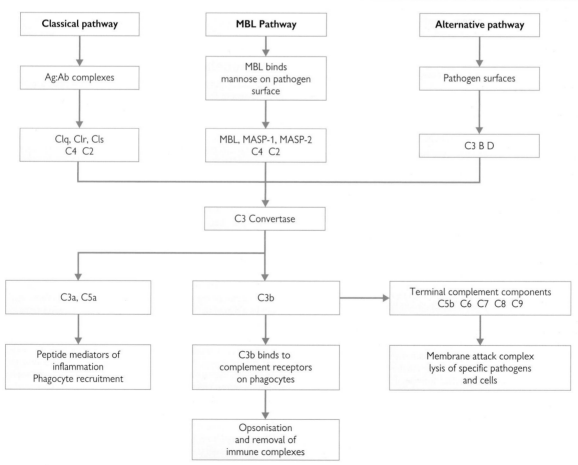

Fig. 14.5 Complement activation pathways. MBL = mannose-binding lectin; MASP = MBL-associated serine protease.

14.3 Response to infection

Imagine that the skin is breached at the site of a central line insertion. Because of a failure of sterile technique, a combination of pathogens from the patient's skin and the overworked anaesthetist's hands passes into the tissues (Figure 14.6).

The first response: the innate immune system

Patterns of molecules (such as repeating sugars or endotoxin) seen on the surface of pathogens are recognized by receptors in the innate immune system. This triggers activation of the complement cascade. In our scenario with multiple pathogens it is likely that all three pathways of complement activation take place, reflecting the different PAMPs (classical and lectin pathway) and the presence of antibody against some components of some of the pathogens that have been previously encountered.

Adaptive response

In addition, activation of phagocytic cells (neutrophils, macrophages, and dendritic cells) occurs directly by recognition of pathogen via their own pattern recognition receptors, and indirectly in response to products of complement activation. Pro-inflammatory cytokines and chemokines are produced, causing swelling, heat, redness, and pain at the site of line insertion, and calling more inflammatory cells to the site of infection.

Phagocytosis causes destruction of the bacteria, and in macrophages and dendritic cells leads to dissection of the bacteria into short peptide fragments that are then presented as antigens to lymphocytes. The process of antigen processing and presentation is highly complex and carefully controlled.

Pathogen-derived peptides are presented as antigens on the surface of APCs by complex molecules—MHC class I or II. Different types of antigens are presented with each:

- MHC class I presents pathogens degraded in APC cytosol (e.g. viruses).
- MHC class II presents pathogens degraded in vesicles.

This distinction is important because the form of antigen presentation is a major factor in determining the nature of the subsequent adaptive immune response.

The MHC molecules themselves are highly variable in structure, and so the target lymphocytes that recognize presented antigen are actually specific for both the presented peptide and the individual MHC molecule. This is termed MHC restriction.

An antigen presented with MHC class I will tend to activate cytotoxic (CD8) T cells, whereas MHC class II will activate CD4 cells. These CD4 cells then develop into either TH_1 or TH_2 types, activating either macrophages and cytotoxic responses (TH_1) or B cells and antibody production (TH_2) as described above (Figure 14.7).

While antigen and MHC recognition are essential steps, they are not sufficient for T-cell activation in isolation. The T cell also has to receive a 'co-stimulatory' signal from the APC in order for activation to go ahead. This is typically in the form of exposure of molecules (called B7.1 and B7.2) on the APC surface to a counter-receptor, CD28, on the lymphocyte.

These combinations of T-lymphocyte-controlled steps mean that additional reinforcements are recruited to the site of our central line. The various different pathogens are cleared by a combination of specific antibody (initially IgM but later IgG) activated macrophages and specific cytoxic T cells. As this response fades and neutrophils clear up all the cellular debris, the adaptive immune system 'files away' small numbers of the specific B and T cells that reacted against these antigens, so that it can readily access them again in the event of similar threat in future.

The description above is obviously only a brief summary, but it does highlight the central role of the antigen presentation step in regulating the specificity and nature of the adaptive immune response. Two extreme clinical examples highlight what happens when this process escapes from the normal control mechanisms.

Toxic shock syndrome

Toxic shock syndrome (TSS) is acute severe illness characterized by high fever, diffuse red rash, hypotension, and evidence of organ dysfunction (diarrhoea, transaminitis, thrombocytopenia, uraemia, CNS disturbance). There is also late desquamation of hands and feet 1–2 weeks later. Hypotension may be profound, and many features are shared with sepsis-induced multiple-organ failure.

The causative agents are molecules termed 'super-antigens'. These are exotoxins, most often secreted from Gram-positive bacteria, that cause direct T-cell activation. These proteins cross-link the MHC II molecule and T-cell receptors, regardless of specificity. Treatment is supportive, and includes pooled immunoglubin to accelerate removal of the super-antigen.

The 2006 clinical trial of a monoclonal antibody to CD28

CD28 is the T-lymphocyte receptor for the co-stimulatory stimulus from APCs (see above). This molecule 'TGN1412' was developed as a 'super-agonist' to CD28, meaning that it activated T cells in the absence of the MHC + antigen binding to the TCR, i.e. in a non-specific and unregulated way.

The hope had been to develop a strategy to mitigate autoimmune and immunodeficiency disease, but what actually happened was dramatic and unselective widespread T-cell activation termed a 'cytokine storm'.

All six healthy male volunteers became critically ill, with pyrexia, tachycardia, erythroderma and severe vasodilatation, and capillary leak with hypotension. All developed respiratory distress, and one developed overt acute respiratory distress syndrome. All eventually survived.

These two examples illustrate the power of the adaptive immune response; but also the extent to which the complex control mechanisms of MHC restriction and need for co-stimulatory signals hold this process in check very effectively in the majority of circumstances.

Recognition of a patient with an immunodeficiency

An increasing number of patients are unable to mount a normal immune response because of congenital or acquired immunodeficiences or therapeutic immunosuppression. This increase has resulted from improved survival from such conditions, and the wider use of immunosuppressive medications.

The suspicion or recognition of immunodeficiency or immunosuppression is usually gleaned from a drug history or analysis of a full blood count.

- Neutropenia ($<1.0 \times 10^9$/ml) from bone marrow failure, most often associated with chemotherapy, is an important finding. It significantly worsens the risk from any episode of infection. For example, during treatment for childhood leukaemia, deaths from septic shock are now as common as deaths from the primary disease, with case fatality rates of around 10–15%, much higher than those seen in healthy hosts.

- Less well recognized is the potential importance of severe lymphopenia ($<1.0 \times 10^9$/ml). While this is a frequent finding during acute viral infections, it can also be an indicator of untreated or severe acquired immunodeficiency syndrome. In young infants, it can be a sign of one of the many causes of congenital severe combined immunodeficiency syndrome. If such a diagnosis is suspected, specialist advice should be sought.

The risks of immunodeficiency or immunosuppression are the rapid onset and increased severity of common infections. Patients on high-dose steroids with septicaemia may not display pyrexia, so even minor symptoms warrant investigation.

A further risk is from 'opportunistic infections'—disease attributable to organisms that are non-pathogenic to a healthy host. A good example is *Pneumocytis jirovecii* pneumonia, which is widely recognized as an AIDS-defining illness but is also seen in many immunodeficient and immunosuppressed states.

Patients who are critically ill with sepsis, trauma, or burns, or following major surgery—especially involving cardio-pulmonary bypass—often have evidence of reduced immune function. A major deficit is often seen in the ability of macrophages/monocytes to produce inflammatory signals in response to danger signals such as endotoxin. This state of 'monocyte deactivation' or 'acquired immunoparalysis' greatly increases the risk of nosocomial infection and poor outcome. It can be recognized by fall in surface expression of the HLA–DR complex.

Therapies for acquired immunoparalysis are the subject of many current studies. The immunomodulatory amino acid glutamine is a potential treatment. Persistent lymphopenia during a period of critical

illness is an additional risk factor for nosocomial infection and death in both adults and children.

Reduced secretions of the pituitary hormone prolactin have been implicated in accelerated lymphoid cell death and lymphopenia. Some combination of glutamine, cytokines, trace metals, and prolactin secretagogues may be employed as immunomodulators in the future, but currently no recommendations can be made other than to recognize the very high risk of nosocomial infection for any critically ill patient. The simple physical barriers to infection must be restored by removing indwelling devices, such as vascular and urinary catheters and endotracheal tubes, as soon as practicable.

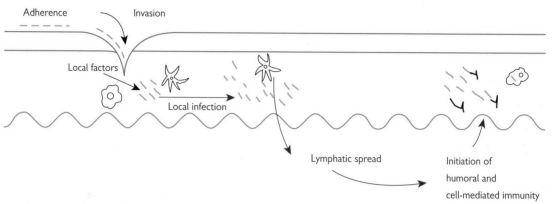

Fig. 14.6 The sequence of events leading to infection. Bacteria first adhere to the skin surface. Following penetration of the epithelium, the bacteria are destroyed by a combination of local factors including antimicrobial peptides, phagocytosis, and complement activation. If this is insufficient, local infection ensues and the immune response is stepped up: further complement activation, stimulation of macrophages, and production of cytokines. NK cells perform innate immunity functions. Dendritic cells follow bacteria to the lymphoid tissue, and there the microbes are phagocytosed. Adaptive immunity is initiated and infection cleared by a combination of specific antibody, cytotoxic T cells, and T-cell-dependent macrophage activation.

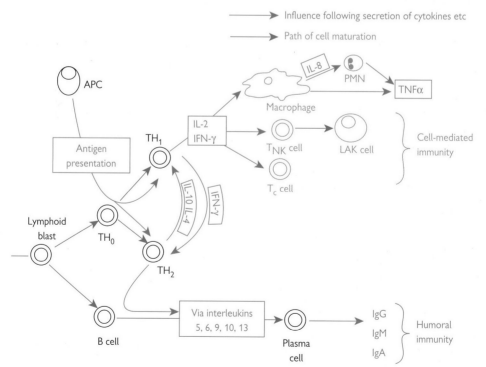

Fig. 14.7 T-lymphocyte differentiation. A major subset of T cells (CD4 cells) are directed to mature in one of two ways according to the nature of the antigen presented to them by macrophages or dendritic cells and the local pattern of cytokines:

- TH_1 maturation supports a series of cell-mediated cytotoxic mechanisms including activation of cytotoxic (T_C, CD8) T cells and NK cells (T_{NK}). There are further stimuli to macrophage and neutrophil activation. Target cell death here is typically achieved by induced apoptosis, which does not perpetuate local inflammation.
- TH_2 maturation leads to production of mediators, which direct B lymphocytes to mature to plasma cells and to produce antibody. Target cell death here is typically by lysis, and may cause further local inflammation.

An immune response that has components of both TH_1 and TH_2 may be most effective.

Acquired immune deficiency syndrome (AIDS) was recognized in 1981, and the causative agent, human immunodeficiency virus (HIV), was first isolated in 1983. Current theory is that the virus was first passed from chimpanzees to humans in the early part of the twentieth century. Human immunodeficiency viruses are now classified as HIV-1 and HIV-2. HIV-1 is more virulent and causes the majority of clinical cases of AIDS.

The majority of the >40 million people infected with HIV viruses live in sub-Saharan Africa, although infection rates are increasing rapidly throughout Asia. The long latent period between infection and symptoms means that many of those who are infected are unaware.

Pathogenesis

HIV is an enveloped, double-stranded RNR virus. It uses a viral enzyme, reverse transcriptase (RT), to transcribe RNA into DNA that becomes integrated in the host cell genome. Infection occurs from contact with blood, semen, vaginal fluid, or breast milk. The target cells in the host are CD4 T cells (and some antigen presenting cells). HIV surface proteins bind to the CD4 molecules and other co-receptor on the host cell surface, often chemokine receptors such as CCR5 on macrophages or CXCR4 on lymphocytes. Different forms of the HIV virus bind to different co-receptors and follow a slightly different clinical course. The importance of this co-receptor mechanism is evident in the fact that some individuals are naturally resistant to HIV infection by virtue of a mutation of CCR5. Around 10% of Europeans are heterozygous and 1% are homozygous for this allele.

Most patients are clinically unwell with a flu-like illness during the primary viraemic phase which occurs within a few weeks of exposure. At this point, CD4 cell counts fall sharply as the virus replicates before adaptive responses are mounted. Cytotoxic T-lymphocyte and antibody responses then reduce the levels of circulating virus, and CD4 counts recover to a variable degree. Patients with lower levels of detectable virus after primary infection have a more favourable subsequent course.

HIV continues to replicate during this latent period, continually eroding immune function and reducing numbers of CD4 cells remaining. Typically, AIDS is seen some 2–15 years later with the development of opportunistic infection or malignancy.

Diagnosis

The standard method for diagnosis of HIV infection remains an ELISA for anti-HIV antibody. Modern forms of these tests are highly sensitive and can detect the different forms of the virus (HIV-1, HIV-2, and subtypes). However, ELISA alone cannot rule out early infection because a patient may not yet have 'seroconverted' (changed from antibody negative to antibody positive).

Seroconversion follows the viraemic phase (Figure 14.8) and this may occur weeks, or rarely months, after exposure. This 'diagnostic window' is a particular problem: patients who are infected but not yet seropositive are typically highly infectious because of the viraemia.

Direct testing for elements of the virus
ELISA for p24 antigen and PCR for HIV RNA offer a way to shorten the diagnostic window, and are being used more frequently in conjunction with antibody testing. Repeat testing is required to definitively exclude HIV in high-risk cases, e.g. in the child of an HIV postive mother.

Treatment

The management of HIV infection is now focused much less on the care of opportunistic infections and malignancies than on direct treatment of the HIV infection itself. The aim to slow or prevent the immune consequences, including loss of CD4 cells, has been achieved with remarkable success in areas where highly active anti-retroviral therapy (HAART) is available. One recent estimate equated the impact of a new diagnosis of HIV on life expectancy with a new diagnosis of insulin-dependent diabetes. This is a dramatic change in the last 25 years. Therefore there are increasing numbers of patients surviving on complex combinations of anti-retroviral drugs. Many of these have important side effects that are of relevance to anaesthetic and intensive care staff, including mitochondrial toxicity. Some of these drugs are summarized in Table 14.1.

Needlestick injuries

All healthcare workers need to be aware of the risks and procedures when a 'needlestick' injury occurs. Recognition of these risks and the development of 'self-sheathing needles' have reduced, but not eliminated, this problem. Needlestick injuries from HIV-positive patients are of particular importance because of the efficacy of post-exposure prophylaxis.

The risk of HIV transmission increases with:
- A deep injury
- An injury with a needle that has been in a patient's blood vessel
- Presence of visible blood on the instrument that breeched the skin
- Injury from a patient with advanced disease or a high viral load.

However, the overall risk for HIV transmission from percutaneous exposure is around 1 in 300.

Immediately following ANY exposure, whether or not the source is known to pose a risk of infection, the site of exposure (e.g. wound or non-intact skin) should be washed liberally with soap and water but without scrubbing. Antiseptics and skin washes should not be used: there is no evidence of their efficacy, and their effect on local defences is unknown. Free bleeding of puncture wounds should be encouraged gently but wounds should not be sucked. Exposed mucous membranes, including conjunctivae, should be irrigated copiously with water before and after removing any contact lenses.

The exposed healthcare worker should be aware of local arrangements for access to urgent advice about occupational exposure and post-exposure prophylaxis (PEP). A risk assessment of the appropriateness of starting PEP needs to be made urgently by someone other than the exposed worker, ideally a doctor designated according to local arrangements for the provision of urgent post-exposure advice. This guidance refers only to the issue of HIV PEP. Consideration should also be given to risk of exposure to hepatitis B (if the exposed worker is not immune) and hepatitis C.

PEP should be recommended to healthcare workers if they have had a significant occupational exposure to blood or another high-risk body fluid from a patient or other source either:
- Known to be HIV infected, or
- Considered to be at high risk of HIV infection, but where the result of an HIV test has not or cannot be obtained, for whatever reason.

PEP should not be offered after exposure through any route with low-risk materials (e.g. urine, vomit, saliva, faeces) unless they are visibly bloodstained. Also, PEP should not be offered where testing has shown that the source is HIV negative, or if risk assessment has concluded that HIV infection of the source is highly unlikely.

A standard PEP regimen is to start the following within 24hr of exposure: zidovudine 250mg or 300mg BD plus lamivudine 150mg BD plus nelfinavir 1250mg BD (or 750mg TDS).

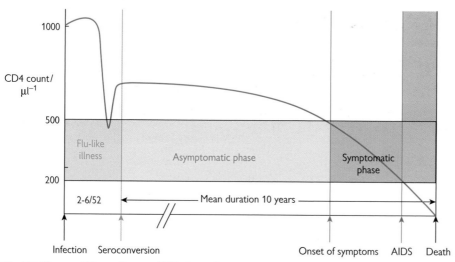

Fig. 14.8 The natural history of untreated HIV infection. Initial infection is followed by a flu-like illness, during which CD4 counts fall. As cytotoxic T-lymphocyte and antibody responses are mounted, detectable circulating virus levels fall and CD4 numbers recover. Viral replication continues, and CD4 counts slowly wane until the patient is unable to resist infection with opportunistic organisms or control the development of malignancies.

Table 14.1 Summary of antiretroviral drugs currently in use			
Trade name	**Abbreviation**	**Drug**	**Mechanism of action and consequent side effects**
Nucleoside analogues or nucleotide reverse transcriptase inhibitors			
Combivir™	CBV	AZT+3TC	Converted to active metabolites after endocytosis. Prevent normal DNA assembly by competitive inhibition with nucleotides. Combinations that target different nucleotides have additional benefit, i.e AZT (competes with thymidine) and 3TC (competes with cytidine).
Emtriva™	FTC	Emtricitabine	
Epivir™	3TC	Lamivudine	Usually well tolerated.
Kivexa/Epzicom™	KVX	3TC+ABC	GI upset; headache; fatigue. Longer term: myelotoxicity; polyneuropathy; myopathy; pancreatitis. *Mitochondrial* toxicity—often tissue specific with long high-dose use causing hepatoxicity, hyperlactataemia (15–35%), and rarely life-threatening lactic acidosis (4/1000 patient years). More frequent and severe in infants.
Retrovir™	AZT	Zidovudine	
Trizivir™	TZV	AZT+3TC+ABC	
Non-nucleoside reverse transcriptase inhibitors (NNRTIs)			
Rescriptor™	DLV	Delavirdine	Direct binding to viral reverse transcriptase near binding site—inhibition of DNA formation.
Sustiva/Stocrin™	EFV	Efavirenz	GI symptoms; rash (15–20%), can be Stevens–Johnson syndrome; liver dysfunction; CNS disturbance (especially first few days after efavirenz).
Viramune™	NVP	Nevirapine	
Protease inhibitors (PIs)			
Aptivus™	TPV	Tipranavir	Inhibits HIV protease, which forms functional viral proteins from gene products. Result is virus that cannot enter target cells and hence is non-infectious.
Agenerase™	APV	Amprenavir	GI symptoms; lipodystrophy and dyslipidemia; UDP-glucuronosyltransferase inhibition, increasing the level of bilirubin in around 50% of patients; nephrolithiasis with indinavir (~10%).
Crixivan™	IDV	Indinavir	
Invirase 500™	SQV	Saquinavir	
Fusion inhibitors			
Fuzeon™	T-20	Enfuvirtide	36 amino acid peptide given by subcutaneous injection which binds to activated form of HIV gp41-protein and inhibits fusion of HIV with the target cell. Local skin reactions at injection site.

Chapter 15

Haematology

During early fetal life, red blood cell (RBC) production occurs predominantly in the liver with some contribution from the spleen. From the fifth month *in utero*, red bone marrow starts to produce blood cells. By birth, the marrow is the main site of haematopoiesis, with lymphocyte production continuing in the spleen and other lymphoid tissue.

Bone marrow initially occupies the cavities of all bones, but from the age of 5–7 years fat begins to replace marrow in the long bones. In adults, red marrow is confined to bones of the trunk, skull, and upper ends of the humerus and femur. The iliac crests and sternum are convenient sites for bone marrow sampling.

Red blood cell production

Renal secretion of erythropoietin stimulates RBC production. Erythropoiesis requires essential dietary constituents, particularly iron, vitamin B_{12}, and folic acid. Depletion of body stores of these substances can lead to reduced or abnormal RBC production.

Erythropoietin

Erythropoietin is a 165-amino acid glycoprotein hormone. It is mainly produced in the peritubular fibroblasts of the kidney, with less than 15% produced in the liver. It acts on immature marrow erythroid cells to increase both differentiation and proliferation.

It is secreted in response to reduced oxygen delivery, and results in increased RBC production until normal tissue O_2 delivery is restored. Local hypoxia causes activation of transcription factors that stimulate mRNA synthesis by the erythropoietin gene on chromosome 7.

Erythropoietin has been synthesized by rDNA techniques and is commercially produced from mammalian cell lines. It is used therapeutically in treatment of the anaemia of chronic renal failure.

RBC structure

The mature RBC is an anucleate biconcave disc 7–8 μm in diameter, 2.5μm thick near the rim and 1 μm thick at the centre. The biconcave shape enhances the diffusion of respiratory gases by increasing surface area. It also increases RBC flexibility, allowing the cells to bend as they squeeze through narrow capillaries.

The membrane is a bipolar structure containing enzymes, antigens, and contractile and structural proteins. Carbohydrates are only present on the cell surface. Four groups of protein provide a structural lattice on the inside of the membrane.

Red cell metabolism

Without organelles, the RBC is only able to produce ATP via the Embden–Meyerhof (glycolysis) pathway (Section 17.6). Two ATP molecules are produced for every glucose molecule metabolized to lactate. Three "shunts" or branches from the Embden-Meyerhof pathway are very important in red cell metabolism (Figure 15.3): the hexose monophosphate (HMP) shunt; the Rapoport-Leubering shunt; and the methaemoglobin reductase pathway.

The HMP shunt (Figure 15.3; also Section 17.6) is also known as the pentose phosphate pathway, and is valuable to all cells. It produces NADPH, essential for the action of glutathione which in turn helps to maintain cell membrane integrity. In erythrocytes, the HMP shunt is essentially the only mechanism for NADPH production. Any defect in the pathway can have profound effects on red cell survival. The inability to produce NADPH leads to accumulation of peroxides, predominantly H_2O_2. This in turn leads to haemolysis as the cell membrane weakens. Peroxide accumulation also increases the rate of oxidation of hemoglobin to methaemoglobin, further weakening the membrane.

Glucose-6-phosphate dehydrogenase (G6PD) converts glucose-6-phosphate into 6-phosphogluco-δ-lactone, and is the rate-limiting enzyme of the HMP shunt. Deficiencies in the level of activity glucose-6-phosphate dehydrogenase (G6PD) can cause haemolytic crises in response to infection or certain foods. G6PD deficiency is, however, associated with resistance to malarial parasites. The weakening of the red cell membrane in G6PD deficiency is such that the erythrocyte cannot sustain the parasitic life cycle.

The Rapoport-Leubering shunt produces the 2,3 DPG essential for the functioning of red blood cells. 2,3 DPG decreases the affinity of haemoglobin for oxygen, regulating its supply to the tissues where it promotes unloading (along with the Bohr shift and acidotic conditions; see Section 13.12).

NADH produced by the Embden-Meyerhof pathway is required by methaemoglobin reductase for the reduction of methaemoglobin (Section 15.2) to haemoglobin. This mechanism is aptly named the methaemoglobin reductase pathway.

Red cell destruction

RBCs have a life span of 100–300 days. They are removed from the circulation by macrophages in the bone marrow, spleen, and liver.

Haemoglobin

Structure

Haemoglobin (Hb) is a protein with a molecular weight of 64.5kDa. It is composed of four subunits, each comprising a haem moiety conjugated to a polypeptide. The synthetic pathway for haem is shown in Figure 15.1. There are two pairs of polypeptides in each haemoglobin molecule. Salt bridges, hydrogen bonds, and hydrophobic interactions bind these four peptide chains to one another. In normal adult haemoglobin (HbA), there are two α and two β chains.

Each haem group consist of a porphyrin ring with a central iron atom. This iron is the site of oxygen binding. It is temporarily oxidized (from the Fe^{2+} to the Fe^{3+} state) when carrying oxygen, forming oxyhaemoglobin. Deoxyhaemoglobin is the form of haemoglobin without bound oxygen.

Oxygen binding

A single oxygen molecule can bind to the iron atom of each haem group, so the molecule as a whole can carry four oxygen molecules (Figure 15.2). Oxygen binding to haemoglobin is a cooperative process; when one subunit becomes oxygenated, a conformational change occurs in the whole complex, increasing the affinity of the other subunits for oxygen (this is known as an allosteric effect). As a consequence, the oxygen dissociation curve (ODC) for haemoglobin is sigmoidal (Section 13.12) .

Effect of CO_2, H^+, and 2,3-DPG

2,3-diphosphoglycerate (2,3-DPG) binds to haemoglobin, reducing its affinity for oxygen. This shifts the oxygen dissociation curve to the right. In acclimatization to high altitude, the concentration of 2,3-DPG in the blood is raised, allowing the unloading of larger amounts of oxygen in the tissues under conditions of lower oxygen tension. This phenomenon (molecule X affects the binding of molecule Y to a transport molecule Z) is called a heterotropic allosteric effect.

Types of haemoglobin

In the human embryo, Hb is made up of two α and two ε residues ($\alpha_2\varepsilon_2$). From 12 weeks' gestation, fetal haemoglobin (HbF) consists of $\alpha_2\gamma_2$. Within 24 weeks of birth, the majority of Hb is adult (HbA $\alpha_2\beta_2$) and less than 3% of consists of $\alpha_2\delta_2$ (HbA2). Gene switches control the changes in subunit production.

Fetal haemoglobin binds oxygen with greater affinity than adult haemoglobin (because it binds 2,3-DPG less avidly). This means that the fetal haemoglobin curve is left-shifted compared with the adult curve. As a result, fetal blood at the placenta is able to take oxygen from maternal blood. Fetal haemoglobin is normally replaced by adult haemoglobin soon after birth.

HbA combines with glucose to form HbA_{1C}. This occurs at a slow rate, and the percentage of HbA_{1C} is representative of glucose levels averaged over a longer time. (The half-life of a RBC is 50–55 days, and the average lifespan is ~120 days). If blood glucose levels are high, the percentage of HbA_{1C} increases. HbA_{1C} levels <6% reflect good long-term diabetic control.

Myoglobin is found in muscle. It is similar to haemoglobin in structure and sequence, but it is a monomer, lacking cooperative binding. It is used to store rather than transport oxygen (Section 8.2)

Iron metabolism

Absorption of iron

Iron is essential for the production of haemoglobin, myoglobin, cytochromes, catalases, and oxidases. Most iron (25mg) used in daily production comes from recycling other iron stores. Only 1–2mg is absorbed each day. The absorption of iron is described in more detail in Section 17.5.

Haemosiderin

Haemosiderin consists of insoluble Fe^{3+} oxide–hydroxide deposits and may cause organ damage. Deposits form after bleeding into tissues. RBC degradation releases Hb into the extracellular space where it is phagocytosed by macrophages and further degraded.

Iron loss

Iron is lost across the placenta to the fetus, and small amounts are lost in hair, urine, and faeces.

Folate and vitamin B_{12}

Vitamin B_{12} is important for the normal functioning of the nervous system and the formation of blood. Every cell utilizes it in DNA synthesis and regulation, fatty acid synthesis, and energy production.

B_{12} is used to regenerate folate, so it is not surprising that most of its effects can be replicated by sufficient quantities of folic acid.

In vitamin B_{12} deficiency, anaemia, and megaloblastosis occur due to defective DNA synthesis. Rather than symptoms of B_{12} deficiency per se, these are actually symptoms of folate shortage, since they disappear when the body has a proper supply of folic acid.

One of the two mechanisms dependent exclusively on B_{12}, methylmalonyl coenzyme A mutase (MUT) is necessary for methylation of myelin sheath phospholipids. Sufficient folic acid does not prevent subacute combined degeneration of the cord or peripheral neuropathy. Because folate masks deficiency of B_{12} by improving megaloblastosis, levels of the latter should be checked before the administration of folate.

Folic acid is used in some countries to fortify cereals, bread, and flour. There is little evidence that high levels are harmful, although they may interfere with the function of anti-malarials and worsen absorption of vitamin B_{12}.

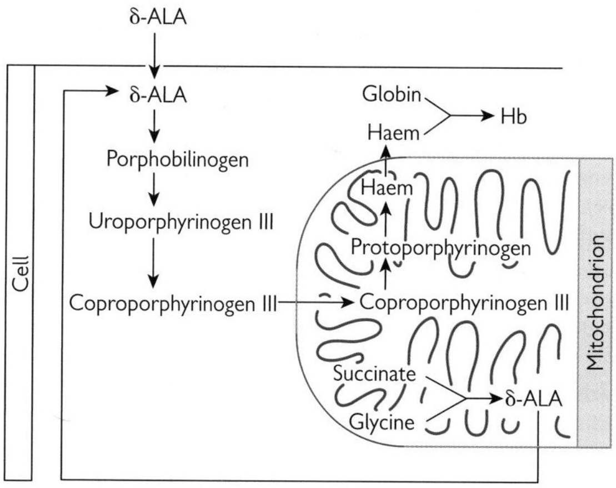

Fig. 15.1 Haemoglobin synthesis involves a number of steps within the cytoplasm and the mitochondrion.

Fig. 15.2 Diagram of haem. Unloading of oxygen pulls apart the globin chains, allowing entry of 2,3-DPG. This decreases the affinity of Hb for oxygen.

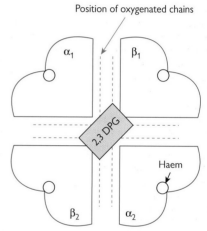

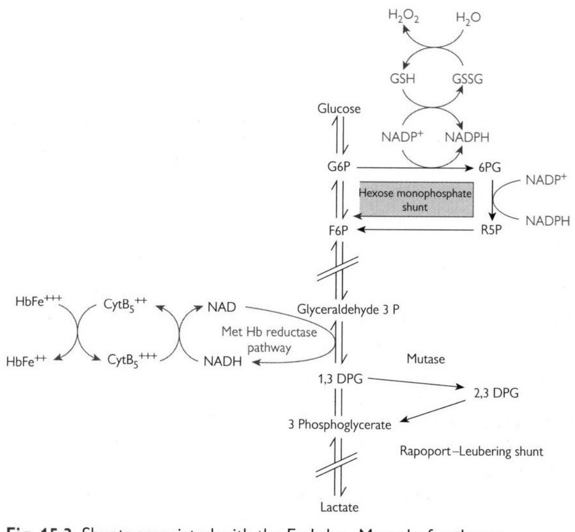

Fig. 15.3 Shunts associated with the Embden–Meyerhof pathway.

15.2 Abnormalities of haemoglobin production

Genetics of haemoglobin production

The globin genes encode the amino acid sequences of haemoglobin polypeptide chains. Each chromosome 16 has two identical α globin genes (four in total in each cell). Each gene is responsible for 25% of α globin production. Each cell has two β globin genes, one on each chromosome 11.

There are two major types of inherited disorders of haemoglobin:
- **Haemoglobinopathies:** abnormal polypeptide chains are produced.
- **Thalassaemias:** the chains have normal structure but production is reduced or absent.

Sickle cell disease

Aetiology
Sickle cell disease has an autosomal recessive pattern of inheritance. Heterozygotes (genotype HbAS) possess sickle trait. Homozygotes (genotype HbSS) have sickle cell disease.

Geography
Common throughout Africa, parts of Asia, and Southern Europe. The sickle cell gene confers immunity to one type of malaria, and in some parts of Africa up to 40% of the population have the sickle trait.

Pathogenesis
A single DNA base change results in substitution of valine for glutamate at position 6 of the β globin chain, giving HbS.

HbS polymerizes and precipitates within RBCs at low oxygen pressures (PaO_2 5–6kPa), producing characteristic sickle-shaped cells. The distorted cells increase blood viscosity, impair blood flow, and cause capillary and venous thrombosis and infarction. RBC life span is reduced (5–15 days) because of chronic haemolysis, which leads to anaemia (5–10g/dl).

The presence of other haemoglobins inhibits the degree of polymerization of HbS.
- Heterozygotes (HbAS) will only sickle at a PO_2 of 2.5–3kPa.
- HbC is less soluble than HbA, and inhibits sickling less well. Heterozygotes for HbSC may sickle at a PO_2 of around 4kPa.

Clinical features of sickle cell disease
Vaso-occlusive episodes (painful crises) cause most of the long-term problems. Multiple episodes of organ infarction are precipitated by cold, infection, dehydration, and/or hypoxia.

Children commonly show delayed growth and development. They are at risk of parvovirus-induced aplastic crises and splenic sequestration, which causes severe anaemia and hypotension.

Acute chest syndrome
This presents with pleuritic chest pain, fever, tachypnoea, hypoxaemia, and pulmonary hypertension. Parenchymal infiltrates are seen on the CXR. The WBC is generally raised. Mortality approaches 10%.

Diagnosis
A sickle solubility test (Sickledex) detects the presence of HbS but provides no information about other haemoglobins. Haemoglobin electrophoresis is required for an exact diagnosis. A blood film demonstrates sickle cells and target cells. Howell–Jolly bodies (basophilic nuclear remnants found in RBCs) are seen once splenic atrophy is established.

Management
General measures include prevention of infection by encapsulated bacteria with pneumococcal vaccine, antibiotics, and folic acid. Analgesia is often required for chronic pain. Acute painful crises are treated with hydration, supplemental oxygen, analgesia, and antibiotics.

Hydroxyurea stimulates HbF production and proportionally reduces the amount of HbS. Bone marrow transplantation has been shown to cure sickle cell disease.

Anaesthetic implications
Preoperative
The extent of complications should be thoroughly assessed. Preoperative starvation should be accompanied by IV fluid administration. Before major surgery, HbS levels can be reduced to 20–40% by exchange transfusion.

Intraoperative
It is important to avoid hypoxaemia, acidosis, hypothermia, and hypovolaemia. Tourniquets should be avoided, and IV regional anaesthesia is contraindicated.

Regional anaesthesia may confer significant advantages: it produces vasodilatation and good perioperative analgesia, and avoids potentially difficult intubation (there may be abnormal facial bone structure).

Postoperative
Adequate analgesia, supplemental oxygen and adequate hydration are essential. Sickle cell patients are not suitable for day-case surgery.

Thalassaemias

Aetiology
A group of inherited disorders involving decreased production of α or β chains.

Geography
Seen in people originating from the Mediterranean, central Africa, and southeast Asia.

Pathogenesis
Four genes control α chain synthesis, and two genes control β chain synthesis. The severity and type of disease depends on the number and type of genes affected.

α-thalassaemias
Deletion of one out of the four genes has no discernible effect.

Deletion of two genes causes **thalassaemia trait**, giving rise to mild anaemia.

Three gene deletions causes α **thalassaemia intermedia**. This causes the following:
- Anaemia and stimulation of erythropoietin
- Production of excess β chains, which form HbH. HbH is insoluble, and causes RBC deformation
- Moderate to severe anaemia secondary to haemolysis.

Deletion of all four α globin genes causes α **thalassaemia major**, a condition incompatible with life.

β-thalassaemias
Deletion of one of the two β globin genes causes β **thalassaemia minor**, a mild iron-resistant hypochromic anaemia.

Deletion of both β globin genes gives rise to β **thalassaemia major** (Cooley's anaemia), where no β globin chains are produced:
- Presents in infancy as HbF levels fall
- Severe chronic transfusion-dependent anaemia
- Skeletal abnormalities secondary to bone marrow hyperplasia
- Hepatosplenomegaly and cardiac failure.

Diagnosis
Diagnosis of thalassaemia is made by haemoglobin electrophoresis.

Management

Transfusion is accompaniedy by chelation therapy (desferrioxamine) to avoid iron overload. Bone marrow transplant is an option.

Anaesthetic implications

These are mainly related to anaemia. Thalassaemia can often be mistaken for iron-deficiency anaemia as it gives a similar hypochromic, microcytic anaemia. However, because of constant haemolysis and repeated transfusions, thalassaemic patients are frequently overloaded with iron, and require desferrioxamine to chelate this excess. Consider the possibility of organ damage from chronic iron overload.

Cross-matching of blood can be difficult.

Bone marrow hyperplasia may be seen in the bones of the head, resulting in a difficult airway.

→ Methaemoglobinaemia

Methaemoglobin (metHb) is produced following the oxidation of the iron atom in haemoglobin from the ferrous (Fe^{2+}) to the ferric (Fe^{3+}) form. RBC methaemoglobin reductase (NADH-dependent) reverses this process (Section 15.1), keeping levels at less than 1% of total Hb.

Methaemoglobinaemia occurs physiologically, via haemoglobin auto-oxidation. Oxyhaemoglobin contains superoxo-ferrihaem ($Fe^{3+}O^{2-}$), and unloading oxygen normally restores the Fe^{2+} status of deoxyhaemoglobin. Failure of this process results in production of a superoxide radical (O^{2-}), resulting in formation of methaemoglobin.

Acquired methaemoglobinaemia is usually due to exposure to toxins or drugs. Patients with G6PD deficiency are particularly susceptible to drug-induced methaemoglobinaemia; while G6PD pathway is relatively unimportant in health, it can compensate for failure of the methaemoglobin reductase pathway. Substances that can cause methaemoglobinaemia include:

- Nitrites/nitrates (inorganic, e.g. fertiliser; or organic, e.g. GTN)
- Local anaesthetics (particularly prilocaine and benzocaine)
- Antibiotics (e.g. sulphonamides, nitrofurans)
- Zopiclone
- Antimalarials (e.g. primaquine, chloroquine)
- Aniline dyes, naphthalene (moth balls), and various other household or industrial agents.

Congenital causes of methaemoglobinaemia include:

- Abnormal Hb;
- Abnormalities of the NADH MetHb reductase process.

Cyanosis requires the presence of at least 5g/dl of deoxygenated haemoglobin but only 1.5g/dl of methaemoglobin. Methaemoglobinaemia can affect the reading of pulse oximeters. In the presence of high levels of methaemoglobin, the pulse oximeter typically reads 85%, regardless of the actual oxygen saturations.

Symptoms and signs of methaemoglobinaemia vary with the fraction of methaemoglobin present (Table 15.1). Acquired methaemoglobinaemia (particularly in the context of intentional self-poisoning) may be fatal.

Table 15.1 Symptoms and signs of methaemoglobinaemia

% methaemoglobin	Symptoms and signs
1–10	Asymptomatic.
10–20	Cyanotic appearance (especially mucous membranes).
20–30	Headache, exertional dyspnoea, anxiety.
30–50	Tachypnoea, fatigue, palpitations, confusion, dizziness.
50–70	Coma, seizures, arrhythmias, acidosis.
>70	Death.

The clinical hallmark of methaemoglobinaemia is fixed hypoxia (unresponsive to administration of high-flow oxygen), in the absence of significant cardiopulmonary pathology.

Treatment

Patients with methaemoglobin levels >20% require active treatment (those with co-morbidities may require treatment at lower levels).

- Removal of the causative agent where possible (e.g. contaminated clothing).
- High flow supplemental oxygen.
- Methylene blue 1–2 mg/kg over 3–5 minutes, repeated at 1 mg/kg every 30 minutes as necessary to control symptoms. The dose of methylene blue should not exceed 7 mg/kg as the agent in itself can cause dyspnea, chest pain, and hemolysis. Methylene blue requires G6PD to work and so is ineffective in patients with G6PD deficiency. Methylene blue can cause bluish discolouration of skin and mucous membranes, and so persistent "cyanosis" may not be associated with failure of treatment.

Exchange transfusion can be considered for those with severe methaemoglobinaemia unresponsive to therapy.

The methaemoglobin reductase pathway is immature in infants, and so they are susceptible in situations of oxidative stress, including dehydration and hypoglycaemia. Treatment in this context is supportive and includes rehydration, correction of acidosis and maintenance of blood glucose. Prilocaine (a constituent of EMLA cream) is avoided in young infants due to the risk of methaemoglobinaemia.

Blood groups

Genetically determined antigens, found on the surface of RBCs, dictate blood group. Blood is grouped depending on which types of antigen are present.

ABO system

The ABO proteins are the most antigenic of all the RBC surface elements. There are three antigens: A, B, and H (Figure 15.5) each with its unique gene and glycosphingolipid. These genes do not code directly for the antigen, but rather for the enzyme that makes it.

A and B antigens are modifications of the H antigen. Those people with only the H antigen are designated blood group O, while those with antigen A, B, or both are blood groups A, B, or AB respectively.

The naturally occurring antibodies are IgM, and do not cross the placenta. They are formed in the first year of life (possibly in response to food or viral challenge).

Rhesus system

Up to four rhesus genes are located at two loci on chromosome 1. There are five potential corresponding antigens (D, c, C, e, and E). Rhesus classification is based upon the presence of D antigen.

There are no naturally occurring rhesus D (RhD) antibodies; these are only formed when a RhD-negative person is exposed to RhD-positive blood, either during transfusion or when a RhD-negative mother bears a RhD-positive child. These antibodies are IgG, and therefore can cross the placenta to cause haemolytic disease of the newborn (Figure 15.4) 85% of the Caucasian population is RhD-positive. 90% of RhD-negative people transfused with RhD-positive blood will develop anti-D antibodies.

Other red cell antigens

There are a total of 21 blood group systems. The importance of a particular antigen relates to the frequency of the development of antibodies to that antigen. Some of the more clinically significant include Kell, Duffy, and Kidd antibodies.

Compatibility testing

The central aim of compatibility testing is that recipient antibodies should not react against donor RBCs. (It should also be remembered that antibodies in donated plasma may damage the recipient's RBCs).

A major cross-match is performed and demonstrates compatibility between the recipient's serum and the donor RBCs. Minor testing (between donor serum and recipient blood) is not usually carried out, since all donated blood is tested for irregular antibodies and if it contains these, it is not issued.

Donor blood is prepared as follows.

- Saline agglutination. This detects anti-A, anti-B, anti-P, anti-M, anti-N, and anti-Lewis antibodies.
- Papain agglutination, which increases the titres of cold agglutinins.
- Low ionic strength saline test for the detection of agglutinating antibodies.
- Coombs' test (Figure 15.6).

Full cross-matching takes up to an hour. Group-specific blood can usually be made available within 20min. Non-cross-matched O rhesus-negative blood is reserved for life-threatening emergencies.

In an exciting development, two bacteria have been engineered to produce enzymes that are able to modify and remove A and B antigens from the RBC membranes. This strategy is currently in the trial phase, but if successful could increase blood supplies to many ABO groups.

Storage of blood

The length of time that any type of blood can be stored is determined following assessment of RBC survival 24 hr after transfusion. The accepted standard is that a minimum of 70% must survive.

Donor blood is preserved by mixing it with a preservative solution at the time of collection, and storing it at low temperature under strict asepsis to minimize the risk of bacterial contamination.

By storing the blood at 2–6°C, cellular metabolism is vastly reduced (<4% the usual rate of glycolysis). Storing at lower temperatures increases the risk of freezing and cell damage. At higher temperatures, 2,3-DPG is lost more rapidly, significantly affecting the function of transfused cells.

Blood products

Approximately 17 million units of blood are donated in Europe each year. 450ml are taken from the donor and 60ml of supplements are added, following which the mixture is cooled to 4°C.

All blood products in the UK are now leucocyte-depleted and are screened for a number of infective agents.

Whole blood

- Volume: 450ml
- Shelf-life: 35 days
- Haematocrit: 0.45
- Stored with A-CPD (adenine, citrate, phosphate, dextrose)

Platelets do not function after 3 days. Whole blood has normal concentrations of albumin and clotting factors (except V and VIII) and is the source from which all other blood products are derived.

Packed red cells

- Volume: 250ml
- Shelf-life: 35 days
- HCT: 0.6
- Stored with SAGM (saline, adenine, glucose, mannitol)

Platelets

There are two sources:

- Pooled: derived from the whole blood of up to eight donors
- Apheresis: obtained from a single donor (platelet pheresis).

Platelets can be stored for up to 5 days at 20–24°C. They must be continually agitated to prevent clumping. One pool of platelets will increment the platelet count by $5–10\times10^9$/L.

Fresh frozen plasma (FFP)

FFP is derived from the plasma of a single donation. The plasma is frozen to −20°C and thawed immediately before use. It can be stored up to a year. Each 150ml bag contains most of the clotting factors, albumin, and gamma globulin. Fibrinogen levels are low.

A usual initial dose is 10–15ml/kg, which raises coagulation factor levels by 12–15%. The aim should be to reduce a prolonged prothrombin time to less than 1.5 normal.

Cryoprecipitate

This is precipitated by rapidly thawing FFP. It is re-frozen, and stored at −20°C. It has a shelf-life up to a year. Like FFP, it is thawed immediately before use. Each unit has a volume of 20–40ml. It is high in factor VIII, fibrinogen, and von Willebrand factor.

Transfusion should be considered if plasma fibrinogen is <0.8g/L. Ten units of cryoprecipitate should increase fibrinogen levels by 1g/L.

Table 15.2 **ABO system**				
Blood group	A	B	AB	O
Frequency	42%	9%	3%	46%
Antigen	A	B	AB	H
Genotype	AA or AO	BB or BO	AB	OO
A_b present	Anti-B	Anti-A	None	Anti-A Anti-B

➜ **ABO blood group compatibilities**

		RECIPIENT			
		A	B	AB	O
DONOR	A	✓	✗	✓	✗
	B	✗	✓	✓	✗
	AB	✗	✗	✓	✗
	O	✓	✓	✓	✓

Note that O is the universal donor, and AB is the universal recipient.

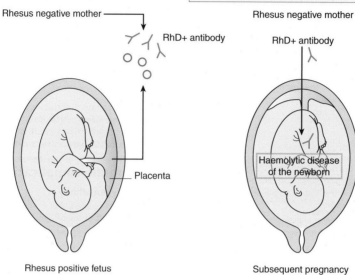

Fig. 15.4 Haemolytic disease of the newborn and anti-D administration.

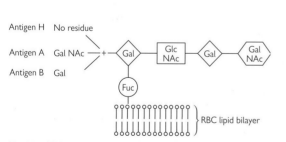

Fig. 15.5 RBC antigens.

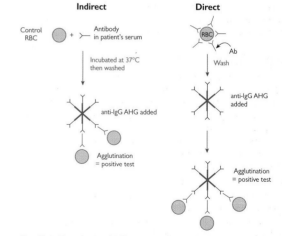

Fig. 15.6 Coombs test. Different specific anti-human globulins (AHGs) can be raised against different RBC antibodies. This is used to diagnose specific causes of haemolytic anaemia (e.g. due to autoimmune disease) and Kidd and Duffy antibodies missed by other forms of cross-matching.

Table 15.3 **Changes in stored blood with time**		
Change	7 days	28 days
RBC survival (%)	98	75
2,3-DPG (%)	99	5
pH	7.0	6.7
Na+ (mmol/L)	166	155
K+ (mmol/L)	11.9	>25
Glucose (mmol/L)	17	12
Free Hb (µg/L)	7.8	29

Storage lesion is the term used to describe loss of functional platelets and RBCs, coagulation factor depletion, reduction of 2,3-DPG, haemolysis, microaggregate formation, and the biochemical changes seen in Table 15.3. Hyperkalaemia usually resolves as the RBCs regain their metabolic activity.

Although the appropriate administration of blood products is often life-saving, it is not without risk. Various complications of blood transfusion are recognised. They can be broadly divided into immune and non-immune mediated phenomena.

Immune complications

Acute haemolytic transfusion reaction

ABO incompatibility is the most common cause of acute haemolytic transfusion reaction (AHTR). It is usually caused by recipient plasma antibodies to donor RBC antigens. It is sometimes caused by antibodies against antigens other than ABO.

Human error is the most common causal factor: mislabelling the crossmatch sample, or failing to check the intended recipient against the blood product prior to transfusion are the most common clinical scenarios. The severity of AHTR depends on:

- The degree of incompatibility
- The amount of blood given
- The rate of administration.

Symptoms and signs include discomfort and anxiety, dyspnoea, fever, rigors, facial flushing, and severe pain (particularly lumbar). Shock, DIC, and renal failure may develop within the hour. Jaundice, due to acute intra-vascular haemolysis, follows later.

For AHTR developing under general anesthesia, there are signs of shock and DIC, including hypotension and uncontrollable bleeding.

The management of a suspected acute reaction is described opposite.

Delayed haemolytic transfusion reaction

A patient may have a negative pre-transfusion antibody screen despite having been sensitized to an RBC antigen: the antibody levels are simply too low to be detected.

After transfusion with this antigen, a delayed haemolytic transfusion reaction will occur, usually within 1–4 weeks. Only transfused RBCs that possess the antigens are destroyed: the haematocrit falls and there is a slight rise in LDH and bilirubin.

This is not usually dramatic, and may be manifest as mild fever with few, if any, symptoms. It is often unidentified and is self-limiting. Rarely, severe symptoms occur.

Febrile non-haemolytic transfusion reaction

Febrile reaction may occur without haemolysis. It is may be due to antibodies directed against white cell HLA from otherwise compatible donor blood. WBCs also release cytokines during storage, and this is another possible cause.

Multiparous women or those who have had multiple transfusions are most at risk of this type of reaction.

Clinically, there is a temperature increase of more than 1°C, rigors, and sometimes headache and back pain. There may also be symptoms and signs of allergic reaction. These shared features of AHTR mandate thorough investigation, although most febrile reactions are treated successfully with paracetamol.

White cell reduced blood might be needed for future transfusions.

Allergic reactions to unknown components

These are common and are usually due to allergens or, less often, antibodies in donor plasma. They occur during or immediately after the transfusion.

Reactions are usually mild, with fever, urticaria, and headache. Rarely, anaphylaxis occurs, particularly in IgA-deficient recipients.

For those who have had such a reaction previously, an antihistamine may be given prophylactically just before a further transfusion.

Graft-versus-host disease

Transfusion-associated graft-versus-host disease (GVHD) usually occurs when immunocompetent donor lymphocytes attack immunocompromised host tissues. GVHD may occasionally occur in immunocompetent patients who receive blood from a close relative (this occurs when the patient is heterozygous for an HLA haplotype for which the donor is homozygous).

Symptoms and signs develop 4–30 days after transfusion, and include fever, skin rash (with bullae), vomiting, and watery and bloody diarrhoea. Lymphadenopathy, pancytopenia (bone marrow aplasia), jaundice, and elevated liver enzymes are also common. It has >90% mortality as no specific treatment is available. GVHD is prevented by irradiation (to damage DNA of the donor lymphocytes) of all transfused blood products.

Acute lung injury

This is an infrequent complication caused by antibodies in donor plasma that agglutinate, degranulating recipient granulocytes within the lung. These antibodies may be either anti-HLA or anti-granulocyte antibodies.

Progressive respiratory distress is accompanied by CXR changes of non-cardiogenic pulmonary oedema. This is the second most common cause of transfusion-related death, although many mild to moderate episodes are missed. Supportive care is required.

Non-immune complications

Altered oxygen affinity

RBC 2,3-DPG is reduced after 1 week and absent after >10 days. This results in left shift of the oxygen dissociation curve, i.e. an increased affinity for O_2 and slower O_2 release to the tissues.

This is clinically significant only in infants, sickle cell patients, and some patients with severe heart failure. 2,3-DPG regenerates in transfused cells within 12–24hr.

Volume overload

The high osmotic load of blood products draws volume into the intra-vascular space, leading to volume overload in susceptible patients. Unless there is bleeding, RBCs should be infused more slowly in those at risk (e.g. those with heart failure or renal failure).

Infectious complications

Bacterial contamination

This is rare, but may be due to poor collection technique or transient asymptomatic donor bacteraemia. Prior to issue, all RBC units are inspected for bacterial growth. Most organisms, including spirochetes, are killed by refrigeration.

Platelet concentrates are stored at room temperature, and so have greater potential for bacterial growth. To minimize this risk, they are not stored for more than 5 days. The risk of bacterial contamination of platelets is 1:2500.

Hepatitis

This is a risk with transfusion of any blood product. Immunological (antibody) tests for hepatitis are required for all donor blood because the viraemic phase is transient. Concomitant clinical illness precludes blood donation.

The estimated risks of transfusion hepatitis are as follows:

- Hepatitis B: 1:200,000
- Hepatitis C: 1:2.6 million
- Hepatitis A: no significant risk.

HIV infection

Nucleic acid testing for HIV-1 antigen as well as HIV-1 p24 antigen is carried out routinely. Additionally, blood donors are asked about behaviours that may put them at high risk of HIV infection. The estimated risk of HIV transmission due to transfusion is 1:2.6 million.

Cytomegalovirus (CMV)

May be transmitted by WBCs, and so is not transmitted through FFP. Immunocompromised patients are at risk of CMV disease and should receive CMV-negative blood products that have been provided by CMV antibody-negative donors.

Creutzfeldt–Jakob disease

New variant Creutzfeldt–Jakob disease is a theoretical risk, and in some parts of the world blood from UK donors is not used.

Malaria

This may be transmitted via infected RBCs; donors may be unaware that they have it. Malaria may be latent and transmissible for up to 15 years, and cold storage does not render blood safe.

Prospective donors must be asked about malaria or whether they have travelled to an area of prevalence. A risk of latent malaria means that donation should be deferred.

Massive blood transfusion

There are a number of definitions of massive blood transfussion:

- Transfusion of 10 units of blood within 6hr
- Transfusion of 5 units of blood within 1hr
- Transfusion of a volume of blood greater than or equal to one blood volume in 24hr (e.g. 10 units in a 70kg adult).

Complications of massive transfusion

- Transfusion of such a large volume may 'wash out' the patient's own blood. Although clotting factor levels usually remain sufficient, factor VIII may become deficient. Tests of coagulation should be performed: FFP and cryoprecipitate may be needed.
- Dilutional thrombocytopenia is a common complication. Platelets in stored whole blood are not functional. 5–8units of platelet concentrate may be required.
- Hypothermia: rapid transfusion of large amounts of cold blood can cause arrhythmias or cardiac arrest. Hypothermia is avoided by using an IV set with a heat-exchange device that appropriately warms the blood.
- Citrate toxicity: patients with liver failure may have difficulty metabolizing citrate. Hypocalcaemia may result but this rarely necessitates treatment. It may also potentiate hypomagnesaemia.
- Transfused blood is hyperkalaemic: K^+ toxicity is usually of little concern, but it may be worsened by hypothermia.
- Hypokalaemia may occur up to 24hr following transfusion since older transfused RBCs (>3 weeks' storage) actively take up potassium.
- There is increased risk of transfusion reaction due to the increased antigenic challenge and the potential for human error when checking blood product registration under pressure.

✚ Methods of reducing exposure to homologous blood

Preoperative
- Autologous blood transfusion: blood is collected preoperatively and stored in glycine at 4°C for up to 35 days.
- Recombinant erythropoietin is often given in conjunction with pre-donation. Iron and folic acid supplements are also required for the production of RBCs. It is expensive. Side effects include seizures, hypertension, and thrombophilia.
- Drugs that adversely effect coagulation should be stopped.

Intraoperative
- Intraoperative haemodilution: infusing crystalloid before blood is spilt reduces haemoglobin concentration. Blood that is lost subsequently contains a lower concentration of RBCs. Postoperative haemoconcentration increases Hb levels accordingly.
- Intraoperative controlled hypotension: caution should be exercised in those patients with cardiovascular comorbidity.
- Red cell salvage is particularly useful for cardiothoracic surgery.
- Pharmacological manipulation: tranexamic acid is an anti-fibrinolytic and may aid the development of clots.
- Meticulous surgical technique by senior surgeon.

Postoperative
- Adherence to transfusion policies.
- Red cell salvage: cell-saver devices are used to re-infuse RBCs following total knee replacement surgery.

✚ When to use irradiated blood

Irradiated blood is given to prevent GVHD caused by WBCs in the transfused blood.

Gamma-irradiation prevents lymphocytes dividing, and all granulocyte transfusions are routinely irradiated. Plasma products do not need to be irradiated.

Patients at risk of GVHD:
- Those receiving transfusions from family members.
- HLA-matched donors.
- Patients with inherited or acquired deficiencies in immunity.
- Treatment with cytotoxic drugs.
- Bone marrow/stem cell transplantation (recipients and prospective donors).
- Exchange transfusions.
- In utero transfusions.

✚ When to use CMV-negative blood

Transfusion-acquired CMV is not a problem for immunocompetent individuals, but can be a serious problem in the immunocompromised, where it causes pneumonitis, chronic hepatitis, gastroenteritis, chorioretinitis, or disseminated disease.

Indications for CMV-negative blood include:
- CMV-antibody-negative pregnant women
- CMV-antibody-negative recipients of allogeneic stem cell grafts
- Transfusions *in utero*
- HIV patients

✒ What to do for suspected transfusion reaction

Early recognition of symptoms suggestive of a transfusion reaction and prompt reporting to the blood bank are essential. The most common symptoms are chills, rigors, fever, dyspnoea, light-headedness, urticaria, itching, and flank pain.

- The transfusion should be stopped immediately and the IV line kept open with normal saline. The remainder of the blood product together with clotted and anticoagulated samples of the patient's blood should be sent to the blood bank for investigation.
- Re-check the sample and patient identifications.
- Diagnosis of AHTR is confirmed by demonstrating intravascular haemolysis with free Hb in the plasma and urine and low haptoglobin levels. Hyperbilirubinaemia may follow.
- The most common complications of transfusion are febrile nonhaemolytic and chill–rigor reactions.
- Further transfusion should be delayed until the cause of the reaction is known unless the need is urgent, in which case type O Rh-negative RBCs should be used.

15.5 Mechanisms of coagulation

Formerly, coagulation was considered as consisting of distinctly separate intrinsic, extrinsic, and common pathways. Both the intrinsic and extrinsic systems were considered to be able to generate the burst of thrombin necessary for the production of fibrin clot. This cascade view supports laboratory measures of coagulation (Section 15.8), but falls short of satisfactorily explaining features of *in vivo* clotting. This view has been superseded by a concept which promotes a central role for tissue factor on cell surfaces, and activated clotting factors on platelet surfaces.

Cell-based model of coagulation

The modern model of coagulation describes three distinct steps. Initiation takes place at a low level in the tissues at all times, keeping the process 'on stand-by'. Amplification takes place when tissue injury occurs, and leads to propagation, which produces the large amounts of thrombin needed for clot formation (Figure 15.7).

Initiation

A low-level of tissue factor (TF) pathway activity occurs outside the vascular compartment at all times. TF is present on many interstitial cells, and the surfaces of these cells are the site for initiation. Factor VII, factor X, and prothrombin are able to diffuse into the interstitial space. On contact with TF, they generate small amounts of thrombin. This does not lead to massive clot formation because the process is separated from other key cellular components by the vessel wall.

Amplication

TF on sub-endothelial cells is exposed following damage to blood vessel walls. Platelets, factor VIII, and von Willebrand factor (vWF) come into contact with the thrombin generated on the TF-expressing cells. This thrombin fully activates the platelets stuck at the exposed site of injury. Thrombin also activates other clotting factors, including:

- Factor V, released from activated platelets, which is able to cleave factor VIII from vWF, and then activate it.
- Factor XI, which binds to activated platelet surfaces.

By the end of this phase, the platelets, activated by relatively small amounts of thrombin, are covered in activated coagulation factors.

Propagation

TF/factor VIIa found nearby on the surface of TF-expressing cells generates IXa. This is able to combine with its cofactor VIIIa on the platelet surface, leading to the activation of factor X. The combination of Xa with its cofactor Va leads to the generation of large amounts of thrombin. Thrombin splits fibrinogen into fibrinopeptides A and B. Weak hydrogen bonds initially form between fibrin monomers. Under the influence of factor XIII, the structure is stabilized by covalent bonding.

Platelets

Platelets are small colourless discs, less than half the diameter of a RBC at 2–3 μm. The usual plasma concentration is 120–450×10^9. They are anucleate and cannot synthesize protein.

Platelet structure

The exterior glycocalyx contains membrane glycoproteins that play a part in adhesion and aggregation. Protein surrounds a lipid and phospholipid bilayer within the plasma membrane. The phospholipid derives factors PAF, arachidonic acid, and platelet factor (PF) 3.

Beneath the membrane lies a microtubular skeleton. An open cannalicular system invaginates through both, resulting in larger area for adsorption of clotting factors. Within the cytoplasm there are:

- Dense tubules: site of prostaglandin and thromboxane synthesis.
- α granules: contain factors used in coagulation, e.g. PDGF, vWF, PF4, thrombospondin, fibrinogen, and fibronectin.
- Dense granules: contain ADP, ATP, and pyrophosphate.

Production

Platelets are derived from megakaryocytes, part of the myeloid cell line. The megakaryocytes divide without mitosis: they enlarge, and platelets bud from the cell membrane. Young platelets undergo a period of maturation in the spleen prior to their release. After a median survival of 10 days, they undergo degradation by reticulo-endothelial cells in the liver or spleen.

Production is controlled by the cytokine thrombopoietin, which acts by binding to specific receptors on the megakaryocyte surface.

Von Willebrand factor

vWF is the bridging molecule that enables platelets to localize and adhere to sites of injury. It facilitates recruitment and aggregation of other platelets. It also forms a non-covalent complex with factor VIII, stabilizing and protecting it from rapid removal from the circulation.

vWF is synthesized in the endothelial cells (where it is stored in Weibel–Palade bodies) and in megakaryocytes (and subsequently stored in the α-granules of platelets). The mature vWF subunit is assembled into multimers, which are required for biological function.

Antigens

Platelets express HLA class I, ABO, and HPA 1-5 antigens. They are a potential cause of transfusion reaction.

The role of the platelet in haemostasis

Platelets are involved in the amplification and propagation stages of coagulation (Figure 15.8).

Adhesion

Platelets are rapidly recruited to areas of endothelial disruption. Adhesion does not require energy. Direct collagen adhesion is facilitated by glycoprotein Ia. Further adhesion occurs via glycoprotein Ib-IX, a platelet surface receptor, which binds to the vWF–endothelial microfibril complex.

This exposes the GP-IIb–GP-IIIa complex, which binds vWF, fibrinogen, and fibronectin: platelets spread across the endothelial surface.

Platelet activation

Activation is induced by:

- Adhesion to collagen
- The action of soluble agonists (e.g. ADP, adrenaline)
- Cell contact during the process of aggregation
- Thrombin from the coagulation process.

Protein phosphorylation via phospholipase C results in an increase in intracellular Ca^{2+}. Subsequent calmodulin- and calcium-dependent reactions change the shape of the platelet.

Release reaction

Both exposure to collagen and the action of thrombin cause platelet degranulation.

- Dense granule release reinforces platelet activation.
- α granule release reinforces platelet aggregation and adhesion. Platelet-derived growth factor (PDGF) released from α-granules stimulates cell division and healing in the vascular smooth muscle.

Aggregation

- Released ADP and thromboxane A_2 cause aggregation at the site of vascular injury.
- Further aggregation releases more ADP and thromboxane A_2.
- ADP also increases fibrinogen receptor numbers on the platelet.
- α granules release fibrinogen and vWF, and these enhance adhesion and aggregation of platelets. Thrombospondin is also released at this time and this stabilizes the aggregate of sticky platelets. This is later strengthened by a fibrin mesh.

Procoagulation

Platelet activation increases pro-coagulant activity. Movement of calcium into the platelet induces conformational change and exposure of membrane phospholipid PF3. This is pro-coagulant and forms complexes with coagulation proteins as described above. Fibroblasts subsequently lay down new collagen, permanently sealing the breach in the vessel wall.

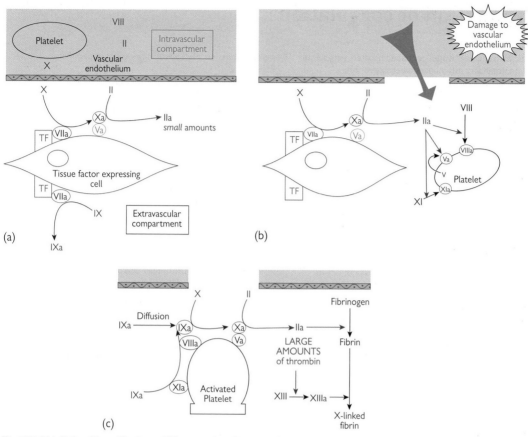

Fig. 15.7 (a) Initiation, (b) amplification and (c) propagation of haemostasis.

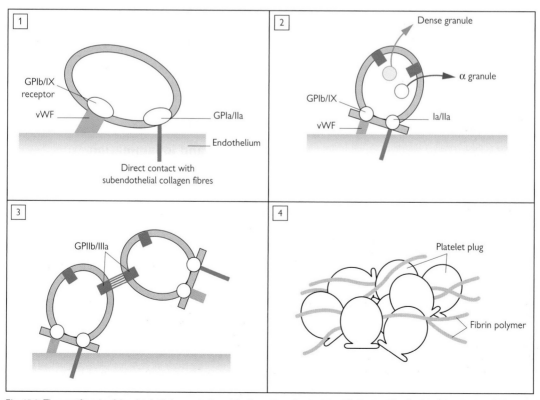

Fig. 15.8 The specific role of the platelet in haemostasis and the formation of cross-linked fibrin clot: (1) adhesion; (2) activation; (3) aggregation; (4) stabilization of the platelet plug.

15.6 Regulation of coagulation

Without inhibition, coagulation would continue unabated. Any stimulus for coagulation simultaneously induces mechanisms that:

- limit production of the fibrin clot by controlling the production and activity of thrombin;
- stimulate fibrinolysis, breaking down fibrin clots.

Control of thrombin levels

Uncontrolled activation of thrombin would lead to widespread clot formation, vascular occlusion and death.

There are three principal mechanisms by which thrombin activity is regulated (Figure 15.9).

- Most circulating thrombin is maintained as inactive prothrombin. Its activation requires the coagulation process, and at every step there are feedback mechanisms that adjust the active and inactive enzyme balance.
- Proteins C and S inhibit activation of factor VIII and V.
- Four specific thrombin inhibitors regulate thrombin activation.
  - *Antithrombin III (AT-III):* this also inhibits the activity of factors IXa, Xa, XIa, and XIIa, and its varied effects make it crucial to regulation of coagulation. AT-III activity is potentiated by the binding of heparin: this alters the shape of AT-III, resulting in a higher affinity for thrombin (and other substrates). Heparan (an endogenous heparin-like substance) and heparan sulphate expressed on the surface of endothelial cells act as the natural activators of AT-III. These molecules help to control the activation of the intrinsic coagulation cascade factors, and this is why heparin prolongs the activated partial thromboplastin time (Section 15.8).
  - *α_2-macroglobulin:* interestingly, this also inhibits plasmin (see below).
  - *Heparin cofactor II* has a direct, albeit minor, antithrombin effect.
  - *α_1-antitrypsin* is the primary serine protease inhibitor but has a relatively minor influence over thrombin. It also inhibits plasmin.

Fibrinolysis

Fibrinolysis is the process whereby fibrin clots are dissolved. Plasmin, a proteolytic enzyme which degrades fibrin, is central to this process. It is produced in the liver as the precursor molecule plasminogen. The conversion of plasminogen to plasmin is particularly stimulated by:

- t-PA: this is released by the endothelium several days after the initial injury. In this way, appropriately formed clot is later lysed.
- Urokinase, found in the extracellular matrix and in plasma.

Plasminogen becomes trapped within the clot as it is formed. It contains specific regions (called kringles) that bind to the lysine and arginine residues of fibrin and fibrinogen. Later, following conversion to plasmin, it removes the lysine and arginine C-terminals, breaking down the fibrin mesh. Plasmin promotes the production of more plasmin through stimulation of both t-PA and urokinase production.

Plasmin hydrolyses both fibrinogen and fibrin to fibrin degradation products (FDPs). FDPs compete with thrombin and slow down the conversion of fibrinogen to fibrin.

D-dimers are cleavage products of cross-linked fibrin (Figure 15.9). Their presence in large amounts in blood indicates active coagulation and fibrinolysis (e.g. in deep vein thrombosis, post-partum, or during convalescence from surgery).

Inhibitors of fibrinolysis

- *Plasminogen activator inhibitor 1 (PAI-1):* a serine protease inhibitor (part of a family of proteases involved in the regulation of coagulation, inflammation, and other 'cascade' processes). PAI-1 is produced by the endothelium and adipose tissue. It is the most important inhibitor of fibrinolysis. PAI-1 also has a role in the development of atherosclerosis, where fibrin is deposited in peripheral tissues. High levels impair effective peripheral fibrinolysis.
- *Plasminogen activator inhibitor 2 (PAI-2):* similar in structure and function to PAI-1. It is mainly secreted by the placenta, and so only found in any quantity during pregnancy.
- *α_2-antiplasmin* inhibits plasmin.
- *α_2-macroglobulin* inhibits plasmin.
- *Thrombin activatable fibrinolysis inhibitor (TAFI):* a plasma zymogen which, when exposed to the thrombin–thrombomodulin complex, is converted to an active form that inhibits fibrinolysis.

Tissue factor (thromboplastin)

Tissue factor (TF) is the principal initiator of the coagulation cascade. It is a very widespread constitutive protein present in most extravascular tissues. It is also expressed in response to injury, hypoxia, and a variety of chemical stimuli including lipoplysaccharide, TNF-α, IL-1, IL-2, IL-6, interferon-γ, lipoprotein, thrombin, and plasmin. It is expressed on the surface of vessel wall smooth muscle cells, macrophages, and fibroblasts, but it is not usually found on endothelial cells or blood cells unless stimulated by inflammation.

TF is a trans-membrane glycoprotein receptor and has a very similar structure to the interferon class of cytokine receptors.

80% of the molecule is extracellular, and contains the factor VII/VIIa binding site. The small intracellular portion promotes intracellular signalling; one such process activates factor VII and affects multiple other pathways.

TFPI feedback inhibition

Tissue factor pathway inhibitor (TFPI) is a dual inhibitor:

- It binds to the TF–factor VIIa complex to prevent it from acting on either factor IX or factor X.
- It directly inhibits factor Xa.

Production of factor Xa is subject to its own negative feedback (Figure 15.9). It combines very tightly with TFPI, and this complex inhibits the TF–factor VIIa complex so that only factor XIa is able to generate factor IXa and factor Xa. Factor XI is generated by thrombin during amplification.

TFPI modulates TF-induced thrombogenesis but its influence over thrombin production is not exclusive. It is an important defence against inappropriate thrombus formation, which could cause myocardial infarction, CVA, or deep vein thrombosis.

Coagulation and inflammation

Initiation of coagulation triggers intracellular inflammation, and activated coagulation factors VIIa, Xa, and IIa (thrombin) interact with cell-surface protease-activated receptors (PARs). These are G-protein-coupled receptors (GPCRs).

- PAR-1, 3, and 4 transmit factor IIa signalling.
- PAR-1, 2, and 3 transmit factor Xa signalling.
- PAR-2 transmits factor VIIa signalling.

PAR activation induces the expression of a variety of inflammatory molecules, including TNF-α, interleukins, adhesion molecules, and growth factors.

TF has an important role to play in inflammation, since the phosphorylation of its cytoplasmic domain leads to pro-inflammatory intracellular signalling. Fibrin is also pro-inflammatory.

Inflammation also promotes coagulation, and a positive feedback loop involving AP-1, Erg-1, and NFkB induces TF expression. This increases the availability of TF for factor VII or factor VIIa binding and so creates a cycle where coagulation and inflammation promote one another.

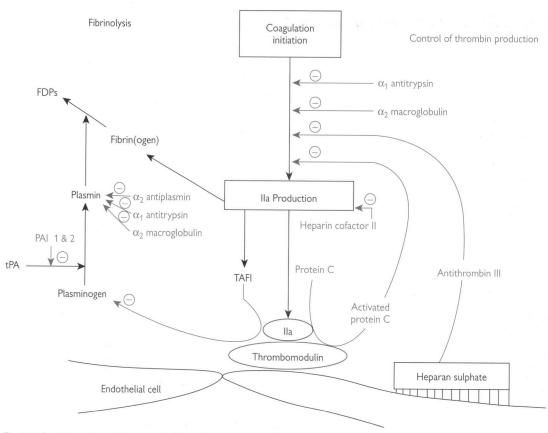

Fig. 15.9 Limitation of coagulation: control of thrombin production and fibrinolysis. Tissue plasminogen activator (tPA) is found on the surface of endothelial cells but secreted following vascular injury. Thrombin-activated fibrinolysis inhibitor (TAFI) binds tightly to plasminogen after it has bound to fibrin, before its cleavage to plasmin. Protein C requires its cofactor, protein S, in order to exert its action as a serine protease inhibitor against the production of thrombin.

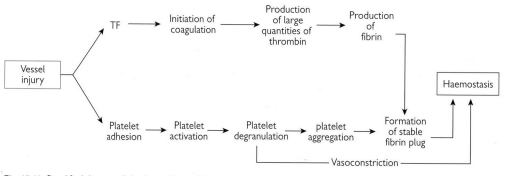

Fig. 15.10 Simplified diagram of platelet activity and haemostasis.

Impaired coagulation

Haemophilia

The haemophilias are a group of congenital coagulopathies. Haemophilia A is due to factor VIII deficiency. It is characterized by spontaneous bleeds into joints and muscles, leading to long-term arthropathies and neuropathies, with disability and deformity.

Haemophilia demonstrates X-linked recessive inheritance. Factor VIII is genetically mapped on chromosome 10, and is produced in the liver, spleen, kidney, and lymphoid tissue. It affects 1:10,000 males.

Symptoms usually correlate with factor VIII activity. In the normal person, 1ml of plasma contains 1 unit of factor VIII activity.

Diagnosis

Family history of bleeding disorder provides a valuable clue. APTT is prolonged but the PT and the bleeding time are normal.

Treatment

Factor VIII replacement treats episodes of bleeding and provides prophylaxis against further episodes. Recombinant factor VIII is the preparation of choice, although FFP or cryoprecipatate is used in emergencies. Use of pooled serum factor VIII risks viral infection.

Anaesthetic considerations

Expert haematological advice should be sought.

Factor VIII concentrate is given 1hr prior to surgery. The aim is to maintain the level at 50% normal until the fourth postoperative day.

Anaesthetic techniques associated with bleeding, or where bleeding may cause severe complications, are best avoided: naso-tracheal intubation is contraindicated; and regional techniques and central lines should be attempted with great care. PCA or morphine infusions postoperatively are associated with fewer bleeding complications than regional catheters.

The anti-fibrinolytic drug aminocaproic acid may be given as an adjunct. DDAVP (a synthetic vasopressin analogue used to improve platelet function in uraemia, von Willebrand disease, and haemophilia) is only of use in cases of minor bleeding.

Haemophilia B (Christmas disease) is due to factor IX deficiency. It behaves clinically like haemophilia A, and is also inherited in an X-linked recessive manner. Specific factor assays are required to differentiate haemophilia A from haemophilia B.

von Willebrand disease (vWD)

vWD is the most common inherited bleeding disorder, seen in approximately 1% of the population. It is due to either qualitative or quantitative defects of von Willebrand factor. It demonstrates autosomal dominant inheritance, with marked phenotypic variation. There are three types: types 1 and 2 are quantitative defects, and type 3 is qualitative and is due to a mutant protein.

vWD may be discovered at any age and in either sex, and is usually associated with easy bruising, recurrent nose bleeds, prolonged postoperative or post-traumatic bleeding, bleeding gums, or menorrhagia.

Diagnosis

The diagnosis of vWD is made with clinical observation, laboratory testing, and family studies, especially in mild forms of the disease. The severity depends on vWF levels.

Treatment

DDAVP is used in mild to moderate disease. It induces the release of vWF from endothelial storage granules, and provides a two-to three-fold increase in vWF levels within 1hr. It lasts for 6hr, and so is given four times daily. Tachyphylaxis may occur. It is useful for minor surgery, e.g. dental extractions.

For major surgery, cryoprecipitate, FFP, or factor VIII concentrate should be used to increase functional vWF levels. Specialist haematological advice should be sought to discuss the exact dosing regimen.

Idiopathic thrombocytopenic purpura (ITP)

This is a post-viral syndrome, where antiplatelet antibodies (IgG) are directed against membrane glycoproteins IIb/IIIa. The resulting complex is phagocytosed in the spleen. Platelet transfusion is ineffective.

Most acute cases are self-limiting and generally occur in children. 10% (mainly young women) develop a chronic disorder with severe sequestration that ultimately warrants splenectomy.

Clinical features

In children, the onset is abrupt. In adults the onset is insidious and includes petechial haemorrhage, easy bruising, and purpura. Menorrhagia is common. Rarely, intracranial haemorrhage is seen.

Diagnosis

The platelet count is reduced (10–50 10^9/L). Increased megakaryocytes are seen in an otherwise normal bone marrow.

Treatment

High-dose steroids improve most cases, although a few require second-line treatment with IV immunoglobulin. Splenectomy may be required for resistant cases, although outcome is variable.

Anaesthetic considerations

Costicosteroid supplementation needs to be considered. IV gamma globulin 1g/kg/day for 2 days preoperatively may help to reduce bleeding. Anaesthetic techniques associated with bleeding, or where bleeding could cause severe complications, are best avoided (naso-tracheal intubation, regional techniques and central lines). IM injections should not be given.

Vaccination against capsular organisms should be provided before splenectomy. Platelets should be available for transfusion, and the platelet count carefully monitored postoperatively.

Thrombophilia

When a patient presents with DVT or PE, the common risk factors should be considered (see box opposite). Their absence suggests a possibility of thrombophilia, features of which are given below. Further investigation is mandatory.

- Thrombosis, first time at age <40 years old
- Recurrent thrombosis (venous or arterial)
- Family history of thrombosis
- Thrombosis in unusual sites

Thrombophilic states share clinical features, and full diagnosis is often made in a specialist centre. The common types are listed in the box opposite). Treatment strategies are based on providing adequate anticoagulation therapy; this is especially important perioperatively. Congenital conditions may require genetic counselling.

Acute episodes of thrombosis are treated according to site and severity. In some cases they may warrant thrombolysis.

→ von Willebrand factor

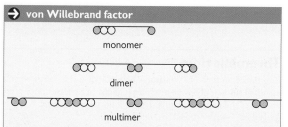

Fig. 15.11

Von Willebrand factor (vWF) is a large glycoprotein monomer produced in the Weibel–Palade bodies of the endothelium, platelet α-granules, and subendothelial connective tissue. Monomers are N-glycosylated and arranged into dimers and multimers in the Golgi apparatus and endoplasmic reticulum. Interestingly, vWF carries ABO antigens. vWF promotes binding to other proteins, particularly factor VIII and it is important in platelet adhesion to wound sites. Its binding to platelet glycoprotein Ib is most efficient under conditions of high shear stress, such as are found in small vessels with fast blood flow.

The vWF peptide is organized into four domains (A–D). Within each domain are functional residues that mediate platelet adhesion and aggregation and protect factor VIII from premature inactivation. Examples include the following:

- The A1 domain binds to type 4 collagen. It contains the binding region for glycoprotein Ibα, part of the platelet GPIbα–IX–V receptor complex and the heparin-binding site.
- The A3 domain binds to type 3 collagen.
- The C domain contains the platelet GPIIb–IIIa complex binding site.
- The D' and D3 domains contain the factor VIII binding site.

→ Common thrombophilic syndromes

Antithrombin III deficiency

AT-III is synthesized in the liver and inhibits the serine proteases of the coagulation cascade. Its activity is markedly potentiated by heparin. Deficiency may be congenital or acquired.

Protein C deficiency

Protein C is a vitamin-K-dependent protein synthesized in the liver as an inactive form. It is activated to protein Ca when thrombin binds to thrombomodulin. It is a serine protease, which inactivates factors Va and VIIIa. Its activity is markedly enhanced by its cofactor protein S. Deficiency may be congenital or acquired.

Protein S deficiency

Protein S is a vitamin-K-dependent factor synthesized in the liver. It is a cofactor of protein C in the inactivation of factors Va and VIIIa.

Factor V Leiden (activated protein C resistance)

Factor Va catalyses the activation of prothrombin to thrombin and the subsequent combination of thrombin and thrombomodulin activates the anticoagulant protein C.

Factor V Leiden is a gene mutation which confers resistance to protein C activation. Arterial thrombosis is not increased.

Antiphospholipid syndrome

The syndrome is made up of two distinct entities:
- Anti-cardiolipin antibodies
- Lupus anticoagulants.

10% of patients with SLE have antiphospholipid antibodies, although others with malignancies, infections, and ITP may also possess them. It is an acquired condition.

→ Risk factors for DVT and PE

- Recent surgical procedure with immobilization
- Obesity
- Malignancy, especially adenocarcinoma
- Previous history of DVT or PE
- Pregnancy (up to 2 months post-partum)
- Long-bone fracture
- Heart failure
- Travel
- Oral contraceptive use

Table 15.4 Severity of factor VIII deficiency according to plasma level

Factor VIII level (IU/100ml)	Bleeding symptoms
50	None
25–50	Significant bleeding after major surgery
5–25	Significant bleeding after minor surgery
1–5	Occasional spontaneous haemorrhage
<1	Spontaneous haemorrhage

15.8 Tests of coagulation

It is acknowledged that older concepts of clotting cascades are inadequate to describe the process of clotting *in vivo*. However, they reflect the *in vitro* processes which are measured by laboratory tests of coagulation. The cascades are shown in Figure 15.12 for reference while considering the laboratory investigations described here.

Prothrombin time

Prothrombin time (PT) is the time required for fibrin clot formation in a citrated plasma sample following addition of Ca^{2+} and tissue thromboplastin (factor III).

It is sensitive in the detection of coagulation factor deficiency due to lack of vitamin K and liver disease.

When the test is used to monitor oral anticoagulant therapy, the results are expressed as an international normalized ratio (INR).

Interpretation

This tests extrinsic and common pathway factors V, VII, and X, prothrombin, and fibrinogen. An abnormal result is may be due to:

* Liver disease (all clotting factors except vWF and tissue plasminogen activator are synthesized in the liver).
* Vitamin K deficiency (factors II, VII, IX, and X).
* Oral anticoagulant therapy.

International normalized ratio

The INR is the ratio of the prothrombin time for the patient's plasma to the prothrombin time for control plasma. The sensitivity of commercially available thromboplastin reagents is variable, and so a correction factor (International Sensitivity Index) is applied to the prothrombin ratio to enable the result to be issued as an INR.

The target therapeutic interval is the level at which the benefit of therapy should outweigh the risk of bleeding (Table 15.5).

Activated partial thromboplastin time (APTT)

This measures the time required for fibrin clot formation following addition of calcium and phospholipid emulsion to a plasma sample. Kaolin is used as an activator. The normal range is usually 25–35, but it varies with reagents and method and so is laboratory specific.

Clinical indications for use

This tests the intrinsic and common pathways. The therapeutic interval for continuous infusion heparin is generally 1.5–2.5 times the baseline or control APTT. It cannot be used to monitor LMWH regimes.

There is little point in using this as a preoperative screening test because of its limited sensitivity and specificity. It can be used as an initial test when:

* There is a history that suggests coagulation factor deficiency.
* There is a history that suggests a coagulation factor inhibitor or a lupus inhibitor.
* There is a need for a baseline result.

Interpretation of results

Coagulation factor levels may be reduced to only 30% of normal before the APTT is prolonged. Therefore mild haemophilia and von Willebrand's disease may not be detected by this test.

The APTT is normal in factor VII deficiency (PT prolonged) and factor XIII deficiency.

Artefactual prolongation of the APTT can be a consequence of heparin contamination, difficult or slow collection, the addition of too small a volume of blood to the collection tube, poor mixing of the blood with the citrate anticoagulant, suboptimal specimen storage, or a delay in testing the sample.

Thrombin time

The thrombin time (TT) measures how quickly a clot forms when a standard amount of bovine thrombin is added to a platelet-poor preparation of the patient's plasma. This typically takes 14–16sec. It is prolonged in:

* Afibrinogenaemia, hypofibrinogenaemia, dysfibrinogenaemia.
* Heparin (corrects with protamine).
* DIC.
* Hepatic disease.
* Excessive fibrin degradation products or paraproteins, when there is partial correction with protamine.

Activated clotting time (ACT)

This test is typically performed at the bedside and is used to quantify the heparin effect, e.g. during cardiac surgery or during renal replacement therapy. Whole-blood clotting time is recorded following addition of the blood to a tube containing Celite. The normal range is 100–140sec.

It is prolonged by thrombocytopenia and warfarin, and is associated with prolongation of both INR and APTT.

Bleeding time

A tourniquet around the upper arm is inflated to 40mmHg and three small cuts are made on the inner aspect of the forearm. The blood from each wound should clot within 9.5min. This is a simple test of platelet function. It is abnormal in von Willebrand's disease and prolonged by aspirin therapy.

Thromboelastography

In contrast with conventional tests of blood coagulation, which look at isolated stages of blood clotting, the thromboelastograph (TEG®) examines the whole process. The measurements are made from the viscous and elastic properties displayed graphically from the beginning of clot formation until fibrinolysis (Figure 15.13).

A small sample of whole blood is placed in a heated oscillating chamber. A plastic pin, immersed in the blood, is attached to a torsion wire. As a clot begins to form, the pin begins to move with the chamber oscillations. The cup is rotated through 4.5° over 10sec with a 1sec rest period at each end. The torque of the cup sample is transmitted to the pin and suspending wire. The movement of the pin is transduced into an electrical signal, which is related to the strength of the clot. The resulting trace gives a measure of the time taken to form the first fibrin strands, the kinetics of clot formation, the strength of the clot, and the dissolution of the clot over time. Examples of thromboelastograph traces are shown in Figure 15.14.

Results obtained by thromboelastometry depend on:
* the activity of the plasma coagulation system;
* platelet function;
* fibrinolysis;
* many factors that influence coagulation, including drugs.

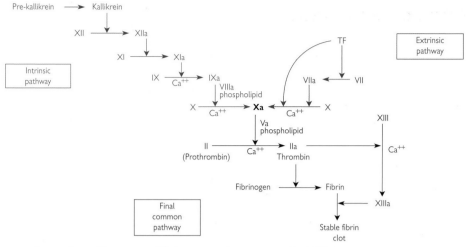

Fig. 15.12 *In vitro* coagulation pathways. The intrinsic and final common pathways are tested by APTT, the extrinsic and final common pathways are tested by the INR, and the final common pathway (from IIa onwards) is tested by the thrombin time.

Table 15.5 Therapeutic intervals for oral anticoagulant therapy	
	INR
Treatment of DVT, PE, transient ischaemic attacks	2.0–3.0
Recurrent DVT and PE; arterial disease including arterial grafts	3.0–4.5
Prosthetic tissue valves • Sinus rhythm • AF	None after 3 months 2.0–3.0 (aortic), 2.5–3.5 (mitral)
Mechanical heart valves	2.0–3.0 (aortic), 2.5–3.5 (mitral)

Table 15.6 Interpretation of APPT and PT		
APTT **Intrinsic and common pathways**	**PT** **Extrinsic and common pathways**	
Prolonged	Normal	Suggests deficiency of factor VIII, IX, XI, or XII, or I, II V, X (common)
Prolonged	Prolonged	Suggests common pathway factor X, V, II, or I (fibrinogen) deficiency, warfarin, or DIC
Normal	Prolonged	Suggests deficiency of factor VII or I, II, V, X (common)
Prolonged Not corrected by *in vitro* addition of normal plasma		Suggests coagulation factor (VIII or IX) inhibitor or lupus inhibitor
Prolonged	Normal (addition of a heparinase is part of the test)	Heparin

➔ Features of the thromboelastograph

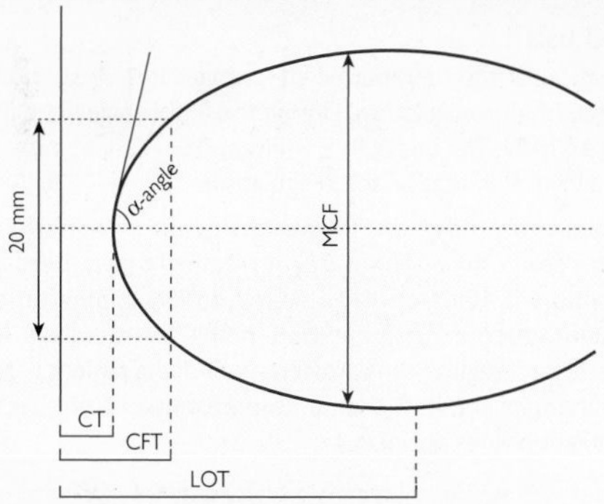

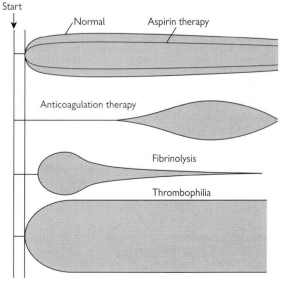

Fig. 15.13 Detail of a thromboelastogram.

Clotting time (CT): the time from start of measurement until the trace becomes 1mm wide. It represents the time taken to form fibrin. It is affected by deficiency of clotting factors, anticoagulants, and thrombocytopenia.

Clot formation time (CFT): the time from initiation of clotting until a clot firmness of 20mm is detected. It is affected by levels of fibrinogen, platelets, and factor XIII.

Maximum clot firmness: the widest point of the trace. It is affected by: quantity and qualitative function of platelets and fibrinogen.

α-angle: the angle between the midline and the tangential line from the 1 mm point. It is affected by low levels of fibrinogen, platelets, and clotting factors and by poor platelet function.

Lysis index 30 and 60: these measure the percentage of lysis at 30 and 60 minutes following MCF. Lysis is due to the entire process of fibrinolysis.

Fig. 15.14 Examples of thromboelastograph traces.

Anticoagulants are used for the prevention and treatment of thrombosis. The choice of drug and degree of anticoagulation required depend on the clinical setting. Generally, anticoagulants are useful when the risk of thrombus is in the slower moving venous circulation, and in the presence of mechanical heart valves.

Heparin

Heparin is a naturally occurring anticoagulant produced by basophils, mast cells, and the endothelium. It is commercially derived from animal mucosal tissues, e.g. porcine intestine or bovine lung.

Medical use

The effects of heparin can be difficult to predict, and the APTT must be monitored in order to achieve appropriate anticoagulation.

Heparin is an anticoagulant, preventing the formation of new clots and extension of existing clots. It does not break down clots that have already formed. It is used for anticoagulation for acute coronary syndromes, atrial fibrillation, DVT, and PE, and within extra-corporeal circuits for cardiopulmonary bypass and renal replacement therapy.

It is also used to form an inner anticoagulant surface on medical devices such as test tubes and renal dialysis machines.

Heparin is used to as a bridge to long-term anticoagulation therapy because its onset of effect is rapid. It is continued until warfarin therapy is established.

Administration

Heparin is given parenterally (IV or SC) based on weight. IM injections lead to the formation of haematomas and so this route is avoided. It must be given frequently or as a continuous infusion because of its short half-life (1hr).

Adverse reactions

- Heparin-induced thrombocytopenia syndrome (see box opposite)
- Alopecia
- Osteoporosis

Mechanism of anticoagulant action

AT-III binds to a specific pentasaccharide sequence contained within the heparin polymer, causing a conformational change in AT-III that exposes its active site. This modification leads to inactivation of thrombin, factor Xa, and the other proteases involved in blood clotting. Heparin binding increases the activity of AT-III 1000-fold.

The conformational change in AT-III alone inhibits factor Xa, although AT-III must also bind to heparin in order to inactivate thrombin. The highly negative charge of heparin attracts thrombin.

In vivo anticoagulation is enhanced by endothelially derived heparan sulphate proteoglycan. Heparin is also stored within the secretory granules of mast cells and released at sites of tissue injury, possibly providing a defence mechanism at these sites.

Low molecular weight heparin

Natural heparin consists of chains of varying molecular weight (5000–40,000Da). Low molecular weight heparins (LMWHs) consist of only short-chain polysaccharides with at least 60% of chains <8kDa. They are obtained by fractionation or depolymerization. LMWHs may have similar *in vitro* activity, but significantly different clinical profiles. These differences are amplified at both high and low body temperature.

Their potency is quantified a measure of anti-factor Xa activity and most have a rating of >70 units/mg, together with an anti-factor Xa-to-anti-thrombin activity ratio of >1.5.

Indications for LMWH

- Prevention of perioperative DVT
- Treatment of DVT and PE
  Acute coronary syndromes
- Prevention of clotting in extra-corporeal circuits

LMWHs permit outpatient treatment of DVT because they can be given subcutaneously and do not require APTT monitoring. The use of LMWHs needs to be monitored closely in patients at extremes of weight or with renal dysfunction in view of their renal clearance.

When specific monitoring of their action is required, anti-factor Xa activity assay is the most appropriate method.

Warfarin

Warfarin is a synthetic derivative of coumarin, found naturally in licorice and lavender. Warfarin inhibits vitamin K reductase, the enzyme responsible for recycling oxidized vitamin K back into the system.

Mechanism of action

Warfarin inhibits the synthesis of the biologically active forms of the vitamin-K-dependent clotting factors II, VII, IX, and X, as well as the regulatory factors protein C, protein S, and protein Z.

In order to bind to phospholipid surfaces on the vascular endothelium, the precursors of these factors require carboxylation of their glutamic acid residues. This is carried out by gamma-glutamyl carboxylase. Vitamin K is a cofactor in the reaction; it can only take place if the carboxylase enzyme is able simultaneously to convert a vitamin K hydroquinone (a reduced form) to vitamin K epoxide. This is then recycled back to vitamin K and vitamin K hydroquinone by another enzyme, **v**itamin **K** ep**o**xide **r**eductase (VKOR) (Figure 15.4).

Warfarin inhibits the VKORC1 subunit of epoxide reductase, ultimately reducing the availability of vitamin K hydroquinone. This in turn inhibits glutamyl carboxylase, prohibiting carboxylation of glutamic acid residues, and preventing coagulation factors from binding to the blood vessel endothelium. The coagulation factor precursors are produced, but they perform poorly. Warfarin's inhibition of quinone reductase is relatively minor.

The initial effect of warfarin is briefly to promote clot formation; production of protein S is also dependent on vitamin K activity, and reduced levels increase the tendency to form thrombus. The co-administration of heparin reduces the risk of thrombosis.

Medical use

Optimization of the therapeutic effect mandates close monitoring of the degree of anticoagulation. During the initial stages, the INR should be checked daily. The target INR will vary from case to case depending upon the clinical indication for coagulation.

It is difficult to predict the pharmacokinetics of warfarin and many algorithms for commencing warfarin treatment have been proposed. One example is 10mg on day 1, 10mg on day 2, 5mg on day 3, and subsequent dose adjustment depending on the INR. Whatever regimen is used, regular clinical assessment of the patient together with measurement of the INR should be performed to ensure that over-anticoagulation does not occur.

Indication	INR
Treatment of DVT, PE, or TIA	2.0-3.0
Recurrent DVT or PE; arterial disease including arterial grafts	3.0-4.5
Prosthetic tissue heart valves • Sinus rhythm • AF	None after 3 months 2.0-3.0 (aortic), 2.5-3.5 (mitral)
Prosthetic mechanical heart valves	2.0-3.0 (aortic), 2.5-3.5 (mitral)

Side effects

Haemorrhage

The only common side effect of warfarin is bleeding. The risk of severe haemorrhage is small but definite (1–2% annually), and any benefit needs to outweigh this risk when warfarin is considered as a therapeutic measure. Risk of bleeding is increased if the INR is beyond the therapeutic range, or if warfarin is combined with antiplatelet drugs.

The risk may also be also increased in elderly patients and those receiving heparin.

Warfarin necrosis

This rare complication occurs shortly after starting treatment in patients with protein C deficiency. The tendency for warfarin to promote thrombosis in the early phase of treatment is enhanced by this inherent deficiency.

Osteoporosis

Several studies have demonstrated a link between warfarin use and osteoporosis-related fractures.

Interactions and contraindications

Warfarin undergoes many drug interactions and its pharmacokinetics and metabolism vary greatly between patients. Therefore dosing is quite difficult and mandates regular monitoring.

Drugs known to interact with warfarin (e.g. aspirin, simvastatin) should be started with caution, since the INR may be affected.

Warfarin is a teratogen which causes deformation of the face and bones, especially if given in the first trimetster. During the third trimester, warfarin often precipitates antepartum haemorrhage. If anticoagulation is required at this time, LMWH should be used instead.

Alcohol reduces the metabolism of warfarin and elevates the INR. Patients are discouraged from drinking any alcohol. Patients suffering alcohol-related liver disease are usually treated with LMWH when anticoagulation is indicated.

Warfarin also interacts with many herbs or dietary supplements, including:

- Ginkgo
- St John's wort
- Ginseng
- Garlic (as a supplement)
- Ginger.

Antagonism

Warfarin can be reversed with the following:

- Vitamin K. For patients with an INR between 4.5 and 10.0, 1mg of oral vitamin K is effective. However, it takes several hours to work.
- FFP is used for rapid reversal (e.g. in cases of severe haemorrhage).
- Prothrombin complex concentrate is becoming more popular as a specific method of reversing the effect of warfarin.

Pharmacokinetics

Warfarin consists of a racemic mixture of two active optical isomers, each of which is cleared by a different pathway. The potency of S-warfarin is five times that of the R-isomer.

Pharmacogenomics

Warfarin activity is partly determined by genetic factors. VKORC1 gene polymorphism explains a third of the efficacy variation between patients; some forms of the enzyme are less susceptible to suppression. This explains why Africans may be relatively resistant to warfarinization. Polymorphism of CYP2C9 (an isozyme of cytochrome P450) alters the rate of warfarin metabolism, causing further variation in dose requirement.

→ Heparin-induced thrombocytopenia syndrome

Heparin-induced thrombocytopenia syndrome (HITS) causes platelet aggregation and consumption of clotting factors. This may lead to both local thrombosis, and generalized bleeding.

HITS can develop following repeated administration of heparin. Immunological testing may aid diagnosis. Confusingly, there is also a benign self-limiting form of thrombocytopenia associated with early heparin use, in which case heparin therapy may be continued.

Table 15.7 Unfractionated heparin vs. low molecular weight heparin (LMWH)

Unfractionated heparin	LMWH
Molecular weight ~20kDa	Molecular weight ~3kDa
Continuous infusion required	Once-daily dosing
Use requires APTT monitoring	Does not require APTT monitoring
	Smaller risk of bleeding
	Smaller risk of osteoporosis
	Smaller risk of heparin-induced thrombocytopenia
Effects are reversible with protamine sulphate	The properties of LMWHs vary; even those prepared by similar mechanisms may have very different chemical, physical, and biological properties

→ Vitamin K

Vitamin K is a fat-soluble vitamin, absorbed in the terminal ileum in the presence of bile salts. It is produced by bacteria found in the gut; a source of dietary vitamin K is not essential for most healthy people. Poor absorption occurs with obstructive jaundice, where absence of bile salts precludes the formation of micelles (Section 17.4).

Vitamin K is responsible for the generation of clotting factors II, VII, IX, X, together with proteins S and C. It acts as a cofactor in the modification of glutamine residues, adding a second carboxyl group. The presence of this second negative charge is required for interaction with Ca^{2+}, and absence of the modification renders the factors inactive.

Note

- Vitamin K is presented in solution with cremaphor, a substance which readily causes anaphylaxis.
- Reversal of warfarin-induced coagulopathy by vitamin K alone takes several hours.
- If a large dose of vitamin K is used (e.g. 10mg), subsequent anticoagulation with warfarin may be difficult to achieve.

Vitamin K and the newborn

Vitamin K does not cross the placenta; neonatal stores are deficient and dependent clotting factors are low. Breast milk contains very low levels of vitamin K, so all neonates in the UK are offered vitamin K injections soon after birth. Bacterial production of vitamin K starts within weeks of birth.

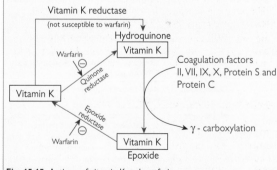

Fig. 15.15 Actions of vitamin K and warfarin.

15.10 Antiplatelet agents

Anticoagulants have limited effect in the arterial circulation. Instead, agents which inhibit platelet function are used in conditions associated with arterial thrombosis. Such diseases include acute coronary syndromes, cerebral ischaemia, and following cardiac or vascular surgery.

Like anticoagulants, antiplatelet agents have implications for anaesthetic practice as they increase bleeding risk. Their effects are more difficult to measure than those of anticoagulants, as specific tests of platelet function are not routinely available. Antiplatelet agents may have significant effects on clotting, despite a normal platelet count.

Currently, the mainstays of anti-platelet therapy are aspirin, clopidogrel, and to a lesser extent dipyridamole. They are detailed in below.

However, newer glycoprotein IIb/IIIa inhibitors (abciximab, eptifibatide, and tirofiban) are available and should be considered (with specialist advice) for the management of unstable angina or non-ST-segment-elevation myocardial infarction (Section 10.11).

Glycoprotein IIb/IIIa inhibitors are recommended for patients at high risk of myocardial infarction or death when early percutaneous coronary intervention is desirable but does not occur immediately; either eptifibatide or tirofiban can be used (in addition to other appropriate drug treatment).

A glycoprotein IIb/IIIa inhibitor is also recommended as an adjunct to percutaneous coronary intervention:

- When early percutaneous coronary intervention is indicated, but is delayed.
- In patients with diabetes.
- If the procedure is complex.

	Name	Aspirin	Clopidogrel	Dipyridamole
Properties	Uses	Treatment of coronary and cerebral arterial thrombosis; primary and secondary prevention in cardiovascular disease, claudication, atrial fibrillation, and following CABG. Analgesic and anti-inflammatory.	Prevention of is chaemic events in patitents with symptomatic ischaemic disease. Acute coronary syndromes (in combination with aspirin). Monotherapy if aspirin contraindicated.	Adjunct to oral anticoagulants in prevention of thromboemboli from prosthetic heart valves. Secondary prevention of ischaemic stroke/TIA (with aspirin)
	Chemical	Aromatic ester of acetic acid. Prodrug for salicylic acid.	Prodrug. The active metablite is a thiol derivative of the parent compound.	Piperidine derivative
	Presentation	Tablets 75–600mg, various compound preparations.	Pink tablets 75mg or 300mg.	Orange tablets 25mg or 100mg; suspension; modified release capsules.
	Primary actions	Anti-inflammatory, antiplatelet, antipyretic, analgesic	Inhibits platelet aggregation	Inhibits platelet aggregation; vastodilator.
	Mode	COX inhibition (irreversible in platelets). May inhibit lipooxygenase pathway.	Inhibits binding of ADP to P2Y12 receptors and prevents ADP-mediated activation of GPIIb/IIIa. Irreversible.	Inhibits platelet phosphodiesterase; inhibits re-uptake of adenosine. Both result in increased cAMP and inhibit platelet aggregation.
	Route/dose	PO: initially 300mg, then 75mg od. Higher doses required for anti-inflammatory or analgesic action.	PO. Prophylaxis: 75mg od. Acute coronary syndrome: 300mg followed by 75mg od (with aspirin)	PO. 300–600mg/day in divided doses. Alternatively 200mg bd as modified release preparation.
Effects	CNS	Analgesia: peripheral and central actions.		Can reduce the incidence of recurrent CVA by up to 20%. Headache.
	CVS	Few haemodynamic effects; main CVS actions are related to platelet inhibition. Bleeding time prolonged due to suppression of thromboxane A2	May worsen cardiac failure; main CVS effects are related to platelet inhibition. Can precipitate TTP.	Vasodilatation and postural hypotension. (Originally used in the treatment of angina.)
	Resp	Uncouples oxidative phosphorylation: increase O_2 consumption/CO_2 production. Central hyperventilation, pulmonary oedema, respiratory failure in overdose.		
	GIT	Gastric ulceration and potentiation of bleeding	Potentiation of bleeding from GI tract (or any other site)	
Kinetics	Absorption	Completely absorbed from upper GI tract. FPM reduces OBA to 70%.	Rapid absorption from GI tract; OBA 50%.	Average time to peak concentration 75 min after oral dose
	Distribution	Rapid hydrolysis to salicylic acid, which is 80–90% plasma protein bound; VD 0.15L/kg.	98% bound to plasma proteins (94% of metabolite).	Highly plasma-protein bound, distribution $t_{1/2}$ 40min
	Metabolism	(Of salicylic acid): 50% to salicylurate; 20% to salicylphenolic glucuronide in liver: saturable (zero-order) kinetics. 15% by first-order hepatic pathways 15% excreted in urine (first-order)	85% by hepatic esterases to inactive metabolites. Only 15% is metabolised (by cytochrome P450 enzymes) to active form	Conjugated as a glucuronide in liver
	Excretion	Metabolites excreted in urine. Due to 70% zero order metabolism, half life changes with dose. Since the action on platelets is irreversible, termination of effect depends on new platelet synthesis.	Metabolites excreted in urine and faeces. Half life of clopidogrel is 6h; the active compound binds irreversibly with a half life of 11 days. Termination of action depends on new platelet synthesis.	Conjugated metabolites exreted in bile. Terminal elimination $t_{1/2}$ 10h.
	Notes	Excessive hypertension should be controlled before aspirin administered. May displace oral anticoagulants and sulphonylureas from plasma proteins, increasing their effect. Overdose may cause metabolic acidosis or respiratory alkalosis; mortality is 1–2%. Removed by haemodialsysis.	CYP2C19 poor metabolizer status is associated with diminished response to clopidogrel. The optimal dose regimen for poor metabolizers has yet to be determined. Concomitant use of omeprazole should be avoided as it is metabolised by CYP2C19.	May counteract the anticholinesterase effect of cholinesterase inhibitors and potentially aggravate myasthenia gravis. IV preparation available for use as an alternative to exercise in coronary perfusion studies.

Chapter 16

Microbiology and infection control

Infectious disease is one of the most common causes of human morbidity and mortality worldwide, and places a high burden on both community and hospital healthcare provision. Globally, infections are a leading cause of death in infants and children. World Health Organization figures show that the four major infective causes of death worldwide are respiratory tract infections, severe gastroenteritis, malaria, and measles.

The discovery that micro-organisms were the aetiological agents for human disease revolutionized both medicine and public health. The germ theory of disease, promoted after pioneering work by scientists such as Louis Pasteur and Robert Koch, paved the way for development of highly specific agents to combat these conditions—anti-microbials and vaccines—arguably two of the most important medical developments in history.

Knowledge of the mechanisms of spread of disease, and the public health and civil engineering measures to prevent them is vital to human health inside and outside the hospital environment. Infections have played a significant role in human evolution and society throughout history. Some of the great pandemics (such as cholera, influenza, and bubonic plague) have shaped the course of history.

Occasionally, a unique syndrome is recognized, attributable to a new pathogen (e.g. SARS coronavirus, HIV). It is inevitable that new pathogens/syndromes will continue to emerge. In addition, well-known causes of infection can re-emerge (TB and syphilis are good examples), necessitating continued vigilance.

The importance of diagnosis

Accurate and timely diagnosis of infectious agents is a prerequisite for optimal management of infections because it allows:

- Appropriate targeted antimicrobial therapy to be given quickly.
- Control measures to be instituted to prevent spread of disease in hospital and community.

In addition, isolation of disease-causing organisms can give invaluable information about the following.

- Pathogenesis: for example, pathogen-specific factors such as presence and function of virulence factors.
- Epidemiology: macro- and micro-evolution of bacterial virulence and antimicrobial resistance both locally and globally.

Modern microbiological laboratories now use a wide range of techniques for both diagnosis and screening for exposure to infectious pathogens. Isolation of a pathogen from normally sterile sites (e.g. blood, cerebrospinal fluid, joints) remains an extremely valuable process for accurate diagnosis.

Increasingly, molecular and proteomic techniques are being used to complement |(and in some cases to replace) culture methods. Rapid high-throughput methods continue to be developed and introduced. However, in some cases, microscopy by a skilled technician on site is still the best way of achieving rapid diagnosis of a number of important clinical syndromes (e.g. meningitis).

However, there are a number of situations where recovery of an organism is unsuccessful and other methods are useful. For example both broad-range and species-specific PCR can be used on tissue and blood. Serological conversion is an often overlooked but important diagnostic test (e.g. in Q fever, leptospirosis, mycoplasma, and legionnaire's disease).

In virology, molecular methods are largely replacing cell culture, microscopy, and even serology in diagnosis and screening. Methods such as real-time PCR can also be used to determine the viral load and mutations associated with antiviral resistance, which can provide essential information about disease progression or response to treatment.

Factors affecting outcome from infections

The last two decades have seen an explosion in knowledge of the biological processes involved in the host response to microbial colonization and infection.

Predisposing factors

- *Premorbid or prediagnosis risk factors*: extremes of age, underlying chronic disease (chronic cardiac, pulmonary, renal hepatic disease); burns and trauma.
- Known *immune deficiency*: primary (rare but important) and, more commonly, secondary to other conditions—malignancy, immune-suppressive treatment (corticosteroids, cyclosporin, methotrexate, cyclophosphamide), bone marrow and solid organ transplant, myelosuppressive drugs, prolonged neutropenia, HIV infection.
- Increasingly, host factors are being recognised as important in determining susceptibility and severity of infections. Such factors may be part of the innate or adaptive response, and are often due to genetic polymorphisms. They include: mannose binding lectin (MBL), natural endotoxin antibody, toll-like receptors (TLRs), cytokines, chemokines, signal transduction pathways, complement, and coagulation.

Nature of the infective agent

Case fatality and/or morbidity rates from infections can vary, depending on the organism. Highly virulent organisms such as *Staphylococcus aureus* and *Streptococcus pyogenes* possess a plethora of virulence mechanisms that are able to circumvent the host immune response and also cause cellular and tissue damage. In some, very specific syndromes can be discerned, such as necrotizing pneumonia with panton valentine leucocidin (PVL) producing strains of *Staphylococcus aureus*.

The host response

It is widely accepted in sepsis syndrome that host-mediated processes have a major role in pathophysiology of this condition. Many of the cellular and physiological processes seen in severe sepsis are a consequence of activation of a number of key cellular and physiological processes. Many of these can be driven by pathogen-specific components (such as endotoxins and exotoxins), but also through networks of inflammatory pathways activated to counteract these products:

- Endothelial activation and function
- Leucocyte activation and induced tissue injury
- Immune paresis following trauma or surgery
- Dysregulated coagulation pathways with microvessel thrombi
- Neuro/endocrine/metabolic dysregulation
- Cellular apoptosis and necrosis
- Hyperproduction of cytokines and chemokines seen in some severe infections (meningococcaemia, toxin-mediated disease).

Traditionally, initial characterization of bacteria is judged by its appearance on **Gram staining**. Typically, the thick peptidoglycan cell wall of Gram-positive organisms traps the purple blue dye (crystal violet), whereas the thin layer of Gram-negative organisms does not, allowing it to be washed away by a decolourant (acid alcohol or acetone) (Figure 16.1). Therefore Gram-positives appear blue/purple whereas Gram-negatives appear red because of the presence of a counter-stain. However, Gram's stain is not a suitable technique for some organisms, notably acid-fast organisms such as Mycobacteria, Nocardia, and some Actinomyces, and cell-wall-deficient bacteria such as mycoplasma.

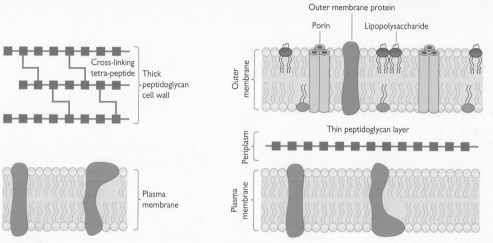

Fig. 16.1 Structures of Gram-positive and Gram-negative bacteria.

Gram-positive bacteria

Capsule

A number of important bacteria produce an extracellular polysaccharide (occasionally polypeptide) polymer matrix layer. **Biofilms** contain extruded viscous material which has been shown to be of critical importance in persistent colonization/infection of medical devices and also in deep-seated infections. When the film is well organized and relatively thick, it is classed as a **capsule**. Pneumococci are typically encapsulated and the structure of the capsule forms the basis of serotyping. The capsule confers resistance to host-mediated attack, particularly phagocytosis and complement mediated lysis.

Cell wall

Typically the surface layer is composed of a thick peptidoglycan cell wall and is responsible for the shape of the bacteria. Peptidoglycans are polymers of N-acetyl muramic acid and N-acetyl glucosamine which in Gram positives are cross-linked by a tetra-peptide bridge. This cross-linking is achieved by enzymes such as transpeptidases, which are the major site of action of B-lactam antibiotics. In some Gram-positives, the cell wall is anchored covalently to the plasma membrane via teichoic and lipoteichoic acid. Both peptidoglycans (including their subunits) and teichoic acid are recognized by the innate immune system via Toll-like receptor 2 (PGN and teichoic acid) and NOD (PGN only) receptors.

Cell membrane

The cell membrane is a single plasma layer composed of a phospholipid bilayer and which also contains proteins.

Exotoxins

Exotoxins are important virulence factors (e.g. toxic shock syndrome toxin of *Staphylococcus aureus*, botulinum and tetanus toxins) which are secreted by many Gram-positive (but also Gram-negative) bacteria.

Gram-negative bacteria

Capsule

Like Gram-positives, a number of Gram-negatives express capsules (e.g. *Neisseria meningitidis*).

Cell wall

In Gram-negatives, the cell wall is thin and exhibits less cross-linking than that seen in Gram-positives. It is located between the outer and inner (plasma) membrane.

Cell membrane

Gram-negative organisms have two cell membranes. The outer layer is asymmetric, with the outer leaflet containing lipopolysacchride (sometimes referred to as endotoxin). This important molecule is an amphipathic glycolipid with a hydrophilic polysaccharide attached to a hydrophobic core or lipid A. The lipid A component is recognized by innate immune receptors, principally toll-like receptor 4 and is partly responsible for inducing the inflammatory responses seen in endotoxaemia. The lipopolysaccharide is also involved in bacterial resistance to phagocytosis and complement. The outer membrane contains many proteins, including porins, which have hydrophilic channels allowing passage of molecules, including antibiotics, into the cell. Porins are also immunogenic and are recognized through host innate immune mechanisms.

Pili/fimbriae

Pili (Figure 16.2) are almost exclusively found in Gram-negative organisms. They are involved in bacterial adhesion to host cells and transfer of genetic information (including resistance and virulence genes).

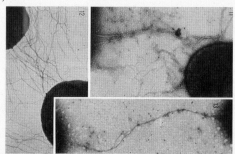

Fig. 16.2 Electron micrograph of pili of Neisseria meningitidis.

16.2 Antimicrobial therapy

Introduction

Before the development of sulphonamide antimicrobials in the 1930s and the discovery and subsequent purification of penicillin in the 1940s, there was little that could be offered as specific therapy against serious infections such as infective endocarditis and meningitis. Diseases such as lobar pneumonia, puerperal sepsis, and soft tissue and wound infections often killed otherwise fit young people.

Antibiotics are arguably the most successful chemotherapeutic agents that have ever been developed in medicine. As antimicrobial therapies have been developed, so too has the ability of microbial world to adapt and become resistant to these drugs.

Key developments in antimicrobial therapy

- *1860–1880:* germ theory of disease—Pasteur and Koch (in 1875 Koch's postulates were used to prove that *Bacillus anthracis* is the causative agent of anthrax).
- Paul Ehrlich used small molecule screening approach to identify molecules that could selectively stain, and therefore could target and kill micro-organisms ('magic bullet').
- *1909:* Arsphenamine (Salvarsan), the first modern chemotherapeutic agent, was used to treat syphilis and trypanosomiasis.
- *1935:* Prontosil was patented—its active agent was a sulphonamide.
- *1928:* Alexander Flemming discovered a substance produced by penicillium mould that killed staphylococci. He called it penicillin, but was unable to purify it in sufficient quantities for therapeutic use.
- *1939–1940:* Florey and Chain purified penicillin for use in patients. The first patients were successfully treated in 1942.
- *1945–1960:* the majority of classes of anti-microbials in use today were characterized and developed for use.
- *1961:* the first report of a methicillin-resistant staphylococcus in Carshalton, UK.
- *1970–1980:* new antibiotics developed by chemical remodelling of existing core (or scaffold) structures. They have improved the spectrum of activity, pharmacokinetics, and stability to resistance mechanisms.
- Linezolid (*2000*) and daptomycin (*2003*) approved by FDA. Both are novel synthetic antimicrobials developed in the 1980s. Both have activity against Gram-positive micro-organisms only. Tigecycline, a novel glycylglycine, obtained FDA approval in 2005 and is active against Gram-negative and Gram-postive organisms, including MRSA.
- Genomics have revealed numerous potential genes encoding products with antimicrobial potential, and equally numerous resistance genes that are cryptically embedded in bacterial genomes, which could evolve into true resistance genes.

Antimicrobial

A term used to describe a compound which either kills or inhibits the growth of microbes. This includes antibacterial, antifungal, antiviral, and anti-parasitic compounds.

Antibiotic

Normally refers to an agent extracted from moulds or other bacteria which kill or inhibit bacterial growth. Examples include penicillin, streptomycin, and vancomycin. Many currently used antibiotics are semi-synthetic derivatives of naturally occurring compounds, in which existing structures have been chemically modified. Examples include flucloxacillin, ampicillin, and meropenem.

Action of antibacterial agents

Antimicrobials act in concert with host defence mechanisms, surgery, and supportive therapy in the management of infections. Antibacterial agents exert their effects by interfering with normal physiological processes and metabolic pathways of bacteria. The exquisite selectivity of antibiotics for bacterial over host cellular processes is important for their safety profile.

The aim of antimicrobial therapy is to prevent ongoing bacterial proliferation and kill existent bacteria, allowing host immune mechanisms to clear bacterial breakdown products. There is good evidence that a high rate of killing of bacteria in early stages of sepsis is critical to outcome. It has also been proposed that optimizing dose and length of therapy will reduce the probability of generating antimicrobial resistance.

The traditional measure of potency of antibiotic against a particular organism is the minimum inhibitory concentration (MIC). Antimicrobials are sometimes described as either bactericidal or bacteristatic. These terms relate to the difference in concentration between the minimum concentration required to inhibit the growth of bacteria (MIC) and the concentration required to kill the majority of bacteria (minimum bactericidal concentration (MBC)) *in vitro*.

In general, bactericidal antibiotics are required in infections where host defence mechanisms are relatively ineffective, such as meningitis and infective endocarditis.

Combination therapy

Combination antibiotic therapy may be indicated in a number of situations:

- Pre-emptive therapy in life-threatening or severe illness where causative organisms are not known and broad but efficacious coverage is important.
- Where antibiotic synergy may be needed. Examples of this include β-lactam–aminoglycoside combinations targeting streptococcal endocarditis. Synergy is also seen in β-lactam aminoglycoside combinations against other organisms, especially *Pseudomonas aeruginosa*.
- Complex polymicrobial infections, such as necrotizing soft tissue infections and cystic fibrosis.
- Use of bactericidal antibiotics and bacterial protein synthesis inhibitors in staphylococcal and streptococcal toxin-mediated disease.

Efficacy of antimicrobials

Factors affecting the efficacy of antimicrobials *in vivo* include:

Disease

Meningitis, osteomyelitis, device-related factors, presence of devitalised tissue.

Pathogen

Ability to persist, form biofilms, production of toxins and virulence factors.

Host

The presence of neutropenia, immune deficiency, effects of chemotherapy (including long-term steroids) and age.

Pharmacokinetic/pharmacodynamic predictors of efficacy of antibiotics

Combination of **pharmacokinetic** data (serum concentrations of antimicrobial over time, e.g. absorption, distribution, and elimination) and **pharmacodynamic** data (relationship between pharmacokinetic data and antimicrobial effect, e.g. inhibition or killing) can be used to assess the efficacy of antimicrobials (Figure 16.3).

The three pharmacokinetic parameters that are most useful for evaluation are:

- Peak serum level (C_{max})
- Trough level (C_{min})
- Area under the concentration–time curve (AUC). The AUC is an index of drug exposure.

When integrated with antimicrobial effect (e.g. MIC) three basic patterns of efficacy emerge, depending on class and mode of action of the antibiotic. This has implications for dosing schedules, route of administration, and length of therapy.

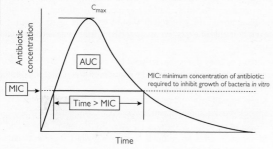

Fig. 16.3 Predicting antibiotic efficacy using pharmacodynamic and pharmacokinetic parameters.

Type I: Peak/MIC—aminoglycosides, quinolones, ketolides

The goal of therapy is to maximize the **concentration** to achieve faster and more extensive killing. Quinolones are sometimes classed as type III antibiotics.

Type II: Time/MIC—penicillins, cepahlosporins, carbepenems, monobactams, lincosamides, linezolid

The critical parameter is the time that antibiotic concentration is above the MIC. Therefore the goal of therapy is to maximize **duration of exposure** of antimicrobial to organism. For example, for β-lactams and erythromycin, a time above MIC of at least 70% is associated with maximum killing. If the time period above MIC is reduced, bacterial killing maybe suboptimal and outcome from infection (e.g. Gram-negative sepsis) may be worse.

Type III: 24hr AUC/MIC—vancomycin, tetracyclines, quinolones, azithromycin

The aim of therapy is to maximize the **total amount of drug above the MIC** over a 24hr dosing period.

PK/PD data can be used to characterize the overall efficacy of antibiotic therapy against certain pathogens in different clinical situations (e.g. bacteraemia, meningitis, and pneumonia). This can lead to changes to dose and frequency recommendations (e.g. treatment of severe *Staphylococcus aureus* infections with glycopeptides).

Site of action of antibiotics

Note: antibiotics in bold are principally bactericidal; others are bacteristatic.

Cell wall synthesis inhibitors	**β-lactams** • **Penicillins** • **Cephalosporins** • **Carbapenems (meropenem, imipenem)** **Glycopeptides (vancomycin, teicoplanin)** **Cycloserine** Fosfomycin Isoniazid Ethambutol
Ribosome function/protein synthesis inhibitors	Aminoglycosides (e.g. gentamicin/amkacin/tobramycin) Chloramphenicol Tetracyclines Macrolides and ketolides (erythromycin, azithromycin, clarithromycin, roxithromycin) Fucidic acid Oxazolidinones (e.g. linezolid) Lincosamides (clindamcyin) Streptogrammins **Glycylcylclines (e.g. tigecycline)**
Nucleic acid/transcription and translation inhibitors/DNA synthesis inhibitors	**Quinolones (e.g. ciprofloxacin, moxifloxacin, levofloxacin)** **Rifampicin** **Novobiocin** **5-Nitroimidazoles (e.g. metronidazole)**
Cell membrane	**Polymixin** **Daptomycin**
Metabolic pathway/folate synthesis	Sulphonamides Diaminopyrimidines (e.g. trimethoprim)

Some antibiotics are bactericidal against certain pathogens but bacteristatic against others. For example, linezolid is bactericidal against streptococci but bacteriostatic against staphylococci and enterococci. Tigecyline, a glycylglycine (derivative of tetracycline), is bactericidal against all Gram-positive organisms except enterococci, and most Gram-negatives except Acinetobacter species.

Even 'bactericidal' antibiotics, such as cephalosporins, are predominantly bacteristatic when duration above MIC is reduced.

In general, antibiotics where the MIC and MBC are close together are bactericidal.

Antibiotic resistance can be defined as the continued growth of an organism *in vitro* in the presence of concentrations of antibiotic that are achievable in the patient without toxicity.

Occasionally *in vivo* responses to antimicrobials do not correspond well to *in vitro* (laboratory) measurements. Clinical resistance is defined when combined laboratory studies, animal models, and clinical trial data are taken into account.

Resistance to antimicrobial agents is increasingly recognized globally and has potential catastrophic consequences for the ability to treat infectious disease effectively. The outcome of infections from multid-rug-resistant (MDR) bacteria compared with the same species of bacteria which are not antibiotic sensitive is often worse in terms of both mortality and morbidity. The reasons are not always related to increased virulence of the bacteria.

- The comorbidities of patients differ: elderly patients have more invasive procedures and more immunosuppression.
- Appropriate antibiotic therapy may be delayed because resistant bacteria are not detected or suspected initially.
- The efficacy of antibiotics used against some resistant bacteria (e.g. glycopeptides for *Staphylococcus aureus* infections) may be less than that of more conventional antibiotics against sensitive strains.

The presence of MDR pathogens also increases healthcare costs because of:

- More limited repertoire of antimicrobials available, some of which are expensive and require monitoring.
- Patients colonized or infected with MDR pathogens require special provision such as source isolation, eradication regimes, and even separate facilities in some cases.

Mechanisms of resistance

The majority of important antibiotic resistance mechanisms are due to the presence and function of genes which affect antibiotic function. Antibiotic usage can act as a selection pressure on genetically adapted organisms. Genetic mechanisms of antibiotic resistance generally involve a whole genetic element containing the following.

- The gene conferring the mechanism of resistance (e.g. a β-lactamase gene).
- Insertion sequences, promoters, and other genes that are also required for bacterial function.

Some of these genetic elements can be horizontally transferred from one bacterium to another, and even between species.

Plasmids

Plasmids are an important way of transferring resistance genes in certain classes of micro-organism.

They are semi-autonomous self-replicating DNA molecules within bacteria that can harbour resistance genes to multiple antibiotics.

Transfer of the plasmid from a resistant donor bacterium to a sensitive recipient bacterium will result in a new clone of resistant bacteria.

Other genetic elements are present within the main chromosome which can transfer and integrate into the recipient's DNA.

Genes conferring resistance to antibiotics are present throughout the microbial world. Even when new antimicrobial agents are developed mechanisms exist that confer resistance to these agents either in pathogenic organisms or in other non-pathogenic species that can act as a source of these genes.

Drug development from initial screening/design to approval is an extremely lengthy and costly exercise and very likely to lag well behind requirements for new agents. Resistance has been detected quite quickly after introduction even to 'novel agents' such as daptomycin and linezolid. Some bacteria are intrinsically resistant to many antimicrobials, including *Stenotrophomonas* and *Burkholderia* species.

Resistance vs. virulence

Antibiotic resistance does not necessary denote that organisms are more pathogenic or virulent.

- Certain strains may have increased efficiency for colonizing the host; or may persist in environments (e.g. epidemic MRSA 15 and 16).
- Antibiotic use may act as a selection pressure to promote colonization in certain patient groups.
- Occasionally sudden appearance of a virulent clone with horizontally acquired resistance genes (e.g. community-acquired PVL-positive MRSA) can occur. In these cases, virulence and resistance factors act in concert and result in increased morbidity and mortality.

Risk assessment

Early effective antimicrobial therapy is essential to improving outcome from severe infections, paticularly sepsis syndrome, meningitis and pneumonia. An assessment should be made as to whether a patient is at risk of exposure to, or suffering from, antibiotic-resistant pathogens.

Antibiotic policies should be designed to optimize therapy for particular patient groups. Information to be considered in assessing the degree of risk includes the following.

- Knowledge of local and regional resistance patterns (e.g. rates of aminoglycoside and β-lactam resistance in coliforms and MRSA).
- Proactive surveillance systems are essential to monitor trends and to decide whether an outbreak is occurring, which may necessitate change to antibiotic policy.

High MDR colonization rates and critical sepsis are seen in the following situations:

- Immune suppressed individuals
- Febrile neutropenia
- ICU/HDU patients
- Specialist burns units
- Cystic fibrosis patients
- Indwelling central venous catheters
- Chemotherapy or total parenteral nutrition
- Those with a recent exposure history:
  - Hospital admission in last 3 months
  - Attended hospital outpatients and received wound care inlast 30 days
  - Resident in nursing homes or long-term rehabilitation facility.
  - Attended haemodialysis units
  - Admission from a country with high prevalence of MDR pathogens
  - Admission from ward/hospital experiencing an outbreak with a particular pathogen.

Mechanisms of antimicrobial resistance

Antibiotic modification

Usually due to a bacterial enzyme which inactivates the antibiotic.

β-lactamases cleave the β-lactam moiety of this class of antibiotics.

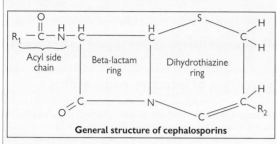

General structure of cephalosporins

Fig. 16.4 General structure of cephalosporins

Examples include:

- *Staphylococcus aureus* penicillinase.
- Many coliforms possess β-lactamases, some of which inactivate many classes of β-lactam antibiotics.
- Chloramphenicol is inactivated by acetyl transferase.
- Aminoglycoside-modifying enzymes add a side chain that renders them incapable of transport across the membrane.

Blockage to antibiotic transport

Antibiotics must gain entry into the bacterial cell in order to act on their target. They use different mechanisms to achieve this.

- Outer membrane proteins called porins facilitate entry of antibiotics across the hydrophilic outer membrane. Loss of expression of porins prevents transport of a number classes of antibiotics rendering them useless. This is seen in *Pseudomonas aeruginosa* resistance to carbapenem and also coliforms.

Efflux mechanisms

Exit and entry of molecules into the bacterial cell is controlled by a number of complex mechanisms, often by active transport. Such efflux pumps can combine with loss of porins to render some bacteria resistant to anti-microbials.

- These combined mechanisms are exemplified by the opportunistic pathogen *Pseudomonas aeruginosa*.
- Efflux pumps are characteristic of tetracycline resistance.

Target modification

Alteration of antibiotic binding sites by steric hindrance or reduction in affinity is seen in a number of important resistance mechanisms.

- β-lactam resistance in staphylococci and penicillin resistance in Streptococcus pneumoniae.

Target overproduction

In some cases, overproduction of target may overwhelm the ability of the antibiotic to affect bacterial function.

- Glycopeptide resistance in staphylococci, sometimes termed vancomycin intermediate strains.

Resistance in some medically important bacteria

Multidrug-resistant enterobacteriaciae/coliforms

- *Extended spectrum β-lactamase (ESBL)*: these target a broad range of β-lactam antibiotics, especially third-generation cephalosporins (e.g. cefuroxime, cefotaxime, and ceftazidime). These are mainly found in enterobacteriaceae (*Escherichia coli* and *Klebsiella* classically but also Enterobacter, Serratia, Proteus). Caution must be observed in use of β-lactam/inhibitor antibiotics (e.g. timentin, augmentin, and piptazobactam) as efficacy in severe infections against ESBL-expressing coliforms can be unpredictable. In these instances, carbepenems are treatment of choice.
- *AmpC cephalosporinases*: these can inactivate cephalosporins. In some bacteria they are expressed all the time, giving obvious resistance. In others, genes are inducible, in that they can be switched on ('de-repressed') during therapy.
- *Metalo-β-lactamases*: this is a diverse group of enzymes present in some environmental bacteria. They confer cross-resistance to all β-lactams, including carbepenems. Treatment options are limited.
- *Aminoglycosides*: combination of aminoglycoside resistance and ESBLs is common in healthcare environments.
- *Fluoroquinolones*: resistance increasingly found in community and hospitals.

Methicillin-resistant Staphylococcus aureus (MRSA)

Staphylococcus aureus possessing a genetic element SCCmec which includes gene mecA. This encodes for an altered penicillin binding protein pbp2' which is low affinity for β-lactams. This is within a genetic region that also permits insertions of other genes that confer resistance to multiple antibiotics, including fucidin, rifampicin, gentamicin, macrolides, and lincosamides.

Possession and expression of this gene confers cross-resistance to the majority of β-lactams including flucloxacillin, cephalosporins, and carbapenems.

Frequently found in healthcare environments, and increasingly in community.

Vancomycin-resistant enterococci (VRE)

Many species of enterococci possess genes that confer resistance to vancomycin teicoplanin or both. Cross-infection is well described.

Acinetobacter species

These are increasingly found in hospital environments, especially intensive care and burns units. They are of low pathogenicity but can cause ventilator-associated pneumonia, skin infections, and septicaemia. Some clones of *Acinetobacter baumanii* are highly resistant to majority of antimicrobial drugs; those with metalo-β-lactamases are particularly troublesome. Some of these are associated with genetic elements that can easily transfer to other bacteria.

Penicillin-resistant Streptococcus pneumoniae

High-level penicillin resistance is uncommon in UK. Penicillin resistance is due to altered PBP structure, reducing affinity for β-lactams.

Primary antibiotic chemoprophylaxis is a key component in effective control of infection occurring after both elective and emergency surgical procedures. Chemoprophylaxis is distinct from early pre-emptive therapy in high-risk situations where infection is anticipated, such as contaminated or dirty surgical site operations. Prophylaxis has been shown to reduce mortality in lower gastrointestinal surgery with primary anastamosis of the colon and to reduce morbidity in total hip replacement. In helping to prevent surgical site infections (SSIs), prophylaxis can reduce length of stay, inconvenience, and discomfort of the patient.

Rationale

The aims of prophylactic administration of antibiotics to surgical patients are to:

- Use antibiotic prophylaxis in specific situations where evidence exists that it is effective.
- Reduce the incidence of surgical site infections.
- Minimize adverse effects, e.g. allergy.
- Minimize deleterious effects on patients' own flora and host defence mechanisms.
- Target likely pathogens, covering MRSA and other resistant bacteria if known or likely to be present.

Choice of antibiotic

Antibiotics given must cover the expected pathogens at the site of operation. For surgery below the waist (e.g. intra-abdominal surgery), adequate Gram-negative and anaerobic cover is necessary. Above the waist (including head and neck surgery), oral anaerobic flora must be covered in addition to *Staphylococcus aureus* and β-haemolytic strepotococci.

Known or likely colonization with resistant flora must be accounted for. For example, if a patient is known to be colonized with MRSA, a glycopeptide such as vancomycin is appropriate. This is especially important in high-risk situations, such as cardiothoracic, orthopaedic, and neurosurgical procedures. Application of topical mupirocin to the anterior nares of patients undergoing these high-risk procedures, who are known to be MRSA colonized or have a high risk of carriage if results are not known, should be considered.

Glycopeptides are indicated when an individual has known β-lactam allergy, although the allergy should be accurately corroborated beforehand.

The safety profile, pharmacodymamic and kinetic considerations (such as antibiotic half-life), and cost also play a role.

Timing and duration of prophylaxis

In the majority of cases, there are few indications beyond giving a single dose of antibiotic(s) at surgery. The principle aim is to achieve high levels of antibiotics in the relevant tissues during maximum risk of microbial contamination. The optimal timing of the antibiotic will depend on the type and route of antibiotic being administered. Classic studies of prophylactic regimens indicated that the most critical period for risk of SSI is the first 3hr after incision or contamination.

- In general, IV antibiotics such as β-lactams (penicillins, cephalosporins) should be commenced 30min prior to incision.
- In the case of glycopeptides (vancomycin, teicoplanin) it has been recommended that administration be given 120–60min prior to incision.

Additional dosing

- In long operations (>4hr) in high-risk situations (cardiac surgery) a second dose of antibiotics is recommended, particularly if the half-life of the antibiotic is short.
- In operations involving cardiac bypass, antibiotics should be given at induction, at bypass, and after bypass has ceased, but should not normally be given for >48 hr in total.

- A 24hr regimen is recommended for arthroplasty operations.
- Additional doses can be given if there is new contamination, a new incision has to be made, and/or the operation is unexpectedly prolonged.
- If there is major blood loss (> 1500ml for adults), additional doses may be required as antibiotics levels can fall below the MIC.

Prevention of infective endocarditis

Antibiotic prophylaxis against infective endocarditis (IE) in at-risk patients is a subject of recent debate. "At-risk" includes patients with an increased lifetime incidence of IE, and those in whom IE would have a very poor prognosis. The risk depends on the type of cardiac defect, with prosthetic material and a high degree of haemodynamic disturbance posing the greatest risk (see box opposite).

Guidance on prophylaxis has changed significantly. In the 1960's, antibiotics were recommended for up to five perioperative days. More recently, the value of giving prophylactic antibiotics at all has been questioned. The risks of complications (such as anaphylaxis on an individual level, and antimicrobial resistance in the wider clinical setting) are not necessarily offset by the potential benefits of prophylaxis against a rare complication.

Factors influencing this change in guidance include: paucity of firm evidence of the efficacy of antibiotic prophylaxis; a general lack of association between confirmed cases of IE and surgical procedures; and the likelihood that transient bacteraemias occur during everyday activities, such as tooth-brushing.

A recent NICE guideline (echoed by the British Heart Foundation and British Society for Antibiotic Chemotherapy) recommends that prophylactic antibiotics should no longer be given to patients undergoing dental, upper and lower gastrointestinal, genitourinary (including obstetric), or respiratory (including ear, nose, and throat) procedures. If a patient at any degree of risk is receiving antimicrobial therapy for a gastrointestinal or genitourinary procedure at a site where there is suspected infection, he or she should receive an antibiotic that covers endocarditis-causing organisms. Additional emphasis is placed on:

- Good oral hygiene
- Education of at-risk patients, with advice to seek medical attention for any febrile illness after surgery
- Consideration of IE, with prompt investigation and treatment of at-risk patients attending with febrile illness after surgery.

American Heart Association guidelines recommend somewhat more liberal prescribing for dental, respiratory, and infected soft tissue procedures, but only in the very highest-risk patients.

These changes in guidance represent a paradigm shift in the approach to those at risk of IE. They have the potential to cause confusion, particularly in patients who are used to receiving antibiotic prophylaxis. The risks and benefits of prophylactic antibiotics should be discussed with patients on an individual basis.

The valvular vegetations of infective endocarditis are pictured in Figure 16.5.

Other routes of administration

Antibiotic impregnated bone cement

Randomized controlled trials have shown that combined IV prophylaxis and antibiotic impregnated cement reduces rates of revision, aseptic loosening, and infected prostheses.

Eye surgery

Intra-cameral cefuroxime reduces endophthalmitis is cataract surgery. Intravitreal antibiotics reduce severe intra-ocular infection in open globe injury.

Antibiotic-impregnated intra-ventricular devices in neurosurgery

Randomized controlled trials have shown a significant reduction in infection rates with antibiotic-impregnated permanent intraventricular devices.

✚ Patients at risk of infective endocarditis

High risk

Previous IE

Prosthetic heart valve, including bio-prosthetic material and homografts

Cyanotic congenital heart disease

Aortic regurgitation or stenosis

Mitral regurgitation

Ventriculo-septal defect

Coarctation of aorta

Surgically repaired congenital heart defects with residual haemodynamic abnormality

Cardiac transplant recipients with valvulopathy

Intermediate risk

Mitral valve prolapse with regurgitant murmur

Mitral stenosis

Tricuspid valve disease

Pulmonary stenosis

HOCM

Bicuspid or calcified aortic valve

Surgically repaired cardiac abnormality with no haemodynamic abnormality

Low or negligible risk

Mitral valve prolapse without regurgitant murmur

Trivial regurgitant valve on Echo without structural abnormality

Secundum atrial septal defect

Cardiac pacemaker or defibrillator

Patent ductus arteriosus

✚ Recommendations for surgical antibiotic prophylaxis

Surgical chemoprophylaxis highly recommended

Prophylaxis has been definitively shown to reduce mortality, major morbidity, and hospital costs for the following procedures, and will also reduce antibiotic consumption.

Appendectomy	Arthroplasty
Colorectal surgery	Open fractures
Caesarian section	Open surgery for closed fracture
Induced abortion	Hip fracture
Transurethral resection of prostate	Cataract surgery

Surgical chemoprophylaxis recommended

Gastro-oesophageal surgery	Vascular surgery
Small bowel surgery	Craniotomy, spinal surgery
Open cholecystectomy/other	Corneal grafts, lacrimal surgery
Bile duct, pancreatic, liver, spleen surgery	Open reduction/internal fixation of mandibular fractures
Percutaneous endoscopic gastrostomy insertion	Facial plastic surgery
Abdominal/vaginal hysterectomy	Head and neck surgery, especially clean–contaminated
Third/fourth-degree perineal tears	Breast surgery (cancer, implants)
Transrectal prostate biopsy	Cardiac surgery on bypass (no more than 48 hr)
Radical cystectomy	Pulmonary resection
Lower limb amputation	

Low or negligible risk

Clean benign head and neck and facial surgery	Urinary tract endoscopy
Tonsillectomy	Arthroscopy
Laparascopic cholecystectomy	Transurethral resection of bladder tumours
Inguinal/femoral hernia repair (with or without mesh), incisional or laparoscopic	

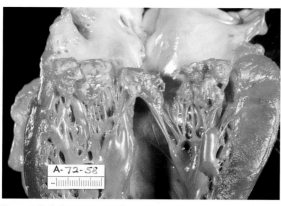

Fig. 16.5 Pathology specimen demonstrating the valvular vegetations of infective endocarditis.

Useful resources and further reading

National Institute for Clinical Excellence (www.nice.org.uk).

British Society for Antimicrobial Chemotherapy (http://www.bsac.org.uk).

Scottish Intercollegiate Guidelines Network (www.sign.ac.uk). Excellent and detailed guidance on antibiotic chemotherapy.

Bratzler DW *et al.* (2004) *Clinical Infectious Diseases* **38**, 1706–15. American Advisory Statement on antibiotic prophylaxis in surgery.

American Heart Association (www.americanheart.org). Includes links to endocarditis prophylaxis schedules.

16.5 Infection control issues

The prevention of spread of infections is critical to effective healthcare in both community and hospital. Healthcare delivery is changing and with it the requirement for robust clear policies and procedures to reduce transmission of microbial pathogens, whether resistant or not. Drivers of change in current healthcare provision which may affect rates of spread of pathogens include the following.

- More rapid turnover of patients because of less invasive surgical procedures.
- More complex surgery: solid organ, bone marrow, and stem cell transplants; implantable devices.
- Changing demographics: increased numbers of immunocompromised or high-risk patients. These include those with conditions such as congenital heart disease or cystic fibrosis surviving into adulthood; and also the increased proportion of elderly patients.
- Imported diseases-migration, travel, immigration.
- Change to ambulatory management of chronic disease: dialysis, home TPN, home intravenous therapy.

Much of prevention of communicable disease is common sense and relatively simple in both theory and practice, but it must be applied rigorously in order to succeed. Therefore infection control has to be deeply embedded in all aspects of hospital policies and procedures including procurement, hospital design, personnel, education, and clinical governance frameworks.

In recent years infection control has become a priority area for governments. In the UK, trust performance indicators relating to infection prevention and control are published. The current Healthcare Act 2006 sets out a code of practice that all healthcare organizations are required to follow.

Compulsory core policies for NHS bodies

- Standard (universal) infection control precautions.
- Aseptic technique.
- Major outbreak plans for communicable disease.
- Source isolation of patients.
- Safe handling and disposal of sharps.
- Prevention of occupational exposure to blood-borne viruses (BBVs), including prevention of sharps injuries.
- Management of occupational exposures to BBVs and post-exposure prophylaxis.
- Disinfection policy.
- Antimicrobial prescribing.
- Reporting of healthcare-associated infections to the Health Protection Agency as directed by Department of Health.
- Control of infections with specific alert organisms, taking into account local epidemiology and risk assessments. These include, as a minimum, MRSA, *Clostridium difficile*, and transmissible spongiform encephalopathies.

Organizational structures

Healthcare providers, such as NHS Trusts and Primary Healthcare Trusts have a responsibility to ensure the health and safety of patients, staff, and visitors. The ultimate responsibility in UK rests with the Chief Executive and Management Board. Normally, the body responsible for preparing and implementing policies and procedures is the Infection Control Team headed by an Infection Control Doctor and an Infection Control Nurse. Most trusts now have a Director of Infection Prevention and Control (DIPC), who manages overall infection control strategy at board level. Key to the success of effective implementation of infection control policies in practice is the link with each clinical unit via a named consultant and senior nursing staff.

The hospital environment

Modern hospitals should be designed and built with infection control in mind.

The operating environment

There should be adequate provision of suites designed for the likely case mix and operation type and throughput of work. This includes the requirement for ultra-clean operating theatres, including laminar flow (where necessary) and provision of highly efficient particulate air (HEPA) filters. The exact number and type will depend on the clinical profile of the department. The performance of operating theatres is usually monitored by Estates and Facilities. Their design and performance maintenance schedule is under guidance set out in the Department of Health's Health Building Note 26 (currently under revision).

There should be adequate provision of source isolation for highly transmissible pathogens and airborne pathogens (e.g. TB, influenza, measles, varicella zoster), enteric pathogens (multidrug-resistant coliforms, Salmonella, Shigella, *Clostridium difficile*) and viruses and pathogens that can easily be transmitted via contact (MRSA and *Streptococcus pyogenes*). This is detailed in Health Building Note 4.

Universal precautions

Good working practice demands the use of universal or standard precautions to prevent cross-contamination with micro-organisms.

Hand hygiene

Transmission of microbes on the hands is a major source of cross-infection of a number of pathogens, including *Staphylococcus aureus*, *Streptococcus pyogenes* (group A streptococcus), coliforms, and viruses (RSV, para-influenza virus). It can largely be prevented by adequate hand hygiene.

- Wash hands according to the standard method if they are visibly soiled, at the beginning of day, and before invasive procedures.
- Cuts and abrasions should be covered with waterproof dressings and changed regularly.
- Use of alcoholic hand gel applied to visibly clean hands between patient contact episodes, including manipulation of devices and ventilator circuits, is effective.

Personal protective equipment

- Examination gloves if at risk of exposure to exposure to body fluids.
- Gowns, aprons, masks, and eye protection where there is high risk of splashing from body fluids. These must be disposed of after each patient episode.

Aseptic technique for insertion of invasive devices

Safe handling and disposal of sharps

- Correct container available at point of care
- NO disassembly of sharps and syringes
- Do not pass from hand to hand
- No overfilling of containers.

→ Modes of spread of infectious material

Knowledge of the different modes of spread and environmental reservoirs and sources of infectious agents is a prerequisite for prevention of communicable disease.

Contact

* Sources can be hands, but also objects ('fomites') and medical devices (urinary catheters, ventilator tubing, IV catheter hubs).

Inoculation

* Needles
* Trochars
* Invasive medical devices
* Rigid endoscopes
* Surgical instruments
* Vascular grafts
* Prosthetic implants

Airborne

* *Droplet-respiratory pathogens:* viruses but also *Neisseria meningitidis, Bordetella pertussis, Haemophilus influenzae, Mycobacterium tuberculosis.* Transmission can be promoted by coughing and exposure-prone procedures such as deep suctioning. Particles are relatively dense and will not travel beyond 1m. For this reason, respiratory protection is recommended for personnel in close proximity to or performing droplet promoting procedures. BBVs can spread via this route.
* *Aerosols:* in certain situations particles become aerosolized (via a reduction in density and size, usually due to evaporation) and such particles can travel much further than droplets. Respiratory protection and containment in these situations is different. Pathogens that can spread via this route include TB (especially miliary), measles and varicella. Occasionally *Legionella pneumophilia* has been associated with a hospital.
* *Other particles:* airborne particles such as skin scales and dust can contain spores of both fungi and bacteria and also some viruses that can survive for surprisingly long periods in the environment. These can be dispersed via air-conditioning vents, fans, and external and internal building works. Norovirus, which can cause rapidly spreading nosocomial gastroenteritis, can be spread via vomitus after projectile vomiting.

Environmental

Surfaces, floors, mops, storage boxes, and beds can all act as sources for potentially infectious micro-organisms, including the spores of *Clostridium difficile.*

Faecal/oral route

This is usually easily prevented by good hygiene.

Food

Close contact

Sexual contact is uncommon in hospitals, but is not unknown!

→ Decontamination

Contamination of anaesthetic equipment during patient use is inevitable via direct contact, splashing of secretions and blood, and handling. The degree of contamination, and the risk this poses for transfer of infection, will depend on the type of equipment and its use, i.e. whether it goes into a body cavity.

The use of single-use equipment is encouraged wherever possible depending on cost, convenience, and availability.

Reusable devices such as specialist diagnostic equipment or surgical instruments must go through a process of decontamination between patients or procedures. This applies to laryngoscope blades.

Decontamination refers to the whole process of cleaning and either disinfection or sterilization that renders a piece of equipment safe for further use. The degree of decontamination required depends on the risk the device and its use poses to the patient.

* *Critical/high risk* Any device that penetrates the skin or mucous membrane to enter a vascular or normally sterile space—single use or sterilization.
* *Semi-critical/intermediate risk* A device that will be in contact with intact skin or mucous membranes or may become contaminated with transmissible pathogens—high-level disinfection/ sterilization.
* *Low risk/non-critical* A device that is in contact with intact skin or not at all—low-level disinfection or cleaning and drying.

Cleaning

The removal of proteinaceous organic matter before either disinfection or sterilization is essential. This can be difficult with complex equipment (such as flexible endoscopes) which may need disassembly for effective cleaning. This is especially critical for reducing risk of prion disease prior to sterilization.

Low-level disinfection

Low-level disinfection will kill the majority of vegetative bacteria and some viruses, but not spores or bacteria such as mycobacteria. Its success depends on bio-load, contact time, concentration, and bioactivity. Examples include alcohol, hypochlorite solutions, and chlorhexidine.

High-level disinfection

High-level disinfection involves the use of heat or chemicals to kill most vegetative microorganisms. There has been a move away from local processing to centrally processed, automated cleaning and disinfection methods. The advantage of this is that it can be performed in a controlled way using well-validated standard operating procedures. The whole process can then be monitored, quality controlled, and audited so that the equipment pathway can be tracked and reconstructed if required.

This also reduces staff exposure to irritant chemicals and pathogens. Many chemical agents that have been used. Peroxide agents are the most widespread after aldehydes (such as glutaraldehyde) have been phased out.

Sterilization

Sterilization is a process that removes and kills all infective material including spores.

* This is achieved by various means and usually at a central sterile services facility (CSSD). It is not suitable for local processing facilities.
* Includes dry and moist heat sterilization (or autoclaving—the preferred method in most hospitals) and gamma irradiation, although this is only done in specialized facilities and rarely within hospitals.

Infections acquired as a consequence of admission to a healthcare institution have special relevance to modern healthcare. Rates of such infections can vary quite widely between hospitals and healthcare institutions.

Terminology

Community-acquired: refers to infections whose provenance and onset occurs outside the hospital setting, and not within 10 days following hospital discharge.

Nosocomial: acquired as a result of admission to a healthcare facility. For surveillance purposes, this usually denotes infection not evident on admission and commencing 48hr after admission and up to 10 days after discharge, except for surgical site infections (SSIs) which occur 30 days after the procedure (or 1 year when a prosthetic implant is present).

Healthcare-associated infections: The term healthcare-associated infection (HCAI) has been proposed to describe situations of increased risk of infection from pathogens more commonly associated with hospitals. These will vary depending on the type of infection (such as central venous catheter (CVC) infection, SSI with implanted prosthetic device); and the risk has yet to be characterized fully for each type. For bloodstream infections, for example, the following were more likely to represent nosocomial infections than community-acquired infections:

- Receiving home intravenous therapy in last 30 days
- Attended hospital or haemodialysis centre in last 30 days
- Hospitalized in acute care facility for ≥2 days in previous 90 days
- Resident in a nursing home.

The possibility of an HCAI will impact on the empirical selection of antibiotic (if required).

There is a necessity for active local and national surveillance systems, plus good communication between primary care and hospital systems, so that unusual patterns of disease can be acted upon early on. Movement of patients between healthcare facilities is an important route of introduction of resistant pathogens, which is why good communication between medical and nursing staff and infection control teams and microbiology departments is so essential.

Factors that contribute to rates of HCAI

Demographics
Age distribution of patients.

Patient factors
Type and complexity of surgical procedures undertaken, presence of high-risk patients such as immunocompromised patients, haematology/oncology units, solid organ and bone marrow transplants, large ICUs and HDUs, renal dialysis units (e.g. high invasive device usage).

Structural
Provision of single-source isolation rooms.

Organizational
High bed occupancy, mixing of colonized and non-colonized patients, inadequate decontamination protocols.

Behavioural
Poor infection control practices, compliance with good working practices such as hand washing, non-touch techniques.

Environmental
Inadequate cleaning of environmental sources of infection.

An HCAI is any infection acquired whilst in, or as a result of being admitted to, a healthcare facility. Many of those that are measured are device- or procedure-related (see below). However, some, such as *Clostridium difficile* infections, are not. Many of these infections are potentially preventable, and at least controllable, by effective infection control policies and procedures, good clinical practice, and adherence to locally formulated antibiotic policies.

Epidemiology

- It has been estimated that at any one time nearly one in 10 inpatients has a HCAI. These are average figures, and individual rates can vary depending on the individual trust and case mix of wards and patients. Rates are highest in intensive care facilities. This amounts to 100,000 patient episodes per year in England and Wales.
- Mortality: it has been estimated that, in the UK, 5000 deaths/year may be directly attributable to HCAIs and it may be a substantial contributor to 15,000 further deaths. (These data were extrapolated from United States studies).
- Morbidity: discomfort and pain, requirement for reoperation, increased length of stay.
- Cost: it has been estimated that HCAIs cost an additional 1 billion pounds per year in the NHS.

Types of HCAI

Urinary tract infections (UTIs) have the highest rates but the lowest mortality. The highest mortality is from bloodstream infections.

Bacterial
- UTI—often catheter related.
- Pneumonia—mainly ventilator related (see box opposite).
- Surgical site infections (SSIs).
- Bloodstream infections—often CVC related (see box opposite).
- Soft tissue/wound infections.
- Other, including *Clostridium difficile* associated disease (CDAD).

Viruses
- Gastroenteritis
- Respiratory tract infections (RSV, influenza)
- Varicella
- Bloodborne viruses (hepatitis B and C, HIV)
- Prion disease

Reducing HCAI: legislation and guidance

Several key documents have been published in the last few years, culminating in the Health Act 2006 Code of Practice for the Prevention and Control of Healthcare Associated Infections:
- Getting Ahead of the Curve
- Winning Ways
- National Audit Office Report on Healthcare
- Towards Cleaner Hospitals and Lower Rates of Infection: A Summary of Action
- The Saving Lives Delivery Programme to Reduce Healthcare Associated Infections.

The last of these details key interventions designed to have maximum impact on reducing HCAIs through maximum compliance with good practice. The key areas of clinical practice highlighted are:
- Prevention of microbial contamination
- Central venous catheter care
- Preventing surgical site infections
- Care of ventilated patients
- Urinary catheter care.

⊕ Lower respiratory tract infections

Pneumonia is the second most common type of HCAI in both adult and paediatric patients. A subset of these infections is termed ventilator-associated pneumonia (VAP); Figure 16.6.

VAP is an important cause of morbidity and mortality in the critically ill and up to 15% of ventilated patients develop it. VAP also increases ventilator time, mortality rates, ICU and hospital stay, and costs.

VAP is defined as occurring at least 48hr after intubation and mechanical ventilation and within 24hr of extubation.

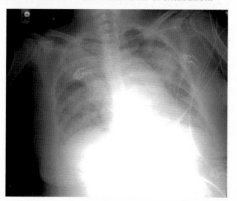

Fig. 16.6 CXR of ventilator-associated right upper lobe pneumonia

Aetiology of VAP

- Overgrowth of oropharynx and stomach with bacteria, including coliforms, exacerbated by higher gastric pH (e.g. due to use of antacids) and enteral feeding.
- Impaired mucociliary clearance and coughing.
- Impedance of glottic closure; pooling of secretions above endotracheal cuffs.
- Micro-aspiration of oropharygeal contents and colonization of the endotracheal tube.

Risk of VAP increases with duration of ventilation, immune suppression, requirement for tracheostomy, re-intubation, neuromuscular weakness, transportation from the ICU or HDU (for surgery, radiography), and being placed in a recumbent position.

Early-onset VAP (occurs within 72hr of admission)
Streptococcus pneumoniae, Moraxella, *Haemophilus influenzae.*

Late-onset VAP

Coliforms, *Staphylococcus aureus* including MRSA, Acinetobacter.

The different groups of organisms alter empirical antibiotic therapy.

There is a current drive to reduce rates of VAP by applying High Impact Interventions (UK). These are measurable quality improvement programmes which combine strict infection control with four components of patient care. The last two are not directly related to preventing VAP but prevent complications of critical care.

- Position of patient: elevation of head of bed to 30–45°.
- Reducing duration of ventilation by sedation weaning, including periodic sedation vacations and reassessing readiness to extubate.
- Gastric ulcer prophylaxis.
- Deep vein thrombosis prevention.

In addition, humidification of inspired air to prevent drying of respiratory secretions, only replacing ventilator tubing when visibly soiled or malfunctioning, and wearing gloves and decontaminating hands before and after suctioning are recommended.

⊕ Bloodstream infections

Although bloodstream infections (BSIs) are less common than other types of HCAI, they have received particular attention because of the mortality and morbidity associated with them and their impact on patient stay and hospital costs.

BSIs represent about 15% of all HCAIs. BSIs can be primary or secondary to another source; however, the majority are related to the presence of CVCs. This has given rise to the definition of catheter-related BSI (CR-BSI). Up to 6000 patients in England and Wales develop a BSI each year. A small proportion is attributable to peripherally inserted venous cannulae. For surveillance purposes, rates are given as the number of CR-BSIs per 1000 catheter days.

Routes of entry for catheter-related infection

The majority of CR-BSIs are related to short-term indwelling CVCs, especially on ICU and HDUs. A significant proportion are from longer-term tunnelled CVCs such as Hickman and Broviac lines, and also Vascath and PICC lines.

The aetiology of catheter-related infections is complex, but the routes of entry of micro-organisms are as follows.

- Contamination of device before insertion (usually at manufacture).
- Skin organisms, including those naturally present, those introduced by healthcare workers, and those invading the wound.
- Catheter hub.
- Infusate contamination: this can be associated with the either the medication or fluids and may also be introduced at manufacture.
- Seeding from a remote infection via the bloodstream.

Early onset infections can occur because of inadequate skin preparation at line insertion or contamination from patient's flora or a healthcare worker's hands. Bacteria can spread on the external surface of the line. This is the most common route of contamination in short-term non-tunnelled CVCs.

Colonization of the hub and intraluminal colonization with bacteria appear to be mainly responsible for infections in tunnelled lines. Certain bacteria, such as staphylococci (both coagulase-negative and *Staphylococcus aureus*) and Candida, adhere to plastic, probably with fibrinous deposits, forming an extracellular matrix or biofilm. Bacteria within the biofilm are inaccessible to antibiotic or host-mediated killing, which is one reason why it is sometimes impossible to treat or eradicate infections from CVCs other than by line removal.

Strategies to reduce the risk of CR-BSIs

- Use single-lumen devices unless otherwise required for patient care.
- Use a subclavian or internal jugular insertion site.
- Use skin asepsis during insertion (alchoholic chlohexidine).

During catheter care:
- Observe insertion site daily.
- Use clean intact dressing at the insertion site, including use of non-stitch securing devices.
- Use aseptic non-touch technique when accessing port/hub, or using alcoholic chlorhexidine wipes.
- Do not routinely change lines if not infected.

→ Classification of type of operation

Clean	No inflammation is encountered and respiratory, alimentary, or genitourinary tracts are not breached. No break in aseptic technique
Clean-contaminated	Respiratory, alimentary, or genitourinary tracts are entered but without significant spillage. Operations involving the biliary tract, appendix, vagina, and oropharynx are included in this category.
Contaminated	Acute inflammation (but NOT pus) is encountered or there is visible contamination of wound. Gross spillage from hollow viscus during the operation or compound open injuries operated on <4hr previously
Dirty	Operations in the presence of pus, where there is a previously penetrated hollow viscus or compound/open injuries. Operated on >4hr previously. Includes old traumatic wounds with devitalized tissue.

→ Criteria for definitions of surgical site infections

Superficial incisional	Infection occurring within 30 days of operation involving skin and or subcutaneous tissue plus one of: • Purulent discharge • Organisms from aseptically taken tissue or fluid
Deep incisional	Infection occurs within 30 days of operation OR within 1 year if implant is in place and is related to operation plus one of: • Purulent discharge from deep incision • Spontaneous dehiscence or deliberately opened by surgeon plus signs of infection • Abscess involving the deep incision found by direct examination during re-operation • Diagnosis by attending physician.
Organ space	Infection occurs within 30 days of operation OR within 1 year if implant is in place and is related to operation AND infection involves any part of the anatomy other than incision (organ or space) which was opened or manipulated during operation AND one of: • Purulent discharge from drain placed into organ/space • Organisms isolated aseptically from organ space • Abscess involving the deep organ space • Diagnosis by attending physician.

→ Factors influencing risk of surgical site infections

Patient characteristics	Operation
Age Nutrition Diabetes mellitus Smoking Obesity Coexistent infections at unrelated site Colonization with high-virulence pathogens, especially *Staphylococcus aureus* Immunosuppression Multiple blood transfusion Anaemia Malignancy	Type of surgical procedure: large bowel resection and limb amputation are high risk Perioperative glucose control (major cardiac surgery and diabetics) Temperature control (normothermia improves rate of SSIs) Skin asepsis Preoperative clipping rather than shaving Preoperative skin preparation Duration of procedure Use of antimicrobial prophylaxis-including coverage for MRSA if colonized and decontamination Operating room function Failure of instrument sterilization Foreign material in surgical site Surgical technique Poor haemostasis Failure to obliterate dead space Duration of surgical scrub Tissue trauma

⊕ High-impact interventions in preventing surgical site infections

Preoperative

MRSA screening for all patients undergoing prosthetic implant, cardiothoracic, neurosurgery, orthopaedic, and vascular surgery.

MRSA decontamination prior to surgery if possible.

Hair removal via clipper but not razor.

Perioperative

Antimicrobial prophylaxis where indicated and at correct dose, type, and timing.

Glucose control: maintaining glucose <11mmol/L in diabetics.

Normothermia.

Maintaining body temperature above 36°C in the perioperative period.

Chapter 17

Gastrointestinal tract and liver

17.1 The upper gastrointestinal tract

This area is important to anaesthetists as it overlaps with the upper airway. Problems here can cause disastrous complications.

The mouth

In the mouth, food is chewed and saliva is added.

Teeth

Teeth consist of three parts: the outer crown, the root, and the neck between the two. The central part of the tooth is the soft pulp, covered by hard dentine. Dentine is 70% inorganic calcium hydroxyapatite, arranged in tubules. In the crown, the dentine is covered by extremely hard enamel—minute mineral rods arranged in bundles, which run vertically onto the chewing (occlusal) surface. In the root the dentine is covered by a thin layer of cement into which the periodontal ligament runs from the bone, firmly fixing the tooth. A neurovascular bundle runs from the end of the root into the pulp, which is very sensitive.

The child has 20 deciduous (milk) teeth, which erupt between the ages of 6 and 30 months. These are shed and replaced by the 32 permanent teeth, in order but at variable ages, between 6 and 12 years. The remuneration expected from the 'tooth fairy' is also variable, and often excessive.

The importance of teeth to the anaesthetist is principally:

- They may obstruct the view or access to the mouth and larynx
- They are vulnerable to damage or accidental dislodgement (particularly if diseased)
- Teeth or fragments may be displaced into the airway with the potential for obstruction, distal collapse, infection, etc.

Saliva

Saliva is hypo-osmolar and alkaline, with high concentrations of potassium and bicarbonate. It protects from mechanical damage and infective agents, and is important in maintaining oral hygiene. It contains amylase and lipase enzymes, which initiate digestion of starches and fats respectively.

Swallowing

Swallowing (deglutition) is a complex series of coordinated movements, initiated voluntarily:

- The mouth contents are moved to the back of the tongue
- The hyoid bone is elevated slightly and fixed
- The palatal arches are brought together and the back of the tongue is pulled backwards.

From here on swallowing proceeds involuntarily:

- The soft palate is tightened and lifted back, closing off the nasopharynx.
- The hyoid bone and larynx are pulled upwards and forwards and the larynx closed off by the aryepiglottic folds and arytenoid cartilages.
- The pharynx is pulled upwards and opened. The back of the tongue acts like a plunger, forcing the bolus down into the pharynx.
- The middle and then the inferior pharyngeal constrictors relax and then tighten, passing the bolus down.
- In the oesophagus, a peristaltic wave moves the bolus into the stomach.

The cranial nerves involved in swallowing are given in Table 17.1. The muscles of the pharynx and oesophagus, together with their resting intraluminal pressures, are shown in Figure 17.1.

Dysphagia

Dysphagia (difficulty in swallowing) is a common problem. Because swallowing is a complex process involving sensation, muscle strength, and coordination, it is susceptible to interference by many diseases.

Failure of normal swallowing predisposes to aspiration and malnutrition. Possible causes include:

Mechanical: foreign body, tumour, abscess, web or stricture, gastro-oesophageal reflux disease (GORD).

Neuromuscular: Diverticuli, pouches, achalasia; myasthenia gravis, motor neuron disease, muscular dystrophy, SLE, dermatomyositis, rheumatoid arthritis.

CNS: stroke (dysphagia in >40%), Parkinson's disease, multiple sclerosis.

Note: an intact gag reflex does not indicate adequate swallowing.

The oesophagus

The oesophagus is a muscular tube with inner circular and outer longitudinal layers. There is a sphincter at each end. Proximally, the upper oesophageal sphincter is a thickened band of striated muscle (cricopharyngeus) 1–2cm long. It maintains a resting pressure in the lumen of up to 60mmHg higher than the surroundings. Distally, the lower oesophageal sphincter (LOS) is anatomically indistinguishable from the rest of the oesophagus; but for a few centimetres the resting pressure is 20–40mmHg higher. Functionally, this protects the oesophagus from the reflux of gastric contents. LOS tone is:

- Increased by cholinergic stimulation, metoclopramide, and gastrin;
- Reduced by β-adrenergic agents, prostaglandin E_1, and most anaesthetic agents.

Whether or not gastric contents reflux into the oesophagus depends on the **barrier pressure:** the LOS pressure minus the intra-gastric pressure.

Gastro-oesophageal reflux disease (GORD)

This is a common condition in the Western world. GORD can cause chest pain, pain on swallowing, oesophagitis, and sometimes less obvious symptoms such as wheezing and 'asthma'. GORD increases the risk of aspiration of gastric contents during anaesthesia. GORD is associated with obesity, excessive intake of alcohol or coffee, and infrequent and large meals. The mechanisms are incompletely understood, but include:

- Mechanical, e.g. hiatus hernia. Normally, the diaphragmatic crura 'pinch off' the stomach from the oesophagus. This cannot occur if part of the stomach is above the diaphragm.
- Functional: low resting tone in the LOS or transient inappropriate LOS relaxations.

Treatment includes:

- Dietary and lifestyle advice.
- Antacids, proton pump inhibitors, or histamine H_2 blockers.
- Occasionally surgery may be indicated.

Table 17.1 Cranial nerves involved in swallowing

Cranial nerve	Name	Action during swallowing
V	Trigeminal	Motor to chewing muscles, tensor veli palatini, mylohyoid Sensory to anterior two-thirds of tongue
VII	Facial	Motor to lips and cheeks, stylohyoid Sensation of taste
IX	Glossopharyngeal	Innervates salivary glands Motor to stylopharyngeus and superior constrictor Sensory to soft palate, posterior tongue, and upper pharynx
X	Vagus	Motor to palatoglossus, levator veli palatini, cricopharyngeus, intrinsic muscles of larynx (recurrent laryngeal nerve) Sensory to posterior and lower pharynx, larynx
XI	Accessory	Motor only to palatopharyngeus, levator veli palatini, uvula
XII	Hypoglossal	Motor to all the muscles of the tongue except palatoglossus

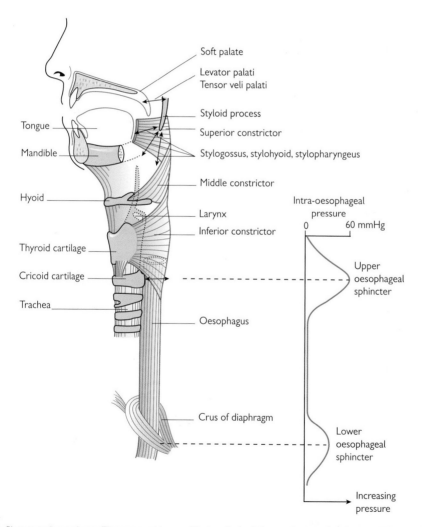

Fig. 17.1 Pharynx and oesophagus. The upper and lower sphincters display higher resting tone than the rest of the oesophagus.

17.2 The stomach, antacids and prokinetics

The function of the stomach, and its alteration by drugs and disease, is of importance in anaesthesia, as it relates to the risk of aspiration of gastric contents. This was first described by Mendelson in 1946 in an obstetric population; it is now known to be a risk to many other groups. Drugs can be used to reduce the likelihood and the severity of the consequences of aspiration.

Gastric secretions

Around 1–2L are secreted daily. There are four main gastric secretions:

- Gastric acid.
- Pepsinogen.
- Mucus (soluble and insoluble).
- Intrinsic factor.

Gastric acid

Gastric acid assists with digestion and the absorption of calcium and iron. It also provides a defence against micro-organisms. It is secreted from the parietal ('oxyntic') cells in the gastric pits of the fundus and body (Figure 17.2). At rest, the cells secrete mainly sodium and chloride. When stimulated, secretion increases and comprises mainly hydrogen ions (up to 150mmol/L; 10^6 x plasma concentration) and chloride.

Acid secretion occurs in three phases, with most being produced in the gastric phase.

Cephalic phase: initiated by the sight, smell or thought of food. The signal is via the vagus nerve; vagotomy completely prevents this phase. Two pathways contribute: a direct cholinergic effect from the vagus on the parietal cells; and vagally stimulated gastrin secretion from G cells in the antrum, mediated by gastrin-releasing peptide (GRP). Gastrin acts in a paracrine manner to stimulate parietal cell acid secretion.

Gastric phase: occurs when food enters the stomach. The acid environment of the stomach normally suppresses gastrin production (negative feedback). Food dilutes the acid, and gastric pH rises, removes this 'brake', and allows gastrin (and therefore acid) to be produced. Gastric distension and digested food (particularly peptides) reflexly stimulate acid production by increasing gastrin and by direct effects on parietal cells. *Long gastric reflexes* relay in the central vagal nuclei; *short gastric reflexes* are confined to the stomach itself.

Intestinal phase: protein products in the duodenum stimulate the release of gastrin. Absorbed amino acids in the blood probably stimulate parietal cells as well.

The stimulus for acid production is amplified by **histamine**, which is released from the enterochromaffin-like (ECL) cells in the gastric lamina propria in response to gastrin and acetylcholine.

Cellular mechanisms of acid production

Gastrin and histamine act on the parietal cell to increase intracellular Ca^{2+} and cAMP, respectively, which drive the highly energy-dependent H^+/K^+-ATPase. This exchanges H^+ for K^+ ions, and can generate a gastric pH as low as 1 (Figure 17.3).

Pepsinogens

These inactive pre-enzymes are cleaved into active pepsin in an acid environment. Pepsin initiates protein digestion. Pepsinogens are secreted, in response to vagal stimulation and an acid pH, from peptic (chief) cells in the fundus and body (type 1), and mucous cells in the pylorus (type 2). As we have already seen, protein digestion stimulates gastric acid production.

Mucus

Soluble mucus is secreted from neck cells in the gastric pits. It lubricates the gastric contents.

Insoluble mucus is produced by surface mucous cells, and forms an alkaline layer, protecting the mucosa from friction, acid, and the action of pepsin.

Intrinsic factor

Intrinsic factor (IF) is a mucoprotein which binds to vitamin B_{12} and allows its absorption in the terminal ileum. It is secreted by the parietal cells independently of acid production. Deficiency of IF leads to pernicious anaemia.

Inhibition of gastric secretions

Inhibition of gastric secretions occurs by a number of mechanisms. **Somatostatin** inhibits gastrin secretion and parietal cell activity, and is released in response to acid in the stomach. Several inhibitory substances known as **enterogastrones** are released from the duodenum in response to the presence of digestive products. These reduce both acid secretion and the rate of gastric emptying, to prevent overload of the duodenum. **Gastric inhibitory peptide**, **secretin**, and **cholecystokinin** are examples.

Gastric emptying

The stomach volume can vary from 0.5 to 3L with little change in pressure because of the plasticity of its smooth muscle wall and vagal reflexes causing relaxation.

There are three layers of smooth muscle: inner oblique, middle circular, and outer longitudinal. Like the rest of the gut, they are innervated by intrinsic and extrinsic (autonomic) nerves and exhibit spontaneous electrical activity (Section 17.3).

Gastric emptying is the result of waves of contraction starting proximally and propagating. The pylorus then has to relax, to allow contents to pass into the duodenum. Not all gastric contractions are expulsive; if the pylorus is closed, they serve to mix and grind the stomach contents, producing **chyme**.

The rate of gastric emptying varies according to the contents.

- **Liquids** start to empty promptly. Under normal conditions, liquids empty from the stomach exponentially, with a half-time of about 20min.
- **Solids** exhibit a lag phase before emptying, typically about 30min. Usually over half a meal will have cleared the stomach after 2hr; <10% remains after 4hr.
- **Chemical composition:** the more extreme the pH, osmolarity, or fat content, the slower gastric emptying proceeds.

Predictions of how much ingested material will remain in the stomach after a given time are extremely unreliable. There is huge individual variation, and external influences may have a marked effect. Some of the factors which affect gastric emptying are given in Table 17.2.

Antacids

Barrier preparations

Alginates (e.g. sodium alginate) are extracted from brown seaweed. These compounds are large polysaccharides and work by providing a floating physical barrier against refluxed acid. They are useful for patients at risk of aspiration due to an increase in abdominal pressure or an incompetent gastro-oesophageal sphincter.

Buffers (neutralize acid)

Magnesium and aluminium salts are good for immediate control of symptoms of acid excess. However, as they are particulate, they are not used prior to anaesthesia as complications are worse following aspiration of particulate material. Magnesium-containing compounds are laxative, whereas aluminium compounds are more likely to cause constipation.

Sodium citrate is a non-particulate colourless solution which buffers gastric acid. The normal dose is 30ml of 0.3M solution. It is given immediately before induction of anaesthesia as it has a short duration of action.

Drugs which reduce acid production

These drugs work to increase the pH of the stomach contents above 2.5. They have no effect on acid already in the stomach, and therefore should be given well before anaesthesia. Two main groups exist: H_2 receptor antagonists and proton pump inhibitors.

H_2 receptor angatonists

This group are competitive antagonists at histamine H_2 receptors; they include *cimetidine* and *ranitidine*. H_2 receptor antagonists generally work within 2hr of oral administration (1hr when administered IV). As well as reducing acidity, these drugs also reduce the volume of secretions produced. They are only partially metabolized in the liver by the cytochrome P450 system, and most are excreted unchanged by the kidneys. The dose should be reduced in renal failure. Cimetidine is a well-known P450 enzyme inhibitor.

Proton pump inhibitors (PPIs)

These include *omeprazole, esomerazole, pantoprazole,* and *lansoprazole.*

PPIs act by non-competitively inhibiting the hydrogen–potassium adenosine triphosphatase enzyme system (H^+/K^+-ATPase) in the parietal cells (Figure 17.3). The rate of gastric emptying is not affected by PPIs.

Drug clearance from the body is unaffected by renal or liver disease. PPIs inhibit hepatic enzymes, and so may potentiate the effects of other drugs.

Prokinetics

The macrolide antibiotic **erythromycin** is probably the most effective prokinetic agent. It is an agonist at gastric motilin receptors. It is given in a dose of 200mg or less. It may show tachyphylaxis and may slow small bowel transit time. Its antibiotic effect may be unwanted.

Cisapride is also effective, and probably enhances bowel transit time as well, but has been withdrawn in the UK because it is prone to cause dysrhythmias, particularly if there is a prolonged QT interval or if clearance is delayed by CYP3A4 inhibition.

Metoclopramide increases gastric motility. It antagonizes peripheral dopamine receptors, improving cholinergic activity. It also directly increases smooth muscle tone. It increases LOS tone, reducing the risk of aspiration significantly. It should also be administered at least 1hr before anaesthesia. More than 10mg may be required. It can cause extrapyramidal side-effects. Domperidone has a similar action but does not penetrate the blood–brain barrier and is less likely to cause adverse CNS effects.

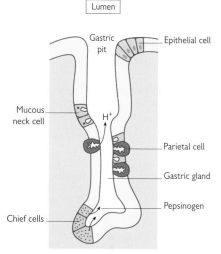

Fig. 17.2 Gastric pit cell types.

Table 17.2 Factors affecting emptying

	Promote gastric emptying	Inhibit gastric emptying
Neural factors (local and central)	Gastric distension	Duodenal distension Ileus Autonomic neuropathy (e.g. diabetes) Pain, anxiety Vagotomy
Mechanical factors		Distal obstruction Supine postion
Drugs	Metoclopramide Erythromycin Domperidone	Opioids Anticholinergics Alcohol

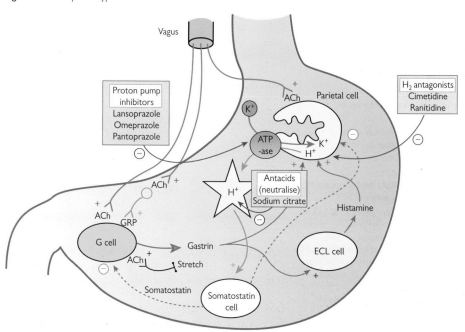

Fig. 17.3 Gastric acid regulation and the effects of drugs.

The regulation of the GI tract affects the type of secretions entering it; the rate at which they do so; the rate at which contents progress through the tract; and the rate of digestive and absorptive processes.

Regulatory substances

Regulation is by endocrine, paracrine, and neurocrine influences. Their interactions are complex and incompletely understood.

Endocrines

An endocrine is a substance carried in the circulation, exerting its effects remote from the site of its production. All the endocrines known to control the GI tract are peptides. So far, five are known as 'full' GI hormones: *secretin, gastrin, cholecystokinin, motilin,* and *gastric inhibitory peptide.* Various other candidate hormones have not yet been fully characterised.

Paracrines

A paracrine exerts its effects close to where it is secreted. The effects of *somatostatin* and *histamine* on the stomach are described in Section 17.2, but they also occur in other parts of the GI tract.

Neurocrines

Neurocrines are released from nerve endings (i.e. they are neurotransmitters).

Vasoactive intestinal peptide (VIP) mediates smooth muscle relaxation via nitric oxide production. *Gastrin-releasing peptide (GRP)* is released in gastric mucosa by vagal activity and promotes the secretion of gastrin. *The enkephalins (leu- and met-)* act on opioid receptors on smooth muscle to cause contraction, raising sphincter pressures and slowing transit.

Motility of the small bowel

Structure and innervation

The smooth muscle is arranged in an inner circular and outer longitudinal layer (Figure 17.4). The circular layer is generally thicker. The innervation is complex, consisting of:

- the prominent **myenteric plexus** of nerves between the muscle layers;
- a smaller **submucosal plexus** inside the circular muscle layer;
- numerous **interneurons** within and between the plexuses;
- **extrinsic innervation** from the autonomic nervous system.

Motility in the small bowel is achieved by smooth muscle contractions. In the fed state, contractions tend to cause segmentations – mixing rather than propelling contents forwards. Mass peristalsis tends to occur during fasting (Figure 17.6).

Electrical activity in the gut wall

Specialized cells (the *interstitial cells of Cajal*) form a network around and through the muscles. These interstitial cells generate and propagate electrical pacemaker activity.

The intrinsic nerves use a large variety of neurotransmitters, including *acetylcholine, serotonin (5-HT), VIP, nitric oxide, somatostatin,* and *substance P.* Often, the same nerve may contain more than one neurotransmitter.

Smooth muscle contractions may be *phasic* (short duration) or *tonic* (sustained). There are several types of electrical activity.

Slow-wave depolarizations occur with a frequency of about 8–12/min in the small bowel. They travel slowly from proximal to distal. Slow waves do not cause contraction; this requires an additional rapid depolarization, the **spike potential,** to reach the threshold required for muscle contraction. Contraction requires both a slow wave and a spike potential (Figure 17.5). The rate of slow-wave depolarization is constant at any given point in the bowel, but the rate of contraction is greatly modified by neural or hormonal influences.

During fasting, the bowel is much less active. A strong peristaltic wave runs the whole length of the gut, about every 1.5hr. This is the **migrating motor complex** (MMC) or myoelectric complex. It stops when a meal is taken. The MMC may help to clear bacteria and indigestible obstructions from the proximal gut.

The **ileocaecal valve** is kept closed by smooth muscle tone. It regulates the passage of contents into the colon, avoiding overload. It also prevents bacterial overgrowth in the small bowel. It relaxes in response to gastric distension, so a meal hastens the transit of the previous one.

Extrinsic neural activity

Parasympathetic efferents originate from the vagus or pelvic nerves, and synapse in ganglia close to the target site. ACh is the predominant neurotransmitter, and tends to promote secretion and motility, and relax sphincters.

The **sympathetic** system mainly has the opposite effect. Sympathetic nerves relay in ganglia remote from the target. ACh is the pre-ganglionic neurotransmitter, and noradrenaline the main post-ganglionic one.

Most of the output of the extrinsic systems is not directly onto the gut itself, but onto the intrinsic nerves innervating smooth muscle, glands, and absorptive cells. Sensory information also travels in the extrinsic system back to the CNS.

Motility of the large bowel

The structural arrangement of the large bowel is similar to that of the small bowel. The longitudinal muscles are gathered into three longitudinal straps (taenia coli). The colon is shaped into a series of sacs by rings of constriction (haustrations). These are not anatomical features, but are areas of increased muscle tone whose position changes. Slow segmentation contractions move the colonic contents gently back and forth. Peristaltic waves from one end of the colon to the other are seen infrequently, typically one to three times a day (the **mass movement**). Transit through the colon generally takes one or two days, compared with a few hours through the small bowel.

There are two anal sphincters. The **internal anal sphincter** is a thickening of circular smooth muscle which is under reflex control. The **external anal sphincter** is striated muscle under voluntary control.

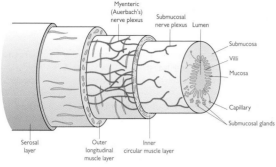

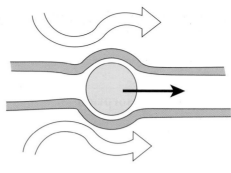

Peristalsis

Fig. 17.4 Structure and innervation of the intestine. The intestinal wall is made up of layers, each with a specialist function. The myenteric plexus lies between the inner circular and outer longitudinal muscle layers.

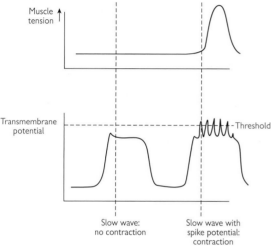

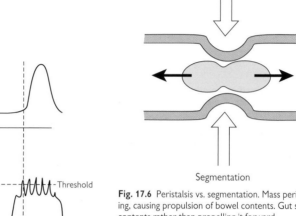

Segmentation

Fig. 17.6 Peristalsis vs. segmentation. Mass peristalsis occurs during fasting, causing propulsion of bowel contents. Gut segmentation mixes the gut contents rather than propelling it forward.

Fig. 17.5 Muscle contraction and membrane potentials of the gut.

➔ Problems with bowel motility

Diarrhoea is the frequent passage of too-liquid stools. Common causes are:

- **Infection**—many agents.
- **Toxins.**
- **Malabsorption** (osmotic diarrhoea).
- **Allergy.**

Severe and persistent diarrhoea can cause dehydration and electrolyte imbalance (particularly in children), most often hyponatraemia, hypokalaemia and acidosis.

Constipation, obstruction, and ileus: constipation refers to the lack of normal passage of GI contents, and may be relative or absolute. Bowel obstruction causes hyperactive bowel initially, but then bowel proximal to the obstruction dilates and becomes flaccid and silent. This effect spreads proximally, causing gastric stasis, nausea, vomiting, and loss of appetite. Ileus often occurs when there is no mechanical obstruction (pseudo-obstruction). This can be due to:

- **Peritonitis.**
- **Surgery:** more likely (and more persistent) if there has been surgery on the GI tract itself, especially the colon. Probably less severe if regional anaesthesia has been used. The new non-absorbable opioid OP3 (mu) receptor antagonist **alvimopan** may reduce the duration of ileus without compromising systemic analgesia.
- **Autonomic neuropathies**, e.g. in diabetes.
- **Hypothyroidism.**
- **Electrolyte** disturbances, especially hypokalaemia and hypercalcaemia.
- **Drugs**, especially opioids and anticholinergics.
- **Hirschprung's disease** is a congenital lack of colonic nerve ganglia causing a functional obstruction. It affects the rectum and distal colon, with proximal gut dilatation. Rarely (but disastrously) it may affect the whole GI tract.

Digestion is the breakdown of food into smaller molecules which can be more readily absorbed.

General principles of absorption in the gut

The structure of the gut is adapted to expose the contents to a large surface area. Most absorption takes place in the small bowel. The lumen of the small bowel is formed into *Kerkring's folds*. The mucosal surface is covered in villi—finger-like projections over which the mucosal cells are arranged. The cells are basically two types: the enterocytes, which are absorptive, and the goblet cells, which are secretory. The cells present a surface of *microvilli* to the lumen—the brush border.

Absorption is not a simple matter of the movement of substances from the gut lumen into blood through the enterocytes. There is a complex interaction of many layers and pathways. From the gut lumen, the layers are:

- The unstirred layer
- The glycocalyx.

Molecules can pass either into the enterocyte or through *tight junctions* between cells into the intercellular space. The cells are arranged on a basement membrane; capillaries run below it. Tight junctions separate the gut lumen from the intercellular space, but they are variably permeable to water and ions. Cells are able to take up substances by:

- Diffusion
- Facilitated diffusion
- Active transport
- Pinocytosis.

The cells influence what goes in and out of the intercellular space by using similar transport mechanisms across the basolateral membrane.

The digestion and absorption of the main classes of dietary components are reviewed below and illustrated in Figures 17.7 and 17.8.

Carbohydrate

About 50% of dietary carbohydrate is starch, and about 30% is sucrose.

Starches are polysaccharides, with glucose subunits joined by $\alpha1-4$ linkages which form a straight chain, and less often by $\alpha1-6$ linkages which form branches. Glycogen is the most branched of the common dietary starches.

Sucrose is a disaccharide consisting of a glucose and a fructose subunit.

The remaining dietary carbohydrates are a mixture of polymers, dimers (like sucrose), and monomers. In the gut lumen the $\alpha1-4$ linkages are cleaved by salivary and (predominantly) pancreatic amylase. However, the $\alpha1-6$ linkages and adjacent $\alpha1-4$ linkages are resistant to amylase, leaving a mixture of saccharides with a lot of $\alpha1-6$ linkages: *α-limit dextrins*.

The enterocyte brush border has numerous membrane-bound **carbohydratase enzymes** (*glucoamylase, sucrase, isomaltase, lactase*, etc.), which break down the remaining polymers and dimers into their constituent hexose sugars (glucose, galactose, fructose). *Isomaltase* breaks most of the $\alpha1-6$ linkages. Most carbohydrate is completely absorbed by the proximal jejunum. The exception is lactose, whose digestive enzyme *lactase* is the only enzyme capable of separating glucose from galactose. In humans (except Europeans), lactase activity declines after infancy, and most adults are lactose intolerant. A large amount of lactose in the diet will cause bloating and osmotic diarrhoea. Lactase activity is concentrated near the tips of the intestinal villi and is easily lost if there is inflammation or gut ischaemia.

The hexose sugars *fructose, glucose,* and *galactose* are too large to enter the enterocytes by diffusion.

- Fructose is absorbed by facilitated diffusion via the GLUT-5 carrier.
- Glucose and galactose are absorbed by a sodium-dependent active transport carrier (SGLT-1). This brings in two sodium ions for every hexose molecule. The sodium is then extruded from the cell by a Na^+–K^+ pump. If sodium accumulates intracellularly to any degree, the carrier is disabled; it depends on a sodium gradient into the cell.

Accumulation of hexoses is prevented by their extrusion via another carrier, GLUT-2, in the basolateral membrane.

The co-transport of sodium and hexose is exploited in **oral rehydration therapy**, where a glucose and sodium solution can be used to treat diarrhoeal water and electrolyte loss. The mixture enhances absorption; water passively follows the solutes.

Protein

Protein breakdown starts in the stomach with the action of *pepsins*. There are at least three isoenzymes, all *endopeptidases* (they cleave internal peptide bonds). They are all acid dependent and so their activity stops as soon as they enter the alkaline duodenum. Further protein digestion is accomplished by *pancreatic peptidases*. These are all secreted as inactive precursors and cleaved into the active form in the gut lumen, either by *enterokinase*, an enzyme secreted at the brush border, or by their own active form (*autocatalysis*).

Amino acid and oligopeptide (2–6 amino acid) digestion products are absorbed into the enterocyte by transmembrane carriers. Each carrier is specific for a particular class of amino acids: one for basic amino acids, another for neutral amino acids, and so on. Some of the amino acid carriers are co-transporters requiring sodium, some co-transport with protons, while others do not require an ion gradient.

Normal protein digestion solution is only 40% single amino acid. Poorly understood mechanisms must exist for the absorption of small peptides, since a solution of mixed amino acids and small peptides results in a faster and higher peak of amino acid concentration in portal venous blood than does a solution of amino acids alone; presumably the amino acid carriers become saturated. In the enterocyte, the peptides are mostly cleaved into single amino acids and transported across the basolateral membrane by carriers similar to those on the brush border.

Lipids

Most dietary lipids are *triglyceride, phospholipid, or sterol esters*. The uptake of lipids into the enterocytes has five main steps (Figure 17.8):

- **Secretion** of lipase enzymes and bile salts.
- **Emulsification** (bile salts).
- **Ester hydrolysis** (lipases).
- Formation of **micelles**.
- **Diffusion** into enterocytes.

Bile salts are formed from cholesterol in the liver and secreted. They have a hydrophilic and a hydrophobic part, and so can interact with lipid in a watery mixture to form an emulsion (a suspension of small lipid droplets). This exposes a lot of lipid to the *lipase* enzymes.

There are a number of lipases. Gastric lipase accounts for only a small fraction of lipid digestion. Pancreatic lipase is secreted from the pancreas in its active form. However, bile salts displace it from the lipid–water interface, so it cannot work without *colipase*, also secreted by the pancreas, which binds to both lipase and the bile salt molecule. This keeps the products of lipolytic action close to bile salts, for micelle formation. Pancreatic lipase hydrolyses triglycerides at the 1 and 3 ester linkages, yielding two *free fatty acids* (FFAs) and a *monoglyceride*.

Phospholipase A_2 is secreted from the pancreas as a pro-enzyme which is activated in the gut lumen. It hydrolyses phospholipids, yielding FFAs and *lysophospholipid*.

Cholesterol esterase hydrolyses cholesterol and triglycerides. It has no specificity for a particular linkage, so it produces FFAs and glycerol.

At a critical concentration, bile salts form small aggregates called **micelles**. The bile salts are arranged so that their hydrophilic parts all face outwards. Small lipids can be dissolved in the inner part of the micelle. The particles formed are much smaller than the droplets in an emulsion (3–10nm vs. 200–5000nm). A micellar solution is completely clear; this extreme water solubility allows the micelles to diffuse into the aqueous layer next to the enterocytes, so the lipids can diffuse into the cell.

Inside the cells, the substrates are re-synthesized into triglycerides. Lipids are packaged with *apoproteins* into *chylomicrons*, which are exported from the cell by exocytosis. They are carried in *lacteals* into the thoracic duct, and from there into the circulation. They are then taken up by the liver.

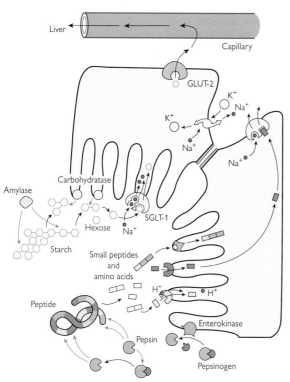

Fig. 17.7 Digestion and absorption of carbohydrates and protein.

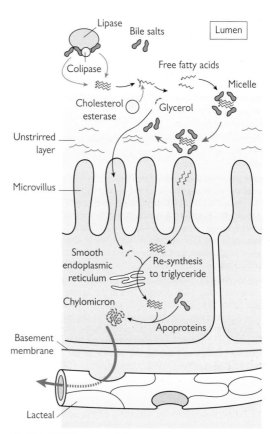

Fig. 17.8 Lipid digestion and absorption.

Water and electrolytes

In the adult about 9L of water a day enter the GI tract; roughly 2L from food and drink, and the rest from GI tract secretions. As the water output in faeces is only about 100ml daily, the rest is absorbed, almost all of it in the small bowel. Water passively follows ions and solutes as they are absorbed both into cells and between the cells into the paracellular space. In the small bowel, the junctions between cells are quite leaky, and water and electrolytes can readily move along their electrochemical gradients. In the colon, the junctions are tighter; the colon can respond to aldosterone by increasing sodium and water absorption and secreting potassium.

Sodium is absorbed in the small bowel by:

- diffusion through the tight junctions into the paracellular space
- co-transport with solutes such as sugars and amino acids
- co-transport with chloride
- exchange for hydrogen ions.

Low intracellular sodium concentrations, favouring inward sodium movement, are maintained by the energy-dependent Na^+/K^+-ATPase on the basolateral membrane.

Chloride is absorbed with sodium and also moves along an electrical gradient, as the basolateral side of the cell is weakly positive with respect to the gut lumen and strongly positive compared with the inside of the cell. The gradient is maintained by the Na^+/K^+-ATPase pump. This exchanges three sodium for two potassium ions, continually generating a net loss of cations. Chloride is also absorbed in exchange for bicarbonate, particularly in the colon, so colonic contents are generally alkaline.

Chloride is secreted by crypt cells into the gut lumen in order to keep the gut contents liquid. (The chloride ions in the lumen draw sodium and water into the lumen through the paracellular spaces). It has to be actively taken into these cells against the electrochemical gradient; the pump exchanges two chloride ions for one sodium and one potassium ion. Chloride is pumped into the gut lumen in response to intracellular calcium and also to the activity of the cAMP-driven *cystic fibrosis transmembrane conductance regulator (CFTR)*. Genetic defects in this channel account for the inability of cystic fibrosis sufferers to secrete chloride from the epithelium of gut, pancreas and airways. The toxins of cholera and other dysentery pathogens cause excessive chloride secretion by activating of the adenylyl cyclase enzyme.

Calcium is absorbed from the gut by a mechanism promoted by vitamin D. Rises in intracellular calcium, which would disrupt essential processes, are prevented by an intracellular binding protein, which allows calcium to be stored in the Golgi apparatus or endoplasmic reticulum. Calcium is extruded from the cell by an ATPase pump.

Iron is absorbed as part of haem in red meat. It is also present as Fe^{3+} in other foodstuffs, but this form is difficult to remove from its organic ligands. It also precipitates in the alkaline pH of the duodenum. Conversion to Fe^{2+} by the acid of the stomach releases it and makes it available for absorption. Overall, it is absorbed in three forms, each of which uses a different mechanism (Figure 17.9):

- **Ferrous ion (Fe^{2+})** is absorbed via divalent metal transporter 1 (DMT1)
- **Ferric iron (Fe^{3+})** is absorbed via mobilferrin–integrin (MFI). However, most is converted to Fe^{2+} by D cyt b on the brush border.
- Absorption of **haem** via a specific haem receptor allows cellular haem oxygenase to liberate Fe^{2+}. This is independent of DMT1.

Duodenal enterocytes control absorption of iron and prevent entry of excessive quantities. Generally, less than 10% of dietary iron is absorbed.

- Within these cells, ferrous iron (Fe^{2+}) binds with apoferritin to form ferritin. In ferritin, it is stored in the ferric state (Fe^{3+}).

- Ferrous iron (Fe^{2+}) is transported across the basolateral membrane by ferroportin. It is coupled to ferrioxidase, and this converts the iron to Fe^{3+}.

Only ferric iron (Fe^{3+}) passes into the bloodstream from the enterocyte. Transferrin carries both absorbed and recycled Fe^{3+}. It binds to its target cell membrane receptors before becoming trapped within the cell by endocytosis. After removal of the iron, the intact transferrin molecule is then returned to the circulation.

Control of absorption

Within the duodenal mucosal cells, apoferritin binds iron to form ferritin. A single apoferritin molecule is able to bind 4000 iron atoms. Absorbed iron influences mRNA for apoferritin to produce more of the protein and increase storage capacity. This relative iron excess is lost as the enterocytes slough off.

Transferrin, the transport protein, has two Fe^{3+} binding sites. Low iron stores result in high levels of poorly saturated transferrin; much of the absorbed Fe^{3+} passes from intracellular ferritin to the plasma protein.

Adequate iron stores result in lower levels of transferrin and so less iron is transferred out of the cell. The level of transferrin is partly responsible for the transfer of iron across the duodenal mucosa.

Vitamins

Vitamins are organic compounds which are essential for metabolic processes, but which cannot be synthesized by humans. Most are assumed to be absorbed by passive diffusion except for those described below.

Thiamine (vitamin B_1) is absorbed in the jejunum by a Na^+-dependent active process.

Riboflavin (vitamin B_2) is absorbed in the proximal small bowel by facilitated diffusion.

Ascorbic acid (vitamin C) is absorbed by an Na^+-dependent active process and by passive diffusion.

Folic acid is absorbed by an active process from the duodenum and jejunum.

Cobalamin (B_{12}) absorption requires binding to intrinsic factor (IF) secreted by parietal cells in the stomach. The IF–B_{12} complex attaches to a specific receptor in the distal ileum. It needs calcium and magnesium ions in an alkaline environment for proper absorption.

Vitamins A, D, E, and K are fat-soluble. They all need to be solubilized in bile salt micelles for effective absorption. Vitamin A is absorbed as β-carotene, which is split into vitamin A in the enterocyte. Vitamins D and E are present in the diet as esters, which are hydrolysed by cholesterol ester hydrolase. Vitamin K exists in two forms, K_1 and K_2. K_1 is absorbed by active transport, and K_2 is synthesized by some gut bacteria and can be absorbed passively from the colon. The fat-soluble vitamins are then incorporated into chylomicrons for transport around the body.

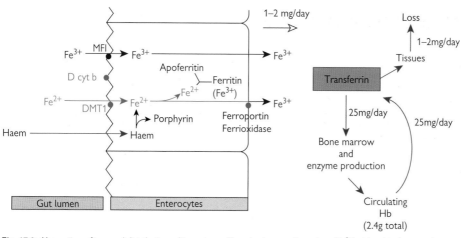

Fig. 17.9 Absorption of iron and distribution of iron stores. Once in the cytoplasm, iron (Fe^{3+}) either binds to apoferritin or is transported across the basolateral membrane into the blood by ferroportin.

17.6 Metabolism

Most of the diet is used to generate or store energy. In mammals, energy production is centred on the glucose molecule. The main pathways for the major classes of dietary intake (carbohydrate, protein and fat) are overviewed here.

In the cell, the currency of the energy economy is the high-energy phosphate bond. Adenosine triphosphate (ATP) is the most obvious example of a molecule with this high-energy bond, but there are many others.

The major biochemical pathways are interlinked and are subject to very precise regulation.

Energy generation

The process of energy generation starts with **glucose**, the basic carbohydrate unit. This 6-carbon compound is converted to pyruvate (3-carbon) by the **glycolytic (Embden–Meyerhof) pathway**. The steps are shown in Figure 17.10. Several of the steps are reversible if substrate concentrations favour it. The irreversible steps allow the process to be regulated. Conversion of glucose to G6P and fructose to fructose biphosphate requires energy. However, later reactions yield more, so there is a net gain of six ATP per glucose molecule.

The glycolytic pathway occurs in the cytosol and does not require oxygen, so can generate energy in anaerobic conditions. In this case, pyruvate is converted to lactate and exported from the cell; this is one of the causes of lactic acidaemia. Lactate can be cleared by the liver if oxygen is available.

If conditions are aerobic, pyruvate dehydrogenase converts pyruvate to acetyl CoA, which enters the next step: the **tricarboxylic acid cycle** (TCA) (citrate or Krebs cycle). This occurs in the mitochondria. The starting point is acetyl CoA (2-carbon, formed from pyruvate) joining with oxaloacetate (4-carbon) to form citrate. The TCA cycle generates a net gain of 30 ATP per glucose molecule. In fact, the yield of ATP is indirect; the cycle actually generates (per glucose molecule): two GTP molecules, six reduced NADH, and two reduced FADH. The energy is used to make ATP by oxidative phosphorylation on the inner mitochondrial membrane.

Oxidative phosphorylation is a series of electron transfers from the reduced compounds NADH and FADH. It is carried out by mitochondrial inner transmembrane lipoproteins: *complexes I–IV, ubiquinone (coenzyme Q),* and *cytochrome c*, which channel electrons (via numerous intermediaries) to molecular oxygen to form water.

Complexes I, III, and IV are *proton pumps*, which drive protons into the intermembrane space, creating a proton gradient. The leak of these protons back into the mitochondrial matrix powers the ATP synthase enzyme which converts ADP to ATP.

The TCA cycle does not require O_2 *per se*; however, oxidative phosphorylation does. Without O_2, substrate concentrations build up and prevent forward movement through the TCA cycle.

A small proportion of glucose is metabolized via the hexose monophosphate shunt, which produces NADPH. This is essential for the action of glutathione, which helps to maintain cellular integrity by reducing membrane and cellular sulphydryl groups. (This mechanism is overwhelmed in acute paracetamol overdose, resulting in hepatic necrosis (Section 17.13)).

Carbohydrate

The human storage polysaccharide is *glycogen*; the pathways by which glucose is converted to and from it are described in Section 17.12.

The preferred substrate for an immediate increase in energy generation is carbohydrate; in the first instance when glucose starts to run low glycogen is the immediate source of extra glucose (as G6P). However, the energy stored as glycogen is limited (typically 2000kcal).

Gluconeogenesis

Gluconeogenesis primarily occurs in the liver, and to a lesser extent in the renal cortex. It is the process which allows glucose to be generated from non-carbohydrate carbon substrates when glycogen stores are exhausted. These substrates include lactate, glycerol, and certain amino acids. All TCA cycle intermediate molecules can be used for the generation of glucose. By convention, pyruvate is the first designated substrate of the pathway.

The enzymes and steps of gluconeogenesis are shown in blue in Figure 17.10. The process is essentially the reverse of glycolysis: most of the enzymes in the pathway operate freely in both directions, depending on the concentrations of substrate available. However, some reactions in the glycolytic pathway are not reversible in this way, and it is these which require different enzymes - and energy - to be undone for gluconeogenesis. The process of gluconeogenesis is very costly from an energy standpoint: glycolysis to 2 moles of pyruvate only yields 2 moles of ATP, whereas gluconeogenesis from 2 moles of pyruvate to 2 moles of fructose-1,6-bisphosphate consumes 6 moles of ATP. The process is worthwhile because some tissues (including the brain) are obligate users of glucose for energy.

Protein

Amino acids can be used as an energy source after deamination in the urea cycle. The products feed into the TCA cycle as pyruvate, acetyl CoA, or other intermediates. It is clearly damaging to lose too much protein in this way. Protein loss is limited initially by using fat for energy production. However since amino acids are an important substrate for gluconeogenesis, a degree of protein loss is inevitable during prolonged starvation.

Lipid

Lipids are the main form of energy store. They have a high energy density (9kcal/g vs. 5 kcal/g for carbohydrate). Also, as they are non-polar, they can be dehydrated: 5kg of fat stores as much energy as over 30kg of glycogen.

Lipids are stored as *triglycerides*. These can be catabolized to *glycerol* and 3 *free fatty acids*. Glycerol can be converted into *triose phosphate*, an intermediate for either glycolysis or gluconeogenesis. Long chain fatty acids can be converted into *ketone bodies*, 2 carbons at a time, by β-*oxidation* in the mitochondria. These can be fed into the TCA cycle by conversion to acetyl CoA. Some glucose is always needed (by the brain, for example) so there will always be a need for gluconeogenesis. An excessive build up of ketones (for example in diabetes) causes ketoacidosis (see Section 18.7).

Regulation of metabolism

Negative feedback

A major part of the regulation of glycolysis is achieved by controlling the irreversible steps in the glycolytic pathway, in particular phosphofructokinase (PFK-1).

PFK-1 activity, and hence the rate of glycolysis, is promoted by high levels of substrate (glucose, F6P), but inhibited by acid, citrate, and ATP (which will rise if there is either a relative lack of oxygen or high activity by the TCA cycle).

The main regulation of its activity is by fructose 2,6,-biphosphate (F2,6BP), which is produced from F6P by the enzyme PFK-2. PFK-2 is itself activated by insulin (and inhibited by glucagon). Therefore the same factors which promote glycolysis will inhibit gluconeogenesis, thus opposing processes are not pointlessly running simultaneously.

Similar mechanisms regulate the activity of pyruvate kinase and phosphoglycerate kinase (promoted by ADP, and inhibited by ATP).

Hormones

Insulin is the main anabolic hormone. It promotes glycogen formation, lipogenesis, glucose uptake, and glycolysis, and inhibits gluconeogenesis.

Glucagon, catecholamines, and the **stress response** promote protein and lipid breakdown and gluconeogenesis.

Metabolic rate

Basal metabolic rate (BMR) describes the energy required by an awake but inactive individual. The process of metabolism produces CO_2 and consumes O_2. The ratio of these two processes is the *respiratory quotient (RQ)*. Carbohydrate produces an RQ of 1.0, protein about 0.8, and fat about 0.7. By measuring O_2 consumption and CO_2 production it is possible to infer which substrates are being used, and whether the individual is in an anabolic or catabolic state. This can be important in providing an appropriate balance of nutrition (e.g in ICU). At rest, about 70% of the energy produced is derived from fat and 30% from carbohydrate. As activity increases, the additional energy is preferentially generated from carbohydrate, and more oxygen is consumed. Eventually VO_{2max} is reached where no more oxygen can be utilized. This is subject to change according to fitness level, see exercise physiology (Section 8.9).

Various factors influence basal metabolic rate; thyroxine increases it, and starvation decreases it, which accounts for the futility of many reducing diets.

Shunts associated with the Embden-Myerhof pathway

At several points along the glycolytic pathway, products are diverted to serve other purposes than feeding into the TCA cycle to produce ATP. These diversions are known as shunts. Not only do they produce substances essential for cell function, they regulate the glycolytic pathway, providing a "blow off valve" for glycolysis.

The hexose monophosphate shunt is described opposite. Its role is to produce NADPH, essential to cellular stability and survival.

The Rapoport-Leubering shunt (Section 15.1) produces the 2,3 DPG essential for the functioning of red blood cells.

The methaemoglobin reductase shunt is described in Section 15.1. It allows conversion of methaemoglobin back to haemoglobin.

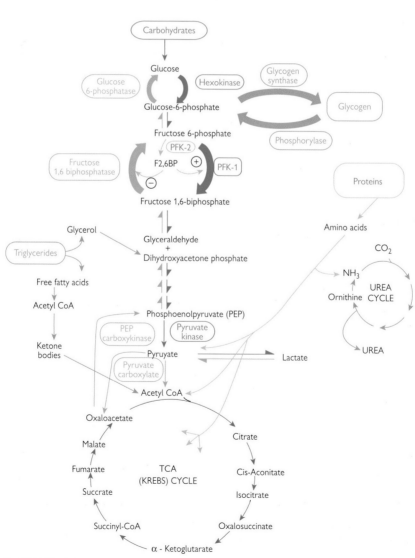

Fig. 17.10 Metabolism.

17.7 Nutrition

Abnormalities of nutrition are an ever-growing problem – with large proportions of the population becoming increasingly overweight whilst others suffer with increasing problems of nutritional neglect.

Control of appetite

Control of diet is multifactorial. The nervous system is more concerned with the coordination of daily intake, whereas endocrine control is more involved with long-term control of body weight and calorific intake.

The arcuate nucleus of the hypothalamus is the coordination centre for hunger and satiety (Figure 17.11).

Appetite stimulation

- Hunger stimulates the release of **neuropeptide Y (NPY)** in the arcuate nucleus. This stimulates Y_1 receptors and increases food intake and calorie storage. The release of NPY has an antagonist effect at receptors involved in inhibiting calorie intake.
- **Ghrelin** (a polypeptide) is produced in the stomach. It acts on the hypothalamus, releasing NPY, and has some direct effects on the vagus, both of which result in an increase in appetite and food-seeking behaviour.

Appetite inhibition

In times of adequate calorie intake, the appetite is suppressed and the rate of metabolism is increased to reduce calorie storage. Cells in the arcuate nucleus contain pro-opiomelanocortin (POMC) which release alpha-melanocyte stimulating hormone (α-MSH), which inhibits hunger via MC4 receptors, providing feelings of satiety. Regulatory factors include the following.

- **Insulin** has a major role in the regulation of glucose uptake and control. A lack of insulin at the hypothalamus results in an increased appetite.
- **Leptin** originates from fat cells and stimulates POMC, inhibiting appetite. (It should follow that obese patients have inhibited appetite because of increased leptin; in fact, this is not the case. The transport of leptin across the blood–brain barrier may be inhibited by excess triglycerides, *reducing* leptin activity in obese patients).
- **Cholecystokinin (CCK)** is released from the duodenum in response to ingested dietary fats and proteins. CCK inhibits appetite and also reduces gastric emptying, causing gastric distension. Both these effects are mediated by the vagus.
- Some of the feedback mechanisms for appetite suppression and stimulation come from the **vagus nerve** (cranial nerve X) via the **nucleus tractus solitarius** in the hindbrain.

Normal dietary intake (Table 17.3)

Carbohydrates

- Make up 45% of nutritional intake (35% as sugar in the West).
- Stored as glycogen (~24hr worth), predominately in the liver and skeletal muscle.
- Glycogen is catabolized in the liver to maintain blood glucose at times of reduced intake.

Lipids

- 50% of daily nutritional requirement, mainly as triglycerides.
- Approximately 20% of total body weight is fat, stored in adipose tissue, which is available for long periods of reduced intake (on average 3 months).

Proteins

- Protein intake should be 10% of daily nutritional requirement, although in the West intake can exceed 15%
- Only used as energy store in extreme starvation—skeletal, myocardial, and liver protein can all be used, but may eventually lead to death.

Clinical abnormalities of nutrition

Obesity

Obesity is an increasing problem in the West, and is particularly prevalent in the USA. Obesity is associated with an increase in morbidity and a twofold increase in mortality. There are a number of implications for patients undergoing anaesthesia (Section 17.9).

Malabsorption

Malabsorption occurs as a result of abnormalities of absorption of nutrition in the face of normal intake. Absorption of energy substrate relies on a number of factors being normal:

- Gut surface area for absorption
- Presence of enzymes
- Carrier molecules.

Various malabsorption conditions exist and can present in various ways depending on the particular condition.

- Short gut syndrome: occurs following surgery when large portions of the small intestine are removed.
- Coeliac disease: gluten intolerance resulting in villous atrophy in the small bowel and malabsorption, which is reversible with omission of gluten from diet.
- Chronic pancreatitis: a lack of pancreatic enzymes results in the inability to digest and absorb digestive fats leading to a deficiency of the fat-soluble vitamins A, D, E, and K.
- Pernicious anaemia: autoimmune damage to gastric parietal cells leads to a lack of intrinsic factor, essential for the absorption of B_{12}.

Malnutrition states

Malnutrition is a deficiency of nutritional intake. This can be a result of:

- Inability to obtain or consume food (e.g. sedation, poverty, handicap, oral/oesophageal pathology).
- Behavioural/ psychiatric disorders, e.g. anorexia.
- Inadequate intake compared with energy expenditure, e.g. catabolic states, burns, sepsis.

Clinical signs of malnutrition

- Reduced albumin <25g/dl
- White cell count <1.5 x 10^9/L
- Weight loss > 10%
- Reduction in skinfold thickness.

A high proportion of patients in hospital have been shown to be nutritionally deficient. For many patients this is a result of disease processes, loss of appetite, and inability to access food of their choice when they want it.

Table 17.3 Normal Daily Nutritional Intake	
Energy	30–40 Cal/kg
Nitrogen	0.2 g/kg
Water	30–40 ml/kg
Sodium	1 mmol/kg
Potassium	1 mmol/kg
Chloride	1.5 mmol/kg
Phosphate	0.3 mmol/kg
Calcium	0.1 mg/kg
Magnesium	0.1 mg/kg
Iron	0.2 mg/kg

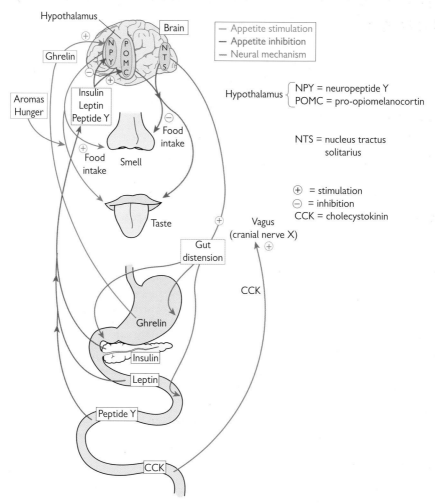

Fig. 17.11 Control of appetite.

In the figure:

- — Appetite stimulation
- — Appetite inhibition
- — Neural mechanism

Hypothalamus $\begin{cases} NPY = neuropeptide\ Y \\ POMC = pro\text{-}opiomelanocortin \end{cases}$

NTS = nucleus tractus solitarius

⊕ = stimulation
⊖ = inhibition
CCK = cholecystokinin

Labels: Hypothalamus, Brain, Ghrelin, Aromas Hunger, Insulin Leptin Peptide Y, Food intake, Smell, Food intake, Taste, Gut distension, Vagus (cranial nerve X), CCK, Ghrelin, Insulin, Leptin, Peptide Y, CCK

Artificial feeding

Enteral nutrition

Enteral feeding involves liquid food being placed directly into the gut via a nasogastric or nasojejunal tube. It is the best choice when normal absorption can take place but intake is problematic. Enteral feeding is relatively free from complications, acceptable to patients, and effective. It reduces the risk of formation of gastric stress ulcers and maintains normal bacterial flora, thus reducing the risk of bacterial translocation. Feeding should start with small volumes and build up gradually. Many feeding regimes involve a 'feeding' break, often overnight, which mimics the normal lack of nutritional intake at night-time. Complications can occur, such as tube blockage, nausea, vomiting, and diarrhoea.

Parenteral nutrition

Parenteral (PN) or IV nutrition is used for those patients who have inadequate gut function or in whom enteral feeding has failed. PN can be used in combination with enteral feeding or as the sole form of nutrition, then called total parenteral nutrition (TPN). PN requires specific IV access, ideally a tunnelled central venous line. Carbohydrate and nitrogen are provided by glucose and an amino acid mixture; trace elements and vitamins can also be added. All elements are suspended in an emulsion of soya bean oil, which provides the fat element of the feed. Complications are far more likely to occur with PN than with enteral feeding regimes. They include:

- Infection (PN is a highly effective culture medium for pathogens)
- Metabolic abnormalities e.g. hyperglycaemia, hypophosphataemia
- Cholestatic liver disease and cholecystitis
- Over- or under-nutrition.

An understanding of the control mechanisms of nutritional intake and abnormalities of nutrition is vital as every body system is affected.

17.8 Obesity

Obesity is a growing problem worldwide, with an incidence of around 17% in the UK. The body mass index (BMI) is used to define obesity:

$$\text{BMI} = \frac{\text{weight (kg)}}{\text{height squared (m}^2\text{)}}.$$

The classification of obesity is shown in Table 17.4.

Obesity occurs as a result of excess nutritional intake. This excess is thought to be due in part to environmental changes, which have ensured constant access to food, and genetic mutations, which result in a loss of control of nutritional intake.

Effects of obesity

Cardiovascular system

- Increased total blood volume although reduction in volume on a ml/kg basis (normally 70ml/kg, but can be as low as 45ml/kg).
- Increased atherosclerosis from hypercholesterolaemia, leading to hypertension and ultimately increased left ventricular work. With time, left ventricular hypertrophy develops and results in myocardial ischaemia and left ventricular failure.
- Increased risk of thromboembolic events (e.g. deep vein thromboses and pulmonary emboli).
- Aortocaval compression can occur, resulting in a reduction in cardiac output.

Respiratory system

- Fat deposits in the soft tissues of the upper airway can make management of the airway more difficult. Upper airway obstruction is more likely to occur with anaesthesia and the supine position.
- Obstructive sleep apnoea (OSA) is more likely to occur in those with obesity when the soft tissues of the pharynx collapse during sleep. This causes intermittent airway obstruction and hypoxia.
- Functional residual capacity (FRC) is reduced whilst awake. This is exacerbated under anaesthesia. In morbidly obese patients, closing volume may exceed FRC during anaesthesia.
- Increased oxygen demand due to an increase in basal metabolic rate (increased tissue mass).
- Increased work of breathing due to reduced thoracic compliance (can be up to 55% reduction) and V/Q mismatch.
- Alveolar hypoventilation syndrome (also known as obesity hypoventilation syndrome): loss of CO_2 drive resulting in hypoxia, which causes hypoxic pulmonary vasoconstriction. This in turn causes pulmonary hypertension and polycythaemia. Pulmonary hypertension can ultimately lead to right ventricular failure.

Gastrointestinal

- Diabetes mellitus is common due to both pancreatic insufficiency ('burnout') and insulin resistance.
- Patients have impaired gastric emptying and an increased incidence of hiatus hernias; hence they are more likely to suffer from gastro-oesophageal reflux. These factors increase the risk of aspiration.
- Gout, hepatic insufficiency, and gallstones are all more likely in those who are obese.

Treatment of obesity

There is no treatment as such for obesity. Reducing diets cut food intake, so there is less 'spare' energy to be stored as fat. A reduction in food intake should be accompanied by an increase in exercise, which will lead to the conversion of fat to energy substrates.

Some pharmacological and surgical treatments are available for the treatment of morbid obesity (BMI >35), but these should not be used in those who have not attempted weight loss programmes.

Pharmacological

- **Sibutramine** acts on appetite suppression pathways to reduce nutritional intake and hence encourage weight loss.
- **Orlistat** inhibits pancreatic enzymes essential for the absorption of fats from the gut.
- **Rimonabant** is a cannabinoid receptor antagonist used successfully in both weight loss and smoking cessation.

Surgical

Surgical procedures are becoming more popular but should be reserved for those who are morbidly obese (BMI >35). Surgical techniques carry risks, e.g. failure, bowel ischaemia, infection, and malabsorption states. Most importantly, a lifestyle change is required of all patients who undergo weight loss surgery; only highly motivated patients should be operated upon.

A variety of procedures exist:

- Jaw wiring has been used in the past, but has been found to be ineffective once the wires are removed.
- Gastric banding surgery is becoming more popular: a band is placed across the stomach to reduce the size of the stomach 'pouch', hence inducing a feeling of fullness with smaller stomach volumes. It can be performed laprascopically or as an open operation. Various methods of gastric band surgery exist.
- Balloons have been inserted into the stomach to reduce its size and hence reduce nutritional ingestion.
- Gastric bypass surgery can be used but has potential complications, e.g. 'dumping', electrolyte disturbance and diarrhoea.

Table 17.4 NICE classification of obesity

Classification	BMI (kg/m^2)
Healthy	18.5–24.9
Overweight	25–29.9
Obese I	30–34.9
Obese II	35–39.9
Obese III ('morbid' obesity)	≥40

➕ Anaesthesia for the obese patient

Preoperative

Pre-assessment several weeks prior to surgery is preferable, to allow identification and optimization of comorbid conditions.

Inform theatres in advance to allow appropriate management of the patient.

Meticulous assessment of the airway. In the morbidly obese it may be helpful to arrange to have two anaesthetists present.

Obese patients should be admitted the night before their operation and should receive preoperative thromboprophylaxis and thromboembolic stockings the night before surgery.

Patients should receive preoperative prokinetics and antacids (e.g. metoclopramide 10mg and ranitidine 150mg) 1hr before theatre. For patients with symptomatic reflux, 10ml of sodium citrate should be given in the anaesthetic room.

Induction, maintenance, and monitoring

Pre-oxygenation is vital. Ideally, position patients with 45° head-up tilt to maintain FRC.

Drug doses are extremely variable in the obese patient. The volume of distribution, drug elimination, and metabolism are all altered, not always in a predictable way.

ECG electrodes should be placed on bony prominences.

Blood pressure monitoring requires correct cuff size: the cuff should be 20% larger than the diameter of the upper arm. Intra-arterial blood pressure monitoring should be used in the morbidly obese and for long procedures.

IV access can be difficult. Central venous access should be considered, and ultrasound imaging used.

Because of the high incidence of hypoxia, FRC reaching closing volume, and reflux, patients should probably be intubated for all but the shortest procedures. The siting of an LMA may be difficult in the obese patient, and hypoventilation is a risk in patients breathing spontaneously. IPPV via an LMA is not recommended as the high pressures required may inflate the stomach, further increasing the risk of aspiration.

The addition of PEEP via an endotracheal tube is a useful tool in overcoming intra-operative hypoxia.

Positioning of patients is vitally important. Most operating tables will take up to 150kg when in the standard operating position, but should be checked for maximum capacity prior to anaesthetizing patients. Transfer devices (sliding sheets, hover mattresses, etc.) should be available for the safety and comfort of theatre staff. Consider anaesthetizing patients on the operating table.

Postoperative

All patients require postoperative oxygen, and early physiotherapy and mobilization to optimize respiratory function.

Some patients may require postoperative CPAP. Any patient with known OSA should have access to their normal respiratory assist devices. Non-invasive ventilation may be required in some individuals.

High-dependency care is advised for those with respiratory and cardiovascular disease. In the morbidly obese, high-dependency care should be considered for up to 3 days postoperatively

Postoperative analgesia can be difficult. Intramuscular injections should be avoided as absorption is unpredictable. Regional techniques can be useful, although they may be difficult to perform.

Perioperative nausea and vomiting (PONV) is a major and persistent problem in anaesthesia, with an incidence of 30–80%. Despite a huge volume of published research there is no definitive answer to the problem.

Definitions

- **Nausea** is the subjective sensation associated with the need to vomit.
- **Retching** is a series of precursor movements which resemble vomiting but do not lead to the expulsion of gastric contents.
- **Vomiting** is the reflexly controlled series of neural and muscular events which lead to the retrograde expulsion of gastric contents through the mouth.

Physiology of vomiting

The series of muscle contractions required to produce vomiting is coordinated via efferents from the motor nuclei of the vagus, phrenic, and other motor nerves to respiratory and GI tract muscles. These originate from the 'vomiting centre', which is not in fact a discrete centre, but rather a complex network of neurons loosely centred on the lateral reticular formation of the medulla (Figure 17.12). In this area is the nucleus tractus solitarius (NTS) containing the nuclei of vagus, glossopharyngeal, and accessory nerves, and this is closely related to the dorsal motor nucleus of the vagus, from where much of the para-sympathetic output to the GI tract originates. There is input to the vomiting centre from the chemoreceptor trigger zone (CTZ) in the area postrema in the floor of the fourth ventricle, a very vascular area which functionally lies partly outside the blood–brain barrier and therefore can be stimulated by a large range of blood-borne chemical agents. The pathways and neurotransmitters of the vomiting centre are illustrated schematically in Figure 17.13.

There are many other stimulatory inputs to the vomiting centre, including the vestibular apparatus (motion sickness), sensory nerves from the GI tract itself (chemical irritants, obstruction) which project to the vomiting centre, the nucleus tractus solitarius, and higher centres (thoughts and emotions). Numerous other stimulants can induce vomiting, including raised intracranial pressure, severe hypotension, ionizing radiation and altered hormonal states, such as pregnancy.

The *reflex of vomiting* often starts with repeated swallowing and quick inspirations. The pylorus closes, and the upper and lower oesophageal sphincters relax. The muscles of the abdominal wall and diaphragm contract to increase intra-abdominal pressure. There are powerful retropulsive contractions of the stomach, expelling the contents. There is no retropulsion of duodenal contents but some may be vomited because of increased tone in the duodenum before pyloric closure, allowing reflux into the stomach. The larynx is drawn upwards and the epiglottis downwards and the glottis closes to protect the laryngeal inlet. There is copious salivation and production of tears. There is a strong learned aversion to the provoking stimulus.

Risk factors for PONV:

- Female.
- History of previous PONV, or motion sickness.
- Non-smoker.
- Opioid analgesia.

Several scoring systems have been used to predict the incidence of PONV in a given patient group. A very simple example is that proposed by Apfel *et al* (1999), in which the presence of the above four risk factors is noted; the predicted incidence of PONV is 10%, 20%, 40%, 60%, and 80% with none, one, two, three, and all four of these risk factors present.

Other factors include the following.

- Children (incidence rises with age, reaching twice the adult level at puberty, and then declines).
- Type of surgery: incidence is increased in gynaecological, abdominal, middle ear, breast, strabismus (squint) correction. It is debatable whether type of surgery is itself a risk factor or merely selects a higher-risk group of patients.
- Duration of surgery: every additional 30min of surgery duration increases the risk of PONV by about 60%.

Risks associated with PONV

- Very unpleasant experience: patients prefer to be in pain than to have PONV.
- Risk of oesophageal rupture or wound dehiscence.
- Risks associated with raised intracranial or intra-ocular pressure.
- Raised venous pressures causing secondary haemorrhage postoperatively.
- Risk of aspiration pneumonitis.
- Common cause of unplanned admission after day-care surgery.

Further reading

Apfel CC (1999) *Anesthesiology* **91**, 693–700.

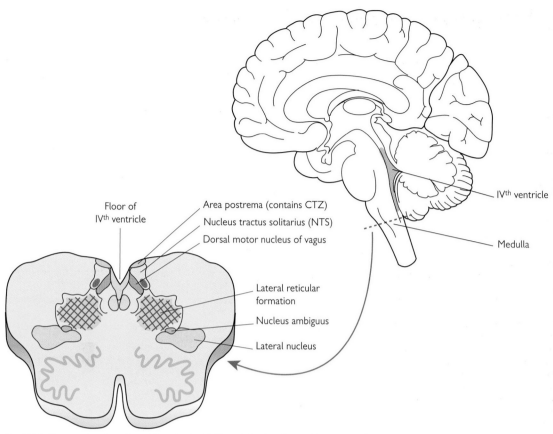

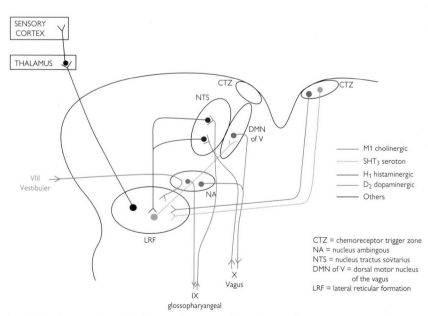

Fig. 17.12 Cross-section through medulla at the level indicated, showing the vomiting centre and its important structures.

Fig. 17.13 Schematic diagram of pathways and neurotransmitters in the vomiting centre

The treatment of PONV is multi-faceted, with both non-pharmacological and pharmacological options available.

Non-pharmacological strategies

Reduce anaesthetic factors causing PONV

- Regional rather than general anaesthesia.
- Total IV anaesthesia with propofol rather than inhalational agent (probably decreases rate of PONV by approximately 25%).
- Avoid/minimize use of opioid.
- Avoid/minimize use of neostigmine (<2.5mg).
- Avoid nitrous oxide.
- Acupressure/acupuncture has been investigated at Chinese P6 and (to a smaller extent) Korean Hand K-K9 points (Figure 17.14). A variety of stimulants including needles, injection of hypertonic glucose solution, and capsaicin has been used. Many studies show efficacy comparable to conventional antiemetics. Techniques do not necessarily require unusual skill or a long time to deploy. They have a generally favourable side-effect profile and are probably under-used.

There are insufficient data to support the use of hypnosis.

Ginger has not been shown to have any efficacy in PONV.

Supplemental oxygen is no longer thought to be effective in preventing PONV.

Pharmacological strategies in PONV

There are very complex interactions between the neuronal areas controlling vomiting and the CTZ with many different active neurotransmitters (>40), and therefore it has not proved possible to develop a single drug to cure PONV. However, 5-HT$_3$ and dopamine D$_2$ receptors are prominent in the CTZ, and cholinergic, muscarinic, and histamine H$_1$ receptors are prominent in the vomiting centres, and drugs particularly directed at these receptors have been widely used.

Antidopaminergic drugs were among the first to be used as antiemetics. The D$_2$ receptor has a major stimulatory effect in the CTZ, and the D$_2$ agonist apomorphine is a potent emetic, but many of the earlier antidopaminergic drugs had significant antagonist activity at muscarinic cholinergic and adrenergic recptors as well. Despite a long history of clinical use (e.g. metoclopramide), the evidence for efficacy can be weak.

Antihistamines have also been used for a long time, but many of them also have anticholinergic activity and are sedatives. Anticholinergic activity is necessary for efficacy in motion sickness (the vestibular afferents are cholinergic).

5-HT (serotonin) receptor antagonists are newer and generally show a clear beneficial effect. 5-HT is released from enterochromaffin cells in the GI tract in response to a range of noxious stimuli, and application of 5-HT to the area postrema provokes vomiting. This effect can be blocked by selective 5-HT$_3$ antagonists (*ondansetron, granisetron, tropisetron, dolasetron*) without much risk of troublesome side effects. Agonists at other 5-HT receptors can also provoke vomiting. 5-HT$_{1D}$ receptors are involved in the vomiting associated with migraine and can be blocked by the selective antagonist sumatriptan, which is an effective treatment in this condition. Antagonists at other 5-HT receptors are either limited by side effects or do not show useful antiemetic activity.

Steroids have been noted to have useful anti-emetic activity by an unknown mechanism. Dexamethasone is most commonly used, but methylprednisolone is an alternative. They are probably better as prophylactic agents than as a treatment for established PONV. The many undesirable side effects associated with corticosteroid use are generally not of any concern with very-short-term use.

Aprepitant is a new anti-emetic which is an antagonist for substance P at the neurokinin-1 receptor, which is found in areas of the CNS important in the control of vomiting. It is given orally before highly emetogenic chemotherapy together with a 5-HT$_3$ blocker and dexamethasone. It appears to confer some extra benefit. It is expensive and is not likely to become routine for use in PONV soon, but clinical trials can be expected.

Efficacy of antiemetic drugs

Accurate and meaningful figures for efficacy are difficult to achieve because the baseline incidence of PONV is so variable, depending on many patient, surgery, and anaesthetic factors.

Drug prophylaxis

Drug prophylaxis is not recommended for routine use. In patients at high risk, the measures described above should be used where possible. For additional drug prophylaxis the best choice at present is probably dexamethasone at the beginning of the procedure and a 5-HT$_3$ antagonist at the end. Each agent independently seems to reduce the risk of PONV by about 25%.

In cases of prophylactic failure, there is little benefit in giving additional doses of drugs already used. A drug from another class should be given.

Cannabinoids may be effective in chemotherapy-induced nausea and vomiting but not in PONV.

Further reading

Rowbotham DJ (2005) *Br J Anaesth* **95**, 77–81.
Gan TJ et al. (2003). *Anesth Analg* **97**, 62–71.
Gan TJ et al. (2006). *Anesthesiology* **105**, A566.

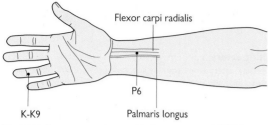

Flexor carpi radialis

P6

K-K9

Palmaris longus

Fig. 17.14 Acupuncture points used in the prevention of PONV.

Table 17.5 Common drugs used in PONV				
Class	**Drug**	**Dose**	**Comments**	**Problems**
Antimuscarinic	Hyoscine	0.4mg	Effective as premedicant	Sedative; central anticholinergic syndrome
Antihistamine	Cyclizine	50mg		Antimuscarinic effects, heart failure after MI, sedation
Antidopaminergic (procainamide derivative)	Metoclopramide	(10mg) 25–50mg	Questionable efficacy, may need higher dose	Extrapyramidal side effects (EPSE)
Antidopaminergic (piperazine phenothiazine)	Prochlorperazine	5–12.5mg	No IV preparation	EPSE, hypotension, neuroleptic malignant syndrome
Antidopaminergic (butyrophenone)	Droperidol	<1mg	Effective at low doses, comparable to 5-HT$_3$ blockers.	Not likely at low doses; withdrawn in UK because of concerns about dysrhythmia (QT prologation)
5-HT$_3$ antagonists	Ondansetron Also: Granisetron Dolasetron	4–8mg 1–3mg up to 12.5mg	NNT 4–7 Higher dose may be more effective	Adverse effects uncommon (headache, constipation, raised liver enzymes)
Corticosteroids	Dexamethasone	2.5–8mg	NNT 4 Unknown mechanism	Unlikely with very short-term use; can cause perineal burning sensation in awake patient
NNT = number needed to treat.				

The liver (Figure 17.15) is the largest solid organ in the body, weighing around 1.2–1.5kg. It lies in the right upper quadrant of the abdomen.

Gross anatomy

The liver has four lobes: the right (largest), the left, and the smaller quadrate and caudate lobes. The quadrate lobe abuts the porta hepatis, a fissure on the inferior surface of the right lobe, while the caudate lobe is posterior, adjacent to the inferior vena cava (IVC) (Figure 17.16).

Relations

- **Superior:** suspended by the falciform ligament; right hemidiaphragm.
- **Inferior:** duodenum; hepatic flexure of colon.
- **Posterior:** upper pole of right kidney; right adrenal gland.
- **Anterior:** ribs and abdominal wall.

Cellular anatomy

There are two terminologies:

- **Lobular** terminology describes histologically visible structures within the liver, with the centrilobular vein at the centre (Figure 17.17).
- **Acinar** terminology describes the functional units of the liver, with the portal tract at the centre.

The functional cells of the liver are called hepatocytes. These are arranged into lobules—hexagonal structures approximately 1mm in diameter. At the centre of each lobule is a central (centrilobular) vein, a tributary of the hepatic vein.

At the corner of each lobule is a portal tract. This contains a portal venule, arising from the portal vein, hepatic arteriole, bile cannuliculus, and nerves. Portal venules and hepatic arterioles bring nutrient-rich and oxygenated blood to the hepatocytes.

Running between columns of hepatocytes are channels called sinusoids. Blood reaches the hepatocytes and drains into the central vein via these sinusoids. Sinusoids do not have a basement membrane, allowing easy movement of solutes between blood and hepatocyte.

The biliary system

Bile is produced in hepatocytes and drains into bile cannuliculi, which fuse to form bile ducts between lobules. The right and left hepatic ducts join to become the common hepatic duct (CHD). This leaves the liver via the porta hepatis, and subsequently joins the cystic duct as it leaves the gallbladder, forming the common bile duct (CBD).

The CBD passes behind the head of the pancreas and joins the main pancreatic duct at the ampulla of Vater. Bile then drains into the duodenum via the sphincter of Oddi.

The blood supply to the bile duct is predominantly from the right hepatic artery.

Nerve supply

Nerve supply is via the hepatic nervous plexus, which enters the liver at the porta hepatis.

- Sympathetic: T7–T10 sympathetic ganglia. These synapse in the coeliac plexus.
- Parasympathetic: right and left vagus nerves.
- Sensory (to capsule): right phrenic nerve (C3,4,5).

Blood flow

The liver receives 25–30% of the cardiac output. It has a dual blood supply from the hepatic artery and portal vein. The vessels enter the liver at the porta hepatis.

Hepatic artery

The hepatic artery arises from the aorta and provides 30% of the blood supply to the liver. Unlike portal venous blood, this is fully oxygenated and so provides about 50% of the liver's oxygen requirement.

The common hepatic artery divides into the right and left hepatic arteries.

Hepatic artery perfusion pressure is approximately 50–70mmHg; arteriolar pressure is approximately 35mmHg.

Portal vein

The portal vein arises from the confluence of the gastric, splenic, superior mesenteric, cystic, and para-umbilical veins. It provides about 70% of hepatic blood flow. Portal vein blood is only 60–70% oxygenated, having already passed through the gut, but it is rich in nutrients. The portal vein is a low-pressure vessel (6–10mmHg).

Control of hepatic blood flow

There are intrinsic and extrinsic mechanisms controlling hepatic blood flow, as well as a reciprocal relationship between hepatic artery and portal vein flow.

Intrinsic control mechanisms

Hepatic artery flow is autoregulated. The artery dilates and constricts in response to changes in blood pressure over the normal range. This mechanism is lost when the systolic blood pressure falls below 80mmHg.

Extrinsic control mechanisms

Many external factors influence hepatic blood flow (Table 17.6).

Reciprocal hepatic artery and portal vein control

Changes in hepatic arterial flow have no effect on portal vein flow, but changes in portal vein flow result in a reciprocal opposite change in hepatic artery flow. This mechanism is thought to be related to fluxes in adenosine, a potent vasodilator.

Venous drainage and lymphatics

Venous drainage is via short hepatic veins. These arise from the posterior surface of the liver and drain directly into the IVC.

Liver lymphatics terminate in small groups of glands around the porta hepatis. Some superficial vessels pass through the diaphragm to reach the mediastinal glands, whereas others accompany the IVC into the thorax and end in a few small glands around the intrathoracic IVC.

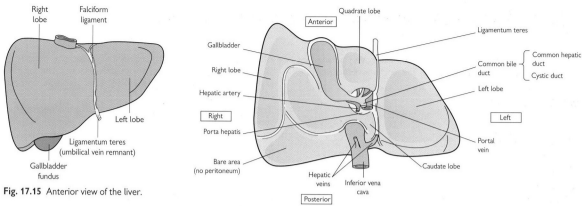

Fig. 17.15 Anterior view of the liver.

Fig. 17.16 Inferior view of the liver demonstrating its four lobes.

→ Hepatic blood flow at the cellular level

Blood flow through the lobule is unidirectional, and so cells closest to the portal tracts are less susceptible to ischaemia than those close to the central veins. As a result, there is variable function between hepatocytes. There are three defined areas:

- **Zone 1:** hepatocytes surrounding the portal area. These receive nutrient- and oxygen-rich blood, and carry out the most oxygen-dependent processes, e.g. gluconeogenesis and urea synthesis.
- **Zone 2:** between zones 1 and 3; intermediate cellular function.
- **Zone 3:** hepatocytes surrounding the central vein. These cells receive blood with the lowest oxygen content, and are therefore more prone to ischaemia. The cytochrome P450 system is most active in zone 3.

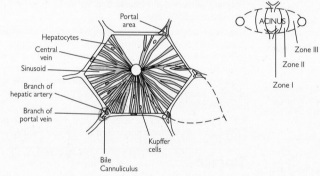

Fig. 17.17 Liver histology. Main picture: lobular histology. Inset: functional zones within the acinar structure (see text).

Table 17.6 Extrinsic control of liver blood flow			
	Anaesthesia	**Drugs**	**Other**

Factors increasing hepatic blood flow	• Hypercapnia
	• Ketamine
		• β-agonists (e.g. salbutamol)
		• Enzyme inducers
		    Phenytoin
		    Carbamazepine
		    Rifampicin
		• Smoking
		• Dexamethasone
			• Eating
			• Glucagons
			• Alcohol
			• Acute hepatitis
			• Brassicas

No change/variable action	• Isoflurane • Sevoflurane • Omeprazole		

Factors reducing liver blood flow	• IPPV
	• PEEP
	• Sympathetic blockade
	  (e.g. spinal /epidural)
	• Thiopental
	• Propofol
	• Hypocapnia
	• Halothane
	• Enflurane
		• Enzyme inhibitors
		    Cimetidine
		    Ketoconazole
		    Spironolactone
		    Chloramphenicol
		• α-agonists
		• β-antagonists
			• Haemorrhage
			• Grapefruit juice
			• Chronic liver disease
			• Surgical manoeuvres
			  (e.g. compression, retraction)

Knowledge of normal liver function is essential to understanding the derangements that occur in liver disease. The functions of the liver can be broadly classified as follows.

- **Synthesis**
  - Proteins (albumin, clotting factors, transport globulins, apoproteins).
  - Fats (especially triglyceride and cholesterol).
  - Bile.
- **Metabolism**
  - Glucose homeostasis: glycogen synthesis and storage, gluconeogenesis.
  - Other newly absorbed nutrients.
- **Storage**
- **Catabolism and excretion**
  - Drug metabolism
  - Urea
  - Bilirubin
- **Immunological/haematological**

Carbohydrate metabolism

The primary purpose of hepatic carbohydrate metabolism is glucose homeostasis.

Storage of glucose

Glycogen is a branched polymer of glucose residues. It acts as a rapidly accessible store of glucose in liver and muscle. Most of the residues are linked by α-1,4-glycosidic bonds. Branches at about every tenth residue are created by α-1,6-glycosidic bonds. Glycogen is synthesized in the liver when glucose is plentiful, a process called glycogenesis:

- Glucose diffuses into cells (non-energy-dependent).
- It is converted to G6P by glucokinase (maintaining a low intracellular glucose concentration, favouring further influx of glucose). G6P is converted to G1P.
- Glycogen synthase uses energy from uridine triphosphate (UTP) to phosphorylate the G1P monomers. These are added to the protein glycogenin to build glycogen polymers.

Mobilization of glucose

When serum glucose levels fall, two processes serve to maintain glucose supply: glycogenolysis (the breakdown of stored glycogen), and gluconeogenesis (the manufacture of glucose from non-sugar substrates; Section 17.6).

During glycogenolysis, G6P is produced from glycogen by the action of phosphorylase. This process uses energy stored in the phosphate bonds of the glycogen itself.

G6P has several possible fates.

- It can feed into the glycolytic pathway for respiration (Section 17.6).
- It can form glucose in the liver (but not muscle).
- It can enter the pentose phosphate pathway to generate reducing capacity (NADPH) and the 5-carbon sugars needed for nucleic acid synthesis.

Regulation of glycogen synthesis and breakdown is by calcium/cAMP-activated protein kinases.

- When stimulated by glucagon or catecholamines, these phosphorylate glycogen synthase, greatly reducing glycogenesis. They enhance the activity of phosphorylase, promoting glycogenolysis.
- Insulin has the opposite effect, promoting both glycogenesis and glucose uptake into liver and muscle.

Protein metabolism

The liver synthesizes the majority of the plasma proteins, and has a key role in the excretion of nitrogenous waste.

- **Albumin:** about 200mg/kg/day. Important in maintaining plasma oncotic pressure. It binds drugs, toxins and hormones. The half-life is 20 days, so plasma levels lag behind decreases in hepatic synthetic capacity.
- **Transport globulins:** a variety are synthesized by the liver, often conjugated to form glyco- and lipo-proteins.
- **Clotting factors:** the liver produces all the clotting factors except factor VIII (vWF; generated in vascular endothelium; Section 15.7). As the half-lives are short (especially factors V and VII), clotting times (PT, INR) or factor levels are sensitive markers of liver synthetic capacity.
- **Excretion of nitrogenous waste:** the liver is the major site for the catabolism of circulating proteins. The deamination of amino acids generates ammonia. This is joined with CO_2 in the urea cycle to form (the less toxic, and more readily excreted) urea.

Lipid metabolism

The key components in the regulation of fat metabolism are **apoproteins,** which form submicroscopic particles with fats. There are five groups, A to E. Apoproteins allow cellular receptors to recognize and manipulate lipoprotein particles.

Bile is a mixture of bile acids, cholesterol, lecithin (a phospholipid), and bilirubin (80% as bilirubin diglucuronide). It is required for lipid digestion (Section 17.4).

Bile acids have polar and non-polar parts, and so can act as detergents. They are secreted and reabsorbed up to 12 times a day in the enterohepatic circulation.

The main product of haem metabolism is bilirubin. It is conjugated with glucuronide prior to excretion in the bile. Failure of bilirubin excretion (either by failure of conjugation, or by obstruction to bile flow) results in jaundice. Unconjugated bilirubinaemia occurs if conjugating capacity is overwhelmed (e.g. by haemolysis; neonates are especially vulnerable as their conjugating enzymes are immature). Biliary obstruction causes conjugated bilirubinaemia.

Bile is a major excretory route for steroids and large molecules. Figure 17.18 shows haemoglobin breakdown and bilirubin metabolism.

Storage

As well as glycogen, the liver stores iron, copper, the fat-soluble vitamins (A, D, E, and K), and vitamin B_{12}.

Detoxification

The effect of hepatic detoxification is often to convert active insoluble compounds into inactive charged (i.e. hydrophilic) substances. These can then be excreted in urine or bile. These substances may be exogenous (drugs, pollutants), or endogenous (many hormones, e.g. thyroxine, aldosterone, vasopressin, and sex hormones. Liver disease can disrupt these systems, with clinical effects).

Phase 1 reactions are electron transfers carried out predominantly by the cytochrome P450 (CYP) enzymes in the endoplasmic reticulum. This is a huge group of iron-containing enzymes (18 families in humans). There is a large variation in the activity of these enzymes between individuals. Most phase 1 reactions are oxidative, but many others occur.

Phase 2 reactions are conjugations with polar molecules: glucuronidation, sulphation, etc. Generally, phase 2 reactions are less prone to disruption by liver disease than phase 1 reactions.

First pass metabolism

First pass metabolism (FPM) can occur when drugs and toxins are taken enterally. The liver is the most important organ of FPM, although the gut wall, and intestinal luminal and bacterial enzymes, can take part. Absorbed substances in the gut enter the hepatic portal system, which delivers them to the liver. Metabolism takes place to a variable extent here: some drugs are completely removed and never enter the systemic circulation, whereas others may be unaffected. Parenteral routes of administration (e.g. intravenous or buccal) avoid this first pass effect.

Bioavailability

First pass metabolism is important in determining the oral bioavailability (OBA) of drugs administered enterally. Bioavailability is the fraction of unchanged drug which reaches the systemic circulation after a dose. By definition, a drug administered intravenously has a bioavailability of 100%. Various factors affect the bioavailability of a drug, depending on the route. These include its chemical properties (e.g. pKa), drug formulations and preparations, adequacy of the local circulation, disease states, and genetic factors.

Immunological and haematological

The liver is a major immunological organ: many patients with liver disease die of sepsis.

60% of the cells in the liver are 'typical' hepatocytes; others include Kupffer cells (fixed macrophages, part of the reticulo-endothelial system), and pit cells (natural killer cells with a role in tumour immunity).

Kupffer cells phagocytose old red and white blood cells. Hepatocytes make fibrinogen, heparin, and prothrombin. The fetal liver is a major site of erythropoiesis.

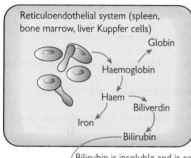

In the reticuloendothelial system, old or damaged red blood cells are phagocytosed. Haemoglobin is released, and is degraded into globin and haem. The haem ring in turn is split, to give iron and a tetrapyrrole, biliverdin. Biliverdin is rapidly reduced to bilirubin.

Bilirubin is insoluble and is carried in plasma bound to albumin.

In the hepatocyte, the unconjugated bilirubin is made soluble by conjugation to glucuronide (80%), sulphate (10%) and other conjugates. The main enzyme pathway is UDP-glucuronosyl transferase. Congenital absence of the activity of this enzyme leads to severe unconjugated bilirubinaemia, incompatible with life. However, 2–7% of the population have reduced levels of enzyme activity: Gilbert's disease. This leads to jaundice (unconjugated bilirubinaemia) during intercurrent illness, but is otherwise benign. The conjugated bilirubin is secreted into the bile.

In the colon, bacterial action converts bilirubin to urobilinogen. Most of this is absorbed, returned to the liver and secreted back into bile. A small proportion is excreted by the kidneys and some is converted to stercobilinogen and then further oxidised to stercobilin, pigmenting the faeces. In total obstructive jaundice, no bile pigments pass into the gut, and the faeces are colourless.

Fig. 17.18 The breakdown of haemoglobin, and metabolism of bilirubin.

Acute liver failure (ALF) requires intensive treatment; even so it carries a high mortality. The most common causes are paracetamol overdose in the UK and viral infection in developing countries.

The main features of ALF are **loss of synthetic function**, **jaundice**, and **encephalopathy**. ALF is classified according to the length of time between the appearance of jaundice and the onset of encephalopathy:

- *Hyperacute*: <8 days
- *Acute*: 8–28 days
- *Subacute*: 29 days–6 months

Features of ALF

Loss of liver function may be sudden and complete, or slow and insidious. If it is very rapid (e.g. huge paracetamol overdose), the patient may not be jaundiced but simply present with coma ± cardio-vascular collapse. Note that portal hypertension is a feature of chronic, not acute, liver failure.

Blood tests typically show **coagulopathy**, **acidosis**, **hypoglycaemia**, and **very high transaminases.**

Effects on individual systems

Jaundice will occur if the patient lives long enough. A variable fraction of the bilirubin may be unconjugated. Even if recovery occurs, the bilirubin falls slowly over many days. A fall in serum transaminases may indicate recovery; conversely, it may signify almost complete liver death.

Central nervous system: encephalopathy is a cardinal feature of ALF. It is graded 0–4.

- Grade 0: minimal hepatic encephalopathy. Subtle changes in memory, intellectual function, and coordination. Asterixis is absent.
- Grade 1: trivial lack of awareness. Patients exhibit shortened attention span, impaired mental processing, sleep disturbances and mood changes. Confusion is mild. Asterixis can be detected.
- Grade 2: lethargy or apathy. Speech is slurred, and asterixis is obvious. There is drowsiness, lethargy. There are gross deficits in ability to perform mental tasks, obvious personality changes, inappropriate behavior, and intermittent disorientation, usually with respect to time.
- Grade 3: somnolent but rousable. Patients are unable to perform mental tasks, disoriented in time and place and markedly confused. There is amnesia, and speech is present but usually incomprehensible.
- Grade 4: coma; response to painful stimuli may be absent.

A major contributor to encephalopathy is a build-up of ammonia. Mercaptans (thiols) produced by bacterial breakdown of proteins in the gut have also been implicated. Neuronal inflammation may play a role. Overactivity of GABA receptors is seen; a temporary improve-ment may sometimes be seen with flumazenil. A secondary effect is cerebral oedema, which causes an increase in intra-cranial pressure. This can cause death due to cerebral herniation (coning). Encephalopathy is confirmed by high-voltage slow waveforms on the EEG.

Circulation: a low (or very low) systemic vascular resistance with a high cardiac output is typical.

Coagulopathy: clotting factors V and VII have the shortest half-lives (hours). Synthesis of factor V does not depend vitamin K; plasma levels or coagulation times (PT/INR Section 15.8) can be used to monitor liver function. Patients are at risk of haemorrhage.

Renal: acute renal failure is usual if the patient lives long enough. The kidneys generally recover if the liver does. NB: *this is* **not** *hepatorenal syndrome.*

Metabolism: hypoglycaemia is inevitable if ALF is severe. Hyponatraemia is common. Serum calcium, magnesium, and phosphate may all be low. There is a marked catabolic state.

Immunology: patients with ALF have impaired immunity, as Kupffer cell function is lost and neutrophil activity is reduced. The risk of sepsis is high; patients are particularly prone to infection by Gram-positive cocci and fungi.

Management and treatment of ALF

Treatment is supportive until recovery or liver transplantation.

Airway and breathing: encephalopathic patients may require intubation and ventilation for airway protection.

Circulation: initially volume resuscitation. The majority of patients eventually require vasopressors to maintain an adequate mean arterial pressure (MAP). Central venous pressure and intra-arterial monitoring are essential.

Metabolism: glucose as an infusion of 20% or 50% dextrose, (via a central vein) to keep blood sugar within normal limits.

Hyponatraemia (sodium <135mmol/L) can worsen increased intracra-nial pressure. Some liver units recommend increasing serum sodium levels to 155–160mmol/L.

Intracranial pressure: all standard measures to reduce the risk of brain injury from raised ICP should be instigated early.

- ICP monitoring may be useful, but insertion of the device can be dangerous in those with a coagulopathy.
- Pupil size and reactivity should be monitored for signs of critically raised ICP.
- Treat acute surges in ICP with mannitol 0.5g/kg (monitor serum osmolarity). Small boluses of hypertonic (30%) saline are sometimes used.

Gastrointestinal: ALF patients are at high risk of gastro-intestinal erosions and bleeding. All patients should be given prophylactic proton pump inhibitors or H_2 antagonists. A reduction in gut motility can result in worsening encephalopathy and therefore prokinetics should be given (e.g. erythromycin, metoclopramide).

Renal: furosemide infusions may maintain an adequate urine output, but clearance of potassium and protons is often inadequate. Renal replacement therapy (Section 12.5) is usually needed.

Infection: broad-spectrum antibacterial and antifungal prophylaxis should be provided.

Coagulation: coagulation status is used to track the evolution of ALF, and so should not be corrected with fresh frozen plasma unless active bleeding occurs.

Drugs: N-acetylcysteine (NAC), a derivative of L-cysteine. It is used in the treatment of paracetamol overdoses. NAC is sometimes used in ALF of non-paracetamol origin. It is thought to act as a free-radical scavenger, and may replenish glutathione stores which are required by the liver for other metabolic functions.

Prognosis

Most patients who die of ALF are killed by sepsis or raised ICP. A few die from haemorrhage.

Spontaneous complete recovery is reasonably common, (generally >50%), but depends on aetiology and many other factors. If there is no possibility of recovery, the only life-saving treatment is liver transplan-tation. Various scoring systems are used to predict which patients have a poor chance of spontaneous recovery and will require transplanta-tion. Most centres expect a patient survival of >60% at 5 years post-transplantation for ALF. Liver support devices have not yet proved useful, despite much research.

⊕ Paracetamol overdose

The metabolism of paracetamol in therapeutic doses is usually by conjugation with glucuronide, sulphate, and cysteine. Conjugates are actively excreted in the urine. A small proportion (10%) is metabolized by the cytochrome P450 enzymes to form a toxic metabolite, N-acetyl-p-aminobenzoquinoneimine (NAQBI). The NAQBI formed under these conditions is in turn conjugated with glutathione, rendering it harmless.

When large amounts of paracetamol are presented to the liver, the usual conjugation pathways are rapidly overwhelmed. This diverts a larger proportion of paracetamol toward the CYP450 system, and significant amounts of NAQBI are generated. Hepatic glutathione is soon exhausted. NAQBI now accumulates, and forms covalent bonds with –SH groups on hepatocellular proteins, disrupting protein function. The result is centrilobular necrosis of liver cells. Renal tubular cells may also be affected.

Presentation

The features of paracetamol overdose vary according to the timing and amount of drug ingested. As little as 7.5g may prove lethal in a high-risk patient (e.g. alcohol overuse, other enzyme-inducing drugs, malnutrition), although in healthy subjects doses of at least 12g (and more usually upwards of 30g) are associated with a fatal outcome.

<24hr: usually asymptomatic, although nausea, vomiting, and anorexia may occur. Very rarely, early lactic acidosis is seen.

24–36hr: symptoms may include vomiting, sweating, erythema or urticaria, mucosal lesions, or evidence of hepatic necrosis (hypoglycaemia, jaundice, and right upper quadrant pain).

36–72hr: liver failure becomes established, with coagulopathy, encephalopathy, metabolic acidosis, and refractory hypoglycaemia. Renal failure with oliguria and rising creatinine may occur ± hepatic failure. Pancreatitis is an occasional feature (again, ± liver failure).

High risk patients

Patients who are particularly vulnerable to the effects of paracetamol poisoning include:

- Chronic alcohol abusers
- Those with established glutathione depletion: HIV infection, eating disorders, cystic fibrosis
- Drugs: rifampicin, phenobarbitone, phenytoin, primidone, carbamazepine, St. John's wort.

Investigations

Paracetamol levels should be measured 4hr post-ingestion (or as soon as possible after that time), and again at 8hr (since delayed absorption may occur). Salicylate levels should also be measured, since many patients who overdose will have taken more than one drug.

U&Es should be measured; early, they provide baseline values, and later may become deranged.

FBC may reveal anaemia (possible evidence of coagulopathy-induced blood loss). Thrombocytopenia is common with severe overdoses and hepatic failure. In G6P deficiency, there may be methaemoglobinaemia and haemolysis.

LFTs: transaminase levels rise early in the course of disease, although do not correlate well to severity of liver damage.

PT/INR is the most reliable index of disease severity. If INR >2.0 24hr post-ingestion, moderate or severe hepatic impairment is likely.

ABG will assess the presence and degree of acidosis.

Urinalysis should be performed to look for haematuria or proteinuria.

Management

Management also depends on the timing of the overdose. If unknown, take the earliest possible reported time. If the overdose was staggered, take the time of first ingestion. In general, err on the side of caution and instigate treatment rather than withholding it. If in doubt, consult a liver unit or poisons information service.

<1hr: gastric lavage and give activated charcoal to limit absorption. Proceed as below.

<24hr: paracetamol levels at 4 and 8 hr (or as soon as possible afterwards). N-acetyl cysteine (NAC), a glutathione precursor, should be given if the level is on or above the appropriate treatment line on the nomogram (Figure 17.19). Levels are less reliable after 12 hr. NAC should be given before levels are known if >10g has been ingested, or if results will be delayed until after 8hr post-ingestion (when efficacy is reduced). Consider a lower treatment threshold (e.g. 7.5g) for high-risk patients. If in any doubt, consult a liver unit or poisons information service urgently.

24–72hr: paracetamol levels should still be taken, but are unreliable. If other investigations are deranged, consider NAC. It may be effective up to 36hr post-overdose.

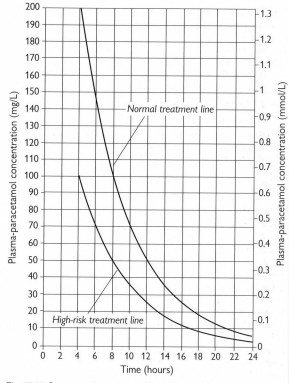

Fig. 17.19 Paracetamol nomogram. (Reproduced with permission from *Oxford Handbook of Acute Medicine* (2nd edn), p. 831.

NAC regimen: 150mg/kg in 200ml 5% dextrose over 15min; then 50mg/kg in 500ml 5% dextrose over 4hr; then 100mg/kg in 1L 5% dextrose over 16hr. If itch or urticaria occurs, give chlorpheniramine and slow infusion. Monitor closely but continue treatment if possible. Severe reaction is an indication to stop the infusion. In cases of NAC allergy, oral methionine (2.5g every 4hr for four doses) can be given as an alternative.

If NAC has been given, admit to hospital and observe for 48hr. Perform daily PT/INR, FBC, U&E, glucose, and ABG. Monitor urine output. Check basal metabolism every 6hr and treat hypoglycaemia.

Indications for specialist advice or referral

Consult a liver unit if:

- Evidence of liver damage: hepatic tenderness, jaundice, hypoglycaemia, coagulopathy (INR >2 or PT >25 and rising), metabolic acidosis (pH <7.3), or encephalopathy.
- Hypotension despite volume resuscitation.
- Renal failure (creatinine >200 and rising, or oliguria).
- Any other concerns.

It is preferable to transfer patients to specialist care before ICU is required.

17.14 Chronic liver disease

Chronic liver disease is an increasing medical problem posing serious risks to patients and to those who have to anaesthetize them. In advanced cases, the liver and other organ systems are jeopardized by even minor interventions. *Any* procedure should be carried out with extreme caution.

Chronic liver disease is characterized by **cirrhosis**, **jaundice**, and **loss of hepatic function**.

Cirrhosis is a histological diagnosis. It is caused by continuing destruction, scarring, and regeneration of liver tissue, leading to fibronodular change. The fibrotic liver offers increased resistance to blood flow, resulting in **portal hypertension**.

There are many causes of chronic hepatitis. Some of the common causes are listed in Table 17.7.

Clinical features of chronic liver disease

Portal hypertension leads to variceal dilatation of veins communicating between the portal and systemic venous systems. **Varices** may rupture with fatal outcome. Portal hypertension may also cause **ascites**, which can be worsened by hypoalbuminaemia.

Most patients have **jaundice**. If obstruction to biliary drainage is a feature then the conjugated bilirubin can be very high; retention of bile salts can cause severe **pruritis**.

Impaired absorption of lipids from the gut can cause **coagulopathy** because of impaired synthesis of the vitamin-K-dependent clotting factors (II, VII, IX, X).

Patients with chronic liver disease are frequently catabolic and often have marked **muscle wasting** and severe **lethargy**.

Often liver epithelial cell (hepatocyte) synthetic function may be well preserved until the end-stage, and so coagulopathy and hypoalbuminaemia may not be severe. Insults such as sepsis, bleeding, hypotension, and drugs can all cause acute decompensation of hepatic function.

Associated effects on other systems

Cardiovascular: patients with chronic liver disease have an increased cardiac output and reduced systemic vascular resistance. There is no associated increased incidence of ischaemic heart disease.

Respiratory: Many patients have a restrictive defect in respiratory function due to splinting of the diaphragm by ascites. Those with ascites are also prone to pleural effusions.

Some patients (<5%) have **hepatopulmonary syndrome** (HPS) and are hypoxaemic because of V/Q mismatch and formation of new intrapulmonary vessels. The correction of hypoxaemia achievable by increasing the FiO_2 is variable, depending on the fraction of true right-to-left shunting.

A few patients have pulmonary as well as portal hypertension (not the same as HPS). It is associated with a high mortality.

Renal: The majority of patients have some sodium and water retention because of reduced renal blood flow and glomerular filtration rate, and increased renin–aldosterone activity. They are at increased risk of acute renal failure.

Some patients with end-stage liver disease develop **hepato-renal syndrome** (uraemia, oliguria, low urinary sodium, and high urine/plasma creatinine ratio). The syndrome is caused by intense renal vasoconstriction rather than by any intrinsic renal pathology. Median survival is <6 months without liver transplantation.

CNS: encephalopathy—as with acute liver failure (Section 17.14). Patients with chronic disease often function with grade 1 encephalopathy. Encephalopathy often worsens with episodes of variceal bleeding or infection.

Hormonal: gynaecomastia and testicular atrophy occur as a result of impaired hormone metabolism. Abnormalities of vitamin D metabolism can result in osteomalacia.

Haematological: Portal hypertension can cause hypersplenism so many patients are thrombocytopenic. Some have pancytopenia.

Cutaneous manifestations: Spider naevi are dilated end capillaries and occur as a result of portal hypertension. Leuconychia (areas of whiteness on fingernails) is a result of low albumin levels.

Effects on drug handling

These are difficult to predict. Phase 1 reactions are carried out by cytochrome P450 (Section 17.13). Their activity may be affected (or not!) in chronic liver disease. Phase 2 reactions (e.g. glucuronidation) tend to be better preserved. If there is biliary obstruction, the clearance of drugs excreted in bile (rocuronium, vecuronium, steroids) may be greatly reduced.

In portal hypertension, portal–systemic venous shunts may allow some oral drugs to escape first-pass metabolism. Drugs with high extraction ratios will then have much higher bioavailability. Clearance of drugs given parenterally which normally have a high intrinsic clearance by the liver may be reduced if liver blood flow is low. If serum albumin is low, drugs normally tightly bound to albumin may have a much higher free fraction (and therefore tissue effect) but may also be cleared faster. Drugs bound to globulins or acute-phase proteins are generally less affected. Volume of distribution may be increased for water-soluble drugs if total body water is high. Drugs metabolized by plasma esterases (suxamethonium, remifentanil) may show decreased clearance. Pharmacodynamic interactions mean that encephalopathic subjects may be very sensitive to the sedative effects of drugs (benzodiazepines, opioids, volatiles) and so they should be anaesthetized with extreme caution.

Treatment of chronic liver disease

Much of the treatment of those with chronic liver disease is about symptom control and organ support, as the process of cirrhosis cannot be reversed and often continues after the provoking stimulus has gone.

Drug therapy

- Antivirals are available for some types of hepatitis.
- Pruritis sufferers take ionic resins and cholesytramine.
- Beta-blockers (or IV terlipressin or octreotide) are used to reduce portal hypertension.
- Diuretics may be given to treat ascites. There is an increased risk of severe hyponatraemia.

Interventional treatments:

- Sclerotherapy or banding of varices can reduce the chance of bleeding and hence the risk of hepatic decompensation or sudden death.
- Transjugular intrahepatic portosystemic shunt (TIPSS). A stent is placed percutaneously between the portal vein and hepatic veins, thus reducing portal vein pressure. Not suitable where liver function is marginal (may decompensate).
- Liver transplantation is the only definitive treatment for end-stage liver disease. Most centres expect 5-year survival rates of 80–90% for patients transplanted for stable chronic liver disease.

Table 17.7 Causes of chronic hepatitis	
Infective	Hepatitis B with or without hepatitis D, hepatitis C (hepatitis A and E do not lead to chronic hepatitis).
Autoimmune	Systemic lupus erythematosus; rheumatoid arthritis. Primary biliary cirrhosis and primary sclerosing cholangitis can mimic chronic hepatitis
Drugs	Alcohol, methyldopa, nitrofurantoin, isoniazid, ketoconazole
Heredity	Wilson's disease, alpha 1-antitrypsin deficiency.
Miscellaneous	Non-alcoholic steatohepatitis.

Chapter 18

Homeostasis and endocrine control

18.1 The cell and mechanisms of hormonal control

The cell is the smallest common unit that makes up all living organisms. A human consists of some 10^{14} cells, all containing the necessary genetic information for cell division and for regulating cell function. The typical size of a human cell is about 10–100µm, but some specialized cells, such as nerve cells, can far exceed this.

Human cell contents are contained within a cell membrane consisting of a lipid bilayer with various proteins embedded in it. Human cells are eukaryotic (the nuclear material is encapsulated within a separate cell nucleus); however, not all cells have a nucleus (e.g. erythrocytes).

Cellular components

Cell membrane
This consists of a selectively permeable phospholipid bilayer containing a wide variety of molecules which serve specific processes such as transport of molecules into or out of the cell. It also maintains the cell resting potential. Cholesterol molecules are incorporated into the bilayer, providing strength and stiffness.

Cytoskeleton
This is composed of microfilaments and microtubules which act to anchor cell contents (organelles) and help during endocytosis (uptake of materials into the cell.

Genetic material
This is contained within the cell nucleus and mitochondria. The nuclear genome consists of 46 linear DNA chromosomes—mitochondrial DNA in a single circular molecule.

Organelles
Cell nucleus: this houses and protects the chromosomes. DNA transcription and RNA synthesis occur here.

Mitochondria are self-replicating organelles which generate most of the ATP needed by the cell via the citric acid cycle. They are also involved in cell signalling, differentiation, and cell growth and death. The number of mitochondria in a cell varies by cell type—liver cells contain many thousands.

Endoplasmic reticulum (ER): a network of tubules, vesicles and sac-like cisternae involved in protein transport and storage of large molecules such as steroids and glycogen. Some drug detoxification occurs in the smooth ER. Rough ER is coated in ribosomes.

Golgi apparatus packages of large molecules made within the cell to prepare them for secretion.

Ribosomes build proteins from the information held by mRNA (Figure 18.1).

Lysosomes house digestive enzymes which would otherwise harm the cell. They are an important defence against viral/ bacterial attack.

Vacuoles are fluid-filled sacs containing food or waste which is utilized or removed by exocytosis.

Hormones

A hormone is a chemical that acts as a messenger between one cell to another. Virtually all tissues produce hormones. The purpose of hormones is to initiate a change in the target cell; this is achieved by acting on specific receptors.

Hormones can:
- Act at distant sites via bloodstream carriage (endocrine)
- Act locally, by diffusing to neighbouring cells (paracrine)
- Have activity within the same cell (autocrine), e.g. interleukin-1 which binds to surface receptors on the cell which secreted it.

Hormone receptors may either be embedded in cell membranes or be intracellular. Typical changes induced by receptor binding include:
- Phosphorylation of proteins
- Changes in ion channels
- Production of second messengers (e.g. cAMP).

Hormonal actions are diverse, but generally serve to regulate metabolic activity. Other actions include:
- Growth regulation
- Control of apoptosis
- Immune regulation
- Control of the reproductive cycle.

Types of hormone
There are three chemical types of hormone:
- Those derived from the **amino acids** tyrosine and tryptophan (e.g. catecholamines, thyroxine)
- **Peptide** hormones made up of small chains of amino acids (e.g. vasopressin, TRH)
- **Steroid** hormones, derived from lipids or phospholipids (e.g. cortisol, testosterone). These act intracellularly.

Feedback mechanisms
Hormones are involved in homeostasis—i.e. the maintenance of a constant internal environment. This allows us to exist in an external environment that is constantly changing. Homeostasis is controlled primarily by negative feedback—endocrine tissue produces a hormone that increases production of a metabolite by the target tissue. This then feeds back to the endocrine gland to reduce further hormone production.

An example of this is shown in figure 1—the hypothalamic-pituitary-adrenal system where corticotrophin-releasing hormone (CRH) released from the hypothalamus acts on the anterior pituitary to increase adrenocorticotrophic hormone (ACTH) release, which in turn causes cortisol to be released from the adrenal medulla. If cortisol levels rise, negative feedback causes CRH and ACTH levels to fall.

Positive feedback can also occur within hormone systems. Here, rising hormone levels drive their own production in a tissue which must then be desensitised or turned over to stop the response. Ovulation is an example—LH from the pituitary stimulates the ovarian follicle to produce oestrogen, which feeds back to increase GRH release from the hypothalamus. This in turn increases further LH release from the pituitary leading to ovulation.

Hormones do not act in isolation—often two or more hormones have synergistic effects leading to a tissue response (e.g. cortisol and adrenaline). Hormones may also have antagonistic effects (e.g. insulin and glucagon).

Hormone receptors
Hormones can only act on cells which have the appropriate receptor for that hormone. There are two types of receptor:
- Cell surface receptors
- Intracellular receptors.

Cell surface receptors
Peptide and amino acid derived hormones are polar molecules, and cannot enter cells, Therefore they act on cell surface receptors. These are G-protein-coupled receptors (Section 9.4).
- They trigger a second messenger system that transmits the signal from the outside to the inside of the cell, often via the activation of protein kinase.
- This leads to phosphorylation of specific proteins.
- This alters protein function.

The second messengers in this system may be cAMP, cGMP, or IP_3.

Intracellular receptors

Since unbound steroid hormones are lipid-based, they are able to cross the cell membrane and gain access to the cytoplasm, where they form complexes with mobile intracellular receptors. The complex moves into the cell nucleus where it acts on DNA to alter gene transcription and affect protein synthesis.

- Type I intracellular receptors bind steroid hormones.
- Type II receptors bind thyroid hormones, vitamin A, and vitamin D.

The receptors are bound to heat shock proteins in the cytoplasm, which render them inert. After hormone binding has occurred, the heat shock protein complex is released. The receptor hormone complex can now move into the nucleus (Figure 18.2).

→ Cell functions

Metabolism

Catabolism is when the cell breaks down large molecules to produce energy (via ATP production). This is by one of two mechanisms: glycolysis does not require oxygen (anaerobic respiration), whereas the citric acid cycle does (aerobic respiration). Anabolism is the reverse, when the cell uses energy to produce complex molecules.

Protein synthesis

This occurs via transcription (produces mRNA from DNA which then binds to ribosomes) and translation (formation of a polypeptide chain based on the information held in the mRNA). This chain folds to produce a 3D protein molecule.

Cell motility

certain cells have the ability to move around the body. This aids in fighting infection, wound healing and remodelling of damaged structures via fibroblast activation. Cell movement may also be detrimental, leading to the spread of malignancies.

Human genome

The 25,000 human genes are encoded in DNA, which is held within 23 distinct paired chromosomes—22 autosomal plus X or Y. Each gene encodes a specific protein which performs a particular function within the cell. The chromosomes also contain vast amounts of 'junk DNA'—up to 97% of the genome. Its function remains largely unknown.

DNA (deoxyribonucleic acid) is formed by nucleotides attached to a backbone of sugars and phosphate groups. Two strands wind together to form a right-handed double helix, held together by hydrogen bonds. Attached to each sugar is one of four organic bases: adenine, guanine, cytosine and thymine.

Mitochondrial DNA

A ring of DNA is found within mitochondria, with 100–10,000 copies per cell. This is always inherited from the mother and encodes the same 37 genes for various proteins, tRNA, and rRNA. This makes it useful for tracing ancestry.

Mutations often occur, and account for such diverse conditions as Wolff–Parkinson–White syndrome and some cases of dementia and diabetes.

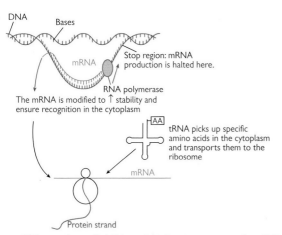

rmRNA recognise specific initiator and attachment sequences on the mRNA. The ribosome holds the mRNA in place initiates the anticodon of the tRNA carrying the specific amno acid & stimulates bond formation between amino acids, resulting in a protein.

Fig. 18.1 The process of protein synthesis from DNA.

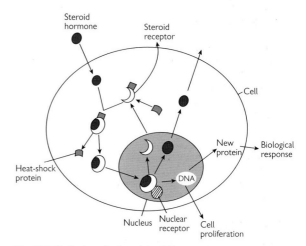

Fig. 18.2 Mechanism of action of steroid hormones.

The hypothalamus

The hypothalamus is part of the limbic system of the brain, and forms the floor of the third ventricle. It lies just behind the optic chiasm and above the pituitary gland, to which it is intimately connected (Figure 18.3).

The hypothalamus synthesizes neurohormones which control the release of hormones from the anterior pituitary gland. These hormones regulate the endocrine system.

Sections of the hypothalamus lies outside the blood–brain barrier and are affected by circulating hormones.

Functions of the hypothalamus

- Synthesis of 'releasing' and 'inhibiting' hormones which control pituitary hormone secretion.
- Production of oxytocin and vasopressin (antidiuretic hormone (ADH)).
- Regulation of water balance by controlling thirst via stimulation of hypothalamic osmoreceptors.
- Control of food intake and satiety in response to stimulation of glucose-sensitive receptors.
- Temperature control via inputs from peripheral and central thermoreceptors. Control of vasoconstriction and shivering via autonomic stimulation.
- Control of behaviour, mood, and sex drive.

The pituitary gland

The pituitary gland sits just below the hypothalamus, linked to it by the pituitary stalk. It is housed within the pituitary fossa of the sphenoid bone. The pituitary has an anterior and a posterior lobe, which are embryologically distinct.

Anterior pituitary

This is derived from Rathke's pouch and consists of glandular epithelium. A portal circulation within the pituitary stalk transports hypothalamic hormones to the anterior pituitary where they exert their effects. This system of communication is an important link between the nervous and endocrine systems.

Six hormones are secreted (Table 18.1). Regulation of secretion is by negative feedback from the target glands, both on the pituitary and the hypothalamus.

Posterior pituitary

The posterior pituitary is derived from brain ectoderm. It is linked to the hypothalamus by axons in the pituitary stalk. The posterior pituitary stores vesicles containing two hormones released by the hypothalamus:

- Oxytocin, produced in the paraventricular nucleus. This stimulates ejection of milk from the breasts and causes uterine contraction following childbirth.
- Vasopressin (ADH), from the supra-optic nucleus. This is released when plasma osmolarity rises, or if blood pressure falls (e.g. during haemorrhage). It acts to promote water reabsorption and causes peripheral vasoconstriction (Section 11.3).

Pathology of the pituitary gland

Pituitary under-secretion

- **Panhypopituitarism** is insufficiency or absence of anterior pituitary hormones. It can be congenital or acquired. Hypothyroidism, short stature, and diabetes insipidus are all features.
- **Sheehan** syndrome occurs as a result of ischaemic necrosis of the anterior pituitary gland following obstetric haemorrhage (the gland is vulnerable to ischaemia during pregnancy because of an expansion in its volume without an increase in blood supply). Hypopituitarism results.

Conditions arising from pituitary over-secretion

- **Acromegaly** is caused by a pituitary adenoma which selectively overproduces growth hormone. It results in soft tissue overgrowth of the hands, feet, and airway. Macroglossia and lower jaw protrusion occur, as do sleep apnoea and heart failure in advanced cases. It can be treated medically with bromocriptine or octreotide, or by surgical removal of the adenoma.
- **Cushing's disease** occurs when excess ACTH is produced. Patients present in a similar manner to those with Cushing's syndrome (Section 18.4).
- **Inappropriate ADH** secretion (Section 11.4) leads to hyponatraemia, with possible confusion, fits, and coma.

Expanding pituitary tumours can cause a classical bitemporal hemianopia if they compress the optic chiasm.

Anaesthesia for pituitary surgery

This is most frequently required for removal of a benign adenoma. Tumours <10mm can be resected via a trans-spenoidal approach; larger tumours may require an open craniotomy. The anaesthetist may be presented with several challenges for this type of surgery.

- Intubation may be difficult in the acromegalic patient.
- Bleeding can be profuse, but is minimized by local adrenaline injections.
- Blood is likely to accumulate in the pharynx and stomach, necessitating care on extubation.
- Diabetes insipidus commonly occurs either intra- or postoperatively, but is usually transient.
- Postoperative swelling is common; dexamethasone is usually given.

Antibiotic prophylaxis is necessary on induction because of passage through the sinuses. Nitrous oxide should not be used as there is a risk of pneumocephalus. The surgery is delicate, so patient movement must be avoided. Sometimes a lumbar intrathecal catheter is placed to drain CSF and improve the surgical field.

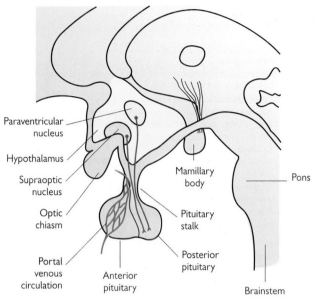

Paraventricular
nucleus

Hypothalamus

Supraoptic
nucleus

Optic
chiasm

Portal
venous
circulation

Anterior
pituitary

Mamillary
body

Pons

Pituitary
stalk

Posterior
pituitary

Brainstem

Fig. 18.3 Anatomical relations of the pituitary gland.

Table 18.1 Hormones secreted by the anterior pituitary		
Hypothalamic hormone	**Acts on**	**Which causes**
Growth hormone-releasing hormone (GHRH)	Anterior pituitary, releasing growth hormone (GH)	Growth in most tissues
Thyrotrophin-releasing hormone (TRH)	Anterior pituitary, releasing thyroid stimulating hormone (TSH)	Thyroid to release T_4 and T_3
Corticotrophin-releasing factor (CRF)	Anterior pituitary, releasing adrenocorticotrophic hormone (ACTH)	Adrenals to release cortisol
Gonadotrophin-releasing hormone (GnRH)	Anterior pituitary, releasing luteinizing hormone (LH) + follicle-stimulating hormone (FSH)	Ovaries to release oestrogens causing ovulation Testes to release testosterone, leading to sperm production
Dopamine	Anterior pituitary, inhibiting prolactin release	Prolactin causes lactation, and therefore dopamine inhibits this
Vasopressin (ADH)	Renal tubules and collecting ducts	Water reabsorption from distal tubules and collecting ducts
Oxytocin	Breasts and uterus	Lactation and uterine contraction

The adrenal glands are situated above each kidney, at about the T12 level.

Structure

The adrenal cortex comprises the outer portion, with an inner core called the adrenal medulla. These two areas are embryologically distinct: the cortex arises from mesodermal cells, while the medullary cells are derived from the embryonic neural crest, so are modified neurons. Blood supply is via the superior, middle, and inferior suprarenal arteries.

The adrenal cortex

The cortex mediates the stress response by producing mineralocorticoids and glucocorticoids. It is also responsible for some androgen production. The cortex can be divided into three distinct zones:

The outermost **zona glomerulosa** lies directly beneath the capsule of the gland. It contains clusters of ovoid cells. These cells secrete aldosterone, which acts on the distal convoluted tubule to regulate sodium and potassium balance.

The central **zona fasciculata** has cells arranged in bundles (fascicles). These cells produce glucocorticoids when stimulated by adrenocorticotropic hormone (ACTH). Small amounts of androgen are also released from this area.

The innermost **zona reticularis** is comprised of cells arranged in a network of fibres (reticulum) and functions similarly to the zona fasciculata, releasing glucocorticoids and androgens. It appears to be stimulated earlier than the zona fasciculata, which only responds to prolonged input.

The adrenal medulla

The medulla is at the centre of the gland, surrounded by the cortex. It can be thought of as a ganglion of the sympathetic nervous system (Section 9.3). However, instead of innervating organs and tissues, the post-ganglionic cells secrete catecholamines into the circulation.

Hormones of the adrenal cortex

Adrenocortical hormones belong to the steroid family and are synthesized from cholesterol. Aldosterone and glucocorticoids are the main cortical hormones.

Cholesterol moves into the mitochondria under the influence of steroidogenic acute regulatory protein (StAR), where it is converted into pregnenolone. These two steps are the rate-limiting factor in the process of adrenocortical hormone secretion. Pregnenolone is then either dehydrogenated to progesterone, or hydroxylated to 17-α-hydroxypregnenolone (Figure 18.4). The first steps of this pathway occur in many tissues, but beyond this point production is limited to the adrenocortical cells.

Renin

Renin is released from renal juxtaglomerular (JG) cells in response to:
- sympathetic stimulation of β_1 receptors on the JG cell surface;
- renal artery hypotension;
- reduced distal tubular sodium delivery.

Renin converts angiotensinogen to angiotensin I (Figure 18.4).

Angiotensin receptors

All are G protein-coupled receptors (GPCRs)

AT1 acts via G protein Gq/11 and Gi/o to stimulate phospholipase C and activation od protein kinase C. This receptor is responsible for the majority of the effects seen in Figure 18.6.

AT2 Acts via Gi2/3. Found in high levels in both the fetus and the neonate. Associated with cell growth and differentiation and neuronal regeneration.

AT3 and AT4 Presently poorly understood

Aldosterone

Aldosterone, a mineralocorticoid, helps to regulate fluid and electrolyte balance (Section 11.4).
- Secretion causes sodium reabsorption in the distal convoluted tubule of the nephron in exchange for potassium and hydrogen ions. This is achieved by activation of principal cell membrane Na^+/K^+ pumps after aldosterone binds to (intracellular) mineralocorticoid receptors. H^+ secretion is also stimulated by a direct action of aldosterone on α-intercalated cells in the collecting duct.
- Sodium retention promotes water retention, and an expansion in extracellular fluid volume.
- Proton and potassium excretion leads to metabolic alkalosis and hypokalaemia.

Regulation of aldosterone secretion
- The major trigger of aldosterone release is angiotensin II, stimulated in response to increased renin levels.
- Secretion is diurnal; more than 70% is secreted between 4 a.m. and 10 a.m.
- Aldosterone is also released in response to stimulation from atrial stretch receptors, which respond to a decrease in blood pressure.

Glucocorticoids

Glucocorticoids have many physiological effects. Cortisol (hydrocortisone) is the most important, and is essential for life. Average cortisol production is about 20mg/day. Glucocorticoid receptors exist in almost all cells.
- The receptors are found in the cytosol and are activated by ligand binding. This complex then moves into the nucleus of the cell and alters gene expression (e.g. the IL-2 gene is inhibited, leading to an anti-inflammatory effect).

Effects of glucocorticoids

Cause hyperglycaemia
- Stimulation of liver gluconeogenesis
- Mobilization of amino acids for use in gluconeogenesis (increased urea production)
- Inhibition of glucose uptake by muscle
- Stimulation of fat breakdown
- Muscle breakdown

Anti-inflammatory effects
- Decrease prostaglandin and leukotriene production
- Decrease cyclo-oxygenase expression
- Decrease cytokine, chemokine, and tissue plasminogen activator release

Immunosuppressive effects
- Suppress cell-mediated immunity
- Inhibit production of IL-1-6, IL-8, TNFγ
- Reduce T-cell production
- Suppress humoral immunity—cause B cells to express fewer IL-2 receptors
- Decrease antibody production
- Decrease phagocytosis

Fetal development
- Lung maturation
- Surfactant production

Mineralocorticoid effects (in high doses)
- Salt and water retention
- Hypertension
- Metabolic alkalosis
- Hypokalaemia

- About 10% of cortisol circulates freely, with the rest bound to plasma proteins (mainly corticosteroid-binding globulin). Only the free portion is biologically active; the bound portion acts as a buffer to prevent sudden swings in cortisol levels.

Regulation of cortisol secretion

Secretion is regulated by ACTH release from the anterior pituitary. ACTH secretion is diurnal (highest in the morning), is increased by stress, and is decreased by negative feedback from circulating glucocorticoids (Figure 18.5).

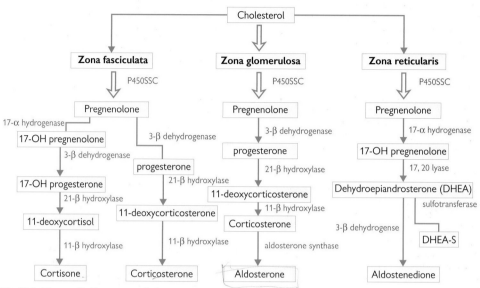

Fig. 18.4 Adrenocortical hormone production.

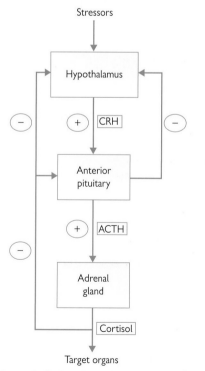

Fig. 18.5 Negative feedback mechanism for release of cortisol.

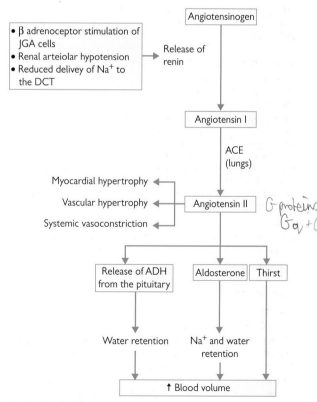

Fig. 18.6 Renin–aldosterone–angiotensin system.

18.4 Disorders of the adrenal glands

Pathology of the adrenal cortex

Adrenocortical insufficiency

- Primary, due to autoimmune destruction of the gland (**Addison's disease**). This results in both mineralocorticoid and glucocorticoid deficiency. Patients present with hypotension, hyponatraemia, metabolic acidosis, hyperkalaemia, weakness, fatigue, hypoglycaemia and weight loss. An 'Addisonian crisis' may present with fever, hypoglycaemia, coma, and circulatory collapse.
- Secondary, due to inadequate ACTH release from the pituitary, inadequate CRH release from the hypothalamus, or insufficient administration of exogenous steroids in a patient who is dependent on them. Mineralocorticoid secretion is usually adequate so electrolyte disturbances are uncommon.

Etomidate causes adrenal suppression which may persist for hours to days following a single dose. The clinical significance of this is unclear, but in critically ill patients it may be prudent to provide exogenous steroids following administration, or avoid etomidate entirely.

Glucocorticoid excess

An excess of glucocorticoids produces **Cushing's syndrome**. It may be due to:

- Adrenal causes such as adenomas
- Pituitary adenomas (Cushing's disease)
- Ectopic ACTH from non-pituitary tumours (e.g. lung).

Regardless of the aetiology, the patient presents with muscle wasting, central obesity, abdominal striae, hypertension, glucose intolerance, and 'moon' facies.

Several factors need to be taken into consideration when anaesthetising such patients.

- They are likely to volume-overloaded and hypokalaemic. This should be corrected preoperatively using spironolactone (an aldosterone antagonist) and potassium.
- Thin skin and osteoporotic bones may be damaged on positioning.
- Muscle weakness may cause increased sensitivity to neuromuscular-blocking drugs.
- Surgery for adrenelectomy can cause significant blood loss, or pneumothorax from diaphragmatic damage.

Mineralocorticoid excess

Hyperaldosteronism (**Conn's syndrome**) can be due to unilateral adenoma, bilateral hyperplasia, or adrenal carcinoma. Other diseases can stimulate aldosterone release via activation of the renin–angiotensin axis (e.g. cirrhosis, congestive cardiac failure, nephrotic syndrome). Clinically, patients present with hypertension, muscle weakness, and polyuria (secondary to prolonged hypokalaemia and loss of the concentrating ability of the kidney). The electrolyte disturbances can be corrected with spironolactone.

Medical uses of corticosteroids

Physiological steroid replacement can be provided by a number of preparations, in a dose that provides approximately the same effects as normal cortisol production. This is approximately 6–12mg/m^2/day (about 20mg/day for an average man).

In supranormal doses steroids may be used to **suppress allergic, inflammatory, and autoimmune diseases**.

Steroids are administered after organ transplant to **prevent rejection**, and are used in graft-versus-host disease.

All the currently used drugs are non-selective in their actions, and so have marked side effects in addition to their beneficial effects. These include skin thinning and bruising, hyperglycaemia, anovulation, muscle weakness, growth failure, and, importantly for anaesthetists, adrenal insufficiency if stopped suddenly.

Synthetic corticosteroids

Because of the wide range of therapeutic uses for corticosteroids, several synthetic molecules have been produced (Table 18.2). They are well absorbed orally, but some may be administered topically, intramuscularly, intravenously, or directly into joints.

Steroid cover during the perioperative period

Patients who have received high-dose steroids for more than a week are at risk of adrenal insufficiency if the steroids are stopped or reduced suddenly. This is because the exogenous steroids suppress endogenous corticotrophin-releasing hormone (CRH) release from the pituitary gland. After prolonged use, the adrenal cortices atrophy—this may take months to recover. Adrenal insuffiency is also likely to occur during times of stress (e.g. during surgery). At such times, an Addisonian crisis may be triggered. In most people the postoperative cortisol surge lasts for 72hr—150 mg of endogenous cortisol may be produced per day after major surgery.

Table 18.3 describes steroid replacement for patients on long-term steroids. If the patient is unable to eat in the postoperative period, replacement steroids must be given intravenously (e.g. hydrocortisone). If the patient can eat, an equivalent oral dose of prednisolone can be given.

Steroid cover should be provided for all patients who have received high-dose steroids in the past 3 months. Adrenal atrophy may still be present so the patient may be unable to mount a stress response.

Hormones of the adrenal medulla

The adrenal medulla is the body's main source of catecholamine hormones. Its main function is to synthesize and secrete adrenaline (70%) and noradrenaline (30%).

Tyrosine is taken up by the chromaffin cells and converted to noradrenaline and finally adrenaline (Figure 9.2). The rate-limiting step in this cascade is the enzyme tyrosine hydroxylase, located in the cytosol of catecholamine-containing nerve cells (Section 9.3).

The catecholamines are stored in granules until their release is triggered by pre-ganglionic sympathetic fibres. 'Stresses' triggering secretion include exercise, trauma, high emotion, and hypoglycaemia. Once released, these catecholamines bind loosely to albumin and other serum proteins for circulatory transport

Pathology of the adrenal medulla

Phaeochromocytoma

These are rare tumours arising from the adrenal medulla which secrete catecholamines.

- They may secrete constantly or intermittently.
- The familial type tends to produce mostly noradrenaline while the sporadic type produce mostly adrenaline.
- Dopamine may also be produced. They may be part of the multiple endocrine neoplasia (MEN type 2) and von Hippel–Lindau syndromes. About 15% are malignant.
- 10% occur in children.
- They may occur bilaterally and up to 25% are extra-adrenal (e.g. in the heart or near the bladder).

Patients usually present with intermittent symptoms of sweating, palpitations, headache, and tremor. These attacks can occur many times on one day or be months apart. Hypertension (often paradoxical) is frequently present.

Diagnosis is made by 24hr urine collection and measurement of urinary metanephrines and vanillylmandelic acid. If available, plasma metanephrines are the most specific test.

Anaesthetic considerations

Surgery is the mainstay of treatment but first the condition must be controlled by medical means. Untreated patients may be significantly hypovolaemic secondary to chronic vasoconstriction. The condition may present in pregnancy.

- α-blockade with phenoxybenzamine is started at least 7–10 days before surgery to allow for expansion of blood volume. Initially 10–20mg/day is given orally, increasing until blood pressure is controlled.
- Only when this is achieved is β-blockade commenced. If this is started too soon, unopposed α-stimulation can precipitate a

hypertensive crisis due to intense vasoconstriction once β$_2$-mediated vasodilatation is obliterated.

- Anaesthetic technique should centre on avoiding hypertensive crises and arrhythmias.
- Epidural anaesthesia combined with general anaesthesia provides good cardiovascular stability, as does the use of remifentanil.
- During surgery, magnesium infusions of 2–4g/h may be beneficial in stabilizing blood pressure.

Table 18.2 Comparison of synthetic corticosteroids

Name	Equivalent dose (mg)	Duration of action (hr)
Prednisolone	5	16–36
Betamethasone	0.750	36
Cortisone	25	24
Dexamethasone	0.750	36
Hydrocortisone	20	8
Methylprednisolone	4	18–24
Triamcinolone	4	24

Table 18.3 Steroid cover during the perioperative period*

Minor surgery (hernias, arthroscopy)	25mg IV hydrocortisone at induction
Moderate surgery (hysterectomy, THR)	Usual preoperative steroids +50mg IV hydrocortisone at induction +60mg/day hydrocortisone for 2–3 days
Major surgery (major trauma, aneurysm repair, prolonged surgery, or surgery where there is delayed oral intake)	Usual preoperative steroids +50mg IV hydrocortisone at induction +100–150mg/day hydrocortisone for 2–3 days Resume normal oral therapy when patient eating normally

*Patients who have received a daily dose of >10mg prednisolone or equivalent in the previous 3 months

449

The pancreas is a gland with both endocrine and exocrine functions. It is a key regulator of carbohydrate metabolism and blood glucose, and is an important source of digestive enzymes.

- It consists of a head, a body, and a tail.
- The pancreatic duct joins the common bile duct to empty into the ampulla of Vater in the second part of the duodenum (Figure 18.7).
- Blood supply is via the superior and inferior pancreaticoduodenal arteries, branches of the gastroduodenal artery, and the superior mesenteric artery. Venous drainage is to the portal vein via the pancreaticoduodenal veins.
- Islets of Langerhans (the endocrine cells which regulate blood glucose) are embedded in the exocrine pancreas, which secretes digestive enzymes. They form only 2% of the weight of the pancreas.

Endocrine functions of the pancreas

The islets contain four cell types.

- β **cells** secrete insulin, which lowers blood glucose. This is the most predominant cell type.
- α **cells** secrete glucagon, which raises blood glucose.
- δ **cells** secrete somatostatin, which inhibits α- and β-cell release.
- **PP cells** release pancreatic polypeptide, inhibiting enzyme release from the exocrine pancreas and stimulating gastric secretion.

Insulin

Insulin, secreted from islet β cells, is the main anabolic hormone. It is produced when C-peptide is cleaved from the precursor, proinsulin. It is formed from two polypeptide chains linked by disulphide bridges. Overall it lowers blood glucose and promotes fat and protein storage. The main metabolic effects are outlined in Section 18.6.

Insulin secretion is increased by:

- Increased blood glucose
- Amino acids
- Glucagon
- β-receptor stimulation
- Drugs, e.g. β-agonists, sulphonylureas, phosphodiesterase inhibitors.

Insulin secretion is decreased by:

- Low blood glucose
- Somatostatin
- α-receptor stimulation
- Drugs, e.g. β-blockers, thiazide diuretics.

Glucagon

Glucagon is secreted from the α cells of the islets. Its main effect is to raise the blood glucose via the breakdown of glycogen in the liver (Section 17.12). Other actions include:

- Stimulation of gluconeogenesis
- Increased lipolysis and ketone formation
- Increased amino acid uptake
- Increased calcium uptake into myocardial cells (positively inotropic and chronotropic).

Generally, glucagon antagonizes the effects of insulin. Secretion is increased during starvation and exercise.

Clinically, it can be used to treat hypoglycaemia (0.5–1mg IV/IM/SC) and also has a role in the treatment of β-blocker overdose (50–150mcg/kg IV).

Somatostatin

This hormone is released from both islet δ cells and the hypothalamus. It is also known as growth-hormone-inhibiting hormone. Effects include:

- Inhibition of growth hormone and TSH
- Reduced gut hormone secretion (e.g. gastrin, secretin, cholecystokinin (CCK))

- Smooth muscle relaxation and decreased gastric emptying
- Inhibition of the release of both insulin and glucagon.

Octreotide is a synthetic analogue of somatostatin. It is used clinically in the treatment of acromegaly, carcinoid syndrome, VIPomas, intractable diarrhoea, and vomiting in the palliative care setting. Its use has also been suggested in the management of variceal bleeding and to decrease the output of enterocutaneous fistulae (unlicensed in the UK).

Exocrine functions of the pancreas

The exocrine pancreas comprises:

- **Centroacinar cells** which secrete bicarbonate ions in response to secretin
- **Basophilic cells** which release digestive enzymes such as amylase and trypsin, in response to CCK stimulation.

Digestive enzymes

These are released at various points throughout the gut, from the oral cavity to the small intestine. Important stomach enzymes are pepsin (a protease) and gastric lipase.

The pancreas releases:

- Trypsin and chymotrypsin (peptidases; break down proteins)
- Elastases (degrade the protein elastin)
- Nucleases (break down nucleic acids)
- Pancreatic amylase (breaks down starch).

Acute pancreatitis

This inflammatory condition, the most common causes of which are outlined opposite, can vary from a self-limiting minor illness to a fulminant life-threatening disease. Assessing severity is difficult, and many scoring systems have been devised. The most widely used is the modified Glasgow system (opposite). A major flaw of these systems is that data are collected over several days, making interpretation difficult in the acute setting. Elevated amylase alone is not sufficient to make a diagnosis.

Patients may present with epigastric pain, nausea, vomiting, and sometimes an acute abdomen. Abdominal distension and flank bruising (Grey Turner sign) may be seen.

Complications are common, ranging from pleural effusions to ARDS and multiple organ failure. Hypocalcaemia is commonly seen. The pancreatic bed can become infected as it becomes necrotic. Eventually a pseudocyst can form.

Treatment

Largely supportive.

- Artificial ventilation may be necessary and careful fluid management is mandatory.
- CT should be performed after a few days to assess the degree of pancreatic damage.
- If gallstones are the cause, urgent ERCP should be performed and antibiotics (e.g. meropenem) prescribed.
- Surgical necrosectomy may be required.
- There is currently no consensus on the use of prophylactic antibiotics.
- Nasogastric feeding should be started early. If this is not tolerated nasojejunal or parenteral nutrition should be used.
- Blood sugar control should be tight. If much of the pancreas is destroyed, the patient may become insulin dependent in the long term.
- Pancreatic enzymes supplements may be needed.

➜ **Causes of acute pancreatitis**

- Gallstones
- Alcohol
- Hypertriglyceridaemia
- ERCP
- Abdominal trauma
- Hypercalcaemia
- Viral infection: mumps, EBV, CMV
- Drugs, e.g. furosemide, azathioprine, antiretrovirals
- Unknown in 25% of cases

➜ **Modified Glasgow scoring system for acute pancreatitis**

- Age >55 years
- White cell count >15×10^9/L
- Blood glucose >10mmol/L
- Urea >16mmol/L
- Arterial oxygen partial pressure <8.0kPa
- Albumin <32g/L
- Calcium <2.0mmol/L
- LDH >600IU/L

A score ≥3 indicates a severe attack.

High-scoring patients should be referred for critical care evaluation.

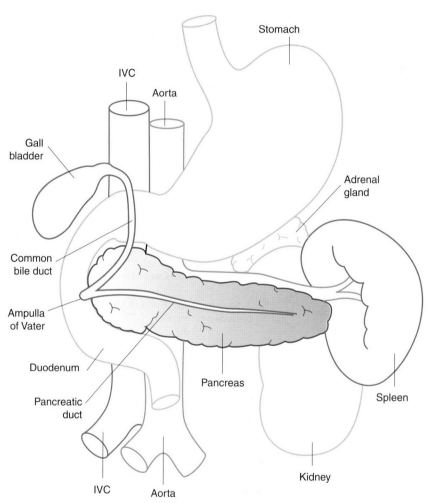

Fig. 18.7 Anatomical relations of the pancreas.

Normally blood glucose is tightly regulated at 3–8mmol/L despite variations in sugar intake. Glucose is either ingested or released by the liver. It is removed from the blood by uptake into muscle and fat cells under the influence of insulin. When blood sugar levels are very high, glucose is excreted in the urine.

Glucose is the sole energy source for erythrocytes, kidney medulla, and the brain.

Blood glucose control after a carbohydrate load

After a meal the following series of events occur to maintain the blood glucose at a normal level.

- Glucose is absorbed in the small intestine leading to a rise in blood glucose level. This rise is detected by β cells in the islets, triggering insulin release. Insulin drives glucose into liver, muscle, and fat cells
- Glucose taken up by the liver and muscle is converted to glycogen. Small amounts are converted into carbon dioxide and water, or used in fatty acid production.
- Glucose taken up by the fat is converted to glycerol and used in the production of triglycerides.
- Blood glucose drops back to normal, and the stimulus for insulin release ends.

Blood glucose control during fasting

During fasting, blood sugar falls to the lower end of normal. Compensatory mechanisms occur to oppose the fall.

- β cells detect the change in blood glucose and inhibit release of insulin.
- Glucose release from the liver increases as glycogen is broken down.
- Glycogen in muscles is broken down to form glucose residues but can only be used locally. It cannot be released into the circulation as muscle lacks glucose-6-phosphatase
- Glucagon release from the α cells of the islets increases.
- Glucagon acts on liver cells to increase cAMP levels. Glycogenolysis and gluconeogenesis increase.

These counter-regulatory mechanisms stop any further drop in blood glucose until liver and muscle glycogen stores are depleted.

Other hormones affecting blood glucose

- Cortisol—increases blood glucose, needed for glucagon to act on liver.
- Adrenaline—increases glycogenolysis in liver and so raises blood glucose.
- Growth hormone—opposes action of insulin on liver and so raises blood glucose.
- Thyroxine—increases gut uptake of glucose.
- Somatostatin—depresses insulin and glucagon release.

Actions of insulin

Muscle and fat

- Stimulates glycose uptake into cells via carrier protein (glucose transporter).
- Decreases fat and protein breakdown.
- Increases fatty acid synthesis and breakdown of triglycerides.

Liver

- Stimulates glycogen production.
- Traps glucose in cells via glucokinase activity.
- Increases oxidation of glucose.

Central nervous system

- Does not cross blood–brain barrier.
- Major effects on brain by altering systemic blood glucose levels: the brain is normally an obligate user of glucose as its energy source.

All cells

- Increases potassium uptake into cells.

Placenta

- Does not cross the placenta.
- Affects the fetus via changes in maternal blood glucose levels.
- Placental hormones inhibit insulin effects, so insulin levels double in late pregnancy

Blood glucose following surgery

Blood glucose tends to rise as part of the stress response to surgery. This is due to impaired insulin secretion, and increased glucose production triggered by raised levels of cortisol and catecholamines.

The greater the surgical insult, the longer the period of hyperglycaemia. There is some evidence that, following major surgery, patients fare better if their blood glucose is tightly controlled in the range 4.4–6.1mmol/L.

Starvation

Starvation describes a state in which there is no dietary intake. If hydration is maintained, most people have sufficient stores to survive a fast of more than 6 weeks, with death usual after about 60 days.

Many adaptive mechanisms occur to cope with this situation. The first is a decrease in metabolic activity to help preserve energy. The brain is an obligate user of glucose, so the priority during starvation is to maintain a steady supply for the brain. Methods of glucose production are detailed in Section 17.12.

Starvation eventually induces a state of ketosis. Ultimately most tissues, including the brain, adapt to using ketones as an energy source. Initially protein catabolism plays a major role in the response to starvation, but later this process slows as ketone bodies become the main fuel. Ketones can eventually supply half the energy requirements. Only red blood cells and the adrenal medullary cells remain obligate glucose users.

Carbohydrate production and utilization during periods of starvation

- Circulating blood glucose adequate for 4–6hr.
- Glycogenolysis until glycogen stores depleted (about 24hr).
- Blood glucose drops.
- Insulin secretion decreases.
- Muscle adapts to using fatty acids as an energy source.
- Liver gluconeogenesis using amino acids (alanine and glutamine) from the breakdown of muscle protein.
- Lipolysis—fatty acids are cleaved to produce acetyl-CoA, leading to ketosis.
- Renal medulla and red blood cells remain obligate glucose users.

➔ **Glucose utilization**

This occurs in two ways.

- **Anaerobic respiration**—this does not need oxygen. Glucose, formed from glycogen, breaks down to form two pyruvic acid molecules which release ATP. This fuels a further 40sec of maximum muscle activity and is used during rapid spurts of activity such as sprinting. Pyruvic acid breaks down further to form lactic acid which can cause fatigue and cramp if it accumulates in the muscle.
- **Aerobic respiration** only occurs in the presence of oxygen. This system is important in endurance sports such as long-distance running. ATP must be produced without the build-up of lactic acid. This is achieved by using oxygen in the breakdown of pyruvic acid, via the citric acid (Krebs cycle), leading to production of carbon dioxide and water rather than lactic acid.

18.7 Diabetes

The term 'diabetes' describes a group of conditions characterized by failure of blood glucose control, leading to hyperglycaemia. Diagnosis is made on a fasting plasma glucose of >7mmol/L (or blood glucose >6.1mmol/L). Impaired glucose tolerance (IGT) describes a fasting plasma glucose of 6.1–7mmol/L. It is an indicator of future diabetes and increased cardiovascular risk.

Type 1 diabetes

This occurs when β islet cells are immunologically destroyed, rendering the pancreas unable to produce insulin. Anti-islet or anti-insulin antibodies may be demonstrated.

The disease is usually rapidly progressive and occurs most commonly in children and young adults, although it may appear at any age. Ketoacidosis is often the first presentation. Patients almost always require lifelong insulin replacement therapy. There is an association with other autoimmune conditions.

Marked insulin deficiency leads to uninhibited gluconeogenesis. The utilization and storage of circulating glucose is also prevented, leading to hyperglycaemia. The kidneys fail to reabsorb the glucose load, causing the osmotic diuresis of glycosuria, leading to thirst and dehydration. Insulin deficiency also leads to increased fat and protein breakdown resulting in weight loss and eventually ketoacidosis (DKA).

Type 2 diabetes

In this form, patients have relative rather than absolute insulin deficiency and there is a peripheral insulin resistance. Both defects must exist; all overweight individuals have insulin resistance, but only those who are unable to increase insulin production will develop diabetes. Up to 6% of the population may be affected.

Hyperglycaemia may be mild and the condition may be undiagnosed for years. There is often a progression from normal to abnormal glucose tolerance to type 2 diabetes. Post-prandial glucose levels are often the first sign of concern. Eventually, fasting hyperglycaemia develops as inhibition of hepatic gluconeogenesis declines.

Obesity or increased intra-abdominal fat are common findings. Insulin resistance occurs with insufficient insulin secretion to compensate. Some patients may have abnormal glucokinase genes, meaning that a higher blood glucose is necessary to trigger insulin release. Patients rarely present with ketoacidosis as this only occurs in the absence of insulin. Instead, hyperosmolar states may occur.

Obesity and type 2 diabetes

About 90% of patients who develop type 2 diabetes mellitus are obese. They are still able to secrete some endogenous insulin, and so are considered to require but not to depend on it. They generally do not develop DKA if exogenous insulin therapy is stopped.

Significant weight loss improves outlook; this often avoids the need for treatment with oral antidiabetic medication or insulin.

Other causes of diabetes

- **Gestational** diabetes occurs in 1% (White) to 14% (African Carribbean) of pregnancies. Older women and those with IGT are at risk. Untreated it leads to fetal macrosomia, hypoglycaemia, hypocalcaemia, and hyperbilirubinaemia. There is an increased rate of Caesarean delivery and mothers have increased risk of chronic hypertension.
- **Drugs** can cause destruction of the β cells (e.g. pentamidine) or impair the actions of insulin (e.g. corticosteroids).
- **Pancreatitis**.
- **Viral infections** (e.g. coxsackie B).
- **Genetic syndromes** such as Down's, Turner's, and Klinefelter's syndromes are associated with diabetes.

Complications of diabetes

These may be acute or chronic.

Acute (Section 18.8)

- Hypoglycaemia following periods of starvation, particularly if diabetic medications continue.
- Diabetic ketoacidosis in type 1 diabetics when no insulin is available.
- Hyperosmolar non-ketotic coma in type 2 diabetics.

Chronic

These are predominantly vascular, due to blood vessel damage from persistently raised blood glucose.

- Microvascular—retinopathy, nephropathy, neuropathy.
- Macrovascular—coronary artery disease, stroke, peripheral vascular disease.

Treatment of diabetes

Oral hypoglycaemics

The aim is reduce HbA_{1c} to <7% to decrease vascular complications. Drugs include those which:

- Increase insulin secretion—sulphonylureas (e.g. glipizide) and meglitinides (e.g. repaglinide).
- Reduce hepatic glucose output (and increase cellular uptake of glucose)—biguanides (e.g. metformin). These should be avoided in renal failure, acute coronary syndromes and cardiac failure, and following the use of IV contrast as lactic acidosis may occur.
- Improve tissue sensitivity but do not increase secretion—glitazones (e.g. roziglitazone).
- Slow gut absorption of starch—α-glucosidase inhibitors (e.g. acarbose). They have no direct effect on blood sugar and can be used in combination with the above agents.

Insulin

Human insulin is produced in the laboratory by inserting human DNA into host cells (*Escherichia coli*) and is now the most common agent used. It is usually given by subcutaneous injection, but an inhaled version is newly available.

Insulin analogues have been created to alter the onset and duration of action, by substituting various amino acids: glargine insulin is long acting whereas aspart insulin is rapid onset.

Perioperative management

Preoperative

Diabetic patients are prone to cardiovascular and renal complications. They should undergo routine blood tests to check renal function and electrolytes and should have a preoperative ECG.

Blood glucose should be measured. If it is poorly controlled, surgery should be delayed where possible. A blood glucose of 6–10mmol/L is acceptable.

Diabetic patients should be placed first on the list to limit long periods of starvation.

Intraoperative

The overall perioperative management of diabetes is outlined in Table 18.4. It is important to decide how quickly the patient will be able to eat and drink postoperatively.

Suspect hypoglycaemia if the patient becomes cold and sweaty.

Standard anaesthetic techniques can be employed but have a low threshold for intubation, or even rapid sequence induction, as diabetic patients are likely to suffer delayed gastric emptying due to autonomic dysfunction.

Hypotension following induction or spinal anaesthesia should be anticipated if the patient has autonomic neuropathy. This can be prevented with slow injection, fluid loading, or the use of vasopressors.

Table 18.4 Perioperative management of diabetic patients

	Type 1 diabetes		Type 2 diabetes	
Type of surgery	Minor	Major	Minor	Major
Preoperatively	Measure BM 4hr and 1hr before surgery First on list Omit breakfast and insulin	Measure BM 4hr and 1hr before surgery First on list Omit breakfast and insulin	Measure BM 8hr and 1hr before surgery First on list Omit breakfast and morning oral hypoglycaemics	Measure BM 8hr and 1hr before surgery First on list Omit breakfast and morning oral hypoglycaemics
Intraoperatively	Measure BM every hour	Measure BM every hour and in recovery 5% dextrose 100ml/hr (+KCl 10mmol/L) in addition to other IV fluids Insulin sliding scale	Measure BM during surgery if >1 hr duration.	Measure BM every hour and in recovery 5% dextrose 100ml/hr (+KCl 10mmol/L) in addition to other IV fluids Insulin sliding scale
Postoperatively	Measure BM every 2hr until eating then every 4hr Normal SC insulin with first meal	Stop insulin infusion when eating Give total preoperative daily insulin requirement as 3–4 doses SC Actrapid insulin Restart normal regime when stable	Measure BM every 2hr until eating Restart oral hypoglycaemics with first meal.	Stop insulin infusion Restart oral hypoglycaemics when eating and drinking

Table 18.5 A typical sliding scale regime*

Blood glucose (mmol/L)	Insulin infusion (units/hr)
<5	0 (give glucose if blood glucose <3.5)
5.1–10	1
10.1–15	2
15.1–20	3
>20	6 (and 3–5IU bolus)

*All such prescriptions must be regularly reviewed in the light of the patient's response.

18.8 Diabetic emergencies

Derangements of blood sugar are common in diabetic patients; at both extremes, they can be life-threatening.

Hypoglycaemia in diabetics is usually due to exogenous insulin administration.

Two distinct hyperglycaemic syndromes occur in diabetics: diabetic ketoacidosis (DKA) and hyperglycemic hyperosmolar state (HHS; the old terminology "hyperglycaemic hyperosmolar non-ketotic coma" has been changed since most patients are not comatose at presentation). Generally DKA is a problem of type 1 diabetics, and HHS a type 2 diabetic complication. However, some cases have overlapping features. In both syndromes, the principles of management are:

- Rapid restoration of adequate circulation and perfusion with isotonic intravenous fluids.
- Gradual rehydration and restoration of depleted electrolytes.
- Insulin to reverse ketosis and hyperglycaemia.
- Identification and treatment of the underlying cause.
- Careful, regular monitoring of clinical signs and laboratory tests to detect and treat complications.

Hypoglycaemia

Hypoglycaemia is the commonest endocrine emergency. Causes of fasting hypoglycaemia include exogenous insulin or sulphonylureas; alcohol; liver failure; Addison's disease; pituitary insufficiency; and (more rarely) insulinomas or other tumours. Post-prandial hypoglycaemia can be seen in type 2 diabetics, or after gastric or bariatric surgery ("dumping" syndrome).

Clinical presentation

Symptoms and signs arise from sympathetic stimulation and direct effects of glycopenia in neural tissues: sweating, tremor, and hunger (sympathetic); confusion, agitiation, lethargy, weakness, seizures, and coma (neuroglycopenia). A review of the drug chart may indicate problems with the patient's diabetic regimen.

Investigations

Finger-prick blood glucose and serum glucose <3.5mmol/L (although clinical hypoglycaemia may occur at higher levels in poorly-controlled diabetes).

LFTs and clotting may indicate liver dysfunction.

Other investigations depend on the clinical picture and likely causes.

> **❗ Immediate management of hypoglycaemia**
>
> If the symptoms are mild and the patient is able to eat, hypoglycaemia can be treated with oral sugar (e.g. a sweet drink or dextrose tablet) and a slower-release carbohydrate meal (bread, rice, etc). Check blood glucose after 10 min and repeat the sugary drink if necessary.
>
> If the patient is comatose or fitting, follow an ABC approach. Establish IV access and give 50ml of 50% dextrose as an IV push (the solution is irritant, so follow with copious flushing of the line).
>
> Glucagon 0.5–1mg (IM, SC or IV) can also be given; the IM or SC routes are useful pending IV access. The effect is temporary (5–10 minutes), so glucagon must be followed by dextrose.
>
> Recheck blood sugar after 10 minutes, and repeat IV dextrose if necessary. An infusion of 10–20% dextrose may be necessary if the underlying cause is slow to resolve.

Ongoing management

Blood glucose should be monitored frequently for at least 24 hours, as rebound hyper- or hypoglycaemia can occur. If the patient is diabetic, their drug regimen should be reviewed in consultation with the diabetic team. Unexplained fasting hypoglycaemia should be referred to an endocrinologist for formal investigation.

Diabetic ketoacidosis

DKA occurs in the absence of glucose and is driven by unchecked gluconeogenesis and failure of cells to take up glucose.

Causes

- Intercurrent infection (particularly UTI)
- Myocardial infarction
- Stroke

- Pregnancy
- Trauma/surgery
- Drug use (e.g. cocaine)
- Missed insulin dose

Clinical presentation

Symptoms include thirst, polydipsia, polyuria/nocturia, weakness, malaise, nausea and vomiting, lack of sweating, changes in appetite, confusion, and/or symptoms of underlying infections or other conditions.

Signs: general signs include dry skin, Kussmaul respiration (laboured, sighing), dry mucous membranes and sunken eyes. The patient is usually tachycardic and tachypnoeic, and may be hypotensive. Hypothermia or pyrexia may be present. Ketotic breath is said to have a "pear drop" smell. The GCS may be reduced and there may be abdominal tenderness.

Investigations

The diagnostic triad comprises hyperglycaemia, ketosis, and acidosis.

Blood glucose is usually very high, but DKA can occur with values as low as 10mmol/L.

ABG: pH is often <7.3; the acidaemia is metabolic, with a raised anion gap. Patients may be markedly hypocapnic.

Urinalysis shows glycosuria and urine ketosis. Most commercially available dipsticks (e.g. "Ketostix") measure acetone and acetoacetic acid. However, beta-hydroxybutyrate is quantitatively more important. As a result, ketosis may paradoxically appear to worsen as the latter is converted into the former during treatment. Specific beta-hydroxybutyrate assays are available. Urinalysis may also reveal evidence of underlying urinary infection.

> **❗ Immediate management of DKA**
>
> ABC approach: assess the airway and breathing. The $PaCO_2$ may be very low to compensate for the acidosis. If the patient requires intubation, respiratory compensation should be maintained with artificial hyperventilation. If not, the acidosis can become extreme.
>
> Establish IV access for fluid and insulin.
>
> The ideal fluid to give in DKA is a subject of debate. While 0.9% saline in large volumes can contribute to metabolic acidaemia (Section 11.13), Hartmann's solution poses theoretical risks of worsening hyperkalaemia, hyperglycaemia, and cerebral oedema (it is slightly hypotonic). The patient is likely to be severely depleted of water, sodium, potassium, and other electrolytes. The key to good management is frequent assessment, and adjustment of fluid regimens to reflect the clinical condition and electrolyte imbalances. A *suggested* regimen for initial management is:
>
> - 1-3L of isotonic fluid over the first hour, depending on the degree of circulatory impairment.
> - If high volumes are necessary, a balanced solution such as Hartmann's, rather than 0.9% saline, may help to avoid hyperchloraemic acidosis.
> - After initial resuscitation, the patient's fluid balance and U&Es should be re-assessed.
>
> Insulin should be started after the first hour's fluid resuscitation, as long as serum potassium is >3.3mmol/L (if less, give 40mmol KCL over 1hr before starting insulin). A loading dose of 0.1-0.15 units/kg may be given, followed by an infusion of 0.1 units/kg/hr. Aim for correction of glucose at a rate of <5mmol/L/hr (reduce the insulin infusion rate if correcting too rapidly).
>
> Total potassium stores may be profoundly depleted despite a normal or even raised serum potassium level. Serum potassium levels can fall precipitously once insulin is given. 20-40mmol of KCl in each litre of IV fluid should be given once the serum potassium falls below 5.5mmol/L (aim for a serum level of 4-5mmol/L).

Ongoing management

Ongoing IV fluid administration should be governed by repeated assessment of the patients' clinical condition and electrolytes. Once the blood glucose has fallen to 11mmol/L, dextrose can be introduced (at this stage, insulin administration must continue, to correct ketosis).

Aim to correct the fluid deficit gradually (over 24-48hr), as too-rapid fluid administration has been implicated in the development of cerebral oedema. This is particularly important in children (see below).

It is not generally necessary to use bicarbonate, as acidosis tends to improve with treatment. It may be indicated in very severe acidaemia (pH <7.0) associated with myocardial depression.

Hourly glucose measurement and an insulin sliding scale should continue until the metabolic disturbance has resolved.

Depending on the severity of the presentation and the response to treatment, the patient may require ITU admission, arterial and/or central lines, an NG tube, and catheter. The mortality of DKA is around 2%.

Further management of the patient's diabetes depends on the clinical scenario. Liaison with the diabetic team is essential.

Cerebral oedema

Cerebral oedema is a life-threatening complication of DKA with a mortality of around 25%. It is more common in newly-diagnosed type 1 diabetics, and young children. Paediatric protocols emphasise prevention of cerebral oedema, and advise slow (48-72hr) correction of fluid deficits and hyperglycaemia. Initial loading doses of insulin are not given.

Symptoms and signs of cerebral oedema include headache, drowsiness, irritability, cranial nerve palsies, and incontinence. Seizures, coma and respiratory arrest are late signs.

Treatment is by prompt administration of hypertonic (3–5%) saline (3–5ml/kg over 30 mins) or mannitol (0.5–1.0 g/kg stat), slowing of IV fluids, and ICU admission for neuroprotective management. Consultant involvement (medical, neurological/neurosurgical, ICU, and paediatric for children) is mandatory.

An early CT should be performed to exclude other intracerebral conditions such as haemorrhage, thrombosis or infarction. Many of the changes of cerebral oedema may be seen late on imaging, and their absence should not delay treatment in cases where clinical suspicion is high.

Ongoing investigation

Ongoing investigations are directed towards diagnosing the underlying cause of DKA, and detecting complications.

U&E: repeat 2hrly during initial treatment. Hyponatraemia can occur due to the osmotic effect of hyperglycemia (extravascular water moves to the intravascular space). There is loss of sodium and potassium. Be aware that high triglyceride levels may lead to artefactual low glucose levels; and high levels of ketone bodies may lead to artefactual elevation of creatinine level.

The FBC may show haemoconcentration (raised RBC count and haematocrit), and evidence of infection (raised leucocyte count).

Serum amylase may be raised, even in the absence of pancreatitis.

Ketonuria may last longer than the underlying tissue acidosis.

CXR may show evidence of pneumonia.

CT scanning: the threshold should be low for obtaining a head CT in patients with altered mental status.

ECG: an ECG can help to assess significant hypokalemia or hyperkalemia, cardiac complications of DKA, and in some cases, reveal a precipitating cardiac event.

Hyperglycaemic hyperosmolar state

Hyperosmolar hyperglycemic state (HHS) is characterized by hyperglycemia, hyperosmolarity, and dehydration without significant ketoacidosis. It less common than DKA, but the mortality is much higher (around 15%). Like DKA, it may be the first presentation of diabetes. It tends to affect older patients with type 2 diabetes, although obesity-related type 2 diabetes is becoming more common and the incidence of HHS reflects this; it has been described in children.

The basic mechanism of HHS is a reduction in circulating insulin with a concomitant elevation of counter-regulatory hormones. Decreased renal clearance and impaired utilization of glucose lead to hyperglycemia. The ensuing hyperosmolarity has two main effects: fluid shifts from the intravascular space (causing intracellular dehydration) and an osmotic diuresis leads to loss of water and electrolytes, compounding the problem.

It is unclear why significant ketosis is avoided in HHS. Type 2 diabetics are usually not completely devoid of insulin, and this may be enough to inhibit ketogenesis but not to prevent hyperglycemia. Hyperosmolarity may decrease lipolysis, limiting ketogenesis. In addition, lower levels of counter-regulatory hormones may be lower.

Causes

In general, any illness that predisposes to dehydration may lead to HHS. A wide variety of illnesses may trigger HHS by limiting patient mobility and free access to water. Pneumonia and urinary tract infections (UTIs) are the most common underlying causes of HHS.

The stress response to any acute illness tends to increase hormones that favor elevated glucose levels. Cortisol, catecholamines, glucagon, and many other hormones have effects that tend to counter those of insulin. Examples of such acute conditions include stroke, MI, and pulmonary embolism.

Patients with underlying renal dysfunction and/or heart failure are at special risk.

Drugs that raise serum glucose levels, inhibit insulin, or cause dehydration may cause HHS. Examples include diuretics, β-blockers, H_2 antagonists, and alcohol. Non-compliance with diabetic therapy may contribute, as can self-neglect.

Clinical presentation

HHS usually develops over days or weeks. Symptoms include polydipsia, polyuria, weakness, lethargy, and weight loss. Signs include those of severe dehydration, and focal or global neurologic deficits. The neurologic features may include sensory or visual deficits, hemiparesis, drowsiness, lethargy, confusion, seizures, and coma.

Symptoms and signs of the precipitating illness, and other chronic illnesses, should be sought. Abnormally high or low temperatures suggest sepsis (hypothermia is a poor prognostic factor).

Investigations

Blood glucose is usually > 30mmol/L.

Osmolality (2[Na^+]+ glucose + urea): patients in coma typically have osmolalities >330 mOsm/kg H_2O. If the osmolality is less in a comatose patient, search for another cause.

Urinalysis: minimal ketonuria

Bicarbonate concentration >15mmol/L.

Initial management

The initial management of HHS is very similar to that of DKA. Airway and breathing should be assessed, and comatose or fitting patients may require intubation and ventilation.

The fluid deficit in HHS is likely to be larger than in DKA: typically 10L for an adult. After initial resuscitation and restoration of circulating volume, similar caveats regarding over-rapid correction of fluid and electrolyte balance apply.

Ongoing management

Again, the ongoing management of HHS is similar to that of DKA. HDU or ICU care is usually appropriate. Fluids and IV insulin infusion should be continued until the metabolic derangement has resolved, and any concurrent conditions should be addressed. Frequent clinical reassessment of volume status, and measurement of blood sugar and electrolytes, guide therapy.

HHS results in a pro-coagulant state with platelet activation. Arterial thrombotic events (e.g. stroke, MI, limb ischaemia) are well-recognised complications of HHS. Aspirin (with a PPI or similar) and prophylactic low-molecular weight heparin should be used.

Further reading

Guidelines for the management of paediatric DKA (including cerebral oedema): www.bsped.org.uk/professional/guidelines

NICE guidelines for management of diabetes (including DKA): www.nice.org.uk:80/nicemedia/pdf/CG015NICEguideline.pdf

Review of HHS: Hyperglycaemic hyperosmolar syndrome. Scott A. *Diabetic Medicine* 2006;23:22-24.

Anatomy of the thyroid gland

The thyroid gland, anterior to the trachea, extends from the thyroid cartilage to the sixth tracheal ring. It is covered by muscle and skin, and moves with respiration. It weighs about 20g and is shield-shaped. An isthmus joins the two lobes (Figure 18.8). Blood supply is via paired superior thyroid arteries (the first branches of the external carotid) and inferior thyroid arteries (from the subclavian arteries). Superior, middle, and inferior thyroid veins drain blood to the left brachiocephalic vein.

The gland is composed of round follicles which absorb iodine from the blood to form thyroid hormones. Each follicle is surrounded by a single layer of epithelial cells which secrete thyroid hormones. Parafollicular cells which secrete calcitonin, important in calcium homeostasis (Section 18.9), are scattered throughout the gland.

Thyroid hormones

Synthesis

- Iodine is absorbed from the small bowel (as iodide) and transported to the thyroid gland in the blood.
- The iodide is actively transported into the follicular cells in exchange for sodium ions.
- It is then converted to iodine (by hydrogen peroxide) and diffuses into the follicular lumen where it is incorporated into the tyrosine residues of the thyroglobulin molecule to form mono-iodotyrosine.
- This reaction is catalysed by thyroid peroxidase.
- Further iodination produces di-iodotyrosine.
- Two of these residues are coupled by oxidation producing thyroxine (T_4).
- If a mono-iodotyrosine molecule is coupled to a di-iodotyrosine molecule, tri-iodotyrosine (T_3) is produced instead.
- The hormones are stored as T_3 and T_4 and only released when the thyroglobulin molecule is taken back up by the follicular cells. This process is triggered by thyroid-stimulating hormone (TSH).
- Any iodine released is recycled.
- Approximately 90% is released in the form of T_4, with the more active T_3 accounting for less than 10%.
- About 100mcg are released per day.
- In the liver and kidney thyroxine is converted into either active T_3 or inactive reverse T_3 (rT_3).
- Only the free portion is metabolically active—the unbound hormones cross cell membranes and bind to intracellular A and B receptors.
- Their effects are modulated via alteration of DNA transcription.

Regulation of thyroid hormone release

- The release of T_4 and T_3 is modulated by release of TSH from the anterior pituitary gland.
- This mechanism is under tight negative-feedback control—as the levels of T_4 rise, TSH production falls.
- TSH production is controlled by thyrotrophin-releasing hormone (TRH) production by the hypothalamus, again under negative-feedback.
- TRH secretion increases when a higher metabolic rate is desirable (e.g. in cold environments).
- TSH secretion is suppressed by high glucocorticoid levels, and high blood iodide levels.

Thyroid hormone production

Effects of thyroid hormones

The major effects of thyroid hormones are as follows:
- Increased basal metabolic rate
- Increased tissue sensitivity to catecholamines, so raised HR and cardiac output
- Regulation of protein, fat, and carbohydrate metabolism
- Important in fetal development, especially the brain.

Disorders of the thyroid gland

Hypothyroidism

This describes a situation when the T_4 and T_3 levels are insufficient. The most common causes are:
- Hashimoto's (autoimmune) thyroiditis
- radio-iodine for the treatment of hyperthyroidism
- iodine deficiency (now rare in the Western world).

Presenting features include bradycardia, hypothermia, slow cognition, hair loss, weight gain, slow reflexes, fatigue, and infertility. Treatment involves the administration of daily thyroxine.

Hyperthyroidism

This is seen when the circulating levels of free T_4 or T_3 are raised. Major causes are as follows:
- Graves' disease (autoimmune)
- Toxic multinodular goitre
- Isolated hyperactive adenoma

Presentation may be with weight loss, palpitations or arrhythmias, dyspnoea, sweating, tremor, and diarrhoea. Exophthalmos or visual disturbances occur with Graves' disease. Diagnosis is made by measuring a low blood TSH. In Graves' disease anti-TSH antibodies may also be found. Treatment may be:
- Surgical, removing all or part of the gland.
- Oral radio-active iodine (destroys hyperactive areas of the gland).
- Drugs—carbimazole or propylthiouracil (PTU) decrease thyroid hormone formation. These act by inhibiting the iodination of thyroglobulin by thyroperoxidase. PTU also blocks the peripheral conversion of T_4 to T_3.
- β-blockers may be used to relieve symptoms.

Thyroid storm

This term describes a life-threatening exacerbation of hyperthyroidism. Onset is sudden and often follows surgery or trauma. Patients present with tachycardia, arrhythmias, cardiac failure, acidosis, and agitation. Eventually coma and cardiovascular collapse occur. Treatment is supportive and best carried out in a critical care facility. Propanolol 1–5mg IV should be given, as should potassium iodide 60mg IV BD. Oral PTU should then be started.

Anaesthesia for thyroid surgery

If possible, thyroid surgery should be delayed until the patient is clinically euthyroid. The airway should be assessed as large goitres can distort normal tracheal anatomy, making intubation difficult. Awake intubation may be required. An armoured endotracheal tube should be used to protect the airway during surgical manipulation.

Postoperative airway compromise is not uncommon. This may be due to haematoma, bilateral recurrent laryngeal nerve palsy (unilateral causes a hoarse voice and mild stridor only), or tracheomalacia.

If haematoma is the cause, the wound should immediately be opened and CPAP applied. Re-intubation may be required.

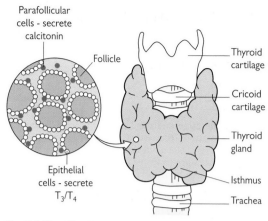

Parafollicular
cells - secrete
calcitonin

Follicle

Thyroid
cartilage

Cricoid
cartilage

Thyroid
gland

Isthmus

Trachea

Epithelial
cells - secrete
T_3/T_4

Fig. 18.8 Thyroid anatomy.

➕ **Emergency anaesthesia in the hyperthyroid patient**

These patients are at risk of cardiovascular collapse and arrhythmias.

Sympathetic stimulation should be avoided and the patient should be premedicated with a benzodiazepine.

β-blockade should be started preoperatively and continued perioperatively unless the patient is in cardiac failure.

Drugs with sympathetic effects (ketamine, pancuronium, and local anaesthetic with adrenaline) should be avoided.

Regional techniques can be employed to reduce sympathetic stimulation further.

Care should be taken to protect exophthalmic eyes.

There are usually four parathyroid glands embedded in, but separate from, the thyroid gland. The glands consist of densely packed cells arranged in nests around abundant capillaries. These cells produce parathyroid hormone (PTH) and contain calcium-sensing receptors that regulate blood calcium levels

Parathyroid hormone

PTH is synthesized in the parathyroid cells and then packaged in vesicles and secreted into the blood by exocytosis in response to low calcium levels. It is a protein consisting of 84 amino acids. It acts to raise blood calcium and lower phosphate levels. This is achieved by three mechanisms.

- Stimulating osteoclasts which resorb bone, releasing calcium.
- Indirectly increasing calcium absorption from the small bowel via increased production of vitamin D by the kidney. This induces production of a calcium-binding protein in the gut which facilitates absorption of calcium.
- Decreasing calcium loss in the urine by stimulating reabsorption.

Hyperparathyroidism

- Primary—due to adenoma, carcinoma (± multiple endocrine neoplasia syndrome), or generalized gland hyperplasia (moderate enlargement of all four glands).
- Secondary—end-organ resistance to PTH, resulting in increased secretion and gland hyperplasia. Seen most commonly in chronic renal failure, but also in vitamin D deficiency and oral contraceptive use.
- Tertiary—follows long-standing secondary hyperparathyroidism and defines autonomous PTH release with loss of feedback control. Severe hypercalcaemia can result.

Anaesthesia for parathyroidectomy

Surgery involves a full neck dissection with removal of either a single gland or, in the case of generalized hypertrophy, removal of 3½ glands. Anaesthesia is as for thyroid surgery, but the airway is less likely to be compromised preoperatively. If the patient is markedly hypercalcaemic, dehydration should be considered and corrected. Postoperative airway complications can occur due to bleeding or bilateral recurrent laryngeal nerve damage.

Hypocalcaemia is commonly seen at 24–72hr postoperatively. Tetany and laryngospasm may occur. Calcium levels should be measured twice daily until stable.

Calcium homeostasis

Calcium is the most abundant mineral in the body, accounting for about 1kg body weight. Blood calcium levels are closely controlled in the range of 2.20–2.55mmol/L. Approximately half is free in the blood—the rest is bound to albumin. If blood albumin levels are abnormal, a corrected calcium level should be used. This is calculated as follows:

Corrected Ca^{++} = Uncorrected Ca^{++} (mmol/L) + 0.02(40 − albumin).

There are three main regulatory mechanisms:

- **PTH** is very important in raising calcium levels as outlined above (Figure 18.9).
- **Calcitriol** is formed in the kidney from vitamin D. It increases intestinal absorption of calcium and hence raises blood levels.
- **Calcitonin** is a 32 amino acid hormone s formed by the parafollicular cells of the thyroid gland. It counteracts the effects of PTH, lowering calcium and raising phosphate levels. It is thought to be of little importance in calcium homeostasis in humans and is not essential for life.

Hypocalcaemia

This is defined as a calcium level <2.2mmol/L (or ionized calcium <1.1mmol/L). The most common causes are primary hypoparathyroidism, vitamin D deficiency, acute or chronic renal failure, and pancreatitis.

Symptoms include paraesthesia and perioral tingling. Tetany and carpopedal spasm occur (Trousseau sign describes carpopedal spasm on sustained inflation of blood pressure cuff) and tendon reflexes are depressed. Chovstek's sign (twitching of facial muscles on repeat tapping over zygoma) may be seen. In severe cases laryngospasm and arrhythmias are seen. Management involves replacing calcium as either IV calcium gluconate or chloride. Oral calcium and calcitriol supplements may be necessary long term. Treatment should be reserved for symptomatic patients or for those with calcium <1.5mmol/L.

Hypercalcaemia

Hypercalcaemia is described as blood calcium >2.6mmol/L, but is not usually symptomatic until the calcium level is >3mmol/L. Symptoms include fatigue, mood change, confusion, diarrhoea, and polyuria. Renal stones can develop. ECG changes include shortened QT interval and arrhythmias. If levels rise above 3.75mmol/L, coma and cardiac arrest occur. Causes of hypercalacaemia are as follows:

- Primary hyperparathyroidism—adenoma, hyperplasia, carcinoma
- Malignancy—breast, lung, kidney, phaeochromocytoma
- Vitamin D intoxication
- Rhabdomyolysis
- High bone turnover—Paget's disease, immobilization
- Drugs—thiazide diuretics, lithium
- Renal failure (secondary hyperparathyroidism)
- Milk alkali syndrome.

Together, malignancy and primary hyperparathyroidism account for 90% of cases.

Treatment of hypercalcaemia

- Rehydration to replace renal or gut fluid losses.
- Furosemide to decrease renal calcium reabsorption and allow further IV rehydration.
- Bisphosphanates (e.g. pamidronate) to inhibit osteoclast activity and bone resorption. This is first line treatment if malignancy is the cause.
- Calcitonin to promote renal excretion and stop bone resorption. It is rarely used except in life-threatening cases.
- Steroids to help in hypercalcaemia secondary to malignancies, sarcoid, and vitamin D intoxication.
- Renal dialysis to remove calcium from the blood.

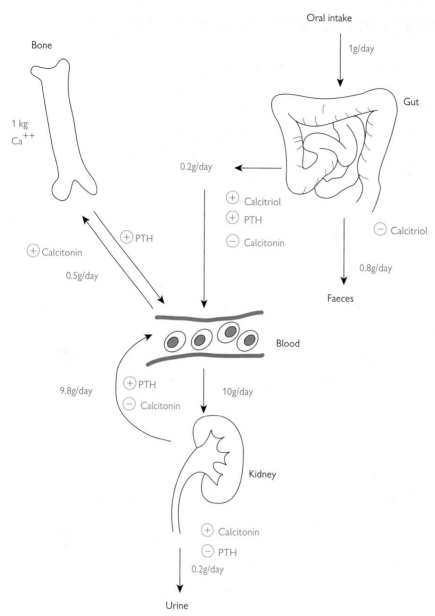

Fig. 18.9 Calcium homeostasis. Hormone actions in green tend to increase serum calcium concentrations; those in red reduce serum calcium.

18.11 Body temperature and its regulation

Body temperature is very closely regulated, varying by only about 1°C throughout the day despite large variations in environment temperature. This tight control is necessary for optimization of enzymatic processes. Temperature is highest in the evening and lowest in the early morning. Reversal of the daily routine leads to reversal of this pattern. Small fluctuations (0.5°C) are also observed during the menstrual cycle. Death is likely to occur if the body temperature rises above 43°C or below 28°C.

Physiological control of body temperature

The body has two temperature compartments—the core which is maintained at 37°C and the peripheral compartment which acts as a heat sink and varies from 28 to 36°C (Figure 18.10). The core is normally the larger compartment, but the size varies markedly with the ambient temperature.

- Temperature is sensed by Aδ fibres (cold) which fire continuously, and C fibres (warm) which only fire during pyrexia. The sensors are found throughout the body, but there are more around the deep abdominal and thoracic structures (i.e. the core zone).
- The signals travel to the preoptic region of the hypothalamus via the spinothalamic tract in the anterior spinal cord.
- The inputs are compared with reference temperatures (the thermoregulatory set-point) and if a difference is detected, thermoregulatory mechanisms are triggered.
- If the warm threshold is exceeded, heat loss responses occur such as sweating, vasodilatation, panting, and behavioural changes.
- If the cold threshold is exceeded thermogenic activities are triggered, e.g. exercise, shivering, and non-shivering thermogenesis.
- Pyrogens, (endogenous or exogenous) act on the hypothalamus to reset the thermoregulatory set-point.

Although autonomic changes occur, thermoregulation relies heavily on behavioural changes to alter body temperature, e.g. turning the heating on, or putting on extra clothes. This is an important concept to understand as general anaesthesia obliterates our ability to affect such change. Temperature regulation is poor at the extremes of age, making the young and elderly prone to hypothermia.

Heat production

Heat is produced by metabolic processes which lead to the breakdown of ATP: 54kJ of energy are produced per mole of ATP. Brain, liver, and skeletal muscle are the greatest producers of heat. Heat production may be doubled by shivering, but this increases the metabolic rate up to sixfold. Non-shivering thermogenesis is important in heat production in the infant but plays little role in adults. It is controlled by stimulation of β_3 receptors in brown fat, which is rich in mitochondria and therefore very metabolically active. It is located mostly between the scapulae and in the mediastinum and rapidly disappears as the infant grows.

Heat loss

Heat is lost from the body by the following mechanisms.

- Conduction is the flow of heat from a warm to a cooler object when the two bodies are in direct contact.
- Radiation is heat lost via the emission of electromagnetic energy (mostly infrared)
- Evaporation is heat lost when a liquid changes phase to a vapour, e.g. by sweating.
- Convection is heat lost to the environment as currents of cool air pass over the body.

Radiation and convection contribute most to heat loss when awake, but conduction becomes a greater contributor during anaesthesia.

Pyrexia

Pyrexia is defined as a body temperature above 37.7°C. The hypothalamic 'thermostat' is reset to a higher level, so heat–generating mechanisms are triggered even though the body temperature is raised.

This leads to shivering and even rigors. It is mediated by pyrogenic cytokines that are released in response to toxins. These cytokines (e.g. IL-6 and TNF) are able to cross the blood–brain barrier and reach receptors in the hypothalamus, causing release of prostaglandins via activation of the arachidonic acid pathway. Prostacyclin (PGE_2) stimulates the endogenous pyrogen receptor (EP3), leading to an elevation in body temperature. Cyclo-oxygenase inhibitors (e.g. aspirin) lower body temperature by inhibiting prostaglandin production.

Fever can be due to many causes other than infection. These are summarised in the box opposite.

Hypothermia

Hypothermia refers to a body temperature below 36°C. This leads to a drop in metabolic rate—up to 10% per degree drop in core temperature. This can provide protection for the brain during times of hypoperfusion and is deliberately used following out-of-hospital VF arrest, and during cardiothoracic surgery.

Perioperative hypothermia is common due to loss of behavioural modification, lack of shivering, and exposure. The physiological effects of hypothermia (see opposite) are widespread. Therefore it is important to monitor temperature during surgery and prevent heat loss where possible.

Hypothermia also commonly occurs during the resuscitation of patients who are critically ill. Haemofiltration can lead to a rapid fall in body temperature if the circuits are not heated.

Thermoregulation during anaesthesia

Normal body function depends on a relatively constant body temperature because many of the enzyme systems have a narrow operating range. Failure to maintain temperature results in hypothermia, which causes a number of systemic effects (see opposite).

An awake person will normally control his/her temperature within narrow limits: usually 37.0 ± 0.2°C. Heat loss is balanced by heat production, with small deviations causing large physiological changes.

Changes in temperature will induce many responses including behaviours. If someone becomes too warm, they will move to a cooler environment, take off clothes and begin to sweat. If they become cold they will move to a warmer area and put on clothes; piloerection will occur, cutaneous vasoconstriction will be induced, and they will start to shiver.

Thermoregulation and general anaesthesia

All anaesthetics impair normal autonomic thermoregulatory responses in a dose-dependent way, with warm thresholds elevated and cold responses reduced. The vasoconstriction threshold is reduced to about 34.5°C, and the shivering threshold to about 33.5°C. Thermoregulation is particularly affected at extremes of age.

The heat loss in an anaesthetized patient can be divided into three phases.

Redistribution phase

The initial temperature drop lasts about 20min and occurs as a result of redistribution of heat. There is peripheral vasodilatation, with increased peripheral temperature and decreased core temperature. The total heat content of the patient is unaffected.

Linear phase

This is a slow decrease in temperature as heat loss exceeds production. There are four modes of heat loss. This heat loss is exacerbated by various factors: physical exposure (of both intact skin and body cavities), cold IV fluids, cold skin prep, cold dry gases from the breathing circuit, wet drapes (if non-waterproof), and being placed on a chilly operating table.

Plateau phase

During the plateau phase, heat loss equilibrates with heat production. Vasoconstriction limits heat loss and temperature stabilizes.

Thermoregulation and regional anaesthesia

Regional anaesthesia leads to peripheral vasodilatation of the blocked areas, with increased heat loss. The block impairs afferent and efferent cold responses; this can lead to failure of the normal shivering response despite a falling core temperature. Spinal and epidural anaesthesia decrease the vasoconstriction and shivering thresholds below the level of the block by about 0.6°C. Hypothermia may actually be worse than under general anaesthesia because of failure to establish the plateau phase of heat loss (normally achieved by vasoconstriction). However, the very important behavioural responses are preserved—an awake patient can ask for a blanket!

General combined with regional anaesthesia

This is, predictably, the worst combination with regard to thermoregulation. It lowers the vasoconstriction threshold to about 33.5°C. Because of this profound suppression of vasoconstriction and shivering, core temperature continues to fall towards environmental temperature. All measures should be taken to prevent heat loss in these patients.

Fluids and heat loss

In an adult, 1000ml of IV fluid at 20°C causes a drop in body temperature of about 0.25°C, and one unit of whole blood at 4°C causes a drop in body temperature of about 0.5°C. All IV fluids should be warmed if it is predicted that the operation will be prolonged, significant amounts of fluid will be given, the patient is or is likely to become hypothermic, or the fluid carries a significant hypothermic load (e.g. blood, FFP).

→ Prevention of heat loss

Theatre temperature

Theatre temperature plays an important role in maintenance of temperature. It has been shown that where the theatre temperature is <21°C all patients become hypothermic, where theatre temperature is 21–24°C 30% of patients do so, and where theatre temperature is >24°C there is a low risk of hypothermia.

Blood/fluid warmers

Heating during administration

Fluids can be warmed as they are being administered by close contact with warm water, placing tubing between warmed metal plates, or by specialist microwave devices.

Warming cabinets

Fluids can be pre-warmed in a thermostatically controlled warming cabinet. Most crystalloids and colloids can be safely stored for at least a month in these cabinets. In the past microwaves have been used to warm IV fluids prior to administration but caution must be used as they can cause uneven heating and it is very easy to overheat the fluid.

Convection heaters

Forced air convection heaters are now very common and very effective. Care should be taken not to overheat the patient, especially in paediatric practice. All patients being warmed in this way should have their core temperature monitored.

Warming mattresses

Mattresses heated by electric currents or warm fluids can be placed under the patient to prevent conductive heat loss and to help warm the patient. There is evidence to suggest that electric mattresses are as effective as forced air convection heaters.

463

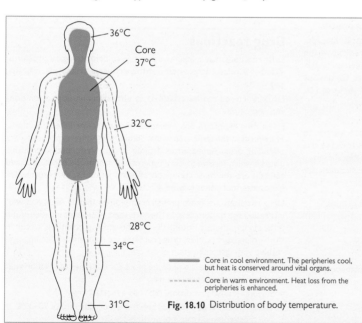

Fig. 18.10 Distribution of body temperature.

Core in cool environment. The peripheries cool, but heat is conserved around vital organs.

Core in warm environment. Heat loss from the peripheries is enhanced.

Effects of hypothermia
- Shivering and increased metabolic demands
- Coagulopathy
- Platelet dysfunction
- Metabolic acidosis
- ↓ Drug metabolism with ↑ duration of action e.g. atracurium
- Decreased tissue oxygen delivery (left shift ODC)
- Reduced MAC inhalational agents
- Decreased wound healing
- Increased infection risk
- Arrhythmias

→ Causes of fever

- Infectious diseases
- Systemic inflammatory response syndrome (SIRS)
- Immunological e.g. inflammatory bowel disease, rheumatoid arthritis
- Pancreatitis
- Tissue destruction: rhabdomyolysis, crush syndromes
- Pulmonary embolus

- Cancer, e.g. Hodgkin's disease, leukaemia
- Neurological, e.g. subarachnoid haemorrhage
- Drugs, e.g. interferon, amphotericin
- Malignant hyperthermia
- Neuroleptic malignant syndrome
- Amphetamine derivatives, e.g. ecstasy (MDMA)

The skin is the heaviest organ in the human body, accounting for about 15% of body weight, and has a surface area of 1.5–2.0m². It is mostly 2–3mm thick, but is thicker in hard-wearing areas such as the sole of the foot. It is richly innervated with 1000 nerve endings per square inch.

Structure of the skin

The skin comprises three layers:

- The epidermis, which acts as a barrier to infection and creates a waterproof outer layer. This layer is devoid of blood cells.
- The dermis, which is comprised of connective tissue and houses hair follicles and nerve endings.
- The hypodermis, or basement membrane.

The epidermis

This is supplied with nutrients by diffusion from capillaries in the upper layer of the dermis. It mostly comprises keratinocytes, but also has melanocytes and Langerhans cells (antigen-presenting cells involved in the presentation of antigens to T-lymphocytes).

The epidermis can be further subdivided into five distinct strata, beginning with the outermost layer: corneum, lucidum (only in the soles of the feet), granulosum, spinosum, basale. Cells move up through these layers, eventually dying due to lack of blood supply. Finally, they slough off after losing their cytoplasm and becoming keratinized. This process takes 30 days. The keratinized layer keeps the skin waterproof, and acts as a natural barrier to infection.

The dermis

This lies below the epidermis and consists of loose areolar connective tissue. Embedded in this are blood vessels, nerves, hair follicles, smooth muscle, and lymphatic tissue. Erectores pilorum muscles connect the epidermis to the hair papilla—when contraction occurs the hairs are pulled taught and 'goose bumps' form, an important mechanism in heat conservation. Sebaceous glands and sweat glands are also present.

The dermis can be divided into two layers. The outermost is the papillary region, comprising loosely arranged layers. Ridging of this region on the fingers and toes gives rise to the unique pattern seen on fingerprinting. A lower reticular layer is denser and becomes continuous with the hypodermis. Most of the structures mentioned above can be found in this layer.

The hypodermis

This is not really part of the skin but is the area that tethers the skin to underlying muscle and bone. Blood vessels and nerves traverse this region. It is rich in elastin and adipose cells which provide insulation.

Functions of the skin

The skin has a variety of protective and immunological functions.

- Protection from penetration by environmental pathogens—a natural barrier to the external environment.
- Langerhans cells form part of the adaptive immune system and present antigens for processing and disposal.
- Heat regulation by vasoconstriction or dilatation of cutaneous blood vessels, sweating and piloerector to trap heat.
- Synthesis of vitamins B and D.
- Storage of water and fat.
- Sensation.
- Psychosocial functions, expression of emotion by flushing.
- Administration route for many drugs, e.g. glyceryl trinitrate, fentanyl
- Elimination of drugs, e.g. volatile anaesthetic agents

Vitamin D metabolism

Skin converts 7-dehydrocholesterol to cholecalciferol (vitamin D₃) under the influence of ultraviolet light. This is converted to 25-hydroxycholecalciferol in the liver and then to 1,25-dihydroxycholecalciferol (the active form of vitamin D) in the proximal tubules of the nephron.

Thermoregulatory control

Heat loss by radiation occurs through the skin. This is regulated by cutaneous vasoactivity. Skin blood flow can increase tenfold during periods of high temperature. Heat loss also occurs by the evaporation of water from the skin via sweating or the heating of water present on hair or skin. Hot and cold thermoreceptors, which feed back the thermoregulatory state to the temperature regulatory zones of the hypothalamus, are present in the skin. Piloerection occurs via contraction of the erectores pilorum muscles during cold periods.

Disorders of the skin

Infection

Skin infections are common, and may be fungal, viral, or bacterial. Intravascular catheters are a major source of skin and soft tissue infection as they breach the natural host defences. Staphylococcal and streptococcal skin infections are most common.

Infections of the skin can be life-threatening, e.g. necrotising fasciitis (commonly caused by group A streptococcus) in which the underlying fascia and muscle become infected. Patients appear septic and unwell with fever and metabolic upset. The skin discolours, becoming violet in appearance with blistering. If the necrotic tissue is not rapidly and aggressively debrided, death is likely to occur. In contrast, cellulitis refers to bacterial infection of the connective tissue below the skin and is usually more limited.

Burns

See Section 23.8.

Drug reactions

Drug reactions may mimic a wide range of dermatological problems, including psoriasis, acne, erythroderma, erythema multiforme, urticaria, and vasculitis.

Drug reactions can be classified as either immunological or non-immunological.

Fixed drug eruptions are examples of immune-mediated reactions. They recur in the same area within 30min to 8hr of re-exposure to the offending drug. Appearances include circular reddened edematous plaques which resolve to leave hyperpigmentation. The hands, feet, and genitalia are the most commonly affected locations. With successive exposures, more sites may be affected.

Drug reactions are more prevalent in women than in men, and with increasing age in both sexes. They are seen in 2–5% of inpatients and >1% of outpatients. Potentially life-threatening eruptions occur in <0.1% of inpatients. Most drug eruptions are mild and self-limiting, and resolve with discontinuation of the offending drug.

Erythema multiforme is one of the more serious types of reaction with significantly higher mortality rates.

- Stevens–Johnson syndrome (SJS) has a mortality rate <5%.
- Toxic epidermal necrolysis (TEN) has a mortality rate of 20–30%. The most common cause of death is sepsis.

History

The first step is to scrutinize a comprehensive medication list. Previous history of adverse reactions to drugs or foods should be noted. Alternative aetiologies, e.g. viral exanthems and bacterial infections, may be more common in children, but most such reactions in adults are due to drugs.

Investigation

History and physical examination are often sufficient for diagnosing mild eruptions. Severe or persistent eruptions require further diagnostic testing.

- Biopsy may reveal neutrophil infiltration.
- FBC often demonstrates leucopenia, thrombocytopenia, and eosinophilia.
- Serum chemistry studies may demonstrate liver involvement especially with hypersensitivity syndromes. Electrolytes and renal and hepatic function indices may vary in those with severe reactions such as SJS, TEN, or vasculitis.
- Antihistone antibodies are found in those with drug-induced SLE.
- Direct cultures may exclude primary infectious aetiology or secondary infection.

Vasculitis may need to be specifically excluded

Treatment

Discontinue the offending medication. This is easier said than done, since individuals are often the most ill patients taking many essential medications. All non-essential medications should be stopped.

Knowledge of the common eruption-inducing medications may help in identifying the culprit.

It is safe to continue to take medicines in the presence of a mild morbilliform eruption since this will often resolve. Often, symptomatic control with NSAIDs and antihistamines is all that is required. Mild exanthematous drug eruptions do not precipitate severe reactions (e.g. TEN). However, such patients should be monitored for mucous membrane blistering and skin sloughing.

Additional treatment of a drug eruption depends on the specific type of reaction produced, e.g. acne, psoriasis or eczema.

Severe reactions (SJS or TEN) warrant care in a specialist unit where attention is paid to infection prevention, nutrition, and fluid balance. Early ophthalmology assessment is mandatory since adhesions may develop, causing blindness.

➕ Immunologically mediated reactions

- Type I (IgE-dependent reactions), causing urticaria, angio-oedema, and anaphylaxis (e.g. insulin)
- Type II (cytotoxic reactions), causing haemolysis and purpura (e.g. penicillins and cephalosporins)
- Type III (immune complex reactions), causing vasculitis, serum sickness, and urticaria (e.g. salicylates, chlorpromazine)
- Type IV (delayed cell-mediated hypersensitivity), causing contact dermatitis, exanthematous reactions, and photo-allergic reactions (e.g. neomycin)

➕ Non-immunologically mediated reactions

- Accumulation
- Adverse effects
- Direct release of mast cell mediators
- Idiosyncratic reactions
- Intolerance
- Jarisch–Herxheimer phenomenon (fever, tender lymphadenopathy, arthraigia, transient macular or urticarial eruptions. Symptoms resolve with continued therapy)
- Overdosage
- Phototoxic dermatitis

➕ Rates of reaction to commonly used drugs

- Amoxicillin: 5.1%
- Trimethoprim sulfamethoxazole: 4.7%
- Ampicillin: 4.2%
- Blood (whole human): 2.8%
- Penicillin G: 1.6%
- Cephalosporins: 1.3%
- Gentamicin: 1%
- Packed red blood cells: 0.8%

➕ Severe reactions

Erythema multiforme (EM)

One classification of erythema multiforme is to categorize both SJS and TEN as EM major (significant illness) but to differentiate them by body surface involvement.

EM minor

Generally a mild disease; patients are healthy, often with target lesions on the extremities. Mucous membrane involvement is similarly mild. Full recovery is usual but relapses are common. Most cases are due to HSV infection, and prophylaxis with aciclovir is helpful.

Stevens–Johnson syndrome (SJS)

This is characterized by large and atypical target lesions, widespremucous membrane and skin involvement (<10%), and constitutional symptoms. SJS can be caused by drugs and infections (e.g. *Mycoplasma pneumoniae*). With SJS/TEN overlap, 10–30% of skin is lost.

Toxic epidermal necrolysis (TEN)

This is more severe and involves a prodrome of painful skin similar to sunburn. This is rapidly followed by widespread full-thickness skin sloughing, typically affecting >30% total body surface area. Most cases are due to drugs. Secondary infection and sepsis are major risks.

Hypersensitivity syndrome

This is characterized by fever, sore throat, rash, and internal organ involvement. Timely recognition and immediate discontinuation of the offending drug are crucial, since the condition is life-threatening and patients may require liver transplantation. Treatment with systemic corticosteroids may be useful.

➕ Features of severe EM or TEN

The following indicate a severe potentially life-threatening drug reaction, such as TEN or hypersensitivity syndrome. These features should always be excluded when drug reaction is suspected.

- High fever, shortness of breath, or hypotension
- Mucous membrane erosions
- Confluent erythema
- Blisters (blisters herald a severe drug eruption)
- Positive Nikolsky sign (epidermis sloughs with lateral pressure)
- Angio-oedema and tongue swelling
- Palpable purpura
- Skin necrosis
- Lymphadenopathy

Stress response describes the hormonal and metabolic changes that occur in the body following an insult such as trauma or surgery. These catabolic changes may be very important in the injured wild animal, but are unnecessary and can be detrimental when they occur following surgery. Much attention has been focused on modifying the responses by the use of general and regional anaesthetic techniques.

Endocrine response to surgery

This involves increased pituitary hormone secretion and activation of the sympathetic nervous system. The main consequences are a catabolic state, and salt and water retention to help to maintain an adequate circulating volume. The following responses bring about these changes.

Sympathetic response: increased secretion of catecholamines from the adrenal medulla results in tachycardia and hypertension.

Hypothalamic–pituitary–adrenal response results in increased ACTH and growth hormone release from the anterior pituitary, and increased ADH and prolactin release from the posterior pituitary.

- ACTH causes increased glucocorticoid secretion by the adrenal cortex within minutes of the onset of surgery, peaking after 4–6hr.
- Negative feedback seems to be impaired, so levels stay raised for some time.
- The effects of growth hormone are mediated via insulin-like growth factors (mainly IGF-1), which promote lipolysis, inhibit protein breakdown, and inhibit glucose uptake by many cells, sparing it for neuronal use.

Decreased insulin secretion: insulin is the main anabolic steroid and its release is inhibited during surgery. This is in part due to α-adrenergic inhibition of β-cell secretion, and results in hyperglycaemia.

Decreased thyroid hormone release is brought about by a decrease in TSH release from the anterior pituitary. This causes the metabolic rate and heat production drop. These hormones fall quickly and take several days to return to preoperative levels.

Metabolic consequences

The overall catabolic effects of the stress response lead to substrates being available for production of energy at a time when the individual is likely to be fasting. This has evolutionary benefits, allowing animals to sustain themselves as their injuries heal.

- Blood glucose levels rise as cortisol and catecholamines augment production, and there is a relative lack of insulin. Hepatic glycogenolysis and gluconeogenesis increase. The greater the surgical insult, the greater is this response; hence there is a more prolonged period of hyperglycaemia following major surgery. Tight glycaemic control following surgery has been shown to decrease postoperative complications and mortality in patients requiring critical care.
- Increased cortisol levels lead to the breakdown of skeletal muscle, which provides amino acids that can be used as energy. This leads to weight loss and muscle wasting. This can be quantified by the urinary nitrogen excretion.
- The increases in growth hormone, cortisol, and catecholamines lead to lipolysis. This produces glycerol, a substrate for liver gluconeogenesis. Fatty acids may be converted to ketones which can be used by almost all cells as an energy source.
- Circulating volume is maintained by a number of mechanisms. ADH acts directly on the kidney to cause water retention, concentrating the urine. Renin secretion is augmented by increased circulating catecholamines. This stimulates the production of angiotensin II, which in turn increases aldosterone levels. This acts to promote water and sodium reabsorption for the distal convoluted tubules of the nephron.

The acute phase response

This describes a series of changes following tissue injury that are mediated by inflammatory cytokines, particulary IL-6. Minimally invasive surgery such as laparoscopy demonstrably decreases levels of the inflamatory mediators when compared with open techniques. However, it is not possible to demonstrate a similar fall in hormones involved in the stress response. Anaesthetic techniques may modulate the stress response but have no effect on the acute phase response as the level of tissue damage is unchanged.

Effects of the acute phase response
- Fever and SIRS response
- Increased IL-1, IL-6, IL-8, and TNFα
- Rise in C-reactive protein
- Rise in fibrinogen
- Rise in caeruloplasmin
- Rise in α$_2$-macroglobulin
- Rise in copper
- Fall in transferrin and rise in ferritin
- Fall in albumin
- Neutrophilia

Anaesthesia and the stress response

Both general and regional anaesthetic techniques have been shown to attenuate the stress response to surgery:

Opioids suppress release of hypothalamic hormones, therefore attenuating the rise in cortisol and growth hormone. The physiological changes associated with major vascular or cardiac surgery are so profound that opioids are unable to block the hypothalamic response completely.

Etomidate blocks the adrenal production of both cortisol and aldosterone. This effect can last for several days after even a single dose. For this reason it is no longer licensed for use by infusion for the sedation of critically ill patients.

Clonidine, an α$_2$-agonist, attenuates the sympathetic component of the stress response.

Epidural or spinal anaesthesia: if an effective block is achieved, this will obliterate the stress response to surgery in the pelvis and lower limb

Systemic responses to surgery
- Activation of sympathetic nervous system
- Salt and water retention
- Endocrine stress response leading to insulin resistance and catabolic state
- Acute phase response leading to SIRS
- Neutrophilia
- Proliferation of lymphocytes

Chapter 19

Obstetric anaesthesia

Normal pregnancy causes major physiological changes due to hormonal, metabolic, and mechanical factors. The main hormone of pregnancy is progesterone; one of its major effects is smooth muscle relaxation. The gravid uterus also causes displacement of other organs with consequent changes in their function.

Airway

Oedema of the airway mucosa can worsen the laryngoscopic view, and restrict ETT size. After 15 weeks, patients are at risk of aspiration (see below) and this necessitates rapid-sequence induction for general anaesthesia. Cricoid pressure may worsen the view at laryngoscopy even further.

Mucosal vessels are engorged and tissues are more friable, so even minor airway trauma can cause bleeding. Breast enlargement can make insertion of the laryngoscope difficult. A short handle or polio blade may help.

The onset of hypoxia is more rapid in late pregnancy (see below); therefore there is a shorter safe time to intubate the mother.

As they are relatively young, most patients will have full dentition. Pregnant women in the UK receive free NHS dental treatment, and so some will have had recent work.

There is a sevenfold risk of failed intubation (approximately 1 in 300 in the pregnant woman at term, compared with 1 in 2230 in the general population). Intubation difficulties, particularly unrecognized oesophageal intubation, have caused maternal deaths (Confidential Enquiries into Maternal Deaths in the UK).

Respiratory

Both components of minute volume increase; the rise in tidal volume (by 40%) by more than the respiratory rate (15%).

The ribs splay, the diaphragm is displaced upwards, and lung volumes are altered. A typical term spirometry trace is shown in Figure 19.1. Note particularly the reduction in FRC. This, combined with increased maternal/fetal oxygen demand, results in swift desaturation during periods of apnoea. The FRC can diminish to encroach upon the closing volume as the gravid uterus splints the diaphragm, worsening desaturation.

The reduced FRC results in faster equilibration of inhalational agents and more rapid onset of anaesthesia (although the increased cardiac output does the opposite).

Because of hyperventilation, there is a decrease in $PaCO_2$ (to ~4.3kPa). This favours offloading of CO_2 from fetus to mother. PaO_2 is normal or slightly increased. Renal bicarbonate excretion is increased, so despite the hypocapnia, pH is only slightly increased (towards the upper end of the normal range).

Despite the reduction in CO_2, the oxygen dissociation curve remains in a normal position (or even slightly right-shifted) because of increased maternal red cell 2,3-DPG. Fetal haemoglobin binds oxygen more avidly than adult haemoglobin, favouring O_2 transfer from mother to fetus. The oxygen dissociation curves are shown in Figure 19.2.

At term, oxygen flux (the product of blood O_2 content and cardiac output, Section 13.12) is about 10% higher than the non-pregnant value, despite a reduction in blood O_2 content because of physiological anaemia (see below).

Cardiovascular

Circulatory changes prepare the pregnant woman for the physical effort and potential blood loss of delivery. Cardiac output increases from 5–6 weeks onwards; at term it has risen by 30–40% to ~6.5L/min. Stroke volume increases by 30%, and heart rate increases by around 15%. The increase in cardiac output can cause benign flow murmurs.

Despite the increase in cardiac output, the blood pressure falls in a normal pregnancy, the diastolic by more (20%) than the systolic (8%). This is due to reduced total peripheral resistance caused by vasodilation in many tissues (skin, kidney, GI, breasts, heart), and placental blood flow. The nadir of blood pressure occurs in the second trimester, increasing towards pre-pregnancy values by term.

The placenta acts as an AV shunt, with flows of 450–600ml/min. Placental flow is not auto-regulated, and is entirely dependent on maternal circulatory status.

Aortocaval compression

From around 13 weeks' gestation, the gravid uterus can compress the IVC when the woman lies supine. This effect worsens as pregnancy progresses, and is almost universal at term. Venous blood is diverted via the vertebral venous plexus to drain into the azygous system. Obstruction of the aorta can also occur, leading to decreased distal flow. This includes placental flow, since the placenta is supplied by the uterine arteries (from the internal iliac arteries). Tilting the patient laterally (around 15° to the left) with a wedge or tilting table will counteract these effects. Alternatively, the uterus can be displaced manually.

The heart is displaced upwards and left by the gravid uterus. As a result, the ECG shows left axis deviation, ST segment depression, and T-wave flattening.

Haematological

There is an increased blood volume (40–45%). Plasma volume increases more than red cell volume, causing a dilutional anaemia, with Hb dropping by 15%. These changes occur by 24 weeks; blood volume then remains fairly constant until term. Despite this increase in volume, the CVP and pulmonary capillary wedge pressure are unchanged as the extra blood is accommodated in capacitance vessels and the placenta.

Overall, pregnancy results in a hypercoagulable state. Coagulation factors II VII, VIII, and IX are increased. Fibrinogen levels double during pregnancy. Platelet counts and function are normal, although turnover is increased. Fibrinolysis by plasminogen is reduced. The prothrombin time (PT) and activated partial thromboplastin time (APTT) are unchanged. The hypercoagulability of pregnancy limits blood loss during and after delivery, but increases the risk of deep vein thrombosis (see opposite).

Plasma protein concentration is reduced (dilutional), reducing colloid oncotic pressure. Albumin is lower (around 35g/l), and plasma cholinesterase decreases by 25%.

The white cell count steadily rises in response to increased levels of cortisol and oestrogen. The adaptive immune response is depressed during pregnancy.

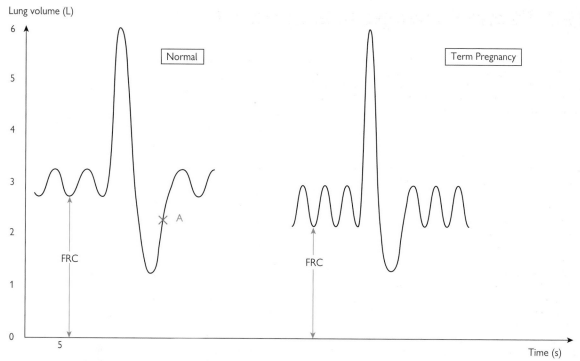

Fig. 19.1 A typical spirograph trace from a normal woman and a pregnant woman at term. Notice particularly the decrease in FRC. If the closing capacity lies at point A, normal tidal breathing at term may result in airway closure.

→ ODCs for maternal and fetal haemoglobin

Despite maternal hyperventilation and alkalosis, increased red cell 2,3-DPG causes a slight right shift of the ODC.

Several mechanisms exist to ensure adequate oxygen transfer to the fetus. Fetal Hb concentration is 50% higher than maternal. The fetal Hb curve lies to the left of normal Hb; fetal Hb binds oxygen more avidly. However, since the functional range of the fetus lies on the slope of the curve ('fully' oxygenated IVC blood in the fetus has saturations of 75%), there is still unloading of oxygen in the tissues.

The Bohr shift describes the rightward displacement of the ODC in the presence of an increased PCO_2 or a decreased pH. At the placental interface, a **double Bohr shift** occurs as CO_2 is unloaded from the fetus to the mother. This transfer acidifies maternal blood, and alkalinizes fetal blood. The maternal ODC moves further to the right, and the fetal ODC shifts further to the left. This widens the 'affinity gradient' between maternal and fetal haemoglobin, favouring oxygen transfer to the fetus.

The Haldane shift is similarly influenced by gas exchange at the placenta. The Haldane effect describes the increased capacity of deoxygenated blood to carry CO_2. **A double Haldane effect** occurs in the placenta. As oxygen transfers from mother to fetus, maternal blood is able to carry more CO_2. The fetal blood receives oxygen, thereby reducing its CO_2-carrying capacity. Overall there is an enhanced CO_2 transfer from fetus to mother.

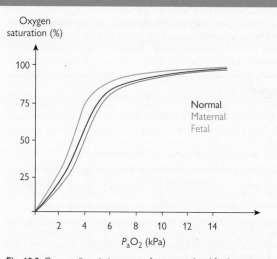

Fig. 19.2 Oxygen dissociation curves for maternal and fetal haemoglobin.

⊕ Thromboembolism and pregnancy

Pregnant women are hypercoagulable and prone to thrombosis. The presence of the gravid uterus causing pressure upon the pelvic and iliac vessels can lead to venous stasis and deep vein thrombosis. The effect is so significant that thromboembolic disease is the leading cause of direct pregnancy-associated death (Section 19.14), affecting 1.94 women per 100,000 pregnancies in 2002–2005.

Obstetric units should have local guidelines in place for thromboprophylaxis in at-risk women. It is important to remember that symptoms of pulmonary embolus may be extremely vague (dizziness or faintness, tachycardia, or flu-like feelings), and the woman may not complain of breathlessness. Several risk factors are on the increase in the pregnant population: obesity, air travel, older age, and Caesarean delivery.

Gastrointestinal tract

Nausea and vomiting are common in early pregnancy. Hyperemesis gravidarum is a severe variant of this, and may cause significant dehydration and electrolyte imbalance.

Progesterone causes relaxation of the lower oesophageal sphincter, and the gravid uterus may increase intragastric pressure. Some researchers have reported a reduction in gastric pH in pregnancy, but this remains controversial. 70% of pregnant women experience heartburn and reflux. An RSI is recommended in all pregnant women at 15 weeks' gestation regardless of symptoms, and earlier if there is symptomatic reflux. The increased risk of aspiration is reduced by premedication, which is designed to reduce the pH and volume of gastric contents.

Pregnancy does not cause a delay in gastric emptying *per se*. However, pain and opioid medication do, so that gastric emptying is severely delayed during labour.

Hepatic albumin production is reduced, leading to an increased free portion of drugs bound to albumin in plasma.

Endocrine

After fertilization, human chorionic gonadotrophin (hCG) is produced (and detected by pregnancy tests). This sustains the corpus luteum for 6–8 weeks. The placenta then takes over, producing progesterone, the main hormone of pregnancy (Figure 19.3). Levels of progesterone increase until term, and control many of the physiological changes of pregnancy (see Table 19.1).

The pituitary gland increases in size, as the number of prolactin secreting cells increases. Growth hormone production decreases during pregnancy.

The thyroid gland hypertrophies, although the levels of free T_3 and T_4 are usually stable as there is an increase in thyroid binding globulin. Parathyroid hormone and serum calcium tend to fall. The level of ionized calcium remains constant though, as serum albumin concentration is reduced.

Renal

Renal blood flow and GFR increase in pregnancy in line with the increase in cardiac output (~50%). However, sodium and water reabsorption also increase, and there is net sodium and water retention. Creatinine clearance increases in line with GFR; the upper limit of normal is 75µmol/L for creatinine and 4.5mmol/L for urea.

The reabsorption thresholds of protein and glucose are reduced, and intermittent proteinuria and glycosuria can occur. Proteinuria >500mg/24hr is abnormal and should prompt further investigation. Glycosuria may be due to pregnancy-induced diabetes mellitus.

The plasma concentrations of urea, uric acid, and creatinine all decrease in normal pregnancy; creatinine should be around two-thirds normal. Creatinine clearance and uric acid measurements are more useful than urea and electrolytes alone.

Progesterone-mediated ureteric relaxation, together with compression of the ureters at the pelvic brim, can lead to urinary stasis and ascending urinary tract infections.

Nervous system

There is a theoretical increase in sensitivity to volatile anaesthetics and opioids (studies on sheep have shown a reduced MAC during pregnancy). In addition, plasma protein levels may alter the free portion of IV induction agents.

Increased intra-abdominal pressure causes engorgement of the epidural veins, with a reduction in the epidural space volume. This also increases CSF pressure (to ~28mmHg) which can rise further (up to 70mmHg) during contractions. CSF density is lower in pregnancy, and there is a progesterone-mediated increase in neuronal sensitivity to local anaesthetic agents. These changes result in changes to the spread and effect of neuraxial blockade, with a much greater effect from a given quantity of agent than might be expected in a non-pregnant patient. The incidence of inadvertent vessel puncture when performing neuraxial blockade is increased (~8%).

Musculoskeletal system

Pregnancy causes a change in the normal lumbar lordosis, softening of ligaments, including the interspinal ligaments, and an increase in oedema and fat deposits over the spine. These changes may make it technically more difficult to perform an epidural or spinal.

Backache is common, affecting half of all pregnant women.

Drug handling in pregnancy

Circulatory changes can affect the distribution and binding of drugs. In pregnancy there is an increase in the cardiac output and therefore volume of distribution for many drugs. There is a decrease in plasma proteins, especially albumin, increasing the apparent volume of distribution for drugs which are highly bound. Other proteins, such as α-1 acid glycoprotein, are relatively unaltered. There is an increase in hepatic metabolism and renal excretion of most drugs.

Thiopental

Thiopental is highly protein bound and therefore has an increased volume of distribution in pregnancy. Doses of 5–7mg/kg are used in general anaesthesia for Caesarean section. It rapidly crosses the placenta; however it is diluted in the umbilical vein and there is some initial hepatic extraction in the fetus.

Suxamethonium

Levels of pseudocholinesterase are lower in late pregnancy. This does not normally prolong the block from suxamethonium in doses of 1–2mg/kg. However, some subclinical variants of suxamethonium apnoea may be unmasked during pregnancy. Suxamethonium does not appear in measurable amounts in fetal blood.

Inhaled anaesthetics

Inhaled anaesthetic agents, including nitrous oxide, have a more rapid equilibration (due to the reduced FRC) and reversal (due to the increase in alveolar ventilation and cardiac output). They freely cross the placenta, and are rapidly excreted via the neonatal lungs after delivery. The amount transferred will depend on concentration and duration of exposure, solubility and placental perfusion.

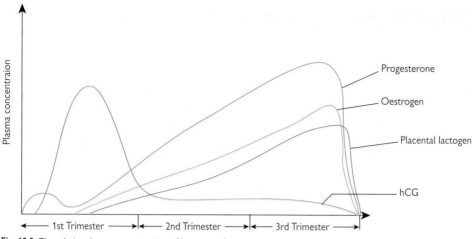

Fig. 19.3 The relative plasma concentrations of hormones during pregnancy.

Table 19.1 **Effects of progesterone**	
Progesterone is a steroid hormone, and a precursor of glucocorticoids, mineralocorticoids, and testosterone. Progesterone receptors are widespread throughout the body and it has effects on all of the major systems	
System	**Effect**
Respiratory	Increased tidal volume and minute ventilation Bronchodilatation: reduced airways resistance Reduced mucus production
Cardiovascular	Vasodilatation in most tissues
Renal	Partial agonist at aldosterone receptors: low concentrations cause net sodium and water loss (as the more potent aldosterone is antagonized); high concentrations cause sodium and water retention (as more receptors are occupied) Reduced ureteric motility
GI tract	Relaxation of lower oesophageal sphincter Relaxation of gall bladder
CNS	Affects synaptic function and myelination; causes fatigue and reduces arousal Reduced apoptosis; possible neuroprotective affect in traumatic brain injury
Reproductive	Prepares uterine lining for implantation Reduces contractility of uterine smooth muscle Thickens cervical secretions Causes breast hypertrophy but inhibits lactation
Immune	Immunosuppressant and anti-inflammatory actions
Metabolic	Mildly catabolic Stimulates appetite Increases core temperature (direct hypothalamic effect)
Musculoskeletal	Softening of ligaments
Fetus	The fetus metabolizes placental progesterone to produce mineralocorticoids and glucocorticoids.

➕ **Multiple pregnancy**

The physiological effects of multiple pregnancy are usually exaggerated compared with singletons. Complication rates increase correspondingly, and there is also a higher incidence of fetal and neonatal problems. Of particular relevance to the anaesthetist is the effect of the gravid uterus on the epidural veins; venous engorgement may be extreme, and the very low volumes of local anaesthetic used in regional techniques may give an extremely high block. Other complications associated more with multiple pregnancies include placenta praevia, pre-eclampsia, anaemia, premature labour, and haemorrhage (both ante- and post-partum). Atony of the over-distended uterus and consequent post-partum haemorrhage is a particular risk.

The placenta is responsible for the transfer of various substances between maternal and fetal blood.

Development and structure

The human placenta has a haemomonochorial structure, with villi of fetal tissue projecting into the maternal tissue to form an extensive network.

Initially, syncytiotrophoblasts, which envelop the implanted blastocyst, erode the spiral arteries of the endometrium. The blastocyst becomes surrounded by small lacunae of maternal blood. The system becomes more organized, with primary, secondary, and tertiary chorionic villi forming a dense vascular network. Further branching increases the surface area, improving diffusion. The total surface area of the villi is around 11m^2.

Multiple fetal villi form a fetal cotyledon; several cotyledons form a placental lobe. At term, the placenta is oval and flat, with an average diameter of 18cm and weight of 500g.

Blood vessels within the villi eventually join the fetal umbilical vessels. Fetal blood passes to the placenta via two umbilical arteries which spiral around a single umbilical vein.

Blood supply to the placenta is from the uterine arteries. It increases from approximately 300ml/min at 20 weeks to 600ml/min at 40 weeks. Placental bloodflow is not autoregulated; it is directly proportional to mean uterine perfusion pressure and inversely proportional to uterine vascular resistance. Reduction in uterine blood flow will cause fetal hypoxia and acidosis.

The metabolic demands of the placenta are comparable to those of the liver and kidney at term.

Functions of the placenta

Respiratory
Maternal blood enters the intervillous space with oxygen saturations of 90–100%. The extensive surface area of the villi and slow passage of maternal blood ensures efficient gas exchange. Blood entering the fetal circulation is 80–90% saturated, since some oxygen is utilized by the placenta itself (Figure 19.4).

The fetal oxyhaemoglobin dissociation curve is shifted to the left, aiding oxygen uptake across the placenta. Other mechanisms enhance fetal oxygen uptake (Section 19.2).

CO_2 readily diffuses across the placenta. The Haldane effect (Section 13.12) augments CO_2 transfer, as deoxyhaemoglobin in the maternal blood has a greater affinity for CO_2.

Hydrogen ions, bicarbonate ions, and lactic acid also undergo passive diffusion.

Endocrine
The placenta synthesizes most of the significant hormones of pregnancy. **Human chorionic gonadotrophin** (hCG) is produced early in pregnancy, initially by the corpus luteum and then by the placenta. It partially blocks the maternal immunological response. The main action of **progesterone** is to cause muscle relaxation, including the myometrium, lower oesphageal sphincter, gastric muscles, ureters, and intestine. It also affects thermoregulation, causing a mild hyperthermia, and increases body fat. **Oestrogen** enhances RNA and protein synthesis, reduces collagen adherence, and aids uterine muscle growth. It also has effects on breast duct and alveolar development. **Human placental lactogen** mobilizes free fatty acids, thereby accommodating increased fetal needs for glucose. The placenta also produces **prolactin** and **renin**.

Nutritional and excretory
The placenta transports nutrients to meet fetal requirements. Most transport processes are active (energy-requiring). Other transport mechanisms include passive and facilitated diffusion, and pinocytosis (Table 19.2).

Table 19.2 Transport mechanisms within the placenta

Passive	Active	Pinocytosis
Oxygen	Glucose	Large macromolecules
CO_2	Amino acids	IgG
H$^+$	Free fatty acids	
Bicarbonate		
Urea		
Na$^+$		
K$^+$		
Lactic acid		

Glucose is the most important energy source, meeting approximately 90% of requirements. Amino acids account for the remaining 10%.

Immunological
The fetus is partially an allograft, with paternal and maternal elements; the placenta plays a role in immunological acceptance of the fetus.

Placental drug transfer

Drugs generally cross the placenta by passive diffusion. The rate of diffusion is governed by Fick's law (Section 7.24). Table 19.3 opposite shows the behaviour of some common anaesthetic agents. Properties governing diffusion include the following.

Lipophilicity Lipophilic drugs readily cross the placenta; hydrophilic drugs less so. Lipophilic drugs include opiates, (fentanyl, pethidine), and local anaesthetics (bupivacaine, lidocaine). Thiopental and propofol rapidly cross the placenta, as do inhaled volatile anaesthetic agents (including nitrous oxide).

Ionization Highly ionized drugs are relatively lipid insoluble so do not pass easily across the placenta, whereas non-ionized drugs pass more freely. Many anaesthetic drugs are weak bases or acids, and will dissociate in an acid or alkali environment, respectively. The pH of the fetus is normally lower than that of the mother. If the fetus becomes more acidotic, weak bases may dissociate, causing 'ion trapping' within the fetal circulation, and lead to accumulation of weakly basic drugs such as local anaesthetics and pethidine. Muscle relaxants are large highly ionized molecules with quaternary ammonium groups. They do not pass easily across the placenta.

Protein binding Only the free portion of protein-bound drugs can cross the placenta. Fetal/maternal protein binding ratios may be of clinical significance for rate of transfer of protein-bound drugs, with the drug distributing preferentially on the side of the placenta where protein binding is more avid.

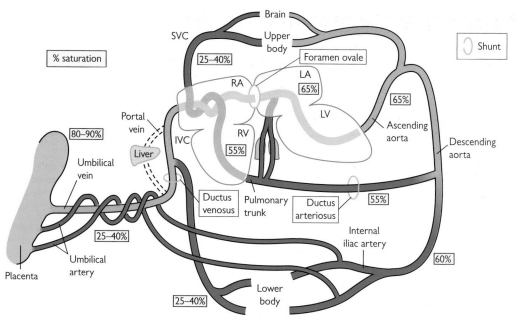

Fig. 19.4 Fetal circulation. The umbilical vein delivers oxygenated blood to the right atrium via the ductus venosus (bypassing the liver) and the IVC. This oxygenated blood streams through the foramen ovale to the left heart, where it is directed to the ascending aorta and the coronary and cerebral circulations. It returns via the SVC to the right atrium depleted of oxygen, where it is streamed down into the right ventricle and pulmonary trunk. The lungs receive only 3–4% of fetal cardiac output; most blood from the pulmonary trunk passes through the ductus arteriosus to the descending aorta, where it supplies the lower half of the body. The umbilical arteries (arising from the internal iliac arteries) return deoxygenated blood to the placenta. For a discussion of changes in the fetal circulation after birth, see Section 20.2.

● Table 19.3 **Transfer of anaesthetic agents across the placenta**	
Inhalational agents	**Intravenous anaesthetic agents**
Transfer is rapid. Risk of neonatal depression dependent on exposure. Nitrous oxide rapidly crosses; however, considered very safe. Eliminated quickly post delivery. Theoretical risk of diffusion hypoxia.	Rapid transfer Neonatal depression. Risk of ion trapping exacerbating effect of thiopental.
Opioids	**Local anaesthetics**
All opioids have the potential for neonatal sedation and respiratory depression: *Pethidine* Rapidly crosses placenta Potential for ion trapping Norpethidine may accumulate in the fetus. *Morphine* Relatively rapid transfer F/M ratio high *Fentanyl* Highly lipid soluble. Rapid transfer; however, no significant neonatal effects with low dose epidural use. *Remifentanil* Constant context sensitive half-life. Rapidly crosses placenta; however, quickly metabolized and redistributed in fetus. Inconsistent data regarding PCA remifentanil for labour analgesia and newborn respiratory depression.	Transfer dependent on dose, site of injection, protein binding, lipid solubility, and ionization. Administration of vasoconstrictors may cause increased fetal levels of bupivacaine. Clinical effect on newborn minimal with therapeutic doses of lidocaine or bupivacaine for labour analgesia and delivery. Prilocaine may cause fetal methaemoglobinaemia. If the fetus is acidotic, there is a risk of ion trapping, with potential for fetal toxicity.
	Muscle relaxants
	Suxamethonium is degraded rapidly by maternal plasma cholinesterase; virtually none reaches the fetus. The percentage of non-depolarizing neuromuscular blocker (rocuronium, pancuronium, atracurium) crossing the placenta ranges from 7% to 22%. There is no detectable clinical effect on the neonate.
	Benzodiazepines
	Cross easily due to lipid solubility Neonatal sedation is significant.

Although extra factors relating to the pregnancy should be considered, the principles of preoperative assessment are the same as for any patient. Senior help should be enlisted at an early stage if problems are anticipated.

The anaesthetic clinic

Some patients are seen antenatally in a dedicated obstetric anaesthetic clinic. This gives an opportunity to discuss options and plan for delivery. Reasons for attendance include:

- High-risk patient or pregnancy
- Planned Caesarean section
- Maternal request (e.g. to discuss analgesic options for delivery such as epidural analgesia).

The anaesthetic clinic is an opportunity to discuss analgesia and/or anaesthesia in detail. Informed consent can be gained for epidurals, rather than waiting until labour when the woman is in pain and may have had sedative drugs. Questions are answered and written information can be provided. Discussions and plans should be carefully documented. Some women will require further investigation, or liaison with other specialties.

History

Previous general or regional anaesthetics Enquire about previous operative deliveries or labour epidurals, including the outcome of the pregnancy. Some women will have had anaesthetic problems in pregnancy and labour, and these should be explored. Problems with regional techniques do not inevitably mean future failures; most patients can be reassured. However, a few will request general anaesthesia for an operative delivery.

Genetic and family history Some women may present with a family history suggestive of malignant hyperthermia or suxamethonium apnoea. Genetic tests are not performed during pregnancy, so as much information as possible should be gleaned from the history, notes (including relatives' notes if possible), and the GP. If this is not possible, assume the worst and make a safe plan on that basis until tests can be carried out post-partum. Involve a senior anaesthetist.

Medical history and health during pregnancy As well as the past medical history, it is important to ask about any change in medical problems during pregnancy. Unexpected or severe worsening of symptoms may require investigation.

Pregnancy may precipitate new problems; pregnancy-induced hypertension and gestational diabetes are relatively common and must be actively excluded. Hypertension and proteinuria are signs of pre-eclampsia and require further investigation if present.

Drugs Most women will avoid medication during pregnancy if possible. For some though, a lesser risk to mother and fetus comes from continuing medications or changing to less teratogenic agents. Diabetics' insulin requirements usually increase. Ask specifically about anticoagulants. In most cases, anticoagulant therapy is interrupted for delivery but there may be issues surrounding the timing of the last dose and epidural or spinal anaesthesia. There should be local guidelines to address this issue.

Allergies Again, investigations may be difficult to interpret during pregnancy, so the history is vital. If a reaction occurs during pregnancy, post-delivery follow-up must be arranged. Local anaesthetic allergy is very rare, but if suspected may significantly affect the anaesthetic plan. Information from the dentist/doctor involved should be sought.

Smoking Most women will attempt to stop or reduce their intake of cigarettes. Reinforcing this is useful.

Examination

As usual, examination centres on the airway and cardiorespiratory systems. Examine the back if an epidural or spinal is intended. Attention to other systems may be appropriate, e.g. neurological examination in MS.

Investigations

All pregnant women are offered regular blood tests during their antenatal care. A recent FBC should be available (a FBC is performed every 4–8 weeks during the second half of the pregnancy). Group and save serum can exclude the presence of unusual antibodies in advance, and should be performed in anaemic patients and those at special risk of obstetric haemorrhage (Section 19.13). Blood cross-matching guidelines vary between units (Sections 15.3 and 15.4) Urea, electrolytes, and uric acid may be appropriate. The ultrasound report will give an indication of the position of the placenta and other features such as fetal size, multiple pregnancy, or polyhydramnios.

Premedication and fasting

Where an operative delivery is planned, antacid prophylaxis is commenced. A typical regimen might be:

- Ranitidine 150mg 12hr preoperatively
- Ranitidine 150mg + metoclopramide 10mg 2–4hr preoperatively
- Sodium citrate (30ml of 0.3M solution) immediately prior to preoxygenation for GA (on table). While some practitioners give sodium citrate prior to regional anaesthesia (in case of conversion to GA), it should be remembered that the duration of action is short (~30min).

Fasting guidelines are as for non-pregnant patients, even though all patients undergoing GA after 16 weeks will have an RSI. High-risk patients may also be advised to fast (or just sip water) during labour.

Assessment on labour ward

Not all pregnant women need or want to attend an anaesthetic clinic. They may meet an anaesthetist for the first time during labour. It is important to remember that a thorough assessment must still be carried out, despite pressure to proceed quickly. The risks and benefits of the procedure must be made clear, and this discussion documented. Occasionally, high-risk patients are admitted without prior review. These should be seen at the earliest opportunity, whether or not anaesthetic involvement is planned. Involve senior anaesthetic and obstetric colleagues early in the care of high-risk patients. In extreme emergencies, there may be very little time. An 'AMPLE' history may be all that is possible: **A**llergy, **M**edications, **P**ast history, **L**ast ate, and **E**vents during pregnancy. An explanation of the anaesthetic technique can be given, and documentation of verbal consent (or in the case of incapacitated patients, treatment in the best interests of the mother) should suffice under these circumstances.

➕ Choice of anaesthetic for Caesarean section

The main anaesthetic choice to be made for a Caesarean section is between regional or general anaesthesia. The majority of elective Caesareans are carried out under spinal anaesthetic. Many women are apprehensive about the prospect of being awake for surgery, and particularly about the possibility of a failed or inadequate block. Proper explanation and reassurance about the technique is often all that is needed, together with a discussion of the steps that can be taken (including converting to GA) if discomfort does occur. Written information should be provided (if time allows) to enable the mother to consider her choices at leisure. The Obstetric Anaesthetists' Association (OAA) publishes leaflets dealing with anaesthesia for Caesarean section and also labour analgesia. A summary of the discussion should be documented on the patient's anaesthetic chart.

Advantages of regional anaesthesia
- Avoids risks of GA
- Avoids neonatal depression
- Reduced blood loss
- Improved early postoperative analgesia
- Birth partner can be present at delivery
- May offer some protection against DVT/PE
- Clear-headed recovery, with early breastfeeding if desired

Disadvantages of regional anaesthesia
- Time to establish block
- Possible discomfort during surgery
- Hypotension, nausea and vomiting
- Itch
- Specific complications, including high block, accidental dural puncture, post-dural puncture headache, nerve damage, infection (superficial or rarely epidural abscess), epidural haematoma (rare)

Pregnancy can affect disease processes throughout the body. Some diseases may be exacerbated, revealed, or precipitated by pregnancy. Others may improve (in which case there is a risk of 'rebound' after delivery). Pregnancy may cause changes in drug handling, or necessitate changes in drug therapy to avoid teratogenesis.

Older parturients may present with diseases of later life (e.g. ischaemic heart disease, cerebrovascular disease). Even lifelong diseases (e.g. type I diabetes) may have progressed much further in these women than in their younger counterparts. Patients with congenital disease are increasingly surviving until adulthood.

Pregnant women with severe disease should have multi-disciplinary management, with midwifery, obstetric, specialist medical/surgical, anaesthetic, and neonatology input. Ideally, pregnancy should be planned. High-risk patients are best cared for in specialist obstetric centres.

Cardiac disease

Cardiac disease is becoming more common in the pregnant population because of older age and improved survival in congenital heart disease. Obesity is more prevalent and is an important contributing factor. There is also a significant incidence of rheumatic valve disease, particularly among the immigrant population. Cardiac problems were the leading cause of death due to intercurrent illness ('indirect' deaths—Section 19.14) in the UK in 2002–2005. Most of these deaths occurred as a result of ischaemic heart disease or thoracic aortic dissection.

Minimally symptomatic women with good ventricular function, normal saturations, and no obstruction of the left heart usually tolerate pregnancy and labour well. Conversely, patients with previous MI or endocarditis, pulmonary hypertension, aortic root disease, or Eisenmenger's syndrome are at very high risk.

Patients with cardiac disease should be reviewed by a cardiologist prior to or early in pregnancy, optimized, and followed up. Appropriate investigations include ECG, echocardiography, FBC, and renal function. Monitoring during labour should include NIBP and continuous ECG, and invasive monitoring in a high-dependency setting should be considered.

Labour analgesia should be considered carefully in the light of the woman's cardiac physiology: an epidural will obtund the sympathetic response to contractions, but will reduce the SVR. It may be necessary to use vasopressor infusions in conjunction with invasive monitoring.

If severe cardiac disease is present, the woman should not be allowed to labour. For operative delivery, epidural or CSE anaesthesia with slow incremental top-ups can be a successful approach. If a GA is used, it is usually opioid based. Again, invasive monitoring is used in order to guide tight haemodynamic control. It is important to consider endocarditis prophylaxis. (Section 16.4)

Thromboprophylaxis is of vital importance in patients with cardiac disease.

Respiratory disease

The most common respiratory disease in the pregnant population is asthma. This often improves during pregnancy. However, care should be taken not to attribute respiratory discomfort purely to the pregnancy. Medication should be continued (although theophyllines may aggravate nausea and reflux). Acute attacks should be aggressively managed, and maternal saturations should be maintained >94% to avoid fetal hypoxia. One in ten asthmatics will need hospital admission for an acute exacerbation during pregnancy.

Respiratory infections should be treated aggressively during pregnancy, with antibiotics, physiotherapy, and oxygen.

In respiratory disease, regional techniques are ideal for both labour and delivery. Care must be taken to titrate the block carefully to avoid unnecessary respiratory embarrassment.

Renal disease

The most common renal disease during pregnancy is urinary tract infection. The incidence of bacteriuria is increased in pregnancy, and this, coupled with relative urinary stasis and dilatation of the upper urinary tracts, predisposes to ascending infection and pyelonephritis.

In chronic renal disease, there is an increased risk of hypertension, pre-eclampsia, premature labour, and fetal death. There is also often a significant deterioration in maternal renal function. Nephrotoxic drugs should be strenuously avoided. If magnesium is used, levels should be carefully monitored. Ergometrine is contraindicated as it is a potent vasoconstrictor, but oxytocin can be used with care.

Epidurals can be used in labour. For operative delivery, careful regional or general anaesthesia can be used. In severe disease, invasive monitoring should be used to guide fluid management.

Endocrine disease

Gestational diabetes mellitus (GDM) is defined as impaired glucose tolerance (of any degree) discovered during pregnancy. It affects around 7% of pregnant women. It carries a risk of macrosomia and neonatal hypoglycaemia. It may require management with insulin, in which case a sliding scale should be used around the time of delivery. Glucose tolerance returns to normal after delivery, and women with GDM are re-tested 6 weeks post-partum. In known diabetics, insulin requirements usually increase during pregnancy, reverting to normal soon after delivery.

Hypothyroidism is treated as normal with thyroxine. Hyperthyroidism is more difficult, as carbimazole and propylthiouracil can cause fetal hypothyroidism (propylthiouracil is preferred as it crosses the placenta to a lesser degree). Radioactive iodine is contraindicated. Occasionally a partial thyroidectomy may be the best therapeutic option.

Neurological/neuromuscular disease

Epilepsy remains the most common cause of seizures in pregnancy. Fit frequency may decrease, increase, or be unaffected by the pregnancy. Control of seizures is important in maintaining maternal and fetal health. However, some drugs are teratogenic, and a pre-pregnancy review should take place with a neurologist. Other causes for seizures should always be considered.

Patients with known intracranial pathology should be managed in conjunction with neurosurgeons. Epidural anaesthesia should be used to prevent hypertension during contractions and to remove the urge to push (which raises intracranial pressure). If an operative delivery is planned, regional or general anaesthesia can be used.

Epidural analgesia during labour is not contraindicated in women with neuromuscular disease (e.g. MS, motor neuron disease, myasthenia gravis, etc.). It has not been shown to affect the progression of any neurological disease and should be offered with the understanding that such diseases are often affected by the pregnancy itself. If there is respiratory involvement, the block should be carefully monitored so as not to impinge upon respiratory muscle function.

Anaesthesia during pregnancy is relatively common, and may be underestimated due to unrecognized pregnancies. Up to 2% of pregnant women will undergo surgery, with the most common procedures being appendicectomy and cholecystectomy. However, any type of emergency surgery may be carried out during pregnancy. Some additional basic principles apply:

- Perform a pregnancy test prior to anaesthesia/surgery in all women of child-bearing age, especially if X-ray imaging is planned.
- Inform the obstetric team.
- Discuss the case with a senior anaesthetist.
- Elective surgery should be delayed until after delivery. If this is not possible, it is still helpful if surgery can be delayed until 10—and preferably more—weeks' gestation.

The increasing use of laparoscopy has led to the development of specific recommendations, including avoidance of laparoscopy until second trimester and limitation of pneumoperitoneal pressures.

General anaesthesia should be avoided during pregnancy. However, it is sometimes necessary and requires careful planning and technique.

Risks to the mother

- Hypoxia (from a combination of difficult airway and swift desaturation).
- Aspiration (due to relaxation of the lower oesophageal sphincter, and often delayed gastric emptying from opioids and pain).
- Awareness during emergency procedures.
- Pulmonary thromboembolism—a significant postoperative risk (Section 13.15).
- Risks specific to the surgical procedure itself.

Risks to the fetus

- Teratogenesis (see opposite).
- Hypoxia secondary to maternal hypoxia or placental hypoperfusion.
- Hypoperfusion from maternal hypoperfusion, mechanical factors, or placental disruption.
- Premature labour: consider the use of tocolytic drugs and steroids to mature the fetal lungs. The cause is multifactorial and it is not known to what extent the anaesthetic contributes. Surgical factors associated with fetal loss and risk of preterm delivery include the nature, severity, and duration of surgery. Intra-abdominal procedures carry increased risk.

General principles

The principles of general anaesthesia during pregnancy apply to obstetric and incidental surgery alike.

- Safety of the mother is paramount (and usually advantageous for the fetus).
- Avoid GA if possible. Use a regional technique or local anaesthesia. However, always assume the worst and prepare for GA (premedication, drugs, equipment).
- Communicate the risks to the mother (including the risks of delaying surgery). In the first trimester, there is a slightly increased risk of spontaneous abortion (increased from 5% to 8%). In the third trimester, the main risk is premature labour (again, increased from 5% to 8%).
- Avoid polypharmacy. Use drugs with an established safety record in pregnancy.
- Fetal heart rate and uterine contraction monitoring should be used where possible (see opposite).

Practical aspects

As pregnancy progresses, maternal physiology changes (Sections 19.1 and 19.2) and this must be taken into account when planning anaesthesia.

Preoperative

A full preoperative assessment (Section 19.4) should be performed. Starvation guidelines are the same as for non-pregnant patients. However, after 15 weeks' gestation, premedication with antacids and prokinetics should be used where possible. Ranitidine (150mg PO or 50mg IV) and metoclopramide (10mg PO or IV) should be given at least an hour before surgery. Sodium citrate (30ml of 0.3M solution) is given immediately before induction.

Induction

Consider on-table induction of anaesthesia to avoid transfers: even brief disconnections from the ventilator risk significant desaturation due to the reduced FRC (Section 19.1). In addition, it is good practice to avoid manual transfers of heavy patients.

Careful and thorough pre-oxygenation should be performed; there is a tendency for pregnant women to desaturate very quickly, combined with a risk of difficult airway.

RSI with cricoid pressure should be used after 15 weeks' gestation, and earlier if there are additional risk factors for aspiration. A difficult airway trolley should be immediately available. Avoid drugs which increase uterine contractility, e.g. ketamine.

The supine position should be avoided after 13 weeks' gestation due to possible aortocaval compression. A wedge or left lateral table tilt (20°) should be used.

Maintenance

Maternal hypoxia leads to uteroplacental vasoconstriction and fetal hypoxia. Increased oxygen during surgery may be required in order to maintain adequate oxygen saturations. Increased airway pressures may be required for ventilation. Anaemia should be treated.

Maternal hypercarbia leads to fetal respiratory acidosis and uterine artery vasoconstriction. Patients should be ventilated to a $PaCO_2$ appropriate for gestational stage.

Maternal hypotension will cause fetal hypoxia and acidosis. Hypotension from whatever cause (peripheral vasodilatation, hypovolaemia) should be promptly corrected with fluids or vasopressors (phenylephrine or ephedrine). Remember to continue left tilt/manual uterine displacement.

Inhalational agents cause uterine relaxation. This is undesirable in many obstetric procedures as it can increase blood loss. However, in incidental surgery, a degree of uterine relaxation may be useful in preventing the onset of pre-term labour.

TIVA can be used to avoid relaxing the uterus.

The MAC of volatile agents is reduced during pregnancy. However, other factors are likely to counteract this. Patients may be particularly anxious; and pain or light anaesthesia will cause catecholamine surges which potentially reduce placental blood flow. Taking all these factors into account, anaesthetic requirements are usually increased compared with the non-pregnant population.

Non-depolarizing agents have a prolonged duration of action. Suxamethonium is not affected.

Postoperative

Postoperatively, mothers should be assessed for pre-term labour: pain, uterine contractions. If there are any signs of labour the obstetric team should be contacted urgently. The use of tocolytic agents may suppress labour.

Pregnant women are hypercoaguable and prone to thromboembolic events. Remember to use DVT prophylaxis such as low molecular weight heparins, thromboembolic deterrent (TED) stockings and intraoperative intermittent pneumatic calf compressors.

✛ Fetal monitoring

The main purpose of monitoring is to detect fetal compromise and pre-term labour. This can be done using an electronic fetal heart rate monitor and uterine contraction monitoring. If monitoring is used, it is the responsibility of the obstetric team, usually a midwife, to set it up and interpret the tracings (NB: anaesthetic agents cause a decrease in fetal heart rate variability because of fetal anaesthesia).

It may be logistically difficult to use monitoring, depending on the site of surgery. Vaginal ultrasound probes have been used as an alternative to the traditional monitors (e.g. during abdominal surgery).

Fetal heart rate monitoring is generally only reliable after 22 weeks' gestation. However, it has been used as early as 18 weeks, so discuss all cases with the obstetric team.

If fetal compromise is detected, simple manoeuvres may improve fetal hypoxia, including increasing maternal oxygen saturations, maintaining adequate blood pressure, and left lateral tilt. If uterine contractions are detected, increasing volatile anaesthetic agents may relax the uterus.

Continue monitoring for 12–24 hr.

✛ Teratogenicity

The risk of teratogenicity is greatest during the first trimester when fetal organs are being formed. Most anaesthetic agents cross the placenta (Section 19.3). However, the study of safety of particular anaesthetic drugs is difficult because of the multifactorial nature of teratogenesis. Other contributing factors are likely to include use of X-ray imaging, the stress response to surgery, and the underlying surgical illness.

Common anaesthetic agents and their known effects on the fetus are shown in Table 19.4.

Table 19.4 Teratogenesis and common anaesthetic drugs

Premedication	Antiemetics
The association between benzodiazepines and cleft lip is controversial and as yet unproven in human studies. However, chronic use during pregnancy may lead to neonatal withdrawal. Metoclopramide and ranitidine are safe in short courses.	Nausea is common during pregnancy and may be exacerbated by general anaesthesia. Metoclopramide is safe. Ondansetron and granisetron have not caused fetal damage in animal studies, and there have been no reports of human fetal abnormalities so far. Cyclizine is thought to be safe.
Induction agents	**Local anaesthetics**
Induction agents such as propofol and thiopental are thought to be safe during pregnancy.	Local and regional anaesthesia, where appropriate, are preferable to systemic analgesics.
Maintenance of anaesthesia	**Analgesics**
Inhalational anaesthetics are thought to be safe at therapeutic levels; however, they may cause a reduction in fetal cardiac output at high levels, resulting in fetal acidosis. Treat hypotension secondary to peripheral vasodilatation. The tocolytic effect of volatile anaesthetics may prevent premature labour. It is probably best to avoid nitrous oxide in the first trimester, as it has deleterious effects on DNA synthesis.	Paracetamol is safe during pregnancy. NSAIDs should be avoided; in early pregnancy there is a risk of fetal loss and fetal renal impairment, and in the later stages of pregnancy they may cause premature closure of the fetal ductus arteriosus. Opioids, such as morphine, are generally safe although they may cause maternal hypoxia and hypercarbia, and if administered prior to delivery may cause neonatal respiratory depression. Codeine phosphate is safe to use, although consider a laxative if prolonged use is anticipated. Long-term use of any opioid will cause neonatal withdrawal symptoms post-delivery.
Muscle relaxants	
Because these are large molecules they do not cross the placental barrier and are safe during pregnancy.	

Pain during labour and delivery (of both fetus and placenta) involves a complex interaction of both physiological and psychological factors. Over 90% of women will experience severe or unbearable pain during labour. The woman's expectations, cultural background, ability to cope, support, fear, and fatigue all contribute to the experience of pain during labour.

Pain pathways of labour

Labour is the process whereby the products of conception are expelled from the uterus after the 24th week of gestation. Pain comes in waves with the contractions. It alters and intensifies as labour progresses. Progesterone may modulate pain pathways, increasing pain tolerance.

Labour pain evokes a generalized neuroendocrine stress response, with physiological effects both on the mother and the fetus.

Labour is divided into three stages:

- First stage: onset of labour (cervix dilated with regular painful contractions) to full cervical dilatation (10cm).
- Second stage: full dilatation to delivery of the baby. Somatic pain from the birth canal is added to contraction pain.
- Third stage: delivery to expulsion of the placenta.

Pain pathways

See also Section 7.22. Pain is transmitted via different pathways during the three stages of labour (Figure 19.5, and Table 19.5). The nature of the pain also changes as labour progresses.

First stage

Pain during the first stage is due to cervical dilatation, lower uterine segment dilatation, and uterine contractions. Pain is transmitted via mainly A-δ and C-fibre afferents. These pass in the sympathetic nerves to the sympathetic chain. The pain is referred to dermatomes T10–L1. This pain is intermittent, visceral, poorly localized, dull, and aching. It is commonly felt in the lower abdomen, but can be felt as backache or in the upper thighs and sacrum. It gradually increases in frequency and severity. Cervical pain is also carried via the parasympathetic pelvic splanchnic nerves (nervi erigentes, from S2, S3).

Pain during the first stage can also be caused by pressure on surrounding structures such as the bladder or rectum.

Second stage

During the second stage, pain is more localized to the perineum. This somatic pain is due to perineal stretching and tearing, in addition to distension and pulling of pelvic structures. Pain is transmitted mainly via A-δ fibres, via the pudendal nerves, to nerve roots S2–S4.

Third stage

Pain during the third stage is due to expulsion of the placenta. The same pathways as for the second stage apply; however, pain is not usually so severe.

In addition to pain pathways relating to the uterus, cervix, and perineum, other pelvic structures may be stimulated during labour. Pain can be transmitted via the ilio-inguinal, genitofemoral, and perforating branch of the posterior cutaneous nerve of the thigh, causing somatic pain in the distribution of L5–S5 dermatomes. The diaphragm may be stimulated, causing referred shoulder tip pain.

Analgesia for labour

Labour is often the first time a woman experiences severe pain. Most labouring women in the UK request and receive analgesia. Analgesic strategies for labour can be classified as non-pharmacological, pharmacological, and regional.

Non-pharmacological

Having a trained assistant and partner present throughout labour is important for advice, reassurance, and comfort. Relaxation techniques, massage, aromatherapy, and warm baths may all help the woman to cope and increase satisfaction.

Acupuncture has been used for labour and delivery. However, no specific acupuncture point is described for labour pain.

Hypnosis can produce analgesia and amnesia in a selected group of patients. It is thought to increase descending pain inhibition. It requires extensive preparation, and is only occasionally used in the UK.

TENS machines: it has been proposed that A-β fibres, which transmit light touch, inhibit pain transmission in the substantia gelatinosa (gate theory of pain, Section 7.27). TENS machines utilize this principle and have been used by labouring women since the 1980s. Electrodes are placed over dermatomes from T10 to L1, and give a low background signal which can be increased with each contraction. They stimulate A fibres, reducing nociceptive C-fibre transmission. They may also increase endorphin release. Some mothers find them helpful in the first stage of labour. However, randomized controlled studies do not demonstrate efficacy.

Pharmacological

The most common systemic drugs used in labour are inhaled agents and opioids.

Inhaled agents

The most common inhaled agent is Entonox, a mixture of 50% N_2O and O_2 (Section 2.3). Its effect is felt a few seconds after inhalation, reaching a maximum in 45sec. It is thought to enhance pain-inhibiting descending pathways. It is rarely contraindicated in labour unless the patient also has a pneumothorax or severe sinus disease. Unfortunately, side effects are common and include light-headedness, nausea, drowsiness, and disorientation.

Recently, small concentrations of sevoflurane or desflurane have been added to entonox. These have shown no advantage over entonox alone, and may increase side effects. Scavenging, for staff safety, is a further concern.

Opioids

Opioids act at multiple sites including the spinal cord, brainstem, and descending pathways. They can be given systemically or adjunctively in regional techniques.

IM pethidine is the most commonly used. In the UK, midwives are allowed to give up to three doses (each 100mg) without a doctor's prescription. This allows a greater choice of analgesia in home deliveries. Pethidine reduces labour pain by approximately 25%. However, it delays gastric emptying and its active metabolite, norpethidine, has convulsant properties (hence pethidine should be avoided in labouring women with epilepsy or pre-eclampsia). It causes more dysphoria than other opioids in current use.

Like all opioids, pethidine crosses the placenta and, depending on the time of injection, may affect the baby on delivery. The highest fetal concentration occurs 2–3hr after IM administration. Neonates are sleepier and slower to establish feeding, despite normal Apgar scores. As it is a weak base, pethidine is more ionized in the fetal circulation and may become trapped there, along with norpethidine.

Morphine (10mg IM) and diamorphine (5–7.5mg IM) are used in some hospitals, and are more effective than pethidine with fewer dysphoric reactions. Again, they both cross the placenta, and concerns have been reported about delayed respiratory depression in the neonate.

Some patients are given IV opioids. Remifentanil can be administered by a PCA, giving an important element of control to the woman. Its rapid onset and ultra-short action are particularly suited to labour. Both mother and baby require close monitoring during labour and after delivery. This technique is usually only used when epidural analgesia is contraindicated.

Table 19.5 Labour stages and pain

Stage	Cause of pain	Nature of pain	Pathway
1	Cervical dilatation Uterine contractions	Visceral	A-δ and C fibres Sympathetic chain (T10–L1)
2	Perineal stretching	Localized	A-δ Pudendal nerves (S2–S4)
3	As above	Less severe than stages 1 and 2	As above

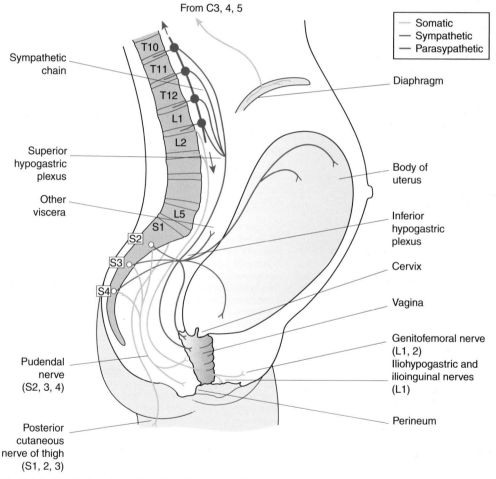

Fig. 19.5 Peripheral pain pathways during labour. Sympathetic afferents come predominantly from T10–L1, parasympathetics from S2–4, and somatic perineal afferents from S2–4 and L1.

Perineal infiltration (for episiotomy), pudendal nerve block (for delivery), and paracervical nerve block (for contraction pain) have largely been superseded by epidural services. Caudal anaesthesia, though tempting on paper, has been associated with rare reports of puncture of the presenting fetal part (usually the head).

Epidural

Epidural (or CSE) is the most effective analgesic for labour, particularly in prolonged or augmented labours. Indications include maternal request, cardiorespiratory disease, hypertension and pre-eclampsia, and multiple births. In women at high risk of operative delivery, a working epidural placed early in labour helps to achieve a smooth progression to theatre if necessary.

Absolute contraindications are maternal refusal, local sepsis, severe bleeding diathesis, increased intracranial pressure, and local anaesthetic allergy.

Relative contraindications are major spinal problems (e.g. spina bifida, lumbar spinal surgery), neurological disease, hypovolaemia, fixed cardiac output, and systemic sepsis.

> **Coagulation and epidurals**
> In otherwise healthy patients, a platelet count above 80×10^9/L is considered safe to site an epidural. If the platelet count is 50–80×10^9/L, further coagulation tests may be required and a discussion of risk vs. benefit in that particular patient made with a consultant anaesthetist. Patients on LMWH pose additional problems.

Placing an epidural

A full anaesthetic history, explanation of the procedure, and patient consent must be carried out in all cases. Increasingly, formal consent forms are being used as evidence of informed consent and local policy should be followed.

Wide-bore IV access (at least 16G) should be gained and a bag of fluid (crystalloid or colloid) attached. The value of preloading all patients with 500–1000ml of crystalloid is debatable. It is more important to consider the individual mother's volume status: hypovolaemia may be unmasked by the epidural, whereas some women will tolerate large volumes of IV fluid poorly (e.g. severe pre-eclampsia, cardiovascular disease).

With the woman either sitting or lying in the lateral position, identify the space. Lower lumbar placement is ideal as the block needs to cover segments T10–S4. The lower lumbar spaces should also be well below the termination of the spinal cord should the needle pierce the dura.

Use strict aseptic technique: hat, sterile gloves, gown, and mask. Prep and drape the back.

It is essential to maintain communication with the mother throughout the procedure. Warn her of any sensations she is likely to experience, and ask her to tell you if she has a contraction or if the urge to move becomes unbearable.

Use about 5ml of 1–2% lidocaine to anaesthetize the skin and subcutaneous tissues.

Introduce the Tuohy needle and advance it into the epidural space using a loss-of-resistance technique. (Saline is common nowadays, but some anaesthetists prefer to use air. The subject is hotly debated; in the absence of clear evidence favouring one or the other technique, either is acceptable.)

Disconnect the loss-of-resistance syringe. There should be no gush of CSF (indicating a dural tap; test with a glucose stick if in doubt) or blood (indicating intravascular placement). Feed the catheter into the epidural space, remembering to note the distance from the skin (using the markings on the Tuohy needle). 3-5cm of catheter should remain in the epidural space.

Aspirate the catheter. Light blood staining which clears on flushing and re-aspiration is acceptable, but persistent frank blood indicates intravascular placement.

A test dose can be given at this stage (see below).

Dress and securely fix the epidural catheter.

Drugs used in epidural analgesia

Test dose

A test dose aims to exclude intrathecal (and, rarely, subarachnoid) placement of the epidural catheter. There are two possible approaches:

Administration of a small volume of high-concentration local anaesthetic (e.g. 3ml + volume of catheter dead space of 0.5% bupivacaine). This dose could be expected to give a swift onset of dense sensory and motor block within 5–10min if given into the intrathecal space. However, it has very little early effect when given epidurally, and so provides no immediate relief for the labouring woman. Later, it may contribute to motor block (3ml of 0.5% = 15mg).

Administration of a larger volume of low-concentration local anaesthetic, which also acts as the first top-up dose (e.g. 10ml of 0.1% bupivacaine). This is less reliable for excluding intrathecal catheter placement, but has the advantage of establishing the epidural faster.

Some anaesthetists use adrenaline-containing solutions to exclude intravascular placement. This approach has low specificity and sensitivity.

Maintenance of analgesia

Various regimens can be used to deliver epidural drugs. Intermittent top-ups have largely been superseded by continuous infusions, with top-ups given via the pump by the midwife as appropriate. Patient-controlled epidural analgesia (PCEA) is increasingly popular; this approach gives the mother the benefits of self-administration and decreases staff workload.

Epidurals usually combine local anaesthetic with an opioid. This combination reduces motor block compared with local anaesthetic alone, improving the ability to push in second stage. Commonly used local anaesthetics include bupivacaine (e.g. 0.1–0.15%), levobupivacaine, or ropivacaine, combined with opioids such as fentanyl (e.g. 2µg/ml) or diamorphine. An anaesthetist is required to give stronger local anaesthetic solutions as these have a greater potential to cause hypotension in the mother with possible fetal compromise. The use of opioids may increase side effects such as itch, nausea, and urinary retention.

Combined spinal/epidural

Combined spinal–epidurals (CSEs) are used in some centres to give faster initial analgesia from the spinal component, followed by the low-dose local anaesthetic and opioid mixture via the epidural catheter. Regimens vary, but typically around 2–3ml of the epidural premixed solution (e.g. 0.1% bupivacaine + 2mcg/ml fentanyl) might be given into the CSF, and the epidural catheter used for additional top-ups when needed.

⊕ Problems with epidurals on the labour ward

Immediate complications
Paraesthesia
Paraesthesia frequently occurs transiently while doing the epidural, especially when the catheter is passed through the Tuohy needle. This is not linked to nerve damage. If the paraesthesia persists, the epidural needle and catheter should be withdrawn.

Bloody tap
A bloody tap is more common in obstetrics (8% incidence) as the epidural veins are dilated. Blood in the Tuohy needle usually requires re-siting of the epidural. Blood in the catheter can often be flushed out, and the catheter pulled back a few millimetres until no blood can be aspirated from it. If this is unsuccessful, the epidural will need to be re-sited.

Dural puncture
The initial management of dural puncture is to establish analgesia for the mother, either by re-siting the epidural one space higher or by putting the catheter into the CSF. **Spinal top-ups must always be given by an anaesthetist.** A full explanation must be given, along with advice regarding headache. Labour can continue as normal.

Post-dural puncture headache (Section 6.15) is likely in young women after a dural puncture (around 70%). Bedrest does not prevent PDPH, although will alleviate symptoms if they occur. Fluids, analgesics (paracetamol and NSAIDs), and caffeine may also help. If the headache does not respond to conservative treatment, an epidural blood patch should be offered.

Early complications (during labour)
Failure or incomplete block
In cases of missed segment or unilateral block, the catheter can be withdrawn so that 2–3 cm remain in the epidural space. A top-up (e.g. 10ml 0.15% bupivacaine with 50mcg fentanyl) is administered with the patient lying on her unblocked side. Failure requires re-siting of the epidural or alternative analgesia.

Hypotension, nausea and vomiting
Hypotension is rare with low-dose local anaesthetics; if it does occur, fluids alone are usually sufficient. Small doses of ephedrine or phenylephrine can also be used. If hypotension is severe, other causes (particularly haemorrhage) must be considered.

Itch
Itch is common, and if troublesome can be treated with small doses of naloxone (40mcg IV). Propofol (10mg IV), or ondansetron (8mg IV) may also help in some cases. Chlorpheniramine is of no value in opioid-induced pruritus.

High block
Most high epidural blocks are due to excessive administration of epidural solution, and can be managed with reassurance, oxygen, and fluids, while stopping the epidural infusion until the block regresses.

Total spinal
With a total spinal (i.e. an epidural dose inadvertently injected into the CSF), the patient will be apnoeic, bradycardic, and hypotensive. This scenario requires intubation and ventilation along with IV fluids and vasopressors (e.g. phenylephrine) to maintain the BP until the block regresses. Patients may be aware, despite being unable to breathe and move, so after initial resuscitation a small dose of anaesthetic agent is required. If the epidural has been inserted for labour, a decision must be made regarding delivery of the baby, with a low threshold for emergency Caesarean section.

Local anaesthetic toxicity
This is sometimes due to excessive doses or intravascular placement of the catheter, but has also resulted from unintended attachment of an epidural solution to an IV cannula. Many institutions use a colour-coding system (e.g. all pumps, syringes, and fluids intended for use with epidurals are coloured yellow).

Late complications
Neurological complications
Nerve injury may be due to delivery alone, and a full assessment is required to determine whether the epidural is the most likely cause. Transient neurological complications (<72hr duration) occur in about 1 in 100 deliveries. One in 2500 women will have neurological complications lasting over 6 weeks. One in 13,000 epidurals is linked to neurological complications.

An epidural haematoma occurs in approximately 1 in 100,000 epidurals. This presents with increasing back and nerve root pain, sensory loss, bladder and bowel dysfunction, and, if untreated, paraplegia. These patients need urgent imaging (spinal MRI) and neurosurgical intervention.

Infection
Infection from epidural insertion is usually superficial, surrounding the insertion site. Very rarely, there is formation of an epidural abscess, which may cause cord compression and requires urgent neurosurgical intervention. It presents in a similar way to an epidural haematoma, although its course may be more indolent. There are often signs of an added systemic inflammatory response.

Further reading
Holdcroft A et al. (1995) Br J Anaesth **75**, 522–6.

Caesarean section is by far the most common obstetric surgical procedure, accounting for up to 30% of deliveries in the UK. In order to decide on the safest anaesthetic technique for mother and fetus, it is essential to know the reason for the operation. The following classification is used.

- *Category 1* requires immediate delivery (<15min) as there is an immediate threat to maternal or fetal life.
- *Category 2* requires urgent delivery (within 30min) as there is maternal or fetal compromise that is not immediately life threatening.
- *Category 3* requires early delivery, but there is no maternal or fetal compromise.
- *Category 4* is an elective delivery at a time to suit the woman and maternity staff.

Practical points

For all Caesarean sections there are some basic rules to follow:

Drugs and equipment: check the anaesthetic machine and emergency equipment at the beginning of every shift. Keep a supply of emergency drugs drawn up and ready for use in the refrigerator. Do not be tempted to raid this supply for less urgent problems!

Antacid premedication: always assume that the patient will need a general anaesthetic, and give antacid premedication accordingly.

Maintenance of BP: fluids, ephedrine, and phenylephrine are used, as they do not cause placental vasoconstriction. The relative merits of ephedrine and phenylephrine are the subject of much debate.

Syntocinon should be given immediately after delivery. An initial 5iu slow IV bolus is given, repeated if necessary. This may be followed by an infusion of syntocinon, e.g. 10iu per hour for 4hr. Only give syntocinon after confirming that all babies have been delivered (in non-singleton pregnancies the ensuing uterine contraction can make delivery of the remaining baby (or babies) extremely difficult, and may cause fetal asphyxia).

Antibiotic prophylaxis (e.g. cefuroxime, co-amoxiclav), if used, is given after delivery of the baby.

Post-operative analgesia: diclofenac and/or paracetamol suppositories are often given at the end of the procedure to provide early analgesia. The mainstays of postoperative analgesia are paracetamol, short courses of NSAIDs (e.g. diclofenac), and morphine (IM or via PCA) as required. Some units cater for the continued use of the epidural.

Thromboprophylaxis: this is a very important issue. In the period 2002–2005, thromboembolic disease was the leading cause of direct maternal deaths (Lewis 2007).

Thromboprophylaxis options include early postoperative mobilization, hydration, graduated compression stockings, intermittent calf compression, and heparin/LMWH. Local guidelines for their use should be in place. Caesarean section in itself is a risk factor for thromboembolism. Other risk factors include weight >80kg, maternal age >35 years, medical complications of pregnancy, systemic disease, para 4+, gross varicose veins, and previous thromboembolic disease.

General anaesthesia

GA for Caesarean section has decreased in frequency because of safety concerns for the mother and fetus. It is still used in some category 1 operations, and in some elective cases where regional techniques are contraindicated. An emergency GA Caesarean is a stressful situation for the patient and it is essential to exhibit calmness and offer reassurance, even if time is very limited and the fullest explanations are not possible.

All patients for Caesarean require a rapid sequence induction. There is an increased risk of airway difficulty in pregnant patients and this is discussed opposite. A failed intubation algorithm for obstetric patients is shown in Figure 19.6. It is essential to be familiar with the contents and whereabouts of the obstetric failed intubation trolley. Classically, RST is performed with thiopental 5–6mg/kg, followed by suxamethonium 1–1.5mg/kg. Atracurium (0.5mg/kg) is given as the suxamethonium wears off. Opioid premedication is often omitted, because of respiratory depressant effects on the neonate.

Maintenance is typically with inhalational agent and N_2O in an FiO_2 of 50%. The theoretical increase in sensitivity to anaesthetic agents must be balanced with the risk of awareness in the mother, who may be anxious and have had no opioid premedication. A short deep anaesthetic before delivery should prevent awareness, with minimal risk to the baby.

After delivery, syntocinon, opioids, and antibiotics (if required) are given, and the FiO_2 and MAC are reduced.

Extubation is performed awake in the left lateral position, after reversing the neuromuscular block and with the mother awake. The anaesthetist is responsible for this, and it is usually done in theatre.

Oxygen and close observation are continued in recovery. Many units keep women nil by mouth for several hours after Caesarean, since occasionally post-partum haemorrhage will necessitate a return to theatre.

Further reading

Lewis G (ed) 2007. *The Confidential Enquiry into Maternal and Child Health (CEMACH). Saving Mothers' Lives: reviewing maternal deaths to make motherhood safer 2003–2005. Seventh Report on Confidential Enquiries into Maternal Deaths in the United Kingdom.* CEMACH, London.

➕ Failed intubation in the pregnant patient

A plan for difficult or failed intubation should be made every time general anaesthesia is planned in a pregnant patient. A failed intubation drill is detailed in the algorithm below.

The reasons for failed intubation include anatomical and physiological changes in pregnancy, the stress of the situation, and in some cases poorly applied cricoid pressure in patients with left lateral tilt. In addition, many Caesarean sections under general anaesthesia are performed out-of-hours by less experienced personnel (i.e. trainees).

There is an increased risk of aspiration of acidic gastric fluid or food, although premedication is given to reduce this risk. In the emergency case the mother may not be fasted and only sodium citrate would have any effect prior to intubation on gastric pH.

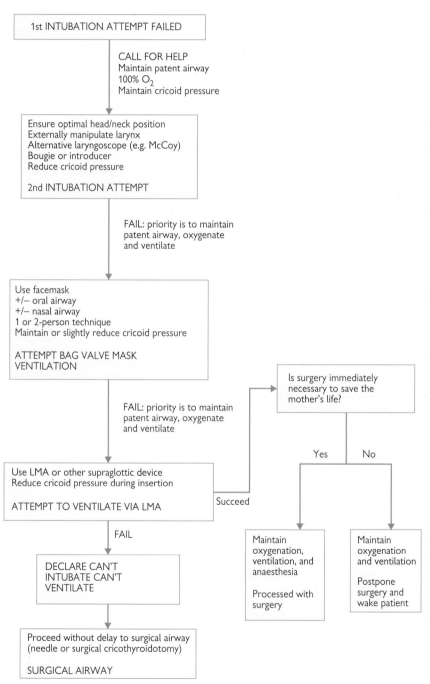

Fig. 19.6 Failed intubation algorithm for obstetric patients.

Regional anaesthesia for Caesarean section can be performed under spinal or epidural anaesthesia, or a combined spinal–epidural (CSE).

Spinal anaesthesia

Spinals are used most commonly both for elective and emergency/urgent Caesarean sections. Small pencil-point spinal needles (26–29G) are used, and a mixture of (usually) heavy bupivacaine (0.5%) and fentanyl (12.5–25mcg) or diamorphine (250–400mcg) injected into the CSF. A total volume of 2.5ml typically gives a block to T3/4 in a patient of average height.

The spinal is usually performed on the operating table itself, to minimize transfers and allow uninterrupted monitoring of the mother (and fetus if appropriate). IV access should be established with a wide-bore fast-running cannula.

The mother may be sitting, or in the lateral position. Some anaesthetists prefer the right lateral position, so that with hyperbaric bupivacaine, there is a rapid spread to the patient's right side. The block becomes complete when the patient is tilted to the left to avoid aortocaval compression. Others report only a marginally lower block on the right when the procedure is performed in the left lateral position or sitting, and the mother tilted to the left for surgery.

The L3/4 interspace is identified just cephalad to Tuffier's line (which joins the iliac crests and passes through L4 vertebra). Using full aseptic technique, 1% or 2% lidocaine is used to infiltrate skin and subcutaneous tissue, and the spinal needle is advanced into the space. Characteristic textures of supra- and interspinous ligaments, and then the ligamentum flavum are felt, followed by a dural 'click.' CSF should be aspirated freely prior to injection of the spinal mixture.

The patient can then be positioned for surgery. Pain-free catheterization is a good indicator that sacral segments have been anaesthetized. The block must be fully assessed before surgery can commence (see box opposite).

The block must reach a height of T4 (nipple level) to light touch before surgery starts. In emergency situations, a swiftly established block to T6 is sometimes taken as adequate, as this is likely to rise higher by the time the peritoneum is reached by the surgeon. In such cases, the mother must be warned of potential discomfort, and an explanation given. Supplemental analgesia (e.g. 50:50 nitrous oxide and oxygen) may be necessary (see below).

'Rapid sequence' spinal

Given the improved safety profile of spinal anaesthesia compared with general anaesthesia in Caesarean section, the concept of a 'rapid sequence' spinal for emergency Caesarean sections has gained acceptance in some centres. Here, IV access and monitoring are established, and sterile precautions are limited to hat, mask, and sterile gloves, and the back is prepped but not draped (the glove packet acts as a sterile surface). Subcutaneous local anaesthetic is omitted. The mother is pre-oxygenated by a trained assistant or second anaesthetist during the *single attempt* at a spinal. Should this fail, there is minimal delay in proceeding to general anaesthetic. The usual contraindications to spinal anaesthesia apply; when the emergency is for severe haemorrhage (e.g. it may not be appropriate).

Epidural anaesthesia

Epidurals can be topped up for Caesarean section where they have been inserted during labour.

Various combinations of drugs can be used successfully to 'top up' the labour epidural for surgery. The important point is that the mother should be fully monitored, IV access verified, and the anaesthetist present, as these top-ups are given. 5-10ml increments of mixture are given at a time, and the block checked after a few minutes. Usually, 10–20ml is required for an adequate block. The amount depends on various factors including the height and build of the mother, the degree of epidural vein distension (greater with twins and polyhydramnios), and any recent epidural solutions given. It must be stressed that even if a low-dose epidural solution appears to have achieved a block of an appropriate height, this block will not be dense enough for surgery and supplemental local anaesthesia must still be given in careful increments.

Usually, the top-up mixture contains a combination of local anaesthetic and lipophilic opioid (e.g. fentanyl or diamorphine). Local anaesthetics include 0.5% bupivacaine, 0.5% levobupivacaine, 0.75% ropivacaine, or combinations of 2% lidocaine (faster onset) with 0.5% bupivacaine.

Some anaesthetists use 1ml of 8.4% sodium bicarbonate to alkalinize the mixture and speed the onset of the block. Some will use adrenaline-containing solutions in order to increase the dose of lidocaine that can be given, and prolong the duration of the block. Any advantages that these drugs confer in terms of speed of onset should be weighed carefully against the time needed to prepare more complicated mixtures, and the potential for drug errors introduced by polypharmacy.

Remember that epidural blockade results in both a lower and an upper sensory level. The block should be checked before surgery commences to ensure that it extends, bilaterally and contiguously from S5 to T3/4. The same principles as for spinal block testing apply (see box opposite).

Epidurals for elective Caesarean section

Epidurals are occasionally used electively for Caesarean section when a more gradual sympathetic block may be desirable, e.g. congenital heart disease or hypertension. It takes longer to establish a block by epidural than spinal. The block is also less dense, so the mother will be aware of more tugging and pulling sensations during surgery.

Combined spinal epidurals

CSEs are used in some centres. These can be performed using a needle-through-needle technique, or by placing a spinal and epidural separately, at different interspaces. CSEs are particularly useful if the epidural component is required for postoperative analgesia, or the procedure is expected to be long or complicated.

Pain during Caesarean section is one of the most common causes of complaint and litigation in obstetric anaesthesia. It is essential to test and document the distribution and extent of sensory and motor blockade prior to surgery. However, there remains considerable debate about what constitutes the height of the block, as there is invariably a zone of partial blockade which may occupy several dermatomes (Figure 19.7). In addition, estimates of dermatomes vary between anaesthetists (and, indeed, textbooks): one person's T7 may be several segments lower or higher than another's!

The modality used to test the block is also controversial: although many anaesthetists use cold (either ice or ethyl chloride spray), evidence is mounting that touch is a more reliable test.

Lower limb motor blockade is classified according to the Bromage score.

- I: no blockade, free movement of legs and feet.
- II: just able to flex knees, free movement of feet.
- III: unable to flex knees, some movement of feet.
- IV: no movement of legs or feet.

Whatever the methods used to assess the block, careful documentation should be used, in order to avoid confusion. 'Block to T4' is inadequate. The use of diagrams may aid record keeping.

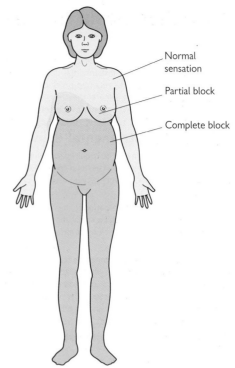

Normal sensation

Partial block

Complete block

Fig. 19.7 Testing the height of the block.

Occasionally, despite careful checking of the block prior to surgery, mothers experience discomfort during caesarean. It is important not to create the expectation of complete anaesthesia from the chest downwards: effective communication prior to and during surgery should help women to tolerate expected sensations (e.g. of firm pressure during dissection, or of pulling and tugging as the baby is delivered).

However, if significant pain occurs during surgery, it must be dealt with promptly and solicitously. Depending on its nature, several strategies can be used to alleviate it:

Inhalational: nitrous oxide 50% in oxygen (the same ratio as used in entonox). Using higher concentrations of nitrous oxide may inadvertently cause general anaesthesia in susceptible patients.

Epidural: if an epidural is in place, it can be topped up with 2% lidocaine (5–10ml) and/or opioids (e.g. fentanyl 100mcg). Surgery should be temporarily halted to allow this to take effect.

Intravenous: short-acting opoids (e.g. 10–25mcg increments of fentanyl or 250–500mcg increments of alfentanil) may be effective for pain.

General anaesthetic: conversion to GA is a last resort but it is sometimes necessary. Sometimes, simply the offer of a GA can help the mother to cope with discomfort as it makes her aware that she has a 'get-out' clause. If a GA is offered and declined, this *must be documented*.

To convert to GA, halt surgery and position the patient appropriately. Sodium citrate should be given if it has not been given in the previous 20min (a straw may help). An RSI should then proceed along the lines outlined in Section 19.9. Beware that the regional technique and possible blood loss from the surgery may worsen haemodynamic instability on induction. Surgery must not restart without the permission of the anaesthetist.

Commonly performed obstetric procedures other than Caesarean section include Shirodkar sutures, instrumental delivery, and manual removal of placenta. Evacuation of retained products of conception (ERPC) frequently appears on the general theatre emergency list; it is important to remember that these patients are obstetric cases.

Anaesthesia for instrumental delivery

A forceps or vacuum extraction may be required for failure to progress in the second stage, especially if there has been concern over the CTG trace. An elective instrumental delivery may be made to avoid pushing, e.g. in cardiac disease.

An epidural may be *in situ* in these patients, in which case it can be topped up for delivery. Alternatively, a spinal may be performed (or rarely a general anaesthetic). The block must extend to T6 for a comfortable delivery.

The obstetrician should decide whether to deliver in the labour room or theatre, as there is a risk of emergency Caesarean section if the instrumental delivery fails. It is acceptable to top up the epidural in the room with close monitoring and access to emergency drugs; cases requiring spinal or general anaesthesia should be done in theatre.

Retained products of conception

Retained placenta

In approximately 2% of deliveries the placenta will be retained (not expelled an hour after delivery of the baby). There are risks of post-partum haemorrhage (immediate or delayed), sepsis, and uterine inversion with attempts to remove the placenta. An operative delivery is required.

If an epidural has been used for labour, this can be topped up for analgesia for manual removal of the placenta. Alternatively a spinal can be performed. The block must reach to T6 for adequate analgesia. This may require an increased volume compared with Caesarean or instrumental delivery (e.g. 3ml), since epidural venous engorgement quickly fades after delivery.

A general anaesthetic is occasionally used where there are contraindications to a regional technique (e.g. severe post-partum haemorrhage). Inhalational agents cause dose-dependent uterine relaxation, which can be helpful surgically. This has to be balanced against the risk of general anaesthetic to the mother and possible increased bleeding.

Post-operatively, an oxytotic infusion is given (e.g. 40iu syntocinon IV over 4hr) to reduce the risk of uterine atony and bleeding.

Very occasionally, a retained placenta will be morbidly adherent (placenta accreta) and a hysterectomy may have to be performed by a senior obstetrician.

Evacuation of retained products of conception

This can occur after a miscarriage, termination, or delivery.

Patients who have miscarried may be offered expectant, medical or surgical treatment. They are usually early in the grieving process and require compassion in their treatment. They are commonly less than 15 weeks pregnant, and so are at low risk of aspiration from their pregnancy alone, but the dates should be ascertained. Surgical treatment is carried out under a general anaesthetic with either TIVA or volatile agent, remembering the potential for inhalational agents to relax the uterus and exacerbate bleeding. An oxytotic agent (e.g. 5iu syntocinon IV) is given at the end of the procedure.

Occasionally, some products of conception (e.g. placental fragments) remain in the uterus after delivery, miscarriage, or termination. These can cause sepsis or haemorrhage and need to be removed surgically. If the patient presents >24hr post-delivery, she is no longer a high risk for aspiration from pregnancy itself. Again, TIVA or volatiles may be used, with oxytotic agents to contract the uterus and reduce haemorrhage. These are usually continued as an infusion post-operatively.

Termination of pregnancy

Terminations may be carried out up to 24 weeks of pregnancy, although are usually performed earlier. Again, the woman has usually made a difficult decision and requires kindness and professionalism. Before 15 weeks, a straightforward general anaesthetic is used; after 15 weeks a rapid sequence induction with premedication as for Caesarean section is required. Again, TIVA with or without a low-dose volatile is used. (In many countries, including the USA, early terminations are carried out without a general anaesthetic.)

Anaesthesia for cervical suture

Women who have had recurrent premature delivery because of cervical incompetence may be offered a cervical suture in subsequent pregnancies. This is usually inserted between 12 and 20 weeks and removed when the mother goes into labour, or electively at 36–38 weeks gestation.

Although it is commonly performed under LA, some surgeons prefer a GA for the procedure because of the uterine relaxation it produces. Some patients may request a GA. If a spinal or epidural is performed, the block must be to T10.

Ectopic pregnancy

An ectopic pregnancy implants outside the uterine cavity (usually in the Fallopian tubes). Most of these patients will be stable enough to await diagnosis by serum β-hCG (positive) and ultrasound (no intra-uterine pregnancy; the ectopic may be seen). In stable patients, laparoscopic surgery is often used. However, there is always a risk of rupture, and wide-bore IV access should be obtained, with fluids ready.

Around 15% of ectopic pregnancies will present as an emergency due to Fallopian tube rupture and arterial bleeding. These patients require an ABC approach; the treatment of C comprises emergency surgery and ligation of the bleeding vessel. Resuscitation should occur simultaneously with transfer to theatre. At least two large-bore IV cannulae should be inserted and blood sent for urgent cross-match. A rapid sequence induction should be performed on the operating table with a cardiostable agent.

The effects of drugs on uterine tone

Several anaesthetic drugs have clinically relevant effects on the pregnant uterus. In addition, anaesthetists are frequently called upon to administer drugs which alter the tone of the uterus in order to aid surgery or to interrupt premature labour. Table 19.6 describes the effects of some of these drugs.

Table 19.6 Effects of drugs on the uterus

Increase uterine tone (reduce bleeding, augment labour)	No effect on uterine tone	Decrease uterine tone (interrupt premature labour)
Oxytocin analogues: syntocinon, ergometrine	Propofol, thiopental, etomidate, nitrous oxide	Volatile anaesthetic agents
Prostaglandins E_2 and $F_{2\alpha}$, carboprost (a $PGF_{2\alpha}$ analogue)	Neuromuscular blockers	β-adrenergic agonists (ritodrine, salbutamol, salmeterol, adrenaline)
α-adrenergic agonists (metaraminol, norepinephrine)	Anticholinesterase inhibitors	Nitric oxide donors (GTN)
Ketamine		Nifedipine
Acetylcholine		Magnesium
Histamine		Oxytocin antagonist (atosiban)
Serotonin		

Gestational hypertensive disease describes a broad spectrum of problems, from mild asymptomatic hypertension to life-threatening eclampsia and HELLP syndrome.

Definitions and clinical features

Pregnancy-induced hypertension (PIH) describes new-onset hypertension (systolic >140mmHg, diastolic >90mmHg, or mean >105mmHg) after 20 weeks' gestation (prior to this, hypertension is virtually always pre-existing). In previously hypertensive women, a rise of 15mmHg diastolic or 30mmHg systolic reflects a pregnancy-induced component.

Pre-eclampsia comprises hypertension (as above) with proteinuria (>0.3g/dL in a 24hr collection, or 2+ on two separate occasions on dipstick testing). Features of severe pre-eclampsia include:

- Severe headache or visual disturbance
- Clonus
- Papilloedema
- Epigastric/hepatic pain or tenderness
- Vomiting
- Platelet count <100 x 10^9/L or rapidly falling
- Deranged LFTs
- HELLP syndrome (see below)

Eclampsia is defined as a generalized seizure occurring during pregnancy or within 7 days of delivery in the absence of other seizure-causing pathology. 44% of eclamptic seizures occur post-partum, and a small proportion of these are later than 7 days. Despite the nomenclature, eclampsia occasionally occurs in the absence of pre-eclamptic features, or precedes them.

HELLP syndrome (haemolysis, elevated liver enzymes, and low platelets) is a life-threatening variant of pre-eclampsia, and an indication for immediate delivery.

Aetiology

Various explanations have been offered. There is a failure of normal formation of placental vasculature, possibly immune-mediated. The reduced placental perfusion appears to cause systemic vascular endothelial dysfunction in the mother, with multi-system effects. There is an imbalance in the arachidonic acid metabolic pathway (Section 7.27), with an excess of thromboxane and a deficit of prostacyclin. This causes vasoconstriction and platelet aggregation. Risk factors include primagravidae, multiple pregnancy, age <20 or >35 years, obesity, and diabetes. 10% of pregnancies are affected, although only 1 in 200 will have severe disease and 1 in 2000 will have full-blown eclampsia.

Pathophysiology

The primary problem in pre-eclampsia appears to be vascular endothelial dysfunction, and multiple organ systems may be affected.

CVS: pre-eclampsia causes vasoconstriction, increased systemic vascular resistance, and hypertension. The vasculature is hypersensitive to catecholamines. Plasma volume is reduced, although CVP is normal or even high.

Renal: proteinuria (>0.3g/dL) is a feature. Reduced GFR causes decreased clearance of urea, creatinine, and uric acid. Renal blood flow is reduced, leading to activation of the renin-angiotensin system. Serum uric acid is used as an indicator for disease severity.

Haematological: loss of plasma proteins leads to reduced oncotic pressure and non-dependent oedema (hands, face, airway). Platelet aggregation is increased. Blood viscosity also rises. Haemolysis may occur and is part of the HELLP syndrome. Severe coagulopathies, including DIC, may complicate the disease.

CNS: cerebral irritation, headaches, and visual disturbances all indicate CNS involvement. Papilloedema may be visible on fundoscopy. Clonus is a sign of impending eclampsia. Intracranial haemorrhage may occur due to the hypertension. Seizures occur in full-blown eclampsia.

GI: nausea and vomiting are common; epigastric pain and hepatic tenderness can be due to liver swelling. Deranged LFTs (raised transaminases) may occur, and may indicate the HELLP syndrome. Liver infarction has been reported.

Respiratory: pre-eclamptic patients are predisposed to develop pulmonary oedema, especially if large quantities of IV fluids are administered.

Management

The management of pregnancy-induced hypertensive disease should take a multidisciplinary approach, involving senior obstetric, anaesthetic, and midwifery staff. The only definitive cure is delivery of the placenta. The risks of prematurity must be weighed carefully against the well-being and stability of the mother. Various strategies are used to reduce the severity of the disease and prolong pregnancy, with the cornerstones of management being control of blood pressure, support of organ perfusion while avoiding fluid overload, and management of complications.

Antihypertensives

Blood pressure of >160mmHg systolic or >110mmHg diastolic is an emergency, and puts the mother at risk of intracranial haemorrhage. IV antihypertensives should be used for initial or short-term control of blood pressure. Agents suitable for use in pregnancy include labetalol (5–10mg increments or 10–200mg/hr by infusion), hydralazine (5–10mg increments, or 5–50mg/hr by infusion), GTN (10–200mcg/min by infusion), sodium nitroprusside (0.5–1.5mcg/kg/min initially, up to 8mcg/kg/min).

Oral antihypertensives are used for medium-term control of blood pressure in pre-eclamptic women. Agents include methyldopa, labetalol, hydralazine, and calcium-channel blockers such as nifedipine (sublingual nifedipine is not recommended as it may cause an exaggerated fall in blood pressure).

Magnesium

Magnesium is the agent of choice in eclamptic seizures and has been shown to be superior to phenytoin and diazepam. It is also useful for seizure prophylaxis, halving the risk of seizures (the prophylactic benefit is probably greater in severe pre-eclampsia).

Magnesium should be given as a loading dose of 4g, followed by an infusion of 1–2g/hr. The plasma concentration and clinical signs of toxicity should be monitored, and infusion rates adjusted accordingly: the therapeutic range is 2–3.5mmol/L. Magnesium is excreted renally, and a reduction in infusion rate is appropriate if urine output is <20ml/h.

Fluid management

Careful fluid management is required. The intravascular compartment is usually depleted, but there is also intense vasoconstriction. Oliguria in this scenario is not overcome by fluid administration, which may cause pulmonary oedema. Current recommendations include fluid restriction (e.g. 80ml/hr or 2L/day). Invasive monitoring should be considered, particularly if oliguria is a feature. Note that fluid restriction is inappropriate in cases of maternal haemorrhage.

Aspirin

Aspirin is sometimes used in high-risk women to prevent pre-eclampsia. It is thought to act via inhibition of thromboxane production. Its use is not universal.

➕ Anaesthesia for the patient with pregnancy-induced hypertensive disease

Regional anaesthesia

Regional techniques can be used safely in the majority of patients. The risks of a precipitous drop in blood pressure after spinal anaesthesia are probably overstated, since the vasoconstriction of pre-eclampsia appears to be induced by circulating rather than neuronal mediators, as well as endothelial damage. Therefore it is only partially reversed by sympathetic blockade. However, extreme care must be taken; a fast-running IV line and immediate access to phenylephrine or ephedrine is mandatory. Some authorities advocate the use of epidural techniques with slow incremental top-ups to improve cardiovascular stability. However, the onset of anaesthesia is slower with this approach.

Regional anaesthesia in severe pre-eclampsia, eclampsia, or HELLP syndrome may be contraindicated by thrombocytopenia and abnormal coagulation. The trend as well as the absolute value is important. In general, a stable platelet count >100 × 10⁹/L poses no problem. Although absolute cut-off values are controversial, platelets <80 × 10⁹/L, 80–100 × 10⁹/L with abnormal coagulation studies, or a rapidly falling trend are usually considered contraindications to regional anaesthesia.

General anaesthesia

General anaesthesia in the pre-eclamptic patient is even more prone to risk than in the general obstetric population. Airway oedema may be severe. Laryngoscopy may provoke exaggerated hypertensive responses. These can be attenuated by continuing existing antihypertensive medication, and administration of IV agents immediately pre-induction (titrated carefully to effect). Short-acting opioids such as alfentanil may also be useful. Antihypertensive agents may also be needed on extubation to prevent further surges in blood pressure.

Post-operative management

Severe pre-eclampsia, eclampsia, and HELLP syndrome should be managed post-operatively on ITU as appropriate, as the clinical situation may deteriorate before it improves. Again, invasive monitoring may be helpful in the management of fluid balance and prevention of overload. If an epidural has been sited, it can be used for postoperative pain relief. NSAIDs should be avoided as they may contribute to renal impairment. Stool softeners should help to avoid straining.

⚠ Eclampsia

Immediate management:

Call for help: senior anaesthetic and obstetric support are needed.

Establish monitoring: pulse oximetry, NIBP, and ECG.

Support the airway and give 100% O₂ by facemask. Beware the risk of aspiration; avoid oropharyngeal airways and bag–valve–mask ventilation if possible.

Avoid aortocaval compression: put the patient in the left lateral position or use a wedge to tilt her 20° to the left.

Establish large-bore peripheral IV access. Take blood for FBC, clotting, U&Es, uric acid, glucose, and LFTs. Group and save serum, as an operative delivery may be imminent.

Do a bedside glucose test and treat confirmed hypoglycaemia with 50ml of 50% dextrose.

Give magnesium 4g over 15min.

Pre-eclamptic seizures are usually brief (<2min) and self-terminating. If the seizure is prolonged, consider benzodiazepines (diazepam or lorazepam 4mg IV), propofol, or thiopental.

In cases of severe hypertension (>160/110mmHg), control blood pressure with IV labetalol (5–10mg increments) or hydralazine (5–10mg increments).

Establish fetal monitoring if undelivered. If there is fetal compromise, an emergency operative delivery is indicated *if the mother is stable enough*.

When able, take a brief history (partner and family may be helpful) and review the notes. Remember that epilepsy remains the leading cause of seizures in pregnant women.

Subsequent management

Continue magnesium infusion at 1–2g/hr; monitor clinical signs and levels, aim for serum magnesium levels of 2–3.5 mmol/L.

Insert a urinary catheter and monitor urine output. Dipstick testing should be performed regularly.

If there is severe hypertension, invasive blood pressure monitoring should be used to guide infusion of antihypertensive agent (labetalol/hydralazine/GTN/sodium nitroprusside).

In the absence of haemorrhage, restrict fluid intake to 80ml/hr. Central venous access may help guide fluid management.

Correct coagulopathy if there is bleeding or if surgery is intended.

Start IV ranitidine (50mg 8-hourly) and metoclopramide (10mg 8-hourly).

Exclusions: epileptic seizure; hypoglycaemia; intracranial haemorrhage; cerebral hypoxia (e.g. haemorrhage, PE); intracranial infection. Consider CT head.

Delivery can be delayed for several hours if there is no fetal compromise, in order to stabilize the mother and establish the diagnosis.

19.13 Obstetric haemorrhage

Haemorrhage is one of the most common direct causes of death in the obstetric population.

Anaesthetists need to have an understanding of the most common causes, be able to recognize haemorrhage when it happens, and most importantly be able to manage it swiftly and appropriately. It is crucial that anaesthetists work closely with the obstetric team when managing maternal haemorrhage.

Ante-partum haemorrhage

Ante-partum haemorrhage (APH) is defined as vaginal bleeding after 28 weeks' gestation. The causes include placenta previa, placental abruption (spontaneous or traumatic), and spontaneous abortion.

Placenta previa

Placenta previa occurs when there is an encroachment of the placenta onto the lower uterine segment or cervical os. It is graded according to the position of the placenta.

- Grade 1—low-lying placenta, but not in contact with the internal os.
- Grade 2—the placenta reaches the os.
- Grade 3—the placenta covers the os; however, the bulk of the placenta is lying to one side of it.
- Grade 4—the placenta sits uniformly on top of the os.

The anterior–posterior lie of the placenta is also important; anterior placentas create increased risk for bleeding during Caesarean section.

Placental abruption

Placental abruption is premature separation of the placenta from the uterus. Bleeding occurs between the placenta and uterine wall. Placental abruption can present with abdominal pain and fetal distress. Bleeding may be occult, contained within the uterine cavity. Abruption can coexist with placenta praevia.

Management of APH

Assessment

Assessment and resuscitation occur simultaneously, and should follow an 'Airway, Breathing, Circulation' format.

History: anaesthetic history; brief obstetric history (with a view to identification of the source of bleeding).

Examination: airway, breathing and circulation are the priorities, in particular looking for signs of hypovolaemia.

Assessment of the degree of blood loss can be very difficult. Even when bleeding is overt, it has been shown that medical staff, including anaesthetists, grossly underestimate the amount. Most obstetric patients are young and healthy, and can compensate for losses of up to 30% of their circulating volume before the systolic blood pressure falls. Pre-existing tachycardia from labour effort and pain may make assessment difficult. Cool peripheries are an ominous sign.

Initial management:

Establish monitoring: pulse oximetry, ECG, and non-invasive blood pressure. Fetal monitoring should also be instigated.

Maintain airway if required.

High flow oxygen (15L/min via non-rebreathing mask).

Left uterine displacement (manual, or with wedge or bed tilt).

IV access: establish two large-bore cannulae. Take blood for:

- Cross-match (6 units)
- Full blood count
- Clotting screen (including fibrinogen)
- Urea and electrolytes
- Glucose
- Uric acid.

Start a rapid infusion of warmed isotonic fluid initially, then blood if required.

Consider arterial blood gas analysis.

Definitive management depends mainly on the cause of the bleeding and the response to treatment. The obstetric team must make a decision about the timing and mode of delivery.

Points to note:

Placental abruption in particular is associated with DIC. Ensure that blood samples are taken early and any abnormalities corrected.

If the mother requires emergency Caesarean section, the options for anaesthesia are general or regional anaesthesia. **Clotting studies and platelets must be assessed prior to any regional anaesthetic.** Other standard considerations (e.g. consent) apply; however, in the presence of haemodynamic instability, a careful general anaesthetic using RSI is the most appropriate choice. Regional anaesthesia may take longer, and risks sympathetic block exacerbating hypovolaemia.

Post-partum haemorrhage

Primary post-partum haemorrhage (PPH) is defined as the loss of >500ml of blood from the vagina within the first 24hr post-delivery (or less, if it causes haemodynamic instability in the mother). Average blood loss is 250–400ml during a normal vaginal delivery, and 500–1000ml durng Caesarean section.

PPH can be sudden and profound. A high index of suspicion should be maintained if a post-parturient shows any evidence of cardiovascular instability. PPH losses are often concealed. Causes of PPH can be classified as follows.

- **Tone:** uterine atony.
- **Trauma:** to cervix, vagina, perineum or other local structures.
- **Tissue:** retained placenta.
- **Thrombin:** i.e. a complication of DIC.

Uterine atony

If the uterus contracts well, it exerts a compressive force on the uterine vessels and prevents bleeding. Uterine atony is failure of this process. It may be associated with overdistension of the uterus (multiple pregnancies, polyhydramnios), prolonged labour, or multiparity. Inhalational anaesthetics also have a relaxant effect on uterine smooth muscle.

Various drugs can be used to increase uterine tone; they are listed in Table 19.6.

Retained placenta

Retained placenta is defined as failure to expel the placenta within 30min of delivery of the baby. It can occasionally cause massive haemorrhage.

Management of PPH

Initial assessment and management is the same as for APH. Assessment and resuscitation occur simultaneously.

Further management:

Retained placenta: manual or operative delivery of the placenta must occur without delay in order to avoid further bleeding. Again, if the mother is haemodynamically unstable a general anaesthetic is preferred.

Uterine atony: in addition to circulatory resuscitation, bimanual compression of the uterus by the obstetrician may reduce ongoing bleeding. Drugs such as syntocinon can be used in consultation with the obstetric team (Table 19.7).

! Major obstetric haemorrhage (MOH)

Definitions vary, but MOH can be defined as blood loss >1500ml.

Recommendations state that a multidisciplinary MOH protocol should be available in all units, and a drill practised at regular intervals.

Obstetric haemorrhage may be overt or concealed. Signs may be non-specific and are often attributed to the pregnancy or labour: tachycardia, tachypnoea, and dilutional anaemia are examples.

A high index of suspicion should always be maintained in obstetric patients, even those without obvious risk factors. In these fit young patients, 35% blood loss (around 2L) can be compensated without a drop in blood pressure. Subtle but ominous signs include cool peripheries (pregnancy usually causes vasodilatation), agitation, and narrow pulse pressure. *Hypotension is a late sign.*

Management of MOH

Call for help. Mobilize team members early.

- Senior obstetrician.
- Senior anaesthetist.
- Anaesthetic assistant.
- Senior midwife.
- Paediatrician if delivery is imminent.
- Porters.
- Alert blood transfusion.

O-negative blood or group-specific blood should be considered if fully cross-matched blood is not immediately available.

Consider early use of a rapid transfuser with warming capabilities; hypothermia exacerbates acidosis and clotting abnormalities.

Clotting abnormalities should be promptly corrected with the appropriate products: FFP, cryoprecipitate, or platelets.

Institute further monitoring in all unstable patients: invasive blood pressure, central venous access, and urinary catheterization. Commence hourly urine measurement and measure temperature.

MOH may require surgical intervention to control haemorrhage if losses are ongoing. These include uterine packing, Rusch balloon, B Lynch suture, internal iliac, uterine, or ovarian artery ligation, and hysterectomy. If the mother has been unstable or shows signs of impaired organ perfusion (metabolic acidosis, decreased urine output, raised lactate, hypothermia), extubation should be delayed and she should be transferred to intensive care. It is always worthwhile seeking input from the intensive care team at an early stage.

493

Table 19.7 **Drugs used to treat uterine atony**	
Syntocinon (oxytocin)	5IU, slow IV Infusion according to local protocol
Ergometrine	0.5mg IV
Syntometrine	Oxytocin 5IU + ergometrine 500mcg, 1ml IM
Hemabate (carboprost)	250mcg IM
PGE$_2$	100mcg intra-myometrial injection
Misoprostol	1g rectal
Gemeprost	1mg pessary intra-uterine cavity

Maternal mortality

Deaths among mothers in the UK are audited by the Confidential Enquiry into Maternal and Child Health (CEMACH). This organization produces triennial reports into the causes of maternal mortality; the most recent of these was published in December 2007 and examined the triennium 2003–2005. Maternal deaths are defined as direct, indirect, coincidental, and late.

Direct deaths

Direct deaths are those due to conditions or complications unique to pregnancy (e.g. obstetric haemorrhage, pre-eclampsia). In 2003–2005, the leading cause of direct death was thromboembolism.

Indirect deaths

Indirect deaths are those due to pre-existing or new medical or mental health problems aggravated by pregnancy. In previous triennia, the most common indirect cause has been suicide, but this has declined. Cardiac disease was the most common indirect cause of death, and indeed the most common overall cause of death, in 2003–2005.

Coincidental deaths

Coincidental deaths are those which occur during pregnancy but are not linked to it. They include deaths due to trauma and to medical conditions which are not exacerbated by pregnancy (such as cancer).

Late deaths

Late deaths occur more than 42 days but less than 1 year after abortion, miscarriage, or delivery. They may be due to direct or indirect factors, or may be coincidental. In 2003–2005, 273 late deaths were reported in the UK.

Anaesthetic deaths

In the report for 2003–2005, the auditors identified six cases in which the death was considered to be directly associated with anaesthesia. It is interesting to note that four of these women were obese, and three of these died from post-operative respiratory failure. There was one case of local anaesthetic toxicity after a bag of 0.1% bupivacaine was administered intravenously in the mistaken belief that the bag contained IV fluid.

It is now common to find lipid emulsion packs ('lipid rescue' packs) on maternal resuscitation trolleys. While the evidence for the use of lipid in local anaesthetic toxicity is scarce, it is encouraging. Anaesthetists are encouraged to report any experiences of the drug at www.lipidrescue.org.

Maternal cardiac arrest

Cardiac arrest is a very rare event during pregnancy, with an estimated incidence of 1 in 30,000 pregnancies. Although it is managed along standard adult advanced life support guidelines, a few important principles need to be considered.

Urgent help is needed from obstetric, anaesthetic, midwifery, and paediatric staff in addition to the arrest team. Senior personnel should be summoned to attend immediately.

If the woman is noticeably pregnant (i.e. a visible abdominal bump), then a left lateral tilt is essential in order to prevent aortocaval compression. This can be performed with a specially designed wedge, but equally a rescuer can manually displace the uterus over to one side.

Oxygen delivery is particularly difficult during resuscitation in the pregnant woman because of reduced FRC and overall reduced respiratory compliance due to the gravid uterus. In addition, oxygen demand is increased during pregnancy. Ventilation breaths during resuscitation are less likely to be effective, and more likely to insufflate the stomach with air (because of the relaxation of the lower oesophageal sphincter). Aspiration is a very real risk. Therefore it is essential to establish a definitive airway as early as possible in the resuscitation of the woman.

Chest compressions are similarly less likely to be effective in the pregnant woman because of the presence of the fetus.

While considering reversible causes of cardiac arrest, give special attention to **h**aemorrhage, **t**hromboembolism (or amniotic fluid embolism), and **t**oxicity (particularly local anaesthetics). Once these have been excluded or treated, move on to the other H's and T's.

Periarrest/perimortem Caesarean

It is recommended that prompt evacuation of the uterus by Caesarean section is considered as a *resuscitative procedure* in the arrested pregnant woman. Ventilation will be improved and oxygen demand reduced. Aortocaval compression will cease, allowing increased venous return and more effective CPR. The woman can be managed in the supine position.

Caesarean section should be commenced within 4min of maternal arrest, and delivery should occur before 5min have elapsed. Moving the mother to the operating theatre is not necessary; and sterile preparation and drapes are unlikely to affect survival. CPR should continue throughout the procedure, and consideration should be given to open cardiac massage once the abdomen is open and the heart can be reached through the diaphragm.

If there is a return of spontaneous circulation, the woman can be moved to the operating theatre to complete the operation. It is essential to consider sedation and anaesthesia at this stage as well as continuing the resuscitation.

Fetal outcome

Once the baby is delivered, it becomes a legal person and merits resuscitation in its own right. Interestingly, 70% of babies delivered within 5min of maternal arrest survive, and the neurological prognosis for these babies is good. The prognosis worsens with delay in delivery.

Stopping resuscitation

If the rhythm is VF/VT, resuscitation attempts should continue while reversible causes are sought.

The decision to abandon resuscitation in a pregnant woman should only be made by senior (consultant) clinicians.

If the mother dies, the coroner should be informed. Meticulous documentation should be maintained.

Further reading

Saving Mothers' Lives: Reviewing Maternal Deaths to Make Motherhood Safer: 2003–2005, December 2007. Available at: www.cemach.org

Chapter 20

Paediatric anaesthesia

495

20.1 Paediatric anaesthesia

Communication with the parents and child

The concerns of the child and its parents will be different and this must be acknowledged in their preoperative preparation. Parental anxiety may be based on their own or others' experience of anaesthesia and surgery, or on what they have learnt through the media. Often, experiences remembered have not been positive. There will also be a certain amount of parental guilt and anxiety about handing over their child to a relative stranger, with a total loss of control. These fears can be allayed in a number of ways.

- Information can be provided at clinic visits.
- A preoperative visit to the hospital (Figure 20.1) may be arranged.
- Preoperative information leaflets and videos can be provided.
- Admission can be arranged for the morning of surgery, where appropriate: this minimizes the duration of hospital stay.
- Admission should be to an appropriate paediatric environment.
- There should be provision for parents to be resident.
- Involvement of a play specialist in preparation for anaesthesia. The child can become familiar with anaesthetic equipment such as 'blowing up the green balloon' on the anaesthetic breathing circuit.
- The anaesthetic visit itself helps establish a rapport, gaining confidence of both the child and its parents.

A child's anxieties will be partly based on its stage of development and partly on the responses of its parent or guardian. This highlights the importance of gaining parental confidence.

An awareness of the various stages of development is important. A small baby will not suffer from separation anxiety provided that it experiences warmth, contact, and food. However, its mother will most probably experience extreme anxiety at having her newborn dependent infant taken away from her.

Toddlers and early school age children experience the most intense separation anxiety. Older children may also suffer separation anxiety, but their fears may centre more on loss of control, loss of identity, and fear of mutilation.

Gaining a child's confidence is important in the conduct of the anaesthetic. The 2–4-year old may communicate best via pictures and drawing, so this can be incorporated in the early preoperative preparation. The 4–8-year old has a concept of reasoning and can express his or her beliefs. This can form the basis for an age-appropriate discussion about the anaesthetic and allow the child a degree of control over it. The older child and adolescent have an increasing perception of what anaesthesia and surgery involves. Figure 20.2 shows a suprisingly accurate recollection of the anaesthetic room from a child after a hospital visit. Again, they should be given an age-appropriate explanation regarding their pathway through anaesthesia and surgery. This age group will also have realistic fears which they should be encouraged to express. The aim is to allay their anxieties, should these be of needles, mutilation, or even death.

Anaesthetists are often involved in anaesthesia for children with learning difficulties or special needs. It is important to gain as much information as possible from the child and its carers about the level of understanding that exists. It is essential never to judge in advance what a child may or may not comprehend.

Psychological aspects of sick children

It should be remembered that a sick child will not necessarily function at an age-appropriate stage of development. Illness can cause regression and increased dependence or, indeed, listlessness and apathy. The sick child may express increased parental dependency, making administration of the anaesthetic difficult. This may be exacerbated by parental anxiety. These difficulties can often be anticipated in the preoperative visit and provision made to reduce their impact.

Issues relating to consent

The child's right to consent is an area that has seen considerable change over the past decade. Many bodies, both nationally and internationally, have produced guidelines on this issue. The UN Convention on the Rights of the Child states that the child should be informed of decisions relating to them directly. It recognizes their right to freedom of expression regarding these decisions, taking into account of course the age and maturity of the child. Issues regarding consent vary from region to region, and with age and circumstance. Key points are outlined below. However, any concern regarding consent in the child should always be discussed with a senior.

Specific rules of consent relating to age

Any person under the age of 18 is considered a child. However, in England, Wales, and Northern Ireland, the 16- and 17-year-old adolescent has a right to make decisions that are of legal standing. In addition, parents can consent on their behalf. However, a court can overrule refusal of treatment by a competent 16- or 17-year-old, if as a consequence they are likely to suffer harm.

Under the age of 16, any child deemed capable of understanding may give or withhold consent. However, a parent, legal guardian, or court may override these wishes, if this is deemed to be in the child's 'best interest'.

In Scotland these rules are different. Children over the age of 16 have the same rights as an adult, and children under the age of 16 have the right to give consent if judged capable by a medical practitioner. This consent is legally binding.

In the Republic of Ireland, the right to consent is legally binding at the age of 18. Irish law is greatly supportive of the rights of the family. As a consequence, the courts are less likely to overrule the wishes of parents in the case of a minor wishing to make his or her own decision.

Who can give consent on behalf of a child who is incapable of doing so?

- Mother, or natural father if married to mother.
- Natural father who is divorced from the mother.
- Unmarried father who has entered into a Parental Responsibility and Rights agreement with the mother. For children born after 1 December 2003, the name of the father must appear on the birth certificate.
- Legal guardian nominated by the parent, in writing, before their death.
- Any person holding a court order with right to consent.
- Person over the age of 16 years who has care and control of the child, unless they are fully aware that the parent would disagree. There are limited rights in this category and they are only utilized for the safeguard of the child's health and welfare.
- A court of law.
- In extenuating emergency situations, if parent or guardian is neither present nor contactable, consent can be obtained from the child if of an appropriate age and understanding. If the child is unable to comprehend the nature of the treatment, or is unconscious, emergency treatment should be administered in his or her best interests.

Consent in anaesthesia

There is still no mandatory process for documentation of consent in anaesthesia. However, the anaesthetist is expected to discuss the nature of the anaesthetic. The parent and child, where appropriate, should be aware of the risks and benefits of regional anaesthesia and/ or major vascular access. It is also advisable to discuss anticipated administration of blood or admission to intensive care. Consent should be obtained for the administration of suppositories. The Royal College of Anaesthetists has produced templates for consent that the anaesthetist can use and include in the notes.

What if the natural mother is under the age of 16?

If the mother of a child is under the age of 16, similar rules apply. It is important to ascertain if she is capable of giving consent, and if she is competent then one can proceed. Alternatively one of her parents or a guardian would have to be involved or, in extreme cases, the court may have to make a decision. Even with a competent mother under the age of 16, it probably is advisable to involve a caring adult such as a parent or guardian.

Consent for transfusion where child's parents are Jehovah's Witnesses

In an emergency situation blood can be administered to save or preserve life. In the elective situation, if parents refuse consent for blood transfusion to save or preserve life, the child can be made a 'ward of court'. Two consultants must declare that administration of blood is essential for life or for the prevention of serious harm.

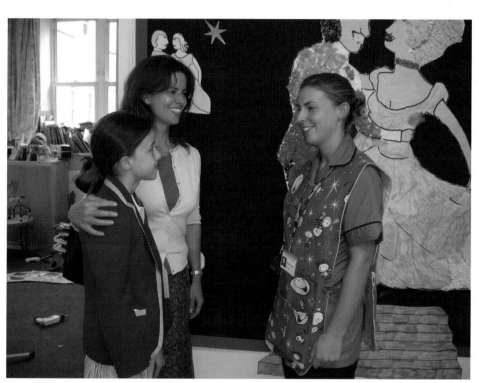

Fig. 20.1 Preoperative hospital visit.

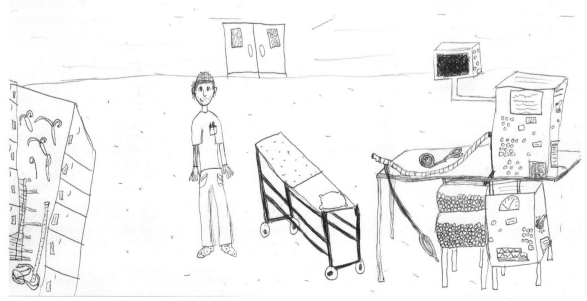

Fig. 20.2 Child's drawing of their impression of hospital care.

Paediatric anatomy and physiology differ in many important respects from those of adults. In addition, paediatric practice encompasses a range of ages with different physiological parameters (Table 20.1). It is important to appreciate these differences in order to understand and identify abnormal physiology and respond appropriately.

Definitions

Terms such as neonate and infant aare used quite specifically, whereas other labels used for children are rather vaguely defined.

Premature: a baby born before 37 completed post-conceptional weeks.
Neonate: a baby up to 28 days old.
Infant: a baby up to 1 year old.
Toddler: an infant or child in the early stages of walking; encompasses the period from around 1–3 years old.
Child: although legally a child is defined as any individual who has not achieved the age of majority (18 in the UK), for practical purposes childhood can be considered to be the period between approximately 3 years of age, and puberty.
Adolescent: broadly defined as a child between puberty and 18 years of age.

Dentition

The first tooth erupts at approximately 6 months, with primary dentition of 20 teeth complete before the age of 3 years. Permanent dentition begins to appear after the age of 6, with loss of the last primary teeth usually by the age of 14 years.

Respiratory

The neonate and infant have narrower airways, which results in increased airways resistance. Airway resistance is greatest from the mouth and nasal passages through to the trachea. Surprisingly, the peripheral airways contribute least to airways resistance as their total cross-sectional area increases dramatically towards the peripheries.

Clinical significance: occlusion of the airway with tubes, secretions, and adenoidal tissue results in considerable obstruction to airflow.

Traditionally the infant airway has been described as funnel-shaped in comparison with the adult cylindrical airway.

Clinical significance: the narrowest part of the infant airway is in the sub-glottic region. This predisposes the intubated infant or child to post-extubation sub-glottic oedema (Figure 20.3).

There are significantly fewer alveoli in the neonatal/infant lung, with each terminal bronchiole opening into a single alveolus or saccule, rather than clusters of alveoli. Hence, the surface area for gas exchange is reduced. Surfactant production beings at 24–26 weeks' gestation.

Clinical significance: an infant born prematurely will develop respiratory distress syndrome in the absence of surfactant production and may require administration of exogenous surfactant.

Breathing is essentially diaphragmatic. The 'bucket handle' movement of adult ribs is not present in the neonate and infant, as the ribs are more horizontally positioned and attached.

Clinical significance: abdominal distension significantly impairs ventilation.

Resting oxygen consumption is higher in the neonate than in the adult. The neonate and infant have a higher respiratory rate than the adult. General musculature is underdeveloped, and minute ventilation is rate rather than volume controlled.

The neonate has a smaller functional residual capacity for volume than that of the adult. In addition, closing volume occurs within tidal ventilation. Tidal volume and dead space reach equivalent volumes, per kilogram, to those of an adult by the end of the first week of life.

Clinical significance: any small reduction in FRC can lead to lung collapse. Oxygen desaturation also occurs more precipitously than in the adult. However, application of CPAP is effective in reducing the work of breathing and recruiting collapsed alveoli in this age group. Respiratory illnesses often result in tachypnoea and fatigue in the neonate and infant, and may require CPAP or mechanical ventilation.

There is increased response to vagal stimulation of receptors in the upper airway of the neonate and infant, and a greater predisposition to laryngospasm.

Clinical significance: bradycardia can occur during induction and intubation secondary to vagal stimulation or as a consequence of hypoxia secondary to laryngospasm.

The rate of onset and emergence from volatile anaesthesia is more rapid due to both increased alveolar minute volume and metabolic rate.

Clinical significance: this affects the conduct of anaesthesia.

Cardiovascular

At birth there is transition from fetal to adult circulation (Figures 20.4 and 20.5). The foramen ovale and ductus arteriosus shunts close, changing the circulation from a parallel to a series system. The placenta no longer performs respiration; this task is now carried out by the lungs.

Systemic vascular resistance increases as the umbilical cord is clamped and the placenta is taken out of the systemic circulation. At the first breath, pulmonary vascular resistance begins to decrease and pulmonary blood flow increases. These mechanisms change the pressures in the right and left atria, functionally closing the foramen ovale; the septum primum is pressed against the septum secundum forming a valvular-competent but potentially patent foramen ovale. These changes raise aortic PaO_2 and within 10–15hr of birth this induces local muscular contraction and functional closure of the ductus arteriosus (DA).

Irreversible closure of the DA usually occurs within 3 weeks in healthy term infants following local fibrosis and formation of the ligamentum arteriosum. Hypoxaemia and acidosis prior to fibrosis are able to reverse or prevent shunt closure. Persistence of fetal circulation occurs when fetal shunting is maintained beyond the transition period in otherwise structurally normal hearts.

It is worth noting that 30–35% of all adults have persistence of a valvular-competent potentially patent foramen ovale. Secundum atrial septal defect accounts for only 7% of all patients with congenital heart disease.

Clinical significance: in some situations the fetal circulation partially persists. This may be to allow mixing of oxygenated with deoxygenated blood in a congenital abnormality or may occur in isolation, requiring pharmacological or surgical correction.

Systemic vascular resistance is low in the neonate and infant, producing systolic blood pressures in the region of 70–100mmHg. Pulmonary vascular resistance falls at birth as oxygenation occurs and pulmonary capillaries open.

Clinical significance: both hypoxia and acidosis will increase pulmonary vascular resistance. This can lead to a right-to-left shunt in the neonate.

As with the lungs, the neonatal ventricles are smaller and less compliant. Normal heart rate in the term infant is 110–150 beats/min. Increases in cardiac output are achieved by increasing heart rate rather than stroke volume, up to rates of 200 beats/min. Figure 20.6 shows the increase in cardiac output from birth up to 16 years.

Clinical significance: at times of stress, there is limited reserve for the newborn to increase cardiac output significantly. Bradycardia occurs in response to hypoxia. Cardiac output cannot be maintained below a rate of 60 beats/min. At this point both administration of oxygen and cardiopulmonary resuscitation should be immediately commenced.

The neonatal ECG shows a right axis deviation, secondary to the predominance of the fetal right heart. This alters gradually throughout childhood, finally developing adult left axis orientation.

→ Approximate circulating volumes in infant and child
Neonate: 90ml/kg
Infant: 80ml/kg
Child: 70ml/kg
A neonate is defined as a baby up to 44 weeks' post-conceptional age.

Table 20.1 Normal physiological parameters in children				
Age	Respiratory rate	Heart rate	Systolic BP (mmHg)
<1	30–40	110–160	70–90
1–2	25–35	100–150	80–95
2–5	25–30	95–140	80–100
5–12	20–25	80–120	90–110
> 12	15–20	60–100	100–120

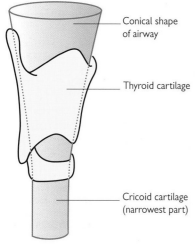

Fig. 20.3 Paediatric airway.

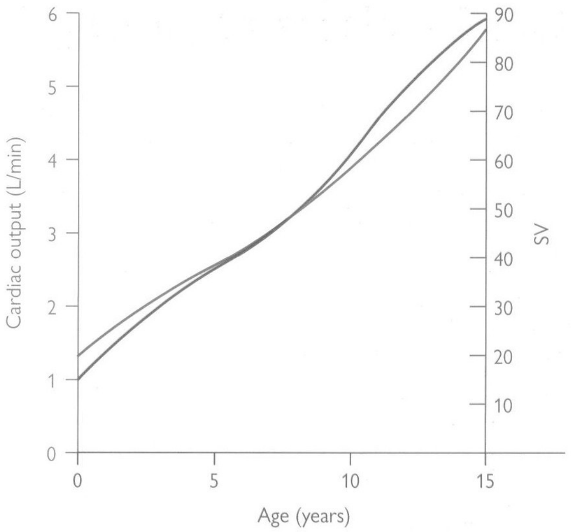

Conical shape of airway

Thyroid cartilage

Cricoid cartilage (narrowest part)

Fig. 20.6 Changes in cardiac output from birth to 16 years.

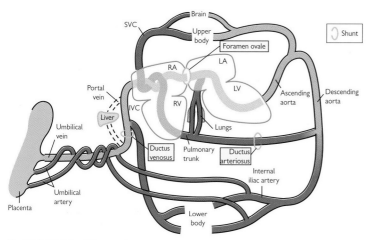

Fig. 20.4 Fetal circulation near term.

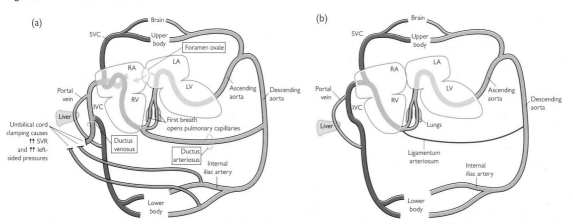

Fig. 20.5 Changes to fetal circulation that occur at the time of birth: (a) transitional circulation less than 1 day after birth; (b) mature circulation. Within three weeks, the neonatal circulation usually demonstrates irreversible change.

Nervous system

Although there is incomplete myelination in the neonate, autonomic function is well developed at birth. The parasympathetic system tends to have a predominant effect in the neonate.

Clinical significance: bradycardia is associated with vagal stimulation and can occur during laryngoscopy, eye surgery, peritoneal traction, and per rectum examination.

Cerebral autoregulation is absent or reduced in the premature neonate and to an extent in the newborn.

Clinical significance: hypotension is associated with cerebral hypoperfusion, potentially leading to significant brain injury. Abrupt increases in pressure can result in intraventricular haemorrhage, particularly in the immature brain. Figure 20.7 shows elastance curves for the neonate, infant, and adult

$$\left(\text{elastance } = 1/\text{compliance}\right).$$

Spinal cord

At birth the spinal cord travels down a much straighter vertebral column than that of an adult. The tip of the dural sac ends at approximately S3–S4 (S1–S2 in an adult), whilst that of the spinal cord ends at L3–L4, rising to L1–L2 at approximately 1 year. In the infant, ossification of the sacral vertebrae is incomplete.

Clinical significance: lack of ossification of sacral vertebrae permits access to this space with caudal anaesthesia. There is a risk of dural puncture or spinal cord injury when performing caudal or epidural anaesthesia.

Gastrointestinal

The pH of gastrointestinal fluid is higher in the neonate but falls to adult values over the first few weeks. However, lower oesophageal sphincter tone is reduced in the neonate and young infant and can lead to gastro-oesophageal reflux.

Carbohydrate reserves are lower in the newborn and infant.

Clinical significance: this can predispose the infant to hypoglycaemia, particularly in times of stress or acute illness.

The neonate may suffer from jaundice in the first few days of life. Contributing factors include the higher haematocrit, shortened red blood cell survival, and immature liver function.

Clinical significance: this is usually benign but must be distinguished from pathological causes of jaundice. In addition, drugs such as morphine are more slowly metabolized in the neonate as enzyme systems are immature.

Haematological

Neonatal vitamin K stores are low, so levels of dependent clotting factors (II, VII, IX, X) are poor in the first few months.

Clinical significance: vitamin K is given at birth, with parental consent, to prevent haemorrhagic disease of the newborn.

Depending on the degree of placental transfusion, newborn Hb concentration is in the region of 18–20g/dl. It falls over subsequent weeks as dilution occurs with expanding circulating volume, reaching a value of approximately 10g/dL at 3 months and 12g/dL at 1 year.

For the first 3 months of life, there is persistence of haemoglobin F in the infant. This results in an increased affinity of haemoglobin for oxygen (Figure 20.8). Although benefical *in utero*, it results in impaired oxygen delivery to the tissues in early infancy.

Temperature regulation

Babies have a large surface area-to-weight ratio, and possess little body fat. As a consequence they lose heat easily. They generate heat by increasing their metabolic rate and by a β-receptor-mediated process of non-shivering thermogenesis. The latter involves metabolism of fatty acids, glucose, and, particularly in the neonate and young infant, brown fat (Figure 20.9).

Clinical significance: under anaesthesia there may be increased vasodilatation, exposure, and subsequent increased radiant heat losses. Hypothermia increases oxygen consumption and leads to hypoxia, acidosis, and hypoglycaemia. Techniques to minimize heat loss are extremely important in the infant and child and will be discussed later.

Renal

The placenta largely maintains intra-uterine homeostasis, although urine production occurs as early as the first trimester. GFR is low in the newborn, achieving adult levels for body surface area by the age of 2 years. Renal function is immature. The ability to concentrate urine in the neonate is approximately 50% that of the adult.

Clinical significance: caution must be exercised with administration of high solute loads, especially sodium, in the neonate.

The infant is capable of diluting its urine. However, excretion of excess water may be limited by the GFR.

Clinical significance: again, caution must be exercised in the administration of fluids. This is particularly important in the sick infant where fluids may be given intravenously. Inappropriate volumes of hypotonic fluid, such as dextrose 5%, can result in life-threatening hyponatraemia and therefore are rarely administered. In fact, 4% dextrose–0.18% saline is no longer in routine paediatric use. Guidelines on administration of IV fluids in the perioperative period have recently been published (see Further Reading). Practice is strongly in favour of the use of isotonic solutions such as Hartmann's solution and isotonic saline.

The total body water (TBW) in the newborn is 80%, with the distribution between intracellular and extracellular being 1:1. In the 16-year-old/adult, the TBW is ~60% with the ratio being 2:1.

Perioperative fluid administration

Fluid management should be aimed at:
- Replacement of specific fluid compartment deficits (Section 11.7)
- Administration of maintenance fluid
- Replacement of ongoing losses.

Fluid compartment deficit

ECF volume

Children presenting for minor elective surgery usually have a minor fluid deficit that does not require correction. Those that are hypovolaemic preoperatively should receive an initial fluid bolus of 10–20ml/kg of isotonic fluid (0.9% sodium chloride or Hartmann's solution) or colloid, repeated as necessary according to clinical signs. In severe blood loss, transfusion will be required.

ICF volume

This is assessed by measuring the plasma [Na^+] and should be undertaken in all children with signs/symptoms of increased thirst or dry mucous membranes. Hypernatraemia results in reduced ICF volume and hyponatraemia results in increased ICF volume. Either may be associated with reduced, normal, or increased ECF volume (Section 11.4) and it is **this** that determines therapy.

Preoperative maintenance fluid requirements

Maintenance fluid requirements for children and infants older than 4 weeks should be calculated according to body weight (Holliday and Segar). It is important to remember that all formulae are merely a starting point, and the clinical response to fluid therapy should guide appropriate adjustments.

Term neonates (>37 weeks' gestational age) will lose up to 10–15% of their body weight in water during the first few days after birth. Their maintenance fluid requirements should be reduced.

Management during surgery

Maintenance fluid should be isotonic and the majority of children may be given fluids without dextrose. Preterm infants and neonates in the first 48hr of life will require dextrose during surgery.

Other losses during surgery

All losses should be replaced with an isotonic fluid or colloid. Blood may be required, depending on ongoing losses. There is no evidence that the use of human albumin solution is better than artificial colloids. Perceived third-space loss is difficult to quantify and should be replaced with isotonic fluid. Normally an estimate is made depending on the type of surgery, e.g.

- 2ml/kg/hr given for superficial surgery
- 4–7ml/kg/hr given for thoracotomy
- 5–10ml/kg/hr for abdominal surgery.

It is important to assess clinical signs (HR, BP, and capillary refill time) for evidence of adequacy of replacement.

Postoperative fluid management

A recent NPSA alert states that hypotonic fluids (e.g. 4% dextrose–0.18% saline) should not be used for postoperative maintenance because of the risk of hyponatraemia. Surgery, pain, and nausea and vomiting all release ADH, resulting in retention of the free water that follows metabolism of the dextrose in the IV solution.

Isotonic postoperative maintenance fluid should be used although some believe that it should contain additional dextrose. Currently, 5% dextrose–0.9% saline is one of the recommended fluids available for such use, although some centres have access to Dextrose-Hartmann's solution.

There is no universal agreement on the rate of maintenance replacement. Some believe that full rates (Holliday and Segar's formula) are appropriate, but others restrict fluid to 60–70% of this rate.

All fluid intake and losses should be recorded on a fluid balance sheet. Ongoing nasogastric or drain losses should be replaced with isotonic fluid. Losses should be measured regularly, and adequate replacement volumes will need to be given to prevent ECF depletion.

When oral intake approximates hourly maintenance rate then IV fluids may be discontinued.

Further reading

www.rcoa.ac.uk/apagbi/docs/Perioperative_Fluid_Management_2007.pdf

NPSA patient safety alert no. 22: Reducing the risk of hyponatraemia when administering intravenous fluids to children. Available at www.npsa. nhs.uk/health/alerts.

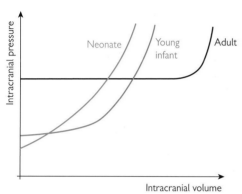

Fig. 20.7 Intracranial elastance graph. The elastance curves for the neonate, young infant (open fontanelles), and rigid adult skull. The neonate produces relatively earlier, albeit less steep, changes in elastance compared with the infant or adult.

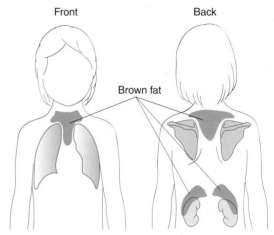

Fig. 20.9 Distribution of brown fat.

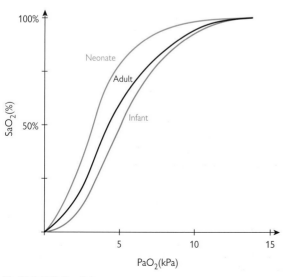

Fig. 20.8 HbF dissociation curve.

> **Oxygen dissociation curves with different oxygen affinities in the neonate, infant, and adult**
>
> Neonates have a lower P_{50} than adults (2.53kPa vs. 3.6kPa) and their higher oxygen affinity results in relatively decreased tissue oxygen unloading. due to the high levels of HbF which does not react well with 2,3-diphosphoglycerate (2,3-DPG)
>
> Infants >3 months have a higher P_{50} than adults (4kPa vs. 3.6kPa) with higher oxygen delivery to tissues at the same PaO_2.
>
> As the HbF proportion declines in the first 2–3 months of life, P_{50} increases rapidly: it is similar to that of the adult by 4–6 months and exceeds the adult value by 8–11 months of age. It remains above the adult value until adolescence. High levels of circulating 2,3-DPG are related to the process of growth and cause the high P_{50}.

The visit by the anaesthetist is of paramount importance. It is essential not only for the assessment of the child but also to establish a rapport with the child and its parents. It gives the anaesthetist the opportunity to discuss previous anaesthetics and any problems encountered. It also allows time for consent to be gained for any intervention or procedure. At this time the parents have the opportunity to ask questions so that they are prepared for events in the anaesthetic room and in the postoperative period.

The anaesthetist should utilize the skills of staff such as play specialists to reinforce the information given to the child and its parents. Through play, pictures, or actual equipment the child and its parents can become acquainted with items of anaesthetic equipment, which might otherwise appear frightening. Often parents will have been provided with information in the form of leaflets prior to coming to hospital.

The preoperative anaesthetic assessment of a previously fit child can be conducted as follows.

History

- Previous general anaesthetic or family history of anaesthetic problems. Any previous issues in the anaesthetic room? Any previous requirement for premedication?
- Neonatal history, specifically seeking information on prematurity, number of days intubated and ventilated on NICU, and any subsequent problems with airway and breathing.
- Medical history of common conditions such as asthma, diabetes, eczema, epilepsy, recurrent colds, or chest infections. Any significant history such as that of asthma should be further explored, with markers such as recent steroid use or hospitalization highlighted. A history of snoring, especially in ENT conditions, may signify the presence of obstructive sleep apnoea. It is also prudent to determine any history of cardiac murmurs. A murmur may be completely innocent, or may signify cardiac pathology (see opposite). The diabetic child requires careful consideration in terms of both preoperative preparation, provision of sliding-scale insulin if required, and re-establishment of his or her normal regime in the postoperative period. Specialist nurses working in areas such as respiratory or endocrine medicine can assist with optimization. Every department will have guidelines to assist with perioperative management.
- A history of recent or recurrent URTI is a subject of much debate (see opposite). In general, a pyrexial child with chest signs should be postponed. Indeed, any unwell child, uninterested in playing and off its food, may need to be postponed. A child with a runny nose, who is well, apyrexial, and without abnormal clinical signs, should not necessarily be rescheduled.
- Drug history in the previously fit child may not be extensive. However, the use of certain drugs such as inhalers or steroids is important and these medications may be required pre- or perioperatively. A child on insulin will need a strict preoperative fasting plan, priority on the operating list, and possibly a sliding scale for insulin.
- Any significant allergies should be noted, and the child and its notes appropriately labelled.
- The child should be appropriately fasted. Local guidelines should be adhered to. A child with reflux or a child in the emergency situation should be discussed with the consultant in charge.
- A dentition check is important, especially in the transition period between loss of deciduous teeth and eruption of permanent teeth.

Preoperative fasting

Adequate preoperative fasting is essential for the administration of a safe anaesthetic and is the subject of much debate. However, prolonged preoperative fasting should be avoided.

After ingestion of a meal, the stomach empties solids in a linear fashion, whereas liquids are emptied in an exponential fashion. Milk behaves as a solid because it separates out, in gastric juice, into a solid and liquid phase. However, breast milk empties faster than formula or cow's milk. It has been shown that the contents of a child's stomach, when clear fluids have been taken up to 2hr preoperatively, are similar to those who have been fasted for significantly longer.

Gastric fluid can reach volumes of 0.4ml/kg with pH values <2.5, yet aspiration in children is rare. However, children at risk include those following trauma or in pain, those who suffer from reflux or neurological disease, and those with an acute abdomen.

Solid food and milk	fasting period 6hr
Breast milk	fasting period 4hr
Clear fluids	fasting period 2hr

Examination

- Formal airway assessment is not always easy in a fasted frightened child. However, the general profile should be noted, with particular attention paid to chin size, neck, and presence of deformity or obesity. State of dentition and mouth opening can usually be easily determined.
- Respiratory system: specifically looking for abnormal chest shape, ventilatory pattern, and presence of added sounds.
- Cardiovascular system: general perfusion, colour, pulse, heart sounds, and presence of murmurs. The identification of a new murmur mandates assessment by a senior paediatrician.
- Temperature should be noted, and the child should be weighed to permit advance calculations.

Investigations

Formal investigation may not be required in the previously fit child.

- A sickle cell screen should be performed in any child of high-risk origin. The parent or guardian should be informed of the result to prevent repeat testing in the future.
- Haemoglobin estimation and routine biochemistry may be required in certain categories of children.

Discussion

- Nature of the anaesthetic: inhalational or intravenous and how this is performed.
- Who will be present and role of the parent before and after the child is asleep.
- Monitoring.
- Use of suppositories, NSAIDs, regional anaesthesia.
- Resolve where possible any parental questions or anxieties, and indeed those of the child.

Document your visit, findings, and details of your discussion with parents and child.

Topical local anaesthesia

EMLA (eutectic mix of local anaesthetic)

- Prilocaine 2.5% and lidocaine 2.5% in oily base
- Application: minimum 1hr pre-cannulation
- Duration: up to 60min after removal
- Disadvantage: risk of toxicity from systemic absorption
- Not recommended <1 month (risk of methaemoglobinaemia)

Ametop gel (Figure 20.10)

- 4% tetracaine (Amethocaine)
- Application: 30–45min prior to cannulation
- Duration: 4–6hr
- Causes localized erythema

→ Premedication

- *Topical anaesthesia* is vital in the prevention of pain associated with intravenous cannulation. *EMLA and AMETOP are generally used.*
- *Sedation* is less commonly used but may still have a role to play. Common situations include the upset child, the child who has had a previous bad experience, the child with behavioural problems, or the older adolescent who may request it. The most commonly used agent is midazolam given orally in a dose of 0.5mg/kg (up to 20mg total) with an onset time of 20–30min. An oral preparation is now available and has a less bitter taste than the IV preparation. Midazolam produces sedation, anxiolysis, and amnesia for up to 60min and therefore has less effect on recovery. Other sedatives less commonly used include temazepam, ketamine, and trimeprazine. Sedation must be avoided in patients with a difficult airway, lung disease, and gastrointestinal disease, or in those with neurological problems, as it is associated with a serious risk of morbidity and mortality.
- *Analgesics* may be given routinely by some anaesthetists up to 1hr prior to anaesthesia. The most common orally prescribed agents are paracetamol 20mg/kg and NSAIDs such as ibuprofen 5mg/kg. Opioids are less commonly prescribed.
- *Anticholinergics* are used to dry secretions in infants and children with difficult airways, especially those undergoing ENT procedures. They may also be used to prevent bradycardia in susceptible infants and children during specific procedures such as eye surgery.
- *Anti-emetics:* it is more common to use anti-emetics intraoperatively or to prescribe them for postoperative use.

→ Features of murmurs in children

Innocent	Pathological
Usually systolic	Pansystolic or diastolic
Heard early	Often end systole if systolic
Quiet	Long/loud
No thrill	Thrill/click often present
No associated cardiac symptoms	Associated cardiac symptoms and signs
Association with fever/exercise	

Referral to a paediatrician is essential if a previously undetected murmur is present.

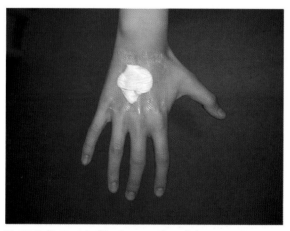

Fig. 20.10 Photograph of Ametop correctly applied.

→ Sickle cell disease (Section 15.2)

Sickle cell disease is an international health issue. It exists in all countries of Africa and in areas to which Africans have migrated. This includes the Americas, the Caribbean, the Mediterranean regions, and the Middle East. The condition has also been reported in India and Sri Lanka.

→ When to postpone: the effect of respiratory tract infections

General anaesthesia in the presence of an acute or recent URTI has been associated with:

- Laryngospasm
- Bronchospasm
- Arterial O_2 desaturation
- Breath-holding
- Coughing.

Significant URTI

Temperature >38°C

Copious secretions

Nasal congestion

Chest signs on auscultation

Parents report child has a bad cold and "not itself"

High risk of adverse events: postpone 2–4 weeks

Mild URTI

Not unwell

Clear nasal discharge

Chest clear

Age <1

Postpone

Age 1–5

Factors in history which increase risk of adverse events:

- Passive smoking
- Child snores
- Prematurity <37 weeks
- Reactive airway disease
- ETT required
- Airway of ENT surgery.

Risk/benefit should be considered on an individual basis. If in any doubt, discuss with consultant.

Age >5

Low risk of adverse events: proceed with surgery.

Preparation

On arrival in theatre, the machine and all anaesthetic equipment should be checked. Drugs should be drawn up by the anaesthetist and clearly labelled. Resuscitation equipment should be checked, present, and in good working order. A skilled assistant experienced in paediatric anaesthesia is essential.

Induction

Anaesthetic induction of the child should always occur in an appropriately equipped, prepared, and staffed room. A decision will have already been made about the mode of anaesthesia. However, a secondary plan should always be made. The choice is generally between a gas and an intravenous induction. This may be determined clinically or by choice of the anaesthetist in conjunction with the child and parent.

Intravenous induction

Drugs should be drawn up in advance, alongside emergency drugs, with knowledge of the child's actual or estimated weight.

Distraction, appropriate to age, allows cannulation to be performed out of sight for the child (Figure 20.11). Monitoring should be attached as tolerated, and if resisted can be attached as soon as sleep commences by the anaesthetic assistant. It is important to proceed with confidence and avoid forcing the child to comply.

IV access for induction

Visible veins should have been identified, and topical anaesthetic applied, on preoperative assessment.

When cannulating small veins, a useful tip is to flush the cannula with saline first, as this enhances the flashback of blood in a narrow gauge needle.

IV cannulation for surgery

Further IV access may be required depending on the procedure being performed. This may be in the form of larger peripheral access or central venous access. Larger bore lines can be inserted once the child is under general anaesthetic. Administration of volatile anaesthesia produces vasodilatation, making cannulation easier.

Emergency care: intra-osseous needle insertion

Repeated attempts at gaining IV access in an acute emergency situation are ill advised, as the infant or child may be in a low cardiac output state. Valuable time may also be lost. After 1–2min in a life-threatening situation, intra-osseous cannulation should be considered. Specifically designed needles are available for this technique (Figure 20.12).

Inhalational induction

Inhalational induction (Figure 20.13) is a technique used more commonly in infants and small children, but may be selected by the older child who is afraid of needles. The parent should be forewarned that the child will wriggle, as a natural resistance and as part of the stages of anaesthesia. They should also be prepared for their child to go floppy and to follow the instructions of the anaesthetist at this stage to lift the child, with assistance, onto the bed. At this point, the nurse involved should lead the parents from the anaesthetic room. It should be remembered that infants and children desaturate quickly, as they are rarely pre-oxygenated and have a low functional residual capacity, so this manoeuvre should be conducted swiftly.

The agent most commonly used is sevoflurane started slowly with oxygen–nitrous oxide. In small infants 100% oxygen and sevoflurane are given alone.

A participating child can hold its own mask and play with 'blowing up the green balloon', but it is advisable for the anaesthetist to keep a supporting hand present. Alternatively, the anaesthetist should either hold the mask or start using a cupped hand until a degree of anaesthesia is achieved.

Maintenance and theatre environment

When the child is transferred to theatre from the anaesthetic room, ventilation should be continued using oxygen via the Mapleson circuit. Once transferred onto the operating table, any additional monitoring should be connected.

All emergency drugs and emergency equipment should be kept in theatre. This includes the Mapleson F circuit, if the child is attached to the anaesthetic machine.

The theatre environment should be warmed in advance. The theatre table should ideally have a heated mattress, and either a radiant heater or warm air blanket should be available. IV fluids should be warm.

In the very small infant, IV fluids may not be attached. Instead aliquots of warmed fluid may be drawn off and given as required since this prevents inadvertent administration of excess fluid. Alternatively fluid should be administered via an infusion pump.

Where possible, the IV cannula should be visible to the anaesthetist: the hand or arm should be positioned appropriately before drapes are applied. Distant access should have an extension line and three-way tap connected; this should also be accessible to the anaesthetist.

Intraoperative fluid replacement

Reduced concentration sodium solutions (<0.9%) with dextrose should be avoided as they can lead to profound postoperative hyponatraemia and death. IV Hartmann's solution is most commonly used intraoperatively, with consideration given to dextrose solutions in the neonate and small infant.

Fluid administration in a child is calculated from full maintenance requirements. Depending on clinical condition or local protocol, fluid may be administered at percentage volumes of full requirement. Additional fluid boluses may be required to compensate for fasting and for ongoing losses, including insensible losses. Several formulae can be used to calculate fluid requirement (see opposite).

The child's position should be checked for correct alignment and all pressure points padded. The eyes should be protected. A temperature probe should be used in any case of significant duration. Lengthy exposure should be avoided, and areas such as the infant's head should be covered to reduce heat loss.

Blood glucose should be monitored during long cases, in the diabetic child, and in neonates and children having extensive regional analgesia.

Surgery should never commence until the anaesthetist is entirely satisfied with the patient's set-up.

Reversal and recovery

All the end of surgery, drugs to reverse muscle relaxation are generally administered. A peripheral nerve stimulator should be used to assess the degree of relaxation present. The recommended dose from 1 month onwards is 0.02ml/kg of glycopyrrolate 500mcg/ml and neostigmine 2.5mg/ml solution. This should be administered slowly.

The child should be extubated awake when cough and laryngeal reflexes have returned. Some experienced anaesthetists will extubate the child deep, especially in procedures where it is particularly undesirable for the child to cough. This technique should *not* be performed in inexperienced hands.

The child should be transferred in the lateral position and cared for by nurses trained in paediatric recovery. Cardiorespiratory instability and the presence of pain, nausea or vomiting should be treated accordingly.

The same attention should be paid to temperature control, glucose monitoring and IV fluid administration as in the theatre.

Once awake, stable, and comfortable, the child can be transferred to the ward environment. The parent(s) usually return to the recovery area once the child is conscious and requesting their presence.

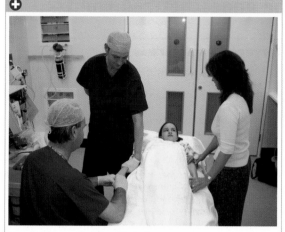

Fig. 20.11 Room set up for IV induction.

Keeping the needle out of sight reduces the child's anxiety. Asking the child to cough as the needle is passed through the skin is a further distraction. Careful fixation of the cannula is essential.

Most common sites for peripheral access, apart from those immediately visible on the dorsum of the hand, are the cephalic vein superficial to the radial styloid and the long saphenous vein. The long saphenous vein lies anterior and superior to the medial malleolus.

Central venous access may be required in the acutely ill child or in a child undergoing major surgery. It should only be attempted by personnel skilled in this technique.

➜ Fluids requirements (from Holliday and Segar)

Body weight	Fluid requirement
0–10kg	4ml/kg/hr
10–20kg	40ml/hr+2ml/kg/hr above 10kg
>20kg	60ml/hr+ 1ml/kg/hr above 20kg

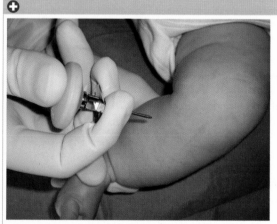

Fig. 20.12 Intra-osseous needle insertion. Tibia: anterior surface, 2–3cm below the tibial tuberosity. Femur: anterolateral surface, 3cm above the lateral epicondyle

Technique

- Gloves should be worn and the site cleaned with alcohol.
- Needle inserted 90° to the skin
- Advanced until a 'give' is felt, indicating cortical penetration.
- Needle should be aspirated and samples taken where appropriate.
- The needle should be flushed and three-way tap attached to permit administration of fluids or drugs.
- Any IV drug or fluid can be administered via this route.

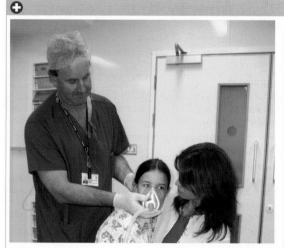

Fig. 20.13 Child on lap of parent for gas induction.

Again, the child can have the anaesthetic administered on its parents lap or whilst sitting on the trolley. With prior explanation, the parent can be helpful in this technique. Their role is to hold the child in a firm cuddle, with one arm under their axilla and the other within their embrace. The child faces away from the anaesthetic machine, where the anaesthetist is positioned behind the parent. This position allows easiest transfer of the child onto the trolley when he/she is asleep.

➜ Estimation of weight

Weight (kg) = (age + 4) × 2 was formerly used. However, the following is a more accurate reflection of today's child and should be used:

$$\text{weight (kg)} = (3 \times \text{age}) + 7.$$

➜ Parents

It is common practice to have a parent present in the anaesthetic room. There are many benefits of having a calm supportive parent available to hold a frightened toddler who will not be reasoned with, or to distract an older child who has a concept of what is happening. However, it is not obligatory.

Good preparation of the parent helps to make this event a smoother process. The environment should be child friendly with a limited number of personnel present. It is important that the anaesthetist proceeds calmly but confidently at induction. Losing the confidence of either the child or its parent can lead to a stressful induction and problems if future anaesthetics are required.

A nurse should always be present with the parent or guardian, ready to lead the parent from the anaesthetic room at the appropriate time.

➜ Factors affecting anaesthesia in infants and children

Induction
- Lower functional residual capacity: more predisposed to rapid oxygen desaturation.
- Higher minute ventilation: faster uptake of volatile agent. More predisposed to hypoventilation or apnoea as a consequence.

Intubation
- Higher vagal tone with increased risk of bradycardia.
- Greater predisposition to laryngospasm and hypoxia.

Maintenance
- Variable MAC depending on age group.

Emergence
- Higher metabolic rate: more rapid emergence.
- Risk of bradycardia and laryngospasm similar to that during induction and intubation.

The airway in the infant and child requires more subtle management than that of the adult.

Anatomy

Skull

The infant has a larger occiput which is apparent from birth and throughout first year of life.

Clinical significance: a pillow is not required for positioning into the neutral position.

Nose and mouth

The neonate and infant have larger tongues, especially in relation to their mandibular space. In addition, for the first weeks of life the neonate is an obligate nose breather.

Clinical significance: because of tongue size, airway obstruction is more likely and is particularly exaggerated in congenital abnormalities such as trisomy 21. Absence of teeth and compression of the soft tissues in floor of mouth can occur when using facemasks. In addition, obstruction of the nasal passages, associated with adenoidal hypertrophy or infection, can lead to significant airway difficulty.

Larynx

In the newborn, the larynx lies opposite C3 (C6 in the adult) and is positioned more anteriorly on laryngoscopy. The epiglottis is larger and somewhat 'omega' shaped. The cricoid ring is the narrowest part of the airway. Traditionally, the subglottis has been described as funnel-shaped although MRI views provide evidence contrary to this.

Clinical significance: it may be more difficult to visualize the vocal cords as the larynx is more anterior. The large floppy epiglottis may also obstruct the view. A straight-blade laryngoscope (Figure 20.14) is frequently used for laryngoscopy as it is less bulky and can be used to lift the epiglottis, providing clearer views. A towel or roll under the shoulders of an infant may also assist in bringing the glottis into view. For the older child, it is appropriate to use a curved blade in a paediatric size (Figure 20.15). Other blades such as the McCoy (Figure 20.16) are also available in paediatric sizes.

The narrow cricoid ring and funnel-shaped subglottis are associated with trauma from endotracheal intubation, especially when excessively large or traditional cuffed tubes are used. Newer specially manufactured cuffed tubes appropriate to paediatric airways are currently under review.

Trachea and bronchial tree

The trachea is 5–6cm long in the newborn with bifurcation occurring at the level of T2. By the age of 1 year the trachea is approximately 8cm long. The alveoli are immature, with the terminal bronchi opening into a single alveolus rather than a cluster of alveoli. The number of alveoli continues to increase until the child reaches the age of 8. Surfactant production from type II pneumocytes does not occur until 24–26 weeks' gestation.

Clinical significance: it is easier to selectively intubate one lung, particularly the shorter and straighter right main bronchus.

Practical application

- The infant airway should be held in the neutral position with chin lift if required. A pillow is rarely required because of the size of the occiput. Hyperextension should be avoided.
- The child's airway should be held, in head tilt–chin lift ('sniffing') position.
- A preselected facemask should be held against the face so that a tight seal is achieved. This also permits delivery of CPAP via the paediatric T-piece. The fingers should rest on the chin and mandible and not over soft tissues as the latter will contribute to obstruction of the airway.
- An oropharyngeal airway may alleviate obstruction.
- The paediatric airway is more predisposed to upper airway obstruction, laryngospasm, and bronchospasm. It is important to achieve a patent airway promptly, using adjuncts if necessary.
- Airway management in trauma is discussed later.

Laryngeal mask airway

The role of the LMA is not as extensive in paediatric practice as in adult practice. This is because:

- An anatomical difference exists in the shape of the smaller paediatric airway
- Down-folding occurs with the larger infant epiglottis, leading to an obstructed ventilatory pattern
- An increased incidence of laryngospasm is associated with its use, particularly in the infant airway.

The original LMA was designed in the early 1980s and is today known as the conventional LMA. It is made of silicone and can be used up to 40 times. Sizes 1, 1.5, 2, 1.5, and 3 are used in children. Size is based on the weight of the infant or child (see opposite).

The LMA does not provide protection against aspiration, so requires careful patient selection. If it does not fit snugly above the glottis in the paediatric airway, it can cause significant problems ranging from gastric dilatation to aspiration or laryngospasm. Therefore its use should be considered with caution and in discussion with an experienced paediatric anaesthetist.

Paediatric sizes of single use, flexible, and ProSeal LMA's are now available.

Paediatric breathing systems

In general, older children and adults can be anaesthetized using adult anaesthetic circuits. However, infants and the smaller child require the use of a paediatric system on induction. The characteristics of a paediatric breathing system should incorporate a low-resistance circuit with minimal dead space. This is achieved by minimizing the presence of valves. Historically, paediatric circuits have been used in children under 20–25kg. However, provided that ventilation is either controlled or assisted in infants, even adult circle systems can be used.

Circle systems are increasingly used in paediatric anaesthesia. Low flow may not be achievable in the presence of a leak around an uncuffed endotracheal tube or indeed in the smaller infant or child. When low-flow anaesthesia is employed, it must be remembered that anaesthetic gas concentrations take longer to reach equilibrium unless high flows are temporarily used. However, the circle system conserves heat, humidity, and anaesthetic gases and reduces environmental pollution. Lightweight 15mm tubing is available for the smaller child. However, sophisticated anaesthetic machines and ventilators can compensate for different types of circuit.

Paediatric ventilation in theatre

Traditionally, pressure-controlled ventilation has been selected as the mode of ventilation in the infant and child. This delivers a preset peak inspiratory pressure with each breath, reducing the risk of barotrauma or pneumothorax. It compensates for leak around the endotracheal tube, as it achieves its preset pressure. However, it does not compensate for changes in lung compliance.

PEEP is generally applied unless there is any contraindication.

Respiratory rate is higher in the infant and small child, and should be set according to the child's age and pathological state.

Volume-controlled ventilation can be used in the younger paediatric patient. Peak inspiratory and expired tidal volume alarms must be set to avoid inadvertent delivery of high pressures, or conversely, low-volume ventilation in the case of an airway leak. However, as in any clinical case, ventilation should be determined according to clinical findings, such as chest movement, air entry, capnography, and oximetry.

For shorter procedures, the Mapleson F circuit (Figure 20.18) can be used in the spontaneously breathing child or, in certain situations, the child can be manually ventilated.

The Penlon ventilator may be used in some centres, particularly in the anaesthetic room. A Newton valve converts this ventilator from a flow generator to a pressure generator. An attachment can be made to the expiratory limb of the circuit to ventilate the child.

→ Tracheal tubes

Tracheal tubes in everyday use are made from plastic and designed for single use. Generally speaking, uncuffed tubes are used in infants and children before adolescence. However, with advances in the design of paediatric endotracheal tubes, there are situations where cuffed tubes can and should be used in the paediatric airway. Cuffed tubes provide more effective ventilation in critical situations and prevent soiling of the airway.

Sizes of endotracheal tube

Age	Weight	Size	Length (oral/nasal)
Neonate	2–4kg	2.5–3.5	8–9cm/11 cm
1–6months	4–6kg	3.5–4	10cm/12 cm
1 year	6–10kg	3.5–4	11–12cm/14cm
1–3 years	10–15kg	4–4.5	13–14cm/16cm
4–6 years	15–20kg	4.5–5.5	14–15cm/19 cm
7–10 years	25–35 kg	5.5–6	16–17cm/21 cm

ETT size = (age in years/4) + 4

ETT length oral = (age in years/2) + 12cm

ETT length nasal = (age in years/2) + 15cm

These formulae are suitable for estimates between ages 2 and 10 years

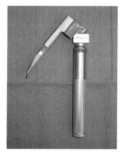

Fig. 20.14 A straight-blade laryngoscope is used in infants under six months old. It is less bulky in the infant mouth and is used to lift the epiglottis so that a clearer view of the glottis is achieved.

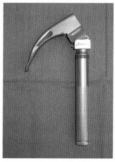

Fig. 20.15 The curved blade laryngoscope is used in the older infant and child. It compresses the tongue into the mandibular space, thus allowing a clearer view of the glottis. Examples include the Mackintosh blade.

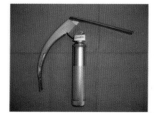

Fig. 20.16 The paediatric McCoy blade is a levering laryngoscope with an angulated tip that can help lift the larger epiglottis upwards in a less forceful action than that of the curved blade laryngoscope.

✚ Securing the endotracheal tube

Once *in situ*, the ETT must be firmly secured. Accidental extubation may be more likely in the lighter, more mobile paediatric patient and in the absence of a cuffed tube. Most centres secure the ETT with tapes rather than conventional ties. This reduces movement of the tube and lessens the risk of trauma to the airway, endobronchial intubation and accidental extubation.

A tie (e.g. 1/0 braid) may be tied to the ETT, thus allowing easier application of the tapes. The tapes are cut in a 'trouser leg' fashion, with one leg anchored to the upper or lower lip whilst the other is adherent to the tube. Two sets of tape are applied on either side of the tube to minimize traction in either direction (Figure 20.17). An oropharyngeal airway may be inserted to stabilize the tube but this practice varies between anaesthetists

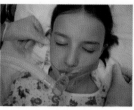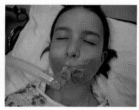

Fig. 20.17 Securing the endotracheal tube.

→ Sizes of conventional LMAs in paediatric practice

Size	Weight	Max. cuff volume
1	Neonate <5kg	4ml
1.5	Infant 5–10kg	7ml
2	Child 10–20kg	10ml
2.5	Child 20–30kg	14ml
3	Child 30–50kg	20ml

→ The Mapleson F circuit

The adaptation of the adult system, made by Ayre in the 1930s, resulted in the production of a paediatric breathing circuit, known as the 'Ayre's T-piece'. It consists of a system with no valves and a fresh gas oxygen flow which is delivered close to the patient. This was modified in the 1950s by Jackson Rees. An open-ended reservoir bag was added to a lengthened limb of tubing. The reservoir bag permits respiration to be observed or assisted. The lengthened arm of tubing reduces entrainment of air, particularly during spontaneous ventilation. Ventilatory assistance can be provided either by delivering PEEP or by controlling actual ventilation. This also permits the anaesthetist to determine lung compliance.

This circuit became known as the Mapleson F circuit. During spontaneous ventilation, fresh gas flow should be 2–3× alveolar minute volume. End-tidal CO_2 should be monitored as close as possible to the patient and flow adjusted accordingly. Scavenging was initially difficult with this circuit because of its open-ended bag. However, recent attachments have been produced with a closed bag, a valve, and a port for scavenging.

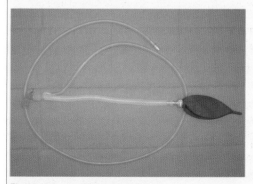

Fig. 20.18 Photo of Mapteson F Circuit.

The management of postoperative pain in children has significantly improved over the past decade. This has come about through the acknowledgement that the service was inadequate and that children were suffering inappropriately. This has led to a reorganization of pain services offered to children in the perioperative period.

As in the adult population, pain in children should be adequately assessed, and this should be appropriate to the child's age and development. The spectrum of ages, and therefore responses to pain, in the paediatric population makes this a more difficult task.

A number of tools have been validated for pain assessment. These are centred on the infant or child's age and development and encompass behavioural and physiological responses to pain. As a child develops it becomes easier to assess the nature and intensity of pain. In addition, the diversity of scoring systems increases, providing the observer with a number of additional tools to use.

It must not be forgotten that parents or carers may quite accurately assess pain, without the use of tools, and that their reports of pain should not be ignored.

Paediatric drug handling

Management of pain in the paediatric population is based on similar principles to that of the adult. Multimodal techniques are recommended to provide balanced analgesia. These techniques combine general and local or regional anaesthesia. However, as in assessment of pain, the challenge of managing pain is complicated by the diversity of ages and stages of development.

Organ development is significant over the first year of life. However, this is an ongoing process throughout childhood and one cannot assume that drugs can just be administered by weight in an adult fashion. Attention must be paid to age-appropriate recommended dose. Restrictions also exist on specific drug usage.

General pharmacokinetic principles of drug distribution apply in infants and children when considering molecule size, degree of ionization, and lipid solubility. However, other factors such as regional blood flow, body compartment size, permeability of barriers such as the blood–brain barrier and subsequent protein binding are less predictable in this population. This results in variable drug prescription regimes.

The elimination of drugs will also be affected by stage of organ development.

- At birth, the GFR is only about 10% of that in the adult. Tubular function is similarly reduced. GFR reaches adult proportions for size by the end of the first year, and tubular function matures similarly in the same period.
- Hepatic function is also reduced, largely as a consequence of immature cytochrome systems and reduced conjugation reactions. These reach levels of adult maturity for age after the first 2 years, but are not entirely static throughout childhood.

It must not be forgotten that this discussion of organ function applies to the healthy neonate and child. Disease alters organ function further, especially if acidosis, hypovolaemia, hypoxia, or hypothermia are present.

Common drugs used in paediatric practice

Analgesics commonly used in paediatric practice include paracetamol, ibuprofen, and codeine. In more severe cases morphine, either orally or via patient-controlled analgesia (PCA) or nurse-controlled analgesia (NCA), is used. Generally speaking, drugs are given orally (PO) where possible, but the rectal route (PR) or intravenous route (IV) are utilized where the oral route is not possible or when under anaesthetic. Drugs are rarely given intramuscularly in the awake conscious child. The most commonly used drugs, their dosage, and intervals of administration are shown in Tables 20.2, 20.3, 20.4, and 20.5.

Morphine for PCA/NCA

Every centre will have its own opioid infusion criteria and it is absolutely essential that protocols are adhered to, in the interests of child safety.

PCA pumps are generally appropriate in any child over the age of 5 who is capable of understanding their use. However, pain, hospitalization, and illness may interfere with the child's ability to manage a PCA pump.

NCA pumps are reserved for those under the age of 5 years, those who have had surgery affecting their ability to use the pump, and those with learning difficulties.

In the child over 50kg, adult PCA and NCA protocols are followed, according to local policy. Separate protocols also exist for neonates and infants <5kg. Subcutaneous infusions for PCA and NCA are also used in specialist centres.

Example of a morphine PCA protocol

- Adequate loading dose is essential prior to commencing PCA.
- Infusion concentration of 1mg/kg morphine in 50ml 5% dextrose or normal saline is prescribed in any child up to 50kg. Maximum concentration 50mg in 50ml.
- The above dilution produces a solution where 1ml = 20mcg/kg.
- Loading dose is generally 2.5–5 ml (50–100mcg/kg) of the above solution.
- Background infusion is generally 0.4ml/hr of the above solution.
- Bolus dose is 0.5–1 ml (10–20mcg/kg).
- Lockout is 5min.
- Maximum dose in 4hr is limited to 20ml.
- Naloxone and anti-emetics are co-prescribed (see below).
- Appropriate patient assessment for pain, sedation, respiratory depression, nausea, vomiting, pruritus, and urinary retention are an absolute requirement. All centres will have standardized protocols to monitor for these side effects.

Example of a morphine NCA protocol

- Adequate loading dose is essential prior to commencing NCA.
- Infusion concentration of 1mg/kg morphine in 50ml 5% dextrose or normal saline is prescribed in any child up to 50kg. Maximum concentration 50mg in 50 ml.
- The above dilution produces a solution where 1ml = 20mcg/kg.
- Loading dose is generally 2.5–5 ml (50–100mcg/kg) of the above solution.
- Background infusion is generally 0.5–1ml/hr of the above solution.
- Bolus dose is 0.5–1 ml (10–20mcg/kg).
- Lockout is 20–30min.
- Maximum dose in 4hr is limited to 20ml.
- Naloxone and anti-emetics are co-prescribed.

Appropriate patient assessment for pain, sedation, respiratory depression, nausea, vomiting, pruritus, and urinary retention are an absolute requirement. All centres will have standardized protocols to monitor for these side effects.

➔ Table 20.2 Dosage (excluding neonates) for paracetamol

Age	Dose	Interval	Maximum dose
1–3months	20mg/kg	8hr	60mg/kg/day
>3months	20mg/kg	6hr	90mg/kg/day
PR loading			
1–3months	30mg/kg		
>3months	40mg/kg		
IV infusion over 15min			
<10kg	Under review		
10–50kg	15mg/kg	6hr	60mg/kg/day
>50kg	1g	6hr	

Note: Duration at maximum dose of paracetamol is 48 hr in 0–3 month age group and 72 hr in >3 month age group.

➔ Table 20.3 Maintenance dosage for NSAIDs

Age	Dose	Interval	Maximum daily
Ibuprofen PO			
>1 months & >5kg	5mg/kg	6hr	30mg/kg
>7 years	5mg/kg	6–8hr	2.4g/day
Diclofenac PO/PR			
>6 months	1mg/kg	8hr	150mg
*Diclofenac IV**			
2–18 years	0.3–1mg/kg	12hr	150mg

*IV route not licensed in children. If administered, review at 48hr.

➔ Table 20.4 Maintenance dosage for opioids*

Age	Dose	Interval	Maximum daily
Codeine PO/PR/IM			
1 month–12 years	1mg/kg	4–6hr	240mg
>12 years	30–60mg	4–6hr	240mg
Morphine PO			
<1 year	80mcg/kg	4hr	
>1 year	200–400mcg/kg	4hr	
Morphine IV			
>1 month	100mcg/kg	4–6hr	
Fentanyl IV			
0–12 years	1–5mcg/kg, then 1mcg/kg as required		
>12 years	50–200mcg, then 50mcg as required		

*BNF recommended doses. Local policy may permit higher/more frequent doses.

➔ Table 20.5 Anti-emetics used in paediatric anaesthesia

Ondansetron	PO/IV	Dose: 0.15mg/kg 8 hourly Max: 12mg/day
Dexamethasone	PO/IV	Dose: 0.15mg/kg 8 hourly

Ondansetron and dexamethasone can be given in combination to higher-risk patients. There is no evidence to support the use of cyclizine in prevention of postoperative nausea and vomiting (APA 2008)

Anaesthesia for ENT and dental procedures

Anaesthesia for ENT surgery encompasses a wide spectrum of procedures. Points of note include the following.

Preoperative assessment

- There may be history of hearing loss, chronic nasal obstruction, or obstructive sleep apnoea (OSA.). It is imperative to check for a history of snoring, apnoea, cyanosis, or daytime somnolence and for evidence of right heart strain. Has a sleep study has been performed? Is a postoperative HDU bed required?
- The child may require a sedative premedication. If there is a history of OSA this should be discussed with an experienced anaesthetist.
- Analgesia premedication may be prescribed for procedures such as adenotonsillectomy (e.g. paracetamol 20mg/kg to a maximum of 1g).
- If there is an associated syndrome this should be addressed with a senior anaesthetist. Management may be required in a tertiary referral centre.

Anaesthesia

- Is a topical nasal vasoconstrictor required?
- Is the child having a gas induction or IV induction?
- Preparation of LMA, or appropriate endotracheal tube, conducive to a shared airway.
- Should topical local anaesthesia be applied to the vocal cords? If so, this should be communicated to recovery staff so that adequate recovery time is allowed prior to drinking.
- Throat packs may be required to prevent airway contamination, especially with nasal procedures.
- Specific positioning in theatre may be required, such as extension of shoulders and neck for adenotonsillectomy.
- Particular attention must be paid with initial instrumentation of the airway, such as insertion of Boyle's gag, as the airway may obstruct at this time. Close observation of chest movement and capnograph are important to detect obstruction early.
- Discuss local anaesthetic infiltration with the surgeon.
- Anti-emetics should always be considered in ENT procedures. Dexamethasone can be utilized as both an anti-emetic and an anti-inflammatory agent.
- Avoid coughing or straining on extubation. Deep extubation may be considered by an experienced anaesthetist.
- Suction of the airway should be performed when the child is under deep anaesthesia. This permits direct visualization of the airway and permits clearance of secretions and blood, especially from the post-nasal space. These can otherwise cause life-threatening laryngospasm. Consider left lateral head down position, to encourage drainage of secretions away from the larynx.

Postoperative care

- Transfer to recovery for appropriate paediatric recovery care.
- Early postoperative bleeding may be a problem. This may manifest itself in a number of ways:
  - Visible bleeding
  - Excess swallowing
  - Vomiting blood
  - Cardiovascular instability.
- The anaesthetist and surgeon must be called immediately if haemorrhage suspected.

Laryngospasm may present during any anaesthesia, but particular risk exists in paediatric anaesthesia especially in association with ENT/airway surgery. It is imperative that laryngospasm is identified and managed immediately (Section 25.4).

Anaesthesia for emergency ENT procedures

Postoperative bleeding following tonsillectomy

Bleeding following tonsillectomy can be immediate or late. Blood loss can be extensive and easily underestimated as much of it may be swallowed. Senior help must be called and initial attention paid to airway, breathing, and circulation. Resuscitation must be commenced in a safe environment before further anaesthesia. The key problems include:

- Hypovolaemia
- Recent anaesthesia in some situations
- Potentially difficult laryngoscopy
- Aspiration risk from blood and full stomach
- Parental and child anxiety.

Anaesthesia can be inhalational or intravenous. Inhalational induction in this situation has been traditionally taught in the left lateral head-down position. This permits blood to drain away from the airway whilst maintaining spontaneous respiration. However, it is an unfamiliar technique to many anaesthetists, and if obstruction occurs the child may lighten and develop laryngospasm.

Rapid sequence induction is a more familiar technique for the trainee anaesthetist and enables early intubation of the airway. However, if the airway is occluded with blood it may be impossible to view the glottis. This risks failure of intubation in an apnoeic patient, and/or aspiration.

Prior to awake extubation the stomach should be emptied. The Hb should be checked, and rechecked in the postoperative period.

Foreign body inhalation

Inhalation of a foreign body may result in partial or complete airway obstruction. In complete obstruction there should be immediate management of airway, breathing, and circulation with a senior anaesthetist and surgeon summoned immediately.

Anaesthesia for partial obstruction of the upper airway is generally performed using an inhalational technique. This keeps the child spontaneously breathing and prevents impaction of the object further into the airway.

Anaesthesia for obstruction of the lower respiratory tract may involve muscle relaxation and rigid bronchoscopy with use of jet ventilation. Dexamethasone is generally administered. Anaesthesia for airway obstruction is generally performed in specialist paediatric centres, unless the patient's condition warrants immediate management in the local centre.

Anaesthesia for general surgery

Anaesthesia for general paediatric surgery such as pyloric stenosis and intussusception is most frequently carried out in specialist hospitals.

Appendicectomy

Appendicitis is a common occurence and the child often presents acutely unwell. Perforation of the viscus mandates immediate surgery, but only following prompt adequate resuscitation.

Airway, breathing, and circulation should be assessed and abnormalities treated. Oxygen may be required, but IV access must be established and fluid administered in order to maintain perfusion and urine output. Antibiotics should be given.

The child will require a rapid sequence induction. An explanation of the sequence of events will be required for the child and its parents. Once intubated, a nasogastric tube may be passed to empty the stomach. This can be removed at the end of the procedure. Analgesia should be administered in a weight-appropriate dosage. Fentanyl is given after induction, and paracetamol and morphine intraoperatively. Local anaesthetic infiltration of the wound may be performed by the surgeon. A PCA/NCA may be required postoperatively.

Anaesthesia for trauma

The child requiring anaesthesia for emergency trauma presents with a variety of issues. Initial mangement consists of he primary survey and treatment of life-threatening injuries. This follows the "ABCDE" approach described in Chapter 23. Cervical spine protection must not be forgotten. The anaesthetist needs to ascertain a number of important factors:

- History of injury and associated injuries
- Time of last meal in relation to time of trauma and therefore duration of fasting
- Presence of pain, nausea, and vomiting
- Administration of opiates

The anaesthetic technique is based on the above findings. If a risk of aspiration exists, the child should be anaesthetized using rapid sequence induction. Analgesia can be regional, systemic, or a combination of both, depending on the site of injury. Fluids will be required if fasting has been prolonged or if resuscitation is necessary.

Regional anaesthesia is a commonly used technique in paediatric anaesthesia. It is rarely used in isolation but as part of a multimodal technique and is usually performed under general anaesthesia. Once established, it permits lighter anaesthesia to be maintained and provides effective early postoperative analgesia. During the early postoperative period other forms of analgesia can be introduced before the effects of the regional block have worn off. It is a useful technique for day surgery as it permits early discharge without the effects of excessive opiate use.

Some of the most commonly used techniques are caudal anaesthesia, ilio-inguinal blockade, and penile blockade. Paediatric epidural anaesthesia is generally performed in specialist centres.

When regional anaesthesia is conducted in adult practice, it is recommended that this is done in an appropriately safe environment. Safety is of paramount importance in the neonatal and paediatric population. There is a significant risk of intravascular or subarachnoid injection in the smaller child as the distance between structures is shorter. Therefore regional techniques should be performed in an environment where the child is fully monitored and has IV access *in situ*. The anaesthetist should have a skilled assistant available and there should be adequate resuscitation facilities.

The subject of regional anaesthesia is a huge topic. Within the context of paediatric anaesthesia, we will discuss the techniques of caudal epidural anaesthesia, ilio-inguinal blockade, and penile blockade.

Caudal epidural anaesthesia

The caudal epidural space is accessible in the infant and child via the sacral hiatus, where there is incomplete fusion of the fifth sacral vertebra. This hiatus reduces in size with age and may be completely inaccessible in adulthood. In the infant and child it consists mainly of loose fatty tissue, which permits spread of local anaesthetic.

Caudal anaesthesia is useful in surgery of the lower abdomen, lower limbs, penis, and scrotum. Contraindications to regional anaesthesia are similar to those in adult practice. In addition, the paediatric anaesthetist may come across an infant with a congenital abnormality of the sacrum or spinal canal where such techniques may be contra-indicated.

Technique
- The child should be fully monitored with IV access in safe environment with adequate resuscitation facilities.
- Position in left lateral position with hips and knees flexed.
- Use an aseptic technique.
- Locate the sacral hiatus by one of three techniques:
  - Palpation of the depression between the sacral cornua.
  - Drawing an imaginary line between the posterior superior iliac spines. This forms the base of an equilateral triangle pointing inferiorly, whose apex overlies the sacral hiatus.
  - Drawing an imaginary line along the midline of the femur, with the hips in 90° degree flexion. This line will cross over the sacral hiatus.

An IV cannula rather than a needle is recommended to prevent damage to nearby structures such as dura, blood vessels, bone, and spinal cord. A cannula gives the anaesthetist a more definite 'pop' as it passes through the sacrococcygeal membrane. It can be advanced over the needle and will only feed in easily if it is within the extradural space. The needle should never be advanced into the space with the cannula.

The cannula is passed via the skin and sacrococcygeal membrane at an angle of 45°. Once in the extradural space it is advanced along the line of the vertebrae at approximately 15°.

Once *in situ* the needle is completely removed. Observation is made for blood or CSF. Injection should be smooth and easy. Negative aspiration should be ensured prior to and throughout injection

Bupivicaine 0.125–0.25% is generally used, although this varies between centres. Again, several techniques can be used to calculate the concentration of anaesthetic to be used. A system known as the Armitage technique for caudal anaesthesia is outlined opposite. It is described for bupivicaine 0.25%. However, similar analgesia can be gained from bupivicaine 0.125%, with less motor block.

The onset of analgesia with plain bupivicaine is around 15min with a duration of 4–5hr. The duration of analgesia can be prolonged by co-administration of other agents such as ketamine or clonidine. This is reserved for those experienced in their use.

Complications of caudal epidural anaesthesia are rare, but are similar to those experienced in adult epidural anaesthesia. However, additional complications include intra-osseous injection, which is similar to IV injection, and potential penetration of the soft cartilaginous sacrum, with visceral injury.

Penile block

The nerve supply to the penis includes two dorsal nerves, the ilio-inguinal nerves and the genito-femoral nerves. Again, several techniques can be used. Described below is blockade of the subpubic space, appropriate for circumcision and distal hypospadias repair.

Technique
- The child should be fully monitored with IV access in safe environment with adequate resuscitation facilities.
- Position supine.
- Use an aseptic technique.
- A short bevelled regional block needle should be inserted almost perpendicular to the skin at a slight caudal and medial slope, 0.5–1cm lateral to the symphysis pubis and immediately below the inferior ramus of the pubic bone. Two 'pops' are felt as the needle tip penetrates the superficial and Scarpa's fascia. The needle should now be within the subpubic space.
- After aspiration, 0.1ml/kg of either 0.25% or 0.5% bupivicaine is injected, up to a maximum of 5ml each side. This is repeated on the opposite side.
- Vasoconstrictors should never be used.

Nerve block for inguinal hernia repair and orchidopexy

Several variations of this technique have been described. The aim is to provide blockade of the ilio-inguinal, ilio-hypogastric, and genito-femoral nerves.

Technique
- The child should be fully monitored with IV access in safe environment with adequate resuscitation facilities.
- Position supine.
- Use an aseptic technique.
- A short bevelled regional block needle should be inserted, one finger's breadth (child's finger) medial to the anterior superior iliac spine at right angles to the skin. A 'pop' is felt as the needle pierces the aponeurosis of the external oblique. Inject 0.75ml/kg of 0.25% bupivicaine above and below the aponeurosis as the needle is withdrawn to the skin.
- The above technique blocks the ilio-inguinal and ilio-hypogastric nerves.
- To block the genital branch of the genito-femoral nerve, insert 1–2ml of 0.25% bupivicaine adjacent to the pubic tubercle above the inguinal ligament.
- Femoral nerve block may occur.

> **Armitage regime for caudal anaesthesia using 0.25% bupivicaine**

Segmental level	Dose
Lumbo-sacral	0.5ml/kg
Thoraco-lumbar	1.0ml/kg
Mid-thoracic	1.25ml/kg

Mid-thoracic block using caudal epidural technique is rarely performed.

Early recognition and prompt treatment of the critically ill child is essential to try to prevent cardiac arrest. Cardiac arrest has a very poor prognosis, particularly if out of hospital. Most children die, and the survivors usually have significant neurological disability.

Aetiology

Children rarely have a sudden cardiorespiratory arrest. Most are secondary to hypoxia and acidosis caused by respiratory pathology (e.g. airway obstruction, infection, or asthma) or neurological pathology (e.g. trauma, infection, epilepsy, or drug overdose). The remainder are due to circulatory failure (shock) caused by fluid or blood loss (e.g. gastroenteritis, burns, or trauma) or fluid maldistribution (e.g. sepsis, anaphylaxis or cardiac failure).

Organization

Resuscitation areas must be fully equipped and checked on a daily basis. All hospital staff (medical and nursing) working with children should be trained in paediatric life support. Regular scenari o training is useful.

Senior help from the multidisciplinary team must be sought early. A structured approach must be adhered to. It ensures better teamwork and less panic.

Primary assessment and resuscitation

Knowledge of normal respiratory and cardiovascular values for age (Section 20.2) is fundamental to being able to recognize the sick child at an early stage. Rapid assessment of ABCDE should identify any life-threatening conditions and these should be treated immediately. The ABCDE approach allows treatment of the most time-sensitive problems first.

If the child is noted to be unresponsive, basic life support and, if appropriate, advanced life support must be commenced without delay (see opposite).

Monitor the child. If unable to weigh the child, estimate their weight in kilograms by the use of a Broselow tape or, if the age is known, use the formula:

weight (kg) = (3 x age) + 7.

Rapid clinical assessment

Airway
Check for signs of airway obstruction and the presence of stridor

Therapy
- Immobilize the cervical spine when trauma is suspected.
- Suction secretions or blood found in the airway.
- Remove foreign bodies but do NOT attempt a blind finger sweep.
- Basic airway manoeuvres may relieve obstruction: head tilt–chin lift (not in trauma) or jaw thrust.
- Airway adjuncts may be required to maintain airway patency.
- All critically ill children require high-flow oxygen (15L/min flow) regardless of the cause of their illness.

Breathing
Assess the work of breathing, respiratory rate, and pattern.

Percuss and ausculate the chest and check for wheeze.

Note the skin colour, and monitor oxygen saturations.

Therapy
- If breathing is adequate, oxygen can be delivered via a reservoir mask.
- Frequent reassessment must be made.
- If breathing is inadequate, ventilation must be assisted with bag and mask until a definitive airway is placed. Mechanical ventilation will be required.
- Life-threatening respiratory pathology must be immediately recognized and treated (e.g. tension pneumothorax, status asthmaticus).

Circulation
Assess heart rate, pulse volume, capillary refill, and skin temperature in order to judge cardiovascular efficiency.

Therapy
- Commence cardiopulmonary resuscitation if there is no pulse, or a pulse less than 60 beats/min with poor perfusion.
- Vascular access must be obtained in the shocked child. An intra-osseus (IO) needle should be used in the arrested child and seriously considered in the critically ill child without IV access.
- Blood should be taken for U&Es, FBC, glucose, blood gases, cross-matching, and blood cultures as appropriate.
- 0.9% saline, Hartmann's, or occasionally colloids may be used for fluid resuscitation. A 20ml/kg rapid bolus (10ml/kg in trauma) is followed by reassessment, and further 20ml/kg boluses (10ml/kg in trauma) as clinically indicated. Trauma patients will require blood after a total of 40ml/kg of crystalloid.
- Adrenaline 10μl/kg (0.1ml/kg 1:10000 adrenaline) IV/IO is given for all arrest rhythms for the first and subsequent doses. High-dose adrenaline of 100μl/kg is now not recommended routinely.

Disability
Assess the conscious level (AVPU) posture, pupils, and blood glucose

Therapy
Remember that A, B or C problems might reduce conscious level.

Decreased conscious level to P or U may require intubation.

Treat hypoglycaemia

Treat prolonged or recurrent fits

Exposure
Examine for signs of injury or skin rash. Check the temperature.

Performance of resuscitation

For resuscitation purposes, an infant is a child under 1 year and a child is between 1 year and puberty. Adult guidelines apply thereafter. Paediatric basic and advanced life support algorithms are shown in Figures 20.19 and 20.20

Initial ventilation will be by bag and mask. Prompt intubation by an experienced operator controls the airway and enables continuous chest compressions.

Pulse check is performed at the brachial artery in the infant and the carotid artery in the child.

The chest should be compressed at the lower third of the sternum, one finger breadth above the xiphisternum, by approximately one-third of depth of the chest. Use 2 fingers or the encircling technique for an infant, or 1 or 2 hands for a child, to achieve appropriate depth of compression at a rate of 100/min. Compression to ventilation ratio 15:2. Chest compressions and ventilation should only be interrupted for defibrillation.

Following primary assessment and resuscitation

After successful primary assessment and resuscitation the child must have a thorough secondary assessment.

This should include history, examination with full exposure, looking particularly for rashes and injuries, appropriate investigations, and radiological imaging.

All intubated children must have an orogastric tube, and the position of the ETT confirmed radiologically.

All major trauma cases should have imaging of the chest, abdomen, pelvis, head and neck as appropriate to their injuries.

The child will be assessed for ongoing dependency, and prompt discussion with the local tertiary referral centre or children's transport team may be required.

514

Paediatric Basic Life Support

(Healthcare professionals
with a duty to respond)

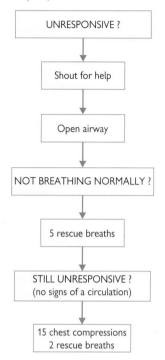

After 1 minute call resuscitation team then continue CPR

Fig. 20.19

Paediatric Advanced Life Support

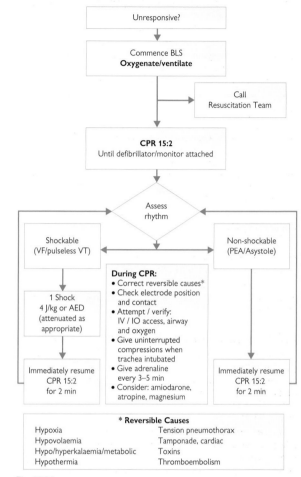

Fig. 20.20

Chapter 21

Geriatric anaesthesia

517

The ageing of the world population has huge implications for anaesthetic practice. More elderly people are presenting for surgery than ever before.

Definitions and terms

Ageing refers to time-dependent post-maturity changes which take place at a cellular level. These changes are progressive and lead to a decline in physiological reserve and functioning. Ultimately, ageing leads to death.

Demographically, three groups of aged people have been described: young-old, aged 65–74 years; mid-old, aged 75–84 years; oldest-old, aged 85 and over. However, this classification does little to stratify risk, and may in fact be seen to promote ageism. To a great extent, 'biological' and 'chronological' age can be distinguished. There is individual variation in the rate at which people age, and disease and environmental factors contribute, accelerating degenerative change. As such, the words 'elderly' 'aged', 'geriatric', etc. are inadequate generalizations.

Physiological changes in the elderly

Respiratory

There is a decline in cartilaginous and muscular support for structures in the upper airway. This may result in collapse of the nares and pharynx during sleep and anaesthesia, and result in airway obstruction. The tendency of the elderly face to 'fall away' from the mask may make hand ventilation more difficult. This effect is exacerbated in edentulous patients.

The elderly lung is less well protected than in earlier life. The upper airway reflexes are preserved, but are less sensitive. They may be affected by degenerative neurological or muscular disease (e.g. Parkinson's disease). Ciliary clearance of secretions is slowed, and the cough may be weakened. A decline in immune function also occurs.

Structural elements in the tracheobronchial tree deteriorate with age. The trachea dilates slightly, leading to an increase in dead space (usually insignificant). Compliance is increased, and this may result in compression and closure of small airways during expiration, leading to air trapping and an increased residual volume. The closing volume of the lung is equal to the supine FRC at age 44 years, and the erect FRC at age 66 years.

The ratio of lung to body weight is preserved in the elderly, and so is the number of alveoli in the healthy aged patient. However, ductectasia (dilatation of small airways and respiratory ducts) occurs with time, increasing dead space slightly and flattening the alveoli so that their surface area is reduced (by ~15% at age 70). The mechanism is thought to be cumulative damage from environmental free radicals; the overall effect is of a mild emphysematous state.

The total lung capacity is usually preserved. Vital capacity decreases. Residual volume and FRC increase due to ductectasia (increased closing volume and air trapping), reduced elastic recoil and respiratory muscle force, and a stiffer chest wall.

Respiratory mechanics is significantly altered in the elderly. There is progressive weakening of respiratory muscles (by 15–35%). Muscle mass and innervation are both reduced, and the contraction–relaxation cycle is slowed as the sarcoplasmic reticulum calcium pump becomes impaired. The functional residual capacity increases, and so the rest length of the inspiratory muscles is decreased; this puts them at a mechanical disadvantage. Malnutrition also contributes, if present. Predictably, FVC and FEV_1 are reduced. With increasing age there is a progressive deterioration in lung function (Figure 21.2a).

There is a reduction in the volume of the capillary bed, and pulmonary vascular resistance increases by as much as 80%. Pulmonary artery pressure increases by up to 30%, but capillary wedge pressure is unaltered if the left heart remains healthy.

Gas exchange worsens with age. There is a loss of functional alveolar/capillary surface area and diffusing capacity. V/Q mismatch results from small airways closure and relatively better ventilation at the apices. Arterial PO_2 is reduced in the elderly, but P_aCO_2 remains constant as CO_2 production tends to decline.

Cardiovascular

Heart The cardiac mass and left ventricular (LV) wall thickness gradually increase with age. Increased collagen and fibrous tissue deposition impair compliance and early LV diastolic filling (diastolic filling may be further reduced with tachycardia, which is poorly tolerated in this age group; Figure 21.3). Preload is increased, and this maintains stroke volume and cardiac output; but overall the heart functions on the flatter part of the Starling curve (Section 10.7) and so there is both less cardiac output reserve and less response to positive inotropes. This is exacerbated by a downregulation of β-adrenoceptors in the face of increased basal sympathetic activity. The system is very sensitive to the effects of anaesthesia, and reduction in cardiac output may be profound. Both systolic and diastolic pressures increase with age (Figure 21.2b).

Peak contractile force is maintained, but prolonged contraction results from impairment of calcium pumps within the sarcoplasmic reticulum.

There is calcific and fibrotic degeneration of conducting pathways, leading to an increased propensity to arrhythmias. Atrial fibrillation is particularly common (affecting 10% of the over-80s). The intrinsic sinus rate (without autonomic influence) is significantly slowed, but overall heart rate is preserved by sympathetic tone (or only slightly reduced).

Valves gradually calcify, thicken, and dilate: mild mitral regurgitation is a common finding.

Vessels Gradual calcification and intimal thickening (exacerbated by atherosclerotic change) in vessels reduces both compliance and elastance (Figure 21.1). The mean arterial pressure is preserved, but the pulse pressure widens. Degenerative changes in the coronary vessels reduce the maximum coronary arterial flow, even in healthy aged hearts. Atherosclerotic change compounds this deterioration.

Baroreceptors in the aortic arch and carotid sinuses become less sensitive, reducing the reflex adaptations to hypotension. This may be particularly noticeable on induction of anaesthesia, when severe or prolonged hypotension is common.

→ **Theories of ageing**

These can be divided into adaptive and non-adaptive theories.

Adaptive theories propose that ageing and death serve the evolutionary needs of the species as a whole, reducing demand on resources and allowing new evolving individuals to flourish.

Non-adaptive theories suggest that ageing is a sign of an imperfect organism which deteriorates over time under environmental stress. It has no evolutionary function.

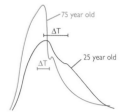

Fig. 21.1 The arterial waveform in the carotid of a 25-year-old compared with that of a 75-year-old. The older patient has:
–higher systolic pressure
–↑ aortic stiffness resulting in ↑ pulse wave velocity
–A reduced time between systolic and diastolic peak pressures (ΔT)

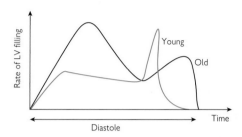

Fig. 21.3 Left ventricular filling with increasing age. The initial peak is due to passive filling but the 2nd peak is due to atrial contraction. The stiffer LV of increasing age accounts for its steeper gradient.

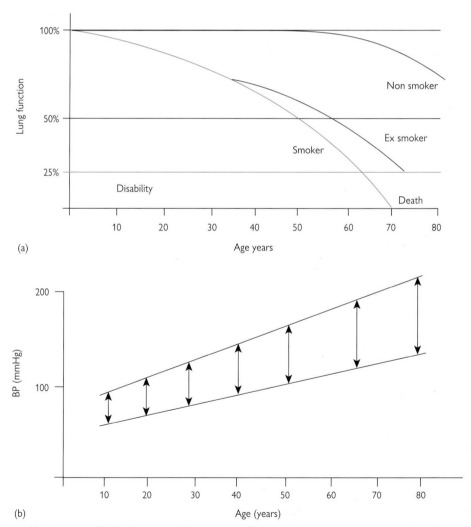

(a)

(b)

Fig. 21.2 Changes in (a) spirometry and (b) blood pressure with increasing age. The expected decline in lung function is worsened by smoking. Giving up reduces the deterioration rate to match that of a non-smoker.

Neurological

Brain There is shrinkage of cortical grey matter but little overall loss of cells. There may be fewer synapses, and a decrease in neurotransmitter concentrations has been demonstrated in animal studies. The white matter volume is well preserved, but myelin sheaths deteriorate, reducing conduction velocity.

Cerebral blood flow decreases, but so does cerebral oxygen demand; autoregulation is well preserved in the healthy ageing brain. However, the incidence of degenerative vascular changes does increase.

The CSF volume increases as the brain atrophies, without a rise in CSF pressure.

Spinal cord

The ageing spinal cord undergoes loss of neurons and reactive gliosis. There is an overall reduction in volume in the spinal cord. This occurs particularly in the ventral horn, thoracic intermediate grey matter, and cervical dorsal columns. The incidence of cervical spondylosis increases with age, and cause myelopathy.

Peripheral nerves

Myelin sheaths degenerate with age, and so conduction velocity in myelinated nerves reduces (by up to 30% in large motor fibres). Some reduction in sensation *or* motor power in the feet is normal in the elderly, and ankle reflexes may be attenuated.

Autonomic nerves

The basal activity of the sympathetic nervous system increases, affecting skeletal muscle and the gut. There is also reduced re-uptake of catecholamines (affecting cardiac nerves), which induces downregulation of adrenoceptors in many organs. Adrenal secretion is reduced overall. The parasympathetic nervous system declines in activity with age. This causes an attenuation of the sinus arrhythmia seen with respiration and reduced response to Valsalva manoeuvres, and contributes to orthostatic hypotension.

Functional impairments may include memory and intellect impairment (40% of over-60s demonstrate impaired memory, but this is by no means universal or inevitable), sleep disorders, impaired hearing and vision, and disturbances of gait, balance, and reflexes.

Renal and fluids

There is a progressive loss of nephrons as the kidney ages, with renal cortical mass reducing by 30%. Distal nephrons form diverticuli, which may become cystic. Cortical bloodflow and GFR are also reduced. This results in reduced creatinine clearance, but serum creatinine remains roughly constant as muscle mass declines. Therefore serum creatinine is a poor measure of renal function in the elderly. Urinary drug clearance is impaired.

Sodium, potassium, and hydrogen ion concentrations in serum tend to remain fairly constant. However, homeostasis may be severely impaired, and the elderly are susceptible to severe electrolyte and water imbalances in the face of illness and IV administration. Nephrotoxic drugs may cause acute decompensation of renal function.

As there are fewer nephrons, the salt load per nephron is greater, and sodium tends to be lost. This is compounded by poor dietary intake and a diminished thirst response. However, the ability to excrete a salt load is also reduced because of deterioration of the counter-current mechanism in the loop of Henle and impaired urinary concentrating ability. Free-water handling is similarly deranged.

There is reduced renin secretion, and this leads to relative angiotensin II and aldosterone deficiency. As well as further reducing urinary concentrating ability, this tends to cause potassium retention, which may be compounded by the use of ACE inhibitors. Elderly kidneys are slow to excrete acid loads, which tends to cause a shift of potassium out of cells.

Problems with continence may result in self-imposed fluid restriction and dehydration.

Gastrointestinal, hepatic, and nutritional

The liver atrophies, and a reduction in size is demonstrable by age 60. Splanchnic and hepatic blood flow decrease. Although there is no change in serum levels of transaminases, alkaline phosphatase, and bilirubin, dynamic function tests (e.g. caffeine clearance) indicate impairments in function.

α_1 acid glycoprotein concentrations rise and albumin concentration falls. This may have implications for the pharmokinetics of drugs administered by single IV bolus. However, it does not affect the pharmacokinetics of more regular medications, as alterations in the plasma free portion are counterbalanced by changes in clearance, establishing a new equilibrium.

Malnutrition is common in the elderly, reflecting decreased appetite, and sometimes difficulties with shopping and cooking.

Endocrine

Glucose homeostasis deteriorates with age, such that 25% of the over-80s are diabetic. There is both dysregulation of insulin secretion and peripheral insulin resistance. Diabetic end-organ damage accumulates with age and may be pronounced in the elderly.

Thyroid function is fairly well preserved, but subclinical derangements are common. There is a reduced clearance of thyroid hormones from the circulation, but this is balanced by reduced secretion.

Thermoregulation

The normal body temperature of elderly patients may be lower than younger individuals, by up to 1°C.

The shivering and vasoconstriction responses to hypothermia are both impaired. Shivering occurs at an average core temperature of 35.2°C in the elderly, compared with 36.1°C in younger patients. Because of reduced muscle bulk, shivering is also less likely to be effective, despite increasing oxygen demand. Shivering (which occurs in the periphery) may paradoxically increase heat loss by causing local vasodilatation and drawing warm blood away from the core.

The febrile response is also blunted in elderly patients. In contrast with younger patients and children, who may become febrile from relatively minor illness, fever in the elderly is almost always a sign of serious infection.

Musculoskeletal and skin

Osteoporosis is common in the elderly. Bone mass declines with age, and bone cortices become thinner, with a reduction in new bone formation and osteoblast activity.

- Osteopenia: bone density 1 standard deviation below that of a 30-year-old white female.
- Osteoporosis: bone density 2.5 standard deviations below that of a 30-year-old white female.

Osteoporosis results in an increased frequency of fractures. Type 1 osteoporosis is typically seen in post-menopausal women. There is disproportionate loss of trabecular bone, and osteoporotic fractures of the vertebrae and distal forearm are common. Type 2 osteoporosis occurs in more elderly men and women (typically the over-75's), and is associated with fractures of the femoral neck, proximal humerus, pelvis, and proximal tibia. Bone healing is slower in the elderly.

The depth of cartilage plates reduces with age, predisposing to joint wear and osteoarthritis.

Muscle mass declines after the age of 30. Both the number and size of muscle fibres diminish. Strength declines, and body composition changes.

Tendons become more brittle and stiff, leading to a reduction in joint mobility.

In the skin, the epidermis, dermis, and subcutaneous fat become thinner. There is reduced barrier function of the skin. There is drying due to reduced sebum production, and loss of elasticity; wrinkles appear. Sweat gland function is reduced. Melanocyte function, and protection against UV light, become progressively impaired. The skin is slower to heal, and vitamin D production is reduced.

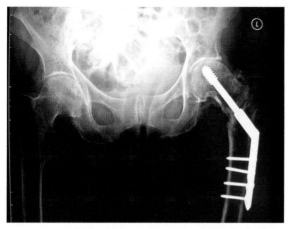
Fig. 21.4 Osteopenic intertrochanteric fracture of the left femur, with dynamic hip screw internal fixation.

Both pharmacodynamic and pharmacokinetic behaviour of drugs may be altered in the elderly. There is a large degree of inter-patient variability in the response to anaesthetic drugs, and this tends to be magnified with age. In addition, polypharmacy is much more common in the elderly and so multiple drug interactions may have to be considered.

Opioids and benzodiazepines generally exhibit enhanced potency in the elderly: a lower effector site concentration is required for an equivalent pharmacodynamic effect.

In terms of pharmacokinetics, several important changes occur with age. The total body water and the size of the intravascular compartment tends to decrease, leading to a smaller volume of distribution and a higher plasma concentration for a given IV bolus dose of drug. Cardiac output may be reduced, and blood flow to tissues (especially muscle) may be slow. This can lead to a delay in distribution, and retention of drug within the central compartment, further leading to increased plasma concentrations. Plasma protein binding is often reduced, increasing the free portion of drug available.

Effector site delivery can be delayed, and drugs may take longer to act. This can present a pitfall for the unwary: a drug may appear not to be taking effect, and so more is given. This leads to an overdose, which when it finally does find its effector site can lead to exaggerated adverse effects. It is important to titrate drugs slowly and carefully in the elderly to avoid this trap.

Clearance of drugs is often impaired in the elderly for various reasons: reductions in GFR and renal bloodflow, hepatic enzyme activity and hepatic bloodflow, and reduced tissue and plasma esterase activity may all contribute. Therefore, many drugs will have a prolonged duration of action which may be compounded by enhanced accumulation of active metabolites.

Specific drugs

Hypnotics and sedatives

Propofol

Propofol displays a reduced volume of distribution (and hence increased plasma concentration) because of reduced total body water and cardiac output. There is also an enhanced sensitivity to the drug. The dose for loss of consciousness, apnoea, and hypertension is reduced accordingly: the induction dose for anaesthesia is 1.5−1.75mg/kg in the elderly. Clearance is also reduced, probably because of a reduction in hepatic blood flow (propofol metabolism in the liver is flow-limited).

The haemodynamic effects of propofol are exaggerated, but delayed in onset.

Thiopental

The dose of thiopental required for anaesthesia is reduced in the elderly. Loss of consciousness occurs at the same plasma concentration as in the young, and so pharmacokinetic factors (rather than increased tissue sensitivity) are assumed to be responsible. These include a reduced volume of distribution due to less total body water and muscle mass. Albumin binding of thiopental is slightly reduced, and may be overwhelmed when the drug is given quickly, further increasing the available plasma concentration.

Etomidate

Like thiopental, pharmacokinetic factors (reduced volume of distribution) reduce the dose needed for equivalent effect in the elderly. There is not an appreciable increase in effector site sensitivity.

Inhalational agents

There is a well-described increase in sensitivity to inhalational anaesthetics, with the MAC to prevent movement to a surgical stimulus declining exponentially with age. Many modern anaesthetic machines can be programmed to take age into account when calculating MAC values.

Although evidence for a significant clinical effect is lacking, inhalational agents have been observed to induce oligomerization and cytotoxicity of proteins associated with Alzheimer's disease.

Opioids

The volume of distribution of morphine is roughly halved in elderly patients, resulting in doubling of plasma concentrations for a given dose. Clearance is also reduced, for both morphine itself and its metabolites. There is also likely to be an increased sensitivity to the drug. Careful titration of dosage to effect is necessary.

The redistribution kinetics of single IV boluses of fentanyl, alfentanil, and remifentanil do not result in significant differences in plasma or effector-site concentrations in elderly compared with young patients. However, the dose required for equivalent effect is roughly halved in the elderly, implying that sensitivity increases markedly in old age. This is compounded by reduced clearance and a prolonged elimination half-life, so that further dose reduction is necessary when using infusions of these drugs (in fact, adjustment for age is much more important than adjustment for body weight). Again, slow and careful titration is required to avoid significant side effects.

Muscle relaxants

Muscle blood flow is reduced in elderly patients, and so muscle relaxants tend to have a delayed onset of action. However, the duration of action is usually prolonged, mainly because of reduced metabolism and clearance. The exceptions are atracurium and cis-atracurium. Atracurium undergoes a mixture of spontaneous Hofmann degradation (40%) and hepatic metabolism. When there is a reduction in the latter, Hofmann elimination becomes more important and the overall clearance is preserved. Cis-atracurium is 83% cleared by Hofmann breakdown.

Local anaesthetics

For peripheral nerve blocks and possibly neuraxial blocks, a reduced dose of local anaesthetic produces the same clinical effect. This is thought to be due to the decrease in myelination in aged nerves and the enhanced availability of cationic binding sites for local anaesthetics. It has been found that the dose requirement for epidural anaesthesia reduces with age, but so does inter-patient variability. There is a reduced clearance of local anaesthetic from the circulation because of reductions in renal, hepatic, and plasma esterase function. The implications for 'one-shot' techniques are minimal; however, when local anaesthetic infusions are used, careful monitoring and titration are required as the reduction in clearance may result in accumulation and toxicity.

Preoperative management

The preoperative assessment of the elderly patient has several aims: to assess physiological reserve, evaluate comorbidity (which increases in incidence with age), and identify any optimization which is required before surgery. Another aim is to stratify risk and plan anaesthesia accordingly. Elderly patients may be more concerned about their level of function after surgery than the mortality risk. It may be appropriate to discuss limitations of therapy, and any advance directives which may be in place.

History, examination, and investigation should follow standard lines, bearing in mind that cardiovascular and respiratory illness may be significantly masked by immobility (e.g. arthritis, blindness, or gait difficulties). Baseline investigations are a little more extensive than in the young patient, as there is a higher incidence of occult disease. A full blood count, urea, electrolytes, blood glucose, ECG, and chest X-ray should be reviewed. Further investigations may be necessary, depending on the rest of the assessment.

Musculoskeletal problems may be aggravated by surgery. It is important to check the movement of the neck and jaw (also considering vertebrobasilar vascular disease, which may be worsened on extending the neck). Ascertain that the position for surgery is comfortable for the patient while awake (e.g. lithotomy, lateral position) and note any restricted joints or movements.

Consent

In order to possess capacity to accept or refuse treatment, a person must be able to understand the relevant information, retain it, and use it to come to a decision. While most elderly patients will retain full capacity, a proportion will not. This may be due to chronic dementia, or may be acute due to delirium or unconsciousness preceding surgery.

Until recently there was no provision for proxy consent for adults under UK law. The Mental Capacity Act 2007 has established a framework for the treatment of adults lacking capacity to consent. The Act grants the power to make proxy decisions about medical treatment to one of two categories of individuals.

- Individuals previously granted a **Personal Welfare Lasting Power of Attorney (LPA)** by a competent patient, to apply in the event of their losing capacity. This person must register their LPA with the Public Guardian. They may not make decisions to refuse life-sustaining treatment unless the patient has specifically authorized them to do so in writing.
- A **court-appointed deputy (CAD)**—a third party granted powers by the Court of Protection in the absence of an LPA. This person may make proxy decisions about treatment but is not empowered to refuse life-sustaining treatment.

In an emergency, the clinician is duty bound to act in the patient's best interests. This should take into consideration any valid advance directives in place which apply to the particular circumstances.

Premedication

Elderly patients vary in their response to sedative drugs. The drug's actions may be unpredictable and they may cause confusion rather than anxiolysis. They must be used with care. If an anti-sialogogue is required, glycopyrrolate is preferable to atropine as it does not cross the blood–brain barrier, avoiding the central anticholinergic syndrome.

Anaesthetic management

General vs. regional anaesthesia

For surgical anaesthesia, both regional and general anaesthesia have their advocates. Neither has been proven to give consistently better results across the board (for mortality or significant morbidity) in the elderly population. Where regional anaesthesia is used as the primary anaesthetic, sedation may also be necessary and this may negate the advantages of avoiding a GA.

It is probably true to say that regional anaesthesia (with or without GA) is associated with better postoperative pain control and fewer short-term complications than the GA—systemic opioid combination. The use of epidural analgesia for thoracic, abdominal, pelvic, and lower limb surgery improves postoperative pain control and reduces the incidence of deep vein thrombosis, cardiac and respiratory complications, and renal failure. However, for a regional anaesthetic to be successful, the patient must be able to tolerate the positioning required for the block and subsequent surgery. Musculoskeletal degeneration may make the block more difficult to perform.

Positioning

Positioning of unconscious patients and insensate limbs must be careful and gentle. Generous padding should be used, as there is a risk of pressure damage to fragile skin.

Thermoregulation

Maintenance of core temperature is of great importance in the elderly patient, whose thermoregulatory mechanisms are likely to be blunted. There are theoretical advantages of renal and cerebral protection during intraoperative hypothermia. However, a fall in temperature of as little as 2°C significantly impairs coagulation and increases intraoperative bleeding. Furthermore, postoperative hypothermia is associated with sympathetic activity, vasoconstriction, and increased plasma concentrations, and significantly increases the incidence of cardiac events in the postoperative period.

The operating-room environment, table, and IV fluids should all be warmed. Forced-air warming blankets, warming mattresses, and passive insulation can be used to maintain temperature intraoperatively.

Postoperative management

Many of the postoperative problems associated with the elderly are due to reduced clearance and prolonged action of anaesthetic drugs. Such residual effects may contribute to airway obstruction, hypoventilation, hypoxia, hypotension, somnolence, delirium, and hypothermia. The use of benzodiazepines (midazolam in particular) has been shown to delay recovery of mental function.

Age per se is not a predictor for postoperative complications. More important is the presence and severity of comorbidity (in particular heart failure, dysrhythmias, and pulmonary and cerebrovascular disease) and preoperative effort tolerance.

Management of acute pain

Management of pain in elderly patients is often suboptimal. This can result in increased cardiorespiratory complications, altered mental states, and progression to chronic pain. Dementia, even if severe, has not been shown to affect complaints of pain, and these should be taken seriously.

Paracetamol is the first-line analgesic of choice for mild and moderate pain in the elderly. Its clearance is reduced, but this does not usually necessitate dose adjustment unless there is a clear indication (e.g. hepatic impairment).

NSAIDs can be effective but must be used with care. They are not suitable for patients with renal disease, coagulopathy (including anti-coagulant therapy), or a history of peptic ulcer disease. When prescribing them for elderly patients, the lowest possible dose for the shortest possible time should be used. Renal function should be monitored. It may be prudent to prescribe gastric protection (e.g. a proton pump inhibitor) concomitantly.

Opioids can be used effectively in the elderly, but the incidence of side effects is increased. Immediate postoperative requirements are comparable with the needs of younger patients. Subsequent opioid requirements of elderly patients are much lower because of reduced clearance; dose reduction is advisable. Patient-controlled devices are suitable provided that the patient can use them effectively.

The intraoperative use of ketamine at subanaesthetic doses may reduce postoperative pain; at these lower doses, side effects are much less severe. Gabapentin premedication shows promise in reducing postoperative pain.

Postoperative delirium

Postoperative delirium (POD) is an acute state of fluctuating consciousness and inattention, not due to dementia, presenting 1–3 days postoperatively. Hyperactive and hypoactive forms exist; the latter are more difficult to spot clinically. Various causative mechanisms have been proposed, including systemic inflammatory response, embolic phenomena, and deranged neurotransmitter metabolism. There is an association between pre-existing dementia and POD, although there is no hard evidence to suggest that POD predicts the subsequent development of dementia.

Postoperative cognitive dysfunction

Postoperative cognitive dysfunction (POCD) refers to a decline in cognitive functioning noticed by some patients (with normal preoperative cognition) after surgery. Any cognitive process can be affected, including personality, memory, motivation, and performance of daily activities. The syndrome is difficult to demonstrate objectively. It does not seem to be linked to general anaesthesia *per se*; it can occur after any type of anaesthetic or surgery.

There is some evidence that patients with subtle cognitive dysfunction preoperatively are at risk of developing POCD. The cerebral function of these patients might be considered to be on the brink of decompensating prior to surgery, but this viewpoint is only speculative at present.

Chapter 22

HDU and ICU care

Intensive care units were first developed in the 1950s following a polio epidemic in Denmark. There were too few 'iron lungs' available, so instead patients received respiratory support in operating theatres and gymnasia with positive pressure ventilation and a tracheostomy. It was noted that the mortality of these patients was only 50% compared with 87% for the 'iron lung' patients. Following this, critically ill patients began to be cared for in specially equipped wards with one-to-one nursing and a multidisciplinary medical team.

Traditionally, ICU was for the sickest patients, those who required at least ventilatory and sometimes other organ support. HDU was for breathing spontaneously patients requiring organ support. However, the Department of Health has promoted a new classification, which focuses more on the level of care required by the individual patient (see opposite).

The critically ill patient

Early recognition of the critically ill patient is important in the prevention of cardiac arrest. Timely resuscitation and early transfer to ICU is associated with improved patient outcome.

- Studies have shown that in the majority of cardiac arrest patients, abnormal observations, and evidence of prior deterioration were documented before further deterioration.
- Scoring systems based on commonly measured physiological parameters were developed to identify patients at risk of deterioration and cardiac arrest.
- High scores, and therefore significantly abnormal physiology, are associated with higher mortality.
- Clearly, identification of at-risk patients is only one aspect of the problem. The response to the ill patient is equally important.

Patients should be assessed using the ABCDE approach. The initial priority is to resuscitate the patient, and not to perform complex diagnostic investigations. These are better performed later, in a live patient!

Admission to ICU

Patients should be admitted to the ICU when they require system support and invasive monitoring in order to prevent or treat organ failure. They should have potentially recoverable conditions, and should be admitted promptly, since treatment delays jeopardize outcome.

Many different types of patient are admitted: there is no upper age limit as it is more important to consider a patient's functional assessment, comorbidity, and quality of life.

If a patient needs intensive care, it is right to expect the referral process to be at a 'consultant-to-consultant' level.

Organization of the critical care unit

ICU provides 1–2% of the total number of hospital beds. There is 24hr medical cover at both junior and senior level, and usually 1:1 nursing for all ventilated patients. Together with capital equipment costs, it is an expensive place to run. Treatment strategies should be the responsibility of senior staff. Ward rounds often take place three times daily, but any patient deterioration should be promptly reviewed.

The admission process

History-taking is as important for intensive care as for any other speciality in medicine. It is vital to obtain as much information as possible from hospital notes and any relevant history from the patient and their relatives or carers. The GP may need to be contacted for further information.

ICU patients are often sedated, intubated, and ventilated, and therefore are unable to participate in clinical examination. The neuromuscular system will be particularly difficult to assess.

On arrival, the patient should be examined in a systematic manner and findings clearly documented. It may be necessary to take photographs of wounds or pressure areas in order to monitor the progression of these lesions. A CXR should be performed to confirm position of the ETT, central line, and nasogastric tube (if present), and to review intrathoracic pathology. A 12-lead ECG will provide a baseline comparision against new dysrhythmias or ischaemic changes.

Ongoing care

Daily blood samples can be used to monitor trends and identify new problems.

Full blood count: a haemoglobin level of 7g/dl is acceptable for most ICU patients and blood transfusion above this level has been associated with poorer outcomes. For those with cardiovascular disease, maintaining a haematocrit of >30% is associated with better outcome.

Urea and electrolytes: renal function is monitored looking at the urea and creatinine. The daily increase in urea is important in determining whether renal replacement therapy will be required. Hypokalaemia and hypomagnesaemia are common causes of cardiac dysrhythmias in intensive care patients. Hypophosphataemia may be present; this is a cause of muscular weakness and hinders respiratory weaning.

Deranged liver function and tests of clotting ability are frequently seen in severe sepsis. The clotting may need to be corrected prior to any invasive procedure.

Discharge from ICU

Patients should have resolution of the condition that necessitated admission to ICU. Ideally they will be self-caring and able to eat and drink independently.

Successful discharge relies on close cooperation between the critical care unit and the receiving ward nurses and medical staff. Clear handover and continuation of care is essential, and special instructions for tracheostomy tubes should be emphasized. Post-discharge review by ICU staff allows early identification of those who deteriorate.

Outcome prediction

Outcome measure may relate not only to mortality, but also to functional outcome and quality of life.

Severity evaluation and outcome prediction have been practised for decades, but are still far from perfect. They maintain false-positive and false-negative rates, and the application of different models for the same patient can conjure very different outcome predictions.

The rationale behind their development is that abnormal physiology will increase the risk of death in a manner proportional to the degree of derangement.

Case mix varies between different ICUs, but the assumption is that outcome prediction models take into consideration most of these characteristics.

Standardized mortality ratio (SMR) is a comparison of the observed mortality against the overall predicted mortality of the ICU.

→ Scoring systems

Randomized controlled trials are difficult to perform in intensive care, and so instead we have to make use of other methods of research. Case-mix-adjusted observational studies are common and allow inferences to be made about outcome between different critical care units.

- Scoring systems are used to assess the severity of illness of a patient. However, they cannot be used to predict outcome for an individual patient.
- They group or stratify patients with a similar severity of illness and thus predict expected outcome for this group.
- Stratification allows creation of a more homogeneous subset.
- They provide a tool to compare outcomes for different treatment groups or outcomes for different intensive care units.

In the 1970s, William Knaus developed APACHE, which scored individual patients according to their physiological abnormalities, chronic conditions, surgical status, and age. APACHE severity scores are converted into an estimate of probability of death.

→ Intensive Care National Audit and Research Centre

The Intensive Care National Audit and Research Centre (ICNARC) Case Mix Programme (CMP) recruits from adult general critical care units. Data are recorded prospectively (by trained data collectors) on consecutive admissions to each participating critical care unit and are submitted to ICNARC in cycles of 6 months. The data are validated locally, and centrally at ICNARC in order to ensure their integrity. Only then are they added to the CMP database.

Participation in the CMP is entirely voluntary, although both the Department of Health and the NHS Executive have recommended that all units should take part.

CMP aims to foster improvements in the organization and practice of critical care. It does this by:

- Promoting local audit of critical care through the provision of comparative data.
- Developing a broad programme of research of relevance to those commissioning, managing, practising, and receiving critical care.
- Improving the quality of audit and research in critical care.
- Promoting the use of evidence in critical care practice and policy.
- Building research capacity in critical care.

ICNARC has recently published a risk prediction model for intensive care that shows better discrimination for UK patients. This will become the standard method of risk prediction used in this country.

→ Quality of life

Describes an individual's functional ability and their pleasure derived from that ability. It describes the fulfilment felt by an individual and how their life is affected by disease, accidents, and treatments.

Quality of life standards cover an extensive range of physical and psychological domains. SIP is an example of such a standard.

Sickness Impact Profile (SIP)

Sleep and rest	Eating
Work	Home management
Recreation and pastimes	Ambulation
Mobility	Body care and movement
Social interaction	Alertness behaviour
Emotional behaviour	Communication

→ Comprehensive critical care

Level 0
Patients whose needs can be met through normal ward care in acute hospital

Level 1
Patients at risk of their condition deteriorating, or those recently relocated from higher levels of care, whose needs can met on an acute ward with additional advice and support from the critical care team.

Level 2
Patients requiring more detailed observation or intervention, including support for a single failing organ or postoperative care and those 'stepping down' from higher levels of care.

Level 3
Patients requiring advanced respiratory support alone or support of at least two organ systems. This level includes all complex patients requiring support for multi-organ failure.

→ Common reasons for ICU admission

Emergency medical
Pneumonia, exacerbation of COPD, generalized severe infection, multi-organ failure, neuromuscular emergencies (e.g. myasthenia gravis, Guillain–Barre syndrome).

Elective surgical
AAA repair, major cancer surgery, reconstruction surgery involving the airway, laparotomy for those with advanced age or significant comorbidity.

Emergency surgical
Multiple trauma, perforated bowel, AAA repair, pancreatitis, massive GI bleeding.

The patient with an altered conscious level often needs prolonged ICU support with mechanical ventilation. They often have associated immunological, metabolic, and psychological problems in addition to the more obvious physiological ones.

Airway

It is important that patients receive analgesia for ETT tolerance. Opiate infusions (e.g. morphine, alfentanil) are commonly used.

Oral hygiene needs to be maintained. Teeth can still be cleaned with an ETT in place, and antifungal preparations are often given to prevent oral candidiasis.

Breathing

Patients with severe lung pathology may be required to be paralysed as well as sedated. This is usually because problems are encountered 'fighting the ventilator'. Unusual ventilatory settings may be used (e.g. reverse I:E ratios), which are difficult for the patient to tolerate without deep sedation or paralysis.

Patients who are intubated and ventilated are often sedated. Their cough reflex may be obtunded or absent. Regular chest physiotherapy and suctioning via the ETT is required to clear secretions.

The ETT should be moved to either side of the mouth regularly in order to prevent pressure sores that might develop at each corner.

The ETT should be carefully secured with tapes, again preventing pressure necrosis of skin contact points.

Circulation

Critically ill patients often require careful administration of inotropes and vasopressors, necessitating invasive monitoring.

Gastrointestinal system

Malnutrition is associated with prolonged ventilation, more infection, and higher mortality. It is also important that critically ill patients receive nutrition as soon as possible to prevent loss of integrity of the gut, which may result in stress ulceration and gastrointestinal bleeding. Stress ulcer prophylaxis may be given if it is not possible to feed the patient enterally.

Most patients should be able to be fed via the enteral route. However, parenteral feeding may be necessary although it is associated with more complications such as line-related infection and hyperglycaemia.

Constipation is a common problem in intensive care patients, often because of the administration of opiates. Aperients and enemas may be needed to regulate bowel movements. Patients may also develop diarrhoea secondary to overflow, drugs, or infection.

Genitourinary

Critically ill patients are catheterized and urine output is measured hourly. If the patient is anuric and receiving renal replacement therapy, the catheter may be removed to prevent it becoming a source of infection.

Musculoskeletal

Critically ill patients lose muscle mass after a long period of being bed bound. Passive movements of limbs are performed in an effort to prevent contractures.

Skin

Patients need to be moved frequently to maintain skin integrity and prevent development of pressure sores. Personal hygiene must also be maintained by regular washing. Specialized beds and mattresses promote good pressure area care and prevent compression neuropathies.

Thrombophylaxis

Critically ill patients are at high risk of deep vein thrombosis. Passive calf movement devices may be used, and in the absence of deranged clotting, fractionated heparin may also be used.

Neurological

Patients are usually sedated; the level varies depending on the severity of illness of the patient. The patient may be comfortable with just an infusion of opioid and therefore able to communicate with others. However, further sedation, such as anaesthetic drug or benzodiazepine infusions may be required. Each unit has its own preferred regimen.

The ICU patient suffers considerable sleep disturbance because of loss of natural sleep patterns. Sedative drugs do not produce physiological REM sleep.

Patients frequently experience hallucinations, and these may be unpleasant and frightening. Anti-psychotic medications (haloperidol or chlorpromazine) or short-term benzodiazepines may need to be administered to alleviate this distress.

Causes of coma

Structural coma

Vascular: bilateral cortical infarcts, bilateral diencephalic infarction, vertebrobasilar strokes.

Infectious: access with mass effect.

Neoplastic

Trauma

Raised ICP

Mass effect

Non-structural coma

Electrolyte imbalance: ↑↓ Na^+, ↑↓ Ca^{2+}, ↓ phosphate, ↓Mg^{2+}.

Endocrine: ↓ glucose, HHS, DKA, myxoedema, Addison's disease.

Vascular: microvasculitis, DIC, TTP, hypertensive encephalopathy.

Toxic: ethanol, CO poisoning, drug overdose.

Infectious disease: meningitis, encephalitis, sepsis, malaria.

Medication effects: Reyes' syndrome, malignant neurolept syndrome, central anticholinergic syndrome.

Deficiency states: thiamine (Wernicke's encephalopathy), niacin (pellagra).

Organ failure: uraemia, hypoxic brain injury, liver failure.

Epilepsy

Temperature derangements

Psychogenic

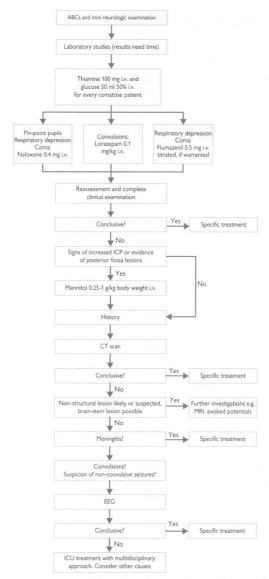

Fig. 22.1 Assessment and treatment of the unconscious patient. (Adapted from European Society of Intensive Care Medicine guidelines).

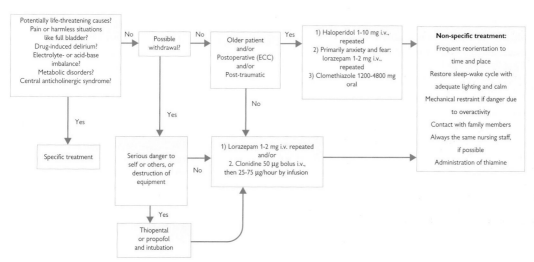

Fig. 22.2 Assessment and treatment of the acutely confused patient. (Adapted from European Society of Intensive Care Medicine guidelines).

Anaesthesia, intubation, and ventilation of critically ill patients can be a stressful and challenging time for the anaesthetist. Patients may require care in remote or low-dependency areas (e.g. hospital wards, A&E, or radiology suites), and they are usually unstable at the time of intubation. The indications for intubation can be summarized as follows:

- Actual or threatened airway obstruction
- Failure to oxygenate
- Failure to ventilate
- To reduce work of breathing, e.g. in pulmonary oedema
- Tissue hypoxia, e.g. carbon monoxide poisoning
- Severe metabolic upset
- Facilitation of IPPV and control of CO_2 (e.g. raised ICP)
- Sedation or reduced level of consciousness to protect airway
- To assist with bronchial toilet.

A critically ill patient might require intubation and ventilation for a combination of reasons. For example, a patient with opiate intoxication may be unconsciousness, may hypoventilate, and may be hypoxic.

Post-induction hypotension

Hypotension is common post-induction and is the result of:

- Unresolved hypovolaemia.
- Positive pressure ventilation, which reduces venous return and therefore cardiac output.
- The action of induction agents. These often cause vasodilatation, antagonizing compensatory vasoconstriction in shock states.
- The sick patient often has a loss of sympathetic tone. Vasodilatation is also induced by nitric oxide, produced as a result of sepsis.

Patients may require fluid boluses, vasopressors, and possibly small doses of adrenaline (10–100mcg) in order to prevent this.

Initiation of ventilation

Non-invasive ventilation

Some patients will respond to CPAP or non-invasive ventilation. However, intubation is usually the safest course of action since it will also allow suction of retained pulmonary secretions that are commonly found with any cause of critical illness. If there is no additional requirement for intubation, a trial of mask ventilation might be reasonable. Generally, suitable patients will be:

- Fully conscious and cooperative
- Cardiovascularly stable
- Not excessively fatigued, and able to tolerate short periods without respiratory support
- Able to take adequate tidal volumes and cough.

Clearly this technique should only be employed in an area where the staff are trained and the equipment adequate. In the early stages of respiratory failure, the signs are often subtle. With worsening clinical conditions, it generally becomes easier to spot. Additional information from ABG analysis is useful. If a patient demonstrates the following then support is indicated:

- Patient exhaustion
- Respiratory rate >35 breaths/min
- Increasing $PaCO_2$
- Respiratory acidaemia with pH <7.30.

Principles of mechanical ventilation

The ventilator is able to support respiratory function by:

- Improving oxygenation
- Controlling excretion of CO_2
- Assisting the respiratory muscles, therefore reducing the work of breathing. This further reduces oxygen consumption.

Ventilator strategy

The pulmonary pathology of a critically ill patient influences gas exchange and determines ventilatory strategy. Common patterns include:

- Pneumonia, consolidation, or lung segment collapse
- Chronic obstructive airways disease
- Acute lung injury/ARDS
- Pulmonary oedema
- Chest wall oedema.

The choice of mode of ventilation will vary according to the patient's problems. There is no evidence that one mode of ventilation is better than all others. However, the common strategy is the avoidance of further lung damage (ventilator-induced lung injury) (see box opposite).

Early use of modes that allow spontaneous respiratory effort may confer some advantage. Critical care ventilators have sensitive flow triggers that respond to patient effort and adapt to patient requirements. This is more comfortable, and less sedation is required for the patient, with fewer side effects. It is important to decide whether the ventilation strategy should be:

- Control of oxygenation with permissive hypercapnia
- Aggressive pursuit of pH and $PaCO_2$ targets.

Using excessive pressures or volumes causes lung tissue trauma, worsening pre-existing lung pathology and causing further impairment of oxygenation and CO_2 clearance. All patients need to be adequately oxygenated to survive, but for the vast majority, CO_2 levels will not influence outcome.

Permissive hypercarbia describes the practice of allowing $PaCO_2$ to climb in an effort to limit ventilator pressures or volumes and ventilator-induced lung injury. For those with raised ICP, however, strict control of $PaCO_2$ may be important.

Satisfactory levels of oxygen and CO_2 are specific for each patient, but generally a previously fit and healthy man will tolerate oxygen saturations down to 88–90%. Pre-existing respiratory disease may mean that even lower saturations are acceptable.

Ventilator settings

The ventilator performs the work of the respiratory muscles. However, with judicious use it can improve gas exchange.

How can we improve oxygenation?

- Increase FiO_2
- Increase mean intra-thoracic pressure:
  - Increase peak inspiratory pressure (PCV)
  - Increase tidal volume (VCV)
  - Increase PEEP
  - Increase inspiratory time, change the I:E ratio

Increased mean airway pressure aids lung recruitment and thus oxygenation. However, excessive use of any measure that increases lung volume or pressure may damage the lungs. There are also CVS effects to be considered: the increase in intra-thoracic pressure reduces venous return, adversely affecting cardiac output. In this way, although PaO_2 may be improved, tissue oxygen delivery may ultimately be made worse. Drainage of pleural effusions or pneumothoraces will also allow lung expansion and more effective ventilation.

How can we improve CO_2 clearance?

Increasing the minute volume will clear CO_2 but this depends on the mode of ventilation and the characteristics of the patient. For most patients 100ml/kg/min (ideal body weight) is a good starting minute volume. A tidal volume of 5–7ml/kg is usually considered safe, although even lower volumes may be appropriate in ARDS. Respiratory rates will usually be 14–20 breaths/min.

→ Modes of ventilation

The most appropriate mode of ventilation for a patient may change during the course of their illness.

Controlled mandatory ventilation (CMV)

A fixed tidal volume or pressure is set at a fixed respiratory rate. No allowance for the patient to take any spontaneous breaths. CMV may be VCV or PCV (see below).

Pressure control ventilation (PCV)

A time-cycled mode of ventilation. Respiratory rate and I:E ratio are determined and each breath is delivered to a set pressure. In the event of compliance or resistance change, the tidal volume delivered will change, since inspiratory pressure is constant.

Volume control ventilation (VCV)

The difference here is that each breath is delivered to a set volume and not pressure. In the event of a worsening of either compliance or resistance, the set tidal voume will still be delivered but at the cost of high airway pressure.

Pressure support ventilation

This is a flow-cycled mode of ventilation. Flow is measured throughout the ventilatory cycle. When inspiratory flow falls to only 25% of that breath's maximum, the ventilator cycles into expiration. In this way the patient determines respiratory rate. The level of pressure support is set by the operator.

Synchronized intermittent mandatory ventilation (SIMV)

The patient is able to breathe spontaneously between fixed breaths. Mandatory breaths might be either PCV or VCV and are set by the operator. The ventilator is able to sense patient effort and is able to provide pressure support for spontaneous breaths in the first 75% of the expiratory phase. On sensing a triggered breath in the last 25% of T_e, the ventilator delivers a full mandatory breath.

BIphasic positive airway pressure (BIPAP™)

BIPAP™ is a trademark term belonging to Drager. Essentially, this is pressure-controlled ventilation with the option of additional pressure support breaths.

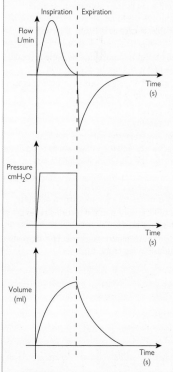

Fig. 22.3 Flow, pressure, and volume during pressure control ventilation.

✚ Adult respiratory distress syndrome (ARDS)

Definition

Bilateral pulmonary infiltrates in the absence of LV dysfunction, but with a known precipitating cause.

$PaO_2(kPa)/F_iO_2$ ratio: <40: acute lung injury (ALI)

<27: ARDS

Pathophysiology

Exudative stage (2–4 days): inflammatory insult to the endothelium and epithelium leads to leakage of fluid, protein, and inflammatory cells from capillaries into alveoli. The resulting shunt causes hypoxia. Reduced lung compliance increases work of breathing.

Proliferative stage: organization of exudate results in 'scar formation'. Proliferation of type II pneumocytes and fibroblasts leads to fibrosis and lung structure damage.

Direct causes

Lung contusion
Pneumonia
Pulmonary aspiration
Inhalation injury

Indirect causes

SIRS (pancreatitis, burns, cardiopulmonary bypass, massive blood transfusion)
Sepsis/septic shock (20–40% of septic patients)
Drug overdose

Treatment measures

Ventilation measures: aim for tidal volumes <6ml/kg and use PCV to reduce the risk of barotrauma.
Aim for appropriate PEEP titrated against tissue oxygenation.
Consider reverse I:E ratio for difficult oxygenation.
Accept oxygen saturations above 85%.
Accept a raised PCO_2 (8–9kPa) or pH 7.15 (this will not be deleterious and will avoid over-ventilation and barotrauma).

Other measures

Prone ventilation*
Inhaled nitric oxide oxide*
Inhaled epoprostenol*
Tracheal gas insufflation with oxygen*

*These manoeuvres may help to improve oxygenation but do not improve mortality.

Steroids may be given in the later proliferative stage to reduce fibrotic changes. They are of no use in the early stages.

Outcome

ARDS: average mortality 60%

Ventilator synchronization with patient effort

In order to synchronize with patient effort, the ventilator needs to be able to sense it. Ventilators do this by:

- Pressure sensing, which responds to the reduction in pressure within the breathing circuit as the patient inhales.
- Flow sensing, which relies on a change in the basal flow of gas that runs through the ventilator breathing circuit. This method is generally more sensitive and produces a rapid ventilator response to inspiratory effort.

This coordination of ventilator action is useful, especially for VCV and PCV modes that supply 'fixed' breaths. During the last 25% of the expiratory phase, the machine will deliver a full fixed breath if it senses patient effort.

In SIMV, detection of spontaneous patient breaths in the expiratory phase allows them to be supported in the manner of pressure support. Again, in the last 25% of expiratory time a fixed breath is delivered in response to patient effort.

Synchronization and a rapid response from the ventilator give better patient comfort and reduce the need for sedation specifically for ventilation. Synchronization will produce less baro- and volutrauma, and less ventilator-induced lung injury.

Inspiratory-to-expiratory ratio (I:E ratio)

The normal I:E ratio is 1:2; it is longer with obstructive lung disease. In patients with poor lung compliance (e.g. ARDS), it may be beneficial to increase the I:E ratio. With VCV this results in lower peak airway pressure, reducing the risk of barotrauma and further lung damage. It improves oxygenation because the prolonged inspiratory time allows alveoli with long time constants to be filled with gas. Patients with increased I:E ratios usually need to sedated and paralysed, as this mode is uncomfortable and not tolerated well.

Positive end-expiratory pressure (PEEP)

This improves arterial oxygenation by increasing FRC and preventing collapse of small airways. It decreases the shunt fraction. The pressure-volume curve may guide the use of PEEP (Figure 22.6).

Although PEEP recruits lung volume, it may also cause over-distension of other alveolar units. To protect against this, tidal volumes should be reduced when high levels of PEEP are used.

PEEP is assessed by its effect on oxygenation. It is usually set at $5-10cmH_2O$, although it may be set higher (up to $18-20cmH_2O$) in patients with severe hypoxia receiving 100% oxygen.

PEEP causes a further fall in venous return leading to a decreased cardiac output and tissue oxygen delivery. 'Best' PEEP is associated with maximum tissue oxygen delivery and minimum reduction of cardiac output.

Weaning and extubation

Weaning is the reduction of ventilatory support and can be started after the first sign of ventilatory or gas exchange improvement. In some patients it takes weeks for completion, and generally the best improvements will be made when the following are satisfied:

- The reason for mechanical ventilation has resolved
- Minimal pain and discomfort
- No acidaemia or metabolic disturbance
- Adequate neuromuscular function
- Respiratory drive minimally depressed by drugs
- Maintenance of adequate oxygenation and CO_2 clearance without excessive work of breathing.

There is no single method of weaning that is demonstrably superior to any other, and therefore the process of weaning should be tailored to the needs of the individual. It should be attempted as soon as the patient's condition allows, but signs of deterioration or respiratory distress necessitate an increase in ventilatory support.

Criteria for extubation are more specific. Patients should:

- Need FiO_2 <0.5
- Have adequate clearance of CO_2 without support
- Be able to cough and cope with volumes of sputum produced
- Be conscious, cooperative, and responsive
- Be in control of their airway reflexes
- Be generally improving and not deteriorating.

Following extubation, they should be closely monitored for signs of deterioration, since some may fail and require re-intubation.

Changing a tracheostomy tube

Tracheostomy tubes often need changing, whether this is to change the type of tube (uncuffed/cuffed or fenestrated/non-fenestrated) or to ensure patency and improve local hygiene.

Manufacturers generally recommend that disposable tubes are changed every 30 days since they are classified as indwelling devices.

A mature tract should have formed before the tracheostomy tube is changed. This usually takes 7–10 days post-insertion, but may be delayed in debilitated or malnourished patients with friable tissues.

Before changing a tracheostomy tube it is important to consider which type is required by the patient. A tracheostomy tube with an inner tube is advantageous: the inner tube can easily be removed and cleaned regularly in order to decrease the risk of tube blockage.

Procedure

- Explain the procedure to the patient and warn them they may experience coughing.
- Always have a skilled assistant present. Ensure that all equipment is present prior to commencing the procedure. This should include the ventilating bougie and patient-monitoring equipment.
- Check that the cuff is patent and lubricate with water-soluble lubricant. Insert the obturator in the lumen. Have a tracheostomy tube one size smaller available, in case of difficulty inserting the tube.
- Correct positioning of the patient is important. The patient should be semi-recumbent on the bed with their neck extended.
- Suction via the tracheostomy tube using a suction catheter. Oral secretions should be removed with a Yankauer sucker.
- Pre-oxygenate the patient.
- Remove the existing tracheostomy tube.
- Insert the new tube, preferably when the patient is exhaling. Direct the tube initially backwards and then downwards to navigate the tract and trachea. Remove the obturator and inflate cuff (if present).
- Feel for exhaled air via the tracheostomy and look for chest movements. Capnography is mandatory for anticipated difficulty.
- Secure the tracheostomy tube. Ensure that the securing tapes are a snug fit to prevent tube displacement.
- Observe the patient for signs of respiratory distress. This suggests airway obstruction or malpositioning of the tube.

→ Tracheostomy tubes

Cuffed tracheostomy tubes

- A cuffed tracheostomy tube should only be inserted if the patient is receiving positive pressure ventilation or is at risk from aspiration.
- If it is not required, change or remove it.

Fenestrated tracheostomy tubes (Figure 22.4)

- A fenestrated tracheostomy tube reduces the resistance of spontaneous breathing, an essential step in weaning a patient from an airway cannula.
- The insertion of the non-fenestrated inner tube enables the patient to receive positive pressure ventilation (Figure 22.5)

Uncuffed tubes

- Allow tracheal toilet with minimal airway resistance increase.

Variable flange tubes

- Anatomical variation sometimes prevents a pre-formed tube from sitting in the tracheal lumen.
- Varying the length of tube inside the trachea overcomes this.

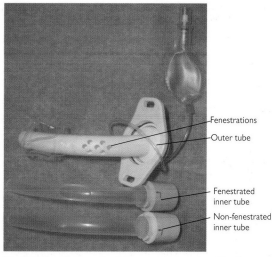

Fig. 22.4 Non-fenestrated and fenestrated inner tubes with a fenestrated outer tube.

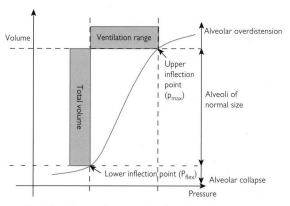

(a) Cuff inflated with non-fenestrated innertube in place. Breathing now occurs only via the lumen of the tracheostomy tube.

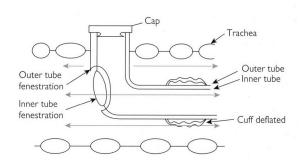

(b) Cuff deflated with cap in place. The patient breathes around the trachy tube and through the fenestrations of both tubes.

Fig. 22.5 Tracheostomy tubes: a) cuff inflated for IPPV and b) cuff deflated with fenestrated inner tube for weaning.

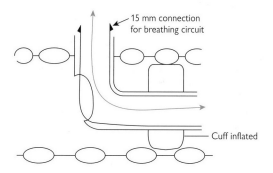

Pflex is the critical opening pressure for the majority of the alveoli. At P_{flex}, lungs lose compliance as alveoli overdistend.

Fig. 22.6 The pressure–volume curve has three zones:

- the lower part corresponds to recruitment, which occurs until the lower inflection point;
- the linear mid-portion represents effective lung inflation.;
- beyond the upper inflection point there is over-distention.

The level of PEEP should be set to above the lower inflection point. This will prevent cyclical collapse and opening of alveoli and attendant shear-stress damage.

PEEP may over-distend other alveolar groups and will also increase the end-inspiratory pressure and so worsen the risk of VILI.

→ Ventilator-induced lung injury (VILI)

Pulmonary pathology results in increased risk of secondary insult from overly aggressive ventilation. Disease does not affect the lungs in a homogenous fashion and positive-pressure ventilation is not conveyed to all parts equally. The normal alveoli are preferentially expanded and, particularly with VCV, this may lead to over-distension with high local lung pressures (volutrauma and barotrauma).

- Alveoli rupture and leak gas, and eventually leak exudative oedema.
- Compliance worsens and tidal volumes are forced into the remaining normal lung tissue, repeating the insult there.
- As units become affected they are more likely to close, opening with successive inspiratory pressures. This cycle results in shear force injury.

Systemic inflammatory response syndrome

Any severe insult (major surgery, trauma, infection) that does not result in immediate death typically results in systemic inflammatory response syndrome (SIRS). SIRS is defined by two or more of the following:

- Hyperthermia or hypothermia
- Tachycardia or bradycardia
- Tachypnoea
- A pathological alteration in white cell count (increased or decreased).

When SIRS is the result of suspected or proven infection, it is termed sepsis.

SIRS and its sequelae represent a continuum of clinical and pathophysiologic severity. Mild to moderate SIRS is probably beneficial. For example, production of mediators such as the cytokines tumour necrosis factor (TNF) and interleukin-1 from macrophages facilitate killing of micro-organisms by both innate and adaptive immunity.

Effects include increasing local vascular permeability and phagocyte recruitment, as well as raising body temperature, which optimizes the function of some microbicidal proteins. These same mediators can cause harm when they are either excessively vigorous or when they spill over.

Sepsis

Approximately 25% of all critical care patients are admitted with a diagnosis of severe sepsis or septic shock. It is the leading cause of death in general ICUs.

Infection triggers a complex network of inflammatory mediators (Figure 22.7), leading to organ hypoperfusion, dysfunction, and ultimately failure. Genetic factors are thought to be involved in the host's response to a septic insult.

Common pathogens of sepsis

Although sepsis is classically described following Gram-negative infection, Gram-positive septicaemia is increasingly common. The incidence of fungal septicaemia is also rising because of excessive or inappropriate use of antibiotics and the increased numbers of immunocompromised patients who present to ICU.

When a site of sepsis is identified, the incidence is as follows:

- 25% lower respiratory tract infection
- 25% urinary tract infection
- 15% soft tissue infections
- 15% GI tract infections
- 10% reproductive organs infection.

In >50% of cases, no organism is identified.

Stages of response

Endothelial response to infection

The response to infection is initiated by the outer membrane components of both:

- Gram-negative organisms (lipopolysaccharide, lipid A, endotoxin)
- Gram-positive organisms (lipoteichoic acid, peptidoglycan).

These outer-membrane components are able to bind to the CD14 receptor on the surface of monocytes. Toll-like receptors signal the cell, leading to the production of the pro- and anti-inflammatory cytokines with their mutually inhibitory effects. Overall, the balance is pro-inflammation.

Different members of the toll-like receptor family can differentiate between various classes of micro-organisms: Tlr4 responds to Gram-negative organisms, while Tlr2 is activated by Gram-positive pathogens and yeasts.

Pro-inflammatory cytokines bind to adhesion molecules on the vascular endothelium leading to endothelial cell activation, production of more cytokines, and induction of nitric oxide synthase.

- Nitric oxide is produced in excess, resulting in vasodilatation and the refractory hypotension of septic shock. Nitric oxide metabolites cause tissue damage.
- Endothelial damage activates the expression of adhesion molecules that attract neutrophils and cleave endothelial heparinoids, resulting in an endothelium that is more likely to support coagulation.
- There is loss of endothelial integrity as gaps appear between cells. Fluid and cells are lost into the interstitium.

Initially IL-1 and TNF help to keep infections localized, but once infection becomes systemic, their effects turn out to be detrimental. High levels of IL-6 are associated with mortality, although the nature of this association is unclear. IL-8 is an important regulator of neutrophil function which is synthesized and released in significant amounts during sepsis. IL-8 contributes to lung injury and organ dysfunction.

Thrombotic response to infection

Tissue factor is the principal activator of coagulation and is released from monocytes and endothelial cells following their cytokine activation. Infection can also directly stimulate coagulation.

The coagulation cascade produces thrombin, which cleaves fibrinogen into fibrin monomers. These polymerize to form clots with RBCs, WBCs, and platelets. The development of intravascular coagulation critically impairs local blood flow, leading to organ failure.

Fibrinolytic response to infection

The activity of inhibitors of fibrinolysis (TAFI and PAI-1) is increased by endothelial injury. PAI-1 inhibits the activity of tPA. (Section 15.6)

The fine balance between coagulation and fibrinolysis in health is disturbed, leading to intravascular occlusion and consumption coagulopathy.

Consequences of the inflammatory response include:

- Increased capillary permeability with interstitial oedema
- Vasodilatation (reduced systemic vascular resistance)
- Redistribution of regional blood flow
- Hypotension (septic shock)
- Multiple organ failure.

Activated protein C

Activated protein C is produced by the binding of thrombin to thrombomodulin on the endothelial surface. It is an important inhibitor of clotting factors Va and VIIIa and promotes fibrinolysis by reducing the effect of PAI-1 and accelerating tPA clot lysis.

Both the level of protein C and its endogenous activation are reduced during sepsis, allowing unopposed microvascular coagulation.

General therapeutic aims for septic shock

- Early recognition of septic shock
- Early resuscitation and continued organ support
- Early and adequate antibiotic therapy
- Control of the source of infection
- Corticosteroids (refractory vasopressor-dependent shock)
- Drotrecogin alpha (if APACHE II >25)
- Tight glycaemic control
- Low tidal volume ventilator strategy in patients with ARDS.

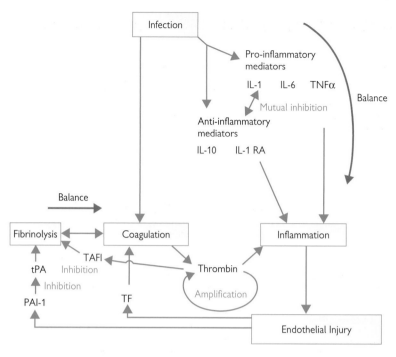

PAI-1	Plasminogen Activator Inhibitor 1
tPA	Tissue-type plasminogen activator
TAFI	Thrombin activatable fibrinolysis inhibitor
TF	Tissue factor
IL	Interleukin
TNF-α	Tissue necrosis factor α

Fig. 22.7 Sepsis pathway: a simplified view of the interaction between infection, inflammation, endothelial injury, coagulation, and fibrinolysis.

→ Definitions

An American College of Chest Physicians/Society of Critical Care Medicine Consensus Conference was held in Northbrook in August 1991 with the aim of agreeing on a set of definitions that could be applied to patients with sepsis and its sequelae.

Systemic inflammatory response syndrome (SIRS)

Manifested by two or more of the following:

- Temperature >38°C or <36°C
- Heart rate >90 beats/min
- Respiratory rate >20 breaths/min
- White cell count >12x10⁹/L or >10% immature neutrophils.

Sepsis

Known or suspected infection plus two or more SIRS criteria.

Severe sepsis

Sepsis with signs of organ dysfunction in more or one of the following systems:

- Cardiovascular
- Renal
- Respiratory
- Hepatic
- Haemostasis
- Central nervous system.

Septic shock

Severe sepsis with hypotension despite adequate fluid resuscitation.

→ Recombinant activated protein C (rhAPC)

rhAPC has anti-thrombotic, profibrinolytic, and anti-inflammatory properties and is therefore able to target the inflammatory and coagulopathic characteristic of sepsis.

The PROWESS (Protein C Worldwide Evaluation in Severe Sepsis) trial was a phase III trial of rhAPC in the treatment of severe sepsis. It produced a 6% absolute reduction and a 19.4% relative-risk reduction in 28-day all-cause mortality compared with placebo ($P = 0.005$).

Most of the benefit occurred in patients at higher risk for death with APACHE II scores >25, early onset of septic shock, and presence of two or more sepsis-induced organ failures at entry into the study.

rhAPC was associated with a greater number of serious bleeding events although this was not statistically significant. It is probably best used in patients with severe sepsis at high risk for death and avoided in patients thought to be at high risk for bleeding.

rhAPC is licensed for use in severe sepsis (NICE 2004).

→ The pro-inflammatory cytokines

- Tumour necrosis factor and interleukin-1 stimulate the release of other cytokines.
- Interleukin-6 stimulates acute phase protein production.
- Interleukin-8 is a neutrophil chemotactic factor.
- Interleukin-1 is a pyrogen and also stimulates T- and B-cell production.

ABC approach

As with any ill patient, the ABC approach is essential.

Airway

Shocked patients often have a reduced level of consciousness, and require airway protection.

Breathing

Evolving sepsis is associated with capillary leak and pulmonary oedema. Cellular aggregates within the alveoli, destruction of type 1 pneumocytes, and neutrophil entrapment amplify the insult to the epithelium and endothelium, leading to the development of ARDS in 40% of those with severe sepsis. Oxygenation becomes more difficult at a time when oxygen requirements increase.

The respiratory rate increses because of worsening acidaemia, oxygenation, and work of breathing, and carbon dioxide levels will eventually rise because of the relatively inadequate minute volume and increased carbon dioxide production. Intubation and mechanical ventilation combat these problems.

Circulation

The clinical signs of shock may be self-evident. Increased capillary permeability and vasodilatation render septic patients hypovolaemic. Fluid resuscitation is imperative—either isotonic crystalloid or colloid can be used. The incidence of pulmonary oedema is not affected by either type of fluid.

The response to volume infusion may be difficult to assess clinically. The response of the central venous pressure or pulmonary artery occlusion pressure to fluid boluses is helpful. A sustained rise in filling pressure of more than 5mmHg after a fluid bolus (250ml) indicates adequacy of filling.

Even after volume resuscitation, vasodilatation often contributes to continuing hypotension. Vasopressors, such as noradrenaline, may be required to increase MAP and perfusion pressure. Cardiac output and invasive blood pressure monitoring allow closer titration of fluids, inotropes, and vasopressors.

After volume restoration, the cardiac output is often high. Tachycardia is an important compensatory mechanism since circulating myocardial depressant factors impair ventricular performance.

Individual organ perfusion also worsens because of intravascular coagulation and microvascular obstruction. Poor peripheral blood flow promotes anaerobic respiration, metabolic acidaemia, and hyperlactataemia. Tissues extract oxygen poorly, a sign of intra-cellular dysfunction. Sepsis may damage mitochondrial electron transfer.

Disability

Circulatory disturbances of septic shock reduce cerebral perfusion and oxygen delivery, which in turn reduce the level of consciousness. If severe, this will cause brain injury. Therapies are directed towards maintenance of cerebral perfusion pressure.

Environment and exposure

Active sepsis can cause pyrexia or hypothermia. The process of infection resets the hypothalamic temperature set-point.

Investigations

Haematological abnormalities and coagulopathies should be corrected. Biochemistry investigations allow quantification of the degree of acidaemia and the need for renal replacement therapy. The tests form the baseline and reference point for all future investigations.

Identification and eradication of infection are also important. A full microbiological screen should be performed, including at least one set of blood cultures, together with saved serum/plasma samples used for more complex investigations, e.g. antigen testing and PCR.

Imaging is often required for identification of the source of infection, assessment of the effects of the disease process, and to ensure that monitoring techniques do not worsen the patient's condition. For example, a pneumothorax is more likely when the central line is inserted in a sick hypovolaemic patient as collapsed veins may be difficult to cannulate.

Antibiotics

Appropriate antibiotics should be given as soon as possible, taking into account the probable source of infection and whether the infection is likely to be community or hospital acquired.

Broad-spectrum antibiotics are given for the first 48hr or until microbiology results are available. It is important that the patient's antibiotic regime is then tailored to the pathogen isolated. Unnecessary antibiotics should be stopped in order to prevent the development of multi-resistant strains.

Further treatment adjuncts

Pathways of cytokine and inflammation Many preparations have been designed to dampen or prevent the inflammatory reaction to a pathogen, including anti-thrombin III, TNF antibodies, and high-dose steroids to name but a few. None of these has been shown to be of therapeutic benefit.

Recombinant activated protein C Details of the PROWESS study are given in Section 22.5.

Steroids

Further management

Patients with severe sepsis frequently progress to develop multi-organ failure. The aim of critical care is to support the failing organs whilst the sepsis process is treated.

Patients frequently develop acute renal failure and require haemofiltration for control of uraemia, acidaemia, hyperkalaemia, and fluid overload. In the majority of septic patients, renal function will return after the disease process has ceased.

Critical illness neuropathy is common, with profound motor and sensory neuronal loss following demyelination. These patients need supportive care whilst myelination is re-established. Patients with severe sepsis frequently stay in ICU for a long time.

Surviving Sepsis Campaign

The Surviving Sepsis Campaign (SSC) was formed in 2002 as a collaboration of the European Society of Intensive Care Medicine, the International Sepsis Forum, and the Society of Critical Care Medicine. It was established to help meet the challenges of sepsis and to improve its management, diagnosis and treatment.

The aim of the campaign is to reduce mortality due to severe sepsis by 25% within 25 years. The SSC has developed a set of evidence-based guidelines for the diagnosis and management of severe sepsis.

These guidelines have taken the form of 'care bundles'. A 'bundle' is a group of interventions related to a disease process which, when executed together, result in better outcomes than when implemented in an *ad hoc* manner.

The full guidelines can be found on the SSC website (www.surviving-sepsis.org).

Sepsis resuscitation bundle

- Serum lactate should be measured.
- Blood cultures should be taken prior to antibiotic administration.
- Broad-spectrum antibiotics should be administered within 3hr of time of presentation for A&E admissions, and within 1hr for non-A&E ICU admissions.

In the event of hypotension and/or lactate >4 mmol/L:

- Deliver an initial minimum of 20ml/kg of crystalloid (or colloid equivalent).
- Apply vasopressors for hypotension not responding to initial fluid resuscitation to maintain mean arterial pressure (MAP) >65mmHg.

In the event of persistent hypotension despite fluid resuscitation (septic shock) and/or lactate >4 mmol/L:

- Achieve central venous pressure (CVP) >8mmHg.
- Achieve central venous oxygen saturation ($ScvO_2$) >70%.

Sepsis management bundle

- Low-dose steroids administered for septic shock in accordance with a standardized ICU policy.
- Drotrecogin alpha (activated) administered in accordance with a standardized ICU policy.
- Glucose control maintained between 4 and 8.3mmol/L.
- Inspiratory plateau pressures maintained <30cmH$_2$O for mechanically ventilated patients.

Table 22.1 Typical pathogens and examples of antibiotic regimens

Source of sepsis	Likely pathogens	Antibiotic regimen	Comments
Respiratory tract	Community acquired: *Streptococcus pneumoniae* *Haemophilus influenzae* *Mycoplasma pneumoniae* Hospital acquired Any community type *Staphylococcus aureus* *Pseudomonas* Coliforms	Benzyl Penicillin 1.8g 6-hourly IV + Clarithromycin 500mg 12-hourly PO/IV Piperacillin + tazobactam 4.5g 8-hourly + Gentamicin IV Add vancomycin by infusion if MRSA suspected	Empyemas common after streptococcal infection—drain urgently if present
Pyelonephritis	Coliforms *Proteus* spp *Klebsiella* spp *Enterococcus* spp	Ciprofloxacin 400mg 12-hourly IV + Gentamicin IV	If pyelonephritis suspected, needs urgent ultrasound scan and drainage
Meningitis	*Neisseria meningitidis* Streptococci	Adults Cefotaxime 2g every 4–6hr IV Change to benzyl penicillin 2.4g every 4–6hr IV if organism proves to be sensitive Children Cefotaxime: paediatric dosing	Do not perform lumbar puncture if patient has raised intracranial pressure
Wound infection following orthopaedic surgery	*Staphylococcus aureus* Streptococci	Flucloxacillin IV 1g 6-hourly Add Clindamycin oral 450mg 6-hourly IV if group A strepococcus infection suspected Add Vancomycin by infusion if MRSA infection suspected	
CVP catheter infections	*Staphylococcus aureus* *Staphylococcus epidermidis* *Candida* spp Coliforms *Pseudomonas* Enterococcus	Vancomycin IV Add Piperacillin + tazobactam IV 4.5g every 6–8hr + gentamicin IV if Gram-negative infection suspected	If a central catheter is considered the source of infection, it must be removed as soon as possible
Intra-abdominal infection	Coliforms Anaerobes *Enterococcus* spp	Piperacillin + tazobactam 4.5g 8-hourly IV + Metronidazole 500mg 8-hourly IV + Gentamicin IV	Frequently seen postoperatively, leaking anastomosis, faecal peritonitis, acute pancreatitis—needs urgent CT scan and drainage or re-laparotomy with washout
Septicaemia Hospital acquired Community acquired	Streptococci, *Staph. aureus*, MRSA Coliforms Group A streptococci *Strep. pneumoniae* *Neisseria meningitidis*	For both hospital and community acquired: Piperacillin + tazobactam IV 4.5g every 6—8hr Add Vancomycin IV by continuous infusion if MRSA suspected Add Gentamicin IV if *Pseudomonas* suspected Add Metronidazole if anaerobic infection suspected	

Average intensive care mortality rates in the UK range from 11% to 31%. Death is often encountered in the critical care unit.

Deaths on the ICU are often sudden and unexpected. This is stressful for the patient's relatives, and providing support for the family of a dying patient is challenging and emotionally draining. It is important that there is support for the medical and nursing staff involved in such situations.

The relatives of a dying patient have various needs.

- Some wish to be with their dying relative.
- They need to be assured that their relative is comfortable and not in distress.
- They need to be able to express their emotions.

End-of-life decisions and withdrawal of treatment

Intensive care techniques can support organ function for long periods without the prospect of recovery. However, the simple prolongation of life in the face of inevitable death is unethical.

Patients are often admitted to ICU for a 'trial of survival' and, unfortunately, there will be a proportion who fail this test. When it is clear that death is unavoidable, withdrawal of support is appropriate. It is worth noting the following points.

- It is more sensible to not start therapies than to withdraw them. Careful prognostic consideration of which patient to intubate or dialyse is always good management.
- Although the wishes of the patient are paramount, those admitted to ICU are often not competent to discuss their management owing to a combination of their disease process and drugs. An appropriately devised advance directive is rare, but legally binding, and helps to guide end-of-life decision-making.
- The decision to withdraw is the responsibility of the medical staff and it is expected that they act as the patient's advocate.
- Regular and open communication with the family is vital. Families often struggle with the concept of futility, and it is a duty to explain clearly the reasons for withdrawal and give time for discussion.
- Difficulties arise when opposing views expressed within families or when families oppose the views of ICU staff. Skillful conflict resolution strategies are required.
- Similarly, referring physicians might request further aggressive therapy, in conflict with the ICU staff.
- Once therapy has been limited, patients should still be cared for compassionately. Pain may be relieved by the use of opiates, whilst agitation or distress may be relieved with benzodiazepine infusions. These doses are to used reduce the patient's suffering and not to hasten death.
- The patient should be nursed in a quiet area or side room, and the family should be given unlimited access.

Later, many relatives find it beneficial to be given the opportunity to meet medical staff to discuss issues relating to the death. Further information, such as post-mortem results, often helps them understand and answers their questions.

The grief response

The stages of bereavement were first described by Lindemann in 1944. Often the feelings and behaviour patterns are manifest before the patient dies, as the relative anticipates the loss. The sudden and unexpected death of a family member leads to an extremely stressful time for the other family members. It is important that relatives receive comfort and support during this difficult time. Many ICUs have staff who specialize in bereavement counselling. The stages are as follows.

- Initial shock and disbelief: crying and yearning are frequently experienced.
- Awareness of loss and its implications: this is often associated with feelings of guilt and anger. This may be seen on the ICU, and relatives may appear aggressive and hostile towards staff.
- Resolution: acceptance of the relative's death and ability to continue with life.

Brainstem death

The brainstem contains many vital structures, including the respiratory and cardiovascular centres, the cranial nerve nuclei, and the reticular activating system. Ascending spinal afferent nerves and descending efferent nerves from the cortex pass through it. Death occurs when an increase in intracranial pressure leads to compression of these vital structures, destroying their function.

The diagnosis of brainstem death is made after clinical examination of cranial nerve reflexes and examination of the response to pain. The conduct of this examination is now well established following guidelines from the Department of Health (1998) and the Intensive Care Society's document on organ donation (1994).

If organ donation is being considered, early involvement of the transplant coordinator is advisable. As with other modes of death for ICU patients, a full and open discussion with the patient's family is imperative.

Clinical prerequisites

Preconditions

The patient should be in unresponsive coma with a known irreversible cause of brain injury.

Exclusions

There should be an absence of:

- Sedative and paralyzing drugs
- Hypothermia (below 34°C)
- Metabolic or endocrine disturbances
- Circulatory disturbances (hypotension).

Testing procedure

- In the UK this must be performed by two doctors, one a consultant and the other at least 5 years post full GMC registration.
- Neither doctor should be part of the transplant team.
- Two sets of tests must be performed by each doctor (together or separately).
- There is no prescribed time interval between the two sets of tests.
- The legal time of death is the completion of the first set of tests.

Test for brainstem reflexes

See opposite.

➕ Tests for brainstem death

Light reflex

Afferent: optic nerve (II)

Efferent: occulomotor nerve (III)

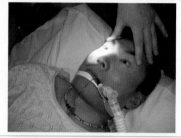

Corneal reflex

Afferent: trigeminal nerve (V)

Efferent: facial nerve (VII)

Stimulate the eye from the side: an approaching object may stimulate via the visual pathway causing them to blink if neurologically intact.

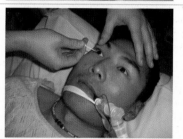

Cold caloric reflex

Afferent: vestibular nerve (VIII)

Efferents: occulomotor (III), trochlear (IV), abducent (VI) nerves.

For the conscious patient, this test would invoke nystagmus with the fast component *away* from the side stimulated.

For the unconscious brainstem-intact patient, this test would invoke slow tonic movement *towards* the side of stimulation (i.e. lacking the fast component of nystagmus).

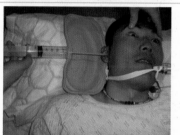

Gag reflex

Afferent: glossopharyngeal nerve (IX)

Efferent: vagus nerve (X)

This is usually performed by moving the ETT against the posterior pharyngeal wall

Cough reflex

Afferent: vagus nerve (X)

Efferent: vagus nerve (X)

This is usually performed by stimulating the carina with a suction catheter

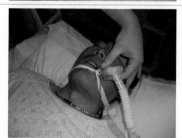

Reponse to pain

Afferent:

- Via the spinothalamic and spinoreticular tracts when pain administered to limbs or trunk.
- Via the trigeminal nerve when pain administered to face.

Efferent:

- Facial nerve (VII)

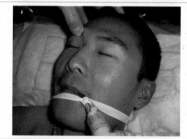

Breathing response to hypercapnia

To confirm the absence of respiratory movements in response to hypercapnia.

- Pre-oxygenate patient with 100% oxygen for 10 minutes. Allow arterial carbon dioxide presure to rise to above 6.0kPa by decreasing ventilation rate on ventilator (confirm with ABG sampling; pH should be <7.4).
- Disconnect from the ventilator and insufflate oxygen via the ETT to prevent hypoxia. Observe and confirm the absence of spontaneous respiration.
- Re-attach patient to ventilator if organ donation is being considered.

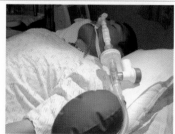

Chapter 23

Trauma

Incidence

Trauma is the leading cause of death under the age of 40 years for both men and women. The legacy of trauma is that for every death, there are three patients left with significant disability.

In the UK the majority of injuries are due to blunt trauma, road traffic accidents (RTAs), falls, assaults, explosions, and self-harm. In 2003 RTAs accounted for 3508 deaths, with 33,707 seriously injured and 253,392 slightly injured. It is worth noting the rising incidence of penetrating injury secondary to knife assaults and gunshot wounds.

Goals

Early resuscitation and reversal of tissue hypoxia reduces mortality and morbidity. Clinical problems should be recognized and treated promptly, with minimal delay in the patient receiving definitive care. Involvement of appropriately skilled senior personnel will help this process.

Precise diagnoses are unimportant: the priority is the detection and treatment of physiological abnormality. Not only will this strategy reduce mortality but it will also minimize morbidity. Getting the simple things right makes a real difference.

What kills trauma patients?

The trimodal distribution of death is illustrated in Figure 23.1. The first peak is for those who die from non-survivable injuries including severe penetrating brain injury, large vessel or myocardial rupture, or very high spinal cord transection.

The second peak of deaths is the group who are potentially saved by good care both at the scene and subsequently in hospital. With appropriate planning and prioritization of care it should be possible to identify and treat all causes of life-threatening injury, including airway injury, tension pneumothorax, pelvic and long-bone fractures, and intracranial haematomas.

Many of those who survive the initial insult are subsequently killed by shock, the inadequate delivery of essential cellular substrate (including oxygen). Tissues with high oxygen requirements (e.g. the brain) are most vulnerable to damage. Shock of only a few hours' duration may cause multi-organ dysfunction and result in prolonged ICU stay and worse prognosis. This is illustrated as the third peak of deaths. Outcome for this group is clearly affected by the management received in the initial stages of resuscitation. Allowing a patient to remain hypotensive with inadequate haemorrhage control and fluid resuscitation will result in organ dysfunction, depressed immunity, and an increased risk of death from sepsis.

Preparation

Effective management of the trauma patient begins with pre-planning for both the ambulance service and the receiving hospital. The treatment strategies of paramedics at the scene should be the same as those applied in the hospital, and the patient should be transferred using predefined transfer agreements. A flow diagram of a typical pre-hospital scenario is shown in Figure 23.2.

Care of the patient begins with protection of the carer: universal precautions (Figure 23.3) should always be used. Preparation in the hospital starts with the design of the resuscitation room. Each bed area should be of the appropriate size and should contain the necessary equipment required for primary survey of the trauma patient. A supply of warmed fluids, O-negative blood, and X-ray imaging should be immediately available.

A single person could assess and treat a trauma patient, but in reality a multidisciplinary team should provide the care. This simultaneous team approach saves time and improves outcome. In the UK, most speciality training programmes encourage attendance at an ATLS®

course. This translates into improved care since everyone at the bedside performs according to the same protocol. Although each member of the team has a predefined role, they should understand the overall objectives. It is important that the team performs under the direction of a nominated team leader.

The anaesthetist's skills make him or her an essential member of the trauma team. He or she is commonly given responsibility for airway management with cervical spine protection. Anaesthetists are accustomed to monitoring physiological parameters and assessing responses to interventions and treatments. Relaying this information to the team leader is useful.

Triage and major incident planning

Multiple casualties may be admitted from one or more incidents and may trigger activation of the major incident plan according to local policy. Staff should be familiar with their role in such an emergency and most hospitals rehearse this escalation regularly. Close cooperation with the ambulance service is mandatory, since the aim is to avoid mass casualties being delivered to one institution.

- Multiple casualties: the available resources of the receiving hospital are not overrun. Patients are triaged according to ABCDE priorities, since most are expected to survive.
- Mass casualties: the receiving hospital has insufficient resources to cope with the number of casualties, and they are treated according to whether or not they will survive. This is the less desirable option.

Sequence

On arrival, the patient is surveyed twice. Life-threatening emergencies are discovered and treated in the **primary survey**. This is performed in a specific order, where the greatest threat to life is assessed and treated first. Any abnormality found must be treated before moving on to the next stage. In practice, even allowing for this emphasis, different members of the team can perform much of the primary survey simultaneously. The primary survey deals with:

- A: airway with cervical spine protection
- B: breathing and ventilation with supplemental oxygen
- C: circulation with haemorrhage control
- D: disability (neurological assessment)
- E: exposure and environment.

Adjuncts and monitoring are used to provide valuable additional information about the patient. The same standards for monitoring a patient in theatre apply in the resuscitation room.

Once the patient is physiologically stable, a detailed 'head-to-toe' secondary survey is performed to screen for additional injuries. Depending on the nature of the injuries, urgent operative care may be required before either the primary or secondary surveys are complete. For example, if the patient is transferred for laparotomy or craniotomy before the secondary survey has been finished, this must be completed later. Failure to do so risks missing potentially life-threatening or disabling injury.

Remember, not all patients will be treated in the local hospital. The extent of their injuries may necessitate transfer to a regional centre for neurosurgical or cardiothoracic care. The decision to transfer should be made early in the treatment pathway, as this will save time and improve patient outcome. Early senior input is imperative (from a clinical and also a medico-legal perspective) and also helps to speed up the process. Once again, it is essential to ensure that the receiving team understand what assessments remain outstanding.

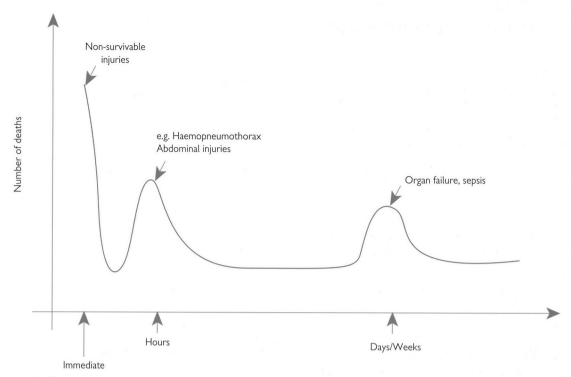

Fig. 23.1 Trimodal distribution of trauma deaths.

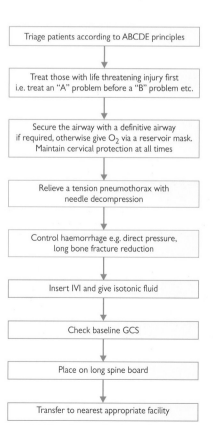

Fig. 23.2 Flow diagram of pre-hospital care considerations.

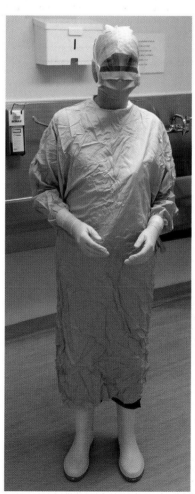

Fig. 23.3 Universal precautions.

The primary survey is a structured rapid assessment of the patient with simultaneous treatment. A look, listen, and feel approach will pick up most immediate life-threatening problems.

Complex investigations at this stage are seldom indicated, and should only be contemplated once physiological normality has been achieved.

Airway with cervical spine protection

From the moment medical care is initiated, the cervical spine should be treated as potentially unstable with an attendant risk of spinal cord injury. Cervical protection is essential. There are two options:

- The combination of an appropriately sized and fitted cervical collar, with lateral blocks and broad tape across the patient's forehead and chin, secured to the spinal board or trauma trolley.
- Manual immobilization: the application of collar, blocks, and tape can be time-consuming and makes it almost impossible to manipulate the airway for intubation. A 'hands-on' approach is often best used until the airway has been assessed and treated. Figures 23.4, and 23.5 demonstrate manual cervical spine protection. Figure 23.6 shows a different method, with the operator at the side of the patient, facing him or her. This latter is useful when airway manoeuvres are being undertaken, to allow more space at the head of the patient.

Is the airway patent?

Ask the patient to speak. A clear spoken voice demonstrates a patent airway *at that time*. It also gives a guide to the efficacy of ventilation and cerebration (although these are not being formally assessed at this stage).

Treatment

- Give high-flow oxygen to every patient. A reservoir mask with 15L/min fresh gas flow can achieve a FiO_2 of 0.85.

Is the airway obstructed?

The presence of noisy breathing or stridor implies that the airway is partially obstructed, possibly by a foreign body, teeth, vomit, or food. Soft tissue swelling may also cause obstruction. In the comatose patient, the anatomy may be normal yet the muscular tone insufficient to maintain airway patency (Figure 23.7).

A completely obstructed airway will be silent, and there may be visible seesaw chest movements.

Treatment

- The airway should be inspected and debris suctioned. Simple manoeuvres may relieve obstruction, but remember that every airway action must be carried out with cervical protection.
- Nasopharyngeal tubes may induce nasal haemorrhage, further compromising the airway. They are contraindicated in those with midface injury or possible basal skull fracture (i.e. those with closed head injuries), since they could penetrate the basal skull and the brain.
- Many patients will not tolerate a Guedel airway and this may induce vomiting, which severely challenges airway and cervical management.
- An inhalational injury or airway burn produces swelling within the larynx and stridor. Swelling may develop over a number of hours and unless the threatened airway is relieved by timely intubation, complete airway obstruction will ensue with death not far behind.

Practical issues

- Senior help may be required, so anticipate problems and communicate in good time.
- Intubation is impossible with well-fitted semi-rigid collar in place. Use a 'hands-on' approach instead. The approach shown in Figure 23.6 is useful here.

- Induction agents will cause hypotension in the trauma patient, so be prepared. Use large-bore IV access and plenty of IV fluid. Anaesthetic agents may not be required for intubation if the patient has a Glasgow Coma Score (GCS) of 3.
- Movement of the patient can dislodge the ETT, and so a quick clinical re-assessment of position should be made after every roll or transfer.
- ETT ties are often impractical with semi-rigid collars *in situ*. Taping the ETT to face and collar with strong fabric tape is an alternative.
- Laryngeal masks have been used in trauma scenarios to good effect in the 'can't intubate, can't ventilate' scenario, but these are a temporary option to allow emergency oxygenation until a definitive airway can be established. They do not protect against airway soiling.

Breathing and effective ventilation

The primary goal with all thoracic conditions is to restore normal gas exchange and perfusion. Chest injuries are found in 25% of trauma calls, and 90% of these can be managed with basic skills (thoracostomy tube insertion) and without surgical intervention. Even in cases of penetrating chest trauma, only 30% require operation.

There are six life-threatening injuries that should be excluded or detected and managed during the primary survey of the airway and chest:

- Airway obstruction or injury
- Tension pneumothorax
- Open pneumothorax
- Massive haemothorax
- Flail segment
- Cardiac tamponade.

These should become evident during a thorough systematic assessment of the chest.

Inspection

This might reveal bruising and swelling, which can signal potential underlying injuries to ribs, lung, and mediastinal structures.

Tracheal position

Deviation of the tracvhea from the midline should raise the possibility of a serious problem within the chest. It is pushed away from a tension pneumothorax or massive haemothorax.

Palpation

A comparison should be made between the two sides. The volume of expansion can be assessed and chest wall defects such as the crepitus of broken ribs or surgical emphysema can be noted.

The percussion note

This should be assessed bilaterally. A hyper-resonant note indicates an underlying pneumothorax, whereas a dull note may illustrate the presence of a haemothorax or diaphragmatic hernia.

Auscultaton

This may reveal normal, reduced, or absent breath sounds. Subtle changes are difficult to assess at the best of times, but with all the activity during a trauma call, these changes are easily missed. An early CXR is indicated.

Clearing the C-spine (removing cervical protection)

The risk of cervical injury should be determined. Potential damage necessitates continued protection. However, early clearance makes ongoing care much easier, especially prior to general anaesthesia or intensive care.

Clinical assessment

The patient should:

- Be cooperative and free from the influence of drugs
- Have a normal GCS
- Be without distracting injury
- Be free of neck pain.

On examination there should be:

- Absence of cervical tenderness on palpation
- Absence of new neurological deficit—dermatomes and myotomes should be entirely normal on neurological examination
- Absence of pain throughout the full range of neck movements (rotation, lateral flexion, and forward flexion and extension). This should carefully be examined last, and only after all other components of the examination have been satisfactory.

If movement provokes neck pain or evidence of neurological deficit, cervical protection should be re-instituted immediately.

If the patient has neck pain or tenderness, neurological deficit, or a high-risk mechanism of injury, imaging of the cervical spine is mandatory.

Imaging

C-spine films

The lateral view will only pick up 85% of cervical bony abnormalities and important time can be wasted trying to get an adequate view from the base of the skull down to the body of T1. Additional AP and peg views are required for a full radiological assessment of the cervical spine, and these are difficult to attain in an intubated patient. CT scanning is now the preferred option.

10% of patients with one fracture will have another in the spinal column, so look for it. This may well necessitate both plain films and CT imaging of the entire vertebral column.

Two-plane X-ray views or CT scanning with reconstruction might provide evidence of bony injury but will not demonstrate cord injury.

The definitive airway

A cuffed endotracheal tube secured in the trachea with the cuff inflated, connected to a supply of oxygen and means of ventilation.

The tube is usually passed via the mouth. Nasal intubation is acceptable if you are certain that there is no threat of basal skull fracture. In some cases a surgical airway is required.

Indications for a definitive airway

- Apnoea.
- Failure of oxygenation by any other means.
- Significant hypoventilation with carbon dioxide accumulation. This is a particular problem for patients with head injuries, where raised carbon dioxide will worsen increases in intracranial pressure.
- Imminent loss of airway, e.g. swelling from inhalational injury to upper airway
- GCS ≤8 defines coma and loss of normal protective airway reflexes.
- Anticipated transfer of patient with potential airway problems. This includes trips within hospital (e.g. to CT scan) as well as between hospitals. When anticipating an inter-hospital transfer (particularly by air), consider elective intubation as there is usually poor access in the ambulance or cabin and motion may make airway manoeuvring almost impossible.

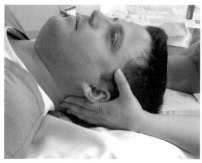

Fig. 23.4 Manual cervical protection. Note that the ears are not covered, allowing the patient to hear as well as possible in a disconcerting and sometimes noisy environment.

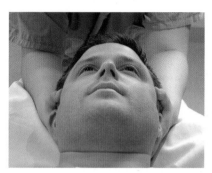

Fig. 23.5 Manual cervical protection (front view).

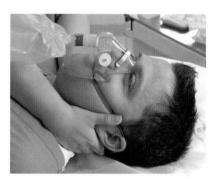

Fig. 23.6 Manual cervical protection (from below). This approach allows easier access for airway interventions.

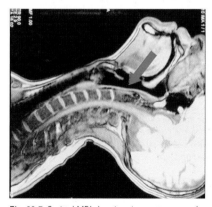

Fig. 23.7 Sagittal MRI showing airway structures. In a patient with a reduced level of consciousness, the large tongue can easily flop backwards (in the direction of the arrow), obstructing an otherwise anatomically normal airway.

Tension pneumothorax

Clinical signs

- Distressed hypoxic patient
- Deviated trachea (away from pneumothorax)
- Hyper-resonant percussion note
- Absent breath sounds on side of pneumothorax
- There may be subcutaneous emphysema.

Figure 23.9b demonstrates the chest X-ray findings of a left tension pneumothorax. Although the X-ray appearances are impressive, tension pneumothorax is a clinical diagnosis, and X-ray confirmation should *not* be sought before treatment.

Treatment

- ABCDE approach.
- Immediate decompression of the pleura with a large cannula placed in the 2nd intercostal space (i.e. just above the third rib) in the mid-clavicular line. Leaving the cannula open converts the tension pneumothorax to a simple pneumothorax. This is a life-saving manoeuvre and time should not be spent using local anaesthetics to numb the skin.
- A formal chest drain must be inserted (in the next few minutes). Complete drainage of the trapped air will relieve distress, allow lung re-expansion and better gas exchange. Figure 23.8 shows the process of chest drain insertion step-by-step. Strict asepsis is mandatory, and local anaesthetic should be used generously in the awake patient.

Massive haemothorax

Clinical signs

- Distressed, tachypnoeic, and hypoxic patient
- Tracheal deviation (away from the haemothorax)
- Dull percussion note
- Reduced absent breath sounds
- Depending on the volume of blood loss, signs of shock.

Figure 23.9a demonstrates the chest X-ray findings of a massive left haemothorax.

Treatment

- ABCDE approach.
- This will need drainage with a formal chest drain, in the same fashion as for a pneumothorax. Re-expansion of the lung will allow improved gas exchange. However, this may take some time to achieve.
- A danger for the patient is that in the presence of continued thoracic bleeding, a chest drain might promote exsanguination. Large-bore cannulae for fluid resuscitation and transfusion and rapid transfer for definitive surgical care offset this risk.
- If the initial loss is >1.5L or ongoing losses are >200ml/hr (in an adult), the patient might require a thoracotomy. Longer term there is a risk of an untreated haemothorax developing into an empyema.

Cardiac tamponade

Cardiac tamponade is usually caused by penetrating injury. The pericardial sac is a fibrous structure which can only hold an additional 20–50ml before the heart is compressed and adequate filling is prevented. The under-filled heart's stroke volume falls dramatically, as does the patient's blood pressure.

Clinical signs

- 'Muffled' heart sounds
- Distended neck veins
- Hypotension unresponsive to fluid resuscitation.

This is known as 'Beck's triad'. It may be difficult to see distended neck veins in the presence of cervical protection or if the patient has untreated hypovolaemia.

Treatment

- ABCDE approach.
- The pericardial sac must be decompressed immediately. This can be done with a long (10cm) single-lumen catheter inserted at a point 2cm inferolaterally to the left of the xiphisternum. The cannula is inserted at 45°, towards the tip of the patient's left scapula.
- ECG monitoring is mandatory and should be observed for ectopics and dysrhythmias suggestive of cardiac irritation or piercing with the needle.
- Aspiration of the cannula is continuous, and once blood is drawn off advancement is discontinued. If >50ml blood is aspirated, aspiration from the ventricle should be suspected and the needle withdrawn.
- Correct placement is confirmed by resolution of the clinical signs following aspiration. The cannula should be left *in situ* as blood may rapidly re-accumulate and further aspiration might be required. Cardiothoracic consultation is mandatory.

Flail segment

A flail segment is a chest wall defect where each of two or more adjacent ribs is fractured in at least two places. The resulting gas exchange problem has less to do with the paradoxical movement than with the underlying contusion. The force required to produce a flail also produces significant underlying lung injury.

Clinical signs

- Respiratory distress, hypoxia.
- Tachypnoea.
- Crepitus over the flail with paradoxical wall movement.
- Central trachea with normal percussion and auscultation.

Treatment

- ABCDE approach.
- Treatment of a flail segment is generally conservative. Analgesia is very important. However, patients often additionally require early intubation and ventilation due to subsequent gas exchange and expectoration problems. It becomes too painful to breathe deeply and cough up sputum.
- Taping of the chest wall theoretically reduces some of the 'floating-rib' movements, reducing pain. This very rarely works in practice.
- IV opiates may work for younger fitter patients, but might depress breathing and compound gas exchange problems. Epidural analgesia provides an alternative.

Open pneumothorax

With a chest wall defect greater than 2cm, or $^2/_3$ the diameter of the trachea, inspiratory effort air is preferentially sucked in from the atmosphere into the pleura with each breath, rather than down the trachea. This leads not only to a pneumothorax but also to massive disruption of air entry to the unaffected lung.

Clinical signs

- Hole in chest wall of >2cm or $^2/_3$ tracheal diameter.
- Respiratory distress.
- Hypoxia, absent or reduced breath sounds on side of injury.

Treatment

- ABCDE approach.
- Cover the hole with an occlusive dressing but only tape this on three sides of the dressing. This forms a flutter valve which prevents further air entry on inspiration, but allows pneumothorax air to escape under pressure during expiration.
- A chest drain should also be placed.
- Early consideration for intubation and ventilation as larger defects will need to be closed in theatre.

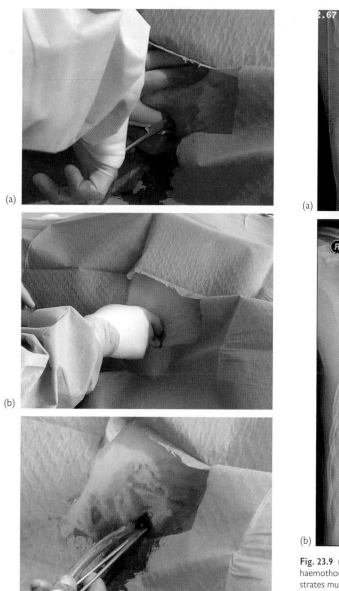

(a)

(b)

(c)

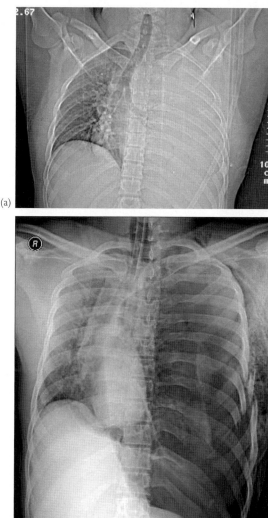

(a)

549

(b)

Fig. 23.9 (a) Massive haemothorax of the left chest. (b) Left tension haemothorax. This was caused by blunt trauma. The CXR also demonstrates multiple rib fractures and subcutaneous emphysema.

Fig. 23.8 (a) With standard asepsis, the local anaesthetic is infiltrated. A 2.5cm incision allows blunt dissection down to the pleura. Chest drain insertion. (b) Once the ribs are spread and the pleura opened by blunt dissection, a finger sweep is performed inside the chest in order to ensure that the lung will not be damaged by introduction of the chest tube (without the aid of a trocar). (c) Successful introduction of the tube is confirmed by 'fogging'. The size of the drain used needs to be suitably large to allow free flow of large volumes of air and or blood. A good guide would be to use a similar size to the appropriate ETT for that patient. The drain should not be clamped. 'Bubbling' of the underwater drain or 'fogging' of the tubing confirms that the drain is functioning.

Aortic disruption

The mechanism of injury is usually one of massive rapid deceleration, e.g. a fall from a great height or a head-on traffic collision at high speed. The aorta is attached to the posterior chest wall and therefore is immobile. However, the heart is relatively mobile, and on deceleration its momentum disrupts the aorta along its arch.

Clinical signs

If the patient survives to reach hospital he/she may demonstrate transient response to fluid resuscitation with profound hypotension and evidence of re-bleeding. However, these patients may be quite cardiovascularly stable, with a contained mediastinal haematoma that is at risk of breaking down. Without a high index of suspicion, this injury can be missed until post-mortem. Figure 23.10 is a line diagram illustrating the chest X-ray changes associated with aortic disruption.

Management

The investigation of choice is a CT aortogram with contrast, once the patient is stabilized (Figure 23.12). Cardiothoracic consultation is required and if the patient cannot be imaged, surgery may be indicated as part of resuscitation.

Oesophageal injury

This injury usually follows a severe blow to the chest or upper abdomen, although penetrating injury may also be responsible. Clinical suspicion should be aroused if there is chest pain out of proportion to the perceived injury.

Clinical signs

Pneumothorax or haemothorax without rib fracture.

Investigations

Mediastinal air is often seen on CXR or CT.

Contrast leaks from the oesophagus following a swallow test.

Subsequent chest drain insertion yields particulate matter.

Treatment

Surgical consultation is mandatory, although late detection of leak warrants conservative management with chest drainage.

Pitfall

Failure to recognize this injury can result in formation of an empyema. This has a high mortality when associated with trauma.

Rib fractures

Ribs 1–3

These ribs are relatively well protected, and the force required to fracture these short strong bones is very high. Anticipate other significant injuries (e.g. great vessel disruption).

Ribs 4–9

Look out for associated pulmonary contusions, pneumothoraces, and haemothoraces.

Ribs 10–12

These ribs cover abdominal solid organs, so investigate the possibility of spleen, hepatic, and renal injuries. Also consider mesenteric disruption with associated bowel ischaemia. A senior surgical opinion should be sought.

Tracheobronchial rupture

Consider this injury if there is a persistent air leak into a chest drain. This will be in phase with inspiration for mechanically ventilated patients. It may be confirmed with bronchoscopy, since over 80% occure within 2.5cm of the carina.

Management

Initial treatment will usually require intubation and ventilation. A double-lumen ETT with independent lung ventilation may be indicated, depending on ease of gas exchange.

More than one chest drain may be required for large leaks. Surgical closure may need to be considered for persistent problems. If left untreated, these injuries often result in bronchial stenosis.

Blunt cardiac injury

This typically arises in association with sternal fractures from rapid frontal deceleration (e.g. following driver impact with steering wheel). Tissue damage includes acute myocardial bruising and swelling, with potential disruption of the coronary arteries and electrical conduction systems.

Clinical signs

There is a wide spectrum of injury, ranging from increased ectopic activity to infarction and arrhythmias with rapid development of cardiogenic shock.

Treatment

This is supportive. The principles are similar to care provided for those with acute myocardial ischaemia, (although, clearly, thrombolysis would almost certainly be contraindicated).

Diaphragmatic rupture

This is usually the result of blunt high-impact injuries to the upper abdomen which produce a large tear in the diaphragm. Penetrating injury tends to leave much smaller holes.

Clinical signs

The force required to produce this injury is significant, so other injuries are certain. The lung is compressed, resulting in respiratory distress, and the patient will be shocked.

These injuries are diagnosed more frequently on the left. The presence of the liver stops visceral migration across a ruptured diaphragm on the right.

Investigations

Diagnosis from chest X-ray is difficult, although a nasogastric tube in the hemithorax (as seen in Figure 23.11) suggests the diagnosis. This is confirmed with administration of contrast for CXR or CT examination (Figure 23.13).

Treatment

Diaphragmatic rupture requires placement of a chest drain and early surgical repair.

Lung contusion

Clinical signs

Distress, tachypnoea, hypoxia.

Contusion results from direct lung trauma, both blunt and penetrating. In young people, more trauma is transmitted directly to lung tissue as ribs 'spring' into the chest.

Hypoxia develops over several hours as fluid fills the alveoli. Early intubation and ventilation should be considered, and continued until the associated local inflammation settles.

The consolidated lung tissue will not always be visible on the first CXR, but repeat films within a few hours often demonstrate diffuse shadowing in the area of chest impact. Traumatized lung tissue leaks fluid and cells, resulting in further local inflammation. Concomitant injuries may require large resuscitation fluid volumes; some of this extra fluid will accumulate in the lung and worsen gas exchange.

A reduced fluid resuscitation regime may sound tempting under these circumstances, but it should not be employed at the expense of an adequate cardiac output and organ blood flow.

Treatment

This is directed towards the maintenance of oxygenation and removal of carbon dioxide. Mechanical ventilation may be required.

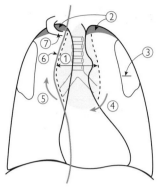

① Widened mediastinum
② Apical capping
③ Fractured scapula
④ Clockwise rotation of left main bronchus
⑤ Clockwise rotation of right main bronchus
⑥ Lateral deviation of NG tube (indications displacement of oesophagus
⑦ Fracture of 1ˢᵗ rib

Fig. 23.10 Line diagram of chest x-ray findings associated with aortic disruption.

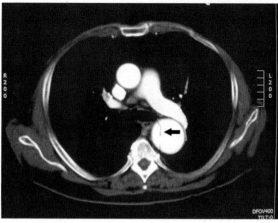

Fig. 23.12 CT of aortic disruption following trauma. The dissection is clearly seen (arrow).

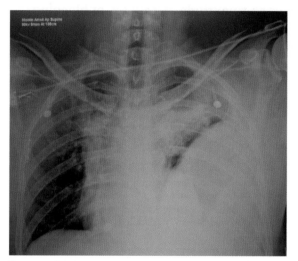

Fig. 23.11 Chest x-ray findings of diaphragmatic rupture. Diagnosis of this type of injury is difficult on plain x-ray evidence alone.

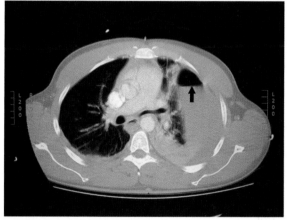

Fig. 23.13 CT findings of diaphragmatic rupture. Within the left hemithorax lies the stomach with its distinctive air/fluid interface (arrow).

23.5 Circulation and control of haemorrhage

The most common cause of shock is hypovolaemia, and this should be assumed to be due to haemorrhage in trauma patients until proven otherwise. There are other causes of shock, but in a trauma patient there may still be an associated element of volume deficit.

The prevention of tissue hypoxia depends, in part, on an adequate circulation. Without an adequate intravascular volume, organ perfusion and oxygen delivery will suffer. Prolonged anaerobic metabolism will affect cell membrane integrity and mitochondrial function. This will eventually lead to endothelial disruption within blood vessels and further intravascular depletion.

Causes of shock in trauma patients

- Hypovolaemia (haemorrhage until proven otherwise).
- Tension pneumothorax.
- Cardiogenic due to either tamponade or myocardial contusion.
- Neurogenic: spinal cord injury interrupts the sympathetic innervation of the vascular system, causing vasodilatation and venous pooling. A high spinal injury also prevents compensatory tachycardia leading to hypotension and shock.
- Septic: this is rare, and is usually associated with late presentation of penetrating trauma.
- Aortocaval compression should never be forgotten in the pregnant woman.

Examination

The aim is to detect hypovolaemia, as evidenced by cool peripheries, tachycardia, prolonged capillary refill time, tachypnoea, and hypotension. Table 23.1 describes the clinical signs associated with loss of progressively larger proportions of the circulating volume. Shock can be classified (I, II, III or IV) according to the amount of blood lost.

Low blood pressure is a **late sign**, and may occur after as much as 25–30% of the circulation has been lost. A raised lactate (>2mmol/L) or base deficit (worse than −2) may highlight a perfusion problem in the absence of hypotension.

Useful adjuncts

CXR, pelvic X-ray, and focussed ultrasound examination of the abdomen (Figure 23.14) will help to determine the source of bleeding. CT scanning should only be performed in the physiologically *normal* patient. Although it provides specific information, a combination of copious bleeding and cardiorespiratory instability make this a very hazardous investigation.

Aims of treatment

Control of haemorrhage

- Apply simple clean pressure dressings to bleeding points.
- Splint long-bone fractures to ease pain and help reduce ongoing blood loss.
- Operation: laparotomy or thoracotomy may be required to control bleeding. *This may take precedence over completion of the rest of the primary survey at this stage.*
- Reduction of a fractured pelvis will limit the space available for bleeding, allowing tamponade to produce haemostasis.

Replacement of intravascular volume

- Establish large-bore (16–14G) IV access, avoiding veins distal to fractures.
- Administer warmed crystalloid (Hartmann's solution) 10–20ml/kg in children and 1–2L in adults as an initial fluid challenge, depending on response.
- Review the response: an adequate volume will lead to resolution of signs of shock. Failure to respond mandates blood transfusion. Remember to seek senior and surgical help early, since only an operation might stop the bleeding.

Pitfalls

- Beware transferring a bleeding patient for CT scanning. This is fraught with danger; rapid decompensation can occur with disastrous consequences.
- Stopping bleeding may require pelvic fixation or laparotomy; remember that the primary survey will need to be completed post-operatively.
- A consumptive coagulopathy may develop rapidly, so anticipate the need for blood products (e.g. fresh frozen plasma, cryoprecipitate, and platelets) since these may take time to be delivered.
- Remember that the bleeding patient bleeds whole blood. The first FBC may demonstrate a normal haemoglobin *concentration* even in the face of extensive volume losses. A repeat FBC after crystalloid resuscitation will highlight red cell deficit.
- Rapid transfusion and volume replacement produces hypothermia. This can contribute to coagulopathy.
- Bleeding into the skull will not cause hypovolaemia or hypotension in adults. Another source of haemorrhage must be actively excluded.

Areas to exclude as sources of bleeding

There are five principal places where blood can accumulate:
- chest;
- abdomen;
- pelvis;
- in soft tissues, associated with long-bone fractures;
- on the floor!

Chest

See haemothorax management (Section 23.3).

Abdomen

This can be extraordinarily difficult to assess with any altered level of consciousness, and palpation can be equivocal. An exploratory laparotomy is advisable for fluid non-responders once other areas of bleeding have been excluded.

In experienced hands, ultrasound scanning picks up even small volumes of peritoneal fluid. Sensitivity and specificity depend very much on operator skill and experience.

Diagnostic peritoneal lavage (DPL), although once a popular technique, is less commonly performed today. It is recommended that it is performed by an experienced operator—the same person who would go on to perform the emergency laparotomy. The test is positive if there is frank blood, >100,000 RBCs/mm^3, or >500 WBCs/mm^3 in the fluid drained from 1L of peritoneal infusate. It is a sensitive test, but cannot specify the source of injury.

Contrast CT scanning can be useful in the *haemodynamically normal* patient. This is especially important when the patient is to be transferred to a specialist centre (e.g. neurosurgery) which does not have general surgery on site. Intra-abdominal injuries with the potential to cause later decompensation can be ruled out in this way. CT is the most reliably sensitive and specific imaging tool when reviewed by experienced clinicians. It also allows assessment of retroperitoneal structures.

Pelvis

Pelvic fractures can be classified into AP compression, lateral compression, and vertical shear. Each type can be open or closed.

Extreme force is required to fracture this strong bony ring, and associated intra-abdominal injury is common (15–30%). It is often likened to a Polo mint, i.e. impossible to break without fracturing in at least two places.

If the pelvis is disrupted, there is potential to exsanguinate from the venous plexus which sits in front of the sacro-iliac joints and/or from major pelvic vessels (e.g. internal iliac).

A *single* assessment of pelvic structural integrity should be performed in the initial assessment. With both hands gripping the anterior superior iliac crests the ring is pushed down firmly and brought together to feel for 'springing'. The intact ring does not normally move. Repeated testing of an unstable pelvis will only serve to dislodge clots and restart bleeding into the pelvis. Asymmetry of the lower limbs may give rise to further suspicion of pelvic fracture.

In the event of a pelvic fracture being found in males, an assessment of the urethra needs to be made prior to urinary catheterization. This includes PR examination of the prostate, and may also necessitate a urethrogram following the secondary survey.

Management needs to be discussed early with an experienced orthopaedic surgeon, who may elect to perform an external fixation of the pelvis in A&E.

Soft tissue and long bones

It is possible to estimate the degree of concealed blood loss from long-bone fractures, which may aid volume replacement strategies.

A closed fracture of the humerus can account for >500ml of blood. A fractured femur may cause loss of blood and fluid in excess of a litre. Bilateral fractured femurs alone can account for loss of 40% of the adult circulation, and put the patient into class III or IV shock. Open fractures of any long bone may result in exsanguination and death.

Splinting will reduce ongoing blood loss and ease the patient's pain.

'Blood on the floor'

Alarming amounts of blood can be missed under A&E trolleys, and in clothes and sheets. Remember to ask the paramedic crew about the amount of blood at the scene.

→ Focused assessment sonography for trauma (FAST)

Properly trained personnel perform FAST in the resuscitation room. It is able to screen for cardiac tamponade and detect free fluid in three other areas:

- peri-hepatic and hepatorenal spaces;
- perisplenic;
- pelvis.

The average time for an experienced operator to perform the examination is 2–3min. As a decision-making tool for identifying the need for laparotomy in hypotensive patients, FAST has an impressive sensitivity of 100%, a specificity of 96%, and a negative predictive value of 100%.

Advantages

- Rapid, portable, non-invasive.
- Low cost.
- Low radiation.
- Repeatable
- Fits in with the process of resuscitation.

Comparison with CT

CT offers a greater diagnostic capability since FAST is not able to give reliable information about solid organ damage. However, beware transferring a physiologically unstable patient to CT—disaster awaits!

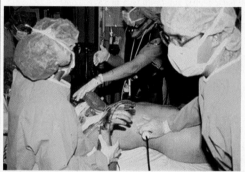

Fig. 23.14 FAST scanning.

→ Evaluation of response to treatment

- Resolution of vital signs towards normal (for age) values.
- Respiration rate and depth improved.
- Improvement in level of consciousness.
- Improving urinary output.
- Skin colour and perfusion improvement.

Table 23.1 Different classes of shock and response to fluid resuscitation

	Class I	Class II	Class III	Class IV
Volume loss	15%	15–30%	30–40%	>40%
Response to fluids	Responder	Responder	Transient responder	Non-responder
Respiration	14–20 breaths/min	20–30 breaths/min	30–40 breaths/min	>40 breaths/min
Heart rate	<100 beats/min	>100 beats/min	>120 beats/min	>140 beats/min
Blood pressure	Normal	Normal	Low	Low, unrecordable
CNS	Normal	Mild anxiety	Confused	Lethargic
Urine output	Normal, >0.5ml/kg/hr	Normal to early oliguric	Oliguric, <0.5ml/kg/hr	Negligible
Treatment fluid	Crystalloid	Crystalloid, consider blood	Crystalloid and blood products, consider operation	Rapid crystalloid and blood products, operation likely

- Rapid responder: fluid bolus quickly fills patient's intravascular compartment and patient remains stable thereafter.
- Transient responder: fluid bolus has a short-lived effect to improve the patients' condition. The patient is usually continuing to bleed from somewhere.
- Non-responder: fluid does not improve the condition, consider operation or exclusion of conditions that cause profound hypotension, with only a component of intravascular depletion, e.g. cardiac tamponade or tension pneumothorax

23.6 Primary survey: disability and exposure

The neurological assessment in the primary surgery comprises:

- Pupil size and response to light. Pupils are normally equal in size (1mm variation is acceptable).
- Evaluation of GCS.

Paramedics will first assess the level of consciousness and this forms the baseline against which subsequent changes may be judged. GCS changes of 2 or more are significant, and signify the need for prompt action. GCS of 8 and below defines coma and is itself an indication for intubation since protective airway reflexes will be lost.

Unilateral fixed dilated pupil with a low GCS

With trauma, this is a sign of increased intracranial pressure (ICP), and usually an expanding lesion will be found on the same side as the dilated pupil. Emergency action is directed at controlling ICP, and CT imaging of the brain will identify treatable lesions requiring neurosurgical intervention.

Bilateral fixed dilated pupils with a low GCS

This is commonly a sign of a significantly elevated ICP. Emergency measures to reduce ICP such as mannitol and hyperventilation may prevent medullary 'coning' and death.

Unilateral fixed dilated pupil with GCS of 15

A normal GCS is not compatible with markedly raised ICP. An additionally dilated pupil is likely to be due to local optic nerve or ocular trauma or instillation of dilating eye drops.

Factors affecting ICP

See Section 7.10.

Skull injury classification

Vault
- Depressed or undisplaced
- Open or closed injuries

Basal skull
- With or without CSF leak
- With or without cranial nerve palsy

Brain injury classification

Focal
- Extradural (epidural)
- Subdural
- Intracerebral

Diffuse
- Cerebral contusions
- Diffuse axonal injury
- Hypoxic injury

Extradural haematoma

This is seen in 2.5–4% of all cases of severe traumatic brain injury (TBI) and is associated with all types of skull fracture. Classically, it is caused by a temporal blow which results in middle meningeal artery bleeding.

Clinical signs

There might be a lucid interval following injury (seen in 38%), with rapid deterioration some hours later as arterial bleeding worsens ICP. Untreated, the patient will develop lateralizing signs with death following soon after.

Management

CT appearance demonstrates a biconcave (lentiform) discrete haematoma at the site of the blow (Figure 23.15). Prognosis can be good if the haematoma is evacuated early: urgent neurosurgical referral is required. Overall mortality is 10%.

Subdural haematoma

Subdural hematoma is seen in 12–29% of severe TBI and has a mortality of 40–60%. It is caused by low-pressure venous bleeding, but can raise ICP and cause a significant mass effect. It is more common in the elderly and alcoholics, as brain tissue atrophy makes shearing of veins more probable.

Management

Morbidity and mortality are worse than for extradural haematoma because it is often associated with greater underlying cerebral damage. CT appearance demonstrates extensive bleeding covering the surface of the brain (Figure 23.16).

Neurosurgical review is mandatory, but surgical intervention only follows careful consideration of the individual case. A more conservative line is often taken for very elderly and those with greater brain injury, since outcome for these groups is generally poor.

Intracerebral haematoma

This is commonly associated with the presence of a subdural haematoma. Typically, development of surrounding oedema over the following few days will produce a mass effect, the size and location of which will dictate morbidity and mortality.

Management

Early neurosurgical review is required, but this is mainly for ICP monitoring and the use of measures to maintain cerebral perfusion pressure (CPP). Occasionally intracerebral haematomas warrant evacuation.

Diffuse axonal injury

This is the result of rapid deceleration and application of rotational forces to the axons of the brain. The axonal disruption causes a functional brain injury lasting for weeks or more.

At the other end of the spectrum are those who suffer an extremely severe neurological deficit and are left in a persistent vegetative state.

Management

There is often a period of raised ICP with compromised CPP. CT scanning may show little abnormality, as the multiple injuries are at a microscopic level (Figure 23.17). MRI is the investigation of choice, but this is rarely appropriate in the acute setting.

Life-threatening spinal injury

High cervical or thoracic injuries are likely have an to adverse effect on ventilation, and necessitate intubation and ventilation.

Management

Optimize oxygenation, ventilation, and organ perfusion.

Immobilize any potential spinal injury until senior experienced assessment can be made.

In blunt spinal injury of <8hr duration, consider IV methylprednisolone. The decision to use steroids should be made after consultation with the spinal injury unit, since evidence supporting their use remains controversial. A typical regimen might be:

- 30mg/kg over 15min;
- 5.4mg/kg over the next 23–48hr.

Environment and exposure

It is essential to inspect all body surfaces, as only two-thirds of the body can be seen when the patient lies supine. 'Log-rolling' the trauma patient off the spinal board at an early stage allows inspection and palpation of the vertebral column and rectal examination. Removal of the hard spinal board also reduces the risk of pressure sores.

Many accidents occur outside and in adverse weather conditions, so the potential for heat loss and hypothermia is great. This is worsened during the process of trauma assessment when clothes are removed; every effort should be made to prevent further patient cooling. Many homeostatic functions are enzyme dependent and hypothermia markedly affects their function (e.g. coagulation, with cold-induced coagulopathy).

- Significant hypothermia (< 34°C) is common following trauma and these patients have a worse prognosis when compared with warm patients of a matched trauma severity.

- Only warmed IV fluids should be given and active warming blankets should be used.

Peripheral cold injury (e.g. frostbite) is rarely seen in the UK. Its development is related to the temperature and duration of exposure, immobilization, the presence of moisture on the affected part, and the presence of pre-existing vascular disease. Once recognized, treatment should not be delayed, clothing should be removed, and the affected part gently re-warmed with dry heat (i.e. blankets). Later care should be aimed at tissue preservation and prevention of infection.

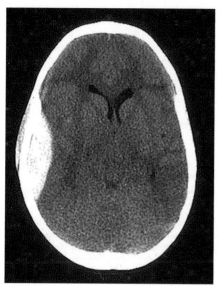

Fig. 23.15 CT of an extradural haematoma. The biconvex right extradural haematoma was associated with signs of raised ICP despite only modest midline shift on this CT scan.

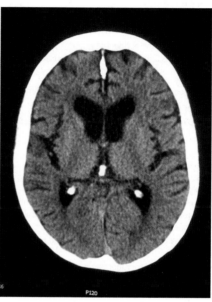

Fig. 23.17 CT of diffuse axonal injury.

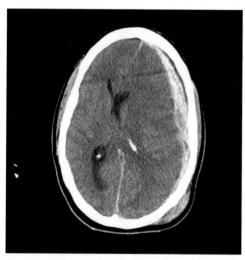

Fig. 23.16 CT of a subdural haematoma. The left subdural haematoma is associated with marked midline shift.

> ➜ **Neurogenic and spinal shock are NOT the same thing!**
>
> *Neurogenic shock.*
> This results from the loss of sympathetic outflow and the resultant vasodilatation further compromises any intravascular depletion. If the outflow is blocked above T1–4 (cardiac sympathetic supply), bradycardia and hypotension are likely. These patients may well be non-responders to IV fluids, and after exclusion of other sources of haemorrhage, vasopressor support should be started.
>
> *Spinal shock*
> This term describes a purely neurological deficit which does not cause haemodynamic compromise. It causes flaccidity and loss of reflexes. Duration is variable.

> ➜ **Classification of different types of cold injury**
>
> *Frost nip*
> Numb white skin that feels stiff to touch. The underlying tissue is warm and soft. Little chance of blistering or permanent tissue damage.
>
> *Frost bite*
> White or yellow skin with a waxy appearance, which turns purplish on re-warming. Underlying tissues are hard. There are usually blood- or fluid-filled blisters, and permanent tissue damage is very likely.
>
> *Non-freezing injury*
> Injury that occurs when blood vessels constrict in response to heat loss. It usually occurs in cold wet conditions and is known as trench foot. Permanent muscle and nerve injury may ensue.

23.7 The AMPLE history and secondary survey

A full history of events and comorbidities is often unavailable. However, make sure that you seek information from the paramedics attending the scene as it will aid the understanding of the mechanisms of injury and help focus investigations.

AMPLE is an *aide memoire* for attaining the key points.

A	Allergies
M	Medications: especially recreational drugs, insulin, and cardiovascular treatments
P	Past medical history/surgery
L	Last meal: significant trauma often stops gastric emptying
E	Events surrounding the accident

Analgesia

Pain relief can be provided by mechanical or pharmacological means.

Mechanical: splinting of fractures

Primarily this is used to aid haemorrhage control but is also effective in reducing pain.

Pharmacological

- Ketamine is often used pre-hospital, because it causes little respiratory depression. However, it produces dissociative anaesthesia and may make neurological assessment unreliable.
- Entonox may be useful for interventions such as fracture splinting, but should not be used if there is a suspicion of a pathological gas-filled space (e.g. pneumothorax, pneumocranium).
- Opiates are the mainstay of analgesic therapy, but need to be given with care.
  - Careful assessment of respiratory function is imperative since they can reduce respiratory drive and increase hypercapnoea and hypoxia.
  - Incomplete volume resuscitation places the patient at considerable risk of hypotension. Reduction of the sympathetic arteriolar tone unmasks the volume deficit.
  - With volume resuscitation assured, small incremental boluses of opiates should be titrated against pain. 10–20mcg boluses of fentanyl or 1mg bolus of morphine are effective, especially prior to painful procedures and manipulations of displaced factures.

Imaging

CXR and pelvic X-rays provide valuable clinical information, but further imaging may be required to fully assess all injuries.

The only patients fit enough to undergo CT examination are those who have physiologically normal and stable parameters. This requires discussion with a senior colleague.

Intra- and inter-hospital transfer

The need for clinical transfer often becomes apparent by the end of the primary survey, and referral should be made without delay. Inter-hospital transfer is most often performed for patients with neurosurgical or cardiothoracic injury. However, no patient should be moved if they are too unstable—bring definitive care to the patient.

Transfer of patients between areas of the same hospital or between different hospitals is a hazardous undertaking. Stabilization is particularly important and the same principles should be applied for both intra- and inter-hospital transfers.

Good transfer performance begins with preparation. The contents of any pre-packed transfer bag, and pathways of care should be established before they are needed.

All equipment used for transferring patients needs to be stored ready for full immediate operational deployment. Portable monitoring equipment should be fully charged, drugs and sufficient disposable items should be in date, and enough oxygen should be taken to last at least twice the expected duration of the transfer.

Transfer personnel (typically an anaesthetist and ODP) need to be sufficiently skilled to cope with adverse events. Mobile phone or walkie-talkie communication with the hospital during transfer is essential. Physiological parameters must be recorded en route.

Knowledge of the exact destination reduces the chances of delay, and it is now commonplace for satellite navigation to be used by the driving personnel. Receiving areas need to be forewarned in order to be ready to receive the patient.

The transfer team need to know who to hand over to. All documentation, X-rays, and cross-matched blood should go with patient, and if images are to be sent on disc it is important to ensure that this can be read by the receiving institution. Continuity of care is important, and the team needs to be fully versed with the patient's clinical details prior to departure.

Any family members should be informed of the transfer and given directions to and the phone number of the destination hospital.

Secondary survey

This is a complete top-to-toe inspection and can only be fully completed with an awake and compliant patient. Occult injuries should be actively sought, as missed injuries are an (often avoidable) cause of pain and disability for patients surviving trauma. However, if the patient deteriorates during this assessment, it is important to revisit the primary survey and review ABCDE.

If a log-roll has not already been performed, it should be completed and documented during the secondary survey. Figure 23.18 shows the correct technique.

Catheterisation and passage of an oro- or nasogastric tube may be indicated, and further invasive monitoring may be required.

In the male patient, urethral disruption must be excluded clinically prior to catheterization for fear of causing further damage. Warning signs include:

- blood at meatus of penis;
- scrotal bruising;
- high-riding prostate on PR examination.

If urethral disruption is diagnosed, a suprapubic catheter will be required.

Early oro- or nasogastric tube insertion is particularly useful in anaesthetised patients. The orogastric route is safest in anaesthetised patients who have sustained any degree of head trauma; it can be replaced with a nasogastric tube later, once basal skull fracture has been excluded. Gastric distension is common, and can impair basal lung expansion.

Musculoskeletal injury and compartment syndrome

Compartment syndrome develops a number of hours after the initial assessment and is associated with prolonged pressure on skeletal muscles or hypotension in the presence of long-bone fractures. It most commonly involves compartments below the knee. Signs include:

- pain out of proportion to injury;
- pain in calf or forearm on passive movement of distal digits;
- paraesthesia;
- pallor;
- paralysis;
- loss of pulses (this is a late sign);
- hard tissues, almost 'wooden' in consistency.

This is a medical and surgical emergency. If it is left untreated, the patient can develop acute renal failure secondary to muscle death (rhabdomyolosis), or irreversible limb ischaemia. Unless fasciotomies are carried out quickly, the limb will be lost.

Spinal cord neurological assessment

The initial assessment should detect life-threatening spinal injury patterns, e.g. high spinal cord transection with shock.

During the secondary survey, more subtle deficiencies are found. Lateralizing signs or spinal levels of neurological deficiency should be noted.

The primary survey is carried with cervical protection at every stage. However, early clinical clearance of the spine and cord, if possible, makes ongoing care much simpler.

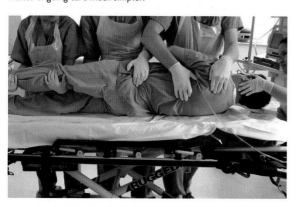

Fig. 23.18 The log-roll. Four people are required to log-roll a patient, and a fifth is required to examine the back and perform a rectal examination. The person controlling the lifting sequence is usually the anaesthetist, who is responsible for airway control and cervical protection. The collar should be removed prior to any movement otherwise the back of the neck will not be seen. The three people performing the rolling should be arranged in order of height, with the tallest at the head end (this end requires the greatest reach). The hands should be arranged as shown; this allows the lifted leg to maintain its position relative to the pelvis and vertebral column, thus preventing further damage at sites of injury. Instructions from the anaesthetist should be clear and concise, for example: 'We will roll on the command of 'ROLL', to 45° and then maintain that position. We will return to supine on the command 'DOWN'. Is everyone ready? Ready, steady, ROLL.'

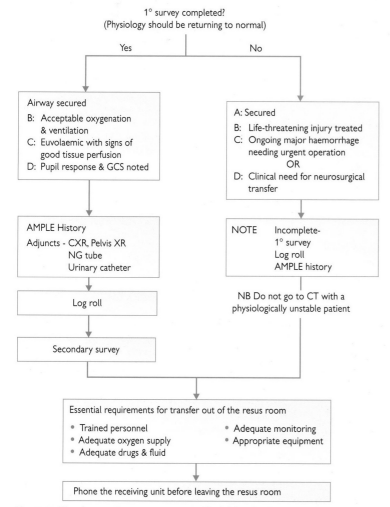

Fig. 23.19 Flow diagram of trauma care pathway. The left hand pathway demonstrates a complete primary and secondary survey in a patient with no life-threatening injuries. The right hand pathway describes the progress of a patient in whom resuscitative surgery is necessary: this takes priority over completion of the secondary survey. Progress through the trauma surveys should be carefully documented and any outstanding examinations or investigations should be handed over to the receiving team.

The same principles of care apply to children, the elderly, and the pregnant patient. However, physiology and compensatory mechanisms in these groups may be different from those in the normal healthy adult.

Children

There are significant differences in the anatomy and physiology of children which affect their care following trauma. Normal values vary with age, and knowledge of these values is important if they are to be used to guide therapy. Smaller patients and unfamiliar equipment also make for more challenging management. However, it is important to remember that the priorities for trauma care remain the same.

Although not usually part of the trauma team, senior paediatric support ensures comprehensive care. It is also vital to ensure parental presence, since this may help calm the anxious child.

Pre-prepared systems of paediatric management (e.g. Broselow) are invaluable. Such systems base equipment, drug, and fluid information on the age or size of the child. When admitted, the child is measured with a colour-coded tape and all resuscitation equipment required for a child of that size is found in the associated colour-coded container. Drug, fluid, and resuscitation doses are similarly colour-coded.

The chest wall is more pliable and there is a greater risk of lung contusion without rib fracture. With a higher metabolic rate and oxygen demand children will subsequently develop hypoxia very quickly.

Children have great cardiovascular reserve and so tolerate the effects of hypovolaemia well. The downside is that medical staff must be aware of this; as the last thing to change, once the blood pressure starts to drop, cardiovascular collapse is imminent.

Small children have fewer long nephrons and cannot concentrate their urine to the same extent as adults. They need to pass more urine per kilogram to clear a urea load.

- 0−3 years 2ml/kg/hr
- 3−5 years 1ml/kg/hr
- 6−12 years 0.5−1ml/kg/hr

SCIWORA (spinal cord injury without radiological abnormality) is more likely in young children because of their relatively large heavy heads and small necks. This, together with 'elastic' spinal ligaments, allows greater spinal movements and cord damage without bony injury or X-ray abnormality.

Children will quickly cool down because of their low body fat and high ration of body surface area to mass.

Children exhibit different age-related patterns of injury. For example, in young children the relatively large abdominal organs are lower riding and easier to damage.

Management issues

- Parental presence may help calm the anxious child.
- Traditionally, uncuffed ETTs are used (although modern low-pressure high-volume cuffs are now being used in many centres). C-spine management can be difficult, as there are no semi-rigid collars that will fit small children. Lateral blocks, tape, and vacuum 'bean bags' may be a temporary solution.
- Fluid volumes: 20ml/kg as initial crystalloid bolus.
- Blood: 10ml/kg as initial blood bolus. A lack of ischaemic heart disease in this group allows for greater tolerance of normovolaemic anaemia.
- Different GCS. Infants will not be able to talk and respond in the same way as adults, and this needs to be reflected in their neurological assessment.
- Early notification of senior paediatric support to help and arrange area for definitive care.

The elderly

Irrespective of health prior to trauma, elderly patients tolerate traumatic insults poorly. Early aggressive intervention is required to prevent long hospital stays from relatively minor trauma. Falls are a major reason for admission.

Comorbidity and polypharmacy are common features. Elderly patients usually require higher perfusion pressures, and without this consideration there is a risk of under-resuscitation and rapid progression to end-organ dysfunction.

Medications may affect responses to treatment, especially ACE inhibitors and β-blockers.

The pregnant patient

Ask **every** female trauma patient: 'Are you pregnant?' Although the aim is to treat both patients successfully, priority should always be the mother. Good care for the mother will give the child the best chance of survival as well.

Again, physiological changes influence management. Hormonal effects increase the chance of aspiration and raise baseline respiratory rates. Maternal blood volumes are increased up to 40% by the third trimester, so they can compensate for longer before becoming hypotensive due to blood loss.

In the first trimester the fetus is intra-pelvic, and is well protected from all but massive pelvic disruption. Trauma at this time carries the risk of spontaneous abortion and rhesus iso-immunization.

In the second and third trimesters, the fetus is intra-abdominal and is obviously more vulnerable, although the mother's viscera are relatively protected. Vaginal bleeding may be a sign of placental abruption, and amniotic fluid loss needs urgent investigation. Early fetal assessment by an obstetrician may help calm maternal anxieties or expedite delivery, if that is appropriate.

Vena-caval compression by the uterus in the third trimester can cause hypotension. Putting a 20−30° lateral tilt on the table, or wedging the spinal board and moving the uterus to the left, can alleviate this.

The burned patient

Despite the often dramatic appearance of the burned patient, the assessment priorities are the same as for any other patient. *Do not be distracted from performing a thorough primary survey.*

Special care should be taken in assessing the airway and potential for stridor and obstruction. This is the result of inhalation of super-heated gases and particles, and occurs in fires within enclosed spaces. Carbonaceous phlegm, soot in the mouth, and facial singeing of hair should alert staff to this potential problem. Early intubation is essential, since this may be almost impossible once swelling has developed.

Classification

Burns are described as partial or full thickness and are assessed for extent with Lund and Browder charts (Figure 23.20).

- Partial burns are very painful and incorporate first-degree (sunburn type) and second-degree (blistering of superficial layers of skin) burns. Pain can be alleviated by covering the burned area with cling film. This also allows ongoing viewing of the area.
- Full-thickness burns, otherwise known as third-degree burns, are painless because nerve endings are destroyed. The skin is tough and leathery, and does not stretch. If circumferential, escharotomies may be required in order to allow limb perfusion or adequate ventilation.

Once flames are extinguished, patients should be nursed in a very warm environment: loss of skin will prevent normal thermoregulatory mechanisms. Although burns may be relieved by cold water, continued washing will cause iatrogenic hypothermia.

Fluid replacement

This must be calculated from the time of the burn.

As an initial guide, 4ml of warmed Hartmann's solution per kilogram per percentage burn to be given in the first 23hr post-burn.

- Half should be given in the first 8hr.
- The remainder should be given in the remaining 16 hr.

As with all critically ill patients, this regimen is a guide and further fluids may be required in excess of this amount. Nothing replaces frequent clinical assessment of the patient's general status and organ perfusion. Preservation of urine output at more than 0.5ml/kg/hr, together with a correcting base deficit, suggests adequate fluid resuscitation.

Who should be transferred?

Each hospital network will have varying transfer guidelines, and early burns specialist consultation is always the aim.

Consideration should be given to:

- 10% burns in <10 years and >50 years.
- >20% in all ages.
- specific areas involved—face, hands, feet, genitalia, and skin over major joints.

→ Estimation of burn size

Rule of nines

This is a method of estimmating percentage burn, which is useful in determining the need for transfer to burns unit and for calculations of fluid requirements in the first hours post-burn.

Pitfall

Burns rarely occur in the same distribution as in the diagram. A rough estimate can be made by taking the patient's palm as 1% and working out burn size in relation to this.

Assessing extent of burns—Lund and Browder charts

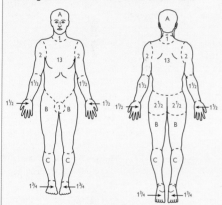

Relative percentage of area affected by growth (age in years)

	0	1	5	10	15	Adult
A: half of head	9½	8½	6½	5½	4½	3½
B: half of thigh	2¾	3¼	4	4½	4½	4¾
C: half of leg	2½	2½	2¾	3	3¼	3½

Adults rule of 9's:	head	=	9%
	each arm	=	9%
	each leg	=	18%
	front of trunk	=	18%
	back of trunk	=	18%
	perineum	=	1%

Infants rule of 5's:	head	=	20%
	each arm	=	10%
	each leg	=	20%
	front of trunk	=	10%
	back of trunk	=	10%

Fig. 23.20

→ Glasgow Coma Scale for paediatric patients

Best eye response (E)

4	Eyes opening spontaneously
3	Eye opening to speech
2	Eye opening to pain
1	No eye opening

Best verbal response (V)

5	Infant coos or babbles (normal activity)
4	Infant is irritable and continually cries
3	Infant cries to pain
2	Infant moans to pain
1	No verbal response

Best motor response (M)

6	Infant moves spontaneously or purposefully
5	Infant withdraws from touch
4	Infant withdraws from pain
3	Abnormal flexion to pain
2	Extension to pain
1	No motor response

Chapter 24

Statistics for the anaesthetist

24.1 Descriptive statistics

Statistical methods allow us to draw inferences about a population by studying a sample from it. In addition, they give us information about the applicability of the results to the population, expressed in terms of probability.

Statistics can be characterised as descriptive or inferential. Descriptive statistics summarize large amounts of data into shorter descriptions. Inferential statistics are used to make inferences about a population by studying a sample from the population.

Types of data

Nominal data Information is labelled according to category. There is no intrinsic order. Examples are gender (male or female) or route of drug administration (oral, IV, IM, etc.).

Ordinal data Information is classified according to category, but there is an intrinsic order. However, the differences between the consecutive levels are not the same, nor is there exact equivalence between subjects. Examples include ASA grade (where ASA 4 cannot be said to be 'twice as unwell' as ASA 2, and where two patients with ASA 2 status may have completely different underlying illnesses); and pain scoring (mild, moderate, and severe).

Parametric data have an intrinsic order, with equal distances between intervals. Every point in the continuous scale is a valid measurement with a definite meaning. Continuous data can be interval or ratio data. The two types can be compared by considering the Celsius and Kelvin scales of temperature:

- **Interval data** have equal differences between numbers, but without a natural zero. In the Celsius scale, 'zero' does not denote a total lack of internal energy; it is an arbitrarily defined point (the freezing point of water).
- **Ratio data** have equal differences between numbers, including a natural zero—a complete absence of the thing being measured. Temperature measured on the Kelvin scale is ratio data: a temperature of 100K indicates twice the energy of a temperature of 50K. 'Absolute zero' implies a complete absence of internal energy.

Estimates and parameters

Statistical tests are conducted on the samples. The values obtained are known as **estimates**. For example, the mean age of the sample is an estimate (of the population mean). A second sample from the same population would give a different estimate of the mean age. The corresponding value in the population is known as the **parameter**. The mean age of the population is the parameter. An estimate is made to try and determine the parameter.

The true parameter can never be known unless the entire population is studied, but the sample can provide a reliable estimate. The question underlying all statistical tests is how close the estimate is to the parameter of interest.

Measures of central tendency

Central tendency is a single value representation of a set of data. Common measures include the following.
- **Mode:** the most commonly occurring value.
- **Median:** the middle value in an ordered list of the data.
- **Mean:** the average value. It is the sum of all the values divided by the number n of data points.

The mean uses all the values in the data, and is sensitive to the influence of outliers.

Neither the median nor the mode use the values of all the available data, and they are resistant to the influences of outliers.

Parametric data can be represented by the mean, median, or mode, whereas non-parametric data are best represented by the median or mode. The choice of the measure is dependent on the data. For example, in a questionnaire-based satisfaction survey, the satisfaction levels of most people (mode) may be more appropriate than the 'average' level of satisfaction, which may be significantly distorted by small numbers of outliers.

Measures of dispersion

Measures of dispersion provide a context for interpreting a measure of central tendency. Two sets of data may have the same mean, but very different spreads. The spread of the data is also known as its **distribution**. Many real-world phenomena occur with in a normal (Gaussian) distribution (Figure 24.1). Common measures of dispersion include the following.

Range The difference between the largest and the smallest values. It is influenced by extreme values and has limited use.

Quartiles express the distribution in quarters. The interquartile range (IQR) is the difference between the first and third quarters. When used with the median, it can show whether the distribution is symmetric about the median. It does not use all the values available (ignores the first and last quarters), but is not affected by outliers.

Variance measures spread in data using all the values available. Measures of variance are based on the difference between the measured value and the central measure. The simplest way is to calculate the difference between each value and the mean and to sum the results. This sum is then averaged. However, in a normal distribution the result would be zero, as half the values are below the central value, giving negative numbers. This problem is overcome by squaring each value before adding them up. Squaring has two effects: it removes the negative sign, and it adds weight to the variance (after squaring, a value further from the mean contributes more to the variance than a value close to the mean). Variance is a very important concept in statistics and forms the basis of other concepts like regression.

Standard deviation (SD) is the square root of variance. As variance is a squared value, it does not have a directly relevant meaning (e.g. if the mean value is measured in metres, then the variance is in square metres). SD converts the variance into appropriate units. In a normal distribution, the SD has a defined relationship to the area under the curve (Figure 24.2), allowing the calculation of *p*-values.

The central limit theorem

If a large number of samples are drawn from a population and the means are calculated, the means would be normally distributed even if the original data were not. This is known as the central limit theorem. In effect, any distribution can be converted into a normal distribution by taking the means of multiple sampling exercises. Such a distribution is known as the sampling distribution, and its raw data comprise a list of means. The mean of the sampling distribution should be equal to the true mean of the population. The standard deviation of the sampling distribution is known as the **standard error of the mean** (SE_m), and quantifies the uncertainty in the estimate of the mean. While the mean of the sampling distribution (the true mean of the population) cannot be determined, the standard error of mean can be estimated from the SD and the sample size n:

$$SE_m = \frac{SD}{\sqrt{n}}.$$

Then, by using the properties of a normal distribution, the true mean can be predicted to lie between two standard errors of means around the sample mean.

When publishing research, means should always be quoted with standard deviations. Some studies quote the standard error of the mean instead. This can be converted to standard deviation if the population size is known. However, by definition, standard error is less than the standard deviation. This results in tighter error bars and better-looking pictures, but is misleading.

The normal distribution

The normal distribution is a bell-shaped curve, symmetrical about a central axis. This central axis corresponds to the mean, median, and mode (Figure 24.1). The normal distribution allows us to make powerful predictions as a result of its symmetry. The normal curve has a consistent relationship with the standard deviation (Figure 24.2). This consistent relationship is important in deriving p-values (Section 24.2).

The standard normal curve has a mean of 0 and a standard deviation of 1. The area under the curve of a standard normal curve is 1. Any normal curve can be mathematically converted to a standard normal distribution. This allows both single-sample comparison (normal distribution of one sample with a known (standard) mean and standard deviation) and two-sample comparison (normal distributions from two populations).

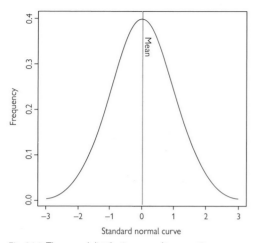

Fig. 24.1 The normal distribution curve. Its properties are:
* symmetric around the mean
* mean = median = mode
* the area under the curve has a predictable relationship to the standard deviation.

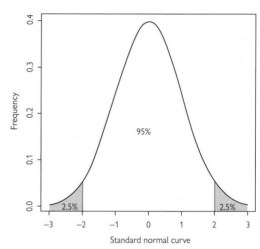

Fig. 24.2 Relationship of the normal distribution curve to the standard deviation.

Skew and kurtosis

Skew occurs when values are clustered around one side and sparse on the other. This results in loss of symmetry, with the curve typically having a peak and a tail. The skew is said to be positive when the peak appears at the left and a long tail on the right (Figure 24.3) and negative when the peak is at the right (Figure 24.4). Most variables in medicine have a skew, with a positive skew much more common than a negative skew. For example, blood pressure is distributed with a positive skew. Most individuals have a normal blood pressure but some have very high pressures. Very low pressures are not as common for obvious reasons. The presence of a skew biases results by altering the fundamental properties of a normal distribution. Skew can be removed by mathematical treatment of the variables. Common treatments include taking the inverse, squaring the variable, or taking the log function of the variable. If one variable in a sample needs treatment for skew, serious consideration should be given to treating all the other variables in the sample in the same way. Not doing so might invalidate the results.

Kurtosis describes the peak of a normal curve. A normal distribution with a sharper peak is leptokurtotic and a blunter peak is platykurtotic. Kurtosis depends on the variance of the sample and the presence of outliers

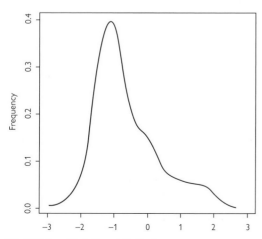

Fig. 24.3 A positively skewed distribution

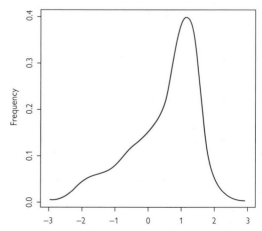

Fig. 24.4 A negatively skewed distribution

24.2 Inferential statistics

Statistical analysis is a tool. It can be put to good use as long as the underlying assumptions and principles are understood. It can also be used inappropriately with poor results. 'Significant' results can be obtained by subjecting random numbers to statistical tests. The usefulness of the analysis is determined by the context of the research, a carefully formulated research hypothesis, the meticulous collection of data, and the application of appropriate analytic processes.

Sample selection

A population is defined as a set of entities for which inferences are to be drawn. The ideal way to answer any question pertaining to a population is to study the entire population. This is completely impractical for almost all questions worth answering, so a compromise is struck by studying a sample from the population. A sample can be considered analogous to a small-scale model of a physical object. Inferences can be drawn by testing and observing the model, provided that the model is representative of the original object. The more accurate the model, the more useful are the inferences. Similarly, the more representative the sample, the easier it is to generalize the results to the population.

The representative quality of the sample can be improved by clearly defining the population to be studied. Any study can only be extrapolated to the population in question. For example, a study about postoperative nausea and vomiting in female patients undergoing gynaecological surgery cannot be extrapolated to patients undergoing chemotherapy.

Important considerations in selecting a sample are randomization, avoiding bias, and appropriate sample size (power analysis).

Hypothesis testing

Formulation of a suitable hypothesis is the fundamental requirement of a well-designed study.

A hypothesis is a predictive statement. Most research starts out with the aim of proving a hypothesis correct, e.g. 'anti-emetic A gives a lower incidence of nausea and vomiting than anti-emetic B'. However, in statistical terms, a good hypothesis is one that can be proved false. This is done by creating a **null hypothesis**. The null hypothesis is exactly the opposite of what needs to be proved. A null hypothesis states that there is no difference between the two populations. The **alternative hypothesis** suggests that there is a difference. So, for the anti-emetic study, the null hypothesis is that the two populations have the same incidence of vomiting. For a study comparing mean blood pressure, the null hypothesis would be that the two populations have similar mean blood pressures despite different treatments.

By using the alternative hypothesis, we start with the assumption that there is a difference between the populations. However, if a difference is not found, it does not automatically falsify the alternative hypothesis. It might just be that there is not enough evidence. By using the null hypothesis, we start with the assumption that there is no difference between the populations. When a difference is found using statistical tests, the null hypothesis is rejected and the alternative hypothesis is accepted. The use of the null hypothesis also allows the determination of probabilities and confidence intervals for the truth of the alternative hypothesis.

p-values

A p-value is the probability of a result occurring by chance, provided that the null hypothesis is true. p-values are determined by applying statistical tests to sets of data (section 24.3).

A lower p-value implies that the null hypothesis is unlikely. For example, in the anti-emetic study, a p-value of 0.05 indicates that there is a 5% chance that the result observed was obtained by chance, i.e. there is no difference between the two drugs and a significant result is seen purely as a result of chance. This means that we can never be *absolutely* sure about any of the results, but the lower the p-value, the more confident we are.

Prior to the start of a study, an α-value must be decided upon to evaluate the significance of the result. If the p-value from the data is less than the α-value, the result is considered significant. The α-value is usually set at 0.05, so a p-value <0.05 is considered significant: the null hypothesis is rejected, giving weight to the alternative hypothesis. A p-value <0.01 is considered extremely significant. However, when the p-value is >0.05, the null hypothesis is not accepted as true; it is merely *not rejected*. This is because the p-value may be high because of other factors such as sample size, difference in effect size etc.

Error

Two kinds of errors are possible in hypothesis testing (Table 24.1).

Type 1 error occurs when the null hypothesis is rejected when it should not be. As we have already seen, the α-value is the probability of a type 1 error.

Type 2 error occurs when the null hypothesis is accepted when it is false. The β-value (see below) is the probability of a type 2 error.

Experimental design and error

Good experimental designs aim to reduce the error in research studies. Error occurs because of:

- random error due to intrinsic variation in samples;
- systematic error, also known as bias.

Bias is defined as a systematic error that results in incorrect estimation of statistical parameters. Increasing the sample size reduces random error, but has no effect on systematic error. The major types of bias are as follows.

- **Selection bias:** a systematic error in selecting patients results in groups that are not comparable. Selection bias is minimized by randomization.
- **Measurement bias:** a systematic error occurs in measuring the variables of interest. Measurement errors can result from equipment error or observer bias. Measurement bias is minimized by blinding and by standardizing the measuring equipment.

Confounding occurs when association between the study factors is distorted because of other variables influencing these factors.

Errors can be reduced by the following methods.

Randomization reduces selection bias. By randomization, any individual in a population has the same chance of being selected for the sample as the other members of the population.

Blinding reduces measurement bias. In a single-blind study the subject is unaware of the treatment administered. In a double-blind study both the subject and the observer are unaware of the treatment administered.

An adequate **sample size** reduces random errors. The ideal sample size for a study is calculated by **power analysis**. The power of a study is the probability of appropriately rejecting the null hypothesis if it is false $(1 - \beta)$. Conventionally, a β-value of 20% is considered an acceptable probability of a type 2 error. This results in a power of 80%. The required sample size will depend upon the following.

- *Effect size* which is the difference in effect between the treatment and control groups. The greater the effect size, the lower the sample size has to be to demonstrate the effect.
- *β-value:* conventionally 20%.
- *α-value:* conventionally 0.05.
- *Distribution* of value measured, i.e. parametric or non-parametric.

Interpreting p-values

The p-value is an important concept in statistics. It is determined by applying statistical tests (Section 24.3) and represents the probability that the observed value occurred by chance. This follows from the relationship between the normal distribution and the standard deviation. In a normal distribution, the mean ±2 standard deviations on either side covers 95% of the observed values. The outliers (the shaded regions in Figure 24.2) each contain 2.5% of the observed values.

If a value is picked randomly from this distribution, there is a 95% chance that it would fall in the unshaded area. In other words, there is only a 5% chance that a value would be obtained from the shaded area. Suppose that a value is picked from another distribution. If this value falls within the shaded area of the first distribution, then there is only a 5% chance that the two distributions are the same. Hence the p-value is 0.05.

Table 24.1 Hypothesis testing

		Null hypothesis	
		True	False
Decision	Accept	Correct	Type 2 error (false positive)
	Reject	Type 1 error (false negative)	Correct

Power and error

The upper panel (Figure 24.5) shows a population which is normally distributed, with a mean of 0 and a standard deviation of 1. The probability of a randomly chosen value falling in the shaded region is α.

The lower panel (Figure 24.6) shows a different population, which is also normally distributed, but has a mean of 1 and a standard deviation of 1.

The question of interest is how to differentiate these two populations. Suppose that the statistical test gave a value indicated by the point marked * in the second population. The corresponding point in the first population is also marked. Since this point falls in the unshaded region of the first population, there is no way of differentiating the two populations (both populations are the same). We accept the null hypothesis even though we *know* the values come from different populations (type 2 error). Therefore any value falling in the unshaded region of the second population would result in a type 2 error given by β. Any value falling in the shaded region of the second population would give a correct result, constituting the power of the study.

Notice the line dividing the regions aligned in the two curves. Changing the significance level (α-value) of the study automatically changes the power (β-value) of the study. The degree of inter-relationship depends on the sample size and the effect size (how closely both the curves overlap).

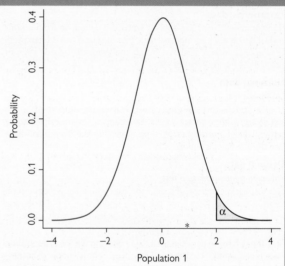

Fig. 24.5

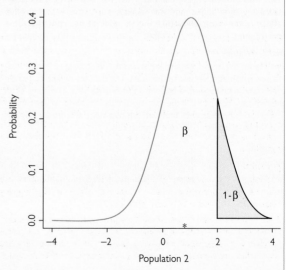

Fig. 24.6

24.3 Statistical tests

Assessing distribution of data

To apply parametric tests, the normality of a distribution must be confirmed either by a test (Kolmogorov–Smirnov test) or graphically using Q–Q plots. Q–Q stands for quantile–quantile, and these plots show the values from the sample plotted against the values expected theoretically if the distribution were normal. In a normal distribution, the dots should fall around a straight line. Any deviation (as shown in Figure 24.7) indicates a non-normal distribution.

Assessing significance of data

Many statistical tests exist to assess the significance of data—i.e. whether the values obtained are due to real effects (differences or similarities) between observed populations or due to chance.

The **p-value** is the probability that the results obtained are due to chance alone, and is an important statistical number. It is obtained by applying one of a number of tests to the obtained results. It is essential that the test applied is appropriate to the type of data otherwise the resulting p-value will be invalid.

Parametric data

Non-parametric tests are applied when the data arise from a non-normal distribution. For nominal data, the chi-square test is often used. Tests applicable to ordinal data include the Wilcoxon signed-rank sum test and the Mann–Whitney test.

Nominal data
Chi-square test
The chi-square test compares observed values (measured in the test group) with expected values. Expected values are calculated by extrapolating known data from a population to the study population (see the example opposite).

Ordinal data
Wilcoxon signed-rank sum test
This test again compares the obtained data with a known population mean. If the data were from the same population, the distribution would be expected to be symmetrical, i.e. as many numbers above the mean as below it.

First, the difference between each data point and the mean population value is calculated. The data are then placed in order (ranked) according to the size of the difference from the mean value. For ranking, the negative and positive signs are ignored.

The ranks of the negative numbers only (i.e. below the population mean) are then added, and this number correlates with a p-value reflecting the probability that the samples came from the same population.

Mann–Whitney test
The Mann–Whitney test (also known as the Wilcoxon rank sum test) is a non-parametric version of the t-test. The data are ranked as a single group, and then separated back into the original sets. The sums of all the ranks are compared: if the data are similar, the sums will be similar. The greater the difference between the two sums, the more likely it is that the data are from different populations.

Parametric data

Parametric tests are applicable to data which are normally distributed. Tests appropriate for parametric data include Student's t-test and Student's paired t-test.

Student's t-test
This test assesses the null hypothesis that the mean value obtained from the sample is identical to the known population mean (i.e. there is no difference between the two). The single-sample test is:

$$t = \frac{\text{(sample mean – known mean)}}{\text{SE of sample mean}}.$$

When the means are the same (i.e. the samples are from the same population), $t = 0$. As the sample mean deviates more from the population mean, the t-value increases and the corresponding p-value (obtained from statistical tables) decreases, i.e. the probability that the data came from two different populations increases.

Student's paired t-test
This test examines paired data (i.e. observations from the same subject before and after an intervention).

With paired data, each observation can be compared with the same previous observation *from the same subject*. The phenomenon of interest is not differences between whole populations, but differences within individuals. The t-value is calculated as follows:

$$t = \frac{\text{(mean difference before and after)}}{\text{SE of difference}}.$$

ANOVA tests
ANOVA stands for analysis of variance. In its most basic form, an ANOVA test can be used to determine whether the estimated means of several samples are equal (from the same population), or different (from different populations). This simple type of ANOVA is an extension of the Student's t-test to include more than two populations.

Complex ANOVA tests can be used to examine differences between several different groups and the effects of many variables (dependent or independent). When there is more than one dependent variable, the test is known as a MANOVA (multivariant analysis of variance).

One or two tails?

A one-tailed test only considers the differences above *or* below the null value. It can ask the question: 'Is this parameter more likely in the study population than in the sample population?' Alternatively, it can ask: 'Is this parameter less likely in the sample population?'

A two-tailed test can evaluate differences in either direction within the study sample. It asks the question: 'Is the likelihood of this parameter different within the sample population?' The difference may be positive or negative.

For example, drug X, an analgesic, is thought to cause less itch than drug Y. The null hypothesis is: 'The incidence of itch is the same whether drug X or drug Y is used'. A two-tailed test must be carried out on the study data, as these may actually reveal that drug X causes *more* itch than drug Y.

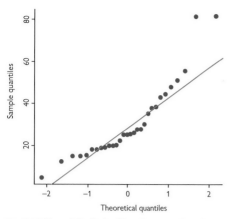

Fig. 24.7 Normal Q–Q plot. Quantiles are points taken at regular intervals from a set of data. If the data is split into a hundred subsets, each quantile is called a percentile; if the data is split into four, the quantiles are known as quartiles. Theoretical quantiles for a normal distribution are plotted against the actual quantiles from the data. Normally distributed data give a straight-line plot. This plot shows non-normally distributed data; in fact this data set is exponential. Using parametric tests (which assume a normal distribution) on such data is inappropriate. Some data may be able to be transformed (e.g. by taking logarithms or inverse values) to give a normal distribution.

Choosing tests

The choice of tests for generating the test statistic and p-value depends on the type of variable and the type of comparison.

Table 24.2 Statistical tests

Comparison	Nominal data	Ordinal data	Parametric data
Two groups	Chi-square test (Fisher exact test for smaller samples)	Mann–Whitney test	Unpaired t-test
Paired groups: one variable measured twice in the same group (e.g. before and after treatment)	McNemar's test	Wilcoxon signed-rank test	Paired t-test
More than two groups	Chi-square test	Kruskal–Wallis test	One way ANOVA
More than two groups with repeated measurements (e.g. before and after treatment)	Chi-square test	Friedman test	Repeated measures ANOVA
Association between two variables	Contingency coefficient	Spearman correlation	Pearson correlation
Quantitative association between two variables	Logistic regression (simple for one variable and multiple for many variables)	Non-parametric regression	Linear regression (simple for one variable and multiple for many variables)

Example: chi-square test

Assume that the incidence of left-handedness in the general population is 10%. In a department of 50 anaesthetists, nine are left-handed. If the population statistic was applied to the anaesthetic department, we would expect only five anaesthetists to be left-handed.

In this study, the null hypothesis would be: 'The incidence of left-handedness in anaesthetists is similar to that in the general population'. This allows us to construct a 'contingency table'.

	Observed	Expected
Right-handed	41	45
Left-handed	9	5

Chi-squared = 3.556. Two-tailed p-value = 0.0593. By conventional criteria (which demand a p-value <0.05), the incidence of left-handedness is not demonstrated to be significantly different in anaesthetists than in the general population. However, remember that the p-value represents the probability of this discrepancy occurring by chance in any sample. Here, the probability is 5.93%. Conventional statistical tests demand a 5% probability or less to 'prove' significance. This particular study is rather equivocal, despite being above conventional p-value cut offs. It is always up to the reader to make up his/her own mind when judging the validity of medical evidence.

Example: Wilcoxon signed-rank sum test

After drug A, the average pain score in a post-surgical population, measured on a visual analogue scale, is 40/100. After drug B, 10 patients were evaluated and gave pain scores as shown in the table. The differences between each score and the expected mean (40) were calculated, and these were ranked (ignoring positive and negative signs for ranking purposes).

Patient	Pain score	Difference from mean (=40)	Rank
A	18	−22	6.5
B	39	−1	1
C	22	−18	4
D	18	−22	6.5
E	42	+2	2
F	6	−34	10
G	7	−33	9
H	14	−26	8
I	59	+19	5
J	24	−15	3

Adding the ranks of the negative values (i.e. pain scores below 40) gives 46. The ranks of the positive values (pain scores above 40) gives 7. The corresponding p-value is 0.04: the test shows statistical significance.

24.4 Presenting data and assessing association

Presenting data

Histograms
A histogram (Figure 24.8) is similar to a bar chart. It presents data in intervals defined by the investigator.

Pie charts
A pie chart is a representation of nominal or ordinal data, according to the percentage incidence in the population of interest. For the chart to make sense, all categories in a pie chart should be mutually exclusive.

Cumulative charts
A cumulative chart (Figure 24.9) is often used when reporting mortality in study populations. The line represents the number of patients remaining over time.

Box and whisker plots
The box and whisker plot (also known a box plot Figure 24.10) is a simple, intuitive, and informative method for summarizing both continuous and ordinal data.

The data are divided into quartiles, each containing 24% of the data. The lowermost horizontal line in the plot is the lowest value. Each horizontal line represents a quartile. Therefore the space between Q1 and the minimum line contains the first 24% of the values, while the space between Q2 and Q1 represents the second 24% of the values and so on. By definition Q2 is the median value.

The central box contains all values from Q1 to Q3 and represents the central 50% of the values. A vertical bar connects the box to the minimum and maximum values. Extreme outliers are represented by dots.

The difference between the maximum and minimum values is the range, and the difference between Q3 and Q1 is the interquartile range.

The boxplot provides a powerful visual representation of:
- The distribution, including its symmetry (the example in Figure 24.10 shows a positive skew)
- Range and interquartile range
- Median
- Outliers.

Measures of association

Correlation and regression are techniques used to study the relationship between two variables (e.g. fall in blood pressure and dose of propofol). The variables under experimental control are the independent variables and the measure of interest is the dependent variable.

Correlation
The **Pearson correlation coefficient r** is a measure of the correlation between two parametric variables. Non-parametric variables are correlated using the **Spearman** β (rho) or **Kendall** τ (tau) correlation tests.

The correlation coefficient takes a value between −1 and 1. The number indicates the strength of association, while the sign indicates the direction of association. A correlation coefficient of 1 indicates a perfect positive correlation, i.e. an increase in one variable is associated with an increase in the other variable. A correlation coefficient of −1 indicates a perfect negative correlation, i.e. an increase in one variable is associated with a decrease in the other variable. A correlation coefficient of zero implies that the variables are unrelated.

The size of the association cannot be estimated by the correlation coefficient, as it is not linear. A coefficient of 0.4 does not mean twice the correlation of 0.2.

The **coefficient of determination, R,** is the square of the correlation coefficient. It is interpreted as the amount of variation in the outcome variable that is explained by the predictor variable. For example, the coefficient of determination for two variables with a correlation coefficient of 0.4 is 0.16 (0.4^2). This means that 16% of the variation in the outcome variable is accounted for by the predictor variable.

Correlation implies association, but not the causation or the direction of the association.

Regression
Regression analysis also examines the relationship between variables, but in addition provides a quantitative relationship between the dependent and the independent variables.

Regression analysis entails the formulation of a mathematical model to explain the data. This is called the generalized linear model.

Simple regression relates one dependent variable to one independent variable. The result is an equation of the form

$$y = ax + b$$

where y is the dependent variable and x is the independent variable. This can be expressed graphically as a line of slope a which intercepts the y-axis at b. In statistical terms, a is the coefficient of x and b is the error factor. The line can be considered to be a prediction of the dependent variable by the model, for any given value of the independent variable.

Multiple regression relates a dependent variable to multiple independent variables. The result will be expressed as

$$y = a_1x_1 + a_2x_2 + \ldots + b$$

where a_1, a_2, etc. are the coefficients and b is the error factor. The interpretation is similar to that for simple regression.

The error of the model is the difference between the predicted value and the actual observed value. The total error is calculated as the sum of the squares of the differences.

For a given set of data, many lines can be drawn, each with its own slope and intercept. Each of these lines forms a model. The best of the many models that can be used to explain the data is the one with the most explanatory power. The best model has the least error. The mathematical technique for determining the regression line uses this principle and is known as the least-squares method.

There are many different types of regression analysis, including the following.
- **Linear regression:** both the dependent and the independent variables are continuous.
- **Logistic regression:** the dependent variable is categorical (e.g. mortality outcome) and the independent variables are either continuous or categorical (e.g. blood pressure or ASA grade).

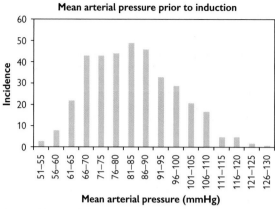

Fig. 24.8 Example of a histogram.

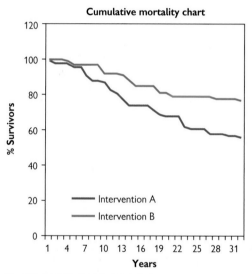

Fig. 24.9 Example of a cumulative display.

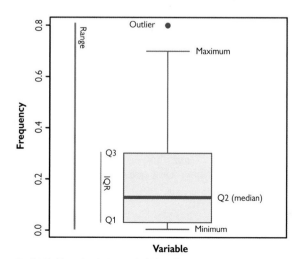

Fig. 24.10 Example of a box and whisker plot.

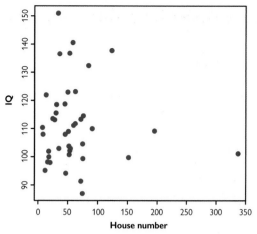

Fig. 24.11 No correlation.

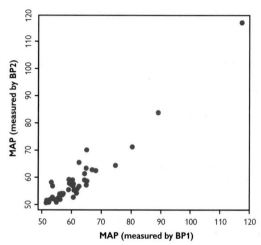

Fig. 24.12 Positive correlation.

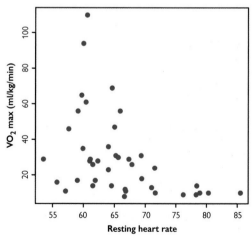

Fig. 24.13 Negative correlation.

Correlation

The relationship between two variables is graphically represented by a scatter plot. Scatter plots are drawn by plotting the value of one variable against the value of the other. Two uncorrelated variables are seen as random points in Figure 24.11. Correlated variables appear to fall along a straight line. In positive correlation increase in one variable is associated with an increase in the other (Figure 24.12), while in negative correlation increase in one variable is associated with a decrease in the other (Figure 24.13). As shown, correlation in the real world is rarely perfect.

24.5 Meta-analysis

Meta-analysis is a statistical method which combines studies addressing similar research questions. By combining many smaller studies, meta-analysis overcomes the problems of their inadequate power, allowing stronger conclusions to be drawn.

The steps in a meta-analysis are as follows.
- Identify a problem and formulate a hypothesis.
- Literature review to identify all previous studies of this problem.
- Review of each previous study identified by a literature search with respect to predefined criteria (sample size, randomization, blinding etc.), ideally by more than one investigator.
- Use statistical techniques to identify the effect size from each of the short-listed studies. The results from each study will contribute to the final effect size. In general, the larger the sample size, the larger the effect size in the primary study, and the smaller the confidence intervals, the greater will be the contribution to the final effect size.
- Summarization and presentation of the results. The results are presented graphically using a forest plot.

Some drawbacks of meta-analysis are as follows.
- **Inhomogenous studies:** primary studies are often different in terms of fundamentals such as inclusion criteria, grouping of subjects, definition of success, etc. This results in two major problems. First, the study population may be different and therefore not comparable. Secondly, the results may actually measure different things and not be suitable for amalgamation.
- **Publication bias:** positive studies are more likely to be published. Studies with negative data are unlikely to be included in the meta-analysis.
- **Inclusiveness:** the identification of appropriate studies is partly subjective and requires familiarity with the study area. Publications in journals not indexed in large databases and in foreign languages are likely to be ignored.
- **Poor quality of studies:** meta-analysis does not account for poor quality of primary studies. A large meta-analysis of many poor-quality studies does not improve the accuracy of the results.
- **Difficulties in interpretation:** although the results of a meta-analysis have a strong statistical background, it is difficult to apply them to the care of individual patients.
- **Statistical limitations:** assumptions made during the analysis (e.g. linearity of regression) may not be valid.

Forest plots

Forest plots are used to represent the results of meta-analysis graphically. The forest plot provides a large amount of information in a concise manner.

The arrangement of a forest plot is shown in Figure 24.14. Modern plots use either the odds ratio or the relative risk for the horizontal scale of the graph.

The forest plot lists each of the shortlisted studies included in the meta-analysis with their references.

The result of each study is shown as a box (blue) with side-arms (light blue). The midpoint of the box represents the estimate for the variable of interest in the study. The width of the box represents the precision of the estimate (standard error). Thus a study with a low standard error has a narrow box. (Some plots represent the sample size by the width of the box, while others quote the sample size in the text together with the references).

The side-arms represent the confidence intervals at 95% drawn to scale. The shorter the arm, the smaller the confidence interval.

The green line is the zero line (odds ratio of 1 indicates no significant difference between the treatment and control groups in the study). If the confidence interval crosses the green line, the study has a non-significant result.

The result of the meta-analysis is shown as a diamond. The centre of the diamond represents the overall estimate, while the tips indicate the confidence intervals. If no part of the diamond touches the zero line, there is an overall significant result.

A greater effect on the result is provided by:
- larger sample size;
- greater effect size (blue box further away from the zero line);
- greater precision (narrower boxes);
- narrower confidence intervals (smaller side-arms).

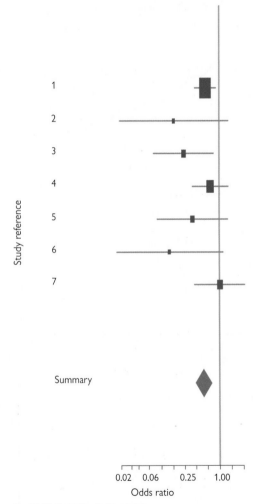

Fig. 24.14 Example of a forest plot.

→ Interpreting tests

Sensitivity is the proportion of patients with a disease correctly diagnosed as positive (true positive). It is the probability of correctly diagnosing the disease when the disease is present.

Specificity is the proportion of patients without a disease correctly diagnosed as normal (true negative). It is the probability of not diagnosing the disease when the disease is absent.

False positive is the proportion of patients without a disease wrongly diagnosed as positive.

False negative is the proportion of patients with a disease wrongly diagnosed as normal.

Positive predictive value is the probability that a person has the disease given a positive test result.

Negative predictive value is the probability that a person does not have a disease given a negative test result.

Risk

In simplistic terms, the risk of an event is the ratio of events occurring in the study group to the total number of events across all groups. It is also called the event rate.

Relative risk of an event is the ratio of risk in the treatment group to the risk in the control group. This implies that having a risk factor increases the chance of having an event by a factor given by relative risk.

Absolute risk reduction is the difference in event rates between the treatment and control groups.

Relative risk reduction is the percentage reduction in events in the treatment group compared with the control group. It is the absolute risk reduction expressed as a percentage. The denominator in relative risk reduction is the event rate in controlled group. The reduction in risk by not having a risk factors is the relative risk reduction.

Attributable risk is the risk attributable to the risk factor. It is similar to relative risk reduction but has the event rate in the treatment group as the denominator.

Odds is the ratio of the probability of an event occurring to the probability of the event not occurring.

Odds ratio is the ratio of the odds of an event occurring in one group to the odds of it occurring in another group. The odds ratio is the probability that the risk factor is associated with the event. An odds ratio of 1 indicates no association.

Number needed to treat (NNT) is the number of patients needed to be treated to prevent one adverse outcome. NNT is the reciprocal of absolute risk reduction, and is a more intuitive way of looking at risk. An intervention with a larger NNT is less efficacious then one with a lower NNT.

Number needed to harm (NNH) is the number of patients needed to be treated to cause one adverse event. A drug with a low NNH has a low therapeutic ratio.

Number crunching: using probability tables

Parameter	Formula					Example					
				Disease						**Disease**	
				Present	Absent					Present	Absent
	Test	Positive		a	b	Test	Positive			30	15
		Negative		c	d		Negative			20	50
Sensitivity	$a/(a + c)$					30/(30+20) = 60% chance of correctly diagnosing disease					
Specificity	$d/(b + d)$					50/(15 + 50) = 76.9%					
Positive predictive value	$a/(a + b)$					30/(30 + 15) = 66.7% chance of having the disease, if the patient has a positive test result					
Negative predictive value	$d/(c + d)$					50/(50+20) = 71.4% chance of not having the disease if the patient has a negative result					
				Outcome						**Nausea**	
				Present	Absent					Present	Absent
	Intervention	Present		a	b	Drug	X			20	50
		Absent		c	d		Control			30	15
Risk	present/(present + absent) for each group					30/(30 + 15) = 0.67 risk of nausea for control 20/(20 + 50) = 0.29 for drug X					
Relative risk	risk in treatment/risk in control					0.29/0.67 = 0.43 Drug X has 43% relative risk of nausea compared with control					
Relative risk reduction	1 − relative risk					1 − 0.43 = 0.57 Drug X (relatively) reduces nausea by 57% compared with control					
Odds	no. of occurrences of event/no. of non-occurrences					30/15 = odds of nausea with control of 2 20/50 = 0.4 for drug X					
Odds ratio	odds 1/odds 2					2/0.4 = 5 Odds of having nausea with control is five times than when using drug X					
Absolute risk reduction (ARR)	risk in control group − risk in treatment group					0.67 − 0.29 = 0.38 A 38% decrease in absolute risk of nausea with drug X compared with control. Notice how relative risk can be larger than absolute risk reduction for the same data (a fact frequently abused by marketing)					
Number needed to treat	1/ARR					1/0.38 = 2.63 2.63 additional patients will have to be treated with drug X to prevent nausea in one patient. NNT allows easy comparison of related drugs					

Chapter 25

Critical incidents

25.1 Critical incidents and risk

A critical incident can broadly be defined as an unexpected event which causes, or has the potential to cause, harm to the patient.* This definition not only encompasses error, equipment failure, and resource problems, but also unexpected patient responses to anaesthetic interventions. By this definition, not all critical incidents are avoidable, but they do require vigilance and active management.

Risk

Risk can be defined as the probability of a negative occurence. Risk can never be eliminated entirely: many anaesthetic interventions do expose patients to it. The emphasis in clinical practice is (a) to identify and minimize risk, and (b) to accept that negative events do occur, and develop strategies to deal with these and limit their consequences.

Identifying risk

Risk identification can be prospective or retrospective. Situations where prospective risk assessment is important include the following.

- Preoperative airway assessment. (Is this patient at risk of aspiration? Will I be able to manage the airway? Do I need extra equipment or skilled personnel?)
- Planning a trip to the CT scanner from ICU. (Do I have enough oxygen? Is the emergency bag stocked? Will the infusion pump batteries last?)

Retrospective risk identification usually occurs in response to a critical incident. The event is analysed to determine, with the benefit of hindsight, if any of its elements could have been prevented.

Critical incident reporting

Modern critical incident reporting has its roots in systems developed around the time of the Second World War. These systems for the voluntary reporting of untoward events were originally used by military and aviation organizations. The potential human and financial costs of mishaps in such industries have led to highly developed systems for both reporting and preventing such events. The medical profession still lags behind these higher-risk industries, but anaesthetists have led the movement to improve safety.

Critical incident reporting can help to identify trends within an organization, target resources to the prevention of the most serious or common events, identify how variations in practice can influence patterns of critical incidents, allow comparisons between different organizations and time windows, and flag up events which are serious enough to warrant further investigation or wider reporting to the medical community.

There is as yet no standard incident-reporting tool across the whole of the medical profession. The Royal College of Anaesthetists and the National Patient Safety Agency (NPSA) in the UK are currently collaborating to develop a specialty-specific incident-reporting tool. In the meantime, NHS Trusts in the UK are required to implement local reporting strategies. Incidents with wider implications are escalated to the NSPA and other authorities as appropriate.

It is important to emphasize that reporting a critical incident does not constitute an admission, or accusation, of liability. Many systems allow anonymous reporting and do not require the identities of persons involved to be revealed.

Root cause analysis

Individual incident reports provide relatively little information about root causes and possible preventative strategies. Often, further investigation is required to identify the causal factors important in any incident. Treating these root causes is more effective than treating their secondary symptoms. This process is known as root cause analysis (RCA). To be successful, RCA must be evidence based rather than assumption based (just because an incident occurred at night does not mean that it was caused by fatigue). Often, a problem has more than one root cause.

Various techniques are used to perform an RCA. The simplest is the 'Five Whys', a technique designed to follow a chain of events backwards. It simply requires the investigator to ask 'Why?' at each stage in the investigation. Identification of the root cause usually requires at least five whys, and often more. More sophisticated techniques have been developed to allow for the multifactorial nature of most critical incidents. One of these is the 'fishbone' analysis (Figure 25.1).

Classification of critical incidents

Classification can be by the type of incident (equipment failure, medication error, etc.) or by its perceived seriousness or probability of recurrence. A common scale for outcome severity is as follow.

1. **Nil:** no adverse outcome or a prevented incident ('near-miss').
2. **Minor:** short-term injury of less than a month's duration.
3. **Moderate:** injury taking up to a year to resolve.
4. **Major:** long-term or permanent disability.
5. **Catastrophic:** resulting in death.

Similarly, a scale for likelihood of recurrence can be constructed:

A. **Almost certain:** expected to occur, and on multiple occasions.
B. **Likely:** expected to occur.
C. **Possible:** not expected to occur.
D. **Unlikely:** may occur (e.g. once in a few years).
E. **Rare:** unlikely to occur in an individual's career.

A 'traffic light' system (Figure 25.2) can be useful for stratifying incidents based on the likelihood of their occurrence or recurrence, and the most serious potential consequences. Such stratification allows an organization to direct its resources towards dealing with the most important problems.

Further reading

Bould MD, Hunter D, Haxby EJ (2006) *Contin Educ Anaesth Crit Care Pain* **6**, 240–3.

http://www.npsa.nhs.uk/patientsafety

---

*It has been suggested that the definition of a critical incident could be widened even further to include any unexpected occurrence, including unanticipated good outcomes. Certainly there are valuable learning opportunities to be gained from positive as well as negative occurrences.

Example of root cause analysis

A 26-year-old woman presents to A&E with lower abdominal pain. An ultrasound scan confirms an ectopic pregnancy and she is placed on the emergency theatre list. She becomes tachycardic and agitated, for which she receives analgesia. She later collapses on the ward; an arrest call is put out and she is rushed to theatre. She is being wheeled into the emergency theatre when the team is redirected to another theatre. A laparotomy reveals intra-abdominal haemorrhage. After salpingectomy and haemostasis she remains tachycardic and becomes hypertensive. The anaesthetist realizes that the vaporizer is empty and administers propofol and midazolam. She is admitted to ICU and makes an uncomplicated recovery. Several days later, on the ward, she complains of nightmares and says that she was aware for a part of the surgery.

Five Why's root cause analysis

Problem: awareness

1st why? Vaporizer ran out of volatile agent.

2nd why? Not noticed that vaporizer was virtually empty at the start of the case.

3rd why? Anaesthetic machine in theatre 13 not checked.

4th why? Emergency case due to be done in theatre 7 but moved to theatre 13 at short notice.

5th why? Theatre 7 unsuitable for use as heating broken.

The Five Whys analysis clearly needs extending to consider why another theatre had not been set up for emergencies, why the heating had broken in theatre 7, and why the anaesthetic team had not been informed. There are clearly other elements of this incident: the anaesthetist's attention was focused on resuscitation from haemorrhage, the second on-call anaesthetist was busy in A&E, initial signs of haemorrhage had been overlooked, and the situation had become an emergency. Ishikawa diagrams (also known as 'fishbone' analyses) pursue more than one avenue of causality, as most critical incidents have more than one root cause. Figure 25.1 is a fishbone diagram for the same incident.

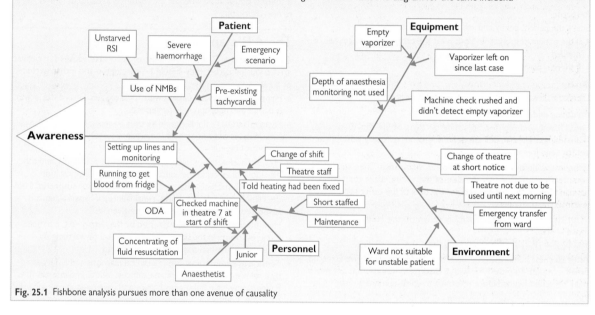

Fig. 25.1 Fishbone analysis pursues more than one avenue of causality

		Most likely consequences				
		None	Minor	Moderate	Severe	Catastrophic
Likelihood of occurrence/recurrence	Almost certain					
	Likely					
	Possible					
	Unlikely					
	Rare					

Fig. 25.2 The traffic light system stratifies incidents based on the likelihood of recurrence, and seriousness of their consequences.

Cardiac arrest requires a swift, co-ordinated response. The principles of management include:

- Establishing a patent airway and ventilating with oxygen.
- Efficient chest compressions with minimal interruptions.
- Rapid DC shock for shockable rhythms.
- Regular boluses of adrenaline to increase myocardial and cerebral perfusion pressure.
- A methodical, structured approach to identifying and treating the cause.

Basic life support

Basic life support (BLS) is the first response to a collapsed patient. It can be performed by a single rescuer in any environment and requires no specialised equipment or skills. The sequence of events is:

Danger?
Make sure you, the patient, and any bystanders are safe.

Response?
Shake the patient gently and ask loudly: "are you all right?"

- If the patient responds, find out what the problem is and get help if needed
- If there is no response, continue

Airway
Open the airway using the head tilt/chin lift or jaw thrust technique.

Breathing and Circulation
Look, listen, and feel for breathing or signs of life for 10 seconds. If breathing is normal, put the patient into the recovery position, and get (or send for) help.

If the breathing is not normal, call for an ambulance. Then start chest compressions: kneeling by the side of the victim, place the heel one hand in the middle of the chest. Put the heel of the other hand on top and interlink the fingers.

With straight arms, press vertically down on the sternum; it should move 4–5cm.

The rate of chest compressions should be 100 per minute.

After 30 chest compressions, open the airway again and give 2 rescue breaths (mouth-to-mouth, or with a mask). Do not attempt any more than 2 rescue breaths before returning to chest compressions.

Do not stop to reassess the victim unless he or she begins breathing normally.

An alternative to giving mouth-to-mouth rescue breaths is to perform chest-compression-only CPR. Compressions should then be continuous, at a rate of 100 per minute.

Advanced life support

Advanced life support follows on from basic life support once the necessary equipment has been assembled. The algorithm is shown in Figure 25.3. It should be started as soon as possible. In particular, defibrillation should not be delayed for chest compressions or other procedures if the rhythm is shockable. Again, the patient should be approached with care and cardiac arrest confirmed.

Airway and breathing
The airway should be opened and 100% oxygen applied via facemask. Breaths should continue at a rate of 30 compressions to 2 breaths while preparing to establish a definitive airway. Once the patient is intubated, breaths can be continued independently of chest compressions.

Circulation
A defibrillator should be attached to the patient and a rhythm check performed (using the paddles if necessary). IV access should be established.

Shockable rhythm
If the rhythm is shockable (VF or pulseless VT), a single shock should be given (360J for a monophasic, and 150-200J for a biphasic defibrillator). CPR should then continue for 2min; only then is the pulse rechecked, and another shock given if necessary (at 360J, or biphasic equivalent).

Adrenaline is only given if VF/VT persists after a second shock, and should be given every 3-4min thereafter (i.e. approximately every second cycle).

Amiodarone (bolus of 300mg) can be given if VF/VT persists after 3 shocks. This can be followed by a further bolus of 150mg, with in infusion of 900mg/24hr if the arrhythmia is refractory.

Non-shockable rhythm
If the rhythm is non-shockable (PEA or asystole), CPR continues for 2min. Adrenaline is given as soon as IV access is established. In asystole or PEA <60/min, atropine 3mg is given as a single dose.

If there is doubt as to whether the rhythm is asystole of fine VF, treat as non-shockable.

The 4 H's and 4 T's

The 4 H's and 4 T's comprise a list of reversible causes for cardiac arrest. During cycles, they should be considered and either excluded or treated.

- Hypoxia: ventilate the patient with 100% oxygen. Ensure the airway is patent and appropriately positioned.
- Hypovolaemia: IV fluids should be used to replace intravascular deficits. In cases of haemorrhage, emergency surgery may be required to control bleeding.
- Hyperkalaemia, hypokalaemia, hypocalcaemia, acidaemia, and other metabolic disorders. These may be detected on investigation (most ABG machines also measure electrolytes) or suspected from the clinical scenario (e.g. burns, renal failure). If hyperkalaemia is suspected, calcium chloride should be given IV.
- Hypothermia: this may be suggested by the history (e.g. a patient found outdoors in the dead of winter). Active re-warming is required and resuscitation may be prolonged.
- Tension pneumothorax: this is a clinical diagnosis and is suggested by a relevant history (e.g. trauma, difficult central line insertion). Patients may have bulging neck veins and have been dyspnoeic prior to arrest. Treatment is by needle thoracocentesis followed by formal intercostal drain.
- Tamponade: cardiac tamponade is rare and difficult to diagnose; because the typical signs (distended neck veins and hypotension) are obscured by the arrest itself. A suggestive history might be of penetrating thoracic trauma, cardiac surgery, or angiography. These may mandate a needle pericardiocentesis or resuscitative thoracotomy.
- Toxic substances: these include drugs as well as poisons. If there is a concrete history or the drug chart gives clues, a specific antidote (e.g. naloxone, digibind) may be available.
- Thromboembolism (pulmonary embolus or coronary thrombosis). The commonest thrombotic cause for circulatory arrest is massive pulmonary embolus. Acute myocardial infarction may also lead to cardiac arrest. Thrombolysis should be considered on a case-by-case basis; ongoing CPR is not a contraindication.

Adult Advanced Life Support Algorithm

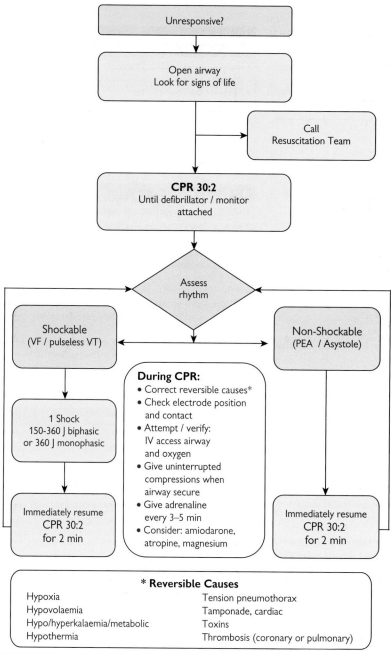

Fig. 25.3 Adult ALS protocol.

25.3 Difficult or failed intubation

Definition

The ASA defines difficult tracheal intubation as that requiring more than three attempts at direct laryngoscopy, or taking longer than 10min.

Failed intubation denotes inability to intubate the trachea during direct laryngoscopy.

Risk factors

Risk factors for difficult or failed intubation include:

- Inexperienced anaesthetist.
- Trauma and obstetrics.
- Predictors of difficult intubation: obesity, reduced mouth opening, reduced cervical spine movement, Mallampati score 3–4, prominent upper incisors, reduced thyromental distance.
- Rheumatoid arthritis.
- Airway pathology or scarring.

Management

In any failed intubation scenario, the priority is to oxygenate. A patient will die of lack of oxygen, not lack of an ETT. Overall, management should be structured as follows (Figures 25.4–25.6):

A   Primary intubation attempt (laryngoscopes ± bougie).

B   Secondary intubation attempt (via LMA or ILMA). Not appropriate in during RSI.

C   Abandon intubation; oxygenate patient; consider awakening and postponing surgery.

D   Can't intubate, can't ventilate. Invasive tracheal access.

⚠ Plan A: Primary tracheal intubation plan

If there are any problems at direct laryngoscopy, call for help.

- Optimize view: neck flexion and head extension; external laryngeal manipulation (BURP—backwards, upwards, rightwards pressure); try alternative laryngoscope (longer-bladed, straight-bladed, McCoy). If an RSI is underway, adjusting or releasing the cricoid pressure may help (be ready to suction the oropharynx).
- If you can see the epiglottis, make two attempts to pass a gum elastic bougie, feeling for the notches of the tracheal cartilages or resistance when the end lodges in a bronchus. Railroading of the ETT is easier if the laryngoscope is left in the mouth and the tube is rotated 90° anticlockwise
- Successful intubation is confirmed by: visualizing the ETT passing through the glottis if possible: bilateral chest rise and fall, bilateral chest sounds on auscultation, and six consecutive normal swings on the capnograph. A fibreoptic laryngoscope can also be used.

If initial tracheal intubation fails, proceed to plan B. Further attempts at intubating at this stage are likely to cause trauma and worsen the state of the airway. If an RSI is in progress, proceed to plan C.

⚠ Plan B: Secondary tracheal intubation plan (not appropriate for RSI: see algorithms)

- Insert an ILMA or LMA. This will re-establish the airway in 95% of cases.
- No more than two insertions.
- Oxygenate and ventilate.
- If necessary, perform fibreoptic tracheal intubation through the LMA or ILMA.

If this fails, revert to facemask (plan C).

⚠ Plan C: Maintenance of oxygenation

- Use facemask, oxygenate, and ventilate.
- One- or two-person mask technique (with oral or nasal airway).
- Consider reducing cricoid force if ventilation is difficult (in the case of RSI).
- If failed oxygenation via facemask try LMA/ILMA. Reduce cricoid force during insertion and proceed to oxygenate and ventilate.
- If this fails, proceed to plan D.
- If you are able to oxygenate and ventilate the patient, and the patient's condition is not immediately life-threatening, postpone surgery and awaken patient
- If you are able to oxygenate and ventilate and surgery is immediately life-saving, continue anaesthesia with LMA or ProSeal LMA

⚠ Plan D: Can't intubate, can't ventilate

Call for immediate help—preferably a senior anaesthetist. Pull emergency buzzer and shout loudly.

Ask for difficult airway trolley/equipment.

Administer 100% oxygen at high flow.

Optimize airway: reposition the head and neck, two-handed jaw thrust, oral/nasal airway, release or reduce cricoid pressure.

Insert LMA: this may provide some oxygenation during attempts at an invasive airway, and improve the route for expired gases during jet ventilation.

If still unable to oxygenate proceed without delay to an emergency surgical airway—surgical cricothyroidotomy or needle/cannula cricothyroidotomy (Section 6.4).

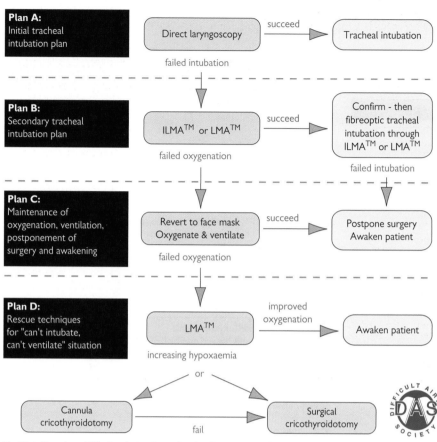

Plan A:
Initial tracheal intubation plan

Direct laryngoscopy — succeed ▸ Tracheal intubation

failed intubation

Plan B:
Secondary tracheal intubation plan

ILMA™ or LMA™ — succeed ▸ Confirm - then fibreoptic tracheal intubation through ILMA™ or LMA™

failed oxygenation

failed intubation

Plan C:
Maintenance of oxygenation, ventilation, postponement of surgery and awakening

Revert to face mask Oxygenate & ventilate — succeed ▸ Postpone surgery Awaken patient

failed oxygenation

Plan D:
Rescue techniques for "can't intubate, can't ventilate" situation

LMA™ — improved oxygenation ▸ Awaken patient

increasing hypoxaemia

or

Cannula cricothyroidotomy — fail ▸ Surgical cricothyroidotomy

DIFFICULT AIRWAY SOCIETY (DAS)

Fig. 25.4 Overview of failed intubation (reproduced with permission).

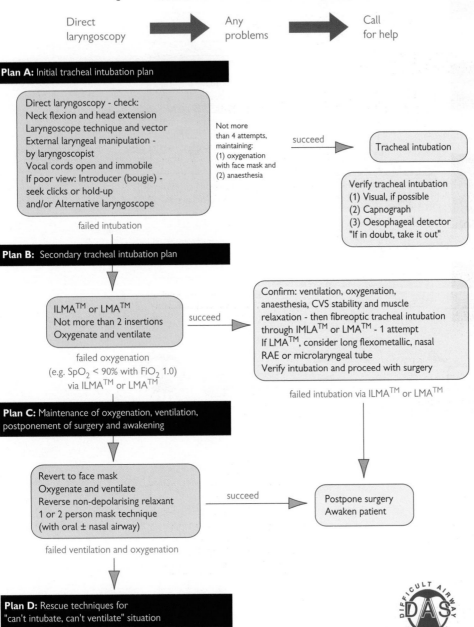

Unanticipated difficult tracheal intubation-
during routine induction of anaesthesia in an adult patient

Direct
laryngoscopy → Any
problems → Call
for help

Plan A: Initial tracheal intubation plan

Direct laryngoscopy - check:
Neck flexion and head extension
Laryngoscope technique and vector
External laryngeal manipulation -
by laryngoscopist
Vocal cords open and immobile
If poor view: Introducer (bougie) -
seek clicks or hold-up
and/or Alternative laryngoscope

Not more
than 4 attempts,
maintaining:
(1) oxygenation
with face mask and
(2) anaesthesia

succeed →

Tracheal intubation

Verify tracheal intubation
(1) Visual, if possible
(2) Capnograph
(3) Oesophageal detector
"If in doubt, take it out"

failed intubation

Plan B: Secondary tracheal intubation plan

ILMA^{TM} or LMA^{TM}
Not more than 2 insertions
Oxygenate and ventilate

succeed →

Confirm: ventilation, oxygenation,
anaesthesia, CVS stability and muscle
relaxation - then fibreoptic tracheal intubation
through IMLA^{TM} or LMA^{TM} - 1 attempt
If LMA^{TM}, consider long flexometallic, nasal
RAE or microlaryngeal tube
Verify intubation and proceed with surgery

failed oxygenation
(e.g. SpO$_2$ < 90% with FiO$_2$ 1.0)
via ILMA^{TM} or LMA^{TM}

failed intubation via ILMA^{TM} or LMA^{TM}

Plan C: Maintenance of oxygenation, ventilation,
postponement of surgery and awakening

Revert to face mask
Oxygenate and ventilate
Reverse non-depolarising relaxant
1 or 2 person mask technique
(with oral ± nasal airway)

succeed →

Postpone surgery
Awaken patient

failed ventilation and oxygenation

Plan D: Rescue techniques for
"can't intubate, can't ventilate" situation

Difficult Airway Society Guidelines Flow-chart 2004 (use with DAS guidelines paper)

Fig. 25.5 Failed intubation—non-RSI (reproduced with permission).

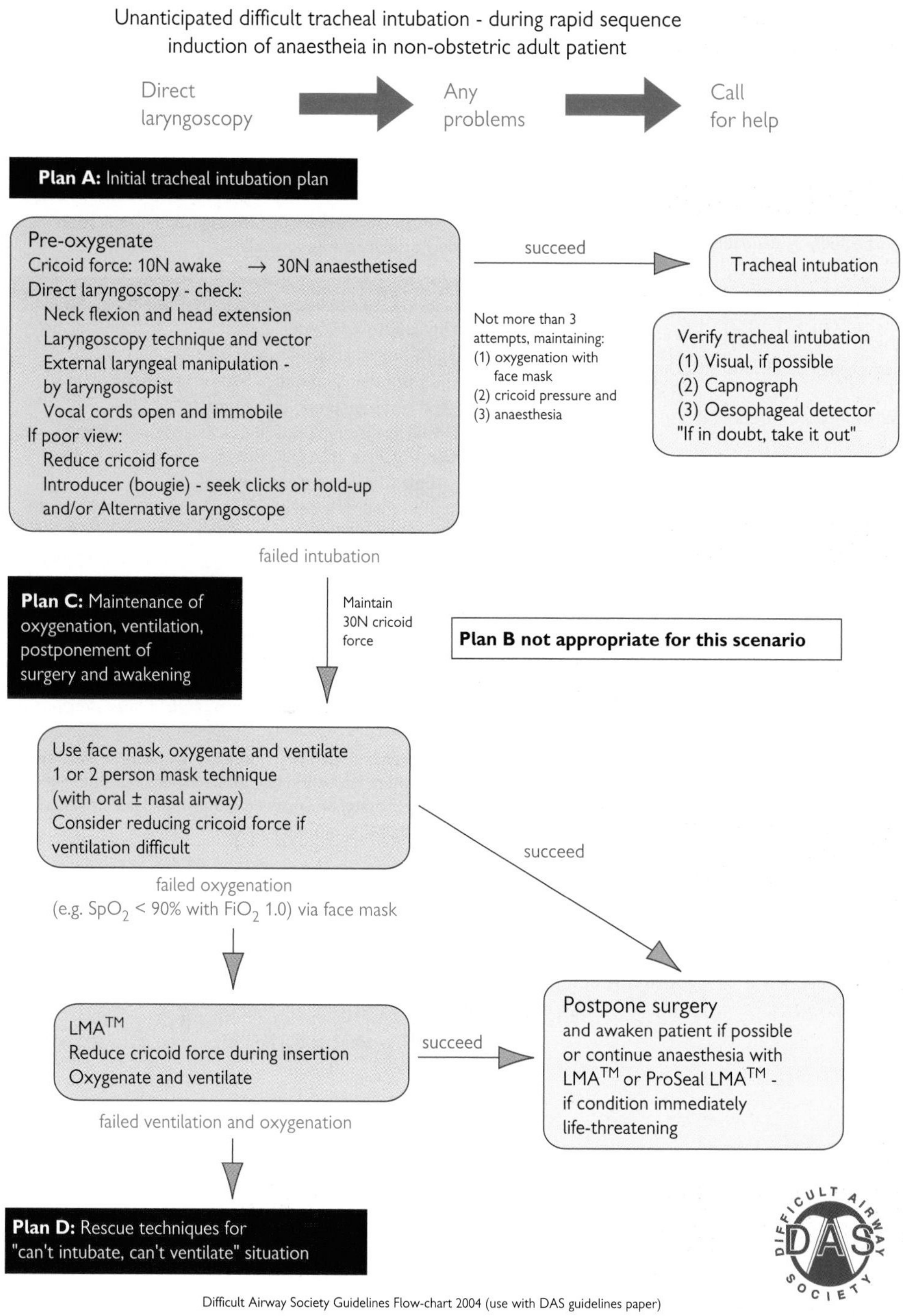

Unanticipated difficult tracheal intubation - during rapid sequence
induction of anaestheia in non-obstetric adult patient

Direct
laryngoscopy

Any
problems

Call
for help

Plan A: Initial tracheal intubation plan

Pre-oxygenate
Cricoid force: 10N awake → 30N anaesthetised
Direct laryngoscopy - check:
  Neck flexion and head extension
  Laryngoscopy technique and vector
  External laryngeal manipulation -
  by laryngoscopist
  Vocal cords open and immobile
If poor view:
  Reduce cricoid force
  Introducer (bougie) - seek clicks or hold-up
  and/or Alternative laryngoscope

succeed

Tracheal intubation

Not more than 3
attempts, maintaining:
(1) oxygenation with
    face mask
(2) cricoid pressure and
(3) anaesthesia

Verify tracheal intubation
(1) Visual, if possible
(2) Capnograph
(3) Oesophageal detector
"If in doubt, take it out"

failed intubation

Plan C: Maintenance of
oxygenation, ventilation,
postponement of
surgery and awakening

Maintain
30N cricoid
force

Plan B not appropriate for this scenario

Use face mask, oxygenate and ventilate
1 or 2 person mask technique
(with oral ± nasal airway)
Consider reducing cricoid force if
ventilation difficult

succeed

failed oxygenation
(e.g. SpO$_2$ < 90% with FiO$_2$ 1.0) via face mask

Postpone surgery
and awaken patient if possible
or continue anaesthesia with
LMA^{TM} or ProSeal LMA^{TM} -
if condition immediately
life-threatening

LMA^{TM}
Reduce cricoid force during insertion
Oxygenate and ventilate

succeed

failed ventilation and oxygenation

Plan D: Rescue techniques for
"can't intubate, can't ventilate" situation

Difficult Airway Society Guidelines Flow-chart 2004 (use with DAS guidelines paper)

Fig. 25.6 Failed intubation–RSI (reproduced with permission).

25.4 Laryngospasm

Definition

Occlusion of the glottis by the action of the intrinsic laryngeal muscles. Laryngospasm is present when inflation of the lungs is hindered or made impossible by unwanted muscular action of the larynx.

Risk factors

Laryngospasm may occur unexpectedly in any patient. Specific causes include the following:

- Airway manipulation during light anaesthesia (especially at induction and emergence)
- Blood and secretions in airway
- Surgical stimulation (e.g. peritoneal traction, anal stretch, cervical dilatation)
- Moving the patient, especially with airway devices *in situ*
- Age <6 years
- Upper respiratory tract infection
- Airway trauma (e.g. difficult intubation)
- Nasal, oral, or pharyngeal surgery
- Obstructive sleep apnoea
- Irritant volatile anaesthetics (desflurane > isoflurane > sevoflurane > halothane)
- Recurrent laryngeal nerve damage (e.g thyroid surgery)
- Hypocalcaemia (may cause neuromuscular irritability).

Presentation

The characteristic crowing sound of inspiratory stridor will be heard during partial obstruction. With complete airway obstruction, no sound will be heard.

In spontaneous ventilation, there will be evidence of respiratory distress with increased inspiratory effort. Tracheal tug and intercostal and suprasternal recession will be evident, accompanied by paradoxical movements of the chest and abdomen. The increase in respiratory effort increases the patient's oxygen demand, exacerbating the resultant hypoxia. Desaturation may be frighteningly swift.

Positive-pressure ventilation may be difficult or impossible, with a flat capnography trace.

Desaturation and bradyardia will develop if laryngospasm is not relieved.

Differential diagnosis

Breathing circuit obstruction.

Breath-holding.

Tension pneumothorax.

Infraglottic airway obstruction (e.g. foreign body, aspiration, clot, sputum, bronchospasm, tracheomalacia).

❗ Immediate management

- Request immediate assistance.
- Dial up 100% oxygen at high flows.
- Stop surgery or other stimulation. Suction secretions.
- A firm jaw thrust may 'break' the spasm.
- Visualize and clear pharynx and airway. Exclude supraglottic obstruction (e.g. base of tongue, foreign body, clot, or tumour).
- Manually apply CPAP with a bag and mask.
- If desaturation continues, deepen anaesthesia with IV anaesthetic agent (20% of induction dose of propofol). Continue CPAP.
- If CPAP fails, give suxamethonium (0.5mg/kg IV; 2–4mg/kg may be given IM or by intra-glossal injection).
- Give atropine (10mcg/kg). About 1 in 20 cases overall—and 1 in 4 infants—will develop bradycardia.

Once airway patency is established, consider whether to continue bag–mask ventilation or use another airway device. Intubation will secure and protect the airway; however, an ETT may precipitate further spasm when it is removed.

Occasionally, hypoxia due to laryngospasm may become life threatening, perhaps where intubation has not been possible. If the patient continues to deteriorate, be prepared to move to a needle cricothyroidotomy or surgical airway—it may be life-saving.

Ongoing management

If the patient has required a definitive airway, a plan must be formed for extubation in a safe environment.

Exclude negative pressure pulmonary oedema.

Complications due to laryngospasm may necessitate intensive care admission.

There is a risk of awareness; this will have to be discussed with the patient after recovery.

Further reading

Pinder A, Dresner M (2003). *Curr Anaesth Crit Care* **14**, 9–14.

25.5 Sudden or progressive difficulty with IPPV

'Difficulty with ventilation' may present with sudden or progressive loss of tidal volume, unexpected increase in peak airway pressure, hypoxia, or changes in $ETCO_2$.

Possible causes can be divided into equipment faults, airway obstruction, increased airway resistance, or reduced chest compliance. Sudden, complete, or intermittent cessation of ventilation is assumed to be obstruction to the breathing circuit or airway until proved otherwise.

Equipment fault

- Incorrect ventilator settings
- Ventilator disconnection, leak, or failure
- Incorrect switch placement between controlled and spontaneous modes
- Failure of pressure regulators or valves
- ETT displacement, kinking, or blockage
- Obstruction in the breathing circuit (foreign bodies, kinked tubing)
- Oxygen flush jammed in the 'on' position
- Closed PEEP valve

Obstruction

- Airway: blood, secretions, foreign body.
- ETT: kinking, displacement, endobronchial intubation, cuff herniation, patient biting.
- Laryngospasm (with supraglottic airway).

Increased airway resistance

- Bronchospasm, excessive secretions, and pulmonary aspiration
- Atelectasis
- Aspiration
- Pulmonary oedema
- Pneumothorax or haemothorax
- Laryngospasm

Reduced respiratory compliance

- Patient breathing against the inspiratory phase of the ventilator.
- Coughing and breath-holding.
- Failure of neuromuscular blockade, inadequate anaesthesia.
- Pulmonary pathology such as pulmonary oedema, infection, fibrosing alveolitis, ARDS, or a pneumothorax.
- Chest wall rigidity (opioids).
- Pneumoperitoneum, massive gastric distension, and patient position (head-down). Patient position: steep head-down.
- Abdominal closure after prolonged surgery.
- Direct pressure from the surgical team.

❗ Immediate management

Follow the ABC approach: correct hypoxia as a priority.

Give 100% oxygen

Call for help if the problem is not swiftly rectified.

Airway

Quick visual sweep of breathing circuit: exclude obstruction, disconnection, ventilator failure, or leak.

Check that the ETT is patent and correctly positioned; reposition or reintubate if necessary. Pass a suction catheter down the ETT to confirm patency. If an LMA is in use, consider intubation.

Breathing

Switch to manual ventilation mode. If ventilation is easy, the problem is in the ventilator circuit. If ventilation remains difficult, hand ventilate the patient with a self-inflating bag with 100% oxygen and monitor chest expansion. Remember to maintain anaesthesia.

Observe the capnography trace (loss of capnograph trace in the presence of sustained cardiac activity is a result of tube displacement until proved otherwise).

Check for bilateral adequate chest expansion. Auscultate the chest.

If wheeze is present, ensure ETT not inserted too far (stimulating the carina). Administer bronchodilators (β-agonists, ipratroprium bromide, and adrenaline in severe cases). Specifically ask: is this anaphylaxis?

If there is blood-stained frothy sputum and dependent crepitations, pulmonary oedema is likely. Treat cardiac failure and fluid overload with diuretics and nitrates. Correct arrhythmias. Continue positive-pressure ventilation.

Unequal chest expansion and breath sounds with tracheal deviation may signify a pneumothorax, haemothorax, lung collapse, or pleural effusion. A CXR will help to differentiate these and guide treatment.

Circulation

Check heart rate, blood pressure, and capillary refill; estimate volume status.

Consider likely causes specific to the patient. Has the patient's position changed? Is there a pneumoperitoneum? Any recent procedure performed, e.g. central line insertion or nerve block?

Paediatric considerations

Bronchospasm, laryngospasm, and endobronchial intubation are more common in paediatric patients. Oxygen reserves are less, so hypoxia develops more rapidly.

Investigations

Further investigations to consider include ABG, CXR (in recovery or on table if necessary), bronchoscopy, and CTPA.

Further reading

Pinder A, Dresner M (2003). *Curr Anaesth Crit Care* **14**, 9–14.

Higgins F (2003). *Update Anaesth* Issue 16, Article 9.

25.6 Hypoxia during anaesthesia

Definition
Inadequate oxygen content in arterial blood.

Presentation
Saturation (SaO_2) below 90%, cyanosis.

Bradycardia in children.

Causes

Failure of delivery of adequate oxygen and/or anaesthetic from machine to the airway device
- Oxygen failure.
- Anaesthetic machine failure.
- Hypoxic mixture (very rare with modern anaesthetic machines, but can occur at very low flows if the inspired O_2 concentration selected is inadequate).
- Ventilator failure.
- Circuit: disconnection, obstruction, or leak.

Failure of delivery of adequate oxygen and/or anaesthetic from the airway device to the patient's alveoli
- Airway device: displacement, disconnection, obstruction, or leak.
- Hypoventilation: central (e.g. opioids) or peripheral (e.g. neuromuscular blockade, diaphragmatic splinting).
- Obstruction: trachea, bronchi, bronchioles (including laryngo- and bronchospasm, and airway soiling).
- Atelectasis.
- Other intrapulmonary problem: pneumo- or haemothorax, collapse.

Failure of delivery of adequate oxygen from alveoli to pulmonary capillaries
- Basal membrane problem
- V/Q mismatch: ventilating underperfused lung
  - Pulmonary embolus
  - Shock (any cause)
  - Severe anaemia
- V/Q mismatch: perfusing underventilated lung
  - Pulmonary oedema
  - Pneumonia
  - Aspiration
  - Atelectasis
  - Endobronchial intubation
- Right-to-left shunts

Failure of delivery of adequate oxygen from pulmonary capillaries to tissues
- Heart failure
- Shock (any cause)
- Severe anaemia
- Increased metabolic demand (e.g. shivering, sepsis)

'Desaturation' may also be caused by a faulty or displaced pulse oximeter or abnormal haemoglobin species. Met-haemoglobinaemia or methylene blue typically give saturations of 85%.

❗ Immediate management

Dial up 100% O_2 at high flows.

Call for help if the problem is not quickly resolved.

Exclude faulty SpO_2 probe (position, diathermy, movement).

Consider causes systematically. If at each stage no cause is found and the difficulty persists, the problem lies further down the sequence.

Exclude failure of delivery to the airway device

Check the oxygen meter. If there is any doubt about the FiO_2, change the oxygen source.

Convert to hand ventilation via the reservoir bag.

Inspect the breathing system; if there is a possible problem, attach a self-inflating bag directly to the ETT (not forgetting to maintain anaesthesia).

Exclude failure of delivery to the alveoli

Continue manual ventilation: watch the chest wall, feel chest compliance, and listen for leaks around airway device. (Take care with high-pressure ventilation through a mask or laryngeal device as it may lead to gastric insufflation, especially in children. This in turn may further compromise ventilation.)

Check capnography trace.

Check the patency of the airway. Ensure the ETT (if in use) is patent, with no leaks, kinks, or obstructions. If necessary, adjust, deflate cuff, pass a suction catheter, or replace.

Consider laryngospasm or presence of foreign body, blood, gastric contents, or secretions. Intubate if necessary; but remember that oxygenation, not intubation, is the goal.

Exclude failure of delivery to pulmonary capillaries

Assess pattern, adequacy, and distribution of ventilation.

Auscultate for bronchospasm, pulmonary oedema, lobar collapse, and pneumo- or haemothorax.

If atelectasis is suspected (elderly, smokers, obese, supine), try alveolar recruitment (CPAP of $30cmH_2O$ for 30sec) or using PEEP with IPPV.

Exclude failure of perfusion

Feel the pulse and evaluate peripheral perfusion, blood pressure, capnograph, and ECG. This may identify an acute circulatory problem such as hypovolaemia, cardiac failure, myocardial ischaemia, or tamponade.

If the problem persists, further investigations may be required (e.g. invasive blood pressure monitoring, FBC, cardiac output monitoring).

Investigations
Further investigations to consider include ABG, CXR, bronchoscopy, and CTPA.

Subsequent management
Depending on the cause of the hypoxia and ease of reversibility, the patient may require postoperative intensive care and ventilation until the cause is resolved (e.g. pulmonary oedema, bronchospasm, aspiration pneumonia).

Further reading
Bamber J (2003). *Curr Anaesth Crit Care* **14**, 2–8.
Morris RW (1993). *Bailliere's Clin Anaesthesiology* **17**, 215–35.
Pinder A, Dresner M (2003). *Curr Anaesth Crit Care* **14**, 9–14.

25.7 Oxygen failure during anaesthesia

Oxygen failure is a rare event, but can have catastrophic consequences. The importance of a machine check cannot be overemphasized: it may not prevent pipeline failure but it confirms the presence of a back-up oxygen supply on the anaesthetic machine prior to induction.

In the event of an oxygen pipeline failure, the priorities are maintenance of oxygenation, ventilation, and anaesthesia. There is also a need to conserve oxygen and to ensure the quality of the gas supply once re-established. However, immediate patient care must come first in all circumstances.

Causes of oxygen failure during anaesthesia

Human error
- Crossed pipelines
- Oxygen tank filled with a different gas
- Oxygen depletion (failure to refill tanks, cylinders, and manifolds)
- Construction damage to pipeline supply
- Unannounced system shutdown

Equipment failure
- Pipeline leak
- Pipeline contamination
- Pipeline obstruction
- Emptying of vacuum-insulated evaporator
- Weather damage to regulators (lightning, freezing, high winds)

Presentation
- Oxygen failure alarm
- Unexplained low FiO_2
- Unexplained low pipeline pressures
- Hypoxic patient
- Ventilator failure
- Notification from other theatres/site manager

❗ Immediate management

As always, do a quick visual sweep of the anaesthetic machine and breathing system. This may identify a disconnection at the wall, breathing system, or patient end.

Check the oxygen meter and pipeline pressure gauges. If these indicate a problem, connect and open the emergency oxygen cylinder.

Call for help. Ask for additional oxygen cylinders.

Notify the surgeon and ask him/her to expedite surgery.

Convert to hand ventilation via the reservoir bag. If there is any doubt about the functioning of the anaesthetic machine, switch to ventilation via a self-inflating bag. However, if oxygen failure is confirmed:

Ventilate the patient. If he/she has become hypoxic, a brief period of increased FiO_2 may be necessary to restore oxygenation.

Conserve oxygen. Once the saturations are ≥95%, use the lowest possible FiO_2 to avoid hypoxia. Close the APL valve on the breathing system, use lowest possible flows, and ventilate by hand via the reservoir bag. Switch off oxygen-driven ventilators. If using a self-inflating bag, room air or low flows of supplemental oxygen should be used.

Continue anaesthesia. If using a self-inflating bag, use TIVA maintenance. If continuing to use the anaesthetic machine, it may be necessary to increase the volatile concentration to compensate for low flows.

Send a spare (third) person to investigate and notify other theatres and the site manager.

Ongoing management

Disconnect the wall oxygen supply. Do not reconnect it until it has been retested (both identity and purity must be confirmed). If there is no other alternative (all other oxygen sources have been spent), use the gas sampling line and oxygen meter to confirm that the wall supply is delivering oxygen and attach a filter to the inspiratory limb of the anaesthetic circuit.

Investigations

As well as reporting and investigating the incident itself, close observation and further assessment of the patient may be needed (e.g. if they have been delivered 'oxygen' from an untested wall supply, or if there has been a period of hypoxia).

25.8 Abnormalities of end-tidal CO$_2$

Rise in end-tidal CO$_2$

Definition
End-tidal CO$_2$ >6.3kPa. Most patients will tolerate moderate hypercapnia. However, it should be corrected when associated with arrhythmias or raised intracranial pressure.

Causes

Increased CO$_2$ production
- Pyrexia: sepsis, malignant hyperthermia, seizures
- Thyroid storm
- Reperfusion injury
- Serotonin syndrome
- Neuroleptic malignant syndrome

Increased CO$_2$ delivery to the lungs
- Abdominal insufflation with CO$_2$
- Injection of sodium bicarbonate
- Release of tourniquet
- Rapid increase in blood pressure or cardiac output

Increased inspired CO$_2$
- Exhausted soda lime (circle) or insufficient fresh gas flow (partial rebreathing system)
- Stuck valve in circle absorber system
- CO$_2$ in fresh gas mixture (modern anaesthetic machines should not carry CO$_2$ cylinders)

Decreased CO$_2$ excretion
- Hypoventilation: respiratory depression, ineffective breathing during spontaneous ventilation, inadequate minute volume with IPPV
- Partial airway obstruction
- Bronchospasm
- Faulty breathing system
- Increased dead space

> **❗ Immediate management**
>
> Increase inspired oxygen to maintain saturations ≥ 95%.
>
> If the patient is mechanically ventilated, ensure adequate minute ventilation; increase tidal volume/rate as necessary.
>
> If the patient is ventilating spontaneously, check depth of anaesthesia. Reduce if necessary. Start assisted ventilation.
>
> Check the system for leaks (compare inspired and expired tidal volumes). Check the ETT cuff pressure.
>
> Look for evidence of rebreathing (a capnography trace which fails to return to ≤0.4kPa). If necessary, replace the soda lime (circle system) or increase the fresh gas flow (other circuits). Disconnections in the breathing system can increase dead space (e.g. internal limb of Bain circuit).
>
> Check for stuck expiratory valves in the circle system.
>
> If there are doubts about the breathing system, change to an alternative means of ventilation, *but maintain anaesthesia.*
>
> If EtCO$_2$ continues to rise despite increased ventilation, consider malignant hyperthermia (Section 25.22) or thyroid storm.

Investigations
ABG to confirm hypercapnia and assess degree of acidosis. Others according to clinical findings.

Fall in end-tidal CO2

Definition
End-tidal CO$_2$ (or *Pa*CO$_2$) <4.5kPa.

Causes

Slow decrease in CO$_2$
- Hyperventilation
- Fall in body temperature
- Falling lung or body perfusion

Sudden drop of end-tidal CO$_2$ to zero
- Extubation, anaesthetic circuit disconnection, or kinked or totally obstructed ETT
- Kinked or disconnected sampling tube
- In ventilated patients, ventilator failure

Sudden drop in end-tidal CO$_2$ but not to zero
- Leak in circuit, e.g. deflated cuff
- Obstruction, e.g. acute bronchospasm
- Leak in sampling tube (drawing in room air)

Exponential decrease in CO$_2$
- Circulatory arrest: cardiac or hypovolaemic
- Pulmonary embolism (gas, thrombus, fat)
- Sudden severe hyperventilation

> **❗ Immediate management**
>
> *No end-tidal CO$_2$*
>
> 100% oxygen. **Confirm a cardiac output.** If cardiac arrest is confirmed, commence advanced life support (Secton 25.2).
>
> Check ETT, monitor, connections, and ventilator. Loss of capnograph trace with a cardiac output is ETT displacement until proved otherwise.
>
> Ventilate by hand with 100% oxygen. Monitor chest expansion. This should exclude disconnection or obstruction. If obstruction of the anaesthetic circuit is suspected, hand ventilate with 100% oxygen using a self-inflating bag. Remember to maintain anaesthesia.
>
> Check the position of ETT/LMA. If in doubt, remove and replace. Exclude laryngospasm or foreign body.
>
> *Low end-tidal CO$_2$*
>
> Check airway patency and connections as above.
>
> Exclude hyperventilation: check the tidal ventilation and respiratory rate. Observe chest expansion and auscultate.
>
> Consider the possibility of a gas/air embolism (Section 25.12).
>
> Check vital signs: pulse, SpO$_2$, BP, temperature. Look for causes of low cardiac output (e.g. caval compression, excessive blood loss, myocardial ischaemia).
>
> Check ABGs to ensure that the end-tidal CO$_2$ correlates with the blood gas.

Ongoing management

Replace equipment for subsequent cases if a problem was detected.

Elderly patients undergoing major surgery may have hypovolaemia, hypothermia, and/or low metabolic rates. Adjust their ventilation to produce normal end-tidal CO_2, as a low $PaCO_2$ will cause cerebral vasoconstriction and further compromise cerebral perfusion.

A rare underlying cause is hypothyroidism; check TFTs if this is a possibility.

Investigations

ABG, others depending on findings (e.g. ECG if suspected myocardial ischaemia, CTPA to exclude PE).

Further reading

Pinder A, Dresner M (2003). *Curr Anaesth Crit Care* **14**, 9–14.

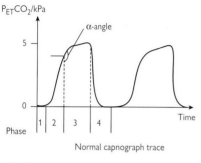

Normal capnograph trace

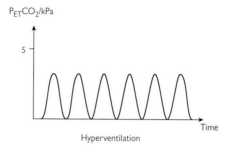

Hyperventilation

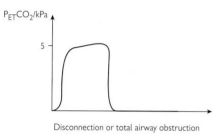

Disconnection or total airway obstruction

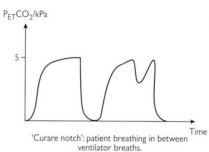

'Curare notch': patient breathing in between ventilator breaths.

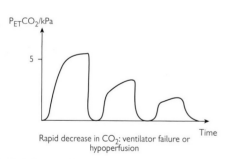

Rapid decrease in CO_2: ventilator failure or hypoperfusion

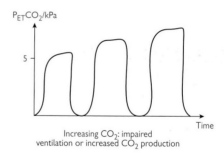

Increasing CO_2: impaired ventilation or increased CO_2 production

Fig. 25.7 Capnograph traces

Bronchospasm

Definition

Bronchospasm is the contraction of the smooth muscle in the walls of the bronchi and bronchioles, causing narrowing of the lumen. It is usually associated with mucus plugging and mucosal oedema.

Bronchospasm in anaesthesia may present in isolation or as part of anaphylaxis. It often occurs in patients with pre-existing respiratory disease such as asthma.

Risk factors

- History of asthma, particularly if poorly controlled
- Upper respiratory tract infection
- Airway irritation, light anaesthesia, tracheal intubation
- Smoking

Clinical presentation

Respiratory signs include tachypnoea, hypoxia, wheeze, cyanosis, silent chest, and hyperexpansion. The patient may also be tachycardic or hypotensive. In the conscious patient there may be difficulty completing sentences, a reduced conscious level, or exhaustion.

During mechanical ventilation, increased airway pressure, rising $ETCO_2$, prolonged expiration, an up-sloping capnograph trace, and a reduction in tidal volume are suggestive of increased airways resistance.

Differential diagnosis

- Misplaced/blocked/kinked ETT or circuit.
- Pneumothorax.
- Aspiration of gastric contents.
- Anaphylaxis.
- Pulmonary oedema.
- Obstruction distal to ETT (such subglottic stenoses might be bypassed with a smaller ETT, but beware of trauma. A fibreoptic bronchoscope can be helpful).
- Drug-induced (e.g. NSAIDs, atracurium).

❗ Immediate management

Request immediate assistance.

Administer 100% oxygen; ensure adequate IV access.

Cease stimulation/surgery.

Deepen anaesthesia. The majority of cases are due to airway irritation from laryngoscopy or intubation.

If intubated, exclude oesophageal or endobronchial placement.

If LMA or facemask in use, consider the possibility of aspiration or laryngospasm.

Give salbutamol 5mg (nebulized).

Give ipratropium bromide 500mcg (nebulized).

In extreme situations, IV adrenaline may be necessary 10–100mcg (0.1–1ml of 1:10,000), titrated to response.

Give hydrocortisone 100mg IV; repeat 6-hourly.

If bronchospasm follows induction, stop all potential precipitants and maintain with isoflurane, sevoflurane, or TIVA.

Ongoing management

This depends on the patient's condition and the underlying cause.

If severe bronchospasm continues, consider a bolus of magnesium sulphate (2g IV over 20min) and an aminophylline infusion.

Volatile anaesthetics (isoflurane, sevoflurane) and ketamine may help.

Severe cases will need further management in ICU.

Investigations

ABG sampling. Rising CO_2 is ominous.

CXR: exclude pneumothorax.

FBC, U&Es (hypokalaemia can be caused by β-agonists).

25.10 Anaphylaxis

Definition

An anaphylactic reaction is an IgE-mediated immune response to a usually innocuous substance. This leads to release of histamine, serotonin, and other vasoactive mediators from basophils and mast cells. These cause the systemic symptoms outlined below. As it is antibody mediated, anaphylaxis requires previous exposure to the substance.

In an anaphylactoid reaction, the clinical symptoms and severity are indistinguishable from an anaphylactic reaction. However, it is the result of direct non-specific histamine release and does not require previous sensitization.

The incidence of these events during anaesthesia is between 1:10,000 and 1:20,000.

Risk factors

- Female predominance (2.7 ♀:1 ♂)
- Atopy
- Asthma
- History of drug or food intolerance

Agents involved in anaphylactic reactions during anaesthesia

- Neuromuscular blocking agents: suxamethonium and rocuronium most commonly
- Latex
- Antibiotics: penicillin and cephalosporins most commonly
- Colloids: gelatins, hetastarch
- Hypnotics: thiopental, propofol, midazolam
- Opioids: fentanyl, morphine, sufentanil

Clinical presentation

Respiratory: bronchospasm, angio-oedema of airway.

Cardiovascular: hypotension, tachycardia or bradycardia, cardiovascular collapse, cardiac arrest.

Gastrointestinal: diarrhoea, nausea, vomiting, cramps.

Cutaneous: erythema, urticaria.

Haematological: coagulopathies.

❗ Immediate management

Stop all potential precipitants (remember skin prep and latex).

Stop surgery and call for help.

Give 100% oxygen at high flows.

Verify and maintain the airway. Intubate as as soon as possible, as airway swelling may worsen the laryngoscopic view if intubation is delayed.

Administer adrenaline 50−100mcg increments IV (0.5−1ml 1:10,000) or 0.5−1mg IM (0.5−1ml 1:1000). Continue administering boluses of adrenaline as required (see Table 25.1 for paediatric doses of IM adrenaline).

The adrenaline will treat bronchospasm and upper airway swelling, but nebulized bronchodilators may also be required.

Assess circulation; commence CPR if cardiac arrest occurs.

If the blood pressure is low, elevate the legs.

Insert two large IV cannulae and rapidly infuse isotonic fluid. Colloid may be used (unless thought to be the cause).

Table 25.1 Intramuscular dose of adrenaline in children

>5 years	0.5ml of 1:1000
4 years	0.4ml of 1:1000
3 years	0.3ml of 1:1000
2 years	0.2ml of 1:1000
1 year	0.1ml of 1:1000

Ongoing management

Antihistamines: chlorpheniramine 10mg IV (H1 blocker) and ranitidine 50mg IV (H2 blocker).

Corticosteroids: hydrocortisone 200mg IV followed by 100−200mg 4−6-hourly. This will take several hours to be effective.

Bronchodilators: treat persistent bronchospasm with nebulized (5mg) or IV (250mcg) salbutamol.

Adrenaline: cardiovascular instability may last several hours and can be treated with an adrenaline infusion (0.01–0.5mcg/kg/min).

Transfer the patient to ICU.

Investigation and reporting

Mast cell tryptase levels: samples should be taken immediately (after treatment), and 1hr and 6hr later. Store at 4°C if the sample can be analysed within 48hr, or freeze at −20°C for later analysis. Serum tryptase is raised in both anaphylactic and anaphylactoid reactions.

The patient should be referred to a regional allergy centre for skin testing and RAST testing.

All incidents should be reported on the Yellow Card found in the British National Formulary to the MHRA (Medicines and Healthcare Products Regulatory Agency).

The patient should be given a written record of the reaction and be encouraged to carry an anaesthetic hazard card or MedicAlert bracelet.

Further reading

Christopher M *et al.* (2000) *Update Anaesth* Issue 12, Article 14.

Laxenaire MC *et al* (2001) *Br J Anaesth* **87**, 549−58

anaphylacticreactions.com/Therapy.asp

25.11 Tension pneumothorax

Definition

A tension pneumothorax is a progressive build-up of air within the pleural space under pressure. This is usually due to a lung laceration or rupture creating a flap of tissue. This flap acts as a valve which allows air to escape into the pleural space but not to return (positive-pressure ventilation may exacerbate the effect). The pressure in the pleural space displaces and distorts the mediastinum and obstructs venous return to the heart. This leads to respiratory and circulatory instability and eventually collapse/arrest if untreated.

Causes

There are many causes, of which traumatic and iatrogenic are the most common. They include the following:

- Spontaneous (associated with asthma or bullous emphysema, or idiopathic).
- Trauma (including iatrogenic):
  - Out-of hospital (blunt or penetrating)
  - Central venous catheter placement
  - Chest compressions during CPR
  - Laparoscopic surgery, thoracic surgery, nephrectomy, percutaneous nephrolithotomy
  - Percutaneous tracheostomy
  - Fibreoptic bronchoscopy with closed-lung biopsy
  - Severely displaced thoracic spine fractures
  - Brachial plexus nerve blocks
  - Colonoscopy and gastroscopy have been implicated in case reports.
- Barotrauma secondary to positive-pressure ventilation.
- Use of nitrous oxide in patients with pneumothorax.
- Clamping of chest drains.
- Unsuccessful attempts to convert an open pneumothorax to a simple pneumothorax, with an occlusive dressing functioning as a one-way valve.
- Diaphragmatic hernia + trauma or visceral perforation.

Clinical presentation

Tension pneumothorax is a clinical diagnosis, which requires urgent recognition and management. Some environments allow access to rapid ultrasound confirmation but this should never delay treatment.

In non-ventilated patients, diagnosis requires a high index of suspicion. There are decreased or absent breath sounds and hyper-resonance on the affected side. There may be distended neck veins and cardiovascular embarrassment, and the trachea may be deviated away from the affected side.

In ventilated patients, peak airway pressures increase. There may be decreased expiratory volumes secondary to air leakage into the pleural space and increased end-expiratory pressure, even after discontinuation of PEEP. Occasionally, the development of a tension pneumothorax may occur hours or days after the initial insult.

Early findings

- Chest pain
- Dyspnoea
- Anxiety
- Tachypnoea
- Tachycardia
- Hyper-resonance over the chest wall on the affected side
- Diminished breath sounds on the affected side

Late findings

- Decreased level of consciousness
- Tracheal deviation away from the affected side
- Hypotension
- Distension of neck veins (may not be present if concurrent severe hypovolaemia)
- Cyanosis

❗ Immediate treatment

Tension pneumothorax is a life-threatening condition that demands urgent management. Use an ABC approach.

Call for help.

Give 100% oxygen.

Perform emergency needle decompression.

After needle decompression, immediately begin preparation to insert a thoracostomy tube (chest drain). Reassess the patient.

Needle thoracostomy

A 14–16G IV cannula is placed in the second rib space in the mid-clavicular line. The needle is advanced until air can be aspirated. The needle is withdrawn and the cannula is left open to air. A rush of air from the needle confirms the presence of a tension pneumothorax. This procedure converts a tension pneumothorax into a simple pneumothorax.

Needle thoracostomy is not without risk. Cannulae are prone to blockage, kinking, and dislodging, allowing a relieved tension pneumothorax to re-accumulate undetected. The needle can cause lung laceration and air embolism, especially if the initial diagnosis was wrong.

A formal chest drain is the definitive treatment of tension pneumothorax and should be performed after an emergency needle thoracostomy.

Ongoing management

Perform a CXR to assess for lung re-expansion and thoracostomy tube position.

Monitor SaO_2 and check arterial blood gases.

Complete the primary survey, gain large-bore IV access and take bloods for FBC and group and save (or cross-match if indicated).

Intensive care may be indicated, depending on the patient's clinical status. High-dependency monitoring is required in the immediate aftermath in case of recurrence.

Further reading

Leigh-Smith S, Harris T (2005) *Emerg Med J* **22**, 8–16

Scott Bjerke H, Carmack B (2006) Tension pneumothorax emedicine topic 2793

Definition

Presence of gas in the venous system, which travels into the pulmonary arteries.

Causes

- IV lines and infusions:
  - Pressurized infusions
  - Infusions with air vents *in situ*
  - Central lines left open to air or during removal.
- Neurosurgery:
  - Posterior fossa and upper cervical spine procedures in the sitting position
  - May occur in other situations, e.g. tumours encroaching on posterior half of sagittal sinus.
- Orthopaedic surgery:
  - Total hip replacement
  - Arthroscopic surgery
  - Long-bone surgery (e.g. intramedullary nailing)
  - Spinal surgery in prone position
  - Polytrauma.
- Other surgery:
  - Surgical point is >5cm above the right atrium (e.g. neck, vascular surgery)
  - Pressurized gas in the operating field
  - Laparoscopic surgery.
- Extracorporeal circulation:
  - Cardiopulmonary bypass
  - Haemodialysis.

Presentation

Situation of risk for air embolism.

Chest pain; sudden hypoxia, and loss of EtCO$_2$ trace.

Hypotension, tachycardia, arrythmias; sudden elevation of CVP. The ECG may show right heart strain and ischaemia.

The first presentation may be a PEA cardiac arrest.

Detection/monitoring

Transoesophageal echocardiography is the most sensitive monitoring device and may detect as little as 0.02ml/kg of air and bubbles as small as 5μm diameter. However, it is relatively invasive and requires expertise to place and interpret.

ETCO$_2$ monitoring is sensitive, easy and in common usage. ETCO$_2$ drops suddenly with air embolism.

Precordial Doppler ultrasound detects small amounts of air by converting changes in blood density into sound. It is sensitive and non-invasive. Its use in combination with ETCO$_2$ is practical and effective.

The precordial stethoscope is very insensitive. The classic 'millwheel' murmur is a late sign and indicates a massive gas embolism with imminent cardiovascular collapse.

Prevention

Minimize elevation of the surgical site above the heart, in particular the sitting position. Consider monitoring in situations of high risk.

Avoid hypovolaemia and consequent low CVP.

PEEP may reduce risk of air embolism.

⚠ Immediate management

Give 100% oxygen at high flows; this will reduce the nitrogen content of bubbles and therefore their size.

Call for help.

Quickly assess the airway (exclude disconnection or obstruction), breathing, and circulation. If PEA arrest has occurred, commence advanced life support.

Stop surgery and prevent further entrainment of gas using techniques most appropriate to the surgical situation:
- Flood the operative field with saline.
- Lower the surgical site below the level of the heart.
- Release any pressurized gas (e.g. pneumoperitoneum).
- Compress open vessels and/or major drainage vessels (e.g. jugular vein during craniotomy).

Increase venous pressure with rapid fluid administration.

If a CVP line is *in situ*, immediately aspirate it in an attempt to retrieve some of the embolus. If there is no CVP line, prepare to site one (although it is likely to have less impact and should not delay resuscitation).

Ideally, the patient should be placed in the left lateral position head down, to try to keep air in the right atrium. This is not always feasible, especially if CPR is in progress.

Ongoing management

Avoid subsequent nitrous oxide, which will diffuse into and enlarge a gas embolus.

Establish invasive monitoring and arrange for transfer to ICU.

Following a large embolus there will be increased pulmonary vascular resistance, right ventricular distension, and deviation of the ventricular septum to the left. The resultant decrease in cardiac output can be treated with dobutamine (Archer *et al* 2001).

Further reading

Archer et al (2001)
Muth CM, Shank SS (2000) *N Engl J Med* **342**, 476–82
Sviri S et al (2004) *Crit Care Resus* **6**, 271–6

Fat embolism syndrome

Definition
Fat embolization is the release of fat droplets into the systemic circulation after a traumatic event.

Risk factors
- Intramedullary nailing and long-bone trauma or polytrauma
- Hip and knee arthroplasty
- Liposuction
- Diabetes
- Burns
- Osteomylelitis
- Blood transfusion
- Haemoglobinopathy
- Renal transplant
- Cardiopulmonary bypass
- Pancreatitis
- Connective tissue disease
- Bone marrow transplants
- Chemotherapy

Presentation and diagnosis
Presentation usually occurs 24–72hr after the initial insult.

Respiratory: tachypnoea, dyspnoea, cyanosis, crepitations and wheeze, often accompanied by tachycardia and pyrexia. CXR may be normal, or show diffuse pulmonary infiltrates.

Central nervous system: headache, irritability and confusion. Coma and convulsions in severe cases. Fundoscopy may reveal retinal infarcts. MRI is more sensitive than CT in identification of cerebral fat embolism syndrome.

Cutaneous: approximately 50% of patients will develop a petechial rash over the chest, neck, axillae, and conjunctivae.

Cardiovascular: ECG sometimes shows signs of right heart strain or ischaemia.

No pathognomic laboratory investigation exists for fat embolism. Fat globules may transiently be found in blood, urine, sputum, or CSF, but the diagnosis is made on clinical grounds and by the exclusion of other diagnoses. Gurd and Wilson (1974) described major and minor signs in the diagnosis of fat embolism syndrome (Table 25.2).

! Immediate management
Immobilization of any causative fracture is essential.

Transfer to intensive care with invasive monitoring.

Correction of hypoxia using CPAP or intubation and ventilation as necessary.

Ongoing management
Use of steroids to treat fat embolism syndrome is not of proven benefit and carries significant potential side effects.

If diagnosed early and aggressively supported, the prognosis is good.

Table 25.2	Gurd and Wilson's diagnostic criteria for fat embolism syndrome
Major	Petechial rash
	Respiratory signs
	Cerebral signs
Minor	Pyrexia
	Tachycardia
	Retinal changes
	Jaundice
	Renal changes
Laboratory	Thrombocytopenia
	Sudden drop in Hb
	High ESR
	Fat macroglobulinaemia

One major and four minor criteria and macroglobulinaemia are required

Further reading
Gurd AR, Wilson RI (1974) *J Bone Jt Surg* **56**, 408–16
Parisi DM *et al* (2002) *Am J Orthop,* 31(9), 507–12

Paradoxical embolism

Paradoxical embolism involves emboli (solid or gas) that have passed into the arterial circulation from the venous system, often with devastating consequences. This may occur where a large gas embolus has overwhelmed the pulmonary circulation, which would normally filter out gas bubbles. Alternatively, it may occur where there is a patent foramen ovale and high right atrial pressures. Cardiopulmonary bypass carries a risk of air emboli directly entering the systemic circulation.

Presentation

In an awake patient, the neurological symptoms may range from headache, minor focal deficits, or confusion to fits, paralysis, and coma. Post-anaesthesia, prolonged impaired consciousness may be the only clue.

Embolization of the coronary arteries results in ischaemia, which may progress to infarction, or cause arrythmias or cardiac arrest.

Diagnosis and treatment

The diagnosis is based largely on patient history. Occasionally, gas bubbles can be seen in the retinal vessels. MRI and CT findings may sometimes support the diagnosis.

Treatment is supportive and, as with venous embolism, high oxygen concentrations help to eliminating bubbles by reducing the nitrogen content and maximizing tissue oxygenation. Consequently, hyperbaric oxygen is the first-line treatment for arterial gas embolism once the patient is stabilized.

Further reading

Voorhies RM, Fraser RAR (1984) *J Neurosurg* **60**, 177–8
Ziser A *et al* (1999) *J Thorac Cardiovasc Surg* **117**, 818–21

Accidental intra-arterial injection

Definition

Injection of an intravenous drug into an artery.

Initial reports of intra-arterial injection of thiopental appeared more than 50 years ago. Although a rare occurrence, the consequences can be devastating for the patient. This is particularly so in the case of thiopental; consequently a test dose should be given first. Early recognition and intervention is vital, to reduce tissue damage.

Risk factors

- Difficult IV cannulation (e.g. obesity, darkly pigmented skin, uncooperative patient).
- Inadequate labelling of arterial port.
- Use of the antecubital fossa resulting in brachial artery cannulation.
- Aberrant anatomy, particularly the radial and ulnar arteries. A number of case reports have involved cannulation of aberrant arteries on the dorsum of the hand.

Presentation

Severe pain radiates along the vessel that has been injected. This sign can be masked by anaesthesia itself. Propofol can cause severe pain on IV injection. During the first few hours, skin pallor, hyperaemia, and cyanosis may occur. Awake patients may experience muscular weakness, paralysis, hypesthesia, or anaesthesia. In severe cases there is profound oedema and, eventually, gangrene.

Pathophysiology

The features of intra-arterial injection are as follows.

- Arterial spasm (direct response to the drug, or caused by local noradrenaline release).
- Direct tissue destruction by the drug. Thiopental concentrations ≥2.5% have consistently been shown to cause endothelial destruction and necrosis, leading to gangrene. Intra-arterial promethazine causes similar effects. Propofol does not cause tissue destruction, but leads to a distal hyperaemia lasting for several hours.
- Release of endogenous substances that result in adverse effects (e.g. thromboxane causing vasoconstriction and thrombosis).

❗ Immediate management

Stop injecting immediately.

It is vital that the cannula is left in situ.

Into the cannula, give:

- saline flush (10–20ml) to dilute the irritant.;
- lidocaine 100mg (e.g. 10ml of 1%);
- papaverine 40mg in 10ml saline.

Obtain alternative IV access. Give systemic analgesia.

Regional blockade of the limb may produce vasodilatation. Similarly, sympathetic block may have the same effect (e.g. stellate ganglion block).

Consider anticoagulation with IV heparin (*after* any regional block).

Subsequent management

Involve a vascular surgeon early.

Arrange for frequent observations of the affected limb including Doppler assessment of pulses.

Other treatments are under evaluation, but are currently at the animal model stage. They include specific thromboxane inhibitors (e.g. methimazole), high molecular weight dextrans (e.g. dextran 40), and arterial vasodilators (e.g. reserpine).

Further reading

Macintosh RR, Heyworth PA (1943) *Lancet* **ii**, 571
MacPherson RD *et al* (1991) *Br J Anaesth* **67**, 546–52
MacPherson RD *et al* (1992) *Anesthesiology* **76**, 967–71

Intraoperative hypotension

Definition
A drop in mean arterial pressure of ≥25% of the usual resting value.

Causes of intraoperative hypotension

Hypovolaemia
- Haemorrhage
- Dehydration (diarrhoea, vomiting, bowel prep)
- Capillary leak

Vasodilatation
- Anaphylaxis
- Excessive dose of anaesthetic agent
- High epidural or spinal block
- Septic shock

Obstructive shock
- Pulmonary embolus
- Pericardial tamponade

Cardiogenic shock
- Ischaemia/infarction
- Arrhythmia

Impaired venous return
- Head-up position
- Raised intrathoracic pressure (mechanical ventilation)
- Aorto-caval compression (late pregnancy)
- Tension pneumothorax
- Pneumoperitoneum during laparoscopy

❗ Immediate management

ABC approach: verify the airway and adequacy of oxygenation and ventilation.

Check BP and ECG (arrhythmias, ischaemic change).

Check depth of anaesthesia. Where appropriate reduce delivery.

Reduce any excessive reduction in venous return:
- Remove head-up angulation
- Increase left lateral tilt in late pregnancy
- Reduce excessive intra-abdominal pressure from pneumoperitoneum.

Look for accompanying signs of anaphylaxis (Section 25.10).

Estimate blood and other fluid losses and assess for signs of hypovolaemia: tachycardia, poor peripheral perfusion, oliguria, and low CVP. If hypovolaemia is likely, bolus with crystalloid or colloid (10ml/kg), assess clinical response, and repeat as appropriate. If hypovolaemia is severe, head-down or legs-up position will provide immediate increase in venous return and cerebral perfusion.

Consider and exclude other possible causes of hypotension:
- Air embolism (Section 25.12) will occur in a situation of risk and be accompanied by a flattening of the $ETCO_2$ trace and hypoxia.
- Tension pneumothorax (Section 25.10) will usually present in a patient with pre-existing chest trauma or following a central line insertion. Signs include high airway pressures, engorged neck veins, and a silent hyper-resonant hemithorax.
- Septic shock should be considered in an appropriate context (e.g. faecal peritonitis). These patients are typically pyrexial, tachycardic and vasodilated with diastolic hypotension.
- Patients with high spinal or epidural blocks are also vasodilated, but usually bradycardic.

If the initial response to fluid bolus is inadequate and vasodilation is present, administer a bolus of vasoconstrictor (e.g. metaraminol 0.5–1mg or phenylephrine 0.25–0.5mg). Where there is bradycardia or low cardiac output is suspected, ephedrine 3–6mg is appropriate.

Ongoing management and investigations
A persistently poor response to fluid and vasoconstrictors indicates the need for central venous and invasive arterial pressure measurement.

Patients with cardiogenic or septic shock are likely to need inotropes. In septic shock, noradrenaline 0.01–0.5mcg/kg/min is the first-line inotrope, whereas in cardiogenic shock dobutamine 5–20mcg/kg/min or adrenaline (0.01–0.5mcg/kg/min) should be used.

ABGs should be sent to identify lactic acidosis indicating inadequacy of oxygen delivery or utilization. Patients with worsening lactic acidosis and/or oliguria require cardiac output measurement in theatres or postoperatively on intensive care.

Postoperative 12-lead ECG and CXR should be performed and cardiac enzymes checked.

Intraoperative hypertension

Definition

Severe hypertension: systolic pressure >180mmHg, diastolic pressure >110mmHg.

Risk factors and causes

- Inadequate anaesthesia or analgeia.
- Untreated essential hypertension. For elective surgery, blood pressure readings greater than 180/110 should prompt consideration of postponement until controlled.
- Pre-eclampsia.
- Aortic surgery (the increased systemic vascular resistance caused by aortic cross-clamping is associated with marked hypertension).
- Family history of multiple endocrine neoplasia (type 2) syndrome.
- Acutely raised intracranial pressure.
- Drugs.

❗ Immediate management

If the hypertension is severe, stop surgery until controlled.

ABC approach: quickly verify airway; increase FiO_2; verify ventilation and oxygenation. Call for help if the problem is not swiftly solved.

Eliminate measurement artefact: repeat measurement; palpate pulse whilst cuff cycles; re-zero arterial line.

Diagnose underlying cause by exclusion. Take into account recent events, e.g. tracheal intubation/extubation or aortic cross-clamping.

Check depth of anaesthesia and anaesthetic delivery (end-tidal volatile, TIVA pump, patency of IV cannula). If in doubt, increase depth of anaesthesia.

Consider analgesia: if in doubt, give a bolus of fast-acting opioid (e.g. fentanyl, alfentanil).

Exclude a drug response, e.g. administration of the wrong drug, or accidental intravascular injection of local anaesthetic containing adrenaline.

If severe hypertension persists, an antihypertensive agent should be given to reduce the risk of stroke or myocardial ischaemia. In the presence of tachycardia (and if not contraindicated e.g. by asthma), a β-blocker is a reasonable first choice. Labetalol can be given in 5–10mg increments. Alternatives are esmolol (0.5mg/kg, followed by an infusion of 50–200mcg/kg/min) or metoprolol (1–2mg).

Vasodilators include hydralazine (5mg every 15 min), GTN (1mg/ml, starting at 3ml/hr and titrating to effect), or sodium nitroprusside (0.5–1.5g/kg/min). These may cause tachycardia.

Ongoing management

Consider an exacerbation of a pre-existing pathology such as pre-eclampsia, thyrotoxicosis, phaeochromocytoma, or a Cushing response to intracranial hypertension. Malignant hyperthermia should also be considered. If any of these conditions is suspected, treat accordingly.

Investigations

12-lead ECG; cardiac enzymes (if possible myocardial ischaemia); others depending on possible causes. Visit the patient postoperatively and exclude awareness as a cause.

Definition

Tachycardia is defined as a heart rate >100 beats/min. The various types of tachyarrhythmia are addressed in turn. Management depends on the underlying rhythm, as well as the presence or absence of adverse features.

! Immediate management of any tachyarrhythmia

In every case, use an ABC approach: verify airway, oxygenation, and ventilation, and give 100% O_2. Call for help if the problem is not quickly solved.

Assess the patient for the presence of a pulse. If there is no output, commence advanced life support.

If a pulse is present, look for adverse features:

- Systolic BP <90mmHg
- Heart rate >150 beats/min
- Signs of heart failure
- Signs of myocardial ischaemia
- Conscious patients: chest pain, altered conscious level.

If the patient is unstable and deteriorating with adverse features, attempt synchronized cardioversion. If this is unsuccessful, amiodarone 300mg/10min can be given before a second attempt, followed by an infusion of 900mg/24hr.

Correct electrolyte abnormalities. Aim for serum potassium in the range 4.5–5.0 mmol/L and magnesium 1.0–1.2 mmol/L.

Determine from the ECG whether the QRS complexes are narrow or broad.

Broad-complex tachycardias (Figure 25.8)

When treating broad-complex tachyarrhythmias, first establish whether the tachycardia is regular or irregular.

Regular broad-complex tachycardia

Regular broad-complex tachyarrythmias can be due to:

- Ventricular tachycardia
- SVT with aberrant conduction
- Atrial flutter with regular ventricular response and aberrant conduction (including pre-excitation).

If there is clear evidence that the rhythm is SVT or atrial flutter with aberrant conduction, treat as regular narrow-complex tachycardia (Section 25.15). *If in doubt, treat as VT.*

! Immediate management of regular broad-complex tachyarrhhythmia

Adverse features

If there is no pulse, treat as VF/pulseless VT with advanced life support and unsynchronized DC shocks (Section 25.2).

In the presence of a pulse, other adverse features (see above) require **synchronized** DC cardioversion with escalating shocks of 100J, 200J, and 360J. If unsuccessful, give amiodarone 300mg over 10–20min before a repeated attempt at cardioversion. This should be followed by an amiodarone infusion of 900mg/24hr.

No adverse features

Give amiodarone 300mg over 20min followed by an infusion of 900mg/24hr.

If adverse features develop or the arrhythmia persists for several hours, electrical cardioversion will be necessary.

Ongoing management

Correct reversible causes: electrolyte abnormalities, hypoxia, hypercapnia. Ensure that no CVP line is inserted too far, irritating the myocardium.

Perform a 12-lead ECG and cardiac enzymes at appropriate intervals. If there is evidence of ischaemia or infarction, an urgent cardiology referral must be made and consideration given to percutaneous coronary intervention.

Patients should be invasively monitored in a high-dependency environment postoperatively.

Irregular broad-complex tachycardia

Irregular broad-complex tachycardia can be due to:

- VT with fusion or capture beats
- Polymorphic VT
- Atrial fibrillation with aberrant conduction (including pre-excitation)
- Atrial flutter with variable AV block and aberrant conduction (including pre-excitation).

AF or atrial flutter with aberrant conduction should be treated according to their respective narrow-complex algorithms (Figure 25.9). Pre-excited AF and atrial flutter should not be treated with adenosine, digoxin, verapamil, or diltiazem because these drugs block the AV node and can increase pre-excitation. If in doubt and the patient is unstable, treat as broad-complex tachycardia.

! Immediate management of irregular broad-complex tachycardia

Adverse features

If there is no pulse, treat as VF/pulseless VT with CPR and unsynchronized DC shocks (Section 25.2).

Other adverse features require **synchronized** DC cardioversion with escalating shocks of 100J, 200J, and 360J. If unsuccessful, give amiodarone 300mg over 10–20min before the next attempt at cardioversion. This should be followed by an amiodarone infusion of 900mg over 24hr.

For polymorphic VT (Torsades de pointes), give 2g magnesium sulphate IV.

If there is no improvement, seek expert advice, as overdrive pacing may be necessary.

No adverse features

Stop all drugs that prolong the QT interval, correct electrolyte abnormalities, and give 2g magnesium sulphate IV. The development of adverse features indicates the need for cardioversion.

Ongoing management

Correct reversible causes: electrolyte abnormalities, hypoxia, hypercapnia. Ensure that no CVP line is inserted too far.

Perform a 12-lead ECG and cardiac enzymes at appropriate intervals. Consider cardiology referral (as above).

Patients should be invasively monitored in a high-dependency environment postoperatively.

Tachycardia Algorithm (with pulse)

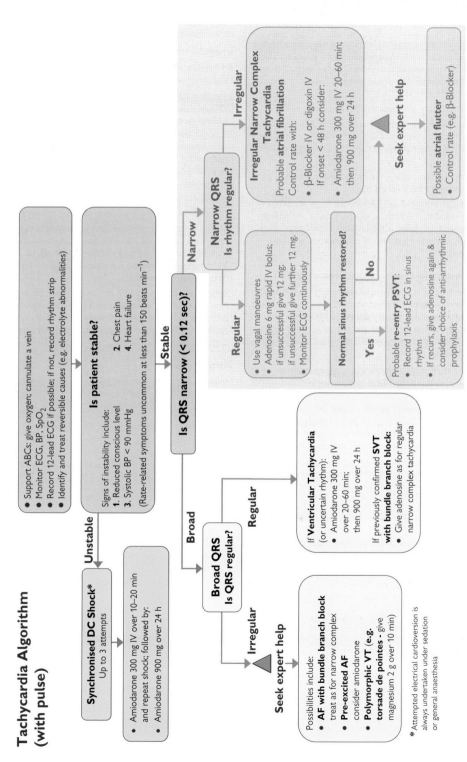

- Support ABCs: give oxygen; cannulate a vein
- Monitor ECG, BP, SpO₂
- Record 12-lead ECG if possible; if not, record rhythm strip
- Identify and treat reversible causes (e.g. electrolyte abnormalities)

Is patient stable?

Signs of instability include:
1. Reduced conscious level
2. Chest pain
3. Systolic BP < 90 mmHg
4. Heart failure

(Rate-related symptoms uncommon at less than 150 beats min⁻¹)

Unstable

Synchronised DC Shock*
Up to 3 attempts

- Amiodarone 300 mg IV over 10–20 min and repeat shock; followed by:
- Amiodarone 900 mg over 24 h

Stable

Is QRS narrow (< 0.12 sec)?

Broad

Broad QRS
Is QRS regular?

Regular

If **Ventricular Tachycardia** (or uncertain rhythm):
- Amiodarone 300 mg IV over 20–60 min; then 900 mg over 24 h

If previously confirmed **SVT with bundle branch block:**
- Give adenosine as for regular narrow complex tachycardia

Irregular

Seek expert help

Possibilities include:
- **AF with bundle branch block** treat as for narrow complex
- **Pre-excited AF** consider amiodarone
- **Polymorphic VT (e.g. torsade de pointes** - give magnesium 2 g over 10 min)

Narrow

Narrow QRS
Is rhythm regular?

Regular

- Use vagal manoeuvres
- Adenosine 6 mg rapid IV bolus; if unsuccessful give 12 mg; if unsuccessful give further 12 mg. Monitor ECG continuously

Normal sinus rhythm restored?

Yes

Probable **re-entry PSVT:**
- Record 12-lead ECG in sinus rhythm
- If recurs, give adenosine again & consider choice of anti-arrhythmic prophylaxis

No

Irregular

Irregular Narrow Complex Tachycardia
Probable **atrial fibrillation**
Control rate with:
- β-Blocker IV or digoxin IV
If onset < 48 h consider:
- Amiodarone 300 mg IV 20–60 min; then 900 mg over 24 h

Seek expert help

Possible **atrial flutter**
- Control rate (e.g. β-Blocker)

* Attempted electrical cardioversion is always undertaken under sedation or general anaesthesia

Fig. 25.8 Tachycardia algorithm: broad complexes.

Narrow complex tachycardias

Sinus tachycardia

Common intraoperative causes of sinus tachycardia are inadequate anaesthesia or analgesia (often accompanied by hypertension), hypovolaemia, hypoxaemia, hypercapnia, and sepsis (often accompanied by hypotension). Rarer causes include pulmonary embolus, malignant hyperpyrexia, and thyrotoxicosis. Treatment should be directed to the underlying cause.

> **! Immediate management of sinus tachycardia**
>
> *Briefly* assess the depth of anaesthesia and delivery of agent. Deepen if necessary. Similarly, consider analgesia and give fast-acting opioids if necessary.
>
> Assess airway, oxygenation and ventilation; correct any problems.
>
> Assess circulation: pulse rate, blood pressure, peripheral perfusion, vasodilatation or constriction, capillary refill. Estimate fluid and blood losses and requirements; give IV fluid (e.g. 20ml/kg) or blood if appropriate.
>
> Specifically consider sepsis, anaphylaxis, pulmonary embolus, and malignant hyperthermia; treat if necessary.
>
> Many patients can tolerate sinus tachycardia, but some are at risk of cardiac ischaemia due to increased oxygen demand. If the likely causes have been treated, there is no cardiovascular compromise, and the problem persists, consider β-blockade (e.g. labetolol 5–10mg increments IV).

Regular narrow-complex tachycardia: presumed SVT

The most common type of SVT is AV nodal re-entry tachycardia. This causes a regular narrow-complex tachycardia, >120 beats/min, without clearly visible atrial activity. AV re-entry tachycardia is seen in patients with Wolf–Parkinson–White syndrome and is also a regular narrow-complex tachycardia. Both are usually well tolerated unless there is underlying heart disease.

> **! Immediate management of presumed SVT**
>
> *Adverse features*
>
> If the patient is unstable, attempt **synchronized** DC cardioversion with escalating shocks of 100J, 200J, and 360J. If unsuccessful, give amiodarone 300mg over 10–20min before a repeated attempt at cardioversion. This should be followed by an amiodarone infusion of 900mg over 24hr.
>
> Adenosine may be given whilst setting up for cardioversion. This may correct a nodal tachycardia, or reveal a diagnosis of AF or flutter.
>
> *No adverse features*
>
> Begin with vagal manoeuvres: carotid sinus massage (in the absence of a bruit); Valsalva manoeuvre.
>
> If the arrhythmia persists, try adenosine as a 6mg bolus. If there is no response, two further boluses of adenosine may be given, this time each at 12mg.

Termination of the arrhythmia with vagal manoeuvres or adenosine is almost diagnostic of AV or AV nodal re-entry. Recurrence can be treated with adenosine or a drug with AV nodal blocking action (e.g. diltiazem or a β-blocker).

Occasionally, fast AF or atrial flutter will appear similar to SVT on the ECG. (Typical atrial flutter usually has an atrial rate of approximately 300 beats/min with a 2:1 block, producing a tachycardia of around 150 beats/min and flutter waves). Fortunately, initial treatment for SVT will either resolve the arrhythmia or unmask the atrial waveform.

Irregular narrow-complex tachycardia: AF or flutter

An irregular narrow-complex tachycardia is most likely to be AF, or sometimes atrial flutter with variable AV block.

> **! Immediate management of AF/atrial flutter**
>
> *Adverse features*
>
> If the patient is unstable, attempt **synchronized** DC cardioversion, with escalating shocks of 100J, 200J, and 360J. If unsuccessful, give amiodarone 300mg over 10–20min before a repeated attempt at cardioversion. This should be followed by an amiodarone infusion of 900mg over 24hr.
>
> *No adverse features*
>
> If there are no adverse features, treatment options are as follows.
>
> *Rhythm control with electrical cardioversion and anticoagulation.* If the patient has been in AF for more than 48hr, there is significant risk of atrial clot formation. Cardioversion should not be attempted until full anticoagulation has been achieved or atrial clot has been excluded by trans-oesophageal echo.
>
> *Rate and/or rhythm control with drugs.* Pharmacological control of heart rate can be achieved with magnesium, digoxin, diltiazem, or β-blockers, alone or in combination. If the AF is of <48hr duration, synchronized cardioversion can be considered or rhythm control using amiodarone.

Further reading

Nolan J et al (2006). *Advanced Life Support Providers Manual* (5th edn). Resuscitation Council (UK), London

Tachycardia Algorithm (with pulse)

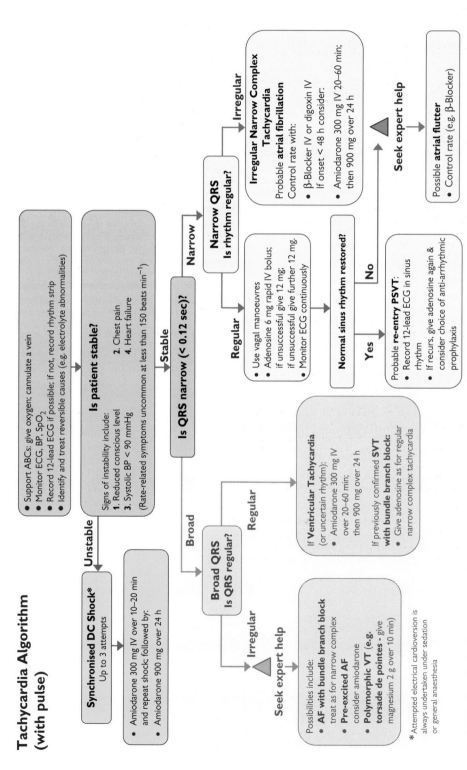

Is patient stable?

Signs of instability include:
1. Reduced conscious level   **2.** Chest pain
3. Systolic BP < 90 mmHg   **4.** Heart failure
(Rate-related symptoms uncommon at less than 150 beats min⁻¹)

- Support ABCs; give oxygen; cannulate a vein
- Monitor ECG, BP, SpO₂
- Record 12-lead ECG if possible: if not, record rhythm strip
- Identify and treat reversible causes (e.g. electrolyte abnormalities)

Unstable

Synchronised DC Shock*
Up to 3 attempts

- Amiodarone 300 mg IV over 10–20 min and repeat shock; followed by:
- Amiodarone 900 mg over 24 h

Stable

Is QRS narrow (< 0.12 sec)?

Broad

Broad QRS
Is QRS regular?

Regular

If **Ventricular Tachycardia** (or uncertain rhythm):
- Amiodarone 300 mg IV over 20–60 min; then 900 mg over 24 h

If previously confirmed **SVT with bundle branch block:**
- Give adenosine as for regular narrow complex tachycardia

Irregular

Seek expert help

Possibilities include:
- **AF with bundle branch block** treat as for narrow complex
- **Pre-excited AF** consider amiodarone
- **Polymorphic VT (e.g. torsade de pointes** - give magnesium 2 g over 10 min)

Narrow

Narrow QRS
Is rhythm regular?

Regular

- Use vagal manoeuvres
- Adenosine 6 mg rapid IV bolus; if unsuccessful give 12 mg; if unsuccessful give further 12 mg.
- Monitor ECG continuously

Normal sinus rhythm restored?

Yes

Probable re-entry PSVT:
- Record 12-lead ECG in sinus rhythm
- If recurs, give adenosine again & consider choice of anti-arrhythmic prophylaxis

No

Seek expert help

Possible **atrial flutter**
- Control rate (e.g. β-Blocker)

Irregular

Irregular Narrow Complex Tachycardia
Probable **atrial fibrillation**
Control rate with:
- β-Blocker IV or digoxin IV
If onset < 48 h consider:
- Amiodarone 300 mg IV 20–60 min; then 900 mg over 24 h

*Attempted electrical cardioversion is always undertaken under sedation or general anaesthesia

Fig. 25.9 Tachycardia algorithm: narrow complexes.

25.17 Intraoperative bradycardia

Definition

Heart rate <60 beats/min, although heart rates in the range 40–60 beats/min are normal for some individuals. Extreme bradycardia of <40/min is rarely well tolerated and usually requires treatment. Less severe bradycardia should be assessed for the presence of accompanying adverse features: hypotension, ventricular arrhythmia and heart failure.

Risk factors

- Surgery causing vagal stimulation, e.g. traction on the eye (squint surgery), anal or cervical dilatation, and peritoneal traction.
- Several drugs may cause bradycardia, including anticholinesterases, rapidly acting opioids (fentanyl, alfentanil, remifentanil), suxamethonium (particularly after repeat doses), and β-blockers.
- Sick sinus syndrome.
- Myocardial infarction.
- Raised intracranial pressure.
- Hypothermia.
- Hypothyroidism.

Further reading

Nolan J et al (2006). *Advanced Life Support Providers Manual* (5th edn). Resuscitation Council (UK), London

---

❗ Immediate management (Figure 25.10)

ABC approach: verify airway, oxygenation, and ventilation. Increase FiO_2 to ensure adequate oxygenation. Call for help if the problem is not quickly and easily resolved.

Young healthy patients may tolerate heart rates of 30–40 beats/min without compromise, but most anaesthetists would treat heart rates <40/min because the risk of asystole or sinus arrest is increased. In all age groups, assess for hypotension and adequacy of perfusion.

Stop surgical or other stimulation.

If adverse features are present, treat with atropine in 500mcg aliquots up to a maximum 3mg or glycopyrrolate 200–600mcg. In the presence of acute myocardial infarction or ischaemia, atropine should be used with caution to avoid tachycardia, since this is likely to worsen ischaemia.

If adverse features are absent, or in a patient who has responded well to initial atropine, the risk of progression to asystole should be assessed. High-risk rhythms are:

- second-degree Mobitz type II heart block;
- third-degree heart block;
- ventricular standstill of duration ≥3sec;
- recent asystole.

If there is a risk of progression to asystole or the patient has not responded to initial atropine, then transvenous pacing should be considered. In the interim, atropine may be repeated up to a maximum of 3mg. Otherwise, give adrenaline 2–10mcg/min. Other drugs to consider include iosoprenaline (0.5–1mcg/min) or, in the case of β-blocker or calcium-channel antagonist overdose, glucagon.

If there is a delay in achieving transvenous pacing in extreme bradycardia or ventricular standstill, transcutaneous pacing or 'fist pacing' can be used.

Bradycardia Algorithm
(includes rates inappropriately slow for haemodynamic state)

If appropriate, give oxygen, cannulate a vein, and record a 12-lead ECG

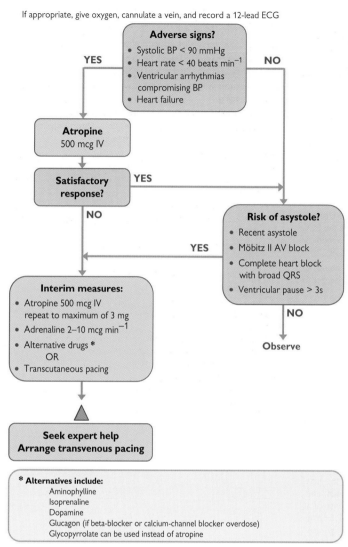

Adverse signs?
- Systolic BP < 90 mmHg
- Heart rate < 40 beats min^{-1}
- Ventricular arrhythmias compromising BP
- Heart failure

YES　　　　　　　　　**NO**

Atropine
500 mcg IV

Satisfactory response?　　**YES**

NO

Risk of asystole?
- Recent asystole
- Möbitz II AV block
- Complete heart block with broad QRS
- Ventricular pause > 3s

YES

NO

Observe

Interim measures:
- Atropine 500 mcg IV repeat to maximum of 3 mg
- Adrenaline 2–10 mcg min^{-1}
- Alternative drugs *
  　OR
- Transcutaneous pacing

**Seek expert help
Arrange transvenous pacing**

* Alternatives include:
Aminophylline
Isoprenaline
Dopamine
Glucagon (if beta-blocker or calcium-channel blocker overdose)
Glycopyrrolate can be used instead of atropine

Fig. 25.10 Bradycardia algorithm.

Definition

Myocardial ischaemia occurs when myocardial oxygen consumption exceeds delivery.

Myocardial oxygen consumption increases with increasing systolic pressure and heart rate. Consequently, hypoxia, anaemia, tachycardia, systolic hypertension, and diastolic hypotension can all precipitate myocardial ischaemia.

Myocardial oxygen delivery depends on arterial oxygen content and coronary artery blood flow. The coronary artery flow, in turn, depends on the duration of diastole (shortened in tachycardia) and the diastolic pressure.

Treatment is directed at improving myocardial oxygen delivery and reducing consumption.

Clinical presentation

During general anaesthesia, the usual symptoms will be hidden. Consequently, this is often a diagnosis based only on the ECG changes. For this reason, patients at increased risk should always have the ECG leads placed in the the CM5 configuration or a five-lead ECG monitor should be used.

The ECG can display ST segment depression, indicating ischaemia, or elevation, indicating an evolving acute myocardial infarction. Ischaemia of the conducting system predisposes to cardiac arrhythmias.

Ventricular impairment may present with hypotension, tachycardia, impaired perfusion, or pulmonary oedema.

> **❗ Clinical management**
>
> ABC approach: quickly verify airway, increase FiO_2, verify ventilation and oxygenation. Call for help if the problem is not swiftly remedied.
>
> Correct hypovolaemia, anaemia, and vasodilatation with fluid, blood, and vasopressors, respectively. A CVP line may be needed to guide fluid replacement and possibly administer inotropes. Vasodilatation with hypotension is best treated with vasopressors (metaraminol, phenylephrine, or noradrenaline), but dobutamine may be required if there is evidence of left ventricular failure,.
>
> Sinus tachycardia should be controlled with analgesia in the first instance. If tachycardia, hypertension, and ischaemia persist, and in the absence of contraindications, bolus with increments of a β-blocker (labetalol 5–10mg increments, metoproplol 1–2mg aliquots, or esmolol 0.5mg/kg followed by 50–200mcg/kg/min). In the context of hypertension and ischaemia, a GTN infusion (1mg/ml starting at 3mg/hr) should be considered since this will reduce preload, afterload and improve coronary arterial blood flow.
>
> Other arrhythmias should be treated as appropriate.

Ongoing management

Postoperatively, the patient should be transferred to HDU/ICU.

A 12-lead ECG and cardiac enzymes should be performed.

Continuing ischaemia should be treated with oxygen, nitrates, morphine/diamorphine, and aspirin (300mg).

Anticoagulation will have to be balanced against the risk of post-surgical bleeding.

The patient should seen by a cardiologist and considered for emergency percutaneous coronary intervention. Thrombolysis will be contraindicated by all but the most minor surgery.

Further reading

Slogoff S, Keats AS (2006) *Anesthesiology* **105**, 214–16.

Definition

A complication of incompatible blood transfusion. The interaction between donor red blood cell antigens and the recipient's antibodies leads to haemolysis.

Pathophysiology

Amongst the most severe transfusion reactions are those characterized by intravascular haemolysis. In an immediate reaction caused by ABO blood group incompatibility, antigen–antibody complex is formed. This causes complement fixation and intravascular haemolysis. The capacity of haptoglobin to bind free haemoglobin in the plasma is rapidly exhausted and there is progressive haemoglobinaemia. The plasma will appear red.

Beyond a plasma haemoglobin concentration of 150mg/dl there is haemoglobinuria. Haemoglobin in the form of acid haematin precipitates in the distal tubule causing mechanical blockage. The nephrotoxic effects may be reduced by increasing urine volume and pH.

Disseminated intravascular coagulation (DIC) occurs because red cell stroma is severed, releasing erythrocytin. This, in turn, activates the intrinsic system of coagulation. 20–60% of patients suffering a severe haemolytic reaction will die. It may take as little as 10ml of blood to precipitate such a response.

Risk factors

The majority of haemolytic transfusion reactions are caused by human error.

- Incomplete request forms.
- Incomplete or hurried checking procedures, e.g. matching the blood to its accompanying form but not to the patient.
- Laboratory labelling errors.
- Failure to replace wrist identification bands removed during induction.

Clinical presentation

Symptoms may develop soon after the onset of transfusion but may be masked by anaesthesia.

In the anaesthetized patient, the earliest signs may be hypotension, prolonged clotting times from DIC, and haemoglobinuria from blood destruction.

In the awake patient there may be head, chest, and flank pain. The patient may complain of nausea, chills, and dyspnoea, and there may be fever, rigors, flushing, and an urticarial rash.

❗ Immediate management

Immediately stop the transfusion. Call for help.

Give 100% O_2 at high flows. Assess for airway, respiratory, and cardiovascular compromise, and support as necessary.

Check identity of patient and blood product documentation to confirm the diagnosis.

Therapy should be directed to ensure an adequate renal perfusion pressure and a urine output of at least 75–100ml/hr.

- Give generous IV fluids (20mg/kg to start, repeated as necessary).
- Give mannitol 50g bolus.
- Vasopressors may be required.
- Alkalinize the urine to pH >8 with boluses of sodium bicarbonate. This may prevent precipitation of acid haematin in the distal tubules.

Investigations

Check the platelet count and a clotting screen to monitor development of disseminated intravascular coagulation.

The presence of haemoglinuria, haemoglobinaemia and elevated levels of lactic dehydrogenase and unconjugated bilirubin lend further support to the diagnosis.

Ongoing management

Inform the blood bank and return the unit of blood together with a post-transfusion blood sample for repeat cross-match. The direct antiglobulin test (Coombs' test) will be positive because the donor red blood cells will be coated with recipient antibody.

A consultant haematologist should be informed and the case reported to the Serious Hazards of Transfusion Scheme (SHOT).

The patient will need to be transferred to the ICU for monitoring and further supportive therapy.

Further reading

Miller RD (2000). Transfusion therapy, In: Miller RD (ed) *Anaesthesia*. Philadelphia, PA: Churchill Livingstone, 1613–44

Perrotta PL, Snyder EL (2003). Blood transfusion. In: Warrell DA *et al.* (eds) *Oxford Textbook of Medicine*. Oxford University Press, 791–800

Seyfried H, Walewska I (1987) *World J Surg* **11**, 25

25.20 Adverse drug reactions

Definition

An adverse drug reaction (ADR) is any noxious or harmful effect of a drug, which is not part of its useful clinical action.

Type A (pharmacological) These reactions are dose dependent, predictable, and based on known actions of the drug. They may have pharmaceutical, pharmacokinetic, or pharmacodynamic mechanisms. They include overdose toxicity, side effects, and drug interactions.

- *Overdose:* toxic reaction linked to excess dose, abnormally high availability, and/or impaired excretion (e.g. airway obstruction due to over-sedation with benzodiazepines, digoxin toxicity in renal impairment).
- *Side effects:* undesirable pharmacological effect at standard doses (e.g. dry cough from ACE inhibitors).
- *Interaction:* action of a drug on the effectiveness or toxicity of another drug (e.g. verapamil + β-blockers can cause asystole, dysrhythmias, and heart failure).

Type B (idiosyncratic) These reactions are non-dose-dependent and immunologically or genetically determined. They are rare and unexpected. They include intolerance, allergy, and metabolic idiosyncracies.

- *Intolerance:* a low threshold to normal pharmacological action of a drug (e.g. very severe gastritis from NSAIDs).
- *Allergy:* an immunologically mediated reaction, characterized by specificity, transferability by antibodies or lymphocytes, and recurrence on re-exposure (e.g. anaphylaxis from penicillins).
- *Pseudoallergic reaction:* a reaction with the same clinical manifestations as an allergic reaction (e.g. as a result of histamine release) but lacking immunological specificity (e.g. anaphylactoid reactions to radiological contrast media).
- *Idiosyncracy:* a genetically determined qualitatively abnormal reaction to a drug related to a metabolic or enzyme deficiency.

This classification is imperfect. For example, type A reactions exhibit huge inter-patient variability. With advances in pharmacogenetics, some reactions which were considered to be idiosyncratic are now predictable. Many reactions have elements of both categories.

Incidence

Type A effects account for around 80% of all ADRs. The incidence of ADRs is estimated at 1 in 6000 during anaesthesia. Up to 20% of hospital inpatients experience an ADR.

Some drug reactions relevant to anaesthesia

Muscle relaxants These are responsible for anaphylactic reactions in 1 in 4500 general anaesthetics.

Opioids These are among the most commonly prescribed anaesthetic drugs. True anaphylactic reactions are rare. Morphine is able to induce histamine release and occasionally leads to an anaphylactoid response. Side effects (e.g. pruritis, nausea, vomiting) and relative overdose (respiratory depression, hypotension) are far more common.

Local anaesthetics Reactions are seldom related to the local anaesthetic itself, but may be linked to preservatives.

Prevention of ADRs

Take a thorough drug history, including non-prescription medications, and consider potential interactions. Ask about previous adverse reactions, or a family history of these.

Never use a drug unless there is a good indication. Prescribe as few drugs as possible, with clear instructions about their use. Regular review and discontinuation of non-essential medications helps to avoid ADRs.

As a rule, a drug responsible for an adverse reaction should not be re-used unless there is an absolute need and no alternative. This is seldom the case.

Presentation and investigation

The clinical signs and symptoms of ADRs are extremely varied. Any system can be affected, and effects can be acute (e.g. bronchospasm due to β-blockers), or chronic and insidious (e.g. pulmonary fibrosis due to methotrexate, nephropathy due to NSAIDs).

Investigations are targeted towards the clinical presentation. The following list is not exhaustive but contains some illustrative examples.

Drug levels (digoxin, phenytoin, aminophylline, gentamicin, vancomycin, paracetamol, salicylates) may be elevated above the normal therapeutic range.

FBC may indicate anaemia (haemolytic anaemia caused by amoxicillin); neutropenia (immunosuppressants), or thrombocytopenia (immune-mediated paracetamol reaction).

Coagulation studies: PT may indicate over-warfarinization; APTT can monitor the effects of unfractionated heparin.

Urea and electrolytes may reveal electrolyte disturbances contributing to the ADR (hypokalaemia exacerbates digoxin effect) or caused by it (hypokalaemia caused by thiazide diuretics). Creatinine may indicate renal injury (gentamicin, vancomycin, ACE inhibitors).

Blood glucose can be reduced by insulin and sulphonylureas, or increased by steroids and thiazide diuretics

ECG may show rhythm disturbances (bradycardia from β-blockade, characteristic signs of digoxin toxicity, hyperkalaemia (ACE inhibitors), or hypokalaemia (thiazides).

CXR may show fibrotic lung changes (amiodarone).

Immunological tests: these include skin prick tests, radio-immunoassays, and tryptase. They are useful in the diagnosis of anaphylactic reactions.

Principles of management

For management of anaphylaxis, see Section 25.9.

Prompt and active management of ADRs is needed in all cases. Provide supportive or symptomatic care as required.

Specific antidotes and remedies exist for some ADRs (e.g. naloxone for opioid-induced respiratory depression; flumazenil for benzodiapine overdose; digibind for digoxin toxicity; N-acetyl cysteine for paracetamol overdose). The National Poisons Information Service or TOXBASE (ww.spib.axl.co.uk) are valuable sources of information and guidance.

Consider re-challenge or desensitization for allergic phenomena. This should only be performed under specialist supervision.

Document and report any suspected adverse drug reaction. Reporting can be carried out via the Freepost 'Yellow Cards' in the back of the British National Formulary or at www.yellowcard.gov.uk

25.21 Local anaesthetic toxicity

Systemic toxicity from local anaesthetics (LA) occurs when plasma levels exceed toxic threshold. This can result from:

- Excessive doses: may occur because of calculation errors, or may be associated with regional catheter techniques where continuous infusions or repeated doses are given.
- Rapid systemic absorption: intravenous regional anaesthesia and intercostal blocks are associated with rapid absorption
- Inadvertent intravascular injection: this may occur due to accidental placement of a regional block needle or catheter in a vessel (e.g. during epidural or transarterial brachial plexus block), or may be a result of a local anaesthetic preparation being mistaken for IV fluid.

Prevention

Recommended maximum doses are a guide, and should always be considered in the light of the proposed technique. Hypoxia, hypercarbia, and acidosis all exacerbate the myocardial depressant properties of local anaesthetics.

When administering local anaesthetics:

- IV access should be secured before administration of LA, and resuscitation equipment should be available and fully functional. A trained assistant should be present.
- Use the least toxic drug, and lowest dose, possible to achieve the desired duration of block. Reduce doses in elderly and sick patients.
- Calculate the dose carefully. (Recommended maximum doses can be found in Table 7.12). Remember that a 1% solution contains 10mg/ml. For epidurals and regional catheters, check the total dose administered within the last 24hr.
- Inject slowly, and divide large amounts indo smaller volumes if possible. Aspirate the needle or catheter prior to injection and at regular intervals throughout injection.
- Maintain verbal contact with the patient and ask them to report any unusual sensations during injection.

Clinical presentation of LA toxicity

CNS: early features include light-headedness, dizziness, tinnitus, perioral numbness/paraesthesia, abnormal taste, confusion and drowsiness. With severe toxicity, tonic-clonic seizures can occur, with progressive loss of consciousness, coma, respiratory depression, and eventual respiratory arrest.

CVS: if the preparation contains adrenaline, tachycardia and hypertension may occur. If no adrenaline is added then there may be bradycardia with hypotension. Severe cardiovascular toxicity is rare: usually about 4-7 x the convulsant dose needs to be injected to precipitate cardiovascular collapse. Collapse is due to the depressant effect of the local anaesthetic acting directly on the myocardium. Severe and intractable arrhythmias can occur with accidental iv injection.

Immediate management

Stop injection **immediately** if the patient shows any signs of toxicity, and **assess**.

Call for help

Confirm a cardiac output. If the patient is in cardiac arrest, commence CPR using standard ALS protocols.

Assess and secure the airway, and give 100% oxygen. Assess the breathing; ventilation may be required (hyperventilation may help by increasing the pH)

Confirm or establish IV access. Assess the pulse and blood pressure. Treat any circulatory compromise with isotonic IV fluid, +/- vasopressors (e.g. ephedrine, small boluses of adrenaline).

Arrhythmias should be managed along standard lines, but may be refractory to treatment.

If there are generalized seizures, control them with small incremental doses of thiopental, propofol or benzodiazepines. Intubation and ventilation will probably be necessary. If the patient is conscious but has CNS features, small doses of intravenous midazolam (e.g. 0.5-1mg increments) can help to raise the seizure threshold.

Use of lipid emulsion in LA-induced cardiac arrest

If cardiac arrest associated with LA toxicity is unresponsive to standard therapy, the use of lipid emulsion (Intralipid®) is recommended (doses are for a 70kg adult):

- Give an intravenous bolus injection of Intralipid® 20% 1.5ml/kg over 1min
- Give a bolus of 100ml
- Continue CPR
- Start an intravenous infusion of Intralipid® 20% at 0.25ml/kg/min
- Give at a rate of 400ml over 20min
- Repeat the bolus injection twice at 5min intervals if an adequate circulation has not been restored
- Give two further boluses of 100ml at 5min intervals
- After another 5 min, increase the rate to 0.5ml/kg/min if an adequate circulation has not been restored
- Give at a rate of 400ml over 10min
- Continue infusion until a stable and adequate circulation has been restored.

Prolonged resuscitation may be necessary: CPR may have to be continued for >1hr. Cardiopulmonary bypass it may be appropriate to consider other options: cardiopulmonary bypass may be appropriate, if available.

Note: propofol is not a suitable substitute for Intralipid.

Ongoing management

Abandon (or expedite) surgery.

Milder cases can be monitored in recovery until their symptoms resolve completely.

For severe cases, establish invasive monitoring and arrange for a transfer to ICU.

25.22 Malignant hyperthermia

Definition

Malignant hyperthermia (MH) is an inherited muscle disorder which, when triggered, produces hypermetabolism, muscle rigidity, and breakdown. Uncontrolled release of calcium from the sarcoplasmic reticulum of skeletal muscle leads to increased metabolism.

The syndrome is usually seen when a susceptible patient is exposed to volatile anaesthetics and/or suxamethonium. When first reported in 1960 the mortality rate was 70%, but with early recognition and prompt use of dantrolene, this has dropped to 5%. The incidence of MH is estimated to be 1:15,000 anaesthetics for children and 1:50,000–1:150,000 anaesthetics for adults.

Genetics of malignant hyperthermia

Clinically, the pattern of inheritance is a heterogenous autosomal dominant disorder with reduced penetrance and variable expression. Early genetic linkage studies found linkage to the locus of the ryanodine receptor gene (RYR1) which encodes the skeletal muscle sarcoplasmic reticulum calcium release channel. However, there is genetic heterogeneity, with results from 30–80% of families consistent with linkage to RYR1. Genomic searches have found loci on several other chromosomes to which MH susceptibility was linked, including one gene encoding for a subunit of the dihydropyridine membrane calcium channel. In short, the current state of knowledge precludes DNA-based diagnosis at present. Instead, diagnosis of the MH-susceptible phenotype uses *in vitro* caffeine–halothane contracture tests.

Risk factors

- Family history of MH.
- History of unexpected death of a relative during anaesthesia.
- Duchenne muscular dystrophy, King–Denborough syndrome, and central core myopathy.
- History of neuroleptic malignant syndrome or past heat stroke.
- Previous masseter spasm during anaesthesia.

Pathophysiology

The critical initial event is a sudden rise in myoplasmic calcium ions. These are released from the sarcoplasmic reticulum via the abnormal type 1 ryanodine receptor. Peak intracellular calcium release rates are three times normal. This results in prolonged actin–myosin interaction and sustained muscle contraction.

Biochemical pathways are activated in an attempt to re-sequester the calcium, leading to breakdown of ATP. This metabolic stimulation leads to increased CO_2 and heat production, with respiratory and lactic acidosis.

The onset of generalized muscle rigidity indicates that the muscle can no longer produce ATP. Without ATP, cell membranes break down, allowing leakage of potassium, calcium, creatine kinase, and myoglobin into the ECF.

Clinical presentation

Masseter spasm following induction may be the earliest sign of MH: it may hinder intubation and continue for several minutes. However, only 30% of cases of isolated masseter spasm will progress to MH. Generalized muscle rigidity may develop alongside masseter spasm or later, during maintenance with volatiles. It restricts circulation to the muscle bed, and indicates that muscle ATP production capacity is nearly exhausted. It is usually associated with a fulminant course. Rhabdomyolysis is confirmed by raised serum creatine kinase and urinary or serum myoglobin. It often causes hyperkalaemia, which may lead to cardiac arrhythmias. It may also result in DIC.

Hypermetabolism generates large quantities of CO_2, resulting in tachypnoea, increased $EtCO_2$, and respiratory acidosis. Oxygen consumption can increase fivefold, with a marked drop in mixed venous oxygen saturation. Lactic acidosis develops, and arterial blood gases show a mixed respiratory and metabolic picture. Sympathetic nervous system activation leads to tachycardia.

Hyperthermia is a late manifestation. However, temperature may increase as rapidly as 1°C every 5min; the body temperature can exceed 46°C.

Whilst in some patients the signs of hypermetabolism will be evident within 10min, in others it may take several hours. Consequently, MH will occasionally present postoperatively. In the investigation of postoperative pyrexia, it should be remembered that the clinical features of MH will be identical, however late the presentation.

Differential diagnosis

Several disorders share features with MH, and should be considered in the differential diagnosis (Table 25.3). Neuroleptic malignant syndrome is triggered by a wide range of neuroleptics and presents with hyperthermia, acidosis, hyperkalaemia, and myoglobinuria. Brain injury can lead to pyrexia and rigidity, whilst some muscle dystrophies and various forms of myotonia predispose to life-threatening hyperkalaemia on exposure to MH-triggering agents.

> **⚠ Immediate management**
>
> Hyperventilate with 100% oxygen.
>
> Discontinue administration of volatile anaesthetics and suxamethonium.
>
> Call for senior anaesthetic help.
>
> Abandon surgery if possible. Otherwise, maintain anaesthesia with safe agents, e.g. propofol TIVA, nitrous oxide, non-depolarizing muscle relaxants, opioids. Ask the surgical team to stay and help.
>
> Immediately mix and administer dantrolene 1mg/kg. Repeat up to 10mg/kg until the signs (pyrexia, hypercapnoea, tachycardia) have abated. Typically 3–5mg/kg will be required but occasionally >10mg/kg is necessary.
>
> Cool the patient using cold IV infusions, cooling blankets, and ice applied to the axillae and groins. Stomach or peritoneal lavage can also be used. Cool to 38°C to avoid accidental hypothermia.
>
> Monitor for cardiac arrhythmias and check U&Es, ABGs, FBC, and clotting.
>
> Treat hyperkalaemia with dextrose and insulin, and severe unresolving acidosis with sodium bicarbonate.
>
> Anti-arrhythmic agents can be used, except calcium channel antagonists which can cause hyperkalaemia and cardiovascular collapse.

Ongoing management

Place CVP and arterial lines, a urinary catheter, and a core temperature monitor. Transfer to ICU.

Check serum CK, and serum and urine myoglobin. Monitor the patient for renal failure. In the case of myoglobinuria, alkalinize the urine with sodium bicarbonate and maintain polyuria using IV fluids and mannitol.

Continue dantrolene 1–2mg/kg 4-hourly for 24–36hr.

Continue observation in the ICU for at least 48hr, as recrudescence occurs in up to 25% of cases.

Refer to the MH investigation unit for *in vitro* muscle contracture tests.

Investigations

MH susceptibility is currently diagnosed using the European protocol for the *in vitro* caffeine–halothane contracture test (CHCT). The CHCT measures abnormal contractures produced in isolated living skeletal muscle fibres on separate exposure to halothane and caffeine. The muscle fibres are obtained from the quadriceps (under femoral nerve block with or without sedation, or anaesthesia free of triggering agents). The CHCT has 99% sensitivity and 93.6% specificity. Patients whose results are equivocal (i.e. only one test is positive) are classified as 'MH susceptible'. A further contracture test using ryanodine appears to have superior specificity, but has not yet been accepted as the gold standard.

Anaesthesia for MH susceptible patients

For uncomplicated elective surgery it is appropriate to screen at -risk patients in advance. Where possible, regional techniques are used. However, anaesthesia using TIVA, opioids, and non-depolarizing neuromuscular blockers is safe (Table 25.4). Triggering agents should be avoided; a vapour-free anaesthetic machine must be used. Dantrolene is not used prophylactically becuse of its side effects.

Further reading

Abraham RB *et al* (1998) *Postgrad Med J*, **74**, 11–17
Ali SZ *et al* (2003) *Best Practice Res Clin Anaesthesiol* **17**, 519–33
Hopkins PM (2000) *Br J Anaesth* **85**, 118–28
Klinger W *et al* (2005) *Neuromusc Disord* **15**, 195–206
Wappler F (2001) *Eur J Anaesthesiol* **18**, 632–52

Table 25.3 Differential diagnosis of MH

Inadequate anaesthesia/analgesia
Thyroid storm
Neuroleptic malignant syndrome
Phaeochromocytoma
Anaphylaxis
Hypoxic encephalopathy
Sepsis
Iatrogenic overheating
Cocaine or ecstasy overdose
Tourniquet ischaemia

Table 25.4 Safe drugs and triggering agents in MH

Drugs contraindicated in MH	Drugs safe in MH
Volatile anaesthetics	IV anaesthetic agents
Suxamethonium	Opioids
Calcium-channel antagonists	Benzodiazepines
	Non-depolarizing neuromuscular blockers
	Nitrous oxide
	Glycopyrrolate
	Atropine
	Neostigmine
	Local anaesthetics
	Inotropes

25.23 Status epilepticus

Definition

Continuous seizure activity for ≥30min or intermittent seizure activity lasting ≥30min, during which consciousness is not regained.

Status epilepticus affects approximately 14,000 people per annum in the UK and carries an overall mortality of 25% (although much of this results from the underlying condition causing the seizures).

Pathophysiology

When seizures continue beyond 30min, cerebral autoregulation fails, cerebral blood flow falls, and intracranial pressure rises. Cerebral oxygen delivery is inadequate to meet demands and seizures continue, but clinically are seen to diminish to muscular twitching or even nothing. Cardiovascular, respiratory, and metabolic derangements combine with excitotoxicity to produce neuronal damage. It is vital to terminate seizures rapidly to reduce long-term sequelae.

Risk factors

- Head injury.
- Ischaemic/hypoxic brain injury (e.g. post cardiac arrest).
- CNS infection.
- Drug overdose (e.g. tricyclic antidepressants).
- Pre-existing epilepsy with poor treatment compliance or recent change of treatment.
- Electrolyte imbalance (e.g. hyponatraemia, hypocalcaemia, hypomagnesaemia, hypoglycaemia).
- Renal or hepatic failure.
- Brain tumour.
- Alcoholism.

Presentation

Loss of consciousness.

Tonic–clonic seizures.

Urinary incontinence.

With prolonged seizures, signs may become more subtle.

❗ Clinical management

ABC approach. Give high-flow oxygen, maintain the airway, and call for help.

Cannulate a vein, and take a blood sample for biochemistry and haematology.

Check glucose urgently with a near-patient kit, and treat confirmed hypoglycaemia (50ml of 50% dextrose).

Give IV lorazepam (0.1mg/kg) or diazepam (0.1mg/kg). Lorazepam is the agent of choice because of its longer duration of action.

If seizures persist after 10min, give phenytoin* (15mg/kg, at a rate of up to 50mg/min) or fosphenytoin† (22.5mg/kg at a rate of up to 225mg/min).

If seizures still persist, further phenytoin (up to a total of 30mg/kg) or fosphenytoin (up to a total of 45mg/kg) may be given.

If the seizures remain refractory, phenobarbital 20mg/kg can be considered. Intubation and ventilation are likely to be necessary at this stage to protect the airway and optimize gas exchange. In any case, general anaesthesia is the definitive treatment for refractory seizures. Propofol or thiopental, with suxamethonium, can be used for induction. Longer-acting neuromuscular blockers should be avoided, as their action may mask continuing seizures.

Anaesthesia is maintained with infusions of propofol (2–10mg/kg/hr) or thiopental (3–5mg/kg/hr; there may be significantly delayed recovery after prolonged usage of thiopental). Ideally, either agent should be used in conjunction with continuous EEG monitoring to minimize the dose used to abolish seizures.

Ongoing management

Search for an underlying cause (see risk factors).

Treat complications, e.g. hyperthermia, rhabdomyolysis, arrhythmias, pulmonary aspiration.

Investigations

ABGs, FBC, U&Es, blood glucose, anti-convulsant blood levels.

CT brain.

Where available, EEG.

Further reading

Chapman MG et al (2001) Anaesthesia, **56**, 646–59

Treiman DM (1999) Curr Treat Options Neurol **1**, 359–69

---

*Phenytoin carries significant risk of hypotension and arrhythmias and the patient should be monitored. There is also a reported 6% incidence of a potentially devastating soft tissue reaction, 'purple glove syndrome', with infusions of phenytoin distal to the antecubital fossa.

†Fosphenytoin is a water-soluble prodrug that is enzymatically converted to phenytoin. Fosphenytoin can be infused more rapidly, has a lower incidence of cardiovascular side effects, and has no adverse effects on extravasation.

Index

611